PRINCIPLES AND PRACTICE OF
Veterinary Technology

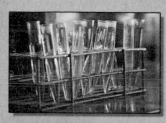

PRINCIPLES AND PRACTICE OF
Veterinary Technology

SECOND EDITION 2

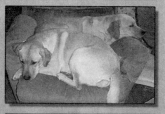

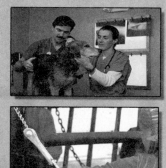

Margi Sirois, EdD, MS, RVT

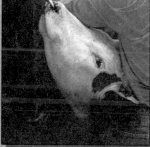

with 575 illustrations, including 32 color plates

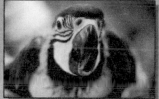

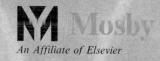

Mosby

An Affiliate of Elsevier

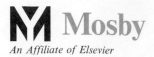
Mosby

An Affiliate of Elsevier

Publishing Director: Linda L. Duncan
Managing Editor: Teri Merchant
Project Manager: Pat Joiner
Production Editor: Sarah E. Fike
Designer: Julia Dummit

second EDITION
Copyright © 2004 by Mosby, Inc.

Previous edition copyrighted 1998.

NOTICE

Pharmacology is an ever-changing field. Standard safety precautions must be followed, but as new research and clinical experience broaden our knowledge, changes in treatment and drug therapy may become necessary or appropriate. Readers are advised to check the most current product information provided by the manufacturer of each drug to be administered to verify the recommended dose, the method and duration of administration, and contraindications. It is the responsibility of the treating veterinarian, relying on experience and knowledge of the patient, to determine dosages and the best treatment for each individual patient. Neither the Publisher nor the editor assume any liability for any injury and/or damage to persons or property arising from this publication.

The Publisher

Mosby, Inc.
An Affiliate of Elsevier
11830 Westline Industrial Drive
St. Louis, Missouri 63146

Printed in United States of America

ISBN-13: 978-0-323-01907-1
ISBN-10: 0-323-01907-2

09 10 11 12   9 8 7 6

For my family—especially Dan, Jennifer, and Daniel

Contributors

Elaine Anthony, CVT, MA
Associate Professor, St. Petersburg College
Pinellas Park, Florida

Michael D. Cross, DVM
Program Coordinator, Veterinary Technology
Baker College, Flint, Michigan;
Owner/Operator, Cross Veterinary Clinic, P.C.
Grand Blanc, Michigan

Harold Davis, Jr., BA, RVT, VTS
Coordinator & Instructor, Clinical Instruction: Hospital
    Practices
Supervisor, Emergency & Critical Care Service
University of California, Davis
Veterinary Medical Teaching Hospital;
Co-founder, Academy of Veterinary Emergency and
    Critical Care Technicians
Organizing Committee Member
Academy of Veterinary Technician Anesthetists
West Sacramento, California

Gael L. De Longe, DVM
Professor of Veterinary Technology (retired)
Blue Ridge Community College
Weyers Cave, Virginia

John T. Ervin, BS, DVM
Colonel, U.S. Army (Ret)
Adjunct Professor, St. Petersburg College
Veterinary Technology Department
St. Petersburg, Florida

Shashikant Goswami, BVSc, PhD
Associate Professor
Veterinary Technology Program
St. Petersburg College
St. Petersburg, Florida

Sheila R. Grosdidier, BS, RVT
Veterinary Management Consultation
Lecompton, Kansas

Connie M. Han, RVT
Co-owner, CH2 Veterinary Imaging Consultants
West Lafayette, Indiana

Guy Hancock, DVM, M.Ed.
Program Director
Veterinary Technology Program
St. Petersburg College
St. Petersburg, Florida

Karen Hrapkiewicz, DVM, MS, Dipl ACLAM
Director, Wayne County Community College
    District
Veterinary Technology Program
Clinical Veterinarian
Wayne State University
Detroit, Michigan

Cheryl D. Hurd, RVT
Co-owner, CH2 Veterinary Imaging Consultants
West Lafayette, Indiana

Bertram A. Lipitz, DVM
Director, Research Animal Facility
School of Osteopathic Medicine
University of Medicine and Dentistry of
    New Jersey
Stratford, New Jersey

Michelle Mayers, VMD
Adjunct Professor
Veterinary Technology Program
Trident Technical College
Charleston, South Carolina

Donna A. Oakley, CVT, VTS
Director of Nursing
Director, Penn Animal Blood Bank
University of Pennsylvania
School of Veterinary Medicine
Philadelphia, Pennsylvania

Sarah Okumura, MA, RVT, CVPM
Veterinary Technology Program Director
Western Career College
San Leandro, California

Stuart L. Porter, VMD
Professor of Veterinary Technology
Blue Ridge Community College
Weyers Cave, Virginia

Rebecca J. Rose, CVT
President, Colorado Association of Certified Veterinary
    Technicians
Gunnison, Colorado

Christine Royce-Bretz, RVT
Veterinary Technologist
Purdue University
West Lafayette, Indiana

Scott W. Rundell, DVM
Coordinator, Veterinary Technology Program
Morehead State University
Morehead, Kentucky

Katie Samuelson, DVM, CVT
Dove Lewis Emergency Animal Hospital
Portland, Oregon

Margi Sirois, EdD, MS, RVT
Program Director
Veterinary Technology
Education Direct
Scranton, Pennsylvania

Sally B. Smith, LVT
Airborne Animals and Companion Pet
   Enterprises
Blairstown, New Jersey

Teresa Sonsthagen, BS, LVT
Instructor, North Dakota State University
Veterinary Technology Program
Animal and Range Sciences Department
Fargo, North Dakota

Kathy A. Sylvester, BA, RVT, VDT
Veterinary Technician Manager
Rutherford Animal Hospital
Rutherford, New Jersey;
Dental Department Coordinator
Bergen Community College
Paramus, New Jersey

Terry N. Teeple, DVM
Program Director
Veterinary Technology Program
Pierce College
Lakewood, Washington

Vivian Tiffany, CVT
Adjunct Instructor
St. Petersburg College
St. Petersburg, Florida

C.L. Tyner, DVM
Professor of Anesthesiology
Department of Clinical Sciences
College of Veterinary Medicine
Mississippi State University
Mississippi State, Mississippi

Preface

Veterinary technicians are increasingly called on to perform advanced diagnostic and treatment procedures in a variety of clinical settings. Since the publication of the first edition of this text, the number and diversity of skills required of veterinary technicians have greatly expanded. This book represents an effort to collect the broad scope of information needed by the practicing veterinary technician. Veterinary assistant and veterinary technology students also will find this a valuable everyday reference. Discussions present the fundamental information veterinary technician students should know and entry-level technicians will find useful. Learning objectives at the beginning of each chapter will help students guide their study, and recommended readings provide additional sources of detailed information on the topics.

This new edition includes updated and expanded information that reflects the latest developments in the practice of veterinary technology. The book is organized so that basic information is presented early on. Communication and practice management chapters have been expanded to include personnel and inventory management, conflict resolution and teamwork, and issues related to the human-animal bond. Discussion of legal and ethical issues related to the practice of veterinary medicine also has been expanded. Practical applications follow with an effort made to keep information relevant for the clinical setting. Clinical laboratory material has been expanded from one chapter to four chapters and reflects the new emphasis on greater point-of-care capabilities in the veterinary clinic. Avian anesthesia topics also have been added.

The contributors to this edition are all involved in education of veterinary technicians. Their clinical and pedagogical experiences are evident in their discussions, which distill complex subjects down to the essentials. It is my hope that this new edition will become an essential reference in the teaching of veterinary technicians and be utilized in their daily practice of veterinary technology.

Margi Sirois, EdD, MS, RVT

Acknowledgments

This volume would not have been possible without the hard work of all the contributors. I sincerely thank them for their efforts. Thanks also to Dr. Paul Pratt and all the contributors to the first edition. Much of their work has been incorporated into this new edition. I owe my special thanks to Teri Merchant for her endless patience and humor and to Sarah Fike, Linda Duncan, Liz Fathman, and Ray Kersey for their support. I will always be grateful to my mentors, Harriet Doolittle, Marianne McGurk, and Doug McBride, and the many other veterinary technician educators that have encouraged and inspired me. And to my students— past, present, and future—I am indebted to you for always teaching me as least as much as I hope have been able to teach you.

Brief Contents

Contents

Contents

PRINCIPLES AND PRACTICE OF
Veterinary Technology

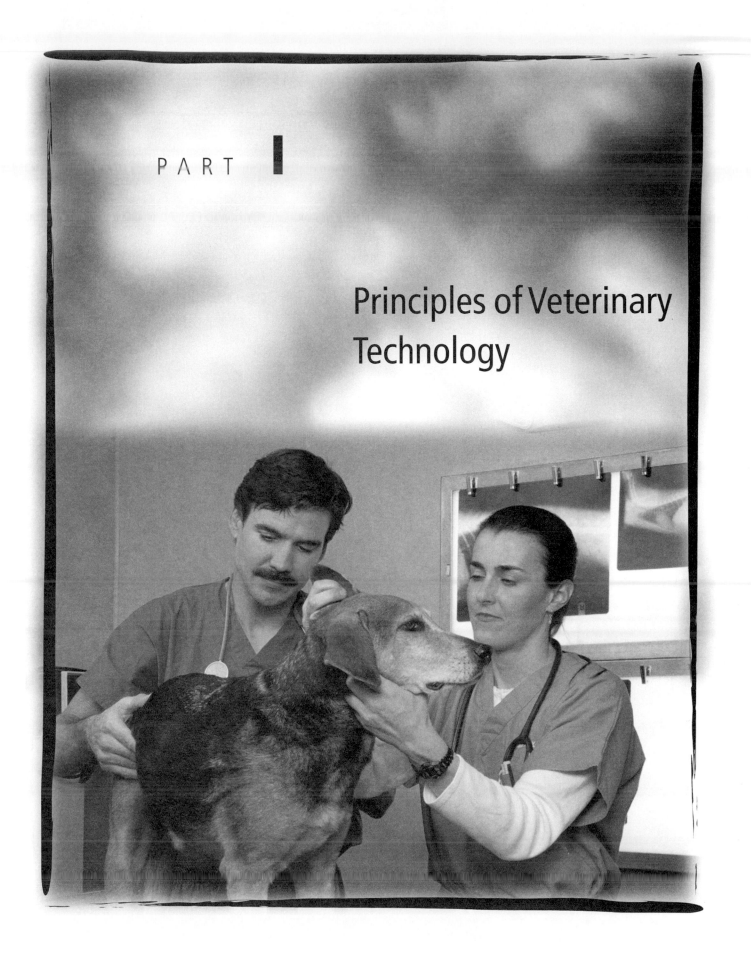

PART I

Principles of Veterinary Technology

Overview of Veterinary Technology

Rebecca J. Rose

Learning Objectives

After reviewing this chapter, the reader should understand the following:
- Education of veterinary technicians
- Nomenclature describing veterinary personnel
- Scope of a veterinary technician's duties
- Certification, registration, and licensing procedures for veterinary technicians
- Career opportunities, salary ranges, and organizations available to veterinary technicians

Veterinary technicians are a relatively new group of paraprofessionals in veterinary medicine, similar in many respects to nurses in human medicine. By the American Veterinary Medical Association's (AVMA) definition, a veterinary technician must be a graduate of an AVMA-accredited college program in veterinary technology and work under a licensed veterinary practitioner (DVM or VMD).

The emergence of veterinary technicians (educated in technician training programs) as members of the veterinary team is an important development for the veterinary profession. This change was in its infancy in the 1960s, in the developmental stage in the 1970s, dynamically changing in the 1980s, and matured in the 1990s. Veterinary technicians will play an increasingly important role in the veterinary profession, such as nurses do in human medicine, into the new millennium.

EDUCATION OF VETERINARY TECHNICIANS

As of this writing, there are 80 AVMA-accredited veterinary technology programs. To attain AVMA accreditation, veterinary technology education programs must meet 11 minimal requirements pertaining to facilities, faculty,

The authors acknowledge and appreciate the original contribution of Roger L. Lukens, whose work has been incorporated into this chapter.

admission requirements, and curricula. All programs are required to provide training in a variety of clinical tasks regulated by the Committee on Veterinary Technician Education and Activities (CVTEA). They must "provide technical skill acquisition strengthened through meaningful experience to enable graduates to not only be a productive employee at entry level for veterinary technician, but also develop the capabilities to perform satisfactorily in a position of increasing responsibility." These curricula must be designed to provide hands-on experience to ensure that each student performs 200 "essential tasks" listed in the *AVMA Accreditation Policies and Procedures Manual*. It is also desirable that an additional 84 "recommended tasks" be performed by each student. Proficiency outcomes for each procedure depend on the program emphasis and the number of times students have practiced these tasks. The CVTEA is continually incorporating the latest scientific knowledge, deleting studies that are no longer useful, and utilizing modern teaching methods. In 1999 in the United States, over 1733 veterinary technician students graduated from 80 AVMA-accredited programs.

NOMENCLATURE DESCRIBING VETERINARY PERSONNEL

"The AVMA recognizes the valuable assistance of veterinary technicians as an integral and valuable component of veterinary medicine in the United States and urges the full utilization of veterinary technicians whenever possible in veterinary research, regulatory, and health care activities. The practice of veterinary medicine is enhanced through efficient utilization of each member of the veterinary health care team by delegation of tasks and responsibilities to the appropriate level of support staff."

AVMA Policy on Veterinary Technology Preamble

The following definitions provide more complete descriptions that encompass the latest developments in the profession from the AVMA.

Veterinary technology is the science and art of providing professional support service to veterinarians. AVMA-accredited programs that educate veterinary technicians are usually called veterinary technology programs.

A *veterinary assistant* is a person with training, knowledge, and skills at the level of a clinical aide, but less than that required for a veterinary technician. Veterinary assistants can be compared with nurses' aides in human medicine. Generally, veterinary assistants are trained on the job, but some graduate from six-month training programs. Duties of assistants may include restraining, exercising patients, feeding, cleaning premises, and other clinical support tasks (non-income–producing tasks). These aides may also be described by the terms *clinical, hospital, technician's, ward,* or *veterinary* combined with *aide, attendant, caretaker,* or *assistant.* They are most appropriately called *technician's assistants* or *clinical aides,* rather than *veterinary assistants.* The physician's assistant has more training and requires less supervision than a registered nurse, in contrast with the clinical aide (nurse's aide).

A *veterinary technician* is a graduate of an AVMA-accredited program in veterinary technology. A veterinary technician's duties are similar to, in human medicine, those of a registered nurse, nurse-anesthetist, operating room technician, dental hygienist, medical laboratory technician, or radiographic technician. Professional nursing-related duties that produce income are delegated to a veterinary technician by a licensed DVM in a fee-for-service veterinary practice. Veterinary technicians may also work in research, education, sales, or governmental positions.

A *veterinary technologist* is a graduate of a four-year, AVMA-accredited veterinary program who holds a baccalaureate degree from veterinary technician study; or a graduate veterinary technician with a bachelor of science (B.S.) degree in another program with studies in supervision, leadership, management, or a scientific area. Duties of veterinary technologists include veterinary technician duties, often in combination with personnel management or hospital management. They may be employed as teachers, research associates, group leaders, sales managers, or clinical technologists in a specialty practice. Their role is sometimes compared with that of the physician's assistant, except veterinary technologists require more direct supervision in treating patients by veterinary practice law.

A *veterinarian* is a doctor of veterinary medicine. A veterinarian is a graduate of a four-year, AVMA-accredited program, such as one of the 27 American or 4 Canadian veterinary medical colleges. To practice veterinary medicine, veterinarians must pass a licensure examination in the states or provinces in which they wish to practice. Most veterinarians graduating today have four years of preveterinary studies, with a B.A. or B.S. degree, in addition to four years of study at a veterinary college, culminating in a Doctor of Veterinary Medicine degree (DVM or VMD).

A *veterinary team* is a combination of doctors, paraprofessionals (veterinary technicians and/or technologists), and support staff (receptionists, managers, technician's assistants, and caretakers).

The AVMA encourages schools, organizations, and regulatory authorities to use the standard terminology described above.

SCOPE OF VETERINARY TECHNICIAN'S DUTIES

Veterinary technicians are often unrecognized by the public and misunderstood by veterinarians. Varying expectations and lack of standardization of employee roles allow businesses to establish their teams by their own criteria. A few visionary veterinary schools are teaching veterinary students to view themselves as the "delegators" and not necessarily the "doers." With advanced practice management skills, veterinarian students learn staff utilization and understand how tasks are delegated to the appropriate employee within the hospital. Doctors of the "old school" are rapidly altering their management style for greater profitability, efficiency, and staff satisfaction through delegation and utilization. Due to the increased utilization awareness and high demand for educated veterinary technicians, students graduating with a degree in veterinary technology have the choice of well-managed, high-tech, high-touch practices offering salaries high enough to keep them in the profession. Technicians who are unhappy with their current job conditions must take a good look at all their options. There are veterinary clinics that offer benefits, appropriate compensation, career advancement, vacation, continuing education, and retirement plans.

Veterinary technicians are now assuming a major role in practice by performing medical and surgical nursing procedures, laboratory testing, anesthesia induction, maintenance, monitoring during recovery, management, staff training, and other clinical procedures. Veterinarians delegate many income-producing procedures to veterinary technicians. This enables the veterinarian to concentrate on prescribing medications, diagnosing, and surgery, and increases his or her productivity (Box 1-1).

BOX 1-1

Scope of Veterinary Technician's Duties

Caring for the Hospitalized Patient

Administering of medication
Sample collection
Physical therapy
Specialized intensive nursing care
Bandage/dressing application
Nutritional management

Clinical Pathology

Specimen collection
Hematology procedures
Microbiology techniques
Parasite evaluations
Biochemical analysis
Cytology examinations
Urinalysis

Outpatient/Field Service

Physical examination
History taking
Client education
Administration of medication
Administration of vaccines
Specimen collections

Radiology

Patient preparation and positioning
Radiation calculations and exposure
Radiation safety
Radiographic film developing
Maintenance of equipment

Anesthesiology

Preanesthetic evaluation
Administration of local anesthetics
Administration of general anesthetics
Monitoring
Patient recovery

Dental Prophylaxis

Examination of oral cavity
Cleaning and polishing

Surgical Assisting

Patient preparation
Instrument/equipment sterilization
Surgical suite preparation and maintenance
Assistance during surgical procedures
Postoperative patient care
Wound management

Office/Hospital Management

Medical supplies inventory control
Bookkeeping and practice management
Supervision of hospital personnel
Training of hospital personnel
Reception duties and client education

Biomedical Research

In addition to the above areas of responsibility, veterinary technicians in research may also:
Supervise operation of technicians in research colonies and facilities
Assist in design and implementation of research projects

Adapted from NAVTA: Veterinary technology: a career dedicated to quality animal care.

A megastudy, sponsored by American Animal Hospital Association (AAHA), AVMA, and Association of American Veterinary Medical Colleges, conducted by KPMG LLC Consulting services in 1999 identified inefficient delivery services (lack of utilization) as one of six areas that practitioners need to improve to increase practice profitability. For many years, consultants have urged veterinarians to delegate technical tasks to technicians. The National Association of Veterinary Technicians in America (NAVTA) considers delegating tasks to technicians a cornerstone in the effective delivery of veterinary medicine.

In a study performed by *Veterinary Economics* (June 2002), data collected from a small animal practice demonstrated that delegation of appropriate tasks to the veterinary technician was more cost-efficient than if the veterinarian performed those same tasks. Simply stated, it is in a veteri-

narian's best interest to delegate appropriate tasks to the appropriate employee.

The average respondent to the 2000 NAVTA survey had more than 10 years of experience; 98% were certified, registered, or licensed as veterinary technicians; and 84% graduated from an AVMA-accredited program. The average yearly salary was $25,500. The previous survey, done in 1994, reported average yearly income as $22,152, an increase of more than 15%.

CAREER OPPORTUNITIES FOR VETERINARY TECHNICIANS

According to the AVMA, 77% of career positions for veterinary technicians are in veterinary practices, with about 59% employed in companion animal practices, about

10% in mixed-species practices, about 4% in equine practices, and about 2% each in food animal and specialty practices. The greatest demand for veterinary technicians is in companion animal practices.

Nonpractice career opportunities (22%) include diagnostic/research laboratories (13%), industry/sales (2%), veterinary technician education programs (2%), government (1%), and miscellaneous (4%). The miscellaneous category includes positions with zoos (especially ion zoos with a hospital and full-time zoo veterinarians), livestock farms (animal health liaison with a consulting veterinarian), wildlife rehabilitation centers, humane shelters, the military, relief technicians, and colleges of veterinary medicine (clinical technicians).

SALARY RANGES FOR VETERINARY TECHNICIANS

The 1999 AVMA reported average annual salary for experienced veterinary technicians was: $20,057 in equine and mixed animal practices, $19,004 in food animal practices, $21,860 in companion animal and government positions, $23,163 in specialty practices, $29,536 in teaching and diagnostic/research laboratories, and $33,644 in industry sales positions. In a 1999 AVMA survey, there were 4,165 job openings on file with 54 job placement programs and only 133 recent graduates seeking a position. Even though some employers list positions with several placement programs, the shortage of veterinary technicians remains significant in many geographic areas. How many of these potential employers were willing to delegate appropriate tasks and pay a salary sufficient to retain a veterinary technician in the profession is unknown.

There is a trend toward group practices (today's practice averages more than two veterinarians per practice in the United States, with many practices having three or more doctors), increased client expectations of quality care, and an economic need to leverage veterinary productivity. These changes have allowed veterinary technicians to play a greater role in providing nursing care and related medical services.

CERTIFICATION, REGISTRATION, AND LICENSING OF VETERINARY TECHNICIANS

Upon graduating from an accredited AVMA program, veterinary technicians are eligible to take the Veterinary Technician National Exam (VTNE). Results of the VTNE may be transferred to other states via the Interstate Reporting Service. The Veterinary Technician Testing Committee, a committee of veterinarians and technicians appointed by various professional organizations, validates the VTNE.

Depending on the state, veterinary technicians are considered certified, registered, or licensed after completing and passing the VTNE; standards vary among states. Contact your local technician association or veterinary state board for further information.

Veterinary technicians are educated to follow specific ethical and legal guidelines while working under the direction and supervision of a licensed veterinarian. The employing veterinarian has the ultimate responsibility for using a technician in an appropriate ethical manner, consistent with state and federal laws. According to veterinary practice acts in all states, only the veterinarian can legally diagnose diseases, prescribe therapy, perform surgery, and issue a prognosis (predicted medical outcome). Chapter 2 presents detailed information on the laws and ethics of veterinary practice.

THE FUTURE OF VETERINARY TECHNOLOGY

For veterinary technology to advance as a profession, veterinary technicians must join state and national organizations to advance the cause for better utilization of veterinary technicians, attain greater professional recognition, develop more effective continuing education programs, and generally represent its members in political, legal, and other related matters. Whereas an increasing number of veterinarians have leveraged their productivity through full utilization of veterinary technicians, few have an incentive to discuss their advantage with other veterinary practices. Therefore, future advance in utilization of veterinary technicians depends on the collective efforts of veterinary technicians and their professional organizations.

VETERINARY TECHNICIAN ORGANIZATIONS

There are many state, local, regional, and national professional associations for veterinary technicians. The National Association of Veterinary Technicians in America (NAVTA) represents the veterinary technician profession nationally in seeking changes that help its members and the profession as a whole. NAVTA has been very successful in many areas, with its current emphasis on representing its members while striving to improve utilization of veterinary technicians, thus improving career opportunities for veterinary technicians.

By viewing the NAVTA (www.navta.net) or AVMA (www.avma.org) websites, you will be directed to the nearest active veterinary technician association. Take a positive step toward networking, upgrading, and improving your professional status by participating in your local association. Never stop learning; knowledge is everything. Being an active member of a professional association promotes you like no other effort.

RECOMMENDED READING

The NAVTA Journal National Association of Veterinary Technicians in America, Battle Ground, Ind.

The Veterinary Technician, Veterinary Learning Systems, Trenton, NJ.

Veterinary Economics, Veterinary Medicine Publishing Group, Lenexa, Kan.

RECOMMENDED VIEWING

The best possible care, Hill's Pet Nutrition, Sue Berryhill, RVT.

NATIONAL ASSOCIATIONS

NAVTA (National Association of Veterinary Technicians in America)
Pat Navarre, Executive Director
PO Box 224, Battle Ground, Ind. 47920
765-742-2216
www.navta.net

AVMA (American Veterinary Medical Association)
1931 North Meacham Road, #100
Scaumburg, Ill. 60173
www.avma.org
AVMA publishes a yearly directory listing veterinarians and hospitals in its association.

Association of Veterinary Technician Educators (AVTE)
Terry Teeple, DVM
Pierce College
9401 Farwest Drive SW
Tacoma, Wash. 98498
www.avte.net
AVTE provides information on educational programs.

VHMA (Veterinary Hospital Managers Association)
Christine Quinn, Executive Director
Albany, N.Y.
www.vhma.com

Association of Veterinary Practice Management Consultants and Advisors
Louis Gatto, CPA
528 Arizona Avenue, # 201
Santa Monica, Calif. 90401
310-393-2434

Academy of Veterinary Emergency Critical Care Technicians (AVECCT)
Veccs.org/technicians/index.cfm

Association of Zoo Veterinary Technicians
Virginia Crosett, Executive Director
Louisville Zoo
PO Box 37250
Louisville, Ky. 40233

REGIONAL, STATE, AND LOCAL ASSOCIATIONS

View listings on NAVTA and AVMA's websites and link to your state Veterinary Medical Association to obtain a current list of technician associations.

WEBSITES

National Association of Veterinary Technicians in America www.navta.net
American Veterinary Medical Association www.avma.org
Veterinary Hospital Managers Association www.vhma.org
Canadian Association of Animal Health Technologists and Technicians www.caahtt-acttsa.com
American Association of Veterinary State Boards www.aavsb.org
Canadian Veterinary Medical Association www.cvma-acmv.org
National Commission for Veterinary Economic Issues www.ncvei.org
NetVet http://netvet.wustl.edu/

2

Ethical, Legal, and Safety Issues in Veterinary Medicine

Bertram A. Lipitz

Learning Objectives
After reviewing this chapter, the reader should understand the following:
- Ethics of the veterinary profession
- How ethics affects the veterinary technician
- General categories of law
- Laws protecting veterinary employees against physical injury, sexual harassment, and discrimination
- Laws relating to ensuring quality veterinary service
- Laws regulating the biomedical industry
- How to avoid hazards in the veterinary workplace
- Hazards of handling animals
- Primary zoonotic diseases that pose a danger to veterinary personnel
- How radiation injury can be avoided
- Hazards of anesthetic and compressed gases
- How to prevent the spread of infectious diseases
- Content and use of Material Safety Data Sheets
- Occupational health and safety of the biomedical industry
- Four biosafety hazard levels and precautions for each

ETHICS

Our lives are governed by rules and laws. As children we are taught the differences between acceptable and unacceptable behavior. Quickly we learn the standards by which to judge the actions of others and ourselves, and easily recognize negative behavior when we encounter it. As adults, we intuitively know what is right, what is fair, and what is honest.

Our society sets specific standards for proper living. An ethical person lives by these standards. Laws set the maximum limits from which we can deviate from the acceptable norm. When someone does something unethical, is it something illegal? Not necessarily. Ethics are usually based on higher principles than the minimal requirements of the law, and as a member of a profession we are expected to adhere to ethical standards above those acceptable for the populous.

Ethics can be defined as "the system of moral principles that determines appropriate behavior and actions within a specific group." Members of the medical profession are expected to adhere to the highest ethical standards. The public accepts without question the decisions and judg-

The authors acknowledge and appreciate the original contributions of Philip J. Seibert, Jr., and Catherine Ann Picut, whose work has been incorporated into this chapter.

ments made by medical professionals because of their education and expertise.

This text was written for individuals who work within the veterinary profession. We serve the public, and most importantly the animal kingdom. A veterinary technician should have a profound commitment to honesty, compassion, proficiency, and hard work. Individuals with high ethical standards fit perfectly.

ETHICS OF WORKING WITH ANIMALS

The use and abuse of animals has been well documented throughout history. Practices such as rat baiting, dog and cockfights, and the pointless slaughter of animals for sport have passed from commonplace to criminal acts. Our culture demands that we treat animals with kindness, respect, and compassion. Animals who were once thought to exist only for our use and pleasure are now considered as individuals with the ability to feel pain and experience stress. Nowhere is this concept more important than in the veterinary profession.

A veterinary technician, either working in the industry or in training, is assumed to be an individual with a strong commitment to the care and welfare of animals. Technicians must make a personal determination concerning the status of the animals with which they share the world. There are many ways to look at this complex situation.

Some people ask if the rights of an animal should be the same as for humans; they believe that animals should not be used for any purpose. People, they maintain, are merely the highest form of animal life, and all life is important and equal. If you would not do something to a person, they argue, then it should not be done to an animal.

Animal rights activists question the use of animals for food, clothing, entertainment, and biomedical research. Some even question the use of animals as pets. They question whether owning a pet is the same as slavery in people. The majority of Americans believe in regulated forms of animal use as long as it is compassionate, humane, and not of trivial importance.

Although the public accepts the concept of animal use, it demands nothing less than exemplary care for animals. This is shown in many ways. The public has no tolerance for a dog owner who criminally starves a pet, a commercial puppy mill that houses puppies in unsanitary conditions, or a biomedical facility that fragrantly violates federal laws that govern the care and use of animals in research. Society considers it a privilege to own an animal and use it for pleasure or profit. This privilege can be taken away if the owner does not adhere to acceptable standards of animal care.

The standards for animal care are continually rising, as well they should. Just as humans have made advances in other aspects of life, our relationship with the animal kingdom also continually improves. The veterinary profession can take credit for many positive changes that have benefited animals, and it will continue to strive for greater advances in the future.

ETHICS OF THE VETERINARY PROFESSION

Questions of ethics within the veterinary community tend to fall into several major categories. We will look at some of these more closely to better understand the ethical challenges that can occur within the veterinary profession.

PROFESSIONAL ETHICS

Medicine will always be an art as well as a science. Professional judgment is the freedom given to all physicians to treat a case in a manner that they think best. Sometimes the choices made by the professional are not those that the others in the profession would commonly choose. There may be a fine line between freedom and responsibility. Who decides the difference?

Professions create peer review boards that evaluate possible violations of acceptable professional behavior. A genuine effort is made, within the veterinary profession, to correct deficiencies in individuals whose methods and choices are consistently not up to accepted professional standards and

whose actions may be detrimental to the public view of veterinary medicine. State and national veterinary medical associations are active in assisting the few colleagues who need help returning to an acceptable practice mode. State licensing boards throughout the country review complaints against veterinarians and their hospitals. These boards may impose penalties or compulsory retraining to avoid future complaints. Suspension of a license to practice is the final weapon that a state board uses to ensure that all individuals are practicing to a high standard.

How does this affect an individual who works within the profession? As an employee, you have an ethical obligation to discuss any matter concerning animal care that troubles you with the veterinarian. Keep an open mind. Often what may appear as inappropriate action by the veterinarian may be satisfactorily explained with a frank dialogue. In most cases, honest discussion will resolve the problem. In extreme cases, technicians may have to address their concerns to another veterinarian, the local veterinary medical associations, or the Board of Veterinary Medical Examiners. Technicians working in the biomedical industry should be able to report any suspected acts of animal neglect or abuse to review boards without fear of reprisals.

ETHICS OF SERVICE TO THE PUBLIC

People who work within the veterinary profession are obligated to serve the public, and in doing so to provide medical care and treatment at a level consistent with the standards of the profession. Members of the profession are morally compelled to report abuses inflicted on animals, and legally responsible for reporting public health problems.

It is well understood that the public pays veterinarians and their staff for their services. In essence, the veterinary hospital enters into a contract with the pet owner, wherein for a certain amount of money, specific services are rendered. The owner is legally responsible for paying the bill, but what are the obligations of the veterinary hospital? Aside from legal obligations of the hospital to competently render the service, the hospital is also morally responsible for treating the animal with care and compassion.

Should the presence or absence of a fee determine if a sick animal is treated? Ethically, the veterinarian and the supporting staff are obligated to provide at least basic life-saving treatment and pain relief whenever possible to any animal in its care. This may include performing euthanasia on a badly injured stray in obvious pain.

Veterinary professionals also act as teachers. There is an obligation to communicate with the public in clear, easy-to-understand language. The subjects may be as diverse as the care of an animal with diabetes, the correct use of dispensed medication, or nutritional tips. We are obligated to communicate and inform.

In the field of biomedical research, the veterinary profession is guided by the concept of the "Three *R*s." The concept was developed by William Russell and Rex Burch in 1959. The Three *R*s stand for *Replacement*, *Reduction*, and *Refinement*. The public has empowered the veterinary profession to ensure that research strictly follows these principles. Because of the Three *R*s, animals are only used when there are no viable nonanimal models, the number of animals used is kept to a minimum, and the comfort of the animal becomes of paramount importance. Every research facility that uses animals must have ongoing veterinary coverage to ensure that the Three *R* principle is applied to all animal research.

OBLIGATIONS TO THE ANIMAL KINGDOM

The primary function of the veterinary profession is to protect the health and welfare of the animals in our care. We are concerned with the treatment of the sick, the prevention of disease, and the general well being of all animal life. We have become the animal's advocate in society. We care, and are proud of our concern. Moreover, we are not hesitant to insist that anyone with animal contact show the proper respect for that living creature. We demand that pain and discomfort always be minimized if not completely eliminated. We understand the bond between animals and humans and foster that bond whenever possible. It is our mission and our duty.

LAW

In the daily practice of veterinary medicine, the veterinarian and veterinary technician are confronted with a wide variety of legal issues that affect their professional or business decisions. Bodies of law governing daily practices occurring within a veterinary clinic often overlap and fall into one of four categories: federal law, state law, local/municipal law, or common law. *Federal, state, and local/municipal laws* constitute legislative or written laws. Relevant governmental authorities and agencies enforce these laws, and violations of such may be punishable by fines and/or jail sentence. In contrast, *common law* is a body of unwritten laws that has evolved from use and customs and by judge-made decisions over many years. Government authorities or agencies do not enforce common law in the same way as legislative laws. Common law is enforced by the judicial system when citizens who may have been injured by a violation of the law file civil lawsuits against the violators.

The laws affecting a veterinary practice can be divided into two groups: 1) laws that ensure the quality of veterinary service to patients, and 2) laws that provide a nonhostile and safe environment for employees, clients, and the public.

LAWS THAT ENSURE THE QUALITY OF VETERINARY SERVICE

Practice Acts

The veterinary practice act of each state is the law prescribing which persons may practice veterinary medicine and surgery in the state, and under which conditions. Although practice acts vary from state to state, they generally define the practice of veterinary medicine, make it illegal to practice without a license, state the qualifications for receiving a license, state the conditions under which a license can be revoked, and establish penalties for violating the act.

The practice acts generally define the practice of veterinary medicine and surgery as diagnosing, treating, prescribing, operating on, testing for the presence of animal disease, and holding oneself out as a licensed practitioner. Embryo transfer, dentistry, and alternative forms of therapy, such as acupuncture and chiropractic and holistic medicine, are generally regarded within this definition of veterinary medicine and surgery.

Allowing only licensed veterinarians to legally practice veterinary medicine may raise questions about the duties performed by veterinary technicians or veterinary assistants. After all, many of the procedures performed routinely by technicians (or assistants) fall literally within the scope of the practice of veterinary medicine and surgery, such as inserting an intravenous catheter, inducing general anesthesia, and extracting teeth. However, as long as the technician is under the direction and reasonable supervision of a licensed veterinarian and the technician does not make decisions requiring professional judgment, the licensed veterinarian and not the technician is practicing veterinary medicine in such instances.

Whether a technician is under the direction and reasonable supervision of a licensed veterinarian is a subjective determination that takes into account the degree of experience and competence of the technician, the task being performed, and the risks to the patient involved with performing the task. For example, reasonable supervision of an untrained assistant inducing anesthesia for the first time would probably mean that the veterinarian should be standing by the assistant's side during the procedure. On the other hand, it may be reasonable for a veterinarian to request by telephone an experienced technician to place an intravenous catheter into an animal patient and start fluid administration. Regardless of how experienced the technician may be, the veterinarian must be on the premises or reachable by telephone or two-way radio communication during and for a reasonable time after any veterinary procedure.

Common Law Malpractice

When a veterinarian agrees to treat a client's animal, common law automatically imposes on that veterinarian a legal duty to provide medical or surgical care to that client's animal in accordance with that of a reasonably prudent veterinary practitioner of similar training under the same or similar circumstances.

A veterinarian's failure to live up to this particular duty constitutes *negligence*, which may also be referred to as *malpractice* or *professional negligence*. For malpractice to be subject to litigation, the plaintiff must prove three elements: 1) the veterinarian agreed to treat the patient; 2) the veterinarian failed to exercise the necessary legal obligation of skill and diligence in treating the patient (negligence); and 3) the negligence caused injury to the patient.

Veterinarians can be found negligent and guilty of malpractice for the injurious actions of a technician or assistant under the common law doctrine of *respondeat superior.* For example, if a technician mistakenly gave twice the recommended dosage of anesthesia to a patient, and this doubled dose caused the death of the animal, the veterinarian may be found negligent and guilty of malpractice as if the veterinarian had given the wrong dosage.

LAWS THAT PROVIDE A SAFE BUSINESS ENVIRONMENT

Federal, state, and common laws exist to help ensure safe and nonhostile working conditions for employees of a veterinary practice, as well as safe conditions for the public.

Occupational Safety and Health Act

Every employer with one or more employees must operate in compliance with the Occupational Safety and Health Act (OSHA).

OSHA was designed to provide a safe workplace for all persons working in any business effecting commerce. The broad judicial interpretation of "commerce" includes the business of practicing veterinary medicine and surgery. OSHA requires that all employers "furnish . . . employment and a place of employment which are free from recognized hazards that are causing or are likely to cause death or serious physical harm."

Common Law Ordinary Negligence

Common law establishes for every business owner a legal duty to provide a reasonably safe work environment for employees, as well as a reasonably safe place for clients. Failure to provide this safe environment may constitute ordinary negligence on the part of the veterinarian/business owner. This ordinary negligence is distinguished from malpractice, which is negligence associated with the rendering of professional veterinary medical services. As with malpractice, however, ordinary negligence is not subject to legal action unless it causes injury to a client or employee. For example, if a practice owner provides poor ventilation in a surgical suite and an employee becomes drowsy from anesthetic gases, the employee could not sue and recover damages from the veterinarian unless he or she experiences injury as a consequence (for example, faints and hits his or her head on the countertop).

A veterinarian, in meeting the obligation to provide a safe environment for employees and clients, has a common-law duty to supervise proper restraint of any animal within the veterinarian's control. When a client's animal is being examined and the client restrains the animal, it is the veterinarian and not the client who is primarily responsible for proper restraint of that animal. A veterinarian may be found guilty of ordinary negligence if he or she fails to use reasonable care to avoid foreseeable harm to the restrainer or to other people in the vicinity. The definition of *reasonable care* or *foreseeable harm* varies, depending on the experience or training of the veterinarian and the animal handler, as well as the procedure done on the animal.

Medical Waste Management Laws

Veterinarians who own or operate a veterinary practice may be subject to the requirements of state law governing management and disposal of medical wastes. Local laws may impose additional restrictions on what types of waste transporters and disposal facilities may be acceptable. Typical waste included under these acts are discarded needles and syringes, vials containing attenuated or live vaccines, culture plates, and animal carcasses exposed or infected with pathogens infectious to humans. State and local law may extend these categories of regulated veterinary medical waste to include all carcasses, animal blood, bedding, and pathology waste.

LAWS THAT MAINTAIN A NONHOSTILE WORKING ENVIRONMENT

There is a body of federal, state, and common law that restricts a veterinarian, as the owner of a business, from engaging in hiring or firing practices that wrongfully discriminate against individuals. Firing an individual for discriminatory reasons constitutes a violation of the federal or state Equal Employment Opportunity (EEO) laws and may provide a basis for the terminated employee to sue the employer under common law for wrongful termination of employment.

According to federal EEO laws, an employer of 15 or more employees may not discriminate against employees in hiring or firing practices (or in any practice, for that matter) on the basis of race, color, religion, sex, or national origin. Sexual harassment and discrimination on the basis of pregnancy or childbirth are forms of sex discrimination made illegal under federal law. Employers also cannot discriminate against individuals in hiring and firing of employees on the basis of age between 40 and 70 years or on the basis of disabilities, including AIDS and rehabilitated drug abuse.

Common law also protects employees because it prohibits an employer from terminating that employee for discriminatory reasons or other reasons violating public policy. Under the common law tort of wrongful termination, an employee can directly sue an employer for firing the employee on the basis of sex, race, or religious discrimination, or on the basis that the employee is a "whistle-blower" (i.e., has complained of sexual harassment or other violations of the law).

LAWS THAT CONTROL THE BIOMEDICAL INDUSTRY

During the past century, the biomedical industry has changed our lives. Every antibiotic we use and every vaccine administered to animals and humans can trace its roots to animal research. The life expectancy of humans and their pets is constantly rising. We are living longer, with a higher quality of life, because of the accomplishments of the biomedical industry. Still, these advances have been achieved at the expense of animal life; something that troubles most caring people.

Everyone hopes that the day will come when animals are no longer used as research subjects. It is the hope of the future and a realistic goal. But the reality of the present is that animal research still represents the best hope of mankind to solve its medical problems.

The vast majority of our population understands this need, but also demands that animal research be preformed under strict rules and regulations that ensure the maximum welfare of animals. Hence, laws have been written to ensure that animal research is conducted to the highest standards.

Almost all federal laws on the care and use of animals within the biomedical industry originate from two sources: the Animal Welfare Act, under the direction of the Secretary of the U.S. Department of Agriculture (USDA), and the Health Research Extension Act, directed by the Secretary of Health and Human Services. The National Institute of Health (NIH), a division of Health and Human Services, enforces the federal law. The NIH, has a subbranch called the Office of Laboratory Animal Welfare that publishes the Public Health Services (PHS) *Policy on Humane Care and Use of Laboratory Animals*. The National Research Council publishes *The Guide for the Care and Use of Laboratory Animals* (known as *The Guide*), which establishes standards for animal care and use. Both the USDA and the NIH require research institutions to conform to the regulations found in that publication.

In very specialized situations, other laws and agencies come into play. Research sometimes requires the capture of animals from the wild. In such cases, other agencies including the U.S. Fish and Wildlife Service and the Department of the Interior must be utilized. Some of the laws enforced by these agencies include the Endangered Species Act, the Lacy Act, and the Marine Mammal Protection Act. International treaties intended to protect endangered species and migratory birds are also invoked to enforce specific requirements in certain research projects.

The Animal Welfare Act and the Health Research Extension Act set specific guidelines concerning review of all animal activities by an Animal Care and Use Committee (ACUC). The laws are very objective. They empower the ACUC to address every aspect of animal use, including a review of the specific research that will be conducted, housing of the animals, specific enrichment plans, pain management, and training of research personnel. Since there is great variation in research projects, each institution is allowed to develop its own animal care policy based on its specific needs and the federal legal requirements. In all cases, the ACUC includes a veterinarian and at least one outside member, a nonscientist with no association with the company or institute of learning. In this way, the law ensures that the ACUC addresses the needs of the animals and the concerns of the general public.

SAFETY

OCCUPATIONAL HEALTH AND SAFETY IN THE BIOMEDICAL INDUSTRY

Many graduates of animal technician programs are employed by the biomedical industry in various capacities. Specific positions offered to graduates of animal technician programs vary with the type of institution, but the majority of technicians function as animal caretakers and are generally responsible for the health, comfort, and safety of the animals used in scientific research. Others work in product development, product testing, regulatory control, and teaching.

The types of biomedical companies and institutions that employ veterinary technicians are as follows:
- Drug and pharmaceutical manufacturers
- Private and public teaching institutions, colleges, and universities
- Manufacturers of animal support equipment and animal feeds
- Breeders and distributors of research animals
- Private research foundations
- Government agencies

OCCUPATIONAL HEALTH AND SAFETY PROGRAMS

Every institution that is considered a part of the biomedical industry should have a written Occupational Health and

Safety Program (OHSP) in place to protect the employees who work with animals. The OHSP must be carefully written for the activities and the functions of each specific institution.

A successful program requires the coordination of management, administration, scientists, and workers to ensure that the program adequately covers the complete scope of activities performed at the facility, and all pertinent personnel. Moreover, the program must be flexible enough to adjust to changes that take place in the institution. If, for example, a university institutes a new study on Tuberculosis, which represents a health hazard not previously encountered, then the program must be amended to accommodate the added risk factors. The program must be a dynamic vehicle that changes as needs change. Specific risks within the institution must be carefully evaluated when writing the Occupational Health and Safety Program. For example, a facility that works with nonhuman primates must write into its program measures that address special risks to people when exposed to these animals. A facility that will never house nonhuman primates does not have to include such precautions in its program.

A successful program includes a complete medical history of each employee, a preventative medicine section, including a vaccination program suitable for the work performed, a system of ongoing medical evaluation, and a clear and standard policy for emergency situations. The program must also evaluate individual risk factors such as degree of exposure for each person employed at the facility. A person who cleans the research facility hallway for one hour per day is handled differently from an attendant who handles animals six hours per day.

STANDARD OPERATIONAL PROCEDURES

Administrative and health professionals in a research facility carefully list all the different activities performed on a regular basis by all employees. Then each aspect of the procedure is written in a sequential form, taking into consideration all safety precautions. A Standard Operational Procedure (SOP) is an official detailed description of how each important procedure should be performed at the facility. An administrator or other responsible official of the research facility signs the document. All employees are expected to adhere to the SOP when performing each activity. A copy of the SOP should be readily available at the work site.

BIOSAFETY HAZARD CONSIDERATIONS IN BIOMEDICAL LABORATORIES

The hazards generally found in practice have been discussed. There are however, special considerations that must be given to hazards that are unique to the biomedical industry.

Biosafety Classifications

The Centers for Disease Control and Prevention has established specific guidelines for the safe handling and management of infectious agents in the biomedical industry. Biosafety levels are graded as I, II, III, and IV. The higher the number; the greater the risk. The following is a brief summary of the precautions for each biosafety level. It should be noted that the requirements for each level increase and that requirements for lower levels are automatically included in higher levels.

Biosafety level I

The agents in biosafety level I are those that ordinarily do not cause disease in humans. It should be noted, however that these otherwise harmless substances may affect individuals with immune deficiency.

Examples of products and organisms found in biosafety level I include most soaps and cleaning agents, vaccines administered to animals, and infectious diseases that are species-specific, such as Canine Infectious Hepatitis Virus.

There are no specific requirements for the handling or disposal of biosafety level 1 materials other than the normal sanitation that would be used in a home kitchen. This always includes complete washing of counters, equipment, and hands.

Biosafety level II

The agents in biosafety level II are those that have the potential to cause human disease if handled incorrectly. At this level, specific precautions are taken to avoid problems. The hazards in this level include mucous membrane exposure, possible oral ingestion, and puncture of the skin. Examples of organisms in this level are *Toxoplasma* and *Salmonella*. Generally, substances in this group have a low potential for aerosol contamination.

Although precautions will vary with the specific substances, these are the general requirements for biosafety level II.

- Limited access to the area, including signs that warn of biohazards
- Wearing of gloves, laboratory coats, gowns, and face shields, and use of Class I or Class II biosafety cabinets to protect against splash potential or aerosol contamination
- Careful use of sharps containers
- Specific instruction for the disposal and/or decontamination of equipment and potentially dangerous materials, including monitoring and reporting of contamination problems
- Physical containment devices and autoclaves, if needed

Biosafety level III

Agents in biosafety level III are substances that can cause serious and potentially lethal disease. The potential for aerosol respiratory transmission is high. An example of an organism in this category is *Mycobacterium tuberculosis*.

At this level, primary and secondary barriers are required to protect personnel. General requirements at this level are as follows.

- Controlled access
- Decontamination of waste
- Decontamination of cages, clothing, and other equipment
- Testing of personnel to evaluate possible exposure
- Use of Class I or Class II biosafety cabinets or other physical containment devices during all procedures
- Use of personal protective gear for all personnel

Biosafety level IV

It is unlikely that persons with limited experience in handing biohazards will ever encounter substances that are included in this level. Agents found in this category pose a high risk of causing life-threatening diseases. Included in this level is the *Ebola* and *Marburg* viruses and other dangerous and exotic agents. Facilities that handle these substances exercise maximum containment. Personnel shower-in and shower-out and dress in full body suits equipped with a positive air supply. Individuals who plan to work in these facilities will undergo extensive training to ensure safety.

OCCUPATIONAL HEALTH AND SAFETY IN VETERINARY PRACTICE

As a veterinary technician, you may be exposed to many hazards in your day-to-day routine and in the performance of nonroutine functions. Hazards can include exposure to pathogenic microorganisms, chemicals, or radiation, in addition to the obvious physical dangers. When properly identified, however, these hazards can be controlled and your risk of injury minimized.

Machinery and Moving Parts

Equipment such as fans and dryers have moving parts that can cause severe injury. Never operate machinery or equipment without all the proper guards in place. Long hair should be tied back to prevent it from getting caught in fans or other moving objects. Avoid wearing excessive jewelry, very loose-fitting clothing, or open-toe shoes. If you become aware of an unsafe condition, report it to your supervisor immediately.

Slips and Falls

You can reduce the chance of personal injury from slips and falls by wearing slip-proof shoes and using nonslip mats or strips in wet areas. Be especially cautious when walking on uneven or wet floors. Never run inside the hospital or on uneven flooring.

Lifting

When lifting patients, supplies, or equipment, remember to keep your back straight and lift with your legs. Never bend over to lift an object. If a motorized lift table is not available, recruit help when lifting patients who weigh more than 40 pounds. Remember to follow sound ergonomic principles when positioning or restraining, especially when working with horses or food animals.

Storing Supplies

Store heavy supplies or equipment on the lower shelves to prevent unnecessary strains. Never use stairways as storage areas. Do not overload shelves or cabinets. Store liquids in containers with tight-fitting lids. When possible, store chemicals on shelves *at or below* eye level. Never climb on cabinets, shelves, chairs, buckets, or similar items to reach high locations; use an appropriate ladder or stepstool.

Toxic Substances

Eat or drink only in areas free of toxic and biologically harmful substances. Keep the staff coffee pot and utensils well away from sources of possible contamination, such as the laboratory or the treatment/bathing tub. Ensure that the cabinets above a coffee or food area contain no hazardous chemicals or supplies that could spill on the area. Store food, drinks, condiments, and snacks in a refrigerator free from biological or chemical hazards; vaccines, drugs, and laboratory samples are all potential contamination sources.

Heating Devices

When using equipment such as autoclaves, microwave ovens, cautery irons, or other heating devices, take time to learn the rules for safe operation. Burns, especially from steam, are painful and serious and almost always can be prevented. Autoclaves also present a danger from the pressure that is used for proper sterilization. When opening an autoclave, first release the pressure with the "vent" device and let the steam rise completely before opening the door fully. Always assume cautery devices and branding irons are hot, and use the insulated handle whenever you handle them. Never place heated irons on any surface where they could overheat and start a fire or where someone could accidentally touch them.

Eye Safety

Become familiar with the locations and use of the eyewash stations. Always use safety glasses and other personal protective equipment when required. By law, an employer must provide this equipment; however, the primary reason the equipment is there is for your protection. In every state and territory of the United States, an employee can be legally disciplined, including being terminated, for failure to follow safety rules for the workplace.

Hazards of Animal Handling

Remaining alert

The first rule to follow when working around animals is to stay alert. Sudden noises, movements, or even light can cause an animal to react. If you are the primary restraint person, focus your attention on the animal's reactions and not on the procedure being performed. Learn the correct restraint positions for each species you handle regularly.

Protective gear

Make use of any available capture/restraint equipment. Wear latex examination gloves and a surgical mask when handling a stray, wild, or unvaccinated animal. Maintain an appropriate distance from the work area or animal; for example, do not place your face very close to the mouth of the animal (see "Zoonotic Hazards" section). Wear protective leather gloves when handling a fractious animal.

Barking dogs can be a threat to hearing, especially in indoor kennels. Noise levels in canine wards can reach 110 decibels (dB). Exposure to these noise levels for a short time, such as going into the kennel to retrieve a patient, poses no serious damage to your hearing, but excessive or long-term exposure can contribute to hearing loss. When working in noisy areas for extended periods (e.g., when cleaning cages), always wear personal hearing protectors rated to filter the noise by at least 20 dB. (The package label indicates the rating.)

Chutes and enclosures

Large animals, such as horses and cattle, can severely injure or even kill you when they try to escape restraint. Never place your hand, leg, or any other body part between the animal and the side of the enclosure or chute; use a hook or pole to pass ropes or belts through the chute. If you must enter a stall or paddock containing a large animal, stay on the side of the animal nearer the door or gate so that you can escape if the situation becomes hazardous.

Hazards of Bathing and Dipping

Ventilation

Always use the ventilation fan when bathing or dipping. This will keep fumes from shampoos and dips at a safe level.

Eye safety

Be sure you know where the eyewash device is before you need to use it (Fig. 2-1). If you splash a chemical in your eyes, *do not rub your eyes with your hands.* Immediately call for help. With a coworker's assistance, go to the eyewash station and flush *both* eyes, even if only one eye is affected. Avoid using the spray attachments for tubs and sinks, because the water pressure is unregulated and the streams of water from these devices can be fine enough to lacerate the cornea.

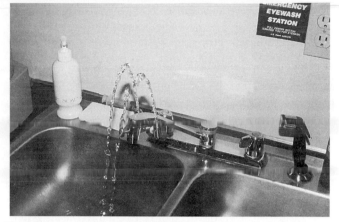

Fig. 2-1 Locate and know how to operate the eyewash devices in your hospital.

Chemical storage

Chemicals used for bathing and dipping animals can be harmful and must be stored properly. Bottles of dips, shampoos, and parasiticides should be stored in a cabinet at or below eye level. The bottle should be properly labeled including contents and any appropriate hazard warning (see "Chemical Hazards" section).

Zoonotic Hazards

When handling such specimens as fecal samples, laboratory samples, or wound exudates, wear protective gloves and *always wash your hands immediately after completing the procedure.* Contamination with these types of materials can usually be cleaned up with paper towels soaked in appropriate disinfecting solution. Latex gloves should be worn and then discarded with the cleaned-up materials.

When treating patients with diseases that are infectious to people or other animals, wear a protective apron, latex exam gloves, and, if appropriate, eye protection. Thoroughly wash your hands with a disinfecting agent, such as chlorhexidine or povidone-iodine scrub, at the completion of treatment. Any clothing that has been contaminated should be changed immediately.

Rabies

Rabies is a very serious, usually fatal viral disease that can affect any warm-blooded animal, including people. Rabies virus is spread by contact with an infected animal's saliva. Usually an uninfected animal becomes infected through the bite of a rabid (infected) animal. The disease has also been transmitted by saliva (even the residue left on a dog's bowl after eating) that contaminates an open wound or contacts the mucous membranes.

The primary barrier to the spread of rabies from the wild animal population to humans is vaccination of pets and other domestic animals. When you must handle an unvaccinated, wild, or stray animal, *always* wear protective latex gloves and perhaps even protective gowns and goggles. A safe and effective human vaccine is available for people who work with animals. Ask your hospital administrator about the availability of this vaccine at your practice.

Bacterial infections

Bacterial infections are certainly possible in the veterinary environment. Aside from the common bacteria that all animals harbor naturally, injury and disease in veterinary patients can expose you to such serious pathogens as *Pasteurella*, *E. coli*, and *Pseudomonas*. Bacteria are most commonly transferred by direct contact with the animal or its excretions, especially if you have cuts or open sores. Some bacteria are easily aerosolized or released into the air, where they can be inhaled and absorbed through your mucous membranes. The best protection from exposure to bacteria is good personal hygiene.

Fungal infections

Ringworm is a superficial skin infection caused by the fungus *Microsporum canis*, among others. Ringworm is very easily transmitted from animals to humans. The most effective protection from ringworm is to wear latex gloves when handling or treating animals with ringworm and to practice good personal hygiene.

Parasitism

When the eggs of common internal parasites, such as roundworms and hookworms, infect humans, they usually do not mature to adult parasites, but they can cause other problems. Some species of roundworm larvae can migrate to virtually any organ in the body and develop into a cyst-like growth causing a condition known as *visceral larva migrans*. These "cysts" are usually not noticeable, but if they develop in a vital organ, such as the eye or brain, they can cause severe problems.

Hookworms can cause a condition known as *cutaneous larva migrans*. This condition particularly affects children who play in areas where pets defecate frequently, such as a sandbox. Unlike the visceral cysts caused by roundworm larvae, the lesions of cutaneous larva migrans are relatively easy to visualize. These usually appear as red, serpentine lines on the skin of the feet or lower legs.

Borreliosis or Lyme disease, a bacterial infection transmitted by ticks, has become a serious concern for pets and people. When an infected deer tick bites a host (animal or person) during feeding, the bacterium *Borrelia burgdorferi* is transferred to the host. Lyme disease in humans is characterized by joint pain, fever, and other flulike symptoms. The best defense against borreliosis is to check your body for ticks after venturing outdoors and remove them promptly.

Mites causing sarcoptic mange can easily infest people. When treating animals with sarcoptic mange, always wear gloves and a protective gown, and wash your hands thoroughly with disinfecting soap immediately after the procedure.

The coccidian parasite Toxoplasma gondii can infect cats and people. Although it is usually not harmful to healthy humans, it might cause serious problems to the fetus of pregnant women. Toxoplasmosis is spread from cats to people usually by ingestion of the infectious oocysts in cat feces. Pregnant women should avoid cleaning cat litter pans.

Biologics

Vials containing biologics, such as vaccines and bacterins, usually are not considered hazardous unless the agent can infect humans. For example, vials containing such agents as canine distemper virus or feline calicivirus are not usually considered a danger to humans, but vials containing biologically hazardous agents, such as brucellosis bacterins, must be treated as potentially infectious during and after use.

Radiation Hazards

Infrequent exposure to small amounts of radiation, such as routine thoracic or dental radiographs, poses little threat to your overall health. However, long-term exposure to small doses of radiation has been linked to genetic, cutaneous, glandular, and other disorders. Exposure to large doses of radiation can cause skin changes, cell damage, and gastrointestinal and bone marrow disorders that can be fatal.

Radiation safety

When using radiographic equipment, never place any part of your body in the primary beam, even a hand wearing a lead-lined glove. Always wear the appropriate protective equipment, such as lead-lined aprons and gloves. Thyroid collars and lead-impregnated glasses are also recommended. Always use the collimator to restrict the primary beam to an area smaller than the size of the cassette. In other words, isolate the area to be radiographed and minimize the scatter radiation.

Portable x-ray machines, such as those used in large animal and mobile practices, can be particularly dangerous because the primary beam of these machines can be aimed in any direction. When using a portable machine, always be sure there is no human body part in the path of the primary beam, even at a distance. Never hold a cassette, whether wearing lead-lined gloves or not; always use a cassette-holding pole. Also, wear a lead-lined apron and gloves.

Everyone involved with radiography must wear a *dosimetry badge*. This badge must always be worn during radiographic procedures to measure any scatter radiation you may receive during the procedure. Your supervisor or hospital administrator will regularly advise you of the readings from your personal dosimetry badge. These reports, required by law, are designed as a warning system to alert you and your supervisor if your exposure to radiation reaches a hazardous level.

Developing chemicals

Radiographic developing chemicals (developer and fixer) can be very corrosive to materials and human tissues. Take extreme care when mixing, transferring, agitating, or transporting these chemicals, and do this only in a well-ventilated area. Always turn on the exhaust fan when you are in a darkroom. Use protective gloves and goggles when mixing or pouring chemicals. For manual processing tanks, stir chemicals with care and avoid splashing. After handling radiographic chemicals, always wash your hands. See Chapter 18 for detailed information on radiation safety.

Anesthetic Hazards

Long-term exposure to waste anesthetic gases has been linked to congenital abnormalities in children, spontaneous abortions, and liver and kidney damage. OSHA has set the safe exposure limit for halogenated anesthetic agents (halothane, methoxyflurane, isoflurane) at 2 parts per million.

According to some sources, as much as 90% of the anesthetic gas levels found in the surgery room during a procedure can be attributed to leaks in anesthesia machines. For this reason, always check for leaks in the hoses and anesthetic machine before use (Box 2-1). Use hoses and rebreathing bags that are the correct size, and inflate the endotracheal tube cuff before connecting the patient to the machine. Start the flow of anesthetic gas after connecting the patient to the machine. Before disconnecting the patient, continue oxygen flow until the remaining anesthesia gas has been flushed through the scavenging system.

A well-designed scavenging system captures excess gases directly at the source and transports them to a safe exhaust port, usually outside the building. This is the most effective means of reducing exposure of waste anesthetic gases in the workplace.

When refilling the anesthetic machine vaporizer, move the machine to a well-ventilated area. Use a pouring funnel and avoid overfilling the vaporizer or spilling the liquid anesthetic. If you accidentally break a bottle of liquid anesthetic, immediately evacuate all people from the area. Open the window and turn on the exhaust fans. Control the liquid with a spill kit absorbent or a generous amount of kitty litter. Pick up the contaminated absorbent or kitty litter with a dustpan, and place it in a plastic trash bag.

Some procedures, such as masking or tank induction, defy collection of waste gases. In such instances, be sure the room is well-ventilated. Exhaust fans for evacuating room air to the outside are recommended. Air-handling systems that recirculate the air can expose others in the hospital. Induction chambers can be connected to the scavenging system or absorption canister to reduce levels of escaping gases.

When changing the soda lime (carbon dioxide absorbent) in anesthetic machines, wear latex gloves. When the soda lime is wet, as it often is from humidity in the patient's breath, it can be very caustic to tissues and some metals.

BOX 2-1 *procedure*

Checking for Leaks in an Anesthetic Machine

1. Assemble all hoses, canisters, valves, or tubes according to the manufacturer's instructions.
2. Turn on the oxygen supply to the machine.
3. Close the pressure-relief (pop-off) valve.
4. Use your thumb or palm to form a tight seal on the Y-piece.
5. Turn on the oxygen flow until the rebreathing bag is slightly overinflated; then close the valve.
6. Observe the pressure in the system on the manometer and watch closely for any decrease. (If the machine is not equipped with manometer, observe the size of the bag closely.) If the pressure remains constant, the machine is considered leak-free. If the pressure drops, there is a leak (or leaks) in the system. The faster the pressure drops, the larger the leak(s).
7. If there is a leak, check the rebreathing bag, hoses, and other rubber or plastic parts for evidence of cracks or deterioration. Replace any parts that are damaged. Check all connections, especially at the vaporizer inlet and outlet. Check the seals at the top and bottom of the soda lime canister and on the one-way valves (clear plastic domes). Tighten any loose connections.
8. After checking all connections and hoses, if there is still a leak, have the machine serviced by a qualified technician before use.
9. When the machine is leak-free, reopen the pressure-relief valve and use the machine normally.

Place used soda lime granules in a plastic trash bag and dispose of it in the regular trash.

If you are a woman and become pregnant, discuss the anesthetic exposure risk with your physician as soon as possible and notify your supervisor immediately.

Hazards of Compressed Gases

Store cylinders of compressed gas (e.g., oxygen) in a dry, cool place, away from potential heat sources, such as furnaces, water heaters, and direct sunlight. Always secure the tanks in an upright position by means of a chain or strap (including small tanks). Transportation carts and floor-mounting collars are also acceptable methods of securing compressed gas cylinders. If the cylinder is equipped with a protective cap (usually the large ones are), it must be firmly screwed in place when the cylinder is not in use. If you must move a large cylinder, do not roll or drag it; always use a hand truck or cart and strap the tank to the cart before moving. Always wear impact-resistant protective goggles when connecting or disconnecting tanks, because air escaping from tanks can cause trauma to the cornea of your eyes.

Hazards of Sharp Objects

The most serious hazard of sharp objects (sharps) in a veterinary environment is from the physical trauma and possible bacterial infection caused by a puncture or laceration. To prevent accidents from punctures or lacerations, always keep needles, scalpel blades, and other sharps capped or sheathed until ready for use. When practical, place the sharp in a red sharps container immediately after use (Fig. 2-2). Do not attempt to recap the needle unless the physical danger from sticks or lacerations cannot be avoided by any other means.

When necessary, needles may be recapped using the "one-handed" method. Place the cap on a flat surface (table or counter). With one hand, "thread" the needle into the cap. The cap may then be firmly seated using both hands. The needle should not be removed from the syringe, but the entire unit should be disposed of in the red sharps container. When full, the sharps container must be sealed and disposed of following the hospital's prescribed policy.

Ordinary plastic milk containers are not appropriate sharps collection containers; a 22-gauge needle can easily penetrate them. The containers made for this specific purpose (usually red and labeled with a biohazard symbol) are the most effective and are usually very economical.

Cutting off the ends of needles before disposal increases the potential for aerosolization of the liquid involved. Collecting sharps in a smaller container and transferring them to a larger container for disposal places someone at an increased risk of exposure. Neither of these practices is recommended.

Never throw needles or other sharps directly into regular trash containers, regardless of whether or not they are capped. Never open a used sharps container. Never insert your fingers into a sharps container for any reason.

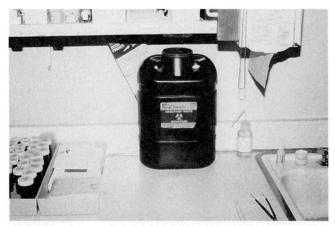

Fig. 2-2 Needles and other sharp objects must be disposed of in specially designed sharps containers.

Chemical Hazards

Many products you use every day can be hazardous. Every chemical, even common ones such as cleaning supplies, can cause harm. Some chemicals can contribute to health problems, whereas others may be flammable and pose a fire threat. The most common chemicals used in the veterinary workplace are insecticides, medications, and cleaning agents.

Veterinary hospitals must follow the guidelines of OSHA's Right to Know law. This law requires that you are informed about all chemicals you may be exposed to while doing your job. The Right to Know law also requires you to wear all safety equipment that is prescribed by the manufacturer when handling a chemical. The safety equipment must be provided by the employer at no cost to you. It is not optional; you must wear what is prescribed.

Hazardous materials plan

A key component of the Right to Know law is the *hazardous materials plan*. This plan describes the details of the practice's *Material Safety Data Sheet (MSDS)* filing system and the secondary container labeling system. The plan also lists the person responsible for ensuring that all employees have received the necessary safety training. You have a right to review any of these materials, so ask your supervisor where your plan is located.

Part of the planning process includes knowing exactly what chemicals are present in the workplace. There must be an up-to-date list of chemicals known to be on the hospital premises. It surprises some people to learn that the average veterinary hospital has over 200 hazardous chemicals present at any time.

Material safety data sheets

More detailed information about every chemical can be found on the Material Safety Data Sheet (MSDS). Ask your supervisor where your hospital's MSDS file is located, and take the time to review it for chemicals you use frequently. MSDSs may look complicated at first glance, but the information that is important to you is easy to find.

Container labels

When you receive a supply of chemicals from the distributor, every bottle is identified with a label containing directions and any appropriate warnings. Always read, understand, and follow these directions and warnings printed on the label. When possible, keep this label intact and readable. Sometimes it is necessary to dilute a chemical or pour it into smaller bottles for use. These smaller bottles are known as *secondary containers*. All secondary containers must have a label that indicates the contents and appropriate safety warnings.

Container caps

Always remember to replace the cap on a chemical bottle after use. Bottles of chemicals should always have tight-fitting, screw-on lids. Always store chemical bottles at or below eye level in a closed cabinet. Never store or use chemicals near food or beverages.

Mixing chemicals

Be very cautious when mixing or diluting chemicals. Always wear latex gloves and protective goggles. Never mix any chemicals unless you know it is safe to do so according to the label or MSDS. Mixing often creates a new, sometimes very dangerous chemical. When making dilute solutions from a concentrate, always start with the correct quantity of water and then add the concentrate. Never add the water to the concentrate, because the chemical may splash or may not react as you expect.

Chemical spills

Minor spills of most chemicals can be cleaned up with paper towels or absorbent, such as kitty litter, and disposed of in the trash or sanitary sewer. However, some very dangerous chemicals, such as formaldehyde or ethylene oxide, require special procedures. Before you use a chemical with which you are unfamiliar, review the MSDS and learn the procedures you must follow for cleaning up a spill. When cleaning up any spill, always wear latex gloves and any other protective equipment specified on the MSDS. Unless prohibited by the instructions on the MSDS, wash the spill site and any contaminated equipment with a detergent soap and water.

Handling ethylene oxide

Many hospitals use ethylene oxide gas to sterilize items that would be damaged by other sterilization procedures. Ethylene oxide is a potent human carcinogen. Take the following precautions:
- Carefully read the MSDS for ethylene oxide.
- Store the ethylene oxide in a safe place.
- Use only approved devices to perform ethylene oxide sterilization.
- Read, understand, and follow all written procedures and safety precautions.
- Know the emergency procedures.
- Be aware of monitoring levels.
- Keep ethylene oxide away from flames and sparks, because it is highly flammable.

Handling formalin

Liquid or gaseous formaldehyde and formalin are serious health hazards in veterinary hospitals. Because formaldehyde is a known human carcinogen, OSHA monitors its use:
- Carefully read the MSDS for formaldehyde/formalin.
- Store formalin containers safely, including specimen jars.
- Use formalin only with good ventilation; avoid breathing vapors.
- Wear goggles and latex gloves; avoid skin and eye contact.

Exposure to formalin can be minimized by use of premixed, premeasured vials of formalin for specimens. Veterinary hospitals that still use bulk formalin for diagnostic laboratory tests (e.g., Knott's test) should consider switching to a newer, less-hazardous method of testing.

Electrical Hazards

Do not remove light switch or electrical outlet covers. Always keep circuit breaker boxes closed. Only persons trained to perform maintenance duties should repair electrical outlets, switches, fixtures, or breakers. If you must use a portable dryer or other electrical equipment in a wet area, it must be properly grounded and plugged into only a ground-fault circuit interruption (GFCI) type of outlet.

Extension cords should be used only for temporary supply applications and should always be of the three-conductor, grounded type. Never run extension cords through windows or doors that could close and damage the wires. Also, never run extension cords across aisles or floors, which creates a tripping hazard. When an extension cord is necessary, it should be adequate for the electrical load. Generally, extension cords longer than 4 feet should not be used for loads greater than 6 amps at 120 volts AC or 3 amps at 240 volts AC.

Equipment with grounded plugs must never be used with adapters or nongrounded extension cords. Never alter or remove the ground terminals on plugs. Appliances or equipment with defective ground terminals or plugs should not be used until repaired.

Fire and evacuation

Always store flammables properly; such materials as gasoline, paint thinner, and ether should never be stored inside the hospital, except in an approved storage cabinet designed for flammables. Some components of specialty dental and large animal acrylic repair kits are also very flammable. Very small amounts of these components can usually be safely stored in an area with good ventilation and free from flames or sparks.

Be alert for situations that could cause a fire. Flammable items, particularly newspapers, boxes, and cleaning chemicals, must always be stored at least 3 feet away from any ignition source, such as a water heater, furnace, or stove. Always use extra care when using portable heaters. Never leave them unattended, and always be sure they are placed no closer than 3 feet from any wall, furniture, or other flammable material.

Know the location of all fire extinguishers on the premises and how to use them (Fig. 2-3). Before you decide to use a fire extinguisher, be sure the fire alarm has been sounded, everyone has left the building (or is in the process of leaving), and the fire department has been called. The

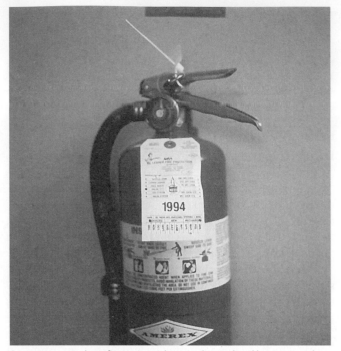

Fig. 2-3 Learn where fire extinguishers are located and how to use them.

National Fire Protection Association recommends that you never attempt to fight a fire if any of the following conditions apply:

- The fire is spreading beyond the immediate area where it started or has already become a large fire.
- The fire could block your escape route.
- You are unsure of the proper operation of the extinguisher.
- You doubt that the extinguisher is designed for the type of fire at hand or is large enough to suppress the fire.

Know where the designated emergency exits are. Make sure emergency exits are always unlocked and free from obstructions. If you must work in a building during non-operational hours (when security warrants that the doors are locked), be sure you have at least two clear exits from the building that can be opened without a key.

Personal Safety

Workers in emergency or 24-hour practices should use the "barriers" that are usually available. Use the buzzer to con-trol access through the front door and one-way locks on the remaining doors. (This lets you out in case of an emergency but keeps the door locked from the outside.) These personal safety techniques are almost essential in these environments.

In any practice, the potential for robbery is always present. In any situation where someone demands money or drugs while threatening your personal safety, *do not attempt to withhold the things they demand.* Cooperate with the demands, but do not go with the person, even to the parking lot. Attempt to remember every detail of the person's appearance and demeanor. This greatly increases the likelihood that the police will locate the person. As soon as safely possible, let everyone else know of the situation. Attempt to contact the police if this can be done safely without the intruder's knowledge; otherwise, do it immediately after the intruder has left the premises.

RECOMMENDED READING

Brody MD: Safety in the veterinary medical workplace environment: Common issues and concerns, *Vet Clin North Am* 23(5):1071-1084, 1993.

Copeland JD: Employer-employee relations, *Vet Clin North Am* 23(5):957-974, 1993.

National Research Council, *Occupational health and safety in the care and use of research animals,* National Academy Press, 1997.

National Research Council, *Guide for the care and use of laboratory animals,* National Academy Press, Washington, D.C., 1966.

Newman E, et al: *Health hazards in veterinary practice,* ed 3, Schaumburg, Ill, 1995, American Veterinary Medical Association.

Office of Laboratory Animal Welfare, *National Institutes of Health, Institutional Animal Care and Use Committee Guidebook,* ed 2, 2002.

OSHA: *Employee workplace rights* (free pamphlet), 1994, U.S. Department of Labor, OSHA, Publications Office, Room N-3101, 200 Constitution Avenue NW, Washington, D.C. 20210.

Renado VT, Ryan G: Technical assistance in radiology, Part 2: Basic considerations and radiation safety, *Vet Tech* 9(10):547-551, 1988.

Seibert, PJ, Jr.: *The complete veterinary practice regulatory manual,* ed 2, Calhoun, Tenn, 1996, Philip J. Seibert, Jr.

Stribling J, Picut C: Food and drug regulatory issues, *Vet Clin North Am* 23(5):991-1005, 1993.

U.S. Department of Health and Human Services, *Biosafety in microbiological and biomedical laboratories,* ed 3, 1993.

Wilson JF: *Law and ethics of the veterinary profession,* Yardley, Pa, 1993, Priority Press.

3

Practice Management

Sally B. Smith

Learning Objectives

After reviewing this chapter, the reader should understand the following:

- Administrative procedures commonly used during a client's office visit and when admitting or discharging patients
- Methods used in billing clients, extending credit, and collecting debts
- Methods used to market veterinary services
- Administrative procedures commonly used in operating a veterinary practice
- Methods used in maintaining and ordering inventory and interacting with vendors
- Uses of computers in veterinary practice
- Procedures used for physically maintaining a veterinary facility

A successful and rewarding veterinary practice is as dependent on practice philosophy and infrastructure as it is on the technical ability to perform medicine and surgery. This chapter focuses on the development of an infrastructure that equips the practice to meet client (and patient) needs.

A customer focus is essential for the success of any small business, and veterinary practices are, by definition, small businesses. It is important to recognize clients as customers, and that customers have a choice of hospitals to use for their pet care services. With proper balance and judicious application of the concepts presented in this chapter, the patient, client, staff member, and practice are all well served.

FRONT OFFICE

In many practices, especially small facilities, the veterinary technician plays an important role in the front office as well as performing technical tasks. These duties include answering the telephone, making appointments, answering pet care questions, selling over-the-counter products, greeting clients as they arrive, and maintaining client records. While some of these duties may seem mundane in comparison to specific technical duties, they are nevertheless extremely important.

Without positive contact, the potential client may go elsewhere, or the established client may be lost. To any customer, the person standing in front of them represents the business. In a veterinary hospital, most clients have no real way to judge the practice's medical standing. They make a judgment based on the perception they develop when dealing with hospital staff by telephone or at the front desk. The average client will not be able to determine how "good" a veterinarian's medical expertise is; they judge whether or not they and their pet like the doctor.

A veterinary technician with positive approach and good people skills can create much good will with clientele. Some clients are more comfortable speaking with a person other than the veterinarian, and the trained veterinary technician can fill this role perfectly.

OFFICE VISIT

As a veterinary technician, your role in the client visit may include several important communication room activities. The initial telephone call and first visit to the clinic are the best times to collect client information. While some practices

The authors acknowledge and appreciate the original contribution of R.A. Goebel, whose work has been incorporated into this chapter.

maintain only computerized client files and verbally ask for information, most will also retain a written or hard copy file. The client information form should ask for information such as the following:

- Breed, age, sex, neuter status, and color
- Past medical problems
- Behavior problems

The practice may also ask for identification information from the client. A driver license and/or social security number is the most common. In the event of nonpayment, it is important to have as much personal information as possible. A collection agency or judge will use this information to track and find a missing client, or to attach judgements to personal credit history.

After escorting the client and patient to the exam room, you have an opportunity to discuss the practice's services as appropriate, to review the reason for the current visit, and to make recommendations for routine services that, by practice policy, would be timely or overdue. You can perform an initial physical examination, including measuring rectal temperature and weight, noting gross physical abnormalities on the record, and obtaining required laboratory samples. You may also note initial findings and client concerns for the veterinarian.

Some practices use a physical examination form that duplicates the information recorded in the medical record to apprise the client of the animal's health. This form should contain lay terminology and document physical examination findings as well as recommendations. This tool helps to formalize recommendations, document information for discussion with the client's family members, and refresh memories of matters discussed during the patient visit. Welcome client questions, and answer them as appropriate. Veterinary technicians can play a major role in client education, as well as in patient care.

As an alternative to traditional office visits, some practices offer drop-off services. Usually this service is only for existing patients. With this service, a client may present the patient, relate any concerns or needs, and retrieve the patient later in the day. You may record pertinent information on a standardized form to obtain an adequate history and authorization for treatment (Fig. 3-1). Obtain the client's daytime telephone or cell phone number, or establish another method to contact the client following the patient's evaluation by the veterinarian. Some practices loan a paging device to clients so that they can be signaled to telephone the practice or return to pick up their pet. Also consider sending an e-mail message, since many people check their e-mail accounts several times a day. Alternatively, you can schedule a tentative pickup time so that the client can be sure a technician or veterinarian will be available to discuss the case at that time.

ADMITTING A PATIENT

If a patient is scheduled for elective surgery, prepackaged folders can speed client check-in. For example, you could assemble a description of the procedure, including cost estimates, procedure authorization and consent form, home care instructions, cage card, and patient identification band, as appropriate for commonly performed elective procedures (Figs. 3-2 and 3-3).

Additional forms can facilitate the communication and authorization process. A *standard consent form* authorizes care to be provided at the practice facility (Fig. 3-4). A *boarding guest registration form* may serve as an authorization form. The boarding guest registration form lists services that should also be offered verbally by the staff member managing the admission process. Owners frequently forget or are distracted when leaving their pet and appreciate these reminders of other services that can be performed conveniently during that pet's stay in the hospital facility. For surgical services, it is imperative to ask when the patient was last fed and watered, or if any snacks were fed before entering the practice. Clients are not aware of the risk of vomiting under anesthesia. Develop a system for marking tumors or growths the pet owner wants removed, since they can be difficult to locate later without the owner present.

As technician, you are frequently involved with not only performing procedures during the patient stay but also providing patient periodic progress reports to the client during the patient's stay.

If a patient must be referred to a specialty practice, the technician can arrange for preparation of such information as referral forms, copies of medical records, laboratory reports, and radiographs. It is essential to properly label and address original radiographs that accompany referrals, as these must be returned to the primary care facility. With all other records, provide copies for the referral practice and retain originals (as legally required) in the referring practice. Finally, the technician may arrange for patient discharge, scheduling of recheck or suture removal visits, and a telephone call to the client for a progress report 48 to 72 hours after release.

DISCHARGING A PATIENT

Complete medical and financial records before the patient is discharged from the hospital. Collect payment in full (or have payment contract signed) and make any follow-up appointment before the patient is brought to the examination room or reception area. Having the essential paperwork completed before the client and patient are reunited expedites the discharge procedure. It also minimizes distractions for the pet owner; once the pet is brought to the discharge room, the owner's attention will focus on the pet,

---

MAGRANE ANIMAL HOSPITAL   (555) 555-5555

What's Wrong with Your Pet?

Please answer the following questions as thoroughly as possible.

Vomiting:
☐ food   ☐ blood   how often? _____   ☐ diet change
☐ eating foreign objects (grass, trash, etc.) _____

Diarrhea:
☐ mucus   ☐ blood   ☐ straining   how often? _____

Sneezing & Coughing:
any discharge? _____ if yes, describe _____
☐ difficulty in breathing   type of cough _____ frequency _____

Urination:
☐ painful   ☐ blood noted   ☐ straining   how often _____

Limping:
which leg(s)? _____ describe problem _____

Skin:
☐ irritation   ☐ any family members itching?   ☐ hair loss   ☐ fleas
☐ applied any shampoos, dips, etc. (explain)? _____ how long? _____

Eyes:
which one? _____ discharge (color, consistency) _____ how long? _____

Ears:
which one? _____   ☐ odor   ☐ discharge   how long? _____

Seizures:
☐ twitching   ☐ any unknown seizure activity (describe)? _____
Any additional information? _____
Any known reaction to medication or vaccinations? _____
Any other pre-existing problems (if new patient)? _____
Currently on any medication and, if so, when was the last dose given? _____
1. At what phone number can you be reached? _____
2. Do you authorize us to do more than an initial exam? _____
3. May we start diagnostic tests or x-rays? _____
4. May we start treating the problem? _____
5. Is there a strict limit on dollars to be spent? _____

*(Unless emergency treatment is required, we intend to thoroughly discuss with you
any involved procedures andlor approximate costs before proceeding.)*

Client's Name _____   Pet's Name _____
Signature   Date

Fig. 3-1 The client is asked to complete a form when dropping off an animal at the clinic for evaluation or treatment.

ANESTHESIA/SURGERY CONSENT FORM

Owner: _____   Patient: _____

Procedure: _____   Phone Number Today: _____

I hereby authorize Magrane Animal Hospital, P.C. and its designated associates to perform the above procedure(s). In addition, in the event that emergency treatment is required and I cannot be reached, I agree to any necessary diagnostic, treatment, or surgical procedures which are required.

In order to maintain a healthy, clean, hospital environment, pets must be free of parasites (fleas, ticks) and be current on vaccinations. If necessary, pets will be updated on vaccinations and treated for any fleas or ticks at an additional charge.

Additional Options/Services

Please initial if you approve any of these additional services

Blood Tests To identify potential health risks we recommend a more comprehensive blood testing to evaluate the liver and kidneys, as well as diabetes (this testing is required on all patients over 7 years of age). The cost is an additional $37.60.

Approve _____

Retained Baby Teeth Occasionally puppies and kittens will not lose their baby teeth on schedule, which results in potential dental problems. We routinely extract these unwanted teeth while the pet is anesthetized. The additional cost is $6.60-$20.20 per tooth.

Approve _____

Fecal Examination We recommend a yearly bowel movement examination for internal parasites (worms). If your pet is overdue we can obtain a sample and test it for parasites while your pet is here for a fee of $11.00.

Microchip Identification We are now able to permanently identify pets using a small microchip implanted beneath their skin. The benefit of microchip identification is the ability to identify missing pets. We offer a $10.00 discount when we implant a microchip during an anesthetic procedure, for a net cost of $26.00.

Approve _____

Approve _____

Nail Trim $6.00

Approve _____

Express Anal Sacs $6.00

Approve _____

I have read and understand this consent form, and I agree to pay for services rendered at the time my pet is discharged or when service is otherwise completed.

Owner or Agent:

Magrane Animal Hospital • 2324 Grape Road • Mishawaka, IN 46545 • (555) 555-5555

Fig. 3-2 Form used to obtain a client's consent to induce general anesthesia or perform surgery.

HOME CARE FOLLOWING SURGERY

Your pet has received a general anesthetic and, as a result, may appear more tired than normal and possibly a little uncoordinated. This is to be expected and the grogginess should disappear in the next day or so.

- To prevent vomiting due to excitement on arriving home, do not give your pet food or water for an hour after returning home. Feed the regular diet lightly today and return to normal feeding tomorrow.
- If your pet becomes listless or refuses to eat the next day, or if vomiting or diarrhea occurs, call the hospital immediately.
- Observe the incision at least twice a day for drainage, excessive swelling, redness, or pain and report any abnormalities immediately.
- Discourage excessive licking or chewing by your pet at the stitches or incision, and call us if it persists.
- Your pet's exercise should be restricted (no free running or jumping) for a week following surgery.
- If your pet is sent home with a bandage or cast, make sure it stays clean and dry. Call the hospital if it becomes wet or heavily soiled.
- If your cat was declawed, use shredded paper towels or newspaper instead of litter for the first 3-5 days at home to help prevent infection.

Future Treatment

☐ Please make an appointment for a recheck in _____ days/weeks.

☐ Please make an appointment for suture removal in _____ days.

☐ Please make an appointment in _____ days for bandage change or removal.

☐ Remove bandage at home in _____ days.

Call the hospital if you have any problems or questions.

Special Instructions

_____

_____

_____

_____

_____

_____

Magrane Animal Hospital • 2324 Grape Road • Mishawaka, IN 46545 • (555) 555-5555

Fig. 3-3 Client handout describing home care following surgery.

STANDARD CONSENT FORM

TO: Magrane Animal Hospital, P.C.; K.T. Neuhoff, DVM; R.L. Doversberger, DVM; K.M. Kline, DVM; T.J. Niemann, DVM; R.A. Goebel, DVM

OWNER'S NAME: _____   NAME OF PET: _____

ADDRESS: _____   SPECIES: _____

BREED: _____

PATIENT NUMBER: _____   SEX: _____

I am the owner or agent for the owner of the above described pet and have the authority to execute this consent.

I hereby consent to the hospitalization of the above described pet and authorize the doctor and his/her staff to administer any medication, tests, anesthetics or surgical procedures that the doctor deems necessary for the health, safety, or well-being of my pet.

I specifically request the following procedure(s) or operation(s):

_____

I understand that during the performance of the foregoing procedure(s) or operation(s), unforeseen conditions may be revealed that necessitate an extension of the foregoing procedure(s) or operation(s) or different procedure(s) or operation(s) than those set forth above. Therefore, I hereby consent to and authorize the performance of such procedure(s) or operation(s) as are necessary and desirable in the exercise of the veterinarian's professional judgement.

I also authorize the use of appropriate anesthetics and other medications, and I understand that hospital support personnel will be employed as deemed necessary by the veterinarian.

I have been advised as to the nature of the procedure(s) or operation(s) and the risks involved. I realize that results cannot be guaranteed.

I understand that all fees for professional services are due and payable at the time of discharge.

I have read and understand this authorization and consent.

ADDITIONAL INFORMATION _____

_____

_____

_____

DATE: _____   Signature of Owner or Agent _____

Witness to Above Signature _____

Fig. 3-4 Form used to obtain a client's consent to provide veterinary care.

not on instructions or follow-up care. For this reason, many practices will issue written instructions and information in addition to speaking with the client.

The final exchange with the client should always include a statement about when the patient's next office visit should be. This serves as a reminder to the client. It also serves as a reminder to you—that you expect the client relationship to continue. Therefore, every time a patient leaves the clinic, there should be some mechanism in place to re-establish contact with the client. For example, schedule an appointment for re-examination and give a reminder appointment to the client. If, for example, there is a blood count and chemistry profile scheduled in 90 days, a staff member can call the client 48 hours before the appointment to remind the client of the appointment. Veterinary practices commonly send *reminder notices* to clients, suggesting an appointment for the animal's annual physical examination (Fig. 3-5). Backup methods must be in place so staff members can follow up on no-shows or lack of response. This maintains the cycle of clients returning to the practice.

Billing, Collection, and Credit Management

Ideally, clients pay in full at the time services are rendered. It is usually best to provide several payment options to clients, including cash, check, credit cards (MasterCard, Visa, Discover, American Express), or medical charge cards (e.g., Care Credit and Health Cap). Medical charge cards can be useful, but common complaints include failure to approve applicant (who may be standing at your reception desk), failure to authorize needed limits of credit, and slow or cumbersome application/approval process.

Many practices extend credit to clients, although sometimes with reluctance. Good credit management procedures protect the practice and serve the clients well. To address potential financial difficulties early, reception staff or others greeting clients and preparing records for the patient visit should simply ask, "How do you intend to pay for today's service? We offer the option of cash, check, or credit card." The client should then be honest in his or her response and indicate the method of payment (ability to pay is implied). If the client will need extension of credit by the practice, it should be apparent at this time.

The financial advantage of extending credit can be twofold. First, if credit is made available, the recommended work can be performed; client and patient are well served and the practice bills additional fees. Second, many clients need more than 30 days to pay and are willing to pay interest on balances extending past 30 days from the time of billing. Some practices charge the client interest at 1.5% per month on an unpaid balance. A billing fee is also assessed to pay for bookkeeping, postage, and other costs related to extending credit. The practice collects interest because the client has use of money owed to the practice. If accounts receivable (money owed by clients) are $24,000

for a three-doctor practice and three fourths of the balance is more than 30 days old, $3,240 in increased revenue would be generated annually by charging interest ($24,000 × ¾ × 1.5% = $270 per month × 12).

Each practice should clearly define criteria for extending credit so that all staff members can understand and implement the practice's policies. Box 3-1 lists sample considerations used in extending credit to clients. Box 3-2 lists factors to be considered when drawing up a payment contract.

It is a good practice for the clinic to mail out monthly billing statements, and to follow up on any past due accounts with a telephone call. Statistically, collection of accounts over 30 or 45 days falls off substantially. Many veterinarians will refuse to see a client with a past due account, unless the account can be brought up to date and paid along with the current office visit fee.

Client Communication

Communication with clients is essential to learn about client/patient needs, to educate clients about animal health needs and their role in meeting those needs, and to remind clients of periodic routine visits, as well as seasonal health needs. A variety of tools can facilitate communication with clients. Examples include newsletters, promotions, client advisory boards, focus groups, client surveys, and posters or signs.

Newsletters

Although newsletters can be somewhat costly and time-consuming to produce and distribute, they are an effective educational tool for clients. Newsletters can inform clients of health services offered by the practice and can introduce staff members. Newsletters produced in-house have the advantage of being more personal than commercially produced newsletters. Columns may include seasonal topics (e.g., heartworm or flea control or heat prostration), behavioral topics, case of the month, staff spotlight (focused on one staff member), and staff updates to introduce new staff or report on recent continuing education experiences. The newsletter may describe new or seasonal services or announce sign-up opportunities for "puppy manners" classes.

Commercially prepared newsletters usually cover seasonal topics. Some companies may personalize them with the practice name, address and telephone number. Some will reserve a small amount of space for a personal message or column from the practice. More and more veterinary facilities are using e-mail to send newsletters to clients wishing to receive them. Since there are no postage or printing costs incurred, e-newsletters are cost-effective and easy to distribute.

Special promotions

Clients can be informed of special events or timely topics using various promotional methods. Examples of special

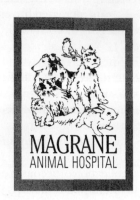

2324 Grape Road • Mishawaka, Indiana 46545 • 555/555-5555 Fax 555-1111

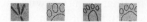

January 5, 1998

Richard Goebel
2601 Darwin Dr.
West Lafayette, IN 47906

Dear Richard,

Rudy's health is very important to us. Our records indicate that it has been more than 18 months since we have given Rudy a complete physical exam. Bringing Rudy in every year for a physical and vaccinations is a step in the right direction on the road to good health. Because dogs and cats age much more quickly than people, a yearly exam for them is the same as a doctor's visit every 6-8 years for us. A lot can change in a year.

Please call us today at 555-5555 for an appointment. We want to help you keep Rudy healthy. Remember it is far less costly to you and your pet to prevent diseases rather than treat them.

If you no longer have Rudy with you, please call to let us know. We would like to know if you have taken Rudy elsewhere for care, particularly if it is because you were dissatisfied with our service or care in any way, since we strive to provide you with the best. Please call and ask to speak with Vikky Warner.

Thank You,

Doctors and Staff of
Magrane Animal Hospital

Fig. 3-5 Letter sent to remind a client of vaccinations past due.

Sample Considerations for Extending Credit

Always request initial payment.

If the animal is ill, treat the animal and check the client's credit rating.

If the procedure is elective and no initial partial payment is made, reschedule the procedure for another time.

If the client has had a relationship with the clinic for more than one year and has always paid his or her bills in the past, establish a payment contract for up to $200 (not to be offered for elective services).

If the client has a history of previous unpaid bills and the account was turned over to a collection agency, do not extend credit with or without a payment contract.

If credit needs exceed $200, call the clinic's designated credit manager to expedite the credit check and negotiate payment terms.

events include National Pet Week, National Dental Health Month, breed rescue events, and humane society projects. Clients can be informed by posters or signs in the practice facility, notices on the outside sign, e-mail, and/or mailings of a special edition of the clinic's letters or postcards (Fig. 3-6). Special incentives can be used to entice clients to participate, such as an open house during National Pet Week or free dental examinations by staff technicians

Considerations When Drawing Up a Payment Contract

Limit the total term of the contract to 90 days or less.

Be sure the client understands that interest will be applied to all unpaid balances extending beyond 30 days.

Be sure the person signing the payment contract is the animal owner or authorized agent and is willing to assume full financial responsibility. The agent must be at least 18 years of age. A minor or child does not have legal authority to enter into a payment contract.

Inspect the client's driver license to confirm information provided (such as name, address, driver license or Social Security number, and photo).

Seek agreement to pay on a weekly (or monthly) basis. Enter the specific details on the payment contract.

Be sure all details are provided in the credit application and payment agreement.

Make telephone calls to verify information provided on the credit application.

Base your decision to extend or not to extend credit on the information provided, negotiated, and verified.

during National Dental Health Month. Some practices use promotions to generate business during predictably slow times of the year. This can help keep staff fully employed and hospital revenues stable if clients respond to the campaign.

Promotions can be announced through special mailings, e-mails, newsletters, and in-house promotion by staff and materials. Signage, handouts, and verbal discussion with clients will encourage their participation.

Client Surveys

Client surveys can help the practice harvest the information needed to determine the level of client satisfaction and to identify unmet client and/or patient needs. You can give surveys to clients when they visit the practice, hand them out to each client for two days per month, or mail them to 1 in every 10 or 20 clients within two weeks following a practice visit. Surveys can also be mailed to a random selection of clients. Develop a random mailing list simply by choosing files or selecting names from a computer-generated list of clients. You can also mail surveys to clients who have not visited the practice in a timely manner in an effort to find out why they no longer request your services.

Surveys should be no longer than one page or 10 to 12 questions. The best results are obtained when answers are placed on a scale rather than as yes/no answers. For example, use the numbers 1 through 5 to represent *never, seldom, sometimes, usually,* or *always.* Leave room for comments at the end of the survey.

Clients respond best if they see the results from their survey participation. Periodic reports in a newsletter or e-mail can highlight survey findings and the action taken by the practice to meet identified needs. Results should also be posted on the clinic website.

Focus Groups and Advisory Boards

Veterinary practices sometimes use focus groups and advisory boards to attract desirable clients. Your favorite clients are likely to refer animal owners like themselves to the practice. It may be in your practice's best interest to cultivate these referrals by first meeting the needs of your clients and asking your favorite clients to refer the friends and family to your clinic. Always express gratitude when referrals are made. The doctors and staff should be able to quickly identify 30 to 50 top clients by any criteria (e.g., they visit the practice frequently, they always comply with instructions, or they really love their animal). Once a long client list is formed, the top 20 can be identified and invited to an evening forum, where a discussion of practice products and services takes place. These favorite clients frequently respond with enthusiasm and are eager to offer constructive criticism and suggestions for the future. Requests for pet pickup/delivery, extended hours, and puppy behavior classes are examples of new services frequently requested

Pet Lines

AAHA
AMERICAN
ANIMAL
HOSPITAL
ASSOCIATION

Special Dental Health Issue

This edition of our newsletter is devoted exclusively to the topic of dental care for your pet. According to the American Veterinary Dental Society, studies show that more than 80 percent of dogs by age three and 70 percent of cats by age three show some signs of gum disease. In this issue you will find articles on the warning signs, free dental examinations, the dental procedure, and home care.

We hope you will keep this newsletter as a future reference as we help to improve your pet's dental health.

Signs Your Pet May Have Dental Problems

by TJ Niemann, DVM

☐ Breath odor
☐ Yellow or brown deposit on teeth
☐ Red or inflamed gums
☐ Gums that bleed easily
☐ Loose or missing teeth
☐ Pain on chewing

If you checked any of the above it may be time to have your pet's teeth checked.

One of the earliest signs of dental problems is the formation of dental tartar (calculus). Dental tartar is that yellow to brown deposit on the tooth surface. It is composed of bacteria, plaque and food debris literally cemented onto the tooth. If not removed it continues to accumulate, eventually migrating down between the tooth, gum, and bone that holds the tooth in place. Left untreated the tooth root can become infected, and/or the tooth falls out due to the weakened attachment between the tooth and bone - either situation is not comfortable for your pet.

Dental Health Examinations

by Carol O'Connor, RVT

Have you looked at your pet's teeth recently? Not sure if what you see is normal? Want to learn how to provide dental care at home for your pet?

Our technicians are trained to perform oral examinations on your pets. They will explain what to look for, what is normal and abnormal, demonstrate home cleaning care, and give recommendations on additional care and tartar-fighting diets.

February is National Pet Dental Health Month. To celebrate this event our technicians will be performing free dental examinations and giving away free pet toothpaste samples and fingerbrushes during the month of February. This is a $21.23 value.

"Pets Need Dental Care, Too". Call 555-5555 to make an appointment for a dental health examination with one of our technicians.

Fig. 3-6 Special issue of a practice newsletter promoting dental care.

and appreciated. This advisory group can also give you feedback for your ideas for new products or services by letting you know if the new idea would be of value to them. Many suggestions can be implemented at little or no cost to the practice. Frequently, the group pleasantly offers affirmation that you are doing a good job meeting client needs.

Depending on your personal practice style and how well you think this process works, you may limit these meetings to occasional use and invite a different group of clients each time. This method would be referred to as a focus group exercise. Box 3-3 lists information gained from a focus group. By contrast, you may want to keep the same group of clients together and meet regularly (quarterly or semiannually) as an advisory board. Some practices have used such advisory boards to assist in putting on an open house celebration or grand opening for a new facility.

Value-Added Services

Offering clients more than they expect to receive can help bond them to your practice. Ways to exceed client expectations may be referred to as *value-added* services. In today's society, convenience and "one-stop shopping" are extremely important. People are constantly striving to do more things within the confines of a 24-hour day.

Some practices have an *Ask-A-Tech* telephone information hotline, on which technicians answer client questions on routine, uncomplicated problems. Many clients use this hotline to ask questions they might have been reluctant to ask the doctor. Others call to obtain advice about animal

care in unhurried conversation with a competent professional. Technicians must always use good judgment in advising clients. Answers should comply with hospital policies and philosophy, even if the technician has other personal feelings. The technician should tactfully recommend an office visit or discussion with the doctor when medical judgment must be made.

Clinic tours for all new or prospective clients will foster good client relations. Tours may also be offered to 4-H, Scout, and school groups. The practice newsletter is a good place to promote tours. Clinic tours offer an opportunity to demonstrate the capability of the clinic's veterinarian(s) and staff to provide a broad range of care for animals. Most clients are surprised at the array of instruments, equipment, drugs, and supply items used to treat their animals. Tours help bond new clients to your practice and encourage others to seek services for the first time or inquire about new services to which they were exposed during the tour. An open house is similar to tours, except the practice is opened up for a set period of time after hours or on a weekend. The public is invited to tour the practice, refreshments are served, and entertainment may be provided.

Presentations for community groups, service clubs, and school groups allow an opportunity to promote your clinic in person. A photographic tour (slides or video) of your clinic can substitute for a clinic tour for your audience. You can also highlight special patient care benefits offered by your clinic as well as seasonal animal health tips. In-house presentations or seminars can also be conducted on a regular basis (monthly or quarterly). The veterinarian, staff, or invited speakers present programs on pet care, specific breeds, or basic grooming or training techniques. Programs should be presented on a regular basis so clients start looking forward to the next presentation. Set up folding chairs in a staff lounge, meeting room, training room, large reception area, or grooming room. Consider what audio-video materials, if any, will be used.

Puppy and kitten socialization classes can be offered free or at low cost to clients who purchase "wellness" packages of services in your practice. Surveys suggest that 30% of all former pet owners no longer own their pet because of unresolved behavioral problems.

Pet selection services are beneficial but not often used. Too many pet owners become owners of new pets as a result of an impulsive decision. Too little thought and advance planning often result in a poor match between new owner and pet. Too often, an unhappy relationship develops and is terminated when the owner puts the animal up for adoption. With some creative thought, your clinic can offer a valuable counseling service to increase the chances of a successful match between the new owner and pet. This has the potential for additional long-term client relationships for your practice. Newsletter articles and public service announcements in your local newspaper advocating

---

BOX 3-3

Sample of Information Gained from a Focus Group

Reasons for Coming to Your Clinic:

"Confidence in staff (know answers or will find them)"
"Congeniality of staff members to each other and to clients"
"Compassionate veterinary care"
"Accommodation of special needs (early drop-off, late office visits, etc.)"
"Staff helps ease the process of euthanasia (flowers, cards, memorial contributions are all appreciated)"
"Excellent newsletters"

Challenges/Opportunities:

"Need improved examination room seating."
"Handrail at front door would be helpful."
"How about computerized record interface with the emergency clinic?"
"More evening appointments requested."
"Note on front page of client's record the best time to call client."

important points to consider in pet selection are well received. Encourage prospective pet owners to seek advice from the veterinarian in considering pet species and breed alternatives.

Grief counseling after an animal's death or euthanasia is essential to maintaining a good relationship with clients. Clients who are supported through this difficult time with your caring attitude, sensitive responses, and assurances on euthanasia decisions respond appropriately. They are likely to own another pet after healing from the grief associated with pet loss and are likely to bring the new pet to your clinic. Chapter 4 contains a discussion of grief counseling.

A hospital website will be a necessary communication tool used in conjunction with brochures, business cards, and other written communications from the hospital. Today's clients are computer-savvy. They want the convenience of going on-line for information, to make appointments, make boarding and grooming reservations, find directions, and learn more about the practice. A website can provide all of this and more. Seasonal information, identification of key staff and introduction of new staff, practice hours, and location should be included. The practice may opt to develop a website, but the use of a professional may prove to be a better choice. The site will need to be kept up-to-date with revisions and new information. If newsletters or a question-and-answer section is included, the information needs to be changed periodically to keep the clientele coming back. The website address should be prominently included in all other written materials, making it easy to find and use for the average client.

Any special event or occasion should be publicized (e.g., hiring of new key personnel or special promotion sales). Send a press release about the event to local newspapers, and as a public service announcement to local radio stations.

CLINIC OPERATIONS

Scheduling of Work

Scheduling of work provides the greatest opportunity for properly managing the practice's single largest investment: its people. Doctor and staff salaries typically make up 40% to 50% of a practice's expense. Managing this expense, therefore, is three times more important than managing the next largest expense: drugs and supplies (13% to 18% of practice expense). To optimize the doctor/staff salary investment, it is best to have a steady and predictable amount of work to do on a year-round basis. Fluctuations in workload are the biggest obstacle for efficient use of staff. Use downtime to complete routine hospital procedures, telephone calls, and cleaning. An employee who can find things to do and use quiet time to accomplish the small tasks is greatly appreciated by the practice owner or manager.

If your clients tell you that both evening and morning hours are important, you face a common but difficult challenge. To avoid scheduling the entire staff for all day and the evening, some staff must work split-shifts or more part-time personnel must be employed. For most practices, this is not an option but rather a necessity for financial survival. Vacation and personal time should be requested in a judicious manner. Time-off requests will most likely to be turned down for peak periods when all hands are busy.

To deal with seasonal peaks and valleys, consider how you can shift the workload from the peaks to fill the valleys. Can you recommend year-round heartworm prevention versus seasonal programs? Can you offer client incentives to purchase elective procedures during slow months, for example by promoting National Dental Health Month in February? Can you slightly reduce or expand the intervals for annual physical examinations (11 months or 13 months) instead of the usual 12 months to increase client visits during the slower months?

Scheduling challenges must consider client needs first, patients' seasonal and illness needs second, and doctor/staff preferences last. Veterinary practice is a service business. For the success of any service business, customer needs must drive priorities. With creative thinking and planning, you may be able to make adjustments to meet the needs of clients, patients, doctors, and staff. It is no longer unusual for a practice to offer evening and weekend appointments in addition to weekday slots.

Teamwork and Hiring the Best

Clients and patients are best served by a team of professionals who are committed to responsive client service and excellent patient care. It can be challenging to assemble, maintain, and grow a successful team.

It all starts with a personnel philosophy that honors the strengths of everyone on the team and fosters mutual openness and respect. The philosophy must recognize that each person has strengths and weaknesses. It is best to focus on strengths and compensate for weaknesses. Allow people to work where they are most likely to be successful and assign to someone else tasks they do not do well. A friendly, accommodating, extroverted person may be suited for receptionist activity; the less outgoing, meticulous perfectionist may be suited to attend the exacting details related to patient care.

Unfortunately, veterinary technicians are often underutilized. The trained technician has the ability to lift some of the work burden off of the veterinarian if the front staff schedules office appointments for heartworm tests, weight checks for obesity programs, blood tests, etc., with a technician rather than the doctor. Often the veterinarian needs be convinced that the technician is capable, and the clientele must be told that the veterinarian will not see the patient for these routine procedures.

Hiring of new employees is important. The cost of hiring and training a new employee to become a dependable daily contributor to the practice can equal at least one year's salary. Selecting an inappropriate person means turnover and a loss of many thousands of dollars to the practice. Staff selection must include a focus on team players. Employees who are team players readily offer help to others when they need it and are equally willing to accept help when needed. This attitude, combined with appropriate cross-training, prepares the team to be responsive to peaks in client demand and patient caseload. It also prepares staff to cover during staff illnesses, vacations, and other absences.

Good hiring practices include utilizing standardized employment application forms, utilizing good interviewing skills, asking for resumes, and checking references. Applications may be purchased, or the practice can devise a personalized form. An attorney should review any forms developed in-house. Ensure that the forms contain no unlawful questions.

Interviewing prospective employees should also follow a standardized format. This is less likely to lead to any discrimination charges. Applicants may be screened with telephone interviews first, and the most likely candidates can then be scheduled for an interview in person. Allow enough time for each interview, usually 30 to 60 minutes when the interviewer can be available and not interrupted. All questions asked should pertain only to the job. Using a job description will give the prospective employee a good picture of what is really required. Never ask personal questions unrelated to the job position. Many good books and seminars are available to hone interviewing and hiring skills.

Attitudes toward teamwork can be detected by carefully questioning applicants about their experience working (or playing) with others. Good team members are neither too independent (lone rangers) nor too dependent (must be told everything to do). Rather, they are interdependent and willing to give or receive help. Although role-playing may be helpful, it is too easy for the prospective employee to guess what the answer should be. It is far better to give the applicant a set of circumstances, and to ask if they have been in a similar situation and what they did. Actions can speak louder than words. If the outcome was not good, ask what they might do differently in hindsight.

Setting expectations and training is also crucial. Many new staff members are slow to succeed because expectations are not clearly communicated. All positions should have a written job description. This description may include the actual list of duties, as well as the overall hospital philosophy. Use it as a guide to teach employees the position. Ideally, a senior employee shadows each new employee for the first week or two until the new employee feels comfortable.

The "big picture" of a practice's philosophy is communicated by a mission statement and is demonstrated by having staff meetings, staff communication, and practice policies in place that drive activities that fulfill the mission statement. Ideally, all employees contribute when writing or updating the mission statement.

Team leaders must define, teach, and periodically measure skill levels. Good performance must be recognized and rewarded. All staff members need assurance that their jobs are important and recognize that they must perform well in their positions to enjoy both personal and professional success. Rewards and recognition should be made as publicly as possible, such as during staff meetings, with posted announcement, or published in newsletters. Performance appraisals may be done quarterly or every six months. This appraisal lets employees know how they are doing, and sets new goals for the coming months. Ideally, there are no surprises during this process, since consistent employee feedback should let them know how well they are performing.

Handle reprimands or corrections in private; nothing can be gained by pointing out a person's shortcomings in public. Such embarrassment undermines trust, erodes confidence, and weakens team bonds.

Employee Record Keeping

The hospital administrator is usually in charge of maintaining employee records. Each employee will have several sets of records. Medical records, which must be maintained separately by law, will include doctor's notes, and any illnesses or accidents related to the job. The personnel file will include all forms from the application process, introductory training for OSHA and the job description, evaluations, notes on any reprimands, written resignations, or firing documentation. Another file may be maintained separately for documentation of training following hiring and during employment. Employees should be asked to sign off on materials included in their files, recognizing that the item has been shown to them or that they did go through the training. This can avoid headaches later in any dispute that may arise.

Medical records

Veterinary practice acts in most states require that medical records be made for each patient, litter, or herd/flock, and that these records be maintained for a minimum period, such as three years. As a practical matter, most practices maintain medical records for a much longer period, often for years after a client relationship is terminated or after the patient dies.

Practical reasons exist for maintaining good medical records beyond the minimal legal requirements. Quality patient care, good client communications, documentation for referrals, and documentation as a legal defense are all valid reasons for maintaining good medical records.

Quality patient care requires tracking and accommodating an animal's wellness and illness needs. An individual patient record should include a master sheet listing species, gender, breed, age, diet, allergies, unique behaviors, and annual vaccination/parasite control documentation (Fig. 3-7). The master sheet should also include a major problem list and prescribed drug list for which refills are indicated. Follow the master sheet with lined pages on which chronological visits, treatments, and client communications are recorded.

Make all entries in permanent ink and enter them promptly to ensure accuracy. Eliminate errors by drawing a single line through the erroneous entry; do not mask by "white out," using correction fluids, or "black out," using a felt-tip marker. This allows a legal observer to note the nature of the error and to be assured that important evidence has not been destroyed. Medical records should contain factual or objective information. Subjective observations must have some basis in fact and not reflect personal opinions of doctor/staff or judgments about the client's truthfulness, credit worthiness, religious or sexual orientation, or other personal characteristics. Treat all records with confidentiality. Do not discuss cases by name with clients; the privacy of owner and patient information must be respected. Clients have a right to review records kept by the practice; copies must be supplied upon demand. Further, medical records can be subpoenaed for legal action and the clinic must comply. Accurate, legible, complete, and contemporaneous record keeping is important.

Careful documentation throughout a patient visit or hospital stay allows caregivers to review such information as previous history, diagnostic and treatment plans, and response to treatment. This review of historical information contributes to the plan for future patient care management. All laboratory reports and imaging interpretations must be included in a complete medical record.

You can weave client communications and summarized telephone conversations into the medical record to document revised estimates, revised treatment plans, and important decisions dictated or declined by the client.

Use the carefully documented medical record when a patient is referred to a specialist. Photocopied medical records should accompany the patient, along with a recent, written summary of the case. Original records should always remain in the practice facility, with one exception. Radiographs are not easily duplicated and are usually sent with the patient. These must be returned to the referring clinic. A log of radiographs removed from the clinic can be maintained in a simple notebook. List the client name, pet name, date of films, and the date removed. Stamp or write the practice name and address on the film file jacket to facilitate the return of the patient radiographs. The practice may also use a form where the client signs for the films, or have them sign the log book.

Some practices include financial documentation in the medical record. This is not a legal requirement and may not be in the practice's best interest. Many practices manage financial documentation in a separate, computerized system. In the latter case, cost estimates and authorizations to treat, as well as transaction totals, may be included in the medical record, but detailed charges (visit slips or invoices) usually are not included in the medical record. Special forms can be used to facilitate record keeping and enhance client communication. For example, a color-coded (by year) vaccination sheet can be developed for easy completion and ready identification within the medical record (Fig. 3-8). Another example is the anesthesia/surgery consent form (Fig. 3-2), which is used to obtain owner authorization to perform elective procedures.

Records format. In the examples shown, the format is an 8½ × 11-inch paper record system designed to be held in a clasp-type file folder. Some clinics find a smaller paper size to be adequate. Other clinics maintain an entirely computerized medical and financial record for each client. Regardless of the format, the record must be accurate, complete, and secure. Storage and retrieval must be convenient and well organized. Various design formats are commercially available to minimize misfiling by incorporating color-coded tabs. If computerized records are used, meticulous accuracy is necessary for all data entry; incorrectly entered computer records may never be retrieved.

Standard operating procedures (SOP) can streamline medical record-keeping detail. Although the medical record requires detailed tracking of all procedures, recording repetitious entries on record after record can become tedious. According to medical record-keeping standards established by the American Animal Hospital Association, simply making the entry by routine procedure name, followed by "SOP," is perfectly acceptable, with one provision. For each SOP, there must be on file in the practice a description of the detailed procedures for each standardized procedure (Box 3-4).

SOP descriptions may be written for all standardized procedures used in the practice, and a loose-leaf binder may be used to store SOP sheets in a central location. SOP descriptions may also be used for front office staff, including what kind of questions may be answered by staff, check-in and release procedures, how to extend credit, and front office record-keeping procedures. Annual reviews and updates of SOP descriptions are important. Once the SOP binder is in place, you may reference all standardized procedures by "procedure name, SOP" as you complete patient medical records.

Inventory management

The pharmacy of a veterinary clinic provides a valuable client service. If the patient needs a prescription item (e.g., an antibiotic) or an over-the-counter nonprescription item (e.g., flea spray), there are numerous advantages in dispensing the item from the clinic's pharmacy. The veterinary

MAGRANE ANIMAL HOSPITAL

2324 Grape Rd.
Mishawaka, IN 46545
(555) 555-5555

PATIENT'S NAME		BREED	OWNER'S NAME		☐ MISS ☐ MR ☐ MRS ☐ DR ☐ MS
DATE OF BIRTH	DESCRIPTION		ADDRESS		
☐ MALE ☐ ALTERED ☐ FEMALE	DOG	CAT OTHER	CITY	STATE	ZIP
BEHAVIOR			HOME PHONE	WORK PHONE	
ALLERGIES			SPOUSE'S NAME	OWNER'S EMPLOYER	
MEDICAL ALERT			SPOUSE'S EMPLOYER	SPOUSE'S WORK PHONE	
X-RAY NUMBER	DIET		REFERRED BY		
FORM OF PAYMENT ☐ CASH ☐ CHECK ☐ VISA/MC		CREDIT ☐ OK	OTHER PETS		

ROUTINE HEALTH MAINTENANCE

YEAR	1997	1998	1999	2000	2001	2002
DA$_2$P						
Reminder						
PARVO						
Reminder						
RABIES						
Reminder						
FVRCP						
Reminder						
FeLV						
Heartworm Test						
Result						
Reminder						
WEIGHT						
FECAL						
Result						

Date Active	Date Resolved	MASTER PROBLEMS	MEDICATION	REFILL

Fig. 3-7 Master record sheet containing a comprehensive record of an animal's medical history.

MAGRANE ANIMAL HOSPITAL
VACCINATION SHEET

DATE _____   PATIENT'S NAME _____

TIME _____   CLIENT'S NAME _____

PROCEDURES _____

PUPPY
DHP-M
PARVO
DHP/PARVO/CORONA
PARVO/CORONA

DOG
DHP/PARVO/CORONA
RABIES # _____
BORDETELLA
HW CHECK _____

CAT/KITTEN
FVT-CR/CHLMY
RABIES # _____
FELV
FECAL _____

CANINE
_____ Behavior   _____ Fecals   _____ Microchip
_____ House Brk   _____ HW
_____ Other   _____ Diet
_____ Spay   _____ Ears
_____ Castrate   _____ Nails/anal sacs
_____ Flea x   _____ Groom
_____ Dental px   _____ Bordetella
_____ Lepto

FELINE
_____ Dental px   _____ FELV   _____ Microchip
_____ Spay   _____ Declaw
_____ Castrate   _____ Chlamydia
_____ Ear Mites   _____ Fecal
_____ Fleas   _____ Diet
_____ Inside   _____ Groom
_____ Outside
_____ GIVE LITERATURE
_____ GIVE HOSPITAL TOUR

TEMP. _____

WT. _____

G.I. _____
    teeth _____
    fecal _____
    anal sacs _____

RESP. _____
    upper _____
    lower _____

EYES _____

EARS _____

C.V. _____
    m.m. _____
    heart _____
    h.w. _____

INTEG. _____
    ext. par _____
    nails _____

LYMPH _____

GEN. UR _____

MUS-SKEL _____

C.N.S. _____

ABD. PALP _____

_____

_____

_____

Fig. 3-8 Sheet summarizing vaccines given and procedures performed. These sheets are often color-coded for easy location in the medical record file.

Sample of Detailed Description of Standard Operating Procedures for Ovariohysterectomy

Procedure: Canine Ovariohysterectomy
Preoperative physical exam
Preoperative blood work: total protein & PCV
Preanesthetic medication: atropine 0.05 mg/kg acepromazine 0.1 mg/kg
Intravenous anesthetic: thiopental 20 mg/kg to effect
Intubate patient
Inhalation anesthesia: halothane 2% to effect oxygen 98%
Patient prep: clip hair, surgical scrub (SOP)

Surgical Procedure

Ventral midline incision
Expose uterus and ovaries
Double ligation of ovarian pedicles and uterine stump
Excision of ovaries and uterus

Three-layer Closure

2-0 chromic gut/muscle wall
3-0 chromic gut/subcutis
3-0 monofilament polypropylene/skin
Terminate inhalant anesthesia; oxygen only for 5 minutes.
Disconnect endotracheal tube from anesthetic machine.
Observe patient; extubate when swallowing reflex regained.
Return patient to housing compartment.
Continue periodic patient observation, and complete the medical record.

technician is often assigned the task of counting out dispensed product or discussing the use of a product with the client. Any prescription product will need to be appropriately labeled to meet legal requirements. A computerized practice will most likely generate a label with a printer that meets requirements and then deducts the product from the inventory log in the system. Handwritten labels are perfectly acceptable, providing all the information is included and written legibly.

Client convenience is very important in the current business environment. "One-stop shopping" saves time and relieves stress for the busy client. Clients appreciate the convenience of having the clinic supply any needed products and services in one visit. Directing a busy client to the nearest feed store or human pharmacy for a needed product is neither profitable nor desirable. Competent professional judgment is required to select the best quality and most appropriate array of pharmaceuticals and biologicals in the practice. Each item dispensed or sold is accompanied by the professional expertise available in the practice. The veterinarian and/or veterinary technician is responsible for prod-

uct selection, instruction for use, cautions about potential side effects, appropriate record keeping, and availability for follow-up information on patient care. The professional expertise related to the clinic's drug and supply inventory make the availability of this inventory more valuable to clients than products purchased from the pet shop, grocery store, or feed store. The veterinary practice is the best source of top quality pharmaceuticals and biologicals for veterinary use.

Internal use or theft of product also plays a role in inventory management. Products used internally usually carry a charge to the client to cover the cost. For example, if a cat is sprayed for fleas, the owner may incur a nominal fee of a few dollars for flea treatment. Employee theft however, probably accounts for the largest percentage of used or missing items from hospital inventory. Employees must realize that not only is the actual cost of the product lost, but also the revenue from the markup to the retail price. The financial loss may only be a few dollars per item, but multiple missing items add up quickly. The products still must be paid for, and both the cost and missing revenue are subtracted from the profitability of the practice. In addition, more cost is incurred to replace the stolen product. Ultimately, less money is available for benefits and raises.

Purchasing guidelines

The veterinarian or veterinary technician must use judgment in selecting a product to be stocked for dispensing (prescription items) or over-the-counter sale (nonprescription). Aside from drugs used for emergency use, which must be immediately available, it makes little sense to invest in inventory that will be used only occasionally. It is better to stock only items that are used frequently and to rely on writing prescriptions or referring clients to other sources for products used only occasionally. Inactive inventory occupies valuable space and ties up capital that could be invested elsewhere. Inactive inventory represents an unnecessary and avoidable practice expense. Each stock item should be assigned a place in the pharmacy where it can easily be found and counted. Keeping inventory in several areas ties up space and makes keeping track of quantities on hand much more difficult.

Damaged goods should be reported to the supplier as soon as possible. Each distributor will have guidelines for returns and damage notifications. In general, the longer the length of time between arrival and the report, the less likely the product will be replaced at no charge. Most companies will have incorrect or damaged products picked up by a carrier at the company's expense.

Economic order quantity. Deciding how much of an item to order is as important as deciding what product to order. If you purchase too little at one time, you risk not having the product available when needed or spending too much time and effort reordering to keep the product in stock. Maintaining excessive inventory occupies storage space and ties up capital in inventory.

A simple equation helps establish the appropriate amount to order for a clinic (Box 3-5). Use of this calculation establishes the correct *economic order quantity (EOQ)*.

$$EOQ = \sqrt{2FS} \div CP$$

where F = fixed cost of placing/receiving/pricing/storing an order, S = annual sales of the item in units, C = carrying cost (usually 25%), and P = purchase price per unit. Consider carrying cost as the cost of investing in inventory (rather than in certificates of deposit or the stock market), cost of outdated products, and the cost of products no longer used when replaced by new and improved products.

Use the EOQ method for all products that are frequently used on a fairly constant (nonseasonal) basis. Do not use the EOQ formula for ordering infrequently used products, such as chemotherapeutic agents, or seasonally used products, such as flea products.

Inventory turnover. Use inventory turnover to measure how well you are managing your inventory. The more often a modest inventory is sold and resold (turned over) each year, the better the financial result. High inventory turnover means that minimum space and capital are tied up in inventory. An easy way to calculate inventory turnover is shown in Box 3-6.

Inventory turnover of less than 5 times per year is considered poor, whereas turnover exceeding 10 times per year is admirable. This simple tool can help monitor how well veterinary practices manage inventory.

A computerized inventory system is included in most software packages. The computer will automatically keep track of product dispensed and subtract it from inventory numbers (assuming it is entered correctly when dispensed). Most software allows for a minimum and maximum level of each product to be established. A list of items to order can

---

Calculating Inventory Turnover

The average value and inventory turnover is calculated as follows:
Average value of product in stock = beginning physical inventory + year-end physical inventory ÷ 2:
$(21,000 + 19,000) \div 2 = 20,000$
Inventory turnover = total value of product purchased annually ÷ average value of product in stock:
$115,000 \div 20,000 = 5.75$
where:
January 1 inventory = 21,000
December 31 inventory = 19,000
Total expenditures = $115,000
Inventory turnover = 5.75

---

then be generated. A physical inventory should verify the computer suggestions before reordering the product.

Drugs and over-the-counter items for returns or credits will also need to be managed. These items are usually returned through your pharmaceutical representative. Each item should be checked upon delivery for a viable expiration date; occasionally items are shipped with short or expired expiration dates. These items should be returned immediately. If a short-dated item can be dispensed and used quickly, then it may be entered as inventory. Otherwise a shortage will exist (as if it had never been ordered and received). Short-dated bottles should not be opened. Most inventory products must be returned unopened and free of tampering in order to be eligible for replacement or credit.

Pricing dispensed products. The pharmacy operation in most practices should be quite profitable. Although some areas of a practice may be only minimally profitable (e.g., surgery or hospitalization), the pharmacy should be making a significant contribution to profitability. Without the profits generated by their pharmacy, some practices would operate at a loss.

Prescription drugs. Prescription drug pricing usually considers *markup* based on drug cost and a *dispensing fee*. Markup is a term commonly used to price a product based on a percentage of cost, such as per tablet, per tube of ointment, or per milliliter. Markup is used to recoup the cost of the drug, the carrying cost, and the ordering cost, and also to generate profit.

A markup of 100% can be illustrated by the following example. An antibiotic purchased for 10¢ and then marked up 100% would sell for 20¢ per tablet. A markup of 50% on the same tablet would result in a selling price of 15¢ per tablet. Most practices have a standard markup established

---

Sample Calculation of Economic Order Quantity (EOQ)

EOQ = $\sqrt{2FS} \div CP$
F   = fixed cost of placing/receiving/pricing/storing one order, e.g., $15
S   = annual sales of the item in units, e.g., 3,000 units of vaccine
C   = carrying cost, e.g., 25%
P   = purchase price per unit, e.g., $2.75 per dose
The square root of $(2)(15)(3,000) \div (25\%)(2.75) = 995$ units
The 995 units should be rounded to the nearest convenient unit. Therefore 1,000 units should be ordered at one time.

for commonly used drugs. The markup ranges from a very low 2% or 3% in a food-animal practice dispensing large quantities of vaccine in a rural setting, to several hundred percent in a small animal practice with high overhead and operating costs (e.g., labor costs, building occupancy costs).

Standard markups may not apply to certain items, such as very inexpensive products (e.g., antihistamine tablets) and very expensive products (e.g., some chemotherapy drugs). In these cases, it is common to have a minimum per-tablet cost, such as 10¢ per tablet, even though the cost of a tablet may by only 1¢ or 2¢ (this would represent a markup of 400% to 900%). If the tablet cost is quite high (e.g., $1.50 to $2.00 per tablet, markups may be reduced to 10% or 20%. The *margin* (difference between selling price and cost per unit) is 8¢ to 9¢ in the low-cost example and 15¢ to 40¢ in the high-cost example. In these exceptional examples, very high markups on very low-cost products actually yield less revenue per unit than very low markups on high-cost products. The objective is to generate enough revenue per unit to cover associated costs and contribute to practice profitability.

Dispensing fee. A dispensing fee is often assessed in addition to the markup to cover the costs of packaging, labeling, and medical and pharmacy record keeping. Significant responsibility and potential liability are incurred in management of the clinic's drug inventory. Potential liability issues include dispensing drugs in child-proof containers; proper documentation of drug dispensing in the medical and pharmacy records; maintaining these records for the required number of years; and proper storage, dispensing, or disposing of controlled substances.

The practice should receive revenue for the cost of handling prescription drugs and also for the responsibility and potential liability (risk) associated with making these prescription drugs available to clients. The dispensing fee, which generates this revenue, might be as low as $2.50 per prescription in some practices and as high as $10 in others (Box 3-7).

Many practices also have a *minimum prescription fee* for situations when only a few low-cost tablets are dispensed. For example, a client may need only two tranquilizer tablets for an anxious pet's car ride. The fee to the client might be $6.50, representing a $5 dispensing fee plus a $1.50 minimum prescription fee, even though the two tablets cost the practice only 25¢.

Over-the-counter products. Over-the-counter (OTC) products, such as flea powder, shampoo, and pet dentifrice, carry less liability and require less labor and less record keeping, and therefore are commonly sold without an associated dispensing fee. These products do not require a prescription and typically arrive in prepackaged form, so the primary product and packaging liability rests with the manufacturer.

Prices of OTC products are typically marked up in a similar method as prescription drugs. For example, a pet flea spray purchased for $6 per unit and marked up 150% would sell for $15 to the client ($6 cost + $9 markup = $15). Price shopping by clients may be more common with OTC products than with prescription products, so OTC products should be priced competitively. Remember, however, that the veterinary professional has carefully selected the best-quality and the most appropriate product and has provided it for the convenience of clients. It is reasonable that a premium should be paid to recognize this value-added client benefit.

In-hospital items. Pricing of products used on hospitalized animals must also be considered. Common methods include charging a flat fee for injections (e.g., $10 per injection) or adding a surcharge for very expensive drugs, such as some postoperative analgesics. In-hospital tablet administration frequently is priced to include drug, labor, and record-keeping costs, such as $3 per administration. Intravenous (IV) fluid administration frequently is priced at one large initial fee (e.g., $15) to capture revenues for setting up the IV drip and for labor related to administering the fluid. An additional per-milliliter fee is commonly assessed, such as 2¢ per milliliter. Using these fees, for example, IV infusion of 1 L of fluids would cost $15 + (1000 ml × 2¢/ml) = $35. This fee would not typically include the cost of catheter placement, which should be charged separately.

BOX 3-7

Example of Prescription Drug Pricing

Twenty 100-mg amoxicillin tablets are to be dispensed. Each tablet costs 10¢, the markup is 150%, and the dispensing fee is $5. The total fee is calculated as follows:
(20 tablets × 10¢/tablet) + (150% × 20 tablets × 10¢/tablet) + $5 dispensing fee = $2 + $3 + $5 = $10 total fee

---

CONTROLLED SUBSTANCES

Handle controlled substances in compliance with state and federal regulations. Controls must be in place so that handling of controlled drugs is careful, deliberate, precise, and secure. This usually means keeping controlled drugs in a locked cabinet or drawer of the pharmacy. Access to controlled drugs by doctors and staff should not be casual and should be limited to doctors and key administrative personnel. Given the increased concern today in society, temptations for abuse may be hard to resist for some practice employees. Practice decision makers must view management of controlled substances as a serious responsibility. Special written inventory requirements for controlled substances include a physical inventory not less than twice per year, as well as dispensing information. Chapter 9 contains more information on controlled substances.

VENDOR TRANSACTIONS

You may view veterinary drug and supply company representatives either as very helpful or as a nuisance. They often appear at inconvenient times to discuss products in which you may have no interest and recommend purchase in quantities far exceeding your potential use. With prior arrangement, the representative can appear at a mutually convenient time to discuss products useful to your practice to be purchased in quantities that fit your economic order quantity and inventory turnover criteria.

A constructive and useful relationship is possible. Ask your reception staff to schedule the initial visit by a company representative for 30 to 45 minutes. During this time, you can get acquainted; take the representative on a tour of the clinic; explain your supply procurement, storage, and dispensing procedures; and relate your practice philosophy. In this way, the representative can gain insight into how your practice is managed and better understand your quality and quantity priorities. The representative can then determine how to best meet your needs with the products and services his or her company has to offer.

You should reasonably expect the sales representative to provide information on the following:

- Current products, including animal health and practice financial benefits. Most companies will provide their representatives with the hospital annual volume of product purchases. Some distributors also have multitiered pricing structures in which the frequent hospital buyer gets a better price than the occasional buyer.
- Trends in the market, such as new drugs, supplies, and equipment
- Practice tips that may have application in your practice
- On-site services, such as checking for outdated products or methods of stock rotation
- Handling drugs or other items being returned for credit or exchange
- Special prices, such as quantity discounts, seasonal or other promotions, or delayed billing
- Benefits related to carrying a "family" of products, such as a line of flea control products for use on the pet (oral and topical), in the home, and in the yard
- Staff and client education materials, such as on flea control, heartworm control, or vaccination programs

USING COMPUTERS

More than 90% of veterinary practices use computers in some manner for practice operations. Many vendors offer hardware and software for veterinary purchases. Operationally and financially, the decision to computerize your practice or to change computer systems can have great implications. The decision maker in your practice should proceed carefully in making this decision. Changing a practice's record keeping to computerized format disrupts the usual routine, but the benefits of computerization far outweigh the initial inconvenience.

Before upgrading to new software or converting from a manual paper system to computers, do some planning in advance. All staff will need training on the new system, and the learning curve will vary with each individual. The beginning of a new year is the best time to consider adding or changing bookkeeping information.

Technology allows the practice to retain information that is more readily accessible than paper files. Computers generate all kinds of reports instantly. However, all data needs to be backed up on a regular (usually daily) basis. Backing up data must be done in order to maintain current information that needs to be available should the system crash or be accidentally destroyed. The decision to use either an off-site backup service or to back up onto disks or a zip drive should be carefully considered. Duplicate in house backup materials should be carried home or kept off site in case of fire or other catastrophic event. Adequate protection with security and virus programs should also be considered and be based on the needs of the practice.

Use of a Computer

Uses of a computer in veterinary clinics include generating the following:

- Financial information (and tracking it)
- Invoices for services rendered
- Reminders and recall notices
- Monthly statements
- Client instructions linked to procedures, vaccination certificates, and prescription labels
- Mailing lists for newsletter, promotional, or informational mailings
- Management data, such as reports on individual and profit center production, trends related to growth or decline of income from various services (e.g., dentistry and hospitalization), cash flow, budgeting, growth or decline in client and/or patient numbers, and owner compliance with wellness recommendations.
- Drug and supply inventory management—calculating turnover rates and generating product orders helps reduce inventory costs.

- Complete patient medical record keeping
- Bookkeeping (general ledger, accounts payable, accounts receivable, payroll processing)
- Medical database references
- E-mail, network access, Internet access, hospital website
- Word processing (letters) and desktop publishing (newsletter)
- E-mail communication with clients, receiving appointment and boarding requests via e-mail, and sending e-newsletters
- Real-time video of boarding pets
- Staff training with CD-ROM programs or Internet classes
- Telemedicine—technology, digital cameras, and computerized records now allow for a second opinion with a specialist without leaving the office.
- Human resource management—maintaining employee time logs, payroll records, etc.

Purchasing a computer

Purchasing a computer for a veterinary practice can be expensive, and its use can affect the daily work routine of many staff members. For these reasons, it may be useful for interested staff to become involved in the decision of which computer system to buy. Consider forming a computer committee.

A computer committee can evaluate the benefits versus the cost before deciding to computerize or to change computer systems. Some software systems may be more appropriate for your practice than others, so develop criteria to match the computer system with your practice's size, type, and philosophy. Although initial price should not be the only consideration, consider how long it will take to cover the cost of purchasing new equipment. Reliability, usefulness, new efficiencies, ease of use, user support, timely software upgrades, installation, and training are all as important as initial price.

Consider computer systems from at least three vendors before any final purchase decision is made. Most companies will be happy to send a representative to demonstrate programs and equipment. Each company should be able to supply an information packet demonstrating various forms and reports for veterinary software. Your accountant may wish to suggest specific programs for bookkeeping.

FACILITY MAINTENANCE

"You never get a second chance to make a first impression." This phrase is particularly pertinent in regard to maintaining a clinic's facilities. Conscientious maintenance of your facility provides many benefits, including increased client satisfaction, improved patient comfort, a pleasant work environment for staff, reduced cost of repair/replacement as a practice expense, and long-term stability of the practice in its current location.

Most clients have a limited ability to objectively judge the quality of medical and surgical care provided by your clinic. They cannot observe much of the clinic, and most have inadequate knowledge to judge medical and surgical quality. The opinion a client forms about your clinic is often based on nonmedical issues, such as consideration shown by staff, expressions of care for the animals, willingness and ability to answer questions, and appearance of the practice facility.

The outside of your clinic should be appealing, readily visible, and useful in guiding people to your practice. Your parking lot should be readily accessible, in good condition, and kept clean. Your building exterior should have a tasteful finish kept in good repair. The signage must be adequate, making the building easy to find.

The air in the reception area and all examination rooms should be odor free (free of masking deodorants as well). The client reception areas and examination rooms should be bright, clean, and orderly. Think about what your clients would see, smell, and hear if you escorted them on a clinic tour right now.

An individual in the practice should be responsible for facility maintenance and repair. Various staff members can take charge of maintenance tasks to spread the workload and attain maintenance/repair goals. Properly trained staff members can complete many interior and exterior maintenance tasks. For instance, front office staff may be responsible for the watering and care of plants in the reception area, and general cleaning there. Maintenance schedules remind those responsible of daily, weekly, and monthly tasks and document completed tasks.

Skilled craftspeople must complete some repairs. Make a list of maintenance and repair personnel so that someone can be quickly summoned in case of an urgent need. This list should include the practice's plumber, electrician, carpenter, lawn service, pest controller, computer supplier, telephone company, and utility suppliers. A supplemental list may include suppliers of major pieces of equipment (e.g., x-ray machine, furnace, air conditioner, blood chemistry analyzer) or systems (telephone or computer system), their telephone numbers, and the model or serial number of the equipment.

Some practices delegate authority for repairs and maintenance to staff according to their area of responsibility. For example, the laboratory technician is responsible for all maintenance and repair of the clinic's laboratory equipment, or surgical technician for the anesthesia machine. Along with this authority goes the responsibility to keep equipment operating in good repair. Provide spending authority by way of an annual budget to maintain major pieces of equipment in addition to a small miscellaneous category. Ward staff may have the authority to manage such

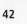

decisions as calling a plumber to repair or upgrade bathing fixtures or unclog a major drain obstruction. The advantage of this delegation is that the problems are resolved by the staff members they immediately affect. Repairs are usually made more quickly and appropriately when the designated employees have a vested interest in the outcome; therefore, staff members are likely to act expeditiously to solve problems in their work area.

RECOMMENDED READINGS

Lukens RL, Landon P: *Guide to inventory management for veterinary practices*, West Chester, Penn, 1993, SmithKline Beecham.

McCarthy JW: *Basic guide to veterinary hospital management*, ed 2, Denver, 1992, American Animal Hospital Association.

Messonnier SP: *Marketing your veterinary practice*, St Louis, 1994, Mosby.

Messonnier SP: *Marketing your veterinary practice II*, St Louis, 1997, Mosby.

Wilson JF: *Client consent forms*, Denver, 1995, American Animal Hospital Association.

4

Human Interaction in the Veterinary Workplace

Sheila R. Grosdidier and Guy Hancock

Learning Objectives

After reviewing this chapter, the reader should understand the following:

- Methods to implement effective communication skills in the veterinary clinic
- Barriers that prevent successful communication exchanges
- Methods to implement effective listening skills to enhance clinical expertise
- Methods to implement assertive communication techniques to understanding with other team members and your practice manager
- Techniques to reduce conflict and manage difficult situations with team members

- Expectations of veterinary clients
- Appropriate ways to interact with clients on the telephone
- Ways to interact with doctors and clients to keep the practice operating smoothly
- Appropriate ways to present bills to clients and to discuss fees
- Stages of grief
- Importance of the human-animal bond to client and co-worker interaction
- Appropriate ways to counsel clients on loss of a companion animal

As a veterinary technician, your success in practice will not be solely based on technical expertise but to a larger degree on the ability to communicate professionally, effectively, and assertively with the veterinary health care team and clients. The advantages of mastering communication skills are improved client interactions as well as a host of personal and professional benefits (Box 4-1). Poor communication is the cause of 80% of failure in the workplace. Fortunately, with the implementation of simple effective communication techniques, it is possible to dramatically reduce the effects of poor communication in the work environment (Box 4-2). Mastering these skills provides a solid foundation that will benefit your career as well as your personal life.

COMMUNICATION PROCESS

If you have ever uttered the words, "This would be a great job if I could just work with patients and not people," you are not alone. It is quite likely that you are like most veterinary technicians. It is easy to apply your technical knowledge and expertise, but the challenging part of your career is interacting with clients and team members. The majority of your time will be spent communicating with others, so the ability to interrelate professionally will define your level of success. Your expertise is most valuable when it can be expressed in a way that is understood. You actively listen to the needs of clients and understand how to serve them, and you are able to build working relationships in cooperation with other team members. Communication occurs through four primary methods: listening, speaking, reading, and writing (Fig. 4-1). Computerization is increasing the reading and writing component through e-mail, furthering the need to be clearly understood in writing. However, person-to-person contact is still the most common form of communication interaction.

Whether you are interacting with clients, supervisors, or coworkers in the workplace, the more senses you use in a positive way, the more likely it is that you will inspire a positive interaction with another person. In the workplace, you can use sight, touch, hearing, and smell to create favorable surroundings, promote positive interaction, and accomplish your tasks.

Communication has several dimensions and occurs simultaneously on many levels. Utilizing more of the different

BOX 4-1

Benefits of Effective Communication in Veterinary Practice

Enhances understanding of employer work expectations
Decreases team conflict
Improves career satisfaction
Strengthens client education and recommendation abilities
Encourages other team members to improve communication
   patterns
Reduces errors that occur due to poor communication

BOX 4-2

Seven Essential Communication Skills that Veterinary Technicians Should Master

1. Use active listening skills
2. Identify and eliminate communication barriers
3. Use assertive communication and be understood
4. Implement conflict-reduction techniques
5. Incorporate problem-solving methods
6. Use collaborative problem-solving skills
7. Assure that written as well as verbal skills are developed

elements in combination will increase the powerful impact when communicating with others. People communicate by verbal (spoken and written) and nonverbal means. Contrary to what most people think, nonverbal communication is more persuasive than verbal and is a substantial part of interaction.

More than 70% of communication is nonverbal. Non-verbal communication involves emotions, which alter the interpretation of a message. It also signals your social and professional position within the workplace (how you relate to supervisors, peers, and subordinates). Nonverbal communication can be likened to the way in which wolves communicate their social position within the pack, using displays of submissive or dominant behavior (e.g., posture, tail carriage, eye contact).

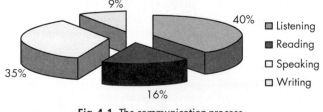

Fig. 4-1 The communication process.

Regardless of the process, the ultimate goal is to be understood. To achieve this goal is not a minor talent. Most people are not well informed on how to communicate as sender or receiver of information. Most communication patterns are based on habit. These patterns often result in the usage of barriers that diminish understanding the message and the chance that an accurate and honest discussion will occur. It is estimated that these barriers are used up to 90% of the time in daily conversation.

Barriers to Communication

Communication barriers are best identified as responses that hold a high possibility for affecting a discussion in a negative manner. These communication obstructions can be particularly damaging when individuals involved are under stress. Used chronically, they have been shown to lower self-esteem and increase defensiveness. Upon reviewing the list of common communication barriers in Box 4-3, they appear to be quite harmless and without negative connotations. However, these barriers have been shown to increase the chance that collaboration will not occur and that a greater distance can exist between the individuals. This is heightened when emotions are running high or the stress level is elevated. This does not mean that when these barriers are used a negative condition will always result; it only suggests that if not considered, a negative result can occur.

Communication barriers can be placed into three primary categories: solution sending, judging, and failure to respond to concerns. While we all use these barriers from time to time, it is essential to fully comprehend their potential in damaging the goal to achieve mutual understanding. In the veterinary practice, any element that detracts from optimal communication must be assessed and controlled to assure the highest quality of medicine is practiced for the patient and superior service is maintained for the client.

BOX 4-3

Common Communication Barriers

Ordering
Excessive questioning
Labeling (name calling)
Falsely praising
Excessive logical argumentation
Advising
Threatening
Excessive reassuring
Diagnosing
Moralizing

Awareness of communication barriers is the first important step in reducing their impact. It is also important to understand that these elements are assumptions based on what you believe about someone. The only assumption that should be made in professional communication is the belief that other people mean well. Review a recent conversation that occurred between you and a client and consider if any of these barriers were used and how they might have influenced your ability to gain mutual understanding. As you build awareness, the next step is to enhance your listening skills to better understand others, avoid making assumptions, and build assertive communication patterns to replace ineffective speech habits and successfully solve conflict situations. Over time, the usage of these barriers will decrease.

Building Effective Listening Skills

"Wisdom is the reward that you get for a lifetime of listening when you would have preferred to talk" — Doug Larson

In the fast-paced environment of a veterinary practice, veterinary technicians are faced with the need to understand and retain information coming from many directions, such as the client, the practice owner, the sales representative, the practice manager, and the other health care team members (Box 4-4). A recent study demonstrated that around 75% of oral communication is ignored. Hearing and listening are very different; hearing is the physiological action of capturing auditory waves. Listening includes engaging the psychological process to evaluate and consider the message of another person.

Active listening requires focus and engagement. The message you are sending is that what the client or peer is saying is important and that you want to understand his or her need (Box 4-5). How do you feel when someone really listens to you? Satisfied, cared about, and rewarded are common outcomes from active listening experiences. Clients who know that someone has taken the time and

made the effort to accurately understand their needs and concerns have a stronger relationship with the practice and are more likely to recommend the practice to other pet owners. Active listening is not just a good idea; it is a critical tool to veterinary technician success in practice.

The entire message is not just in words but in the tone of voice and the body language as well. Body language and tone of voice are particularly effective in conveying the total message of the words spoken. This means that in a telephone conversation with a client, it is even more important to tune into what is being said as clues through body language are not available.

To adapt better listening skills, it is vital to understand the three steps to active listening and to take a proactive position to build this skill over time (Box 4-6). This breakdown of listening stages may appear very elementary, but unfortunately the process is not followed in many clinics. Messages are missed, frustration continues to grow, clients become dissatisfied when their needs are not met, and team members find themselves in stressful situations that could have been avoided.

BOX 4-4

Benefits of Effective Listening

Demonstrates respect
Enables strong working relationships
Diminishes conflict
Reduces miscommunication
Demonstrates empathy
Positions individuals for greater understanding of one another
Enables and is essential to veterinary technician career success

---

BOX 4-5

Active Listening Traits

Strong eye contact
Positive head nodding
Thoughtful silence
Appropriate environment
Paraphrasing ("What you are saying is....")
Meaning reflection ("If I understand you....")
Avoiding distracting behavior
Facing or leaning toward speaker

BOX 4-6

Three Steps to Active Listening

1. *Receive the message:* Listen and look for the total visual and auditory message. Listen for the entire message. If you are thinking about what to say, you are not actively listening.
2. *Process the message:* Evaluate and analyze. Ask yourself, "What does the speaker want me to know?" This takes concentration and focus; as emotions escalate, this becomes even more essential.
3. *Respond to the message:* Let the speaker know you have not only heard, but you understand the visual message as well. Be sure to avoid responses that are based on communication barriers (Box 4-3)

The active listener is most often the controller of a conversation. Listening skills such as direct eye contact and focused attention convey interest and a desire to understand. This is acknowledgement to the speaker that he or she is not merely being listened to, but deeply understood. This advanced level of listening lessens the chance of misunderstanding and increases the chance that additional information will be shared (Box 4-7). When someone interrupts you while you are speaking, what you are about to say is lessened and decreased in importance. Your intention is to share your thoughts and ideas. The person possibly makes barrier-creating remarks or states unimportant opinions. The chance of continuing to share your message is virtually eliminated. This situation is an excellent example of the damage that can occur and the valuable information that can be left unsaid.

Each individual has a goal in listening. Development of listening skills is topically very elementary, yet its application can be very complex if not a bit uncomfortable. As skills are used over time, the advantage becomes evident and the ability to utilize them assumes the form of habit.

Along with effective listening skills is the development of empathetic listening. This is a critical skill, particularly in the veterinary practice. Clients are faced with a broad spectrum of emotions surrounding the serious illness or loss of their pet, and empathetic listening is a less intimidating way to establish a respectful and understanding environment. Judgment must be eliminated in communication with clients in these emotional situations, as this type of response will most often cause alienation at a time when common understanding is vital to assist the client. Ms. Jones may say, "I can't believe Rascal is gone. I don't know what we will do without him." The empathetic listener would be able to respond, "Your family is going to miss Rascal and it is hard to be without him." The exchange is free from judgment; it demonstrates focused listening, caring, understanding, and empathy.

Implementation of valuable listening skills will consistently facilitate strong communication in the workplace with clients, coworkers, and employers. As these skills are developed, they create the foundation to expand and improve oral communication expertise. Your effective interaction with clients and coworkers radically expands the ability to triumph in the veterinary clinic, develop strong business and client relationships, and reduce conflict. Listening will always remain the cornerstone of successful communication skills.

Assertive Communication Strategies

Words alone are imprecise. Often in the veterinary clinic, the ideas we want to express do not fit well into words and sentences. This lack of precision requires skilled communicators to gain an understanding of a speaker's "secret code." We have spent a lifetime developing our own code, and it is just as important to realize that it is true for our team members and clients. The behavior we see is a visible representation of the speaker, but emotions and thoughts are not as easily observed (Fig. 4-2). A client's or coworker's thoughts are not effortlessly understood and even less often are the feelings identifiable. In addition to other benefits, assertive communication is proven to increase the understanding of thoughts and feelings and help "break" the secret code of others (Box 4-8). This style of communication also influences how others receive and interpret your messages. The focus in this style is on speaking in a positive, proactive manner and sharing your concepts and issues in the most effective way.

There are eight steps to integrating assertiveness into your communication style. These steps are part of the DISCOVER method (Box 4-9).

1. *Decide what you want:* Before you get what you want, you must first know what you want. Accuracy in conveying thoughts, ideas, and concerns is based on having a goal and an innate understanding of the end point (what you want). Without close consideration of what the goal is,

---

BOX 4-7

Implementing Active Listening Skills

Focus on what the other person is saying, not what you want to say.

Listen *carefully* to things that others share.

Make a goal to listen twice as much as you speak and to speak less than half the time in a conversation.

Decide that listening is your key to success in the practice.

Use short responses when a person is expressing something very important to him or her; let the person communicate the message.

Identify if the person is talking to you about feelings or facts. This helps to determine your response.

Nod your head or show positive facial expressions when a person is sharing information and you do not know how to respond.

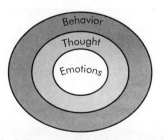

Fig. 4-2 The speaker's "secret code." Behavior is visible; the emotions and thoughts are not as easily observed.

Benefits of Assertive Communication

Expresses needs and ideas more clearly
Enhances self esteem
Improves confidence level
Increases respect for other points of view
Is self-enhancing
Decreases sense of guilt or anxiety
Enables one to be direct without being blunt
Increases constructive over destructive communication patterns
Identifies how to be positive without "sugarcoating" messages
Identifies what you can do, not what you cannot do

BOX 4-9

The DISCOVER Method

Decide what you want
Identify negative tendencies
Substitute positive statements
Choose a technique
Own the situation
Victory celebration
Evaluate the experience
Remember that you are human

---

there can be a continual problem and no solution. How to proceed and what to say will be dependent on the desired outcome of a conversation, business relationship, or situation.

2. *Identify negative tendencies:* With 70% of daily thoughts being negatively based; it is easy to understand how these thoughts can influence the outcome of a conversation or situation. Remember when you had a disagreement with a coworker that resulted in tension. Although you want to try and resolve the issue, your thoughts are, "Why does this always happen to me?" "I know they will never be nice to me again," or "Things never change, so why try?" Soon these repetitive thoughts defeat the belief that a situation can change. To change this process, you must first be aware of negative statements and the barrier they create in meeting your goals. Studies show that relationships are actually stronger after resolving a conflict situation than if the conflict never occurred.

3. *Substitute positive statements:* It's time to challenge and replace negative statements. When you realize that a negative monologue is occurring, exchange the thoughts with "It's fortunate that I have the skills to resolve this situation" or "If it is to be, it's up to me." It is a daunting challenge to change these thoughts because they are a lifetime habit for most people. By identifying the thoughts, replacing them, and reinforcing your choices, the habit is broken.

4. *Choose a technique:* After you have replaced the negative statements, it is time to determine how to establish assertive communication with the other individual that meets your goal. In most situations, using the tips and techniques in Box 4-10 will work well. When conflict, emotion, or stress is at a high level, it is advisable to practice what you want to say. Role-play with a friend, write down the important points you want to use, or practice discussing it in front of a mirror to check your expression and body language to assure an assertive, positive position.

5. *Own the situation:* Mr. Johnson is coming in to pick up his pet, Casey. The medical record indicates that Casey needs to have a teeth cleaning. Dr. Anders has asked that you speak with the client about the procedure. Ownership of the situation means that you determine what needs to be said; set your goal and take the initiative to make the interaction maintain an assertive style. When you speak with Mr. Johnson, your opening statement after shaking hands and making strong eye contact is, "It was a pleasure boarding Casey with us while you were away, Mr. Johnson. Dr. Anders noticed that Casey has advanced dental disease and this is what is recommended..." The speaker is respectful, positive,

---

BOX 4-10

Tips and Techniques to be Assertive

Use tact; express emotions verbally, not nonverbally.
Give others the opportunity to respond.
Respect everyone; you don't have to agree with what is said, but respect their right to say it.
Use the word *I* instead of *you* to reduce the inference of blame.
Stay assertive; passivity creates frustration and allows problems to build.
Deal with situations as they arise except if you need to "cool off" before speaking.
Remember your goals.
Minimize negative inner thoughts.
Express your thoughts, ideas, and feelings directly.
Encourage others by example.

direct, and assertive. The speaker owns the exchange. Even when a client declines a recommendation, assertive communication maintains a positive note and leaves the door open to future opportunities.

6. *Victory celebration:* It doesn't matter if your implementation of assertive communication was a total triumph or a miserable failure; the victory is in taking the risk, challenging yourself to use a different approach, and developing your skills. Remember how good it feels to take action and learn from an experience. Pat yourself on the back, do a victory dance, and revel in the feeling of being in control of your communication future.

7. *Evaluate the experience:* After celebrating your success, review what happened and what you can learn from this interaction. What would you do differently? Perhaps, if appropriate, ask the other person for feedback on your communication style. Consider what you would do differently and what you will continue to do in the future.

8. ***Remember that you are human:*** Be kind to yourself. Having adapted this process to your style, your communication training will most likely exceed the training of 90% of your team members. While no one makes these types of changes overnight, it is plausible to achieve a smooth, positive, effective, and assertive communication style over time with continued implementation, close examination, and demonstrated mutual respect.

Conflict Management

The single most common reason that you will leave your job at the veterinary practice is conflict. The idea of conflict to many team members in a clinic brings to mind angry words, heated exchanges, name calling, tension, and hurt feelings. With all of the potentially damaging elements to the workplace environment, little formal training is given to new employees about how to manage and reduce conflict situations. How coworkers respond to conflict situations can ultimately define their success in the veterinary practice. Sadly, it is all too often that the hardest working and most caring individuals in the clinic will become the first casualties when conflict runs rampant through the workplace (Box 4-11).

Fortunately, it is no longer obligatory to feel powerless in a cycle of heated outbursts, damaged business relationships, and unbearable tension. By facing and managing conflict directly, it is possible to eliminate tension and angry emotions along with strengthening coworker relationships. Conflict is based on different perspective in a situation. The listener *supposes* that the individual speaking has greater value than what is actually being presented. Remember, the emotional reaction of what is occurring supercedes and escalates the situation. If an angry coworker shouts something at you and you feel it is for no reason, you may feel outrage and anger at having been treated in this manner. It is not what is said, but is what is perceived.

BOX 4-11

Benefits of Conflict Resolution

Builds personal development
Strengthens work relationships
Reminds us that "different" does not mean "bad"
Enhances self-esteem
Lessens stress level
Heightens job satisfaction
Improves the ability to look at different perspectives
Gains appreciation of others

Perception becomes reality. This is an important point to remember when a client is explaining what he thought he heard about how to administer a prescribed medication.

Conflict is everywhere, and early in our work experiences we learn that it is best avoided. While it is a positive strategy to reduce the occasions of conflict, it is not realistic to believe that avoiding conflict is a successful way to deal with this issue. The foundation of conflict resolution is to accept the idea that discord is not always negative but can be positive, perhaps even enlightening if effectively handled with easily learned skills and techniques. Once the aversion to conflict has been resolved, it is time to master the skills of conflict management. As you review this process, think of a conflict situation you have faced in the past that did not end well and consider how you could have used these steps to have changed that outcome.

Day after day, veterinary health care teams face situations that exhaust their energy, create stress, and lessen job satisfaction. These situations usually involve team interactions and conflict, not patient care. On Saturday, Mary shouted, "If I have to work one more Saturday because Sarah can't get her butt out of bed on time, I swear I'm going to quit!" A statement such as this nearly guarantees that there will be a conflict between Mary and Sarah at some point. Let's decide that we are going to counsel Mary on how to manage this issue for a positive, successful result. Decide what the desired outcome should be, and have a plan on how to resolve the situation. This will dramatically improve the level of success. As a follow-up to the initial step, it is equally important to recognize potential barriers that will hinder the plan. Most commonly, the biggest obstacle is the use of inflammatory remarks or statements; any phrase that will likely impart a negative response needs to be avoided. Review the barriers to communication seen earlier in this chapter along with Box 4-12 to identify potential barriers. Avoidance of these common phrases and barriers will allow the discussion between Mary and Sarah to focus on issues as hand and strengthen their understanding of one another. Full utilization of active listening skills

BOX 4-12

Inflammatory Statements/Phrases to Avoid When Resolving Conflict

"You never/always...." is an extreme statement; things are rarely all or none.

"But...." can be read as negating everything said prior to it; try substituting the word *and* instead.

"You make me so...." places blame.

"You should...." places blame.

is also an essential part of the resolution strategy. Keep in mind that "Your ears protect your mouth from your feet."

To bridge the gap, explore and understand the perception of the other person. The other person's perception is reality to him or her. While you want to believe that you always maintain composure and listening skills in a disagreement, evidence shows this is often not the case. In situations involving heightened emotions, your mind engages what you want to say while the other person is speaking. If you are thinking about what to say, you are not listening. You will miss important information that is being shared and lose the chance to understand the other person's position. You can incorporate *the three-second rule* to solve this problem. Before replying to the other person, wait three seconds after they have stopped speaking and utilize that time to create your response. It is even a good idea to let the other person know that you are listening carefully to what they say and to best understand their feelings you will be hesitating before responding. This sets a foundation of focusing on resolving an issue and not escalating a conflict.

The mindset to consider listening as an attitude to use in all team interaction has been shown to reduce misunderstandings and develops a greater appreciation for the perspective of coworkers. The ability to reduce and resolve conflict improves dramatically with just this single step. Now we can explore a five-step plan that will work out the majority of conflict circumstances in the veterinary practice. **CASE EXAMPLE:** Janet and Shawn work on the same veterinary health care team at Golden Veterinary Center. Janet is the head receptionist, and Shawn is the surgery technician. During the last few months, tension has increased between the receptionists and the technicians regarding scheduling of surgeries. Several technicians have told Shawn that they are tired of the way the people at the front desk handle schedules. Shawn decided to speak with Janet about the situation. Unfortunately, the conversation ended with Janet accusing the technicians of being lazy and Shawn accusing the receptionists of being poorly trained. Since that meeting, tension has escalated to the point where the only communication between the receptionists and technicians is

along the lines of angry stares and rolling eyes. What can be done to resolve this situation?

Building a solution

Before initiating the five-step plan for resolution, it is essential to remember that in these situations it is not about who is right and who is wrong; but rather what can be done to help return the team to a working, cohesive group. To obtain the most desirable results, each step of the plan must be completed to its fullest potential before moving to the next step. Failure to resolve a situation is most often a result of not completing a step before moving forward. It is not unusual for these situations to appear to worsen at the early stages of resolution. We can illustrate this with the following analogy. A dog has a small erosion around a tooth. Upon further examination, the tooth and gingival are far more damaged below the gumline than what appears topically. This analogy shows that we must look deeper to understand issues of conflict and resolve them effectively.

Step 1: Create a solution setting. In the rush to correct a conflict, it is easy to disregard the importance of an environment in which resolution can flourish. Building the right solution environment will also reduce the chance of recurrence of the issue. Think about a good location to speak with someone regarding a problem. It is inappropriate to speak with someone about a problem in front of coworkers. Choosing the correct time is also of consideration. Friday at 5:30 P.M. after a grueling day of back-to-back appointments and a full hospital ward is not a conducive time to calmly air the issues. Choose a comfortable time and place that is agreeable to all people involved and allows the amount of time necessary to come to a common agreement (Box 4-13). It may be best to choose a location outside the office to reduce interruptions and distractions. This may not always be possible, but conflict resolution should be a priority. Conflict is the primary reason people leave jobs, so resolution is worth the time.

To create the right environment for Janet and Shawn, they decided to go out to lunch together on Wednesday.

BOX 4-13

Create the Right Environment for Resolution

Pick the right time.
Pick the right place.
Choose to listen.
Point out the goal and the benefits of resolution.
Make it private.
Reduce interruptions.
Focus on the issues, not the personality.

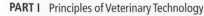

They discussed the need for privacy and lack of distraction with their practice manager, and she agreed that an extended lunch was a good idea. The practice manager also stressed that while the situation was certainly stressful for everyone involved, the resolution would benefit everyone in the clinic. They also agreed that they would spend an hour on the issue and then set another meeting if they were unable to reach an agreement. Engaging in a marathon resolution session will increase stress and decrease the ability to stay on the topic at hand. It may take a few meetings to come to a favorable conclusion. However, during the process individuals can see that the problem is being resolved. This will reduce the tension in the environment.

The location, time, and demonstration of commitment create a positive resolution environment by all parties involved. The individuals need to show interest in resolving the situation and understand the problem from other perspectives. This may not always be possible, but the person who assumes the leadership role in managing the conflict must communicate that the focus will be on fixing the *problem*, not the *person*.

Step 2: And the problem is . . . . Our attitudes come from a lifetime of experiences, learning, and expectations. These attitudes directly influence our perceptions and give us a unique perspective on events. Everyone involved has the same base of experience and will likely draw upon their personal knowledge to view the conflict. Understanding different perspectives will identify the core of the problem. People will have dissimilar points of view in a situation coupled with an array of emotions. To begin the process and identify the problem, it is necessary to clarify each person's view. Be sure to first understand their view of the problem before proceeding. Ask questions to verify that you understand their point of view and to encourage them to focus on the problem and not the emotion. Individuals involved in conflict often feel it influences *all* aspects of the professional relationship they have with coworkers. This is not so. We can illustrate this with the following analogy. If a pet has an ear infection, it does not mean that the pet's entire health is poor. This analogy shows that we must let coworkers know that conflict is just a component of the total work relationship and not the entire team connection.

Understanding different perceptions about a situation also highlights all parts of an issue and allows identification of what needs to happen to see resolution. Clarification and acknowledgement of each person's frustration, miscommunication, and feelings is essential in verifying that their point of view is completely understood. Each coworker involved also knows now that he or she is valued and considered in developing a plan to end the issue.

Janet and Shawn each expressed their thoughts and issues about the problem. They both used active listening and did not try to dispute the feelings of the other. They also looked for what they had in common in the situation.

Both Janet and Shawn were very unhappy about the tension and the backbiting that had been occurring among the team members. They felt this common ground would assist them in ending the unpleasant situation.

Step 3: Develop a plan. To develop a plan for a true and lasting resolution, everyone needs to focus on the present and agree to let go of past experiences. From the past, we can learn what might have prevented the current problem. But it will not assist in providing an overall end to the issue. Evaluate all possible ways to resolve the situation. Start with brainstorming. Ask coworkers to create a list of all parts of the plan. Encourage all ideas to be expressed. Agree that ideas will not be evaluated; they are only to stimulate the group to focus on resolution.

When the list is complete, identify the top ideas that everyone feels can resolve the situation. Everyone is encouraged to participate. When the top ideas have been identified, the next step is to build action steps to implement the ideas. Create action steps by listing exactly what must happen to complete an idea (Box 4-14). A list of all action steps forms the plan. The group must then decide a timeline for implementation of these steps as well as who will be working to complete the tasks. Everyone should be involved in resolution, as this builds commitment to the plan.

After discussing their perceptions and concerns, Janet and Shawn decided to brainstorm to identify ways to end the problem and prevent it from occurring again. The steps they created included discussing the situation with their teams, highlighting that no one wants to continue the current tension, and communicating that they are working together to help resolve the situation. The receptionists and technicians would rotate through the other team's area on a regular basis to better understand what it was like to do the other position. There would also be cross-training to better understand the needs of each position. It was also brought up that the receptionists were often understaffed

---

BOX 4-14

Qualities of Effective Action Steps

Effective action steps:
Are measurable: You know when they are completed.
Show action with the use of verbs: "We will *develop*...." "*Create* a...."
Illustrate an understanding of the team's needs and desired outcome.
Are time-bound: When will the step be completed?
Are neutral and do not favor one team member over another.
Encourage everyone to contribute.
Build a partnership for resolution.

and that newly hired people may have unknowingly contributed to the situation. The team would work together to build a point system for the surgeries. Each type of surgery would be given a point value, and a certain amount of points would be allotted for each day. Janet and Shawn would work more closely to address issues as soon as they occur. They would remember that the team works together to provide the best veterinary health care for its patients and that communication is the key to their success.

Step 4: Implement the plan. Action steps are assigned to team members for implementation and are given dates for completion. The steps are placed into a logical order, clearly defined, and methodically implemented. Communication on how steps are progressing and any issues that arise are essential in assuring that the plan moves forward. Be sure to keep everyone informed on progress. Sometimes the list of action steps appears huge and the movement forward appears slow. Emphasize the outcome, the benefits the team will see by reducing the recurrence of the problem, and the skills that are learned during the journey toward resolution.

Janet and Shawn created a graph that showed progress on the different steps of their plan. They communicated with their coworkers and practice manager the strides that the team was making. The communication between Janet and Shawn improved considerably, enabling the handling of concerns to occur quickly and completely.

Step 5: Celebrate. Resolution of a conflict is ample reason to celebrate. It is essential to emphasize that the team was successful in realizing the issues, taking action to correct the problems, and working together to create a pleasant, effective work environment. The skills learned in these situations enable team members to become more effective in their positions and less likely to leave their job due to frustration and inability to change undesirable issues in their career.

When everyone had cycled through the cross-training process, Janet and Shawn had a surprise breakfast for the team to celebrate their success and highlight the benefits. Each group was given an opportunity to discuss the information they had learned from the experience. The team showed remarkable progress. While there was still some residual animosity, positive changes were quite visible. The tension in bringing the two groups together was dramatically lowered.

Summary

Communication is a foundational element in the success of veterinary technicians in practice today. It is no longer effective to have only technical expertise. Communication skills must also be present. The practice benefits from the well-being of patients, the well-being of the team, and superior service to clients. These benefits nurture and develop the communication proficiency of the health care team.

SEXUAL HARASSMENT

The courts and EEOC guidelines define *sexual harassment* as any unwelcome sexual advances or requests for sexual favors, or any conduct of a sexual nature that renders harm through work interactions when
- Submission is made explicitly or implicitly a term or condition of initial or continued employment.
- Submission or rejection is used as a basis of working conditions, including promotion, salary adjustment, assignment of work, or termination.
- Such conduct has the purpose or effect of substantially interfering with an individual's work environment or creates an intimidating, hostile, or offensive work environment.

As employers, veterinarians are not immune to claims of sexual harassment. As an example, in a recent case, a female veterinary technician won a suit in a state court in which she claimed her veterinary employer's offensive conduct created a hostile work environment. State law applies to all employers within a state. Federal law applies only to employers with 15 or more full-time or part-time employees. However, suits are often filed in both state and federal courts.

Sexual harassment can occur in veterinary practices because the care-giving aspect of practice brings people together emotionally as well as physically. In many veterinary practices, small teams of animal health care professionals frequently work long hours, under arduous conditions, and in isolated treatment and surgical rooms in close proximity. In rural practices, emergency calls, especially after hours, and time-consuming treatments and nursing procedures require team members to maintain close quarters well into the night and early morning. In these types of close-contact conditions, employees tend to form more tight-knit groups than employees of larger, less personal businesses.

Unresolved legal issues remain concerning the amount and kinds of proof required to establish certain elements of sexually harassing conduct by someone other than a managing or supervisory employee. Problems also arise in applying the law to the factual circumstances of a specific case, testing the credibility of the parties' claims and proof, conceptualizing relief, and valuing damages.

When the conduct in question does not directly involve the abuse of authority, an employer may be liable for the acts of its employees (supervisory and nonsupervisory) and perhaps others visiting the business premises on a regular basis (including nonemployees, such as sales representatives). Liability is incurred when the employer knows or should have known of the conduct and fails to take prompt and effective remedial action.

One of the most effective ways for a veterinary employer to avoid claims of a hostile environment is to confront the issue openly and adopt a sexual harassment policy for the practice. This policy can be stated in the employee handbook or presented in another such mechanism. Repeated use of offensive language on the job creates legal grounds for a complaint. A coworker can file a complaint against you, as well as against an employer, for such conduct.

If you as a supervisor or employer's representative are faced with a situation in which employees in your work group are using inappropriate language, one recourse is to diplomatically point out that this behavior offends both men and women and is not appropriate for use in a business environment. Inform them that if they continue to use offensive language, they are subject to the same type of disciplinary action as that for violating other work rules (which, depending on your employer's policies, may include or contribute to termination). Document the counseling session in the employee's file, inform your supervisor, and make a record of the incident for your own files, in case of your later involvement.

In general, unless you know someone well, other than the traditional handshake, don't hug, don't pat, and definitely do not kiss. Treat others the way you want to be treated. Even then, be careful and respectful. The same applies here as with other offensive things: If it looks, feels, sounds, or seems offensive, it probably is offensive.

CLINIC COMMUNICATION

Telephone Etiquette

Initial contact with most new clients is by telephone. Also, most established clients call before coming to the clinic. Be prepared to field a variety of calls.

This preparation starts before you arrive at work. On your way to work each day, make a mental note of anything that could be a problem for a client driving to your clinic. For example, clients may encounter traffic problems caused by road construction, parades, or store openings.

Keeping a laminated map of your area on the front counter is a good idea for two reasons. You can put adhesive notes on it to indicate areas with traffic problems noticed by the staff members on their way to work. This information can be relayed by telephone to clients coming in for an appointment that day. It is also helpful for new receptionists who may not be familiar with the immediate area around the practice so that they can give clients accurate directions.

When directing clients to the clinic, remember that people navigate in many different ways. Some people understand how their city is laid out and can comprehend directions of *north*, *south*, *east*, and *west*. ("Drive south 2 miles, then turn west on Highway 210.") Other people better understand *left* and *right*. ("Go 2 miles and turn left on Highway 50.") Directing people left or right means that you have to visualize left and right from *their* vantage point. Other people know the names of area streets and avenues, still others navigate by landmarks. ("Turn left at the 7-11 on the corner.")

On your way to work, it can be useful to note the distances driven on some streets and from certain landmarks to the clinic. This will help people who navigate by driving distance. ("Go 2 miles and turn left onto Center Avenue.") With a thorough knowledge of your area's streets and landmarks, you can offer new clients clear directions.

Keep notepads and pens near every telephone. Be sure all of the pens work. Keep the appointment book in the same place so that all staff members can quickly locate it.

To select accurate appointment times, you must be familiar with the doctors' schedules. Check each doctor's schedule for the day and the next two or three days. You will sound more intelligent to callers if you actually know which doctors are working on certain days and when they are available. Do not assume you know a doctor's schedule because you have memorized it. There is no such thing as a consistent, permanent schedule or even a temporary one to which doctors adhere. Review the schedules of each doctor every day.

Answering promptly

Ideally, the clinic's telephone must be answered before it rings three times. The receptionist may not always be able to pick up the telephone before the third ring. Every member of the veterinary health care team should be sensitive to the sound of a ringing telephone. Someone must be designated to serve as backup for the receptionist in answering the telephone. This backup person should answer the telephone before the end of the third ring. If the backup person repeatedly has to answer the telephone, the receptionist must be alerted and the problem discussed.

Greeting a caller

There is a simple way to clear your mind and prepare your voice as you are about to answer a call. As you reach for the telephone, get in the habit of forcing yourself to smile. A smile changes your voice and can be perceived over the telephone. Callers expect the following things from a person answering a call:

- They want a greeting that is friendly and professional. Say "good morning" or "good afternoon" with a smile on your face.
- They want to know that they have reached the correct telephone number. Confirm this by saying the name of your clinic.
- They want to know if they are talking to an answering machine or a person. Some answering machines are very clear and can be mistaken for a live person's greeting. Give the caller your first name and offer to be of assistance.

- They want you to offer to help them. After giving your name, ask how you can be of help.

Putting it all together, an appropriate greeting may sound something like this: "Good morning, ABC Animal Hospital. This is Mary. How may I help you?"

This four-part greeting takes about five seconds.

Putting a client on hold

It is sometimes necessary to put a client on hold. Before doing this, always ask the client's permission first. "Good morning, ABC Animal Hospital. May I put you on hold?" The caller must have an opportunity to respond. The call may involve an emergency.

When a caller wishes to speak to a doctor but a doctor is not available, give the client a choice. Offer to keep the client on hold until the doctor can pick up the telephone or offer to have the doctor return the call as soon as possible. If the caller chooses to wait on hold, get back to the caller every 60 to 90 seconds to see if he or she still wants to hold. If the caller wants the doctor to return the call, be sure to get a number at which he or she can be reached at the time the doctor is expected to return the call. When you get back to a caller left on hold, thank the caller for his or her patience, give your name, and offer to be of assistance. "Thank you for waiting. This is Mary. How may I help you?" Even though you gave your name when first answering the call, repeat it when you come back on the line.

After the greeting

After you have greeted the client, identified yourself, and offered to be of assistance, you must learn how you can help the caller *and then do it*. The caller has a question to be answered or a problem to be solved. You were hired to answer questions and solve problems.

Your ability to answer questions and solve problems is directly related to your ability to listen. You may be able to answer most questions, but for others you may need to ask another staff member. You may be able to solve many problems, but others are more complicated. In either case, your success in helping the caller depends on how well you listen to the question or described problem.

Most people listen very poorly. To do it well requires a great amount of concentration. Most people are unable to avoid being distracted, and must concentrate well to become good listeners.

Depending on the amount of activity around you, you may find it necessary to close your eyes or face a blank wall away from distractions while speaking to a caller. It is better not to do something else while you are talking to a caller. You may be unable to concentrate on the call, and the caller will sense that you are not listening. Failure to listen to a caller is insulting and damages any relationship you may have with a client. If you can, use the client's name and/or the animal's name in the conversation. This helps avoid the embarrassment of forgetting to whom you are talking. Also, acknowledge the caller's questions and occasionally ask questions to indicate that you are listening.

Answering questions

When answering a caller's questions, keep your answers positive. This takes a good deal of thought, but there is a positive answer to most questions. For example, a caller asks if you can bill for services rather than collect at the time the services are rendered. Instead of saying, "We don't bill," it would be better to say, "For clients who wish to be billed, we accept a variety of credit cards."

"Is there anything I can do for my animal at home?" may be the most common question that receptionists hear. The answer is, "Yes, I'm sure there will be something for you to do at home. The doctor will explain what you will need to do when she sees you. Would you like to come in today or tomorrow?"

When you are asked a question you do not know how to answer, avoid getting yourself in trouble by guessing. You have two choices. If a staff member who can answer the question is available, you can say, "Just a moment please. I'll have someone who can answer your question speak with you," or "Please give me a number where I can reach you this afternoon. I'll get the answer to your question and call you." If you use the second answer, be sure to write down the question as well as the caller's name and telephone number. Having made that promise to the caller, follow through with it.

When it comes to solving problems for clients, keep in mind that the place to solve medical problems is in the clinic. The telephone is not a medical instrument. Veterinarians who try to practice medicine over the telephone can make serious mistakes. It is best if receptionists and technicians do not try to do things that even veterinarians cannot do well.

Making appointments

Because the solution to the client's problem can be found in the clinic, the client will need an appointment. Some practices still see clients on a drop-in basis, but this is becoming less common. Most clients expect to be told they will need an appointment.

When making an appointment, offer the client a choice of no more than two appointment times. For example, "Would you like to come in today or tomorrow?" "Which is better for you: 2:40 or 4:00?" "If neither of those times is good, do you want the appointment earlier than 2:40 or later than 4:00?" Limiting the choices to only two appointment times makes your work easier and reduces the decision-making stress for the caller.

When making an appointment, obtain a telephone number where the caller can be reached in case you need to cancel or change the appointment.

Controlling the conversation

Anyone who answers the telephone in a veterinary clinic is aware of what it means to lose control of a conversation. Some callers have ample time and delight in giving you the life history of their beloved pets or their own life story. This is time-consuming, and the information is of no use to the clinic.

Asking the appropriate questions can control most of these calls. Try to limit questions to those that can be answered with a yes or no. "Would you like to bring Charlie in today?" or "It sounds like the doctor should see Penny as soon as possible. Can you bring her in this afternoon?"

Asking the question, "What happened?" will open the floodgates and give you more information than you want to know. "How did it happen?" is another open-ended question that allows talkative clients to talk forever.

After one of these occasional nonstop telephone calls, try to determine how you lost control of the conversation. By knowing what questions to avoid and knowing how to formulate yes and no questions, you can minimize this problem.

PREPARING FOR THE VISIT

Your clinic is listed in the telephone book. You have a sign in front of the building. You answered the telephone and invited the caller to come to the clinic. Your invited guests expect you to be ready for their visit.

Clinic Exterior

Preparing for guests takes some preparation. At least once a week, someone on the staff should evaluate the clinic sign, landscaping, parking lot, and building. In some clinics, the employees enter through a back door and may not notice the front of the clinic for weeks.

The owner or manager of the practice and not the staff is ultimately responsible for the exterior of the building. However, remember that clients who are turned off by the appearance of the clinic will stay away and jeopardize your income. Take it upon yourself to mention any problems with the clinic's exterior to your manager. Practice owners appreciate employees who take an interest in the practice. Mention what needs correcting, but do not nag. Nagging is irritating and counterproductive.

Every week a different employee can be assigned the task of inspecting the sign, landscaping, parking lot, and building. If it is a lighted sign, the illumination should come on at sundown and go off after sunrise. Make sure that none of the bulbs are burned out and that there is no graffiti on the sign. The lettering should be intact, and the sign should be checked for any needed repairs.

Someone should be keeping up with the landscaping. The clinic's landscaping must be well maintained to convey a good impression.

The parking lot must be in good repair and clean. A client should be able to walk from his or her car to the front door without ruining a pair of dress shoes. Newspapers, other trash, leaves, and dog droppings must be picked up at least once every day (preferably morning and afternoon).

The clinic building should be inviting and appear well maintained. There must be no peeling paint and no missing molding from the front of the building. In the evening, there should be light shining inside, giving evidence of life and activity in the building. In addition, the walk and parking lot should be well lit.

Having the hours posted in large type on a sign that can be read from the parking lot is a nice touch. This reduces the frustration of finding the clinic closed after getting out of the car.

Clients are invited guests that deserve all of the attention and graciousness you would bestow on any guest you would invite to your home.

Reception Area

The first thing a client sees when entering the clinic is the reception area. If clients must wait to see the doctor, the reception area must at least be comfortable. One associate veterinarian sat for 30 minutes in the reception area of the clinic where he worked to test its comfort level. He noticed several shortcomings and decided on some changes. He threw out old magazines, organized brochures, removed some pictures and posters, put up new wall hangings, discarded dead or dying plants, and purchased new plants.

Every member of the support staff should occasionally spend at least part of a lunch period (not eating) in the reception area. Also, when friends or relatives come to the clinic to meet an employee, ask for their assessment of the reception area. When they walked in, did they immediately feel comfortable? Was it too cold, too hot, too bright, or too dark? The comfort of clients waiting to see the doctor is very important.

Clients' facial expressions may indicate an unpleasant odor in the waiting room. Take the hint and ask them if they smell anything unpleasant. Also, ask salespeople to let you know if they smell anything unpleasant when they come in from outside. Veterinary staff members become accustomed to odors very rapidly and sometimes fail to notice them.

A great way to create an inviting smell in a reception area on a cool day is with hot cider and cinnamon. Some clients might object to an artificial room deodorizer, but few people will object to the wonderful smell of cider and cinnamon, especially if they are offered some. The smell of fresh coffee is also appealing to many people. Be careful with flowers in the reception area. Some clients may have allergies to flowers. Also, employees should avoid wearing heavy perfumes or too much cologne in consideration of clients with allergies.

Clients waiting to see the doctor need some form of distraction. Though some clients are content to simply watch the receptionist and other activities in the office, others prefer to have more to do. Provide other options. Adults can read and children can read or play.

The clinic's brochure, newsletter, or product brochures can be placed in the reception area. If you want clients to read the brochures, do not make available other reading material.

Magazines are appropriate reading material in reception areas if they are carefully selected. Clients probably will not have time to read long articles. Offer magazines with lots of pictures and/or short articles.

For children there is *Ranger Rick,* the National Geographic children's magazine, and others like it. Again, the need is for many pictures and short stories.

Picture books are great for adults and children. One of the best picture books you can have is a photo album of the clinic. It is a good idea to have a professional photographer take the photos. However, many clinics have at least one staff member who is an amateur photographer who would welcome the opportunity to show off his or her ability.

Instead of or in addition to a photo album, a bulletin board can display photos of staff members. A little biographical information with each staff member's photo is a nice touch. Knowing where staff members grew up, what their interests and hobbies are, and how long they have been with the practice is interesting to clients. Photos of clients and their pets also can be very entertaining.

THE VISIT

Maintaining a Professional Demeanor

Some clients waiting in the reception area would rather observe the front desk staff than look at photographs of the staff. These clients listen as you answer the telephone and speak with other clients. They are more interested in your tone of voice and body language than in what you are saying. They picture themselves on the other end of the telephone line and are interested in your reaction to the caller. Depending on what they see and hear, either they will feel comfortable the next time they call or they may never call again.

You may feel better after making faces at the telephone and making disparaging remarks about a caller after you hang up the telephone, but such actions make nearby clients very uncomfortable. If you say anything, make only positive comments about the caller.

When speaking within earshot of clients, be very careful of the conversation between you and other staff members. You may have very good reason to be critical of your boss, one of the veterinarians, or a coworker, but it is wrong to voice criticism where clients can hear. Save any negative comments you may have about clients or co-workers for a time when clients are not present. Negative comments can undermine a client's confidence in the practice. Also, whispering in the presence of another person is very rude.

It is important to always be pleasant while assisting clients. Tasteful humor is a part of being pleasant and also is an important part of maintaining a good attitude in the workplace. However, be sure your humor is appropriate for the audience. Much of the humor in veterinary practices is inappropriate for clients.

In addition to watching the receptionists and technicians, clients tend to observe other clients and animals as they leave the clinic. They observe the animal's appearance and the manner in which the animal is returned to its owner. Make sure every departing animal is clean and smells good.

If you are the person bringing the animal to its owner for discharge, always have something nice to say to the owner about the animal. It shows that you really cared about the animal while it was in your care. It may be difficult to think of something nice to say about a dog that tried to bite you or about a particularly unattractive cat or dog; however, this gives you an opportunity to be creative. Try something like, "Baxter is really happy to see you!" It is worth the effort, because it is important to the animal's owner and to clients in the reception area watching your interaction with the departing client.

Informing the Client

Keep clients informed about how long they can expect to wait until they see the doctor. Offer refreshments if the wait is likely to be long. Also ask if they need any help with their animal. Do they need a carrier for their cat or a leash for their dog? Minutes seem like hours when waiting, so do everything possible to make the wait more comfortable. Be observant and aware of the client's needs, such as pointing out the location of restrooms. Have tissues handy and offer them when needed.

Ensuring Punctuality

It is inconsiderate when a doctor is not on time for appointments. A client's time is worth just as much as a doctor's. A doctor has no right to waste a client's time. Also, a doctor's tardiness for appointments makes the support staff's job more difficult and uncomfortable.

Of course, emergencies and unexpected developments with other patients can cause the doctor to be late. Clients are usually very understanding of such a situation. The more common reasons for delays are telephone conversations with other clients, extended conversations in the examination room, poor scheduling throughout the day, or just not being aware of the time. Another big problem is scheduling appointments every 15 minutes but spending an average of 25 minutes on each appointment.

Try the following things to keep the doctor on schedule:

- Review this part of the chapter with the doctor or doctors at a staff meeting.
- Point out to the doctors that one of the reasons clients are not on time for their appointments is because they do not expect the doctor to be on time.
- Remind the doctors that they would have fewer irritable clients and staff members to deal with if they would be on time.
- Have new clients arrive 15 minutes before their scheduled appointment so that they can be processed and in the exam room on time. Getting a new client into the exam room 15 minutes late can upset a whole morning or afternoon schedule.
- Time the doctors when they are unaware that they are being timed to determine the average time they spend with an appointment. Some doctors need 20 minutes, whereas others may need 30 minutes.
- Be aware of time requirements. Do not schedule two appointments for complicated cases or sick animals one right after the other. Alternate short appointments for suture removals, rechecks, or vaccinations with appointments that are likely to take more time.
- When making 20-minute appointments, schedule appointments every 30 minutes until the day is full, then go back and insert another one in each hour as needed.
- Group appointments in clusters. If you only have three or four appointments for the morning, schedule them one after another. If you allow too much time between appointments, doctors are likely to become otherwise occupied and may be unavailable when the next client arrives.
- Schedule a time during the late morning and late afternoon for doctors to return telephone calls. Ask callers where they can be reached at the scheduled time. Then give the information to the doctor to return the call. Organize the callbacks on the doctor's desk.
- Study the reasons why the doctor tends to be late for appointments and discuss it with him or her. Work together in solving the problem. Staying on schedule is important to the doctor, to you, and of course to the client.

Preparing the Examination Room

Make sure the examination room is empty and clean. It may not be your job to clean the exam rooms, but if you are putting clients in the room, it is your job to make sure it is clean. There is no excuse for putting a client in a dirty exam room.

Consider the client as a guest and yourself the gracious host. A client with a 70-lb dog, 2-year-old child, and an infant in her arms needs help; provide whatever assistance is needed. An elderly client may also need assistance.

If the client is early, and the doctor is treating an emergency case or is likely to be a few minutes late, provide the client with reading material.

Each exam room should have framed copies of the license, diplomas, and any award certificates belonging to any staff doctor that might be using the room. Most clients like to know as much as possible about the doctor who will care for their animal.

Another good idea is to have a reasonably current picture of the doctor and his or her family, including pets. Pictures showing a doctor's outside interests are also sometimes appropriate.

Keep a waiting client informed of any unavoidable delays. Remember, minutes seem like hours to a waiting client, so do not ignore the client, even though the wait may be only five minutes. Some people have claustrophobia, so consider leaving the door to the reception area open. If the client appears to be distressed for any reason, ask what you can do to make him or her more comfortable. Be aware of your guest's comfort level.

Hospitalizing a Patient

The end result of some appointments is that the animal must be admitted for treatment or diagnostic procedures. At that time there are two very important things you can do: provide a written estimate and give postoperative instructions.

Written Estimates

Before a client leaves after an animal is admitted, give the client a written estimate of the charges. A written estimate eliminates most of the questions about charges that clients often ask when the animal is discharged. It may not be the receptionist's or technician's responsibility to give the estimate, but someone must be sure the client has a written estimate.

A written estimate can list two estimated dollar amounts. The first amount is the doctor's estimate. The second estimate, added by the receptionist, is 20% higher than the doctor's estimate. It is a good idea to circle both numbers with a felt-tip pen and draw a line connecting them.

Tell the client that the first figure is what the doctor anticipates the charges will be. Explain that the fee could be as much as 20% higher if complications develop. Also tell the client that the charges will not exceed the second figure unless he or she is contacted and agrees to a higher figure.

Written estimates must be provided with the doctor's permission and cooperation. It is also important that the receptionists take some responsibility in seeing that this is done.

Postoperative Instructions

If the animal is being left for surgery, this is the time to give the client a sheet of postoperative instructions. Ask the client to read the sheet and offer to answer any questions when the client returns to pick up the animal. Clients often ignore instructions given verbally or sheets given to them when they return for the animal.

Status Report

Clients typically are very concerned about the status of their animal hospitalized for surgery or other treatment. Clients can be told a specific time to call for an update on their animals, or they must be asked where they can be reached by a staff member's telephone call. Ask the doctors to tell clients, "Let the receptionist know where you can be reached between 10:00 A.M. and noon tomorrow, and we will call to let you know how your animal is doing."

Before you or the doctor calls the client the next day, the status report must be reviewed. This report contains the following information regarding hospitalized animals:
- The owner's name and telephone numbers
- The animal's name and gender
- A one-word description of why the animal was hospitalized (e.g., ovariohysterectomy or fracture)
- Columns for functional status, such as body temperature, pulse rate, respiratory rate, and whether the animal ate, drank, urinated, or had a bowel movement
- Remarks (often coded), such as: doctor must talk to owner; animal can go home in the afternoon or when the owner wants to pick it up; animal is doing better but still has a fever; or call owner again this afternoon

With this information, the doctor or other staff member can make the telephone calls as necessary and as time permits. These calls can also be made on telephone lines that do not tie up the incoming lines. This reduces the number of busy signals that callers get and minimizes the time they are kept on hold.

Calling clients to discuss their animal's status is preferred to asking a client to call. When clients call, they have to wait while someone to discuss their animal's condition is located. This conveys an image of chaos and inefficiency.

Discharge of Hospitalized Animals

When you tell a client his or her hospitalized animal is ready to go home, be prepared to state the total fees due. If the animal is ready for discharge, treatment has been completed, and medication has been packaged for dispensing, the total fee can be calculated before the owner is called. If the client elects to pay by credit card, you can obtain the credit card number and complete all paperwork before the client arrives to claim the animal.

To avoid the 4:00 to 6:00 P.M. rush of clients picking up animals, ask owners if they would like to pick up their animals in the morning or early afternoon. Many can do so and appreciate the opportunity to avoid the afternoon traffic.

If all charges have not been calculated when you speak with the client over the telephone, have the final fee calculated when the client arrives. It is important to take care of all financial arrangements before the client and animal are reunited.

The Bill

When presenting a bill to a client, *what* you say and *how* you say it are very important. Your tone of voice and body language are equally as important as what you say. If what you say, your tone of voice, or your body language is defensive or gives any hint of apology, you can expect to be challenged regarding the charges.

Remember that the client has agreed to pay the fee mentioned in the estimate; the amount is no surprise and there is no need to apologize. If the charges are more than the estimate and the client has not been informed of the increase, present this news with a positive twist. "This is your lucky day. We did $300 worth of work, but you only owe us the $250 mentioned in the estimate." (Be sure to get the practice owner's permission before you do this.) When the practice owner and the doctors become aware that they did $300 worth of work but were only paid $250, the doctors soon learn to give more accurate estimates. It is not advisable to charge a client more than the original estimate unless he or she has agreed to pay a higher amount.

Complaints About Charges

The number of complaints about charges can help identify the cause of the complaints. If there are several complaints about charges (two or three per day or more than 10% of client visits) the reasons are probably one of the following:
- Poor communication, such as not providing estimates when extensive work is done
- Presenting bills in a manner that invites challenges from clients
- Attracting a clientele by advertising or reputation that will complain about charges, no matter how low the fees

Ways to combat the first two problems have already been discussed. Provide accurate estimates, understand the reason for the charges, and be careful in how you present them to clients.

If your clinic has developed a reputation for low fees, you may want to recruit clients with a higher socioeconomic status. Increasing your entire fee schedule brings in higher revenues for the practice. This problem, however, may be deeply imbedded in the practice owner's "cut rate" philosophy and therefore will not be easy to change.

The best way to deal with a large number of complaints is to find the underlying cause and eliminate it. Dealing with each complaint on an individual basis is time-consuming and depressing for the whole staff. Prevention is the answer.

An occasional complaint (two or three per week or less than 5% of clients seen) usually comes from a bragging client or a client who does not understand the basis of the charges.

These complaints, when merely occasional, must be dealt with on an individual basis. Complaints from bragging clients are easy to identify, once you become aware of them. Such complaints are almost always made in front of an audience of fellow clients. It sounds like this: "Oh my goodness, $1,500 for just a dog. That's more than it costs to take a child to the doctor." The translation is, "Look at me. I can afford to spend $1,500 on my dog. How about that! Don't you wish you were rich like me?"

Your response to such a complaint may be, "Barney sure is lucky to have you for an owner. Many dogs have owners that don't love them as much as you obviously love Barney." The usual response to this acknowledgment of the client's wealth and love for the animal is, "Thank you." The client acted and you applauded. This is one of the few acceptable ways in which people can brag about their wealth; do not deprive them of the opportunity.

The more serious type of complaint is made in the form of a question: "Why am I being charged for this?" "Why are these charges so high?" "What do these charges mean?"

The answer to all three questions is the same: "What is it that you don't understand about the charges? I'll try to explain it for you." Ask this calmly, with no defensiveness in your tone of voice, facial expression, or body language.

When clients tell you they do not understand the reason for the charges, provide an explanation of each fee but do not try to bluff if you do not know the answer. Tell the clients you will have a doctor answer their questions. Ask them to step into an empty exam room and ask a doctor to speak with them.

Hospital Policy

It is not acceptable to answer a client's question with, "It's hospital policy." To simply tell a client that something is or is not hospital policy actually means that you do not know the reason for the directive or there is no plausible reason. For example, if a certain client wants to visit his hospitalized animal and it is against hospital policy, tell the client why he or she cannot visit the animal. Clients usually are not allowed to visit their hospitalized animals, because it would be disturbing to other patients.

There is a reason for every hospital policy. Know the reason and use it to answer client inquiries. If you do not know, have someone who does know the reason speak with the client. Then learn the reasons behind the policies you do not understand.

Completing the Transaction

After fees have been paid and the client has his or her animal (if it was an outpatient visit) or is about to be reunited with the animal after discharge, a few more things must be done.

Ask the client if he or she has any questions concerning the animal. Common concerns of clients include the following:

- "Did I cause the problem?"
- "How can I keep it from happening again?"
- "If it happens again, how can I recognize it before it progresses?"
- "Can I expect this condition to get worse? Will it keep recurring?"
- "Have I done the right thing for my animal?"

Do not forget to make an appointment for recheck, suture removal, or any other kind of follow-up examination that may be necessary.

Make sure that every client has several of the clinic's business cards when he or she leaves. If you have refrigerator magnets, make sure each client gets one. It is important that they have the clinic's telephone number handy to call for an appointment without having to use a telephone directory. If they open the telephone directory to the listing for veterinarians, some clients may be tempted to call another clinic if they get a busy signal or are put on hold when calling your clinic.

Let clients know that even though the clinic may seem busy, you would welcome any friends they may refer to the practice.

Finally, always *thank the client for coming to your clinic*. Remember that every client brings in part of your paycheck. When you say thank you, say it like you mean it.

Client Departure

If it is raining when clients leave the clinic, hold an umbrella over them as you walk to their car. If it is not raining, ask if you can help carry any pet food, flea products, or their animal to the car. At least hold the clinic door open for clients if their hands are full.

FOLLOW-UP

It is important to maintain contact with the owners of animals that have been presented for medical treatment or that had surgery. This is done with follow-up telephone calls to inquire about the animal's condition.

The client's name can be flagged on the clinic's computer for addition to the follow-up call list. Some practices use 3-by-5-inch index cards, stored in a small file box, to maintain a list of clients to be called. On the index card or in the computer file, record the client's name, telephone number, animal's name, and any pertinent information you will need when you contact that client.

Follow-up calls are made for medical reasons. There may be a problem that clients are reluctant to call about. Be sensitive to any hesitancy in clients' responses when you ask how their animals are doing. Encourage them to bring the animal back to the clinic if you suspect a problem. Sometimes the client does not know what to expect after surgery or treatment and may wait too long to seek follow-up care for an animal that is not recovering as expected. Occasionally, such a call can save an animal's life.

The other reason for making these calls is to enhance client relations. Most clients are very impressed by the clinic's concern. Few other service or retail businesses care enough to follow up and see if their client or customer is satisfied. Many clients will talk to their friends about the call they received from your clinic.

Some clinics call clients again in six months to let them know the clinic is there if needed. Even if clients think you are making the call to bring in more business, they will be pleased. These six-month calls are usually made only during slow times of the year or on slow days. They are good for client relations, and there is also a good chance that after six months the animal may need veterinary attention.

File Purging

The ideal way to purge files is to start at one end and work to the other end and then start over. Call any client who has not come to the clinic for the past 15 to 18 months. These clients have ignored their vaccination reminder notices.

When you call, say you are reviewing the files and notice they have not brought their animal in for the recommended vaccinations. Ask if they still have their animal and confirm their current address. If they still have the animal and might be back sometime in the future, note the date of the call and maintain the client's file in your active files.

If you are told that the telephone number is no longer in service or another person now has the number, you can assume that the client has moved. Send a first-class letter to the address listed in your files. If it is returned, with or without the new address, you will know the client has moved. If the client has moved, pull the file and store it with your inactive files.

Importance of Persistence

Always remember that clients can obtain veterinary service for their animals from other clinics. Some of these clinics may be closer to a client's home than your clinic. If you want clients to continue patronizing your business, ensuring your paycheck and job security, you must do something to impress them by doing things for them that are unexpected. Keep your mind active, and continually search for new ways to impress clients. Ask coworkers to join you in an unending search for ways to add more perceived value to your clinic's already superior service. Take care of your clients, and they will take care of you.

THE HUMAN ANIMAL BOND
Guy Hancock

The American Veterinary Medical Association's Committee on the Human Animal Bond developed a definition that has been officially adopted and published in *Journal of the American Veterinary Medical Association* 212(11):1675, 1998. It states...

> "The human-animal bond is a mutually beneficial and dynamic relationship between people and other animals that is influenced by behaviors that are essential to the well being of both. This includes, but is not limited to, emotional, psychological, and physical interactions of people, other animals, and the environment. The veterinarian's role in the human-animal bond is to maximize the potentials of this relationship between people and other animals."

Clients are responsible for opening the profession's eyes to the human animal bond as veterinary medicine has changed from predominantly food animal to companion animal orientation. Pets have moved from the backyard to the house to the bedroom, and are perceived as members of the family. We need to continue to listen to and learn from clients in order to serve their needs as well as those of their animals. Client expectations are changing as medicine changes and as more is learned about the human animal bond.

Clients who are not well informed about the human animal bond may not take into account the impact on household members when making decisions about veterinary care. If there is little bond with the animal, decisions may be influenced more by financial considerations. This is particularly troubling when the decision maker is not as bonded to the pet as other household members. It has been reported that children who are left out of life and death pet care decisions or who are not told the truth by their parents hold lifelong resentment. It is therefore critical for the veterinary team to help the decision maker understand the impact of the human animal bond and how it may affect household members. It is equally important to involve household members in decisions about pet care. Hospitals should continuously document the relationships and bonds within the household in client records so that all members of the veterinary team can use this knowledge to assist clients and animals.

During a patient's health care crisis, it is a delicate matter to help clients who face difficult decisions. Clients are best served if they consider the human animal bond in their decisions, but they must not be made to feel guilty or inadequate if financial realities keep them from doing everything that can be offered. The veterinary team's responsibility is to help the animal and prevent suffering, as well as serve the client. This points out the benefit of prevention; by educating clients about the human animal bond long before there is a crisis, and by encouraging them to have pet health insurance, you help ease the difficult passages.

The opposite extreme from clients who have little appreciation for the human animal bond is clients that are extremely bonded. These clients are well aware of this bond. They may seek or demand services that have never been requested and that the hospital is not prepared to deliver. Clients such as these actually lead the profession to offer new levels of service and veterinary care. The services that your veterinary team performs only for this special client today will be the norm in a few years. Examples are home care by assistants or technicians, respite care, hospice care, and high-technology services such as CT scans and MRI.

Clients consider companion animals to be members of the family or household, in a role very similar to children. They are perceived as helpless innocents who are dependent on the adult people in the house for nurturing and protection. Your goal is to be a partner with the client in helping maintain the bond between them. Part of nurturing the bond is to help clients have realistic expectations of behavior in relation to the species and breed of pet. In addition, you must help clients understand animal behavior and learn to communicate with the animal. Of pets relinquished to animal shelters, the largest number is there because of behavior problems. These problems are mostly preventable or treatable with client education and animal training. Behavior that went uncorrected for too long either prevented the human-animal bond from forming, or broke the bond and resulted in the pet being given up. An important service you can provide to clients and pets is to be a knowledgeable resource on behavior and training. Recognizing and correcting problem behaviors early in a relationship can literally be lifesaving for the pet.

It is important to recognize and honor the bond between the client and pet by treating the pet as an individual, not as an example of a particular species or breed. You should try to build on the bond the pet has already established with the client, and form your own bond with the animal. This can be challenging, because animals are often stressed just by coming to the hospital and can be more interested in avoiding you than bonding with you. Animals are not all equally lovable and friendly, but as a professional you have an obligation to try to give them all your best care. Remember that the way the animal interacts with the client at home may be completely different from the way it interacts with you in the hospital. The careful use of gentle but firm physical restraint, and chemical restraint when needed, will protect you and the animal. It will also reassure the client that the pet is precious to you as well.

Assistance animals such as guide dogs and hearing ear dogs require special care on the part of the veterinary team in recognition of both the dependency of the client on the animal and the very deep bond between them. You must ask the human companion to direct you and be forthright about any questions or concerns. You must be prepared to alter some of your routine policies and procedures to best serve assistance animals. Avoid separating the person and the animal if at all possible. You must also discuss in great detail any procedure that may temporarily incapacitate the assistance animal and prevent it from working. Sedation or tranquilization of any kind will make it unsafe for the animal to work until it has fully recovered.

Hospitalization, which is a routine to people who work in animal hospitals, is stressful to clients who are highly bonded to their pets. They not only miss their pet's companionship, but also worry about them just as parents worry and are distressed by having a child in the hospital. The veterinary team can relieve this strain on both the patient and the client by making patient visits possible and convenient. Frequent calls to give progress reports also help ease the client's mind.

As pets approach the end of life, clients may begin to recognize how strongly they are bonded and anticipate the loss they will experience when the pet dies. This realization makes the pet's remaining days more precious than ever. The mission of the veterinary team is to prevent suffering and support the highest quality of life possible during this time before the pet dies or is euthanized. Human hospice offers a model of how to achieve these goals. Hospice endeavors to keep patients in their homes, surrounded by family and friends, pain free, with their symptoms controlled, so that their last days can be good ones. The patient and family are supported with skilled nursing, respite care for caregivers, as well as spiritual, psychosocial, and bereavement support. Veterinary hospitals can offer these services by having staff provide home care under the direction of the veterinarian, and by finding credentialed psychosocial and spiritual counselors to offer services as needed.

Clients can be assisted in the bereavement process by suggesting ways to memorialize and honor the unique individual and the special relationship with it. Funeral and burial ceremonies, donations, clay paw prints, pictures, and plantings are all ways of recognizing a special and meaningful relationship. Clients who are most bonded with their animals are at risk of suffering the most grief over their loss.

These clients will not get new animals until their grief is resolved, and these are exactly the clients who will provide the best homes for animals and the best veterinary care. It is in the best interest of the client, the animal, and the veterinarian to help clients through their bereavement and become ready to welcome another animal into their homes.

GRIEF COUNSELING

Clients anticipating or experiencing loss of a companion animal are emotionally vulnerable. The hospital is also vulnerable. What you do or say to a client while he or she is experiencing the loss of a companion animal can encourage or discourage his or her future relationship with the practice. At such a time, you have the opportunity to provide the best service your hospital has to offer.

The bonds people form with their pets may be as deep or deeper than those formed with friends or family members. Pets make us feel better when we are ill, comfort us when we are lonely, accept us when we have made a mistake, and love us unconditionally. This human animal bond can be broken in many ways. The pet may die of natural causes, run away, or be stolen, killed accidentally, or euthanized. Clients with a deep emotional attachment to their pets can expect to grieve when they lose them.

It is important to respect the feelings of clients experiencing such loss. To do this, you must first understand the stages of grief and determine the significance of the loss to the client. Elizabeth Kubler-Ross, MD, was the first to outline predictable stages of the process of grieving in her book, *On Death and Dying*. Although she wrote about human loss, the stages can be applied to the loss of pets as well.

Loss of a pet elicits a wide range of emotions in clients; these can be associated with certain stages of the grieving process. You can assist the client's smooth transition from one stage to another. The grieving process is not a steady, linear ascent from depression to joy; rather, it can be likened to a roller coaster ride, with ups and downs at every turn. At the end of the ride is a state of resolution and acceptance, in which the client is at peace with what went before.

By familiarizing yourself with the characteristics of each stage, you will recognize at what point your client is in this process and be able to shape your responses appropriately. These responses can facilitate the smooth transition from one stage to the next in the process of grieving.

STAGES OF GRIEF

The stages of grief include denial, bargaining, anger, guilt, sorrow, and resolution. These stages frequently occur in this order, but they can occur in other sequences. Some stages may be repeated.

Denial

Denial, the first stage of grief, may be played out during the first 24 hours if the animal's death is sudden, or for several days if a terminal illness has been diagnosed. Denial is a coping mechanism that cushions the mind against the shock it has received.

Bargaining

Clients may bargain with God or another higher entity for the life of a pet, or bargain with the pet itself, trying to make it live. They may offer the pet vitamins, tempt it with its favorite foods, and promise never to scold or neglect it again. Bargaining is a way of keeping hope alive and buying time to fully accept the outcome of the situation. When bargaining does not yield the desired results, anger is a natural response.

Anger

When faced with the loss of a treasured pet, clients may become angry with the veterinarian, technician, office staff, family, friends, and themselves. The veterinarian who has failed to "save" the pet, or who has made the diagnosis, may be the initial recipient of the wrath. More often, it is the reception staff members who bear the brunt of the anger, either directly or indirectly. Clients may be fearful of alienating the practitioner on whom they have come to rely. If clients are angry with themselves for overlooking clinical signs or waiting too long to seek care, this self-directed anger, once dissipated, gives way to guilt.

Guilt

Guilt is an unproductive, debilitating emotion that often inhibits progress toward resolution of the loss. It is the enemy of healing and closure and, if excessive, may require the attention of a mental health professional. When guilt subsides, it opens the door for sorrow.

Sorrow

Sorrow, or deep sadness, is the core of the grieving process. Though it can be kept at bay during the early stages through the intensity of denial, anger, and guilt, sorrow eventually settles in and permeates all aspects of life.

Sorrow is, in fact, a healing emotion. This is the time when tears flow freely. Clients feel relief and release from the pent-up emotions of previous days or weeks. Tears may come at work, in the supermarket, or while driving down the freeway. Clients may report sleep and appetite disturbances at this time. The practitioner may want to remind them, soon after a terminal illness is diagnosed, that adequate rest and nutrition are important. With time, sorrow dissipates, and everyday tasks begin to dominate awareness.

Tears no longer break through into daily activities but can surface at more convenient times, such as in the evening after work. Clients then feel more in control and are able to see an end to the intense pain that is true sorrow.

Resolution

In the resolution phase of grieving, clients realize that the pet is gone, that no amount of wishing will make it different, and that they will survive the loss that previously seemed engulfing. Now they can look at photographs of the pet and smile rather than cry; they can remember walks in the park in the summer, instead of anxious trips to the veterinarian; anniversaries and holidays can be recalled with tenderness rather than despair. During this stage of grief, clients may consider sharing life with another pet for the sheer pleasure of having something warm and furry to hug again.

Loneliness

Regardless of how a loss occurs and how well prepared a client is, all clients feel their lives touched by loneliness. This can occur in the presence of family and friends, as well as in the company of remaining pets at home. The client shared a relationship with the departed pet that was special and separate from other relationships. Although other pets, family members, and friends can provide company and comfort, they cannot fill the space left by the departed pet. Loneliness arises from this space, and the space fills slowly as the grief process unfolds. Clients may express anger at losing this particular pet while others to whom they are less attached are healthy and well.

An appropriate response from the staff or veterinarian may be, "Even though you have other pets at home, you may still be lonely for Taffy. While you are healing from this loss, your other pets will still be there to love you."

REPLACEMENT

The decision to replace a deceased pet with a new one should be left solely to the individual experiencing the loss. The veterinary staff should not influence the decision in any way. Some pet owners choose to bond with new pets before their elderly pets die. Others decide that the presence of a new pet in their home would be stressful for the older pet and decide to wait. Some clients may never again adopt new pets. Everyone involved must consider the client's needs, as well as the needs of the current pet. It is important to try to not "fix" the client's loss by suggesting replacement.

If a client is trying to avoid the experience of loss by finding a replacement for the pet, bonding with the new pet usually does not occur. The new pet is not accepted as a unique being if the owner wants it to be just like the deceased pet. Often, these new pets are given away or neglected. Owners may comment that the new Max is nothing like the old Max. Occasionally, a client who had taken good care of a previous pet brings in a pet that has been neglected. This client probably has not bonded successfully with the new pet and may need support in deciding whether to keep it or find a new home for it. The client may not have resolved the loss of the previous pet and may need to see a counselor or support group that deals with pet loss issues.

ASSISTING BEREAVED PET OWNERS

Clients grieve in a variety of ways. Some demonstrate their emotions openly, whereas others may show little if any feeling in your presence. Do not assume that a stoic display means the client is not grieving.

Assess your client's feelings to determine how much support you should provide. When clients show reluctance to accept concerned overtures from you, take a minute to let them know that you care about their well-being. By acknowledging their sadness, you open the door for them to experience their emotions, giving the simple message that it is acceptable to grieve.

Veterinary staff members are in a position to encourage healthy coping skills in their clients. Clients look to the veterinary staff for support, assurance, understanding, and validation when facing a loss. If you can assist your clients in this way, you are building the foundation for natural resolution of the loss. In doing so, you continue to maintain their respect and solidify your working relationship. Recognizing the different stages of grief assists you in providing your clients with the type of support they need.

ACKNOWLEDGING THE LOSS

What a client needs and values most from the staff is their time and presence. In being present with clients during a loss, you help to legitimize the grief reaction and give them permission to verbalize their feelings. Many pet owners go to great lengths to appear stoic in the presence of others. In our society, death is often dealt with through denial, so it is vital that you validate the client's loss. The most beneficial thing a veterinary staff member can do for their clients is to let them know that grieving for the loss of a pet is perfectly normal.

Sending a card, personal note, or flowers to the client are all ways of expressing condolences. What clients will remember the most is how they were cared for during their loss. Being cared for and acknowledged is something a client will remember long after the flowers have wilted and the note or card has been discarded.

Veterinary staff members may feel uncomfortable in attending a grieving client. Some pet owners attribute unrealistic powers of control over life and death to their veterinarians. This is especially true for "last hope practitioners," veterinarians who are specialists in their fields. A client whose pet has cancer and who has been referred to an internist for treatment may have a strong need to believe that this doctor with specialized skills will be able to help the pet. This can place the veterinarian in the difficult position of conveying the limitations of treatment to the client.

Being with a client who is very tearful or angry can be an uncomfortable experience. You may worry that you will do or say the wrong thing. You may find it easier to hide behind the professional role and keep the client emotionally at a distance. This often leaves the client feeling neglected and abandoned. A client is less likely to return to an emotionally nonsupportive veterinary facility, even if the very best treatment was provided for the terminally ill pet.

Your responsibility is not to work in the capacity of a therapist or counselor. However, learning and using a variety of counseling and communication skills can enhance your relationships with your clients. By communicating effectively with your clients, you help them to accept and resolve their losses sooner than pet owners whose losses have not been properly acknowledged.

Useful skills and techniques that can be used to assist your clients include attending, effective listening, reflection, and validation.

Some clients are easier to help than others, and you must make an extra effort to support the more difficult ones. Demonstrate that you are attempting to understand what the clients are expressing by responding at appropriate intervals to their comments. Avoid using clichés or telling them that you know exactly how they feel; you don't.

Try saying, "What I hear you saying is...." Let the client tell you what the loss means to her. Ask the client, "How can I help you? What things have you done in the past that have supported you through a difficult time?"

Reflection

Summarizing what the client is expressing is called *reflection*. When you reflect their underlying concerns, clients feel that you understand what they are saying. In addition, you can reframe the experience of loss and hopelessness into one of hope and possibility.

By establishing open communication, you will be in a position to offer the kind of help that clients need. Some clients may only need to hear that they did the right thing and want to be informed of disposing of the remains. Others need emotional support and may be referred to a group or private therapist.

Validating the Loss

When your clients tell you what the loss means to them, it is important to let them know that you understand the relationship they have shared with the pet. In validating the loss, you will discover that a pet can fulfill many needs of pet owners. Be alert for key comments, such as, "We never had any children. Kelsey was like our child," "Buttons was my whole life," or "How will I ever feel safe alone at night without Cole?" A pet may have served as a child to some, a best friend to others, or even as a bridge to the past. It may have accompanied the owner from college to career, to marriage, and on through other important life stages. It may have been a source of comfort during a stressful time: a divorce, loss of a loved one, a move, or a change in jobs.

Attending

Without realizing it, you can make it difficult for clients to express their feelings and concerns. The way you sit, stand, look at, or speak with them can inhibit or enhance communication.

An open posture with uncrossed arms and legs demonstrates to your clients that you are available and ready to listen. Facing them directly while maintaining comfortable eye contact sends the message that you are interested in what they have to say. Avoid standing behind the counter, desk, or exam table when clients are expressing their feelings about their pet to you.

Effective Listening

Listening effectively is much more than hearing what a client is saying. Listening effectively means giving your complete attention and allowing time for the client to ramble, cry, and show anger. You should learn to tolerate periods of silence from the client. You may feel a strong desire to fill in the silence with words; refrain from doing so. The client needs you to be there silently.

By recognizing the different components of grief, you can accept a client's expressions of anger and denial, and be empathetic about the guilt and deep sadness. Whether the client's initial reaction is overt despair or quiet shock, your interactions set the stage for the grieving process that follows.

The current loss can trigger remembrance of past losses, particularly for the elderly client. This compound effect may threaten to overwhelm the client. Clients can be reminded that this is a common reaction to the loss of a pet.

Use your own words to convey messages of understanding and empathy toward your clients. The idea is to listen and then respond to clients by expressing the core significance of the loss. Validating the loss helps the client feel special and cared for by the veterinarian and the hospital staff.

Achieving Closure

The perfect way to end a conversation with a grieving client is to give a directive. For example, "I would like you to go home, get some rest, and then think about the options we discussed." Or you can inform the client about a support group in your area for bereaved pet owners. For example,

"There is a place you can go and meet with other pet owners who are sharing similar feelings to yours." You can give the client a brochure or offer to make an appointment for him to talk with the support group leader.

Make clients take comfort in thinking about ways in which to honor their pets. For example, clients can donate to a charity in honor of a pet, plant a rosebush near the burial site, or create a scrapbook of memories shared with the pet (Box 4-15).

EFFECTS OF PATIENT LOSS ON STAFF

As difficult as the loss of a pet may be for a client, the loss of a patient may be difficult for the staff and veterinarian as well. Because euthanasia is an acceptable and legal means of terminating an animal's life, veterinary practitioners and their staff face a stress that is unknown to most other medical practitioners.

Each member of the staff has a personal set of beliefs and feelings regarding the issue of loss. Some may feel awkward attending a grieving client. Others may have unresolved feelings about pets they have lost themselves. Most people in the veterinary field have a love for animals and want to help them. Few consider the effect of the loss of a patient upon themselves.

When assisting bereaved pet owners, staff members may feel emotions similar to those the client experiences. Learn how to empathize and assist in a caring manner while still maintaining emotional distance (Box 4-16).

When a client is facing the crisis of losing a treasured pet, you can play a positive role in guiding the client through an emotionally difficult time, thereby solidifying your working relationship with the pet owner. Clients who respect the veterinarian and staff will speak highly of them to others, refer other pet owners to the practice, and return with new pets. Pet loss is an opportunity for everyone concerned to grow emotionally and to solidify working relationships.

COMPOUNDED LOSS

When faced with loss of a pet, the owner is often reminded of losses from the past, both human and animal. A compound loss can feel so overpowering that a client may respond in a way that seems out of proportion to the current facts. When this occurs, you might say, "I can see that you are troubled and concerned about Woody. Have you had other experience with loss?"

Sometimes an invitation to talk about a previous pet loss elicits information regarding past loss of family and friends, the demise of a relationship, or loss of a job. If the informa-

---

BOX 4-15

Suggestions to Help Clients Achieve Closure

- Provide facial tissues.
- Schedule appointment times to allow additional time to be spent with a bereaved pet owner or one whose pet is seriously ill.
- Create a brochure that includes all available support information (pet loss support groups, private therapists, hotlines, burial information, literature on pet loss, etc.). Make the brochure available to clients anticipating a loss as well as to those experiencing one.
- Send a sympathy card or flowers immediately after the loss. Late arrivals can be painful reminders for clients.
- Collect any fees owed before the euthanasia procedure is performed. A client will find it awkward to have to regain composure and pay a bill after the emotional experience of saying goodbye to a beloved pet.
- Let clients know that you and the rest of the staff are available to assist them, before and after the loss of a pet. Most pet owners have questions regarding their pets' illness and need reassurance that they did the right thing.
- If possible, maintain a private area in which clients can say goodbye to their pet, grieve, or regain composure. If such an area is not available, consider allowing extra time in the examination room before or after the loss.
- When attending to the patient, make certain that the owner can tell that the pet is comfortable and cared for. A simple gesture, such as placing a towel on a cold examination table, can demonstrate your compassion for the patient. If you send a final bill to the client, make sure it does not arrive on the same day as the sympathy card or flowers.

BOX 4-16

Helping Staff and Clients Deal with Loss

- Take a team approach to cases in which euthanasia is an option. This can alleviate some of the feelings of failure and grief regarding loss of a patient.
- Create and participate in a support group for veterinary staff. This is a forum for airing private feelings and receiving feedback from peers.
- Refer pet owners to a pet loss support group. This provides clients with a safe place to share feelings and validates the fact that loss of a patient is a real and important consideration for everyone involved.
- Encourage open communication among staff members, confrontation of personal feelings and beliefs surrounding death, and self-examination regarding the emotional reaction to loss of a patient.

tion is forthcoming, you can tell the client, "I know that when faced with the loss of a pet that you love, you can be reminded of other previous losses, and this can hurt more than if you were dealing with a single loss. Don't be surprised if you are suddenly recalling sad times from the past. Just know that it is very natural, at a time like this, to remember family and friends who are no longer with you. Try talking things over with a close friend, or, if you'd like, I can give you some referrals for counseling that might help you get through this difficult time."

Recognizing and Responding to Signals

A client may convey feelings of deep despair either verbally or though body language. Such statements as, "Muffin is the only friend I have in the world. I don't know how I can face another day without her by my side," or "Nothing matters now that Jake is dying. It will kill me to bring him in for euthanasia. I might as well be dead, too," should alert you to the need for outside professional evaluation and treatment.

You must determine if these clients have a reliable, concerned friend or relative who can stay with them, particularly if you have doubts about their safety if left alone. Make appropriate referrals and offer to call for an appointment before they leave the office. Do this openly to encourage trust and open communication. Knowing that an appointment has been arranged can have a calming and reassuring effect. Make every effort to secure the first appointment available and, if possible, telephone the client the next day for a "welfare check" and reminder of the appointment date and time. Extract a promise from the client that he or she will contact the crisis intervention hotline if he or she experiences overwhelming loneliness and sadness. Make certain you know the telephone number and that the client leaves your office with it.

If the client refuses any referrals or assistance and you sense that the client is a danger to himself or herself, you may need to resort to police escort of this client to a local psychiatric clinic for evaluation and treatment. This may be an extreme measure, but it could save a life. Let the veterinarian know about any concerns you may have regarding a client. Develop a protocol for clients experiencing emotional problems surrounding the death or illness of a pet. You might say to the client, "I know that you do not want to accept a referral for help, but I am so concerned about you that I will notify the police for assistance in getting you the help you need. I really do care about you and don't want anything bad to happen to you." Remember that extreme actions displayed by a client sometimes call for extreme reactions by the staff.

Referring to Mental Health Professionals

Clients experiencing intense anger, despair, and guilt often benefit from professional intervention outside of your office. Maintain a list of counselors and support groups for referral of clients experiencing grief associated with pet loss. A pet loss support group can provide a client with a safe place to express his or her feelings. It offers clients the opportunity to meet with like-minded pet owners with whom to share their fears, tears, memories, and finally, smiles.

When making referrals for group or individual counseling services, you might say something like, "I know you are very sad about Mitzi's ailing health. Here is some information about a support group for people who are struggling with the loss of a pet. This may help you to sort out some of your feelings."

Your local mental health department can assist you in compiling a list of mental health professionals and support groups. The Delta Society in Renton, Washington, maintains a list of pet loss support counselors and groups throughout the country. It also can provide you with additional books and videotapes on grief counseling. Assembling a community referral file for your clients takes time and effort, but this special service conveys the hospital staff's concern for their safety and well-being.

RECOMMENDED READINGS

Communication

Adler M: *How to speak, how to listen*. New York, 1983, Collier Books.

Allessandra T, Hunsaker P: *Communicating at work*, New York, 1993, Simon & Schuster.

Bacal R: *Dealing with difficult employees*, Madison, Wis, 2000, CWL Publishing.

Bolton R: *People skills*, New York, 1979, Simon & Schuster.

Bourdeaux D: *12 Steps to personal and professional development*, Mill Valley, Calif, 1993, Wildflower Press.

Deep S, Sussman L: *What to say to get what you want*, Reading, Mass, 1992, Addison-Wesley.

Fuller G: *The workplace survival guide*, Englewood Cliffs, NJ, 1996, Prentice Hall.

Griffin J: *How to say it at work*, New York, 1998, Prentice Hall.

McCurnin DM, Bassert JM: *Clinical textbook for veterinary technicians*, ed 5, St Louis, 2002, WB Saunders.

Siress R: *Working woman's communication survival guide*, Englewood Cliffs, NJ, 1994, Prentice Hall.

Tingley JC: *Say what you mean, get what you want*, New York, 1996, American Management Association.

Sexual Harassment

Burns SE: Issues in workplace sexual harassment law and related social science research, *Journal of Social Issues*, 51:195, 207, 1995.

Farnham A: Are you smart enough to keep your job? *Fortune*, Jan 15, 1996:34-37, 1996.

Graen GB: *Unwritten rules for your career*, New York, 1989, John Wiley & Sons.

Lacroix CA, Wilson JF: Avoiding sexual harassment liability in veterinary practices, *J Am Vet Med Assoc*, 208:1664-1666, 1996.

Lieber RB: How safe is your job? *Fortune*, April 1, 1996:72-104, 1996.

Clinic Communication

AAHA: *Commonly asked questions reference guide*, Denver, 1993, American Animal Hospital Association.

McCurnin DM: *Veterinary practice management*, Philadelphia, 1988, JB Lippincott.

Messonnier SP: *Marketing your veterinary practice*, St Louis, 1994, Mosby.

Messonnier SP: *Marketing your veterinary practice*, vol 2, St Louis, 1997, Mosby.

Human-Animal Bond

Guntzelman J, Reiger M: Helping pet owners with the euthanasia decision, *Vet Med* 88:26-34, 1993.

Guntzelman J, Reiger M: Supporting clients who are grieving the death of a pet, *Vet Med* 88:35-41, 1993.

Hart LA, Hart BL: Grief and stress from so many animal deaths, *Companion Animal Practice* 1:20-21, 1987.

Kay WJ, et al: *Euthanasia of the companion animal*, Philadelphia, 1988, Charles Press.

Kubler-Ross E: *On death and dying*, New York, 1969, Collier Books.

Pettit TH: *Hospital administration for veterinary staff*, St Louis, 1994, Mosby.

Ross CB: Pet loss and the human/companion animal bond. Master's thesis, Sonoma State University, 1987.

5

Veterinary Medical Terminology

John T. Ervin

Learning Objectives

After reviewing this chapter, the reader should understand the following:
- How to construct medical terms from word parts
- Rules used to construct medical terms
- Meanings of common prefixes and suffixes used in medical terms
- Combining forms used to refer to various body parts
- Terms for direction, position, and movement
- Terms used for common surgical procedures, diseases, instruments, procedures, and dentistry

Veterinary medical terminology is the "language" of the veterinary profession. This language is used in everyday speech, recorded in medical records, and used in journal articles and published textbooks for veterinary technicians and veterinarians. The most important part of this chapter is to learn correct pronunciation and proper spelling of medical terms. Next, you will learn to memorize word parts and their meanings. Then, you will be able to recognize and use medical words correctly. To assist the reader with correct pronunciation, accented syllables are printed in UPPERCASE LETTERS. Syllables that are not accented are in lowercase letters. In multisyllabic words with primary and secondary accents, the syllable with the primary accent is in **BOLDFACE UPPERCASE LETTERS,** and the syllable with the secondary accent is in UPPERCASE LETTERS. Unaccented syllables are in lowercase letters. Words of one syllable are in lowercase letters. Multisyllabic words, in which all syllables receive equal stress, are in lowercase letters.

INTRODUCTION TO WORD PARTS

Prefix

A *prefix* is a syllable, a group of syllables, or a word joined to the beginning of another word to alter its meaning or create a new word. The prefix may provide position, time, amount, color, or direction to a root word. A prefix is not often used as a word alone unless a hyphen is inserted between it and the following word.

Example: *Pre-* is a prefix meaning "before, in space or in time." When joined to the root word *natal*, meaning "birth," the result becomes the medical word: *PREnatal. Prenatal* means "before birth." The prefix *Pre* used alone means nothing to the reader.

Root Word

A root word is the "subject" part of the word consisting of a syllable, group of syllables, or word that is the basis (or word base) for the meaning of the medical word.

Example: *CARdi-* is a root word meaning "heart." The root word used alone means nothing to the reader, as shown in the following example.

Example: The patient was diagnosed with *CARdi*. Now add the suffix *itis* (meaning "inflammation") to the end of the root word. The sentence begins to make sense with this addition. The patient was diagnosed with CARditis or inflammation of the heart.

Combining Forms

A combining form is a word or root word that may or may not use the connecting vowel *o* when it is used as an element in a medical word formation. The combining form is the combination of the root word and the combining vowel. It is generally written in the following manner:

Example: CARdi/o: the combining form for the heart (root word plus combining vowel)

See *combining vowel*.

Combining Vowel

A combining vowel is a vowel, usually an *o*, used to connect a word or root word to the appropriate suffix or to another root word.

Combining Vowel Added to a Suffix

A suffix is a syllable, a group of syllables, or a word added at the end of a root word to change its meaning, give it grammatical function, or form a new word. Suffixes normally do not stand alone as words. When they are used alone, a hyphen is used preceding and attached to the suffix.

Example: -*gram* is a suffix meaning "a recording by an instrument." A cardiogram is a recording of heart movement made by an instrument.

Compound Word

A compound word is two or more words or root words combined to make a new word.

Example: *Horse* and *fly* combine to form the word *HORSEfly*.

USING WORD PARTS TO FORM WORDS

Use of the Prefix

A prefix is attached to the beginning of a root word to form a new word.

Example: Prefix + Root Word = New Word

Prefix	Root Word	Combined	Definition
de-	horn	*DEhorn*	To remove the horns
Semi-	PERmeable	*semiPERmeable*	Allowing only certain elements or liquids to pass through a membrane

Suffix

A suffix is attached to the end of a root word to form a new word.

Example: Root Word + Suffix = New Word

Root Word	Suffix	Combined	Definition
TONsil	-itis	TONsilLItis	Inflammation of the tonsils
THYroid	-ectomy	THYroidECtomy	Removal of the thyroid gland

Compound Word

Two words are joined together to form a new word.

Example: Root Word 1 + Root Word 2 = New Word

Word 1	Word 2	Combined	Definition
lock	jaw	LOCKjaw	Common name for the disease tetanus
blood	worms	BLOODworms	Worms (nematodes) that inhabit a main artery of the intestines in horses

There are certain rules peculiar to the use of combining forms and the combining vowel o. These rules are as follows:

- If a suffix begins with a consonant, use the combining vowel *o* with the root word (the combining form), to which the suffix will be added.
  Example: *CARdi/o* (combining form for heart) plus the suffix *megaly* (meaning "enlargement of"), forms *CARdioMEGaly*, meaning "enlargement of the heart." Note the combining vowel *o* is retained.

- Do not use the combining vowel *o* when a suffix begins with a vowel.
  Example: *HEPat/o* (combining form for liver) plus the suffix *osis* (meaning "a condition, disease, or morbid process"), combine to form *HEPaTOsis*, meaning "a disease occurring in the liver." Note the combining vowel *o* is not used.

- If the suffix begins with the same vowel with which the combining form ends (minus the combining vowel *o*), do not repeat the vowel when forming the new word.
  Example: *CARdi/o* minus *o* is *CARdi-*. *CARdi-* plus -*itis* (meaning "inflammation of"), combines to form *carDItis*, meaning "inflammation of the heart." Note, as the rule states, this word may have only a single *i* as the medical root word joins the suffix.

Combining Forms	Suffix	Combined	Definition
cardi/o	-logy	CARdiOLogy	Study of heart diseases
mast/o	-itis	masTItis	Inflammation of the mammary glands

Prefix and Suffix

In this situation, no root word is used. The prefix is added directly to the suffix.

Prefix	Suffix	Combined	Definition
dys-	-uria	dysUria	Trouble urinating
POLy-	-phagia	POLyPHAgia	Eating to excess

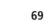

Prefix, Root Word, and Suffix

Words are formed by adding both the prefix and suffix to the root word.

Prefix	Root Word	Suffix	Combined	Definition
un-	sound	-ness	unSOUNDness	A form of physical dysfunction
PERI-	cardi-	-al	PERICARdial	In the area surrounding the heart

DEFINING MEDICAL TERMS USING WORD ANALYSIS

Analyzing words teaches you to think logically and makes words easier to remember. The process of word analysis is the reverse of word construction. When analyzing a word, start at the *end* of the word (the suffix) and work toward the beginning (prefix). Analyze the components in sequence.

Example: oVARioHYSterECtomy =

ovari/o/hyster/ectomy

4 3 2 1

1. The suffix *-ectomy* means to surgically remove.
2. The root word *hyster* refers to the uterus.
3. The *o* is the combining vowel for the previous root word.
4. The root word *ovari* refers to the ovaries.

Thus, *ovariohysterectomy* means "excision (surgical removal) of the uterus and ovaries." Note that steps 3 and 4 may be combined into one step, using the combining form *ovari/o*, which refers to the ovaries.

COMBINING FORMS FOR BODY PARTS

Following is a list of body parts and their respective combining forms. This is not a complete list of combining forms, but it represents some used often in veterinary terminology. To learn these words and their meaning "requires memory." Students should utilize handheld flash cards with the combining form on one side and the meaning or body part on the other.

Combining Form	Body Part
abdomin/o	abdomen
adren/o, adrenal-	adrenal gland
angi/o	vessel
arteri/o	artery
arthr/o	joint
blephar/o	eyelid, eyelash
cardi/o	heart
cervic/o	cervix or neck of an organ
chol/o, chole-	bile

cholecyst/o	gallbladder
chondr/o	cartilage
col/o	colon
crani/o	cranium, skull
cyst/o	bladder
cyt/o	cell
dent/o	tooth, teeth
derm/o, dermat/o	skin
encephal/o	brain
enter/o	intestines
epididym/o	epididymis
esophag/o	esophagus
gastr/o	stomach
gloss/o	tongue
hem/o, hemat/o	blood
hepa-, hepat/o	liver
hyster/o	uterus
kerat/o	cornea or horny tissue
lapar/o	flank, abdomen
lip/o	fat
lymph/o	lymph
mast/o, mamm/o	mammary glands
mening/o	meninges
metr/o	uterus (special reference to inner lining)
muscul/o, my/o, myos-	muscle
myel/o	bone marrow or spinal cord
nephr/o	kidney, nephron
neur/o	nerve
ocul/o	eye
odont/o	tooth, teeth
onych/o	claw, hoof
ophthalm/o	eye
orchi/o, orchid/o	testes
oste/o	bone
ot/o	ear
peritone/o	peritoneum
phleb/o	vein
pneum/o	lung, air, breath
proct/o	rectum
pulmo-, pulmon/o	lung
ren/o	renal (kidney)
rhin/o	nose
spondyl/o	vertebra, spinal column
thorac/o	thorax
thyr/o, thyroid-	thyroid gland
tonsill/o	tonsil
trache/o	trachea
tympan/o	tympanum (middle ear), tympanic membrane, eardrum
urethr/o	urethra
ur/o	urine
uter/o	uterus
vagin/o	vagina
ven/o	vein
ventricul/o	ventricle
vertebr/o	vertebra
vulv/o	vulva

Remember, words for some body parts have more than one combining form. Examples from the previous list are the following:

mouth = or/o, stomat/o; teeth = dent/o, odont/o

There are no general rules for when one or the other is used. This must be learned by listening and reading to be aware of how these combining forms are used. You already know some of them. For instance, you know that there is oral medication, not stomatal medication. Often, the different combining forms refer to a specific part of a structure or a specific use of the structure. *Or/o* often refers to the mouth as the first part of the digestive system, whereas *stomat/o* refers to the lining of the oral cavity or the opening to the oral cavity (e.g., stomatitis, stomatoplasty).

SUFFIXES FOR SURGICAL PROCEDURES

Following is a list of suffixes for surgical procedures. Using the rules for word construction, you can form words to describe a variety of surgical procedures on various body parts, or define these words using the word analysis technique previously described.

Suffix	Meaning	Example and Definition
-ectomy	to excise or surgically remove	CHOLecysTECtomy = surgical removal of the gallbladder
-tomy	to incise or cut into (making an incision)	LAPaROTomy = surgical incision into the abdomen
-stomy	to make a new, artificial opening in a hollow organ (to the outside of the body), or to make a new opening between two hollow organs	CoLOStomy = surgical creation of a new opening between the colon and the outside of the body GAStro-DUodeNOStomy = to create a new opening between the stomach and the duodenum
-rrhaphy	to surgically repair by joining in a seam or by suturing together	HERniORRhaphy = surgical repair of a hernia
-pexy	fixation or suturing (a stabilizing type of repair)	GAStroPEXy = fixation of the stomach to the body wall
-plasty	to shape, the surgical formation of, or plastic surgery (meaning "to	CHEIloPLASty = plastic repair of the lips (to improve looks and function)

Suffix	Meaning	Example and Definition
	improve function, to relieve pain, or for cosmetic reasons")	
-centesis	to puncture, perforate, or tap, permitting withdrawal of fluid, air, etc.	AbDOMinocenTEsis = surgical puncture of the abdomen to remove fluid from the peritoneal cavity

SUFFIXES FOR DISEASES OR CONDITIONS

The same rules and procedures used to form and analyze surgical words can be used with suffixes that refer to diseases or conditions to describe a problem affecting a particular organ or body part. Following is a list of these suffixes:

Suffix	Meaning	Example and Definition
-iasis	infestation or infection with, a condition characterized by	AcaRIasis = infestation with mites lithIasis = condition characterized by formation of calculi
-ism	a state or condition, a fact of being, result of a process	HyperCORtiSONism = condition resulting from excessive cortisone
-itis	inflammation of	TONsilLItis = inflammation of the tonsils
-oma	tumor	LEIomyOMa = tumor of smooth muscles
-osis	abnormal condition or process of degeneration	NePHROsis = degenerative disease of the kidneys

PREFIXES FOR DISEASES OR CONDITIONS

Following is a list of prefixes used to create words indicating a specific problem within the body or a body system.

Suffix	Meaning	Example and Definition
a-, an-	without or not having	aNEmia = not having enough red blood cells

Suffix	Meaning	Example and Definition
anti-	against	AntibiOTic = drug that acts against bacteria
brady-	slow	BRAdy**CAR**dia = excessively slow heart rate
contra-	against, opposed	CONtra**IN**diCAted = something that is not indicated
de-	remove, take away, loss of	deHYdrated = excessive loss of body water
dys-	difficult, troubled	DysPHAgia = difficulty eating or swallowing
hyper-	high, excessive	HYper**THER**mia = body temperature higher than normal
hypo-	low, insufficient	HYpo**THER**mia = body temperature lower than normal
mal-	bad, poor	MALo**CCLU**sion = poor fit of upper and lower teeth when jaws close
poly-	many, much	POLy**PHA**gia = excessive eating
py/o-	pus	PYo**THO**rax = pus in the thoracic cavity
tachy-	fast, rapid	TACHy**CAR**dia = excessively fast heart rate

-ma	-mata or -mas	ENema, ENeMAta or ENemas
-um	-a	Ovum, Ova
-ur	-ora	FEMur, FEMora
-us	-i	Uterus, Uteri

PLURAL ENDINGS

It is important to understand the methods for converting singular forms of medical words to their plural forms, and vice versa. Following is a list of common singular endings and their corresponding plural endings:

Singular	Plural	Example
-a	-ae	VERtebra, VERtebrae
-anx	-anges	PHAlanx, phaLANges
-en	-ina	LUmen, LUmina
-ex, -ix	-ices	Apex, Apices; CERvix, CERvices
-is	-es	TEStis, TEStes
-inx	-inges	MENinx, meNINges

SUFFIXES FOR INSTRUMENTS, PROCEDURES, AND MACHINES

Below is a list of suffixes that, when added to a combining form of a body part, form a word pertaining to an instrument, procedure, or a machine that looks into, cuts, or measures a body part.

Suffix	Meaning	Example and Definition
-scope	instrument for examining, viewing, or listening	OtoSCOPE = instrument for looking into the ears
-scopy	act of examining or using the scope	LAPaROScopy = procedure of using a laparoscope to view the abdominal cavity
-tome	instrument for cutting, such as into smaller or thinner sections	MicroTOME = instrument for cutting tissues into microthin slices or sections
-graph	instrument or machine that writes or records	ELECtro**CAR**diograph = machine that records electrical impulses produced by the beating heart
-graphy	procedure of using an instrument or machine to record	ELECtroCARdi-**OG**raphy = procedure of using an electro-cardiograph to produce an electrocardiogram
-gram	product, written record, "picture," or graph produced	ELECtroCARdiogram (ECG, EKG) = graphic tracing of the electrical currents flowing through the beating heart
-meter	instrument or machine that measures or counts	TherMOmeter = instrument used to measure body temperature
-metry -imetry	procedure of measuring	doSIMetry – act of determining the amount, rate, and distribution of ionizing radiation

TERMS FOR DIRECTION, POSITION, AND MOVEMENT

Following is a list of words used to describe direction or the position of a body part relative to other body parts.

CRAnial: Pertaining to the cranium or head end of the body, or denoting a position more toward the cranium or head end of the body than another reference point (body part) (see Fig. 6-1, p. 78). Example: The head is cranial to the tail.

CAUdal: Pertaining to the tail end of the body, or denoting a position more toward the tail or rear of the body than another reference point (body part) (see Fig. 6-1, p. 78). Example: The tail is caudal to the head.

ROStral: Pertaining to the nose end of the head or body, or toward the nose (see Fig. 6-1, p. 78). Example: The nose is rostral to the eyes.

DORsal: Pertaining to the back area of a quadruped (animal with four legs), or denoting a position more toward the spine than another reference point (body part) (see Fig. 6-1, p. 78). Example: The vertebral column is dorsal to the abdomen.

VENtral: Pertaining to the underside of a quadruped, or denoting a position more toward the abdomen than another reference point (body part) (see Fig. 6-1, p. 78). Example: The intestines are ventral to the vertebral column.

MEdial: Denoting a position closer to the median plane of the body or a structure, toward the middle or median plane, or pertaining to the middle or a position closer to the median plane of the body or a structure (see Fig. 6-1, p. 78). Example: The medial surface of the leg is the "inside" surface.

LATeral: Denoting a position farther from the median plane of the body or a structure, on the side or toward the side away from the median plane, or pertaining to the side of the body or of a structure (see Fig. 6-1, p. 78). Example: The lateral surface of the leg is the "outside" surface.

peRIPHeral: Pertaining to or situated near the periphery, the outermost part, or surface of an organ or part. Example: The enamel of a tooth is peripheral to the dentin and central root canal.

CENtral: Pertaining to or situated near the more proximal areas of the body or a structure; opposite of *peripheral.* Example: The spinal cord is central to the sciatic nerve.

SUperFIcial: Situated near the surface of the body or a structure; opposite of deep. Example: The skin is superficial to the muscles.

deep: Situated away from the surface of the body or a structure; opposite of superficial. Example: The muscles are deep to the skin.

adJAcent: Next to, adjoining, or close. Example: The tongue is adjacent to the teeth.

PROXimal: Nearer to the center of the body, relative to another body part, or a location on a body part relative to another, more distant, location (see Fig. 6-1, p. 78). Example: The humerus is proximal to the radius.

DIStal: Farther from the center of the body, relative to another body part or a location on a body part relative to another closer location (see Fig. 6-1, p. 78). Example: The tibia is distal to the femur.

obLIQUE: At an angle, or pertaining to an angle. Example: The vein crosses obliquely from the dorsal left side to the ventral right side.

reCUMbent: Lying down; a modifying term is needed to describe the surface on which the animal is lying. Example: An animal in dorsal recumbency is lying on its dorsum (back), faceup.

SUpine, SUpin**NA**tion: Lying faceup, in dorsal recumbency. Supination is the act of turning the body or a leg so that the ventral aspect is uppermost.

prone, proNAtion: Lying facedown, in ventral recumbency. Pronation is the act of turning the body or a leg so the ventral aspect is down.

PALmar: The caudal surface of the front foot distal to the antebrachiocarpal joint; also pertains to the undersurface of the front foot (see Fig. 6-1).

PLANtar: The caudal surface of the back foot distal to the tarsocrural joint; also pertains to the undersurface of the rear foot (see Fig. 6-1).

abDUCtion: Movement of a limb or part away from the median line or middle of the body (Fig. 5-1).

adDUCtion: Movement of a limb or part toward the median line or middle of the body (Fig. 5-1).

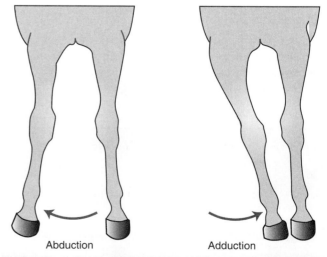

Fig. 5-1 Terms denoting limb movement: abduction and adduction. (From Colville T, Bassert JM: *Clinical Anatomy and Physiology for Veterinary Technicians,* ed 2, St. Louis, 2008, Elsevier.)

FLEXion: The act of bending, such as a joint (Fig. 5-2).
exTENsion: The act of straightening, such as a joint; also, the act of pulling two component parts apart to lengthen the whole part (Fig. 5-2).

DENTAL TERMINOLOGY

The teeth have their own set of positional terms listed below.

ocCLUsal: The chewing or biting surface of teeth; toward the plane between the mandibular and maxillary teeth (Fig. 5-3).

BUccal: Toward the cheek; tooth surface toward the cheek (Fig. 5-3).

LINGual: Pertaining to the tongue; tooth surface toward the tongue (Fig. 5-3).

CONtact: Tooth surface facing an adjacent or opposing tooth (Fig. 5-3).

MEsial: Tooth surface closest to the midline of the dental arcade.

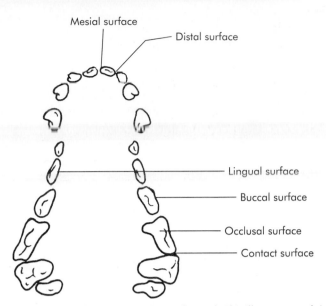

Fig. 5-3 Positional terms pertaining to the teeth. This illustrates teeth in the upper dental arcade, as seen from a ventral view. (From Cochran PE: *Guide to veterinary medical terminology,* St Louis, 1991, Mosby.)

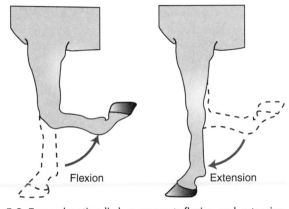

Fig. 5-2 Terms denoting limb movement: flexion and extension. (From Colville T, Bassert JM: *Clinical Anatomy and Physiology for Veterinary Technicians,* ed 2, St. Louis, 2008, Elsevier.)

RECOMMENDED READING

Austrin G, Austrin BA, et al: *Learning medical terminology,* ed 9, St Louis, 1999, Mosby.

Christenson D: *Veterinary medical terminology,* St Louis, 1997, Saunders.

Cochran PE: *Guide to veterinary medical terminology,* St Louis, 1991, Mosby.

Cohen BJ: *Medical terminology,* ed 4, Philadelphia, 2003, Lippincott.

Leonard PC: *Quick and easy medical terminology,* ed 3, Philadelphia, 2000, Saunders.

McBride DF: *Learning veterinary terminology,* ed 2, St Louis, 2002, Mosby.

Mosby's medical, nursing & allied health dictionary, ed 6, St Louis, 2002, Saunders.

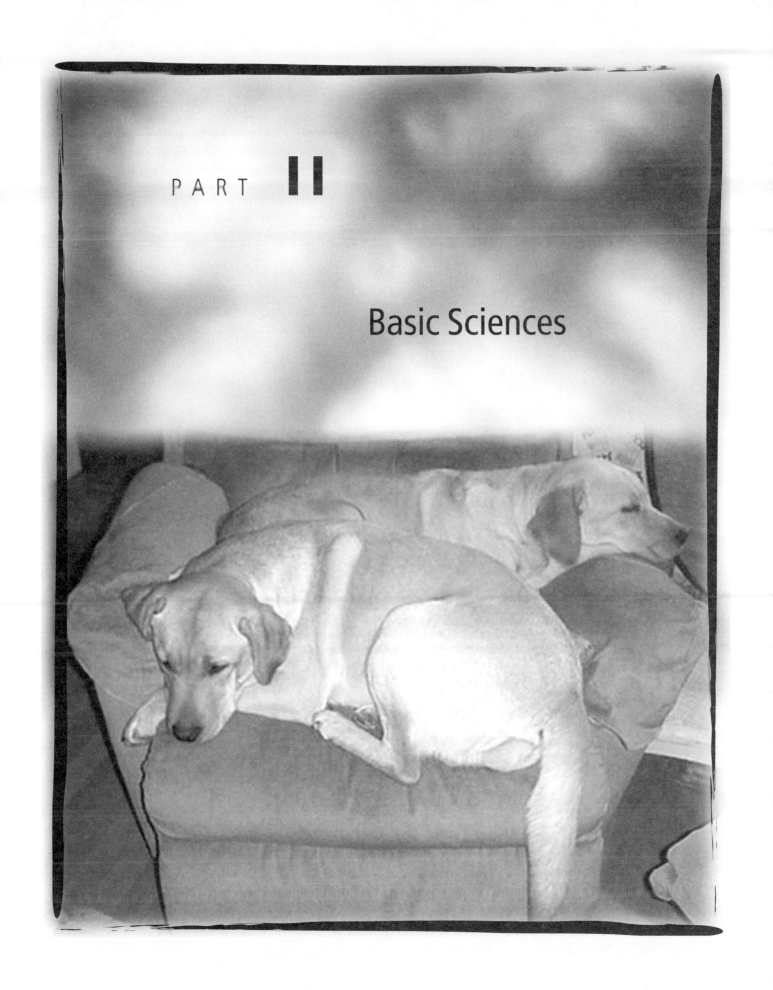

PART **II**

Basic Sciences

Anatomy and Physiology

Shashikant Goswami

6

Learning Objectives

After reviewing this chapter, the reader should understand the following:

- Types of cells and tissues of the body
- Names of organs and structures that make up the various body systems
- Ways in which organs and body systems function and interact
- Differences in the digestive tract of ruminants and monogastric animals
- Various general and special senses of the body and their functions
- Differences between exocrine and endocrine glands
- Features and functions of the male and female reproductive tract
- Normal reproductive cycles of female domestic species
- Ways in which pregnancy is diagnosed
- Stages and events of parturition
- Ways in which males are evaluated for breeding soundness
- Techniques of artificial insemination
- Necropsy procedures for domestic animals

Studying anatomy and physiology will help you better understand the wonderful machine that is the animal body. *Anatomy* is the study of normal structure of various body organs and their location. It tells about the basic similarities or differences within the species. *Physiology*, on the other hand, describes the mechanism and steps of how the body and its various components function. Although anatomy and physiology are two different sciences, studying them together gives a clearer picture of how the body is organized and how its various components function in a complex, interrelated fashion.

GENERAL TERMINOLOGY

There are two approaches to studying anatomy. The first approach is systemic anatomy. The second approach is topographic anatomy. In *systemic anatomy*, the body is divided into systems depending on their function. Examples are the digestive system, respiratory system, and nervous system. To study physiology, the same systemic approach is followed. A *system* consists of many organs that perform similar functions.

Topographic anatomy is the study of locating organs in relation to each other. To describe the positions and rela-

tionships of body parts, topographic terms must be used. Common words, such as *up*, *down*, *front*, *back*, *top*, and *bottom* are not useful, because their meanings depend on the orientation of both the animal and the viewer. To be useful, the meanings of directional terms used to describe anatomy must be clear and independent of the body's position and the angle from which it is viewed (Fig. 6-1).

Many directional terms come in pairs that mean they are opposite of each other. Most terms are relative terms that mean they are used in relation to other parts. *Left* and *right* always refer to the animal's left and right. *Cranial* refers to direction toward the head of an animal, and *caudal* refers to direction toward the tail. *Dorsal* refers to direction toward the backbone, and *ventral* refers to direction away from the backbone (toward the belly). *Superficial* structures are located toward the surface of the body or part, and *deep* structures are located toward the center of the body or part.

Some terms are used only for particular parts of the body. Although the terms *cranial* and *caudal* are useful on most of the body, when speaking of the head, *cranial* loses its meaning. *Rostral* refers to direction toward the tip of the nose and is used only when describing structures on or in the head. *Proximal* and *distal* are used to describe relationships on extremities. *Proximal* refers to direction toward the body (the attachment site of the extremity).

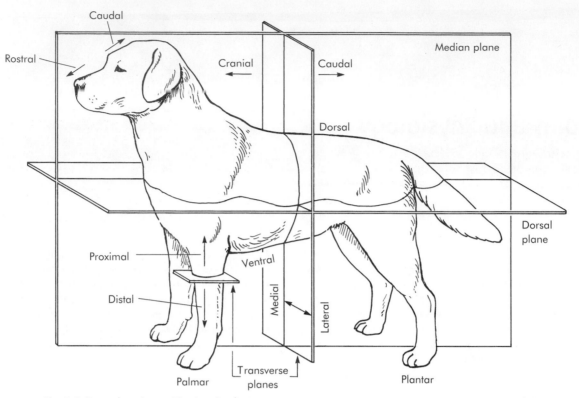

Fig. 6-1 Terms denoting position in animals. *(From McBride DF:* Learning veterinary terminology, *St Louis, 2001, Mosby.)*

Distal refers to direction away from the body (toward the tip of the extremity).

Four basic planes can be used to divide an animal's body and give reference points for other descriptions. A *median plane* or *midline* is an imaginary line that divides the body into equal left and right halves. Any plane parallel to midline is called a *sagittal plane*. A *transverse plane* or *cross-section* divides the body into cranial and caudal parts, and a *dorsal plane* or *horizontal plane* divides the body into dorsal and ventral parts. *Medial* and *lateral* are terms used to describe positions of structures relative to the median plane or midline. A medial structure is located closer to the midline of the body. A lateral structure is located away from the midline, toward the side of the body.

CELLS

Cells are the basic structural and functional units of life. All living things are composed of cells. An animal's body is composed of many different types of cells, each with its own place and function. Each cell relies on the rest of the body to meet its nutritional and waste elimination needs, and the whole body relies on the contribution of all of its cells for its support. This relationship can be summarized by the following formula:

cell health ↔ tissue health ↔ organ health ↔ system health ↔ body health.

Note that the arrows point in both directions. The health of the cell depends on the health of the tissues of which it is part. In turn, the tissues depend on the health of the cells that make them up, *and* the organs they are part of, and so on up the line. The degree of health at each level determines whether the body as a whole is healthy.

Unlike single-celled animals, complex (multicelled) organisms have specialized cells that allow the whole body to operate. Groups of specialized cells make up tissues. Four basic types of tissues make up the animal body: *epithelial tissue, connective tissue, muscle tissue, and nervous tissue.* Functional groupings of tissues make up organs, such as the kidneys, that contain elements of all four basic tissues. Systems are groups of organs that are involved in a common activity. For example, the salivary glands, esophagus, stomach, pancreas, liver, and intestines are all parts of the digestive system.

EPITHELIAL TISSUE

Epithelial tissue covers the interior and exterior surfaces of the body, lines body cavities, and forms glands. Its function includes protection from physical wear and tear as well as penetration by foreign invaders, selective absorption of substances (e.g., by the intestinal lining), and secretion of various substances. All epithelial tissues share three common features:

- They consist entirely of cells.
- They do not contain blood vessels. Epithelial cells derive nourishment from blood vessels in the connective tissues beneath them.
- At least some epithelial cells are capable of reproducing. Epithelial tissue cells must be capable of compensating for wear and tear, as well as injuries.

The covering and lining of epithelial tissue can be either simple (one cell-layer thick) or stratified (more than one cell-layer thick), and it can be composed of several different cell types. Depending on the shape and arrangement of cells, the epithelial tissue is further classified as *simple* and *stratified*:

Simple epithelium: squamous, cuboidal, columnar, and pseudostratified columnar

Stratified epithelium: squamous, cuboidal, columnar, and transitional

Simple epithelial tissues are the following:

Epithelium	Cell Shape	Example
Squamous	Flat, platelike	Blood vessel lining
Cuboidal	Round or cuboidal	Kidney tubules
Columnar	Cylindrical	Intestinal lining
Pseudostratified columnar	Irregular; nuclei not uniform in position	Upper respiratory tract lining

Glandular epithelium cells are specialized cells that secrete substances directly into the bloodstream or out onto a body surface. The "ductless" glands that secrete directly into the bloodstream are the *endocrine glands* (e.g., pituitary gland, thyroid, testes, ovaries, and adrenal gland). They produce hormones. *Exocrine glands* secrete substances through ducts. They can be simple, with a single duct (e.g., sweat glands), or compound, with a branching duct system (e.g., mammary glands).

Stratified epithelial tissues are the following:

CONNECTIVE TISSUE

Connective tissue holds the different tissues together and provides support. It contains few cells and more fibers as compared to epithelial tissue. If the body consisted entirely of cells, it would lie like a puddle of gelatin on the ground. Cells are very soft in consistency. Firmer connective tissue is necessary to support the cells and allow the body to assume an efficient shape and overall structure.

The cells of most connective tissues produce nonliving, intercellular substances that connect and give support to other cells and tissues. These intercellular substances range from various types of fibers to the firm, mineralized matrix of bone.

Six main types of connective tissues are present in the body: *adipose connective tissue, loose connective tissue, dense connective tissue, elastic connective tissue, cartilage,* and *bone.* Blood is also a connective tissue; it will be discussed with the rest of the blood vascular system.

Adipose connective tissue consists of collections of lipid-storing cells, what we commonly refer to as fat. It represents the body's storage supply of excess nutrients. When the dietary intake of nutrients exceeds the body's needs, adipose connective tissue proliferates. In leaner times, when the dietary nutrient intake is insufficient, the lipid stored in the adipose connective tissue can be mobilized to meet the body's nutritional needs.

Loose connective tissue is found throughout the body wherever cushioning and flexibility are needed. It is commonly found beneath the skin and around blood vessels, nerves, and muscles. Its main components are fiber-producing cells, fibroblasts, and three types of fibers (*collagen fibers, reticular fibers,* and *elastic fibers*). Collagen fibers are predominant and are very strong to provide strength to the organs. Reticular fibers form supportive framework. Elastic fibers are a minor component and provide some degree of elasticity. Both sets of fibers are intertwined in a loose mesh that provides cushioning and flexibility in virtually all directions.

Dense connective tissue has the same components as loose connective tissue but is much more densely packed. One variety of dense connective tissue has the fibers arranged in

Epithelium	Characteristics	Example
Stratified squamous	Thick and tough deepest cells reproduce, pushing daughter cells toward the surface. They gradually die and assume a flattened shape as they move farther from their nutrient source in the underlying connective tissue	Skin
Stratified cuboidal	Rare in the body	Ducts of sweat glands
Stratified columnar	Rare in the body and usually seen where one type of epithelium is blending into another type of epithelium	Junction of oropharynx and nasopharynx
Transitional	Capable of considerable stretching	Urinary bladder lining

parallel bundles. This type of tissue is regularly arranged. It makes up *tendons*, which attach muscles to bones, and *ligaments*, which attach bones to other bones. The other type of tissue is irregularly arranged. It is like a densely compacted version of loose connective tissue. It is found in the capsules that surround and protect many soft internal organs.

Cartilage consists of a few cells, called *chondrocytes*, and various types and amounts of fibers embedded in a thick gelatinous intercellular substance, the *matrix*. Cartilage is firmer than fibrous tissue, but not as hard as bone, and contains no blood vessels. Nutrients for chondrocytes must diffuse through the matrix from the periphery of the cartilage. This limits how thick cartilage can become. Hyaline cartilage is smooth and glossy in appearance. It contains more chondrocytes and a few collagen fibers. It is found in the tracheal rings and the articular (joint) surfaces of bones. Fibrous cartilage contains large numbers of densely arranged collagen fibers in its matrix and few chondrocytes, making it very durable. It makes up the majority of the intervertebral disks, which cushion the vertebrae. Elastic cartilage contains large numbers of both elastic and collagen fibers, giving it more flexibility than the other two cartilage types. It makes up parts of the larynx and most of the earflap (pinna).

Bone is second only to the enamel of teeth in its hardness. It is composed of a few cells, the *osteocytes*, embedded in a matrix that has become mineralized through a process called *ossification*. It is important to note that, despite its hard, dead appearance, bone is living tissue with an excellent capacity for regeneration and remodeling.

SKELETON

The skeleton is the framework of bones that supports and protects the soft tissues of the body. Some bones, such as the bones of the skull, which enclose and protect the delicate brain, surround sensitive tissues. Most of the bones of the skeleton, however, form the scaffolding around which the rest of the body tissues are arranged.

Types of Bones

Long bones

The bone shaft where the primary growth occurs is called the *diaphysis*. The area of the bone where secondary growth forms is called the *epiphysis*. Between each end of the diaphysis and each epiphysis is a zone of growth called the *metaphysis*, which contains a hyaline cartilage or growth plate. A small portion of long bone between epiphysis and diaphysis at both ends is *metaphysis*, which contains a hyaline cartilage or growth plate. It is the part where bone grows in length on both extremities. A long bone contains a medullary cavity filled with a bone marrow. Examples of long bones are the humerus, radius, ulna, metacarpals, femur, tibia, fibula,

and metatarsals. Bone marrow contains the stem cells, which produce the blood cells. Bone marrow collection is very valuable to diagnose the diseases of blood, especially when blood shows abnormal cells.

Flat bones

Flat bones are expanded in two directions to provide maximum area for muscle attachment. Examples of flat bones are the scapula, skull bones, and pelvis.

Small bones

Small bones are cuboidal or approximately equal in all dimensions located at complex joints such as the carpus and hock joint. Examples of small bones are the carpal and tarsal bones.

Irregular bones

Irregular bones are bones with irregular shape, such as the vertebrae.

Sesamoid bones

Sesamoid bones are tiny bones found along the course of the tendons. These bones reduce the friction and change the direction of a tendon. Examples of sesamoid bones are the patella and fabellae. The patella, or kneecap, is the largest sesamoid bone.

Pneumatic bones

Pneumatic bones contain air spaces to make the skeleton lighter. Most of the bones of a bird's skeleton are pneumatic bones.

Common Bone Features

- An *articular surface* is a surface in which a bone forms a joint with another bone. It is usually very smooth and is often covered with a layer of hyaline cartilage.
- A *condyle* is a large, convex articular surface usually found on the distal ends of the long bones that make up the limbs.
- A *foramen* is a hole in a bone through which blood vessels and nerves usually pass.
- A *fossa* is a depression in a bone usually occupied by a muscle or tendon.
- A *facet* is a flat and smooth articular area, such as the surface of a tarsal or carpal bone.
- A *bone head* is a spherical articular projection usually found on the proximal ends of some limb bones.
- The *neck of a bone* is the often-narrowed area that connects a bone head with the rest of the bone.
- A *process, tuber, tubercle, tuberosity*, or *trochanter* is a lump or bump on the surface of a bone. It is usually the site where the tendon of a muscle attaches to a bone. The larger the process, the more powerful the muscle that attaches at the site.

Axial Skeleton

The axial skeleton is composed of the bones located on the axis or midline of the body. It is composed of the bones of the skull, the spinal column, the ribs, and the sternum (Fig. 6-2).

The skull is composed of many bones, most of which are held together by immovable joints called *sutures*. The skull bones can be divided into the bones of the cranium and the bones of the face (which extend in a rostral direction from the cranium). The bones of the cranium house and protect the brain, and the bones of the face house mainly digestive and respiratory structures.

The spinal column is composed of a series of individual bones called *vertebrae*. The vertebrae form a long, flexible tube called the *vertebral canal*. The vertebral canal houses and protects the spinal cord. The vertebrae are divided into five groups, and each vertebra is numbered within each group from cranial to caudal (Fig. 6-2). The *cervical* vertebrae (C) are in the neck region. The first cervical vertebra (C1) is the *atlas* that forms a joint with the skull. The *thoracic vertebrae* (T) are dorsal to the chest region and form joints with the dorsal ends of the ribs. The *lumbar vertebrae* (L), which are dorsal to the abdominal region, are fairly large and heavy, because they serve as the site of attachment for the large sling muscles that support the abdomen. The *sacral vertebrae* (S) in the pelvic region are fused together into a solid structure called the *sacrum*, which forms a joint with the pelvis. The caudalmost vertebrae, the *coccygeal vertebrae* (Cy), form the tail. The number of vertebrae in each region varies with species. In the box that follows is the vertebral formula of different species.

> Dog: C 7, T 13, L 7, S 3, Cy 20-23
> Cow: C 7, T 13, L 6, S 5, Cy 18-20
> Horse: C 7, T 18, L 6, S 5, Cy 15-20

The ribs support and help form the lateral walls of the thorax or chest (Fig. 6-2). Their number varies with the species, but the number of rib pairs is usually the same as the number of thoracic vertebrae. They form joints with the thoracic vertebrae dorsally and are continued ventrally by rods of hyaline cartilage, the costal cartilages. The costal cartilages of ribs at the cranial end of the thorax are connected directly to the sternum at their ventral end. The costal cartilages of the caudal ribs do not reach the sternum; they connect to the costal cartilage cranial to them. The spaces between ribs are referred to as *intercostal spaces*.

The sternum forms the ventral portion of the thorax (Fig. 6-2). It is composed of a series of rodlike bones called *sternebrae*. The manubrium sterni is the first (cranialmost) sternebra, and the xiphoid process is the last (caudalmost). These two bones are often used as external landmarks on the animal.

Appendicular Skeleton

The appendicular skeleton is composed of the bones of the limbs (*appendages*). The forelimb is referred to anatomically

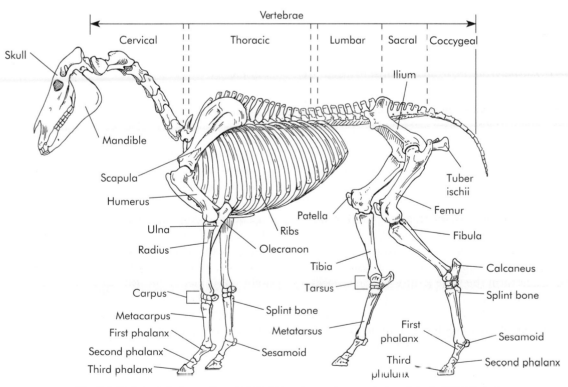

Fig. 6-2 Skeleton of a horse. *(From McBride DF:* Learning veterinary terminology, *St Louis, 2001, Mosby.)*

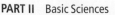
as the *thoracic limb*, and the hind limb is termed the *pelvic limb*.

From proximal to distal, the bones of the thoracic limb are the *scapula, humerus, radius* and *ulna, carpal bones, metacarpal bones,* and *phalanges* (Fig. 6-2). The scapula is the "shoulder blade." It is a flat bone with a shelflike spine on its lateral surface. At its distal end, it has a shallow cavity called the *glenoid cavity* that forms the shoulder joint with the humerus (the long bone of the brachium or upper arm). The proximal end of the humerus is composed of the *head,* the smooth articular surface that forms the shoulder joint with the scapula, and the *greater tubercle,* where the powerful shoulder muscles attach. The distal joint surfaces of the humerus, the *condyles,* form the elbow joint with the radius and ulna, the bones of the antebrachium or forearm.

The *radius* is the main weight-bearing bone of the antebrachium, and the ulna forms much of the very snug-fitting elbow joint with the condyle of the humerus (Fig. 6-2). At the proximal end of the ulna is the olecranon process, the point of the elbow where the powerful triceps brachii muscle attaches. In animals such as cows and horses, the radius and ulna are fused together.

Located between the radius and ulna and the metacarpal bones is the *carpus* (Fig. 6-2). It is composed of two rows of short bones and is equivalent to the human wrist. Just distal to the carpus are the metacarpal bones, equivalent to the bones of the human hand between wrist and fingers. The phalanges are the bones of the digits, equivalent to human fingers. Dogs and cats have five digits (toes) in each forelimb. Cows, sheep, and goats have two digits (split hooves), and horses have one digit. Each digit is composed of either two phalanges (proximal and distal), as in the human thumb, or three phalanges (proximal, middle, and distal), as in human fingers.

The bones of the pelvic limb, from proximal to distal, are the *pelvis, femur, patella, tibia* and *fibula, tarsal bones, metatarsal bones,* and *phalanges* (Fig. 6-2). The *pelvis* is composed of three pairs of bones that are fused in the adult animal: the *ilium,* the *ischium,* and the *pubis.* The cranial part of ilium is the *iliac crest,* which is one of the sites to aspirate bone marrow. At the junction of the three bones on each side is a deep cavity, the *acetabulum,* which is the socket portion of the ball-and-socket hip joint.

The *femur* is the long bone of the thigh region (Fig. 6-2). The head of the femur forms the ball portion of the hip joint, and the *greater trochanter* is the site of attachment for the powerful gluteal (rump) muscles. At its distal end are the condyles, which form the stifle joint with the tibia, and the *trochlear groove,* in which the patella rides.

The *patella,* or kneecap, is the largest sesamoid bone in the body. Sesamoid bones are located in tendons that change direction sharply at joints. The patella helps distribute the force of the quadriceps femoris muscle, the main extensor muscle of the stifle joint.

The *tibia* is the main weight-bearing bone of the distal leg. The fibula is thin and runs along the entire length of the tibia in dogs and cats. In other species, such as cows and horses, the fibula is a very small, sometimes incomplete bone that is primarily a site of muscle attachment (Fig. 6-2).

The *tarsus* is equivalent to the human ankle, and it consists of two rows of short bones. The tuberosity of the large calcaneus or fibular tarsal forms the point of the hock joint, equivalent to the human heel bone. The metatarsal bones and phalanges of the pelvic limb are similar to the metacarpal bones and phalanges of the thoracic limb.

Visceral Skeleton

The bones of the visceral skeleton, when present, occur in soft tissues of the body. The *os penis* of the dog is a well-developed bone in the penis. The *os cordis* forms part of the supporting structures in the heart of cattle. The *os rostri* helps strengthen the snout of swine.

Joints

Bones come together at joints. Our usual image of joints is that of freely movable joints, such as the elbow or hip. However, joints can be any of three main types: *fibrous joints* are immovable, *cartilaginous joints* are slightly movable, and *diarthrodial* or *synovial joints* are freely movable.

Fibrous joints hold bones together but do not allow movement at the joint site. The sutures that hold many of the skull bones together are immovable joints. Cartilaginous joints allow a slight rocking movement. The cartilaginous intervertebral discs and the symphysis that unites the pubic bones of the pelvis allow a slight amount of movement.

Synovial joints are what people usually think of when they think of joints. They allow free movement between bones in several directions. Synovial joints usually have smooth articular surfaces covered by articular cartilage, and a fibrous joint capsule. The inner side of the joint capsule is lined by synovial membrane, which secretes the synovial fluid that is oily in nature and covers and protects the articular cartilages from wearing against each other. The normal synovial fluid is clear, sticky, slippery, and viscous. When the joint is inflamed, the fluid becomes thin and less slippery and cannot protect the cartilage anymore. Many joints also have fibrous ligaments that hold bones together. Most ligaments are *extracapsular* (located outside the fibrous joint capsule), such as collateral ligaments. Some ligaments are *intracapsular* (located inside the joint cavity), such as cruciate ligaments that connect the distal end of the femur to the proximal end of the tibia.

Synovial joints allow some combination of six potential joint movements: *flexion, extension, adduction, abduction, rotation,* and *circumduction.* Flexion decreases the angle between two bones; extension increases the angle. Adduction moves the extremity toward the median plane, and abduction moves it away from the median plane. Rotation is a twisting movement of a part on its own axis. The shaking of the head of a wet dog is a rotation movement. Circumduction is a movement in which the distal end of an extremity describes a circle.

INTEGUMENT

The *integument* is the outer covering of the body. It consists primarily of the skin, hair, claws, or hooves and horns. In nonmammalian species, it also includes such structures as feathers and scales. In addition to its obvious protective role, the integument has several other important functions. Its multitude of sensory receptors makes it one of the most important parts of an animal's sensory system. Integument also helps in regulating body temperature through its ability to adjust blood flow to the skin, adjust the position of hairs, and secrete sweat. The integument also produces vitamin D and secretes and excretes a number of substances through various types of skin glands.

Skin

The skin is the largest body organ. It consists of two main layers: the superficial epithelial layer *(epidermis)*, and the deep connective tissue layer *(dermis)*.

The *epidermis* is composed of keratinized stratified squamous epithelium. The surface layer of the epidermis dries out and is converted to a tough, horny substance called *keratin*, which also makes up the bulk of hair, claws or hooves, and horns (antlers).

Within the deepest layers of the epidermis of most animals are *melanocytes*, cells that produce granules of the dark pigment melanin. This pigment gives color to the skin, hair, and other integumentary structures. An albino animal has a total lack of melanin, resulting in pale, white skin and hair, and unpigmented irises in the eyes.

The *dermis* layer of skin is composed of collagen, elastic, and reticular fibers. It contains hair follicles, *sebaceous glands, sudoriferous glands,* and *arrector pili muscles*. In addition, this layer also contains various sensitive nerve endings and blood vessels. The sebaceous glands are the oil glands of the skin. They secrete oily sebum, which helps waterproof the skin and keep it soft and pliable. Sebum is secreted directly onto the shafts of hairs in the hair follicles. Sudoriferous glands are the sweat glands, which primarily help cool the body. Some animals, such as horses, have sudoriferous glands spread over their entire body. Others, such as dogs and cats, have only a few, clustered in the footpad and nose areas.

The *hypodermis* or *subcutis* is a layer of loose connective tissue just below the dermis, which connects the skin to underlying muscles. It also contains some fat cells. The subcutaneous injection is administered in this layer by lifting a fold of skin.

Hair

Hair covers most of the body surface of most animals. Hair is composed of densely compacted keratinized cells and produced in glandlike structures called *hair follicles*. Hairs are constantly shed and replaced. The visible part of each hair is referred to as the *hair shaft*. The portion within the skin is called the *hair root*. The color of hair results from granules of melanin that are incorporated into the hairs during the course of their development. At the base of some hair roots, a tiny muscle, the arrector pili muscle, attaches. When it contracts, it pulls the hair into a more upright position. This produces "goose bumps" or "raised hackles." The purpose of erecting the hair generally is to retain heat when an animal is cold, by fluffing up the haircoat, or to make the animal look larger and more fearsome as a part of the sympathetic nervous system "fight or flight" response.

Claws and Hooves

Claws and hooves are horny structures that cover the distal ends of the digits. They are composed of parallel bundles of keratinized cells organized into an outer wall and a bottom sole.

Horns

Like claws and hooves, horns are composed of bundles of keratinized cells. They are organized around bony "horn cores," outgrowths of the frontal bones of the skull.

CIRCULATORY SYSTEM

The circulatory system is primarily a transport system in the body. It transports a variety of substances throughout the body, such as cells, antibodies, nutrients, oxygen, carbon dioxide, metabolic wastes, and hormones. Its two main divisions are the *blood vascular system* and the *lymphatic vascular system*.

Blood Vascular System

The blood vascular system consists of a closed system of tubes through which a fluid connective tissue is propelled by a muscular pump. The fluid connective tissue is blood; the tubes are blood vessels; and the pump is the heart.

There are three types of blood vessels: *arteries, capillaries,* and *veins*. Arteries carry blood away from the heart to the capillaries. Arteries are quite large near the heart and gradually branch into smaller and smaller vessels as they course throughout the body. From the arteries, blood passes into the extensive networks of very tiny capillaries located throughout the body.

Capillaries are very porous, composed of a single layer of endothelium and permit substances to move freely between the extracellular fluid (fluid surrounding cells) and the blood. The basic purpose of most of the blood vascular system is to deliver blood to the capillaries, where nutrients, waste products, gases, hormones, and other substances can be exchanged. Such substances as oxygen (O_2) and nutrients move out of the blood and into the cells. Metabolic

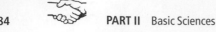
wastes and carbon dioxide (CO_2) move out of the cells and into the blood. From the capillaries, the CO_2-laden, waste-filled blood passes first into small venules and then into veins for the return trip to the heart. Many veins contain tiny one-way valves along their length. These one-way valves, assisted by movement of muscles in the area, help propel the blood back toward the heart.

Blood Circulation Pathways

Systemic circulation

During systemic circulation, blood moves from the heart to the body tissues and back to the heart. The *aorta* (the largest and main artery) originates from the left ventricle of the heart and carries oxygenated blood to various body tissues. The veins take the blood back to the heart and to the cranial and caudal venae cavae, which open into the right atrium of the heart.

Pulmonary circulation

During pulmonary circulation, blood moves from the heart to the lungs and back to the heart again. The pulmonary artery carries CO_2-rich blood from the right ventricle of the heart to the lungs for purification (oxygenation). The pulmonary veins bring oxygenated blood from the lungs to the left atrium of heart.

Heart

The heart is a muscular two-way pump that propels blood around the body and receives it back. It consists of dense accumulations of cardiac muscle cells and connective tissue organized into two side-by-side pumps that together are composed of four chambers (two *atria* and two *ventricles*) and four one-way valves (Fig. 6-3).

The heart has four chambers: two atria (right and left atrium) and two ventricles (right and left ventricles).

- *Right atrium:* The right atrium lies just above the right ventricle and receives CO_2-rich blood from cranial and caudal venae cavae.
- *Left atrium:* The left atrium lies just above the left ventricle and receives oxygenated blood from pulmonary veins. It is separated from the right atrium by an *interatrial septum.*
- *Right ventricle:* The right ventricle receives blood from the right atrium through the *right atrioventricular opening* (A-V opening), which is guarded by a *tricuspid valve.* The pulmonary artery originates from the right ventricle, and its opening is guarded by pulmonary semilunar valves.

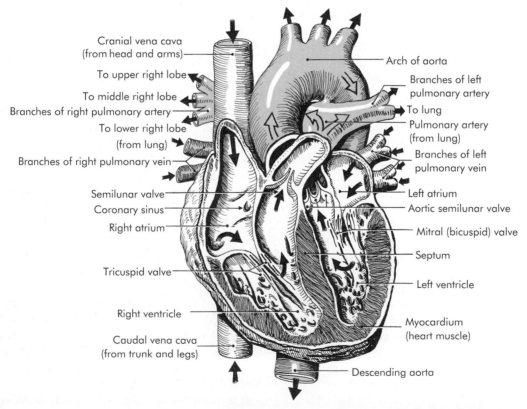

Fig. 6-3 Frontal view of the heart, with cutaway showing the heart chambers, valves, and major blood vessels. *(From McBride DF:* Learning veterinary terminology, *St Louis, 2001, Mosby.)*

- *Left ventricle:* The left ventricle receives blood from the left atrium through the *left atrioventricular opening*, which is guarded by a *bicuspid valve* or *mitral valve*. The aorta originates from the left ventricle, and its opening is guarded by aortic semilunar valves.

Cardiac cycle

The cardiac cycle interprets the series of events happening during one heartbeat. It includes relaxation of heart chambers (*diastole*) to receive the blood and contraction of heart chambers (*systole*) to pump the blood into body tissues and lungs. The receiving chamber of the right side of the heart is the right atrium. Blood flows into it from the venae cavae, the large systemic veins. When the right atrium contracts, it pumps blood through a large one-way valve, the *tricuspid valve*, into the right ventricle. The tricuspid valve gets its name from its three flaps, or *cusps*. When the right ventricle contracts, the tricuspid valve closes and blood flows out through the one-way pulmonary valve into the pulmonary artery, which carries blood to the lungs. When the right ventricular contraction is complete, the pulmonary valve closes, preventing blood from flowing back into the right ventricle.

The dynamics are similar on the left side of the heart (Fig. 6-3). Blood flows into the left atrium from the pulmonary veins. When the left atrium contracts, it pumps blood through the mitral valve into the left ventricle. The mitral valve is named for the resemblance (in an ancient anatomist's eye) of its two cusps to the miter worn by high-ranking Catholic clergy. When the left ventricle contracts, the mitral valve closes and blood flows out through the aortic valve into the aorta, the beginning of systemic circulation. When left ventricular contraction is complete, the aortic valve closes to prevent flow of blood back into the ventricle.

Specialized areas and bundles of cardiac muscle cells initiate each heartbeat, but the rate of heartbeat is controlled by the autonomic nervous system. By its nature, cardiac muscle contracts without needing external stimuli, but the activity of the many millions of individual cardiac muscle cells must be coordinated for the heart to contract in an organized, efficient manner.

Blood

Blood is a specialized connective tissue composed of fluid and cellular portions. The fluid portion is *plasma*, and the cellular portion is composed of *red blood cells, white blood cells,* and *platelets*.

Plasma is composed of 92% water, 7% protein molecules, and 1% other substances and electrolytes. It serves to suspend the blood cells and dissolve the many substances that are transported in the blood. If removed from blood vessels, plasma clots. *Fibrinogen* is one of the proteins in plasma. Fibrinogen is converted through a complex series of steps to strands of *fibrin*. The fibrin strands form a mesh-work that traps the rest of the cellular components and forms what is recognized as a *blood clot*. This blood-clotting process serves to temporarily obstruct leaking blood vessels and minimize blood loss caused by injury.

Red blood cells (RBCs), also called *erythrocytes,* are the most numerous of the blood cells, typically numbering in the millions per microliter of blood. In mammalian species, RBCs do not normally contain a nucleus and are shaped like biconcave discs resembling tiny pillows. In birds, reptiles, and fish, they are normally nucleated and elliptic. The protein hemoglobin, which gives erythrocytes their red color, also gives them the ability to carry large amounts of O_2 to the body's cells.

White blood cells (WBCs), also called *leukocytes,* typically number in the tens of thousands per microliter of blood. They are divided into *granulocytes (neutrophils, eosinophils,* and *basophils)* and *agranulocytes (lymphocytes* and *monocytes).* Granulocytes have stainable granules in their cytoplasm; agranulocytes lack cytoplasmic granules.

Platelets are not whole cells, but are fragments of cytoplasm from large cells (*megakaryocytes)* in the bone marrow. Their function is to help minimize blood loss from damaged blood vessels by adhering to the injured area and initiating the blood clotting process.

Fetal circulation

A fetus developing in the uterus leads a parasitic existence. It derives all of its nutrition and O_2 from the mother's blood and sends its metabolic wastes and CO_2 back to the mother's blood for elimination. The *placenta* is the life support system of the fetus that makes this possible. The fetus is connected to the placenta by the umbilical cord. The placenta surrounds the fetus and attaches to the wall of the uterus so that placental and maternal blood vessels are in close proximity to each other. There is normally no direct mixing of fetal and maternal blood.

The umbilical vein carries nutrient-rich, freshly oxygenated blood from the placenta to the fetus. The fetal heart then pumps the blood throughout the developing fetus, where the blood releases its nutrients and O_2 and picks up wastes and CO_2. The umbilical arteries return this waste-filled blood to the placenta, where it exchanges its wastes for nutrients and O_2.

Because the fetal lungs are essentially nonfunctional until birth, the fetal blood vascular system has two major modifications that divert most of the blood away from the lungs. The *foramen ovale* is a hole in the interatrial septum of the heart, the wall between the left and right atria. This foramen allows some of the blood returning from the systemic circulation to flow from the right atrium directly into the left atrium, bypassing the lungs. The *ductus arteriosus* connects the pulmonary artery with the aorta. Most of the blood pumped out of the right ventricle flows through the ductus arteriosus into the aorta, and into the system circulation, again bypassing the lungs. The developing lungs need only a

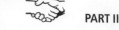

small amount of blood flow to meet their metabolic needs. At or soon after birth, both the foramen ovale and ductus arteriosus close in response to the sudden pressure changes created by the functioning lungs. *Patent ductus arteriosus* (PDA) is a common congenital abnormality in dogs, when the ductus arteriosus fails to close and persists even after birth. In dogs, another vessel called the *ductus venosus* connects the portal sinus to the posterior vena cava, diverting the blood away from the liver until birth. Its lumen is obliterated after birth forming the *ligamentum venosum*. If this duct persists after birth, it creates a *porto-systemic shunt*.

Lymphatic Vascular System

The lymphatic vascular system basically serves to return excess tissue fluid to the blood vascular system. Along the way it filters the tissue fluid, examines it for foreign invaders, and manufactures defensive cells and antibodies to help keep the body healthy.

At the blood capillary level, more fluid flows out of the porous capillaries than returns to them. If not somehow removed, this excess fluid would accumulate in body tissues and cause progressive swelling. Lymph capillaries begin peripherally as blind-ended vessels that pick up this excess fluid, called *lymph*, and move it toward the thorax. The small lymph vessels merge to form larger vessels. These larger lymph channels contain small one-way valves, similar to the valves in veins. Combined with body movements, these one-way valves help propel the lymph to the thorax, where it is deposited back into the bloodstream.

Along the network of lymph vessels are small lumps of tissue called *lymph nodes*. These contain large accumulations of one type of white blood cell, lymphocytes, organized into collections called *lymph nodules*. The lymph nodes filter the lymph, removing debris and foreign invaders, and produce antibody-producing cells that are important components of the body's defense mechanisms.

Lymph nodules are also found in areas of the body other than lymph nodes. The spleen, a large, tongue-shaped organ located near the stomach, is a blood-storage organ, but it also contains large accumulations of lymph nodules. The thymus is a lymphoid organ, located in the caudal cervical/cranial thoracic region. It is of importance primarily in young animals. It helps "jumpstart" the immune system and then gradually shrinks and disappears around the time of sexual maturity. Accumulations of lymph nodules are also found in the tonsils and scattered in the lining of the intestines.

RESPIRATORY SYSTEM

The primary function of the respiratory system is to exchange O_2 in oxygenated blood for CO_2, which is produced as a waste product by the cells. Secondary functions include vocalization (e.g., barking, mooing), body temperature regulation, and acid-base regulation.

Respiration occurs at two levels in the body. Internal respiration involves gas exchange between the blood and the body's many cells and tissues, and it occurs at the cellular level throughout the body. Oxygen (O_2) carried in RBCs is exchanged for carbon dioxide (CO_2) produced by tissue cells. External respiration involves exchange of gases between blood and the outside air, and it occurs in the lungs. Carbon dioxide in the blood is exchanged for O_2 from the air.

The respiratory system is composed of the upper respiratory tract, which consists of a series of tubes that connect the lungs with the external environment, and the lower respiratory tract, which consists of structures within the lungs.

Upper Respiratory Tract

The upper respiratory tract starts at the tip of the nose. Inhaled air enters the nostrils and passes back through the nasal passages. The lining of the nasal passages contains extensive networks of blood vessels, and a ciliated epithelium that is coated with watery mucus. Blood circulating throughout the nasal lining warms the incoming air, the watery mucus humidifies it, and the cilia sweep foreign material that has become trapped in the mucus out of the nasal passages. These functions form a conditioning system that supplies the lungs with relatively pure, warm, humidified air.

From the nasal passages, inhaled air passes through the *pharynx*, or throat. This is a common passageway for both the digestive and respiratory systems. Through a series of intricate reflexes, the pharynx and larynx help prevent swallowed material from entering the lower respiratory tract.

The *larynx*, commonly called the "voice box," is a short, irregular tube of cartilage and muscle that connects the pharynx with the trachea. In addition to its voice-producing function, it also acts as a valve to control airflow to and from the lungs. At the junction of the pharynx and the larynx is the *epiglottis*, a flap of cartilage that acts as a "trap door" to cover the opening of the larynx during swallowing.

Carrying air from the larynx to the lungs is the *trachea*, or "windpipe." The trachea is composed of several C-shaped incomplete rings of hyaline cartilage, which prevent it from collapsing during inhalation. At its caudal end, the trachea divides into the left and right bronchi, which enter the lungs.

Lower Respiratory Tract

The bronchi enter the lungs and branch into smaller and smaller air passageways that eventually lead to tiny grapelike clusters of thin cells called *alveoli*. The alveolus is the actual site of gas exchange in the lungs. Each alveolus consists of a tiny, extremely thin-walled sac surrounded by elastic fibers and a network of capillaries.

Respiratory Mechanisms

The process of external respiration depends on physical mechanisms that allow air to move in and out of the lungs and control systems that set limits on and adjust the process.

Thorax

The area referred to as the *thorax* is located between the neck and the diaphragm. Normally there is negative pressure (partial vacuum) in the *thorax*. Combined with the elasticity and pliable nature of the lungs, this causes the lungs to conform to the size and shape of the thoracic cavity. A small amount of pleural fluid lubricates the lung surfaces and the thoracic (pleural) lining. A puncturing wound or gunshot in the thoracic cavity can deteriorate the negative pressure leading to collapse of the lungs.

Inspiration

Inspiration on inhaling is the process of drawing air into the lungs. It is accomplished by contractions of diaphragm and other muscles. The diaphragm is a dome-shaped sheet-like muscle that completely separates the thoracic cavity from the abdominal cavity. The contraction of diaphragm pushes the abdominal organs down and increases the volume of the thoracic cavity. The lungs expand passively as the thoracic cavity enlarges, and air is drawn into them through the upper respiratory passages.

Exchange of gases

Air that is drawn into the alveoli during inspiration contains high levels of O_2 and low levels of CO_2. Blood passing through the capillary networks around the alveoli contains low levels of O_2 and high levels of CO_2. Both gases move from areas of high concentration to areas of low concentration by a process called *diffusion*. Oxygen diffuses from the alveoli to the blood in the alveolar capillaries. Carbon dioxide diffuses in the other direction (from the blood of the alveolar capillaries to the alveoli).

Expiration

Air rich with carbon dioxide from the alveoli must be eliminated from the lungs so that a fresh breath of O_2-rich air can be inspired. Expiration occurs as muscular contractions compress the thoracic cavity and elastic lung tissue comes back to its original shape, expelling air from the lungs.

Control of breathing

Two systems control the process of respiration: a mechanical control system and a chemical control system. The mechanical control system sets normal limits on inspiration and expiration to allow rhythmic, resting respiration. The inspiratory center in the brain initiates impulses at regular intervals. These impulses travel to the diaphragm, allowing it to contract and the lungs to inflate. Stretch receptors in the lungs sense when the preset limit of inflation has been reached. They initiate impulses that travel to the respiratory centers in the brain, stopping inspiration and starting passive expiration. The chemical control system monitors the chemical composition of the blood. If it senses fluctuations in O_2 and CO_2 levels or pH, it initiates adjustments in respiration necessary to restore normal values.

DIGESTIVE SYSTEM

The digestive or alimentary system converts food eaten by an animal into nutrient compounds that body cells can use for metabolic fuel. The digestive system consists of a tube running from the mouth to the anus, with accessory digestive organs attached to it. Food moving through the tube is broken down into smaller, simpler compounds through the process of digestion. These simple compounds then pass through the wall of the digestive tract into the bloodstream through the process of absorption for distribution of nutrients to body cells.

The structure of a species' digestive system is largely dependent on its diet. Nutrients in the plant-matter diet of herbivores, such as horses and cattle, are largely incorporated within hard-to-digest cellulose. Herbivores depend on the help of microorganisms, such as protozoa and bacteria, to help break down cellulose through a process called *microbial fermentation*. At some point in their digestive tract, herbivores have a large "fermentation vat," where cellulose can be broken down into usable nutrients. In cattle this is the *rumen*, and in horses it is the much-enlarged *cecum*, part of the large intestine. The digestive system of carnivores (meat eaters), such as dogs and cats, is much simpler. Carnivores depend on enzymes to break down easy-to-digest animal-source nutrients through the process of enzymatic digestion. Therefore, no large fermentation vat is needed. Omnivores (species eating a mixed diet), such as pigs, are somewhat intermediate. They depend primarily on enzymatic digestion, with a minor amount of microbial fermentation occurring in their large intestine.

Mouth

The mouth is where food is chewed and mixed with saliva in preparation for swallowing. Four types of teeth, arranged into upper and lower dental arcades, begin the process of digestion by cutting and crushing the food. The most rostral teeth are the *incisors* (I). Ruminants, such as cattle and sheep, do not have upper incisors. They have a firm, fibrous "dental pad" instead. The four *canines* (C), if present, are located at the rostral lateral corners of the mouth, adjacent to the incisors. The *premolars* (PM) are the rostral cheek teeth, and the *molars* (M) are the caudal cheek teeth.

Each tooth is composed of three different kinds of very firm connective tissue. The exposed portion, the *crown*, is

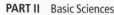
covered by *enamel*, the hardest substance in the body. The bulk of the tooth is composed of a dense material called *dentin*. The root, which helps anchor the tooth in its bony socket, is covered by *cementum*. The fibers that connect the cementum to the bony socket are called *periodontal ligaments*. *Periodontitis* is the inflammation of these ligaments from accumulation of plaque and bacterial toxins in gum pockets. It is the most common tooth problem in dogs and cats over 5 years of age.

Dental formula

A dental formula places the teeth in the upper arcade in the numerator position and the teeth in the lower arcade in the denominator position. To determine the number of teeth in the entire mouth, multiply by 2. See the following box.

Dog:	2 (I 3/3, C 1/1, PM 4/4, M 2/3) = 42
Cat:	2 (I 3/3, C 1/1, PM 3/2, M 1/1) = 30
Cow:	2 (I 0/4, C 0/0, PM 3/3, M 3/3) = 32
Horse:	2 (I 3/3, C 1/1, PM 3/4, M 3/3) = 40

Once the food has been chopped and ground by the teeth and moistened with saliva, it is swallowed. Muscular movements of the tongue and pharynx move the bolus of food back through the pharynx to the opening of the esophagus, where it begins its journey to the stomach and through the remainder of the digestive tract.

Esophagus

The *esophagus* is a muscular tube that connects the pharynx with the stomach. Food passes through it quickly on its way to the stomach; no significant digestion or absorption occurs in the esophagus. The size of the opening of the esophagus into the stomach is regulated by the *cardiac sphincter*. This muscular ring functions as a valve to seal the esophagus off from the stomach. In the normal digestive process, the cardiac sphincter opens only to allow swallowed food to pass into the stomach. It also relaxes to allow food to pass back up the esophagus in species that can vomit or ruminate.

Stomach

The stomach is an enlarged chamber where swallowed food is mixed with hydrochloric acid and digestive enzymes. In simple-stomached animals, such as horses and dogs, significant digestion of food begins in the stomach (Fig. 6-4). In animals with ruminant forestomachs, such as cattle and sheep, microbial fermentation begins before the material reaches the true stomach (abomasum).

Simple stomach

The simple stomach of monogastric animals is a single chamber lined with large folds, the rugae, and dense accumulations of gastric glands. The gastric glands secrete hydrochloric acid and various digestive enzymes, which begin the digestion process, and mucus, which coats the stomach lining and keeps it from being digested along with the food. Very little absorption of nutrients occurs in the stomach. The stomach serves mainly to mix the food with the acid and enzymes to begin digestion. By the time the food leaves the stomach through the pyloric sphincter to enter the small intestines, it has been converted into a semiliquid, homogeneous material called *chyme*.

Ruminant stomach

The ruminant stomach has four compartments: *rumen, reticulum, omasum,* and *abomasum*. The last chamber (abomasum) is called "true stomach" because it is the chamber in which most enzymes are produced. Food swallowed by ruminants passes through three chambers before it gets to the true stomach. These chambers are called the *forestomachs* (Fig. 6-4).

The esophagus opens into the largest forestomach, the *rumen*. This compartment makes up about 80% of the total stomach volume of ruminants and almost completely fills the left side of the abdominal cavity. Its main function is microbial fermentation. It is the main chamber where microorganisms break down the swallowed foods into simpler substances for absorption. Some breakdown products are absorbed into the bloodstream directly through the wall of the rumen, but the majority of nutrient absorption takes place in the intestines.

The *reticulum* is the smallest, most cranial forestomach (Fig. 6-4). It makes up about 5% of the total stomach volume of ruminants and lies against the diaphragm. Its opening is positioned directly ventral to the esophageal opening. Any heavy foreign material that is swallowed by the animal, such as wire, nails, or screws, usually drops directly into the reticulum. The honeycomb-like folds that line it serve to trap foreign material that enters the reticulum. This can irritate the reticular lining, and lead to traumatic reticulitis, commonly called "hardware disease." Normally the reticulum acts as a small fermentation vat also. Its food contents can move freely to and from the rumen.

The *omasum* is a dehydrating, grinding vat that makes up about 7% of the total stomach volume of ruminants. Positioned between the reticulum and the abomasum on the animal's right side, the omasum is lined by large muscular folds. Material entering the omasum from the reticulum has a very fluid consistency. Much of this fluid is absorbed from the omasum, and the muscular folds serve to further grind the food particles.

From the omasum, food enters the true stomach of the ruminant, the *abomasum*. Making up about 8% of the total stomach volume, the abomasum lies ventral to the omasum on the animal's right side. It corresponds to the simple stomach of a monogastric animal and has the same functions.

The stomach of a ruminant functions differently from the stomach of a monogastric animal. When ruminants graze, they swallow food that has received only a cursory

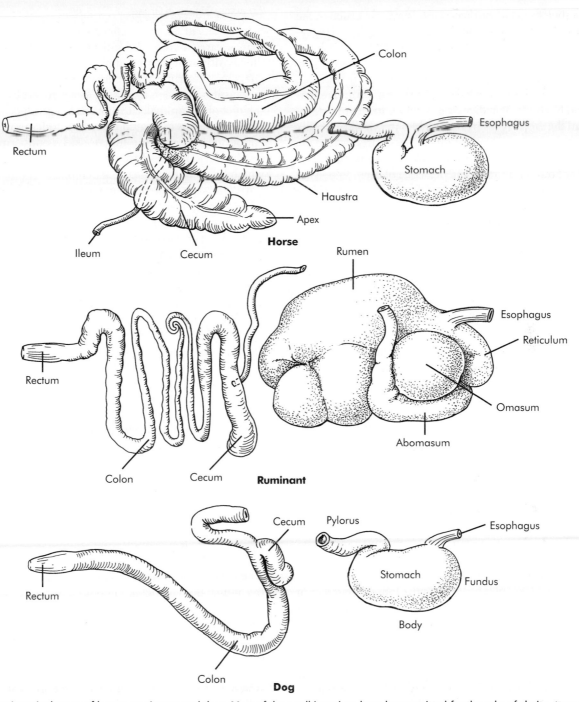

Fig. 6-4 Gastrointestinal tracts of horses, ruminants, and dogs. Most of the small intestines have been omitted for the sake of clarity. *(From McBride DF: Learning veterinary terminology, St Louis, 2001, Mosby.)*

chewing. In the rumen, this coarse material floats on top of the finer material. Once grazing is completed, the coarse material is periodically regurgitated back up into the mouth, mixed with saliva, chewed thoroughly, and reswallowed. This process, called *rumination*, occurs in about 1-minute cycles and is commonly referred to as "chewing the cud." The reswallowed material is then more finely ground and sinks into the ventral portions of the rumen, where microorganisms proceed with fermentation. In addition to releasing nutrients, the microbial action produces large quantities of gases, such as methane. These gases must be eliminated by the animal through a process called *eructation* (belching). If this gas is not regularly eructed, the rumen becomes distended with gas, resulting in a dangerous condition called *rumenal tympany*, or bloat.

Newborn ruminants, such as calves and lambs, essentially function as monogastric animals while they are nursing. Fermentation of the swallowed milk in the rumen and reticulum would likely result in digestive upsets. Closure of a structure called the esophageal groove enables the swallowed milk to bypass the rumen and reticulum, and pass directly into the omasum and abomasum. Closure of the groove is stimulated by the act of nursing, and by the presence of milk. When the maturing animal begins eating solid foods, the groove does not close, and the swallowed food enters the rumen and reticulum for microbial fermentation, as in adult animals.

Intestine

After leaving the stomach, chyme enters the tubelike intestine. Moved along by muscular contractions, the chyme is further digested by mixing with secretions from the pancreas, liver, and glands in the intestinal wall. Most absorption of nutrients takes place in the intestines. The large surface area of the intestinal lining aids nutrient absorption. Countless tiny, fingerlike processes called *villi* cover the lining. Each villus contains tiny blood and lymph vessels at its center, into which nutrients are absorbed through the simple columnar epithelial covering.

The first portion of the intestine is the small intestine, so named because of its relatively small diameter. It has three segments: the *duodenum, jejunum,* and *ileum.* (Note the similarity in name, but difference in spelling, to one of the pelvic bones, the ilium.)

The *duodenum* is the first, relatively short segment of the small intestine. It receives the chyme through the stomach's pyloric valve. Ducts carrying bile from the liver and digestive enzymes from the pancreas enter the small intestine lumen (interior).

The next segment, the *jejunum,* is the longest segment of the small intestine. This is where the majority of nutrient absorption takes place. The ileum is the last, relatively short segment of small intestine. It leads to the large intestine.

The large-diameter large intestine receives undigested and unabsorbed food material from the *ileum.* It absorbs water from the chyme and absorbs any nutrients not previously absorbed by the small intestine. The first segment of the large intestine is the *cecum* (Fig. 6-4). This blind-ended sac is small in carnivores, such as dogs, and very large in monogastric herbivores, such as horses. Next is the longest segment of the large intestine, the *colon* (Fig. 6-4). The final intestinal segment is the rectum, which carries its contents, called *feces,* to the anus for discharge from the body or *defecation.*

The *anus* is the caudal opening of the digestive system to the outside world. It is surrounded by ringlike sphincter muscles that allow the animal to consciously control defecation.

Accessory Digestive Organs

Several sets of *salivary glands* produce saliva, a watery fluid that is carried from the salivary glands to the mouth by ducts. Although saliva contains small amounts of digestive enzymes, its primary function is to moisten and lubricate food as it is chewed, making it easier to swallow. The drier the diet of the animal, the more saliva produced.

The *pancreas* is located near the duodenum and has both endocrine and exocrine functions. Its endocrine functions involve production of two hormones, *insulin* and *glucagon,* which help control glucose metabolism in the body. These hormones are discussed later with the endocrine system. The exocrine secretion of the pancreas, called *pancreatic juice,* is involved with digestion. Pancreatic juice is carried to the duodenum through the pancreatic duct(s). The main components of pancreatic juice are sodium bicarbonate, which helps neutralize the very acidic chyme entering the duodenum from the stomach, and a variety of digestive enzymes.

Located just caudal to the diaphragm, the *liver* is the largest gland in the body. Three important functions of liver are detoxification, storage, and modification of nutrients. It is an important "factory" that assembles simple nutrient molecules into larger compounds that can be used by the body's cells. The portal vein, which carries nutrient-rich blood from the intestines directly to the liver, supplies the raw materials for the factory. The liver also secretes bile, a greenish fluid that carries waste products of hemoglobin metabolism out of the body, and aids in breakdown and absorption of fats and fat-soluble vitamins from the intestine.

NERVOUS SYSTEM

The nervous system is a complex communication system in the animal body. It detects and processes internal and external information and formulates appropriate responses to changes, threats, and opportunities that the animal continually faces. Nearly all conscious and unconscious functions of the body are controlled or influenced by the nervous system.

The basic structural and functional unit of the nervous system is the nerve cell, the *neuron.* Neurons are specialized cells that respond to stimuli and conduct impulses from one part of a cell to another. Two types of fiberlike processes extend from the cell bodies of neurons: *dendrites* and *axons.* Dendrites are often multiple, and they conduct impulses received from other neurons toward the nerve cell body. Axons are usually single, and they conduct impulses away from the cell body, to other neurons or the effector organs, such as muscle cells. The junction of an axon with another nerve cell is called a *synapse.*

The branched end of an axon is called the *telodendron.* When a nerve impulse reaches the telodendron, it causes release of tiny sacs of chemicals called *neurotransmitters* into the narrow synaptic space. When neurotransmitter molecules diffuse across the synapse to contact the cell membrane of the adjacent nerve cell, they induce a change in the other nerve cell. Enzymes in the synaptic space then quickly inactivate the neurotransmitter molecules.

Neurons have three unique physical characteristics: they do not reproduce, their processes are capable of limited regeneration if damaged, and they have an extremely high oxygen requirement. Their lack of reproductive ability means that any loss of neurons, as from disease or injury, is permanent. Their dendritic and axonic processes sometimes regenerate if the nerve cell body is intact; this may restore function of reattached digits or limbs under some circumstances.

The high oxygen requirement of neurons makes them among the most delicate cells in the body. They begin to suffer permanent damage if deprived of blood supply for more than a few minutes. This is why cardiopulmonary resuscitation must begin within just a few minutes after cardiac arrest if there is to be any chance of complete recovery. The main divisions of the nervous system are the *central nervous system*, the *peripheral nervous system*, and the *autonomic nervous system*.

Central Nervous System

The central nervous system consists of accumulations of nerve cell bodies, nerve fibers (axons), and supporting cells in the brain and spinal cord. The brain, consisting of the *cerebrum*, *cerebellum*, and *brain stem*, is housed in the skull (Fig. 6-5). The spinal cord is housed in the vertebral canal formed by the vertebrae. Together they form the main control systems for the rest of the body.

Cross-sections of the brain and spinal cord reveal two distinctly different-colored areas: the gray matter and the white matter. Areas containing accumulations of nerve cell bodies appear grayish and make up the gray matter. Areas containing large accumulations of nerve fibers appear pale and make up the white matter.

The cerebrum is the largest, most rostral part of the brain (Fig. 6-5). It consists of two large lateral cerebral hemispheres separated by a deep cleft. Its surface area is increased by systems of folds termed the *gyri* and grooves termed the *sulci*. The cerebral cortex, or outer layer of the cerebrum, consists of gray matter. The medulla, or inner portion of the cerebrum, consists of white matter. The functions of the cerebrum are very complex and poorly understood. It is the center of higher learning and intelligence, and it functions in perception, maintenance of consciousness, thinking and reasoning, and initiating responses to sensory stimuli.

The cerebellum is located just caudal to the cerebrum (Fig. 6-5). Its surface folds are small and packed closely together, giving it a wrinkled appearance. As in the cerebrum, the cerebellar cortex is composed of gray matter and its inner medulla is composed of white matter. The cerebellum does not initiate movements but serves to coordinate, adjust, and generally fine-tune movements directed by the cerebrum.

The brain stem is the most primitive part of the brain (Fig. 6-5). It forms the stem to which the cerebrum,

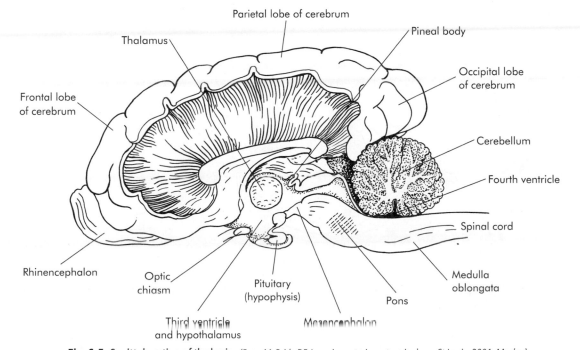

Fig. 6-5 Sagittal section of the brain. *(From McBride DF: Learning veterinary terminology, St Louis, 2001, Mosby.)*

cerebellum, and spinal cord are attached. Color distinctions between gray and white matter are difficult to observe in the brain stem. Functionally, the brain stem maintains the vital functions of the body. Centers in the brain stem control respiration, body temperature, heart rate, gastrointestinal tract function, blood pressure, appetite, thirst, and sleep/wake cycles. Severe damage to vital centers in the brain stem usually results in immediate death.

The spinal cord is the caudal continuation of the brain stem. On cross-section, the gray matter forms a butterfly-shaped area in the central area of the spinal cord (Fig. 6-6). The white matter forms the outer cortex. Spinal nerves exit and enter the spinal cord between each set of adjacent vertebrae. They carry information to and from the peripheral portion of the nervous system.

Peripheral Nervous System

The peripheral nervous system consists of cordlike nerves that run throughout the body. The nerves are actually bundles of axons that carry impulses between the central nervous system and the rest of the body. Nerves that carry only information toward the central nervous system are called *sensory nerves*. Those that carry only instructions from the central nervous system out to the body are called *motor nerves*. Most nerves are *mixed nerves*, a combination of both sensory and motor nerves. The peripheral nervous system includes *cranial nerves* and *spinal nerves*.

Spinal nerves

Spinal nerves originate as two roots, the dorsal root and the ventral root, on either side of the spinal cord. These two roots combine together to form spinal nerve proper. The spinal nerves mainly innervate the striated muscles. Some spinal nerves also carry nerve fibers of sympathetic and parasympathetic fibers, which innervate smooth muscle fibers (organs). Spinal nerves from the thoracic and lumber regions of the spinal cord carry sympathetic nerve fibers. Spinal nerves from the sacral region carry parasympathetic nerve fibers.

Cranial nerves

There are twelve pairs of cranial nerves mainly arising from the ventral surface of the brain. The cranial nerves are designated both by their names and numbers (Roman numerals). For example, the first cranial nerve is called the olfactory (I) nerve, while second cranial nerve is called the optic (II) nerve. Cranial nerves usually innervate to the structures in the head and neck area. The exception is the vagus (X) nerve, which is the longest cranial nerve that innervates many organs of the body.

Autonomic Nervous System

The autonomic nervous system is the "self-governing" portion of the nervous system. It operates independent of conscious thought to maintain *homeostasis*, a constant internal

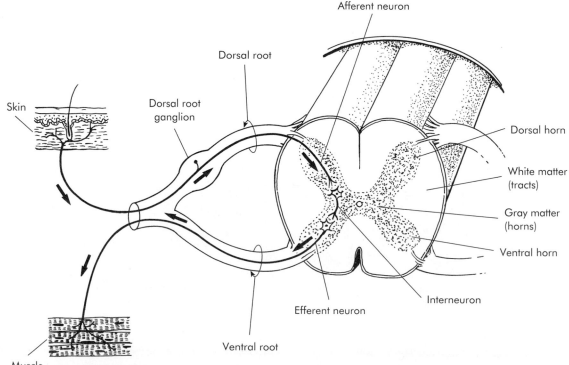

Fig. 6-6 Cross-section of the spinal cord, showing a reflex arc. *(From McBride DF:* Learning veterinary terminology, *St Louis, 2001, Mosby.)*

environment in the body. Primarily a motor system, the autonomic nervous system consists of two parts, the *sympathetic system* and the *parasympathetic system*, which have opposite effects and are in constant balance with each other.

The sympathetic system produces the "fight or flight" reaction in response to real or perceived threats. In a time of crisis or physical threat, the heart rate and blood pressure increase, the air passageways in the lungs and the pupils of the eyes dilate, digestive tract activity decreases, and the hairs stand on end, producing "raised hackles." The net effect is to prepare the body for intense physical exertion and to make the animal look larger and more threatening.

The parasympathetic system has the opposite effect. It is the "rest and restore" system. It predominates during relaxed, routine, business-as-usual states. The heart rate and blood pressure decrease, the air passageways in the lung and the pupils of the eyes constrict, and digestive tract activity increases. The net effect is to allow the body to relax and rejuvenate itself.

MUSCULAR SYSTEM

The general function of muscle is to move the body, both internally and externally. The nervous system gives the orders, and the muscular system is among the most important systems that carry them out. There are three distinctly different kinds of muscle in the body: *skeletal muscle, cardiac muscle,* and *smooth muscle*. All these muscles have the property to contract and relax, which help them to perform various functions.

Skeletal Muscle

Skeletal muscle derives its name from the fact that it moves the skeleton. It is also known as *voluntary striated muscle* because it is under conscious control, and its cells, at the microscopic level, have a striped or striated appearance.

Skeletal muscle cells (*myocytes*) are shaped like long cylinders or fibers. These very large cells usually have multiple nuclei. Most of their mass is composed of smaller myofibrils composed of smaller protein filaments. The net effect is an intricate arrangement of filaments that can slide over each other, shortening the muscle cell when it contracts.

Skeletal muscle fibers respond to impulses delivered by nerves. The "connection" of a nerve fiber with a skeletal muscle fiber is called the *neuromuscular junction*. Each nerve fiber supplies more than one muscle fiber. A motor unit is composed of a nerve fiber and all of the muscle fibers it supplies. If there is a small number of muscle fibers per nerve fiber, fine, delicate movements are possible. The muscles that move the eyeball fall into this category. On the other hand, muscles that must make very large, powerful movements, such as the leg muscles, have a large number of muscle fibers supplied by each nerve fiber.

Skeletal muscles are usually attached to bones at both ends by tendons. The more stable of the muscle's attachments is called its *origin*. The more movable of the attachments is called the *insertion*.

Cardiac Muscle

Cardiac muscle is found only in the heart. It is also known as involuntary striated muscle because it is not under conscious control and its cells are striped, or striated.

Cardiac muscle cells have no characteristic shape. Rather, they form an intricate branching network in the heart. They are firmly attached to each other, which allows considerable force to be generated as they contract.

Cardiac muscle cells each have an innate contractile rhythm that does not require an external nerve supply. The rhythmic contractions of the heart chambers are coordinated by a system of specialized cardiac muscle cells. The heart does have an autonomic nerve supply, but it does not initiate contractions of the muscle cells: it serves to modify them. Sympathetic stimulation increases the rate and force of cardiac muscle contractions. This is part of the fight or flight response. Parasympathetic stimulation has the opposite effect; it decreases the rate and force of contraction. Through this autonomic stimulation, the rate and force of cardiac contractions can be adjusted according to the body's needs.

Smooth Muscle

Smooth muscle is found mainly in internal organs. It is called "smooth" because its cells do not show any stripes or striations under magnification. It is involuntary muscle because it is not under conscious control.

Cells of smooth muscle are spindle-shaped, being wide in the middle and tapered at the ends. Depending on their location, they may be short and thick or long and fiberlike. Two types of smooth muscle are found in the body: *visceral* smooth muscle, found in hollow abdominal organs, and *multiunit* smooth muscle, found where fine contractions are needed.

Visceral smooth muscle occurs in large sheets in the walls of the gastrointestinal tract, uterus, and urinary bladder. These muscle cells are linked, so entire areas of cells act as a large unit. Nerve supply is autonomic and serves mainly to modify contractions. Sympathetic stimulation (fight or flight) decreases activity, whereas parasympathetic stimulation (rest, rejuvenation) increases it.

Multiunit smooth muscle consists of individual muscle units that each require specific nerve stimulation to contract. Unlike visceral smooth muscle cells, these muscle cells are not linked, so their contractions are localized and discrete. Multiunit smooth muscle is found where fine, though involuntary, movements are needed, such as in the iris and ciliary body of the eye, the walls of blood vessels, and the walls of tiny air passageways in the lungs.

SENSES

The senses are the means by which the body monitors its internal and external environment. Sensory receptors are specialized nerve endings that convert mechanical, thermal, electromagnetic, and chemical stimuli from the environment into nervous impulses. When sensory impulses reach the central nervous system, they are perceived as such sensations as smell, taste, or sight.

Various sensations are received and interpreted by the central nervous system. The five senses we usually think of (hearing, smell, taste, touch, and sight) are not the only sensations perceived by the central nervous system. For our purposes, nine sets of sensations will be discussed. They are the following:

General Senses
Tactile sense
Temperature sense
Kinesthetic sense
Pain sense
Special Senses
Gustatory sense
Olfactory sense
Auditory sense
Vestibular sense
Visual sense

General Senses

The *general senses* are so named because they are distributed generally throughout the body or over the entire skin surface. Their receptors are fairly simple modified nerve endings. The tactile sense, or the sense of touch, perceives mechanical contact with the surface of the body. The temperature sense is a thermal sense that perceives hot and cold. The position of the limbs is monitored by the kinesthetic sense, a mechanical sense that provides information on the position of joints and the relative force exerted by muscles and tendons. The sense of pain can be set off by overloads of mechanical, thermal, or chemical stimuli.

Special Senses

The *special senses* are so named because their sensory receptors are concentrated in certain areas, rather than being generally distributed. All receptors for the special senses are located in the head. Also, in several cases, the sensory receptor cells are aided by sophisticated accessory structures.

Gustatory sense

The *gustatory sense*, the sense of taste, is a chemical sense. It detects chemical substances in the mouth and dissolved in saliva. The receptor cells are located in tiny taste buds found mainly on the tongue. Each taste bud has an opening on its surface, the *taste pore*. Hairlike microvilli from the receptor cells project into the taste pore. When dissolved chemical substances enter the taste pore, their molecules interact with the microvilli, generating impulses that travel to the brain and are interpreted as various tastes.

Olfactory sense

The olfactory sense, the sense of smell, is also a chemical sense. It detects chemical substances in inhaled air. The receptor cells are located in the epithelium of the nasal passages. Hairlike microvilli from the olfactory cells project up into the mucous layer that overlies the nasal epithelium. When chemical substances dissolve in the mucus, the microvilli are stimulated and information about odors is transmitted to the brain via the olfactory nerve.

Auditory sense

The auditory sense is the sense of hearing. Through a complex set of auditory passageways and ear structures, mechanical vibrations of air molecules are converted into impulses that the brain decodes as sounds. Sound waves from the environment are collected by the external ear structures, amplified and transmitted through the middle ear structures, and converted to impulses in the inner ear. Most of the ear structures are located in the temporal bones of the skull (Fig. 6-7).

The external ear is composed of the *pinna* (ear flap), *external auditory canal*, and *tympanic membrane* (eardrum). The pinna is a cartilaginous funnel that collects sound waves and directs them medially into the external auditory canal, which leads to the tympanic membrane. The tympanic membrane is a thin, connective tissue membrane that is tightly stretched across the opening into the middle ear. Sound waves cause the membrane to vibrate.

Medial to the tympanic membrane is the air-filled middle ear cavity, which transmits vibrations of the tympanic membrane to the inner ear via three tiny bones called *ossicles*. The first bone, the *malleus*, is attached to the medial surface of the tympanic membrane. It forms a tiny joint with the second bone, the *incus*, which forms a joint with the third bone, the *stapes*, which is in contact with the cochlea of the inner ear. Vibrations of the tympanic membrane are transmitted by the ossicles to the inner ear. Air pressure within the middle ear must equilibrate with the atmospheric pressure of the external air to prevent undue bulging of the tympanic membrane. The *eustachian tube*, which links the middle ear with the pharynx, accomplishes this pressure equilibration as the animal swallows.

The inner ear contains three structures: the *cochlea*, *vestibule*, and *semicircular canals*. The cochlea is responsible for the sense of hearing, while the vestibular part and

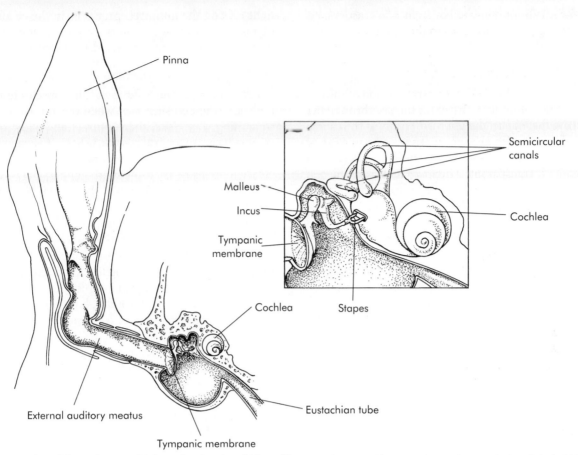

Fig. 6-7 Cross-section of the canine ear, with inset showing the middle and inner ear. *(From McBride DF:* Learning veterinary terminology, *St Louis, 2001, Mosby.)*

semicircular canals help in monitoring balance and head position.

The cochlea is a fluid-filled space shaped like a hollow spiral snail shell. Running along its length, like a ribbon, is the *organ of Corti*, which contains the receptor cells for hearing. When sound wave vibrations are transmitted to the cochlear fluid, the fluid movements distort the microvilli on the receptor cells on the organ of Corti. This generates impulses that are carried to brain via the cochlear nerve.

Vestibular sense

The vestibular sense, also a mechanical sense, monitors balance and head position. Its receptors are contained in two structures of the inner ear: the vestibule and the semicircular canals. Together with the cochlea, these structures make up the inner ear. The vestibule consists of two fluid-filled spaces in each inner ear that contain patches of sensory epithelium on their floor. The sensory cells have hairlike microvilli that project into an overlying coat of gelatinous material. This gelatinous layer contains tiny crystals of calcium carbonate, the *otoliths*. Any tilting or linear motion of

the head causes movement of the otoliths, which distorts the microvilli, generating nervous impulses. These vestibular impulses carry information to the brain about changes in the position and linear motion of the head.

The semicircular canals are three fluid-filled canals of semicircular shape on each side of the head (Fig. 6-7). Parts of the semicircular canals are oriented in different planes, at right angles to each other, much like two walls and a ceiling join at a corner. At one end of each canal are the receptors, which contain sensory cells that are very similar to those of the vestibule. Hairlike microvilli of the sensory cells project into an overlying layer of gelatinous material. Rotation of the head in any plane moves the fluid in a semicircular canal and stimulates its sensory cells. The resulting impulses carry information to the brain about rotary motion of the head.

Visual sense

The visual sense (sight) is the only well-developed electromagnetic sense of mammals. Its receptor organ, the eye, has a complex organization of component parts that function together to gather and focus light rays on photoreceptor cells (Fig. 6-8). When stimulated by light, the sensory cells of the inner eye generate impulses to the brain through the optic nerve. The brain interprets these impulses as light.

The outer covering of the eyeball or globe is a dense fibrous connective tissue layer that supports it and gives it shape. The clear "window" on the rostral portion of the eye is the *cornea* (Fig. 6-8). Light rays enter the eye through the cornea and are focused on the photoreceptors at the caudal portion of the eye. Although the cornea is composed of fibrous connective tissue, it normally contains just enough water to render it transparent. The *sclera* makes up the rest of the fibrous outer layer of the globe. Because of its white color, the sclera is commonly referred to as the "white" of the eye.

Caudal to the cornea is the fluid-filled space called the *anterior chamber*, and the colored *iris* (Fig. 6-8). The watery fluid that fills the anterior chamber is called *aqueous humor* and is produced by cells caudal to the iris. The iris is a muscular diaphragm that controls the size of the aperture at its center, the pupil. In bright light, the parasympathetic system stimulates the iris to contract, reducing the size of the pupil to protect the sensitive photoreceptor cells. In dim light, the sympathetic innervation relaxes the iris muscles, enlarging the pupil to allow more light to enter.

Caudal to the iris is a transparent, biconvex, elastic, crystalline structure called the *lens* (Fig. 6-8). The lens is responsible for the process of accommodation, focusing the light rays on the photoreceptor cells in the caudal portion of the eye to allow for near and far vision. Around its periphery, the lens is connected to the *ciliary body* by tiny suspensory ligaments. The ciliary body contains the muscles responsible for changing the shape of the lens as required to focus the light rays. The muscles in the ciliary body are oriented such that when the animal is looking at something very close, they contract and allow the lens to assume its more natural rounded shape, focusing the close-up image on the photoreceptors. For distant objects, the ciliary muscles relax, allowing the globe's natural elasticity to pull the lens into a flattened shape more appropriate for distant vision.

The area caudal to the lens is filled with a transparent, gelatinous substance called the *vitreous humor* (Fig. 6-8). The light rays pass through this substance on their way to the photoreceptor-containing layer, the retina.

The retina is where visual images are formed. It is a complex, multilayered structure that lines most of the interior of the eye caudal to the lens. It is composed of photoreceptor cells termed *rods* and *cones*, and several layers of nerve cell bodies and synapses that integrate and relay information from the receptor cells to the brain. The rods and cones have different shapes and different functions. The rods are long and narrow, and are more sensitive to light than the cones. They do not, however, detect colors or detail well. They are the receptors for dim light vision. The

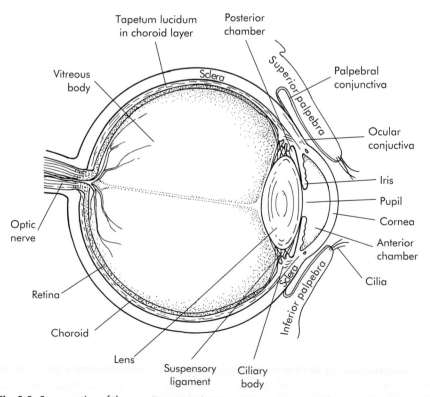

Fig. 6-8 Cross-section of the eye. *(From McBride DF:* Learning veterinary terminology, *St Louis, 2001, Mosby.)*

cones are somewhat flask-shaped, and detect detail and colors well. The area of the retina where nerve fibers converge to form the optic nerve is called the *optic disc*. No rods or cones are present there; it is the "blind spot" of the eye.

The eye is a very sensitive organ that is protected by accessory structures. These include the *conjunctiva*, the *eyelids*, and the *lacrimal apparatus*.

The conjunctiva is a thin membrane that lines the underside of the eyelids and covers the outer aspect of the eyeball. Its transparency allows the sclera of the globe and the blood vessels of the eyelids to show through. Examination of the conjunctiva can easily detect abnormalities such as anemia or jaundice.

The eyelids are dorsal (upper) and ventral (lower) folds of skin lined by conjunctiva that cover and protect the eye when the animal blinks or sleeps. The medial and lateral junctions of the eyelids are the *medial canthus* and *lateral canthus* of the eye, respectively. The third eyelid, or membrana nictitans, is a plate of cartilage covered by conjunctiva located medially between the eyelids and the eyeball. The clinical problems related to eyelids include inversion (lids roll in) and eversion (lids roll out).

The lacrimal apparatus is concerned with production and drainage of tears from the surface of the eye. The lacrimal glands, which produce tears, are located dorsal to the lateral canthus of the eye. Tears flow down over the surface of the eye, aided by blinking movements of the eyelids. At the medial canthus of the eye are the lacrimal puncta, two small openings, one in the upper lid margin and one in the lower lid margin, that drain tears from the eye. From the lacrimal puncta, the tears drain into the lacrimal sac and then the nasolacrimal duct, which carries the tears into the nasal cavity. The ducts may become blocked due to swelling and mucus accumulation, leading to an overflow of tears. The fluorescein dye test is performed to detect blockage in the naso-lacrimal duct and coreal abrasions or ulcers. The overflow of tears may also be result of overproduction of tears by lacrimal glands. The Schirmer's tear test is done to detect the overproduction of tears by the lacrimal gland.

ENDOCRINE SYSTEM

The endocrine system consists of glands in various parts of the body that secrete minute amounts of chemical substances called *hormones* directly into the bloodstream, rather than through ducts. These hormones circulate throughout the body and bind to their respective target cells, causing changes in the activity of those cells.

The endocrine system and the nervous system are partners in regulating and controlling functions in an animal's body. The nervous system operates on a short time scale, it can respond rapidly to changes but is not well-suited to sustained, long-term activity. The endocrine system does not respond as rapidly as the nervous system, but it can maintain secretion of hormones for very long periods.

Recent studies about the functioning of animal bodies show that they are even more complex than earlier thought. Nowhere is this more apparent than in the endocrine system. Hormones, of one sort or another, are produced throughout the body. Some work locally, whereas others circulate to distant parts of the body. For purposes of clarity and brevity, this chapter deals only with the major endocrine glands.

Hypothalamus

The hypothalamus is a part of the brain stem. Together with the pituitary gland, it controls many of the other major endocrine glands. It is extensively connected by nerve fibers to various parts of the brain dorsally, and by nerve fibers and blood vessels to the pituitary gland ventrally. It is a vital link between the nervous system and the endocrine system.

The hypothalamus influences the pituitary gland by two different mechanisms. It produces hormones, called *releasing factors* and *inhibiting factors*. These hormones travel down to the anterior part of the pituitary gland through short blood vessels. There they cause release or inhibition of the anterior pituitary gland's various hormones. The hypothalamus also produces two hormones that are carried down through nerve fibers to the posterior portion of the pituitary gland for storage and release.

Pituitary Gland

The pituitary gland is often called the "master endocrine gland," because many of the hormones it produces direct the activity of other major endocrine glands. The pituitary is a pea-sized gland connected by a stalk to the hypothalamus. In reality it is two separate glands, the anterior and posterior pituitary glands. These glands are physically joined into one structure.

Anterior pituitary gland

The anterior pituitary gland produces and releases six hormones: *growth hormone* (GH), *prolactin*, *thyroid-stimulating hormone* (TSH), *follicle-stimulating hormone* (FSH), *luteinizing hormone* (LH), and *adrenocorticotropic hormone* (ACTH).

Growth hormone, as its name implies, stimulates growth in young animals. It also plays an important role in the general metabolism of body cells in animals of any age.

Prolactin has a known effect only in females. It helps initiate and maintain milk secretion in the mammary glands.

Thyroid-stimulating hormone, as its name implies, stimulates the thyroid gland to produce and release hormones.

Follicle-stimulating hormone derives its name from its effect in females, in which it stimulates production of follicles in the ovary. In males, it stimulates production of spermatozoa in the testes.

Luteinizing hormone also derives its name from its effect in females, in which it promotes ovulation of a mature ovarian follicle and the follicle's conversion into a corpus luteum. In males, it stimulates the testes to produce testosterone.

Adrenocorticotropic hormone stimulates the cortex of the adrenal gland to produce and release its hormones.

Posterior pituitary gland

The posterior pituitary gland does not produce any hormones, but it stores and releases two hormones produced in the hypothalamus.

Antidiuretic hormone (ADH), also called *vasopressin*, causes the kidneys to conserve water, producing more concentrated urine. It acts on the distal convoluted tubules and collecting ducts of kidneys and increases water reabsorption.

The primary effects of *oxytocin*, the second hormone stored in the posterior pituitary, are to promote uterine contractions at parturition and milk letdown from a lactating mammary gland.

Thyroid Gland

The thyroid gland consists of two lobes that may or may not be connected. One lobe is located on either side of the larynx in the neck region. The thyroid gland produces two hormones: *thyroxin* (T4) and *calcitonin*. Thyroxin produces an effect similar to that of growth hormone; it is necessary for normal growth, and it helps regulate metabolism in the cells of animals of any age. The other thyroid hormone, calcitonin, regulates the blood calcium level and is secreted when blood calcium levels are abnormally high.

Parathyroid Glands

The parathyroid glands are several small nodules located in, on, or near the thyroid gland. The effects of the hormone they produce, *parathormone*, oppose those of calcitonin. Parathormone acts to regulate the blood calcium level and is secreted when blood calcium levels become too low.

Adrenal Glands

The adrenal glands are located near the kidneys. They consist of two parts: *cortex* and *medulla*. The adrenal cortex, the outer part of the gland, produces three groups of hormones: *glucocorticoids, mineralocorticoids,* and *sex hormones*. The adrenal medulla, the inner part of gland, produces two hormones that are very similar to each other: *epinephrine* and *norepinephrine*.

Adrenal cortical hormones

Glucocorticoid hormones are the basis for cortisone-type drugs. Their primary effects are to increase the blood glucose level through a number of mechanisms, decrease inflammation, and affect metabolism of fats (mobilization), proteins (catabolism), and carbohydrates (glucose production).

Mineralocorticoid hormones, primarily aldosterone, work mainly in the kidney to promote the retention of water and sodium, which the body needs in large amounts. It does this by promoting elimination of potassium, which the body cannot tolerate in large amounts.

Sex hormones, both estrogens and androgens, are produced in the adrenal cortices of both sexes. The amounts produced are relatively minor.

Adrenal medullary hormones

The hormones of the adrenal medulla, epinephrine and norepinephrine, are released under control of the sympathetic nervous system as part of the body's fight or flight response.

Pancreas

The pancreas is mainly an accessory digestive organ that serves as an exocrine gland as well as an endocrine gland. The exocrine part of the pancreas contains acinar cells that produce enzymes. The enzymes are released in the duodenum through pancreatic ducts. The endocrine part of the pancreas mainly contains small nodules of endocrine cells, the *islets of Langerhans*. Two hormones are produced within the islets: *insulin* and *glucagon*. Insulin is necessary for the body's cells to use glucose for fuel. It prevents abnormally high blood glucose levels and allows glucose to enter the cells for use. A defect in insulin secretion or action leads to diabetes mellitus, characterized by abnormally high blood glucose levels and many metabolic difficulties. The other pancreatic hormone, glucagon, has the opposite effect, and tends to increase the blood glucose level.

Gonads

The gonads are the sex-cell–producing organs. The male gonads are the *testes* and the female gonads are the *ovaries*. In addition to their sex cell production, the gonads are also endocrine organs.

The main hormone produced in the testes is the male sex hormone, *testosterone*. Its *Leydig's cells* produce testosterone at a fairly constant level throughout the year. Very small amounts of the female sex hormone, estrogen, are also produced in the testes by *Sertoli's cells*.

Two main hormones produced by ovaries are *estrogen* and *progesterone*. Levels of the hormones produced by the ovaries fluctuate in a cyclic fashion, linked to the development of follicles and corpora lutea. Under stimulation of FSH from the pituitary gland, follicles develop in the ovaries. The developing follicles produce the hormone estrogen, which is responsible for the signs of "heat," or estrus. After LH from the pituitary gland has caused the follicle to rupture and release its ovum, it then stimulates the empty follicle to develop into a solid corpus luteum, which produces progesterone. Progesterone is necessary for maintenance of pregnancy. If the animal is pregnant, the corpus luteum is retained. If the animal is not pregnant, the corpus luteum lasts for only a short time and then regresses.

URINARY SYSTEM

The many metabolic reactions that take place in the body's cells generate a variety of chemical by-products. Some of these substances are still useful to the body and are recy-cled, but others would be harmful if allowed to accumulate in the body. These harmful waste products must be eliminated. The urinary system is the primary means by which waste products are removed from the blood.

The urinary system consists of two *kidneys*, two *ureters*, the *urinary bladder*, and the *urethra*.

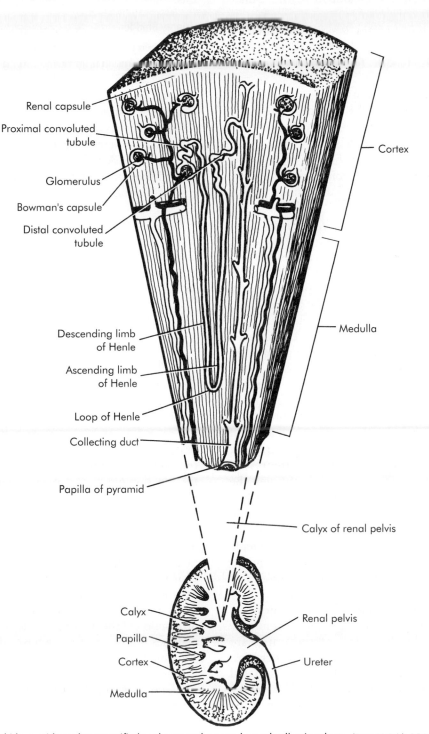

Renal capsule

Proximal convoluted tubule

Glomerulus

Bowman's capsule

Distal convoluted tubule

Cortex

Medulla

Descending limb of Henle

Ascending limb of Henle

Loop of Henle

Collecting duct

Papilla of pyramid

Calyx of renal pelvis

Calyx

Papilla

Cortex

Medulla

Renal pelvis

Ureter

Fig. 6-9 Cross-section of the kidney, with wedge magnified to show renal corpuscles and collecting ducts. *(From McBride DF:* Learning veterinary terminology, *St Louis, 2001, Mosby.)*

Kidneys

The left and right kidneys are located in the dorsal part of the abdominal cavity, just ventral to the most cranial lumbar vertebrae. Most animals have smooth, bean-shaped kidneys. The right kidney of the horse is heart-shaped. Bovine kidneys have a lobulated appearance. Blood and lymph vessels, nerves, and the ureter enter and leave the kidney through the indented area, the *hilus*.

A rough-appearing outer cortex is wrapped around a smooth-appearing inner medulla. The area deep to the hilus region is the renal pelvis, the funnel-like beginning of the ureter.

The work of the kidneys is done at the microscopic level, in tiny waste-disposal units called the *nephrons*. Depending on the animal's size, each kidney may contain from several hundred thousand to several million nephrons. Each nephron is a tube with several bends. This tube has different names because the shape and function of its cells change as it passes through different levels of the kidney matrix. The nephron (tubule) has the following parts: *renal corpuscle*, *proximal convoluted tubule*, *loop of Henle*, *distal convoluted tubule*, and *collecting tubule* (Fig. 6-9).

Renal corpuscles are blood filters, located in the renal cortex. Each renal corpuscle is composed of glomerulus surrounded by a Bowman's capsule. The glomerulus consists of tufts of capillaries interposed between the arterioles entering and leaving the renal corpuscle. A saclike structure called a Bowman's capsule, which is a blind end of each tubule, surrounds the glomerulus. Cells of the glomerulus and Bowman's capsule together make a filtration membrane, which is highly permeable. When blood enters the renal corpuscles, a portion of the plasma, along with its wastes, is filtered out through this filtration membrane into the next portion of the tubule, the proximal convoluted tubule. The balance of the blood that was not filtered out passes into the capillary network surrounding the rest of the nephron. The filtered fluid passes slowly through the rest of the nephron and is modified as it moves along. From the proximal convoluted tubule, the contents pass to the loop of Henle, which dips deep into the renal medulla. Passing superficially out of the medulla, the loop of Henle continues as the distal convoluted tubule, and finally dumps its fluid contents into the collecting tubules, which carry the solution, now called *urine*, to the renal pelvis.

As the fluid that was filtered out in the renal corpuscle passes through the tubules of the nephron, it is chemically altered. Useful substances, like most of the water, are resorbed back into the blood of the capillary network. Waste products that were resorbed initially are secreted from the capillaries back into the tubules. By the time the fluid in the nephron reaches the collecting tubules, it has become urine. Collecting tubules of all nephrons drain urine into the renal pelvis (the funnel-like opening of the ureter in the kidney).

Ureters

From each renal pelvis, urine is transported to the urinary bladder by the ureters, muscular tubes that conduct the urine by smooth muscle contractions. The ureters enter the bladder at oblique angles, forming valvelike openings that prevent backflow of urine into the ureters as the bladder fills.

Urinary Bladder

The urinary bladder is a muscular sac that stores urine and releases it periodically to the outside in a process called *urination* or *micturition*. The kidneys constantly produce urine. As urine accumulates in the urinary bladder, the bladder enlarges and stretch receptors in the bladder wall are activated when the volume reaches a certain point. A spinal reflex then initiates contraction of the smooth muscle in the bladder wall. A voluntarily controlled sphincter muscle around the neck of the urinary bladder enables conscious control of urination.

Urethra

The urethra is the tube that carries urine from the urinary bladder to the outside of the body. In females it is relatively short, straight, and wide, and has a strictly urinary function. In males it is relatively long, curved, and narrow, and serves both urinary and reproductive functions.

REPRODUCTIVE SYSTEM

The reproductive system is very different from other body systems. Whereas most other systems contribute to the survival of the individual animal, the main function of the reproductive system is to help maintain the species. It influences other organ systems, but most parts of the reproductive system are not essential to life. Also, successful functioning of the mammalian reproductive system requires two animals, a male and a female.

Male Reproductive System

The male reproductive system is organized to produce male reproductive cells and transmit them to the female. Its main components are the *testes*, the *epididymis*, the *vas deferens*, the *accessory sex glands*, and the *penis*.

The testes are the male gonads. Their functions include production of the male reproductive cells (*spermatozoa*) and male sex hormones. Before birth, the testes develop in the abdominal cavity. At or soon after birth they descend through slits in the abdominal muscles called the *inguinal rings*, into a sac of skin called the *scrotum* (Fig. 6-10). The scrotum houses the testes and helps regulate their temperature. To produce viable spermatozoa, the testes must be maintained at a temperature slightly lower than body temperature. A muscle in the scrotum, the *cremaster muscle*, acts to raise or lower the testes to adjust their temperature. A network of veins, *pampiniform plexuses*, surrounding the cranial part of testes also helps lower the temperature of arterial blood coming to testes.

Within the testes, spermatogenesis occurs in the seminiferous tubules. Each U-shaped tubule is connected at both ends to efferent ducts. When development of spermatozoa is complete in the seminiferous tubules, the spermatozoa move through the efferent ducts into the epididymis, a long convoluted tube lying along the surface of the testis. Spermatozoa are stored here until ejaculation. If spermatozoa are not expelled from the epididymis, they die there and are absorbed.

Leading from the epididymis proximally up to the pelvic portion of the urethra is the vas deferens. This muscular tube carries both spermatozoa and the fluid they are suspended into the urethra for emission as a component of semen.

Also entering the pelvic portion of the urethra are several types of accessory sex glands. The accessory sex gland found in all common mammals is the prostate gland. Other glands, such as the seminal vesicles and bulbourethral glands, are present only in certain species (Fig. 6-10). Each is responsible for adding components of semen to the spermatozoa that are delivered by the vas deferens during ejaculation.

The penis is the male organ of copulation. It consists of roots, which attach it to the brim of the pelvis; a body, which consists primarily of erectile tissue; and the glans, which is the distal free end of the penis that is richly supplied with sensory nerve endings. The erectile tissue is composed of spongy networks of vascular sinuses surrounded by connective tissue.

With appropriate and adequate sensory stimulation, the penis becomes erect and ready for copulation. Through

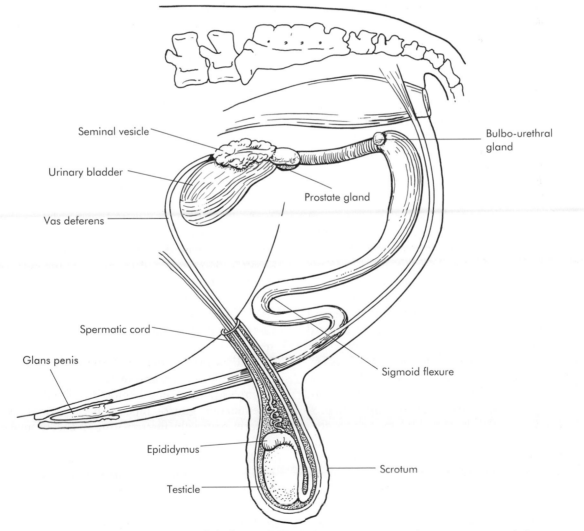

Fig. 6-10 Reproductive system of a bull. *(From McBride DF: Learning veterinary terminology, St Louis, 2001, Mosby.)*

several mechanisms, more blood enters the erectile tissue than leaves it. The result is engorgement and stiffening of the penis, called *erection.*

Continued stimulation of the penis can produce ejaculation, the reflex expulsion of semen from the urethra. Ejaculation occurs in two rapidly successive stages. First, spermatozoa and seminal fluids are moved into the urethra. Second, semen is expelled from the urethra by rhythmic contractions of the muscles surrounding the urethra.

Breeding Soundness Examination of Males

Breeding soundness examination of males should include a good physical examination, evaluation of the reproductive organs, and examination of the ejaculate's quantity, percentage of motile sperm, and percentage of normally shaped sperm. Procedures used in such examinations vary with the species (Table 6-1). Semen can be collected by electroejaculation in the bull, ram, tom, and anesthetized boar. An artificial vagina can be used in the dog, bull, tom, boar, and stallion. Manual stimulation of the penis is effective in producing an ejaculate in the boar and dog and some stallions. After collection of a semen sample, be careful to prevent the sperm from becoming cold or heat shocked, which decreases motility and produces large numbers of secondary abnormalities in the sperm.

Sperm motility is evaluated subjectively as soon after semen collection as possible, using prewarmed slides, preferably on a microscope stage warmed to about 37° C. The motility score is the percentage of individual sperm with rapid progressive motility when examined under high power. Ruminant semen is very concentrated and should be diluted with saline or sodium citrate to see individual motile sperm. After evaluating motility, stain a smear of the semen and evaluate it for morphologic abnormalities. A smear for morphologic evaluation can be made by staining the sperm with any number of stains, such as eosin-nigrosin, Cassarett's, or fine-grain India ink (positively silhouettes sperm). Smear the stained sample onto a slide to produce a thin layer of sperm so individual cells can be seen in their entirety for counting. Examine several hundred sperm and categorize them as normal or affected by a primary abnormality or secondary abnormality (Fig. 6-11). Record the percentage of each type of sperm. Acceptable levels of these abnormalities for each of these species are listed in Table 6-1. *Primary abnormalities* of sperm occur in the testis. *Secondary abnormalities* are produced in the extra-testicular ducts (epididymis) or are artifacts produced by careless semen-handling techniques. Primary abnormalities are predominantly abnormalities of the head and midpiece, but include some tail abnormalities (Fig. 6-11).

After morphologic evaluation, the concentration of sperm in the sample should be evaluated in all species except the bull. In bulls, sperm production is estimated by measuring scrotal circumference. In the other species, the concentration of sperm in the sample is determined by counting the sperm with a hemacytometer, Coulter counter, Spectronic 20 calibrated for sperm, or densimeter. When using a hemacytometer, an RBC pipette can be used for concentrated samples and a WBC pipette for more dilute semen; a Unopette WBC platelet chamber can be used, but care must be taken to be sure the proper dilution factors are used when calculating the concentration.

Artificial Insemination

Successful artificial insemination (AI) depends on accurate determination of the appropriate time to breed, use of high-quality semen, and careful attention to semen-handling and insemination techniques.

Cows

Cows' behavior should be properly observed so as to determine the optimal time of breeding. It is advisable to take at least 30 minutes twice a day, early and late in the day, for observing cows for heat. Cows in heat stand to be mounted by other cows, are usually less interested in eating, act nervous, and vocalize frequently (see Fig. 6-13 later in the chapter). A long strand of clear mucus is commonly seen draining from the vulva or smeared on the tail or perineum. Although standing heat is the time to breed naturally, AI requires use of the "AM/PM rule." That is, cows first seen in heat in the morning should be inseminated that evening and vice versa (see Fig. 6-13 later in the chapter).

Handle frozen semen carefully to avoid killing or damaging the sperm in the insemination straw or ampule. The thawing procedure varies and should be carried out in accordance with the recommendation of the company packaging the frozen semen. In general, ampules of frozen semen are thawed in ice water for 10 minutes. The straws (0.5 cc) are thawed in warm water (32.2° to 35° C) for 45 seconds. However, follow the recommendations of the company processing the semen. Because thawing and refreezing damage the sperm, straws or ampules not being used should not be raised above the "frost line" in the neck of the tank of liquid nitrogen used to store the frozen semen.

Once semen is out of the storage tank and thawed, deposit it in the cow within 15 minutes to ensure viability. Dry the straw or ampule before loading the semen into the insemination gun or pipette, because water kills sperm. Before artificially inseminating the cow, make sure the vulva is wiped clean and dry.

Placing a plastic-sleeve–covered hand just inside the rectum, apply ventral (downward) pressure to open the labia. This helps prevent contamination of the pipette and semen during passage of the pipette into the vagina. Once the pipette is 3 to 4 inches into the vagina, extend the hand in the rectum cranially (forward) to identify and grasp the

TABLE 6-1

Semen Evaluation in Various Domestic Species

	COLLECTION METHODS							
	Manual	Electro-Ejaculator	Artificial Vagina	Volume (ml)	Concentration (Million/ml)	Sperm per Ejaculate (Billion)	Scrotal Measurement	Progressively Motile Sperm (Minimum % Acceptable)	Abnormal Sperm (Maximum % Acceptable)
Dog	Yes	No	40-42° C	10 (1-25)	125 (20-540)	1.25	Yes‡	70%	20%
Stallion	Yes	No	41-50° C	70 (30-250)	120 (30-600)	8.4	Yes‡	70%	35%
Boar	Yes	Yes*	45-50° C	250 (125-500)	150 (25-1000)	37.5	Yes‡	85%	30%
Bull	Yes†	Yes	40-52° C	4 (1-15)	1200 (300-2500)	4.8	Yes‡	30%§	30%§

* Must be anesthetized.

† By rectal massage of prostate and seminal vesicles.

‡ Scrotal width and testes dimension measured by caliper.

‖ Scrotal circumference measured with tape: 30 cm at ≤ 15 mo.; 31 cm at 15-18 mo.; 32 cm at 18-21 mo.; 33 cm at 21-24 mo.; 34 cm at > 24 mo. old.

§ General oscillation or better.

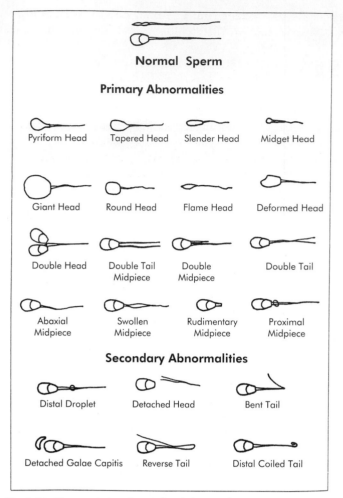

Fig. 6-11 Characteristics of normal and abnormal sperm. Primary abnormalities are of testicular origin. Secondary abnormalities occur during epididymal transport or ejaculation or subsequent to poor semen-handling techniques.

cervix, a firm cylindrical structure. Encircle the cervix with the hand or hold it against the pelvis with the fingers, and extend the vagina to its full length to eliminate any folds in it, which could interfere with passage of the pipette through the cervix. Use your fingers as a guide to make sure the pipette is in the cervix and not in the fornix (along the thinner vaginal wall, beside the cervix).

The pipette must pass through three to five constrictions in the cervix. While passing the pipette through these "rings," always keep your fingers in contact with the end of the pipette to guide it, as well as to protect the uterine wall from being punctured as it enters the uterus. After the pipette enters the uterus ¼ inch or so, depress the plunger slowly, depositing the semen. Withdraw the pipette and examine for pus or blood.

Mares

Artificial insemination of mares is not as widely practiced as in cows, because of breed regulations and the limited avail-

ability of frozen equine semen. However, AI may be used in addition to natural breeding to "reinforce" a service (breeding) in Thoroughbreds and some other breeds. In Quarterhorses, Standardbreds, and a few other breeds, AI is used when several mares must be bred at one time, and the stallion's ejaculate can be diluted and still have sufficient numbers of viable sperm. Regulations for most breeds that allow AI require that the stallion and the mare be on the same farm at the time of AI. In Hanoverians and some other breeds, freezing and shipping of semen to other locations for AI are permitted. Overnight shipping of cooled, extended (diluted) semen is allowed by some breeds, as long as strict recording and animal identification standards are met. Starting on day two of heat and breeding every other day until the mare goes out of heat produces satisfactory results with natural breeding or fresh extended semen that is artificially inseminated. However, use of cooled, extended, or frozen semen requires close attention to the time of insemination and should be used in conjunction with follicle checks to ensure that insemination precedes ovulation as closely as possible. Frozen semen works best if inseminated within six hours before ovulation.

Semen is collected with the aid of an artificial vagina. The temperature inside the vagina should be about 40.6° C at the time of collection. A mare in heat or a "dummy" that the stallion is trained to mount is required to collect semen.

Fresh semen samples should be kept as close to 35° C as possible to ensure sperm viability. The collection container is often equipped with a filter to assist in separating the gel from the remainder of the semen. Raw semen can be placed in a warm syringe and deposited into the mare's uterus through an infusion pipette, or a semen extender can be added to the semen if desired.

Extending (diluting) the semen allows more mares to be inseminated and protects the sperm for a short time until deposition into the uterus. There are several acceptable commercially available semen extenders. They often contain antibiotics to help control any bacteria that have contaminated the semen during collection or that may have been introduced into the uterus during insemination. The semen can be diluted 1:1 or 1:4 with the extender, depending on the sperm concentration in the semen. It is desirable to have 100 to 500 million live normal sperm per insemination dose. Extended semen can be stored or shipped for use several days later.

Stallion semen may be frozen in 0.25-cc to 5-cc straws, in plastic pouches, or as pellets. Follow meticulously the handling precautions mentioned for bull semen and the thawing instructions provided with the semen.

Sows

Sows can be inseminated with fresh or frozen semen. AI is growing in acceptance in commercial swine production. Some reasons for reluctance of the swine industry to extensively use AI are a lack of reliable means of synchronizing heat in gilts and sows, the amount of time and work involved, and the high level of management required. Heat detection and record keeping must be very accurate.

The optimum time to artificially inseminate sows depends on the heat detection techniques used. Sows checked for heat once daily should be bred every day they stand to be mounted, for at least three days. If heat detection is used twice daily, sows should be inseminated 12 and 24 hours after the onset of heat.

After estrus is detected, semen is collected in an artificial vagina or directly in a prewarmed thermos by manually massaging the boar's penis. Semen can be collected while the male is mounted on an estrual female, or boars can be trained to mount dummies constructed for this purpose. The semen can be extended 1:4 or 1:5. One ejaculate usually contains enough sperm to inseminate six to eight females. A minimum of 2 billion live normal sperm is needed for adequate conception and large litter sizes. Frozen extended semen is available from at least one commercial source in the United States and one in Canada.

When AI is used, relatively large volumes (50 to 100 ml) of semen are deposited with the aid of a spiral-tipped pipette or an infusion pipette that has the last (distal) inch bent at a 30-degree angle. These pipettes are actually "screwed" into the cervical rings of the sow.

Bitches

Artificial insemination in the dog is usually carried out with fresh, undiluted semen. However, in the last few years, the American Kennel Club has approved registration of litters using shipped, cooled, extended, or frozen dog semen when collection, storage, transfer, and insemination are done under very strict rules and regulations.

Canine semen is usually collected by manual massage of the penis. Most dogs do not require an estrual bitch present when this is done; however, some timid males may need teasing by a bitch in heat before collection. Collect semen in a quiet room, with good footing for the dog and no distractions. Aerosol bitch scent containing pheromones may be helpful in stimulating the male. The male can also be allowed to smell the vaginal swab from an estrual bitch.

The dog ejaculates in three fractions. The first fraction is clear and contains no sperm; discard this. Collect the second fraction, the sperm-rich fraction. The third fraction (prostatic fluid) is clear. Collect a few drops and discard the rest. There may be a 15- to 60-second delay between passage of fractions.

The semen is protected from cold and heat shock and transferred to a prewarmed syringe and deposited in the cranial vagina through a 6- to 12-inch infusion rod. The rear of the bitch should be elevated during and for a few minutes after insemination. Some veterinarians prefer to introduce the index finger, covered with a sterile, powder-free glove, into the vagina with the infusion rod. The finger is left in the vagina a few minutes and the dorsum of the vaginal vault is stroked gently to simulate the coital tie between the male and female. It is thought that this induces waves of uterine and vaginal contractions that help the sperm move into the uterus.

Canine sperm is usually not diluted because of a lack of ability to synchronize heat in females. Bitches are usually artificially inseminated because the selected male has either a lack of ability or desire to copulate. Bitches should be inseminated on the first, third, and fifth day of standing heat or as determined by vaginal cytology and progesterone determination, if available.

Female Reproductive System

The female reproductive system is organized to produce female reproductive cells, accept male reproductive cells (spermatozoa), allow one sperm cell to unite with each female reproductive cell, and then shelter and nourish the resulting developing fetuses until birth. The organs of the female reproductive system are *ovaries*, *oviducts*, *uterus*, *cervix*, *vagina*, and *vulva*.

The ovaries are the female gonads (Fig. 6-12). Ovaries produce the female reproductive cells (ova) and hormones. Unlike spermatozoa, ova are not continually produced. At or soon after birth, the ovary contains all of the ova it will ever contain. They remain in an immature state until activated by cyclic hormonal cycles.

Under the influence of FSH and LH from the pituitary gland, a few ova at a time develop in the *follicles* of the ovary. A single layer of flattened follicular cells surrounds the immature ova. When a particular follicle becomes activated, the follicular cells become more cuboidal and multiply to form many layers around the ovum. Spaces gradually form between follicular cells through secretion of fluid. By the time the follicle is mature, the ovum sits on a tiny hill of follicular cells and is surrounded by the fluid-filled antrum of the follicle. The mature follicle is a large, blisterlike structure that protrudes from the surface of the ovary. As it develops, the follicle secretes increasing amounts of estrogen, which causes the physical and behavioral signs of heat or estrus. Release of the ovum, called *ovulation*, usually occurs as a result of falling FSH levels and peaking LH levels. Ovulation is characterized by physical rupture of the follicle surface. As the fluid of the antrum rushes out, it carries the ovum with it. After ovulation, the collapsed follicle fills with blood and becomes a *corpus hemorrhagicum* (CH), which is converted quickly to a *corpus luteum* (CL), under the influence of LH. The corpus luteum starts producing progesterone, which is necessary for maintenance of pregnancy. If an animal becomes pregnant, the CL stays on the ovary throughout the pregnancy. If there is no conception and the animal does not become pregnant, the CL

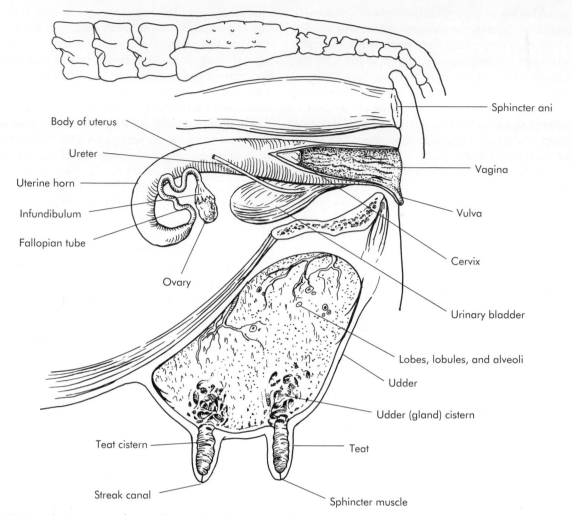

Fig. 6-12 Reproductive system of a cow, also showing the mammary gland. *(From McBride DF:* Learning veterinary terminology, *St Louis, 2001, Mosby.)*

regresses and becomes a nonfunctional *corpus albicans* just before the next heat.

Partially surrounding each ovary, but not physically connected to it, are the oviducts, which are convoluted, tubular extensions of the uterus. At its ovarian end, each oviduct is flared to form the funnel-like *infundibulum*, which "catches" ova as they are released from the follicles.

The uterus is a hollow, muscular organ that is continuous with the oviducts cranially, and opens, via the cervix, into the vagina caudally (Fig. 6-12). In most common domestic mammals, the uterus consists of two cranial uterine horns that unite in a caudal uterine body.

The cervix is a powerful smooth muscle sphincter that functions to close off the lumen of the uterus from the lumen of the vagina most of the time. The only times the cervix is relaxed and partially dilated are at breeding and parturition.

The vagina is the canal from the cervix to the vulva. It receives the erect penis during copulation and is the birth canal for the newborn at parturition.

The vulva is the external portion of the female genitalia. It consists of the *vestibule*, the short space between the vagina and the labia where the urethra opens; the *clitoris*, a small, sensitive erectile body homologous to the penis of the male; and the *labia*, which form the outer boundary of the vulva.

FEMALE REPRODUCTION PHYSIOLOGY: NONPREGNANT ANIMALS

Unlike women and other female primates that have *menstrual cycles*, with variable levels of sexual receptivity, mammals commonly dealt with in veterinary medicine have an *estrous cycle,* in which the period of sexual receptivity, *estrus (heat),* is concentrated during a short period lasting from one to several days. During the reminder of the estrous cycle, the female does not accept the male's sexual advances nor allow mating.

The estrous cycle is composed of four or five stages, depending on the species and whether the animal is *polyestrous (cycles repeatedly)* or *monestrous (cycles only once* during the breeding season). The stages of estrus are *anestrus, proestrus, estrus, metestrus,* and *diestrus.*

Anestrus

Anestrus is the period of ovarian inactivity, with no behavioral signs of heat or estrus.

Proestrus

Under the influence of gonadotropin-releasing hormone (GnRH) produced in the hypothalamus, FSH is released from the pituitary to act on the ovary to cause initial follicle development. These growing follicles produce estrogen, which causes the genital and behavioral changes that attract the male and prepare the female's reproductive tract for mating. Although the proestrus female may show signs of interest in the male, she will not allow mating.

Estrus

Estrus is the period of true heat, during which the female allows mating. The estrogen levels peak early in estrus and cause the pituitary to release LH, which further matures the follicles and results in release of the egg(s) at ovulation.

Metestrus

Metestrus is the short stage during which the female may still attract males but no longer allows mating. During this stage, ovulated follicles metamorphose into corpora lutea, which begin to secrete progesterone. Metestrus is so short in some species that it is not even discussed as a separate stage and is included in diestrus.

Diestrus

Diestrus is a stage of ovarian activity without signs of heat. The CL develops fully and produces maximum levels of progesterone to ready the uterus for the conceptus and maintain pregnancy.

If the female does not become pregnant, prostaglandins are released from the uterus, destroying the CL and stopping progesterone production. The female then either enters anestrus (if it is a monestrous species, such as the dog) or reenters proestrus (if it is a polyestrous species, such as the cow). Some polyestrous animals cycle throughout the year (cow), whereas other animals are seasonally polyestrous (mare, ewe, and doe) in response to changing day length. Seasonally polyestrous animals enter anestrus at the end of the breeding season.

Reproductive Physiologic Patterns

Cows

The normal cow is a polyestrous animal that cycles throughout the year (Table 6-2). Heat lasts about 18 hours of the 21-day cycle (range 18 to 23 days). The signs of approaching heat in cows include nervousness, vocalization, and attempting to mount and ride other animals. A cow in true heat stands to be ridden by other cows. A thick, clear, tenacious string of mucus can often be seen hanging from the vulva of cows in heat. Unlike other animals, cows ovulate about 12 hours after going out of heat. Cows that are to be bred artificially should be bred 12 hours after heat is first detected, if the herd is watched 20 to 30 minutes twice daily for estrual animals (Fig. 6-13). Obviously, cows to be bred naturally must still be in standing heat. Cows often show metestrus bleeding in the mucus one to two days after they have ovulated. It is too late to breed cows that have evidence of metestrual blood in their vulvar mucus.

Mares

The mare is a seasonally polyestrous animal (Table 6-2). Most mares stop cycling (become anestrual) during winter; however, a few mares continue to cycle during winter. The mare's natural breeding season is in late spring and summer. However, breed registration rules require breeding mares in February and March. During the natural breeding season (May through August), the mare's estrous cycle is about 21 days long. They are in standing heat for about 5 days and then out of heat for 16 days.

Estrual mares (in heat) seek out the stallion. They squat and urinate frequently in the presence of the stallion, raise the tail to the side, and evert (wink) the clitoris. Estrual mares stand to be mounted by the stallion. Mares that are not in heat squeal, kick, switch the tail from side to side, pin their ears back, and may attempt to bite the stallion.

Mares enter and leave the natural breeding season with very erratic cycles. They often have prolonged or erratic heats in the early spring. These early-season erratic periods result in extra labor and ineffective breedings. Rectal examinations by a veterinarian can be used to predict the optimum time for breeding. Mares usually ovulate 24 to 36 hours before going out of heat. The best time to breed a normally cycling mare is on the second day of heat and again every other day until she goes out of heat. In the early spring, when mares have prolonged heats, breeding all mares every other day may exhaust the stallion.

The veterinarian can predict ovulation, based on changes in the follicles, as palpated rectally, and on changes in the cervix. The follicles become large and soft before ovulation and the cervix changes from a dry, firm, tight, pale organ to a very pink, edematous, soft, amorphous mass on the floor of the vagina before ovulation. Ultrasonography helps

TABLE 6-2

Reproductive Data for Various Domestic Species

	Cycle Pattern	Cycle Length	Heat Length	Ovulation Time	Natural	AI	Gestation Length	Puberty	Age to First Breeding
					TIME TO BREED				
Cow	Polyestrous	21 days	18 hours	12-18 hours after heat	Heat	12 hours after first see heat	280 days	6-16 months	14-22 months
Mare	Seasonally polyestrous (long day)	21 days	5 days	24-36 hours before end of heat	Day 2 and every other day of heat	Same as natural	330 days (320-360 days)	18 months	2-3 years
Sow	Polyestrous	21 days	2-3 days	36 hours after onset of heat	Daily when in heat	Same as natural	115 days	7 months	8-9 months
Bitch	Seasonally monestrous	4-7 months	7-9 days	Day 2-3 of heat	Days 1, 3, and 5 of heat	Same as natural	62-64 days	7-24 months	6-24 months
Queen	Seasonally polyestrous	21 days	4-10 days	Induced	In heat	In heat	63 days	7-12 months	12-18 months
Ewe	Seasonally polyestrous (short day)	17 days	1-1.5 days	Toward end	In heat	In heat	150 days	6-16 months*	6 months
Doe	Seasonally polyestrous (short day)	21 days	1-3 days	12 hours before end of heat	In heat	In heat	150 days	6-16 months*	6 months

* Lambs and kids born early in the year may reach puberty at their first breeding season. Those born late may wait until the next year's breeding season.

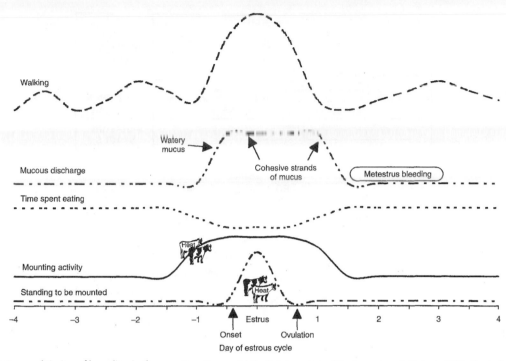

Fig. 6-13 Signs of estrus and timing of breeding in the cow. (From Youngquist-Threlfall: Large Animal Theriogenology, 2, St. Louis, 2007, Elsevier.)

predict ovulation. The follicular wall thickens and its shape changes from round to pointed.

Sows

Gilts (young females) reach puberty at about 6 to 7 months of age, although this varies with the breed and time of year they are born (Table 6-2). Pigs are nonseasonally polyestrous animals; however, in hot, humid climates they may show a reduction in cyclicity during the summer. Pigs are unique in that they show an early postpartum heat but do not ovulate during this heat. They then undergo a true lactational anestrus, at which time they do not resume cyclicity until the litter is weaned. After resumption of cycling, the sow demonstrates heat for 2 to 3 days every 21 days (range 18 to 24 days). Heat is recognized in sows by a slightly swollen, reddened vulva. They are restless, seek out the boar, and assume a characteristic braced stance when the boar mounts. The "riding test" uses this stance to detect sows and gilts in heat. A female in heat assumes the same braced stance if pressed on the back by a person.

Sows ovulate in the last half of heat. They should be bred on the first day of heat and 24 hours later for maximum conception rate and litter size.

Bitches

The bitch (female dog) is a seasonally monestrous animal with a definite anestrous period between cycles (Table 6-2). Most bitches come into season about once every six to seven months. The heats can occur at any time of the year;

however, they seem to be concentrated in spring and fall. Some female dogs may cycle only once a year, as is the case with the Basenji breed. Other individual dogs may cycle every four months and still be considered normal. Bitches reach puberty at 6 to 24 months of age, with an average of 10 to 12 months. Small breeds usually reach puberty earlier than large breeds. Vaginal smears can be used to determine the stage of the cycle (Fig. 6-14). Owners say a bitch has come into heat when they notice attraction of males and dripping of blood from the vulva. This is actually proestrus, not estrus.

Proestrus. This stage is characterized by increased vulvar swelling, a bloody vulvar discharge, attraction to males, and courtship play, such as spinning, crouching in front, nuzzling, and even mounting the male. However, proestrus females do not stand to be mounted by males. The vaginal smear at this stage shows a variable amount of RBCs and WBCs, and initially contains predominantly small, round parabasal and small intermediate vaginal epithelial cells (Fig. 6-14). Parabasal and small intermediate cells are distinguishable by their round shape and relatively large nucleus in proportion to the amount of cytoplasm.

As the bitch progresses through proestrus, the number of RBCs in the smear remains variable. The number of WBCs declines, and vaginal cells increasingly tend toward large intermediate and superficial cells, both of which are thin, large, and angular cells, having small pyknotic (dense) nuclei or no nucleus at all. The vaginal cells are becoming keratinized or cornified. The vulva is still large and edematous at

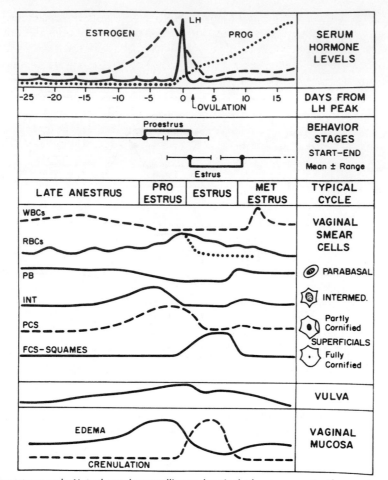

Fig. 6-14 Events during the canine estrous cycle. Note that vulvar swelling and vaginal edema are greatest in proestrus and reduced in estrus. As the vaginal edema subsides, wrinkling (crenulation) of the vaginal mucosa can be detected with vaginoscopy. *(From Kirk RW:* Current veterinary therapy VIII small animal practice, *Philadelphia, 1983, WB Saunders.)*

this stage. Proestrus lasts an average of 9 days (range 3 to 17 days). By the end of proestrus, more than 50% of the vaginal cells are anuclear (no nucleus) keratinized superficial cells (Fig. 6-14). A short-lived LH peak causes progesterone levels to begin to rise at the end of proestrus, or early estrus before ovulation. Kits are available to detect the LH or progesterone rise and predict the time of ovulation for maximum breeding efficiency.

Estrus. The onset of estrus is marked by the bitch standing to be mounted by the male. Estrus averages 9 days in the bitch but can be as short as 3 or as long as 21 days. During estrus, the bitch lifts the tail and deflects it to the side, arches the back, and elevates the vulva.

The vulva is less turgid than in a proestrus; this facilitates copulation (mating). The estrual vulvar discharge may remain red or become straw colored. As mentioned earlier, the estrual vaginal smear consists almost entirely of superficial and large intermediate cells (Fig. 6-14). The WBCs are no longer present in the smear; RBCs may or may not be present. The presence or absence of RBCs is not a significant finding when trying to determine the stage of the cycle.

Bitches ovulate early in estrus. The best time to breed a bitch is on the first, third, and fifth days of standing heat. Breeding bitches on the ninth and eleventh or eleventh and thirteenth days after the onset of vulvar bleeding is less than satisfactory because of the variable duration of proestrus and estrus. Breeding bitches on these predetermined days assumes the owner noticed the first day of vulvar discharge. However, this is often not the case. Breedings based upon the preovulatory rise in LH or progesterone levels are the most effective. The kit directions (mentioned earlier) should be followed for predicting the most fertile period, because the exact days on which to breed vary with the kit.

During breeding, it is important to be sure that the stud (male dog) has inserted the penis completely and that the bulbus glandis (enlarged portion of the penis) is completely inserted into the vagina, producing the coital lock or "tie."

The tie is important for stimulating contractions that help move the semen into the uterus and up the oviducts. A normal tie can last 15 to 30 minutes. The dogs should not be disturbed at this time. Efforts to physically separate the bitch and stud may injure the penis or the vagina. At the end of estrus, the bitch no longer accepts the stud dog, even though he may continue to show interest in her. The bitch then enters metestrus.

Metestrus. Metestrus is a short stage, marked by the female's refusal of the male's sexual advances and reappearance of WBCs and noncornified parabasal and small intermediate cells in vaginal smears. Vulvar swelling and discharge decrease rapidly during this stage. Metestrus rapidly progresses into diestrus. The wide range of days during which breeding can take place in the dog makes accurate prediction of whelping difficult. The whelping date can be predicted to occur 56 to 58 days after the vaginal smear reverts to predominantly noncornified small intermediate and parabasal cells typical of diestrus.

Diestrus. This is the longest stage of the canine estrous cycle; it lasts about 60 days, which is nearly the same length as a normal pregnancy. There is no vulvar discharge after the first few days of diestrus. The vaginal smear contains predominantly noncornified parabasal and small intermediate cells, with a few WBCs.

Toward the end of diestrus, about the time a pregnant bitch would be ready to whelp, the nonpregnant bitch often shows *pseudopregnancy*, or "false pregnancy," as progesterone levels decline. The abdomen may enlarge and the mammary glands may swell and fill with milk. The bitch may start building a "nest" and even undergo a false first stage of labor (Table 6-3). Pseudopregnant bitches often "adopt" socks, stuffed toys, or kittens as their surrogate puppies. They may have a behavior change at this time and become aggressive if attempts are made to remove their "puppies." Pseudopregnant bitches have been known to raise an orphaned litter of kittens. Not all bitches show clinical signs of pseudopregnancy; however, they all undergo the same hormonal changes that could make them exhibit these signs.

Anestrus. After diestrus or pregnancy, the uterus undergoes a period of regeneration or repair during anestrus. Anestrus may last 1 to 11 months, depending on the breed, with an average of 4 to 5 months. The vaginal smear at this time consists of primarily noncornified parabasal and small intermediate cells, with variable numbers of WBCs. At times, WBCs can be quite numerous, making it difficult to rule out infection. Anestrous females do not attract males, nor do they allow courtship or mating behavior by the stud. After anestrus, the bitch reenters proestrus and the cycle repeats itself.

Queens

The queen (female cat) is different from other animals previously discussed in that the others are spontaneous ovulators. That is, they release their eggs at a predetermined time in their cycle, after the appropriate hormonal changes. The queen, on the other hand, is an induced ovulator, meaning coitus (mating) is necessary to stimulate ovulation. The queen is a seasonally polyestrous animal (Table 6-2). If not induced to ovulate, she will have several cycles of sexual behavior before either being bred and induced to ovulate, or having the follicles regress. Queens have a short anestrus period between October and January, but they then cycle regularly the rest of the year if they do not conceive. Because the cat is an induced ovulator, the CL is not produced unless coitus has occurred. The cycle lasts about 14 days and is composed of 1 to 2 days of proestrus, 3 to 6 days of estrus (heat), and about 7 days of metestrus before proestrus occurs again.

Estrus. Estrus in queens is recognized by behavioral changes. They become more affectionate, vocalize, and rub up against inanimate objects and people. When petted, they arch their back, elevate the hindquarters, and laterally displace the tail. Treading of the hind feet is often evident at this time.

Queens do not show the vulvar bleeding as do dogs, but they have similar changes in vaginal cells. Reappearance of WBCs in the smear marks the end of estrus and the beginning of metestrus. Natural breeding can successfully take place at any time during estrus, because the eggs are not ovulated until breeding. Many owners find the recurrent estrous behavior of their cat annoying. Owners can stop the behavior by inducing ovulation and pseudopregnancy after a sterile mating or false mating using a glass rod (e.g., a sanitized rectal thermometer) to gently stimulate the queen's vagina. Ovulation can also be induced by injection of the appropriate LH or releasing factor. Overaggressive probing for a vaginal smear for estrus detection can also stimulate ovulation. Induced ovulation should keep a queen out of heat for 40 days or longer if winter is approaching.

Ewes and does

Ewes (female sheep) and does (female goats) are photosensitive, seasonally polyestrous animals (Table 6-2). They begin to cycle in response to shortening of the day length and thus are fall and winter breeders. Some breeds of sheep and goats vary from this pattern and can be bred at other times of the year. Estrus in the ewe is often not apparent, and a ram wearing a mount marking harness is usually necessary to detect ewes in heat. Does, on the other hand, are more demonstrative of their sexual receptivity. They bleat frequently, approach the male, wiggle their elevated tail, and may urinate in the male's presence. The odor of the buck (male goat) often stimulates cycling and estrous behavior. Does in estrus can be detected by their teasing a male or by exposing a doe to the male's odor on a rag rubbed in his scent glands near the horns.

TABLE 6-3

Stages of Labor in Various Domestic Species

Stage	Cow	Mare	Sow*	Bitch*	Queen
I	1-4 hours (longer in heifers); restless; off feed; isolates self; allantois protrudes	1-4 hours; colic; sweats; isolates self; defecates; urinates; placenta ruptures	2-12 hours; 1-2° F drop in rectal temp; builds nest	6-12 hours; 1-2° F drop in rectal temp; builds nest	2-12 hours; 1-2° F drop in rectal temp; builds nest
II	½-4 hours; abdominal straining; amnion ruptures; calf delivered	5-40 minutes; forceful abdominal straining; amnion ruptures; foal delivered	1-5 hours; amnion ruptures; straining; pigs delivered	3-6 hours; amnion ruptures; pups delivered	3-6 hours; amnion ruptures, kittens delivered
III	½-8 hours; uterine contractions; passes placenta	½-3 hours; rests between uterine contractions; ± mild colic	⅓-4 hours; eats; drinks	½-1 hour; greenish-black fluid passed	½-1 hour; brownish fluid passed

* Several fetuses may be passed before a placenta is passed.

Although these small ruminants are similar in size and seasonality, their estrous cycles are very distinct. Does have a cycle length similar to the cow's, ranging from 19 to 24 days, with an average length of 21 days. The cycle is often shorter in the early part of the breeding season. Unlike cows, does ovulate 12 hours or so before the end of heat. Heat lasts an average of 28 hours, but it may be as long as 3 days. The doe should be bred on the days she is in heat.

The ewe's estrous cycle is shorter than the doe's and cow's. Ewes cycle about every 17 days (range 14 to 19 days). Heat averages 26 hours in length (range 20 to 36 hours), and the ewe ovulates toward the end of heat. It is best to breed on the day the ewe is noted to be in heat.

Gestation lasts about 150 days for both the doe and ewe, and parturition (birth) is followed by a period of anestrus until the next breeding season.

Fertilization and Pregnancy

At copulation, semen is usually deposited in the proximal vagina. Spermatozoa rapidly move through the cervix, into the uterus, and up the oviducts through a combination of their own swimming actions and contractions of the female reproductive tract. Normally the spermatozoa arrive at the oviduct before the ovum has entered it. They must spend some time maturing there to improve their capacity to fertilize the ovum. This final maturation process is called *capacitation*.

When the ovum arrives in the oviduct, spermatozoa swarm around it, but only one sperm cell is allowed to penetrate the ovum and fertilize it. Once a single spermatozoon has penetrated the ovum, entry of all others is blocked. Very soon after fertilization, the nucleus of the ovum and the nucleus of the spermatozoon fuse or combine. The fertilized ovum now has the full complement of chromosomes and is called a *zygote*.

The zygote immediately begins the process of cell division, called *cleavage*, as cells lining the oviduct slowly move it distally toward the uterus. The single cell divides into two cells, the two cells to four, and so on. Cleavage proceeds so rapidly that the cells do not have time to grow larger between divisions. The overall size of the dividing zygote does not increase appreciably during this initial period. When it reaches the uterus, the zygote has formed into a hollow ball of cells, the *blastocyst*, which is ready to implant itself into the wall of the uterus.

Following implantation, the *placenta*, the life-support system of the developing fetus, develops. The placenta is a multilayered, fluid-filled sac in which the embryo develops. It attaches to the uterine wall so that its blood vessels and the uterine blood vessels are intertwined. Nutrients and gases are exchanged between these maternal and fetal blood vessels. There is normally no direct mixing of fetal and maternal blood. The developing fetus is linked with the placenta via the umbilical cord, through which blood in the umbilical arteries and vein flows to and from the fetus.

Pregnancy Diagnosis

One of the indicators of pregnancy in large animals is failure to return to heat after breeding during their breeding season. However, this is not true for dogs because, as seasonally monestrous animals, they will not return to heat for 4 to 7 months, even if they fail to conceive after mating. Mated but nonpregnant cats will not return to heat for several months after breeding. Seasonally polyestrous animals do not return to heat at the end of their breeding season. Traditionally, animals are examined for pregnancy by palpation (manual examination) of the uterus through the abdominal wall or by rectal palpation. Various histologic, chemical, electronic, ultrasonic, and radiographic techniques can also be used to identify a pregnant animal.

PARTURITION

After the preparatory changes of late pregnancy, which ready the dam and fetus for birth, parturition begins. Parturition has several common names, depending on the species involved. The terms *calving, lambing, kidding,* and *foaling* are self-explanatory. However, parturition in the sow or gilt is called *farrowing*, and in the bitch, it is called *whelping*. In the cat, it is called *kittening* or *queening*.

Parturition is divided into three stages (Table 6-3). Stage 1 is preliminary to expulsion of the fetus. During this stage, the uterine muscles undergo rhythmic contractions, which reposition and advance the fetus toward the cervix. In response to these contractions and the pressure of the fetus, the cervix relaxes fully and dilates. The dam in first-stage labor often is anxious and restless and shows evidence of abdominal cramps. Stage 1 ends with delivery of the fetus into the pelvic canal and rupture of the fetal membranes.

Stage 2 is the stage of expulsion of the fetus from the birth canal. Uterine contractions are stronger and accompanied by abdominal straining to help expel the fetus. The importance of abdominal straining versus uterine contractions in the birth process varies among species. Abdominal pressing is very important in foaling, but uterine contractions are relatively more important in farrowing. With successful delivery of the fetus, the dam completes stage 2 and rests during the first part of stage 3.

Stage 3 of parturition is characterized by expulsion of the placenta. Uterine contractions continue but are not as severe as those in stage 2. The uterus begins to shrink toward its nonpregnant size. In polytocous (litter-bearing) species, the cycle of stages 1 to 3 repeats itself with each fetus. Stages 1 and 2 may occur several times and result in passage of several fetuses before a placenta is passed in stage 3 in these species.

After delivery of the fetus, the dam rests and begins to care for the newborn. She licks it dry, which helps stimulate breathing. She chews off any amniotic membrane remaining on the fetus. The bitch and queen usually chew the umbilical cord to sever the placenta. The cord usually ruptures spontaneously during delivery of the calf or during the mare's or foal's efforts to rise.

Calves and foals are usually delivered front feetfirst, in a "diving" position. Most pigs, pups, and kittens are delivered headfirst, but frequently one or both front legs are retracted alongside the body. However, in these small species, rear-end (breech) delivery is common and results in normal, live offspring. Most dams deliver while lying down, but occasionally a cow or mare may deliver while standing up. This can be dangerous to the fetus.

It is often difficult to tell when a dam has finished delivering all of the offspring. Prepartum radiographs made one week before the due date can determine the exact number of pups or kittens in the dam. Twins in mares and cows are uncommon and can be detected by manual exploration of the vagina and uterus. However, this is not as easily accom-

plished in sows, bitches, and queens, so other signs or tests may be necessary. The bitch's abdomen may be palpated for more pups, or a finger in a sterile glove may be introduced into the vagina to feel for another pup. Radiographs of the abdomen may be necessary. Some bitches and queens eat their neonatal pups, so care must be taken to differentiate fetuses in the stomach from those in the uterus. Sows often get up to drink and may eat some feed after a period of rest once the last pig is delivered.

One of the most difficult situations encountered in theriogenology is to decide when parturition is not proceeding normally and the dam is in *dystocia* (difficult birth) and requires assistance. Box 6-1 contains helpful guidelines.

Milk Production

The mammary glands are specialized skin glands that produce secretions that are essential for nourishment of the newborn (Fig. 6-12). Mammary glands are found in both males and females, but the hormone environment necessary for their full development and milk secretion only occurs near the end of pregnancy in females. The process of

BOX 6-1

Guidelines for Intervention in Dystocia in Various Species

Bitch, Queen

Intense straining that does not produce a pup or kitten in 30 minutes
Weak, intermittent straining that does not produce a pup or kitten in 2-3 hours
An interval of over 4 hours between pups or kittens, without further labor
Illness in the dam
A bloody, malodorous or greenish vulvar discharge
Prolonged pregnancy (overdue)
Obvious difficulty in delivering the pup or kitten (e.g., a fetus halfway out)

Sow

Prolonged pregnancy (over 115 days)
Malodorous or bloody vulvar discharge
Expulsion of fetal feces (meconium) without expulsion of a fetus
Weak labor or cessation of labor before delivery of all fetuses
Incomplete expulsion of a fetus

Cow

First-stage labor lasting more than 6 hours, without abdominal pressing
Second-stage labor, with abdominal pressing, lasting over 2-3 hours without progress

Rupture of the waterbag (amnion) without expulsion of the calf within 2 hours
Fetal malposition (backwards, legs retained, etc.)
Fetal monstrosity (malformed fetus)

Mare

Parturition, especially stage 2, in mares is quicker and more violent than in other species. Furthermore, foals seem more susceptible to the adverse effects of dystocia than other neonates. Therefore, differentiation between a normal birth and dystocia is especially important in mares. Delivery should be assisted when any of the following occur:
Appearance of the red unruptured placenta at or outside the vulva at the start of second-stage labor, with evident straining
Failure of the clear amnion to appear soon after the start of second-stage labor
Failure to locate the foal's head and legs in the pelvic inlet at the beginning of second-stage labor
Rolling, repeated getting up and down, and reversing of the recumbent position by the mare, without progressing through stage 2 of labor and delivering a foal
Repeated straining without delivery of a partially expelled foal
Fetal malposition (backwards, legs retained, etc.) or other abnormality in delivery
Fetal fecal (meconium) staining on the foal

milk production, called *lactation*, begins toward the end of pregnancy. Several hormones are involved, chiefly prolactin. The initial mammary secretion after parturition is called *colostrum* and differs from normal milk in composition and appearance. Colostrum has a laxative effect on the newborn and is important in transferring antibodies from the mother to the offspring. The intestine of the newborn can absorb only the large antibody molecules in the colostrum for a few hours after birth, so it is important that a newborn suckle colostrum as soon as possible after birth.

Suckling or milking stimulates continued production of milk. Sensory stimulation of the teat or nipple, either by the offspring's suckling or by milking, causes continued production of the hormones necessary to support lactation. Stimulation of the teat or nipple causes immediate release of oxytocin from the posterior pituitary gland. Oxytocin has the effect of squeezing milk out of the alveoli and small ducts of the mammary gland, into the large ducts and sinuses, where the newborn can extract it by suckling. The immediate effect of suckling or milking is called *milk letdown*. Cessation of suckling or milking results in the cessation of milk production; the mammary gland "dries up."

NECROPSY PROCEDURE

Necropsy (postmortem examination) is an excellent diagnostic tool that should be used as often as possible, when an unexpected death occurs in a cattery, kennel, or herd situation. The course of a disease can be better understood if a necropsy is performed. In addition, the knowledge gained from a necropsy can be applied to future circumstances involving similar conditions or disease processes. If there is a possibility of litigation, or an animal dies while under veterinary care, a necropsy should be performed by a qualified laboratory or institution. A written consent form signed by the owner authorizes a postmortem examination.

Before beginning a necropsy, it is important to make sure that all instruments and required materials are readily available (Fig. 6-15). Obtain a complete clinical history. This information should include the owner's name and address, and complete identification of the animal, including species, breed, age, sex, weight, and name or number. The cause of death, if known, dictates which tissues to collect for testing. Develop a checklist and follow it (Box 6-2). In addition to the tissues listed on the checklist, any abnormal tissue must be collected with attached adjacent normal tissue. Label the appropriate vials and bags with the tissue type, date collected, and animal identification.

Beginning the Necropsy

Using a dog as an example, the following is one method of postmortem examination. The necropsy should begin with a thorough external physical examination. If broken bones

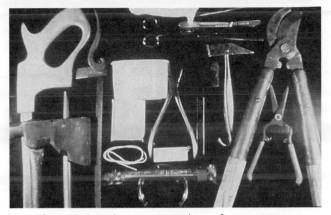

Fig. 6-15 Some instruments used to perform a necropsy.

BOX 6-2

Sample Checklist for Tissue Collection at Necropsy

Primary incision
- ☐ Peripheral lymph node
- ☐ Muscle

Abdominal cavity
- ☐ Liver with section of gallbladder
- ☐ Kidney (cut left kidney longitudinally and right kidney transversely)

Thoracic cavity
- ☐ Thyroid glands with parathyroid gland
- ☐ Esophagus (can remain attached to trachea)
- ☐ Upper trachea
- ☐ Thymus
- ☐ Bronchial lymph node (collect with section of trachea)
- ☐ Lung
- ☐ Right atrium
- ☐ Right ventricle
- ☐ Left ventricle

Adrenal glands
- ☐ Spleen
- ☐ Stomach
- ☐ Duodenum with attached pancreas
- ☐ Jejunum with attached mesenteric lymph node
- ☐ Ileum with cecum
- ☐ Colon
- ☐ Urinary bladder
- ☐ Ovary
- ☐ Uterus
- ☐ Testis

Other
- ☐ Brain with hypophysis
- ☐ Femoral bone marrow

Optional
- ☐ Eyes
- ☐ Tonsils
- ☐ Prostate
- ☐ Spinal cord

---

or gunshot are suspected, radiographs should be obtained to identify these sites. Note the overall body condition, skin and haircoat condition, mucous membrane color, and normal anatomic associations. With the animal in left lateral recumbency, use a knife to make a ventral midline incision, cutting through the skin from the mandibular symphysis, around any external genital organs, to the area of the pubis. Next, cut the pectoral muscles of the accessible (right) front leg. Continue to cut through these muscles until the leg can be reflected dorsally and is resting without support. This cut exposes the axillary lymph nodes (Fig. 6-16). Repeat this technique with the accessible (right) rear leg while disarticulating or separating and exposing the hip joint at the round ligament. Note any joint fluid and its color. Also note the smoothness of the joint surface.

From the ventral midline incision, reflect the skin dorsally from the right side of the animal. Note any changes or abnormalities in the underlying subcutaneous tissue, such as hemorrhage, jaundice, or edema. Next, reflect dorsally the skin from the neck and face. Be careful not to cut the jugular vein in this area. This exposes the prescapular and mandibular lymph nodes; note their size and color. At this point, the body should be completely skinned over its right lateral side, with both accessible (right) front and rear limbs reflected dorsally, exposing the axilla and hip joint. The next step is to open the abdominal cavity.

Abdominal cavity

Make a vertical cut (dorsal to ventral) through the abdominal muscles, parallel to the last rib. Next make a midline incision from the point of the xiphoid cartilage to the pubis. When making this cut, remember to stay shallow so as not to puncture the intestine or stomach. Continue this cut dorsally along the pelvis. Next, reflect this muscle wall dorsally, exposing the abdominal viscera. Note the placement and condition of all abdominal organs. Note any fluid within the abdominal cavity and its color. Before further examination of the abdominal cavity, open the thoracic cavity.

Thoracic cavity

Before opening the thoracic cavity, puncture the diaphragm with the tip of a knife. Under normal circumstances, this causes the lungs to collapse. As this occurs, the negative pressure within the thoracic cavity is neutralized, causing the diaphragm to outpouch.

Using pruning shears, remove the right side of the rib cage. With the shears, cut from the point of the xiphoid cartilage to the thoracic inlet (cranially). Using the shears, begin cutting at the point of the last rib just a few centimeters from the vertebrae, toward the thoracic inlet. During this procedure, use a knife to cut away any soft tissue that may interfere with the cutting action of the pruning shears. To free the rib cage from the thorax, cut away the diaphragm.

Note the placement, color, and condition of all thoracic organs, including the lungs, pericardium, and mediastinum. The *mediastinum* is the mass of tissue that separates the two halves of the thoracic cavity in the area of the thoracic inlet. Note the color and volume of any fluid. With both the thoracic and abdominal cavities open and before any tissue is handled, all specimens for microbiologic testing should be collected at this time. Next, examine the costochondral junctions (area on each rib where bone and cartilage meet).

Often the thoracic organs are removed intact as a group to maintain normal anatomic orientation. This method is often preferred over removing one organ at a time. Begin by inserting a knife at the mandibular symphysis. Incise on either side of the tongue. Free the tongue of all its attachments. Next, grasp the tongue and pull in the direction of the thoracic inlet (caudally) while cutting all dorsal attachments. As this is done, gradually strip the larynx, esophagus, and trachea away from the neck. As these are being stripped, you will encounter the hyoid bone at the base of the tongue, which supports the larynx. Use a knife to cut the hyoid bone at this cartilaginous joint on both sides of the larynx. Continue to strip out the larynx caudally. Note the condition of the tonsils within the dorsal wall of the pharynx (Fig. 6-17). While pulling caudally on the tongue, continue dissecting caudally down the neck. As the dissection continues, salivary glands, deeper lymph nodes, and the thymus can be seen.

Continue pulling the tongue caudally while cutting away any dorsal attachments. This frees the lungs, pericardium, heart, aorta, and vena cava. This large mass of tissues can be completely free from the cavity once it is cut away from the diaphragm. This mass or group of tissues is often referred to as the "thoracic pluck" and includes the tongue, esophagus, trachea, thyroid glands, lungs, heart, great vessels, and thymus.

In examining the thoracic viscera, follow a consistent routine, beginning with the tongue. Examine the surface or mucosa of the tongue for ulcers and areas of necrosis or dead tissue. Next, incise the tongue transversely, noting any color changes within the muscle. Then examine and remove the thyroids, parathyroids, and thymus. In most

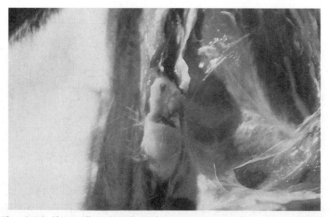

Fig. 6-16 The axillary lymph nodes are exposed when the accessible front leg is reflected laterally.

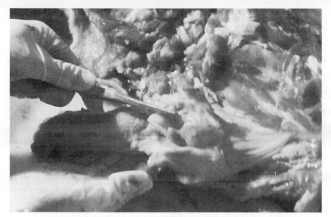

Fig. 6-17 The condition of the tonsils is noted while removing the thoracic pluck.

animals, the thyroid and parathyroid glands lie adjacent to the trachea, just caudal to the larynx, at the point of the fifth or sixth tracheal ring. The thyroid gland appears ovoid and is reddish brown. The parathyroid gland lies so closely to the thyroid that it is often difficult to differentiate; it is somewhat paler than the thyroid and much smaller. The thymus is a lymphoid organ located in the mediastinum. The thymus should be examined for its size in relation to the age of the animal. The thymus is relatively large in young animals but is usually very difficult to identify in older animals.

Use scissors to open the entire length of the esophagus. Examine its mucosal surface for parasites, ulcers, and marked changes in color. Next, incise the dorsal wall of the larynx with a knife. Use scissors to extend this incision into the trachea caudally as far as the two main bronchi of the lung. Examine the contents of the trachea. Often, if death was agonal (not sudden), large amounts of foam are noted along the entire length of the trachea.

Next, make a visual inspection of the lungs, noting their color. Carefully palpate all lobes of the lungs for firmness, crepitation, foreign bodies or abnormal masses, and weight. Going back to the main bronchus, use scissors to extend the incision into the bronchioles as far as possible. Incise into as many bronchioles as possible, looking for such abnormalities as excessive fluid and any lung parasites that may favor these terminal airways.

After the lungs have been completely examined, examine the heart. Carefully assess the transparency of the pericardium and its fluid content. Under normal circumstances, a small amount of clear fluid is present within this sac. Pericardial fluid of abnormal color and/or consistency or present in large volume is a significant finding. Next, incise into the pericardial sac and remove this covering from the heart (Fig. 6-18). Examine the heart, along with its vessels, for size, symmetry, color, and hemorrhage. Palpate the heart for firmness. The right and left sides of

the heart can be differentiated by the thickness of the ventricular walls. The right side is much thinner and more flaccid than the left.

The heart is most often examined by tracing the flow of blood. Begin on the right side and cut into the right auricle using a pair of scissors. This exposes the right atrium. Cutting parallel to the ventricular septum, continue this cut into the right ventricle, cutting toward the apex. Rotate the heart so that this cut can be directed parallel to the coronary groove. Continue to cut in this direction and cut through the tricuspid valve. Continue cutting past the tricuspid valve and into the pulmonary artery. Remove any clotted blood that may be present. Rotate the heart back to its original position and carefully examine the endocardium, valve leaflets, and major vessels. Trace the pulmonary artery, looking for heartworms.

Examine the left side of the heart by first cutting into the left auricle, exposing the left atrium. Next, make a single cut through the center of the left ventricular wall in the direction of the apex. With the apex oriented toward you, identify the septal leaflet of the atrioventricular valve. Cut through this leaflet and proceed through the bicuspid valves and into the aorta. Once again, carefully examine the endocardium, valves, and great vessels. After examining the heart, make several incisions into the myocardium, looking for any changes in color or texture.

Once the thoracic cavity has been completely examined and all necessary tissues collected, examine the abdominal cavity. Examine the liver first. Examine for size, color, and firmness. In addition, note the borders of the liver lobes. These borders should have sharp edges, as opposed to rounded edges. Next, gently squeeze the gallbladder. As you squeeze the gallbladder, bile should flow freely through the bile duct and into the duodenum. If this does not occur, there may be some type of biliary obstruction. Note any resistance to the outflow of bile. Next, remove the liver from the abdomen. Examine the hepatic parenchyma by making multiple parallel incisions (like slicing bread) into

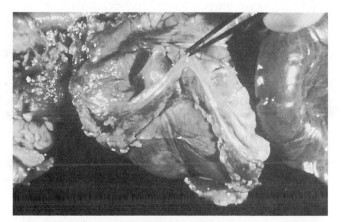

Fig. 6-18 Before examining the heart, remove the pericardial sac.

each lobe. There should be a lobular pattern throughout the liver.

Next, remove the spleen by cutting it away from the stomach. Examine the spleen for size, shape, color, and texture. Keep in mind that if the animal was euthanized with a barbiturate, the spleen will be somewhat enlarged. As with the liver, make multiple parallel incisions throughout the length of the spleen.

Before continuing with the kidneys, it is best to remove the entire alimentary tract from the abdominal cavity. The intestines should be set aside and examined later in the necropsy procedure. Now locate each kidney. The ovoid adrenal glands are often buried in fat and can be located by palpating dorsal and medial to the cranial poles of each kidney. The left adrenal gland is situated somewhat lateral to the aorta, while the right adrenal gland is situated near the dorsolateral aspect of the caudal vena cava. Carefully dissect through the fat and remove both adrenal glands. Make a transverse incision through each gland and examine for color, size, and shape. In addition, note the proportion of the tan adrenal cortex to the reddish-brown adrenal medulla.

Examine the kidneys next, noting their size, shape, and color. Before removing the kidneys, use blunt dissection to locate the ureters. Follow the ureters and examine distally to the point where they enter the bladder. Examine for stones, hydroureter, constrictions, and hemorrhage. Remove the left kidney and make a longitudinal incision through the entire organ with a knife. Examine the renal cortex, medulla, and pelvis. From the cut surface of the kidney, peel away its closely adhered transparent capsule. This capsule must be removed from the kidney to allow for fixation. This cut surface will demonstrate pinpoint indentations or tears, which represent normal vasculature. Examine the subcapsular surface. Repeat the same procedure for the right kidney.

Inspect the urinary bladder and its contents. The contents of the bladder may be withdrawn using a needle and syringe or expressed into a beaker. Incise the thick-walled bladder and examine its mucosal surface. Make impression smears of the bladder if you suspect canine distemper. These smears can be examined for inclusion bodies. Examine the reproductive system next. In the female, locate the oviduct and follow each uterine horn. Note the size of the ovaries and presence of follicles, corpora lutea, and cysts. Next, use the pruning shears and make a cut through the pubis. Separate these bones to expose the underlying vagina and rectum. Cut between the vulva and anus to free the caudal end of the vagina. Gently pull the vagina ventrally while severing the connective tissue that lies between it and the rectum. Continue to carefully dissect the area of the cervix while cutting away at its dorsal attachments.

In the male, incise the scrotum and examine both testes for comparable size and tumors. Note any cryptorchid testis. Also examine the tail of the epididymis and the prostate gland (Fig. 6-19). As in the female, use the pruning shears to cut through the pubic bones and expose the urethra and rectum. Open the urethra, beginning at the penile orifice, and trace it proximally to the prostate and into the bladder. Examine all serosal and mucosal surfaces.

Intestinal tract

To better visualize the segments of intestine, cut the entire mesentery at the point of the mesenteric lymph nodes, close to their attachment to the intestines. Note the size of these lymph nodes. This procedure frees the loops of the intestine from each other, allowing them to be laid out as one, long, tubular structure. Examine the serosal surface of the entire length of the intestines. Then, beginning at the esophageal opening, use a pair of scissors and cut along the greater curvature of the stomach. Examine the stomach contents as well as the mucosal surface of the stomach. Depressions on the mucosal surface may be erosions or ulcers. Also examine for parasites and foreign bodies. Next, remove the pancreas from the duodenum and note its color and size. Examine the pancreas for tumors or hemorrhage.

If sections of intestine are to be cultured, tie them off and remove these unopened segments before any further examination. As the remainder of the small and large intestines is opened, carefully examine their mucosal surfaces. Using scissors, continue cutting from the greater curvature of the stomach into the duodenum, followed by the jejunum, which makes up most of the small intestine. Continue this cut into the ileum and its attached cecum. This comma-shaped, blind sac marks the beginning of the large intestine. Continue cutting into the colon and proceed into the rectum. Collect any fecal samples at this terminal end.

Central nervous system

Every necropsy should include examination of the central nervous system. The clinical history dictates whether both

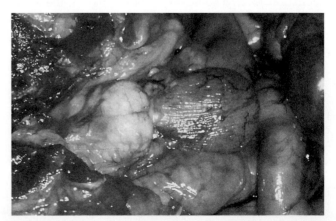

Fig. 6-19 In males, always examine the prostate gland as well as the urinary bladder.

the brain and spinal cord should be examined or the brain alone. Remove the head by using a knife to make a transverse cut through the muscle immediately caudal to the occipital protuberance and deep enough to expose the atlanto-occipital joint. Disarticulate the atlanto-occipital joint and detach the head from the body by cutting the loose muscle and skin.

Once the head is separated from the body, cut and reflect all remaining skin toward the eyes, completely exposing the skull. Cut and remove the temporal muscles on either side of the skull. To remove the *calvaria* (skullcap), up to three cuts are needed. Using a hammer and chisel, make a single transverse cut just caudal to the eyes, extending to both lateral margins of the orbits. At the lateral termination of this cut, make a second cut that extends caudally to the foramen magnum. Repeat this cut at the other lateral termination of the first cut. This third cut frees the calvaria from attachment so it can be easily removed. The exposed dura mater on the surface of the brain is visible as a semitransparent film. Carefully examine for opacity and hemorrhage. Use scissors to remove the dura mater covering both cerebral hemispheres and the cerebellum (Fig. 6-20). Next, examine the surface of the exposed brain for hemorrhage and tumors.

Use extreme care when removing the fragile brain. Begin by making a transverse cut across the olfactory lobes. Next, tip the skull so that the nose is pointed toward the ceiling and the head is resting on its occipital condyles. Allow gravity to pull the brain out of its cavity. Beginning at the olfactory lobes, use the handle of the scalpel to scoop out the brain. Once the optic nerves are visible, use the scalpel blade to cut them. With careful scooping, allow the brain to continue to fall out of its cavity. Remove the hypophysis, or pituitary gland, as intact as possible and attached to the brain. It can be removed from the fossa in which it sits with careful dissection using the scalpel blade. This takes some practice to achieve. As the brain continues to fall away, cut any nerves and attachments that prevent complete removal. At the point of the cerebellum, support

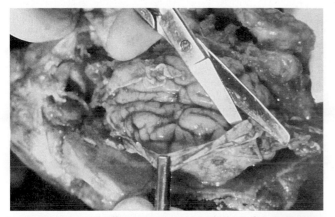

Fig. 6-20 Remove the dura mater to expose the brain for examination.

the brain with one hand to prevent it from falling to the floor. Examine the freed brain for size and shape. Unless indicated otherwise, fix the brain whole in formalin and do not section it.

If the spinal cord is to be examined, it can be removed by performing a dorsal laminectomy. Once the vertebrae are removed, the nerves must be cut to free the spinal cord. Before fixing the spinal cord in formalin, open the dura mater to expose the cord.

ANATOMIC VARIATIONS

Pigs

The two thyroid glands are somewhat fused, giving the appearance of one large gland. The deep purple thyroid glands of pigs are located in the area of the thoracic inlet. The tonsils of pigs are diffuse and located in the area of the epiglottis. This tissue is important for testing if pseudorabies is suspected. Always examine the nasal turbinates for evidence of atrophic rhinitis.

Cattle

The kidneys of cattle are lobulated and embedded in large amounts of fat, termed *capsula*. As mentioned earlier, the four stomach compartments of cattle and other ruminants are the rumen, reticulum, omasum, and abomasum. The rumen occupies most of the left half of the abdominal cavity. It is the first stomach compartment, where food is temporarily stored while undergoing fermentation before regurgitation and remastication. The rumen wall has folds called *pillars* that divide it into muscular sacs. The reticulum is the second of the four stomach compartments. It is the most cranial and the smallest. It has the appearance of a honeycomb. The omasum is the third compartment. From the greater curvature of the omasum extend hundreds of longitudinal folds. The abomasum is the fourth or "true" stomach of ruminants. The heart of cattle contains a bony structure called the *ossa cordis*. These bones develop in the aortic fibrous rings.

Horses

The guttural pouch is a ventral diverticulum of the eustachian tube, which drains the middle ear. This is often the site of mycotic or bacterial infections. Horses do not have a gallbladder. The large intestine of horses is divided into several anatomic areas. The cecum, about 120 cm in length, is curved somewhat like a comma, and is located to the right of the median plane. Four longitudinal bands along the cecum form four rows of sacculations. The great or large colon begins at the cecocolic orifice (located at the lesser curvature of the cecum) and terminates at the small colon. *In situ* (in the normal position), the great colon is

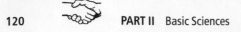

folded and divided into four portions, all of which are identified according to their position. The cranial mesenteric artery should be examined for possible strongyle migration.

RECOMMENDED READINGS

Alden CL: *Color atlas for small animal necropsy*, Lenexa, Kan, 1981, Veterinary Medicine Publishing.

Colville T, Bassert JM: *Clinical anatomy and physiology for veterinary technicians*, St Louis, 2002, Mosby.

Dyce KM: *Textbook of veterinary anatomy*, ed 3, Philadelphia, 2002, WB Saunders.

Feldman EC, Nelson RW: *Canine and feline endocrinology and reproduction*, ed 2, Philadelphia, 1996, WB Saunders.

Frandson RD et al: *Anatomy and physiology of farm animals*, ed 6, Philadelphia, 2003, Lippincott Williams & Wilkins.

Hafez ESE, Hafez B: *Reproduction in farm animals*, ed 7, Philadelphia, 2000, Lippincott Williams & Wilkins.

Hayes KEN: *The complete book of foaling*, ed 1, New York, 1993, Howell Book House.

Jones TC, Gleiser CA: *Veterinary necropsy procedures for the dog and cat*, Philadelphia, 1954, Lippincott.

McBride DF: *Learning veterinary terminology*, ed 2, St Louis, 2002, Mosby.

McKinnon AO, Voss JL: *Equine reproduction*, Philadelphia, 1993, Lea & Febiger.

Ruckebusch Y, et al: *Physiology of small and large animals*, St Louis, 1991, Mosby.

Siegal M: *Book of dogs*, ed 1, NY, 1995, HarperCollins.

Smith MC, Sherman DM: *Goat medicine*, ed 1, Philadelphia, 1994, Lea & Febiger.

Strafuss AC: *Necropsy: procedures and basic diagnostic methods for practicing veterinarians*, Springfield, Ill, 1988, Charles C. Thomas.

7

Nutrition

Sheila R. Grosdidier

Learning Objectives

After reviewing this chapter, the reader should understand the following:

- Basic energy-producing and non–energy-producing nutrients
- Considerations for feeding young and adult dogs
- Considerations for feeding young and adult cats
- Fundamentals of exotic pet diet considerations
- Nutritional peculiarities of livestock
- Methods used in feeding livestock

ENERGY-PRODUCING NUTRIENTS

The most common question in veterinary practices today is, "What should I feed my pet?" This common inquiry compels all members of the veterinary health care team to maintain a high level of current knowledge about the best feeding recommendations for pets. Veterinary clinical practice continues to successfully integrate the application of nutrition to include both the healthy and the ill patient. The quality of a pet's life can be dramatically influenced by the intake of nutrients balanced to its lifestyle and state of health.

A *nutrient* is any constituent of food that is ingested to support life. The six basic nutrients are proteins, fats, carbohydrates, water, vitamins, and minerals. *Energy-producing nutrients* have a hydrocarbon structure that produces energy through digestion, metabolism, or transformation. Energy is used for all metabolism, cell rejuvenation, maintenance of homeostasis, and production of new cells. *Non–energy-producing nutrients* play an important role throughout the body system and are often called the "gatekeepers of metabolism" (Box 7-1).

Proteins

Dietary protein is used to build body tissues. Amino acids, the building blocks of protein, are categorized into essential and nonessential types. *Essential amino acids* cannot be synthesized in the body and so must be supplied by the diet. *Nonessential amino acids* are synthesized in the body (Box 7-2). The proportion of essential and nonessential amino acids largely determines the quality, or biologic value, of a particular protein source. A protein's biologic value is reflected by the amount that is retained by the body after ingestion. A protein with a 100% biologic value is entirely retained by the body after ingestion. A protein of very low biologic value, such as 5%, is almost entirely excreted by the body after ingestion.

Fats

Vegetable and animal fats, oils, and lipids are composed of fatty acids and contain more energy per unit of weight than any other nutrient. There is a direct correlation between fat content and caloric density in a diet; the more fat there is in a diet, the more calories it contains. Cats require three essential fatty acids in their diet, whereas only two are essential in dogs (Box 7-3).

Carbohydrates

Carbohydrates are classified as *soluble* or *insoluble*, based on their digestibility. Mammals cannot digest insoluble carbohydrates, such as fiber, although bacteria can degrade fiber in the stomach of herbivores. Fiber decreases a diet's digestibility and caloric density. Fiber is added to a diet for treatment of obesity or management of gastrointestinal disorders. Soluble carbohydrates, such as sugar and starches, can be readily digested and are metabolized for energy needs.

The authors acknowledge and appreciate the original contribution of R. J. Van Saun and J. A. De Jong, whose work has been incorporated into this chapter.

Nutrients

Energy-producing

Fats
Carbohydrates
Proteins

Non–energy-producing

Water
Vitamins
Minerals

Essential Amino Acids

Arginine
Histidine
Isoleucine
Leucine
Lysine
Methionine
Phenylalanine
Threonine
Tryptophan
Valine
Taurine (cats; conditionally essential)

Essential Fatty Acids

Dogs

Linolenic
Linoleic

Cats

Linolenic
Linoleic
Arachidonic

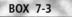

NON–ENERGY-PRODUCING NUTRIENTS

Water

Water provides the foundation for metabolism of all nutrients in the body. Minor alterations in the body's water content and distribution can result in dramatic alterations in nutritional requirements. Water balance in the system affects the ability to excrete waste into the urine by the kidneys. Water is also essential for absorption and metabolism of water-soluble vitamins B and C. Access to fresh, clean water is imperative for all animals. An animal's water needs may not be met if the water source freezes during inclement weather or if the water container is tipped over. It is important to educate clients on providing access to fresh, clean water in all seasons.

Vitamins

Vitamins play a very important role in maintaining normal physiologic functions. These organic molecules are required only in minute amounts to exert their function as coenzymes, enzymes, or precursors in metabolism. *Water-soluble vitamins* are passively absorbed from the small intestine, and excess amounts are excreted in the urine. *Fat-soluble vitamins* are metabolized in a manner similar to fats and stored in the liver. Because of this storage mechanism, toxicity from excessive intake of fat-soluble vitamins can occur. A deficiency of fat-soluble vitamins is not as common as with water-soluble vitamins (Box 7-4).

Minerals

Within the body, minerals are often distributed in ionized form as a cation or anion electrolyte. In this form they are involved with acid/base balance, clotting factors, osmolality, nerve conduction, muscle contraction, and a variety of other cellular activities.

Vitamins

Water-soluble

Thiamin
Riboflavin
Niacin
Pyridoxine
Pantothenic acid
Folic acid
Cobalamin
Vitamin C
Choline
L-carnitine

Fat-soluble

A
D
E
K

Deficiencies or excesses in mineral intake can lead to problems through imbalances. Minerals are closely interrelated, and an imbalance in one mineral can affect several others. Dietary minerals include calcium, phosphorus, potassium, sodium, chloride, magnesium, iron, zinc, copper, manganese, selenium, iodine, and boron.

FEEDING CONSIDERATIONS FOR DOGS

Contrary to popular belief, domestic dogs do not need variety in their diet. Frequent changes in diet have few positive effects, encourage finicky eating, and precipitate digestive disorders. It is best to consistently feed a diet formulated to meet the animal's needs at each stage of life. Regular assessment of weight can help determine the amount of feed. Weight loss or gain indicates a need to re-evaluate the amount being fed or diet selection. Body condition scoring is a valuable way to assess the appropriate amount of food; a review of the body condition scoring system can be found in Fig. 7-1.

Feeding Methods

Portion control

Portion control is currently the most popular way to feed dogs. After determining the animal's nutritional requirements, the daily portion is offered to the animal, either in a single feeding or divided into several portions offered several times per day. The animal is then allowed to consume the food throughout the day or during 5 to 10 minutes for each divided portion.

Free choice

In free-choice feeding, the animal is allowed access to food 24 hours per day. The food supply is replenished as needed. It may be difficult to detect subtle changes in food intake with this method. Free-choice feeding is not recommended for puppies and obese dogs, but it works well for cats.

Time control

In time-controlled feeding, a portion of food is offered and the animal is allowed access for only 5 or 10 minutes. Any remaining food is taken away after that time. Puppies are commonly fed in this manner.

Feeding the Gestating or Lactating Dog

The daily energy requirement during gestation in the bitch increases during the length of the pregnancy. While clients may have the impulse to dramatically increase food consumption, it is important to educate them on how to feed an appropriate amount. Excessive weight gain in the gestating bitch can make parturition more difficult and affect the overall health of the dog. The goal is to increase food intake gradually assessing weight gain carefully during the pregnancy. In the lactation phase, many dogs will require free feeding as they will need to eat smaller meals more frequently to reduce their absence from the puppies during this critical growth phase. Fig. 7-2 shows the relationship between body weight and food intake during lactation and gestation in the dog.

Feeding Puppies

With puppies born by cesarean section or if the bitch has no milk, the veterinary technician must intervene and provide nutritional support to neonatal puppies. Fortunately, they can be raised successfully on canine milk replacer. Cow's milk is not an acceptable substitute because it contains inappropriate levels of protein and lactose. Initially, it may be necessary to use orogastric intubation or a feeding syringe and then gradually adopt a regular small-animal feeding bottle as the puppies begin to thrive. Daily or twice-daily weighing and physical examination of the puppies helps identify problems early enough to adjust feeding protocols or begin other therapeutic measures to avoid mortality. Puppies typically gain 2 to 4 g/kg of anticipated adult weight each day; any variance in weight demands closer investigation. Some neonatal puppies fail to gain weight when nursing the bitch because they cannot compete with siblings for a nipple. Puppies in this situation tend to be restless and whimper inordinately. Normal weight can be restored by allowing such puppies to nurse the bitch without competition three to four times daily.

Weaning begins around 3 to 4 weeks of age in large-breed puppies and at 4 to 5 weeks of age in smaller breeds. To facilitate the transition to solid foods, begin by making a gruel or "slurry" of a growth type of diet. A gruel is created by mixing equal parts of food and water together to form a homogeneous consistency. The mixture should have the texture of cooked oatmeal. Puppies initially may play with or walk through the slurry, but eventually they consume it in increasing volumes. Gruel should be offered three to four times daily during the weaning process. Feed the puppy increasing amounts until the puppy can be maintained without nursing, at 5 to 7 weeks in large-breed puppies and at 6 to 7 weeks in smaller breeds. Once weaning is complete, decrease the volume of water added to the mixture until the puppy is eating the desired diet and voluntarily drinking water.

Feeding Adult Dogs

As a dog matures, be sure to monitor activity level and predisposition to obesity to preserve a neutral energy equilibrium. Reassess feeding methods, because inappropriate techniques commonly result in excessive nutrient intake and obesity. Review feeding habits with clients to preclude future problems (Box 7-5).

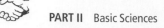

BODY CONDITION SCORING SYSTEM

Body condition assessment will assist the veterinary technician in determining if the puppy or kitten is growing appropriately and if the correct amount of food is being offered. Proper growth can reduce risk for obesity and growth related skeletal disease.

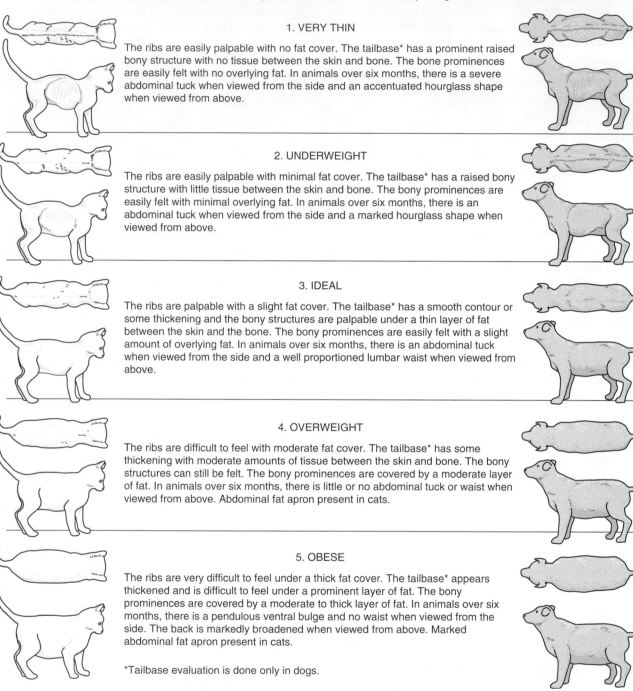

1. VERY THIN

The ribs are easily palpable with no fat cover. The tailbase* has a prominent raised bony structure with no tissue between the skin and bone. The bone prominences are easily felt with no overlying fat. In animals over six months, there is a severe abdominal tuck when viewed from the side and an accentuated hourglass shape when viewed from above.

2. UNDERWEIGHT

The ribs are easily palpable with minimal fat cover. The tailbase* has a raised bony structure with little tissue between the skin and bone. The bony prominences are easily felt with minimal overlying fat. In animals over six months, there is an abdominal tuck when viewed from the side and a marked hourglass shape when viewed from above.

3. IDEAL

The ribs are palpable with a slight fat cover. The tailbase* has a smooth contour or some thickening and the bony structures are palpable under a thin layer of fat between the skin and the bone. The bony prominences are easily felt with a slight amount of overlying fat. In animals over six months, there is an abdominal tuck when viewed from the side and a well proportioned lumbar waist when viewed from above.

4. OVERWEIGHT

The ribs are difficult to feel with moderate fat cover. The tailbase* has some thickening with moderate amounts of tissue between the skin and bone. The bony structures can still be felt. The bony prominences are covered by a moderate layer of fat. In animals over six months, there is little or no abdominal tuck or waist when viewed from above. Abdominal fat apron present in cats.

5. OBESE

The ribs are very difficult to feel under a thick fat cover. The tailbase* appears thickened and is difficult to feel under a prominent layer of fat. The bony prominences are covered by a moderate to thick layer of fat. In animals over six months, there is a pendulous ventral bulge and no waist when viewed from the side. The back is markedly broadened when viewed from above. Marked abdominal fat apron present in cats.

*Tailbase evaluation is done only in dogs.

Fig. 7-1 Body conditioning scoring system. *(Courtesy Hill's Pet Nutrition, Inc., Topeka, Kan.)*

Most dogs are managed efficiently through time-restricted meal feeding. Some dogs nibble throughout the day when offered food free choice. Daily energy requirements have been outlined in Fig. 7-3. Care should be taken in these situations to ensure that optimal body condition is maintained, with weight neither lost nor gained.

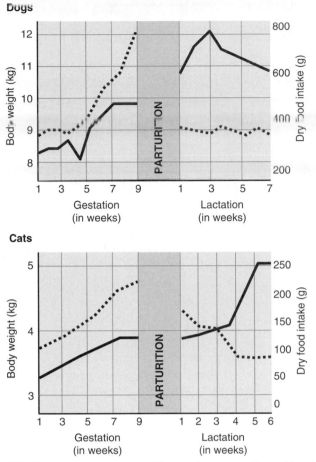

Fig. 7-2 The pattern of normal weight gain during gestation and loss in the postpartum and lactation periods differs between cats and dogs. *Solid line* indicates food intake. *Dashed line* indicates body weight. *(Courtesy Hill's Pet Nutrition, Inc., Topeka, Kan.)*

Feeding Active Dogs

Active dogs require energy to sustain hunting, obedience trial, or other activities. The diets for active dogs must have enhanced levels of fat, the most energy-dense nutrient, as well as increased total digestibility. Dogs that are only slightly more active than others need slightly more food, but working dogs with significant energy demands require a substantial increase in food portions. Any increase in food portions, to condition a dog for work, should be gradually instituted over a 7- to 10-day period. Hunting dogs should be fed just before a period of increased activity so as to avoid hypoglycemia.

Feeding Geriatric Dogs

Older dogs are less able to adjust to prolonged periods of poor nutrition. Any changes in an older dog's diet should be based on careful patient assessment and not solely on the

Recommended Feeding Practices for Dogs and Cats

Match the diet to the animal's stage of life
Feed for the ideal body weight
Measure the amount of food fed
Adjust the amount fed to the animal's body condition
Don't feed table scraps
Don't overfeed
Don't change the diet frequently
If the diet is to be changed, do so gradually over 3 to 5 days
Don't feed multiple animals from a single bowl
Treats should not comprise more than 10% of the diet
Use dry food ("kibble"), ice chips, and vegetables as treats
Deduct the amount fed as a treat from the total amount fed daily

dog's age. Dietary protein should be of high biologic value to reduce the level of metabolites that must be excreted through the kidneys. Dietary fats must be sufficiently digestible to provide adequate levels of essential fatty acids without an excess that could lead to obesity. Because of its detrimental effects on the kidneys, dietary phosphorus should be limited. Increased levels of zinc, copper, and vitamins A, B complex, and E may be required in the diet of older dogs.

Feeding Overweight Dogs

Obesity is the most common nutritional disorder of pets. Obesity places significant stress on the body system and may predispose to diabetes mellitus, cardiovascular disease, and skeletal problems. Early counseling of owners can alert them to weight gain. Educate clients on the potential adverse effects of weight gain. Additional considerations for feeding overweight pets can be found in Box 7-6.

A review of nutritional considerations for different life stages in the cat and dog can be found in Table 7-1.

FEEDING CONSIDERATIONS FOR CATS

Feeding Kittens

Kittens that are orphaned or born to queens unable to nurse must be hand-fed. Weaning should not commence until 7 weeks of age. Kittens can be gradually introduced to a diet by first offering a slurry of canned food mixed with kitten milk replacer. As with puppies, the amount of liquid is gradually reduced. Later they can be offered a dry diet if preferred.

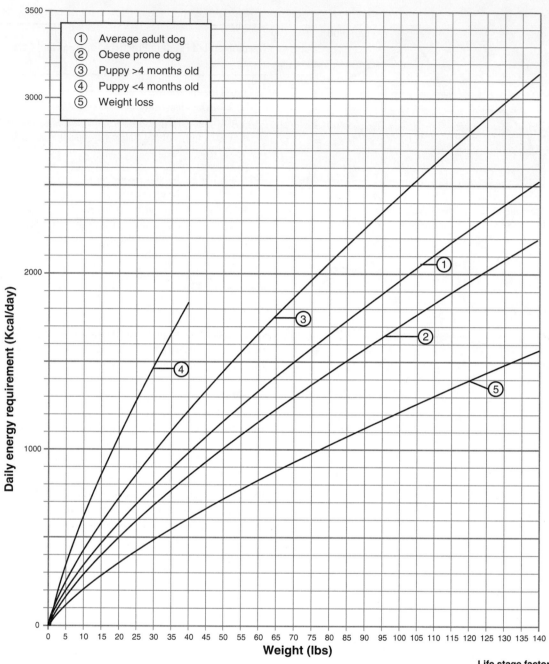

Figures calculated based on RER and life stage factor.

RER = 70 × (Wt [kg])$^{0.75}$

Daily energy requirement (Kcal/day) = RER × life stage factor

	Life stage factor
Average adult neutered dog	1.6
Geriatric dog	1.4
Obese prone	1.4
Weight loss	1.0
Early gestation	1.8
Late gestation	3.0
Lactation	Ad lib
Growth <4 months	3.0
Growth >4 months	2.0
Light work	2.0
Moderate work	3.0
Heavy work	4.0-8.0

Fig. 7-3 Canine daily energy requirements. *(Courtesy Hill's Pet Nutrition, Inc., Topeka, Kan.)*

BOX 7-6

Feeding

Match the diet to the animal's stage of life.	**Overweight Pets**
Feed for the ideal body weight.	Divide the total daily amount fed into multiple feedings throughout the day.
Measure the amount fed.	
Adjust the amount fed to the animal's body condition.	Use ice chips, carrots, celery, or weight-control diet kibble for treats.
Do not feed table scraps.	
Do not overfeed.	Treats should be less than 10% of dietary intake and counted as part of the daily caloric allowance.
Do not change the diet frequently.	
If the diet is to be changed, do so gradually, over 3 to 5 days.	Increase exercise.
Do not feed multiple animals from a single bowl.	Weigh the pet twice per month.
Treats should not comprise more than 10% of the diet.	Keep the pet out of the kitchen during meal preparation.
Use dry food ("kibble"), ice chips, and vegetables as treats.	Even a small amount of weight gain can affect a pet's well-being. Prevention is best.
Deduct the amount fed as a treat from the total amount fed daily.	

Feeding Adult Cats

Adult cats typically eat several small meals throughout a 24-hour period. Unfortunately, many clients provide food to their cats in unlimited amounts, filling the food dish each time their cat empties it. Such free-choice feeding predisposes to obesity. Overfeeding can be prevented by offering limited amounts of food throughout the day. This gives the cat the opportunity to nibble throughout the day while avoiding excessive caloric intake.

Caution owners against offering a constantly changing diet, such as various brands and types of commercial diets, because this can result in undesirable eating behavior.

Feeding Cats With Lower Urinary Tract Disease

Feline urinary tract disease is a complex disease characterized by bouts of frequent painful urination, bloody urine, and, in males, possible urethral obstruction. It tends to occur more often in obese, sedentary cats. Factors other than diet are involved in lower urinary tract disease, but careful attention to the diet of affected cats can help prevent future episodes.

Depending on the type of uroliths (small stones composed of cellular debris and mineral crystals) present in the urinary tract (struvite or calcium oxalate), prevention involves manipulation of dietary mineral, fiber, and water intake. Special commercial diets are available for dietary management of feline urologic syndrome.

Feeding Geriatric Cats

Because aging can diminish the senses of smell and taste, it is sometimes necessary to enhance the aroma and taste of foods to improve their palatability for aged cats. Successful techniques include warming canned food to body temperature in the microwave to improve the aroma, applying gar-lic powder to canned food before it is warmed, and addition of aromatic foodstuffs, such as clam juice or bits of canned fish.

Feeding the Gestating and Lactating Cat

Food intake for the gestating queen is not as dramatic as that found in the canine. Allow the queen to have free access to food during the last 30 days of gestation. Assess weight gain and body condition on a weekly basis to reduce the occurrence of excess weight gain. Free food should be available to the queen throughout lactation to assure ample milk availability to the kittens. Fig. 7-2 shows the relationship between food intake and body weight during lactation and gestation in the cat. Feline daily energy requirements have been calculated in Fig. 7-4.

PET FOOD CONSIDERATIONS

When a nutritional assessment is made for a pet, the need of fulfilling dietary requirements is only partially met by the veterinary health care team. To fully gratify all the dietary needs, it is also necessary to understand the broad assortment of types, classifications, and varieties of diets available commercially today. Often questions arise regarding effective techniques in comparing diets. The effective veterinary technician must be able to answer these questions with insight and full understanding of the pet's nutritional need.

To accurately appraise commercial diets for dogs and cats, it is consequential to obtain accurate information about the common pet foods that clients consider feeding and that are recommended by the veterinary practice. Attention by the veterinary technician should be made to

TABLE 7-1

Nutrient Considerations for Different Life Stages in Cats and Dogs

Life Stage	Food Characteristics	Comments
Cat Kittens 8 weeks to: year Gestation/lactation	Metabolizable energy 4.5 Kcal/g dry matter Digestibility < = 80% Protein 35%-50% Fat 17%-30% Fiber > = 5% Calcium/phosphorus ratio 1.0-1.8 to 0.8-1.5 Magnesium < = 20 mg/100 kcal	Transition the queen to a growth diet at 3 weeks of gestation.
Adult cat	Metabolizable energy 3.75 Kcal/g dry matter Digestibility > 78% Protein 0%-45% Fat 9%-25% Magnesium < 20 mg/100 Kcal	Ad-lib feeding is acceptable to kittens and queens. Free feeding adults may result in overnutrition.
Obese-prone cat	Metabolizable energy 3.50-3.75 Kcal/g dry matter Digestibility >75% Protein 30%-45% Fiber 7%-12% Fat 9%-25% Magnesium < 20 mg/100 Kcal	Feed multiple times (3-4) daily. Fiber provides satiety and decreased caloric density.
Geriatric cat	Metabolizable energy 3.75 Kcal/g dry matter Digestibility > 80% Protein 35%-45% Fiber 7%-12% Fat 9%-25% Magnesium < 20 mg/100 Kcal	Watch excess sodium and energy intake. Increased palatability may be needed.
Dog Puppies Gestation/lactation	Metabolizable energy > 3.9 Kcal/g of diet Digestibility > 80% Protein 27%-30% Fiber < 4% Fat 8%-20% Calcium/phosphorus 1.0-1.8 to 0.8-1.6	Avoid excessive weight during pregnancy. Puppies reach skeletal maturity at approximately 12 months of age.
Adult dog	Metabolizable energy > 3.5 Kcal/g of diet Digestibility > 75% Protein 15%-25% Fiber > = 5% Fat 7%-15%	Food and feeding consistency encouraged.
Obese-prone dog	Metabolizable energy < 3.5 Kcal/g of diet Digestibility > 80% Protein 15%-25% Fiber >5% Fat 6%-10%	Free feeding can contribute to obesity.
Increased activity or stressed dog	Metabolizable energy > 4.2 Kcal/g of diet Digestibility > 82% Protein 25%-32% Fiber < 4% Fat 23%-27%	
Geriatric dog	Metabolizable energy = 3.75 Kcal/g of diet Digestibility > 80% Protein 14%-21% Fiber > 4% Fat 10%-12% Control sodium	The average small-medium breed dog is considered geriatric after 7 years. Giant and large breeds are geriatric at 5 years of age.

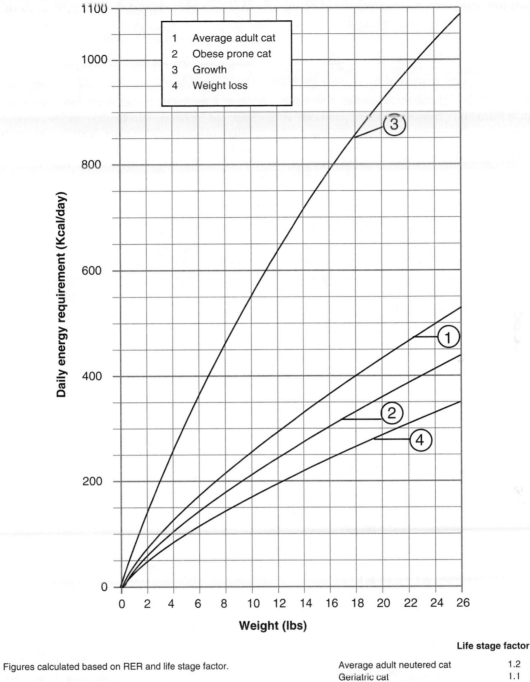

	Life stage factor
Average adult neutered cat	1.2
Geriatric cat	1.1
Obese prone	1.0
Weight loss	0.8
Early gestation	1.6
Late gestation	2.0
Lactation	Ad lib
Growth	2.5

Figures calculated based on RER and life stage factor.

$RER = 70 \times (\, Wt \, [kg] \,)^{0.75}$

Daily energy requirement (Kcal/day) = RER × life stage factor

Fig. 7-4 Feline daily energy requirements. *(Courtesy Hill's Pet Nutrition, Inc., Topeka, Kan.)*

build a comprehensive collection of information to have available when clients' questions originate.

Occasionally, clients inquire regarding their potential to produce a homemade diet. This presents a multifaceted dilemma due to the difficulty in maintaining balance from batch to batch. Most homemade diet recipes have not been analyzed for adequacy, possess ingredients often hard to come by, and are hard to reproduce consistently. Clients should be alerted to these concerns and reminded of the reliability and convenience of many commercial pet foods available today.

Assessing pet food begins with making an overview of general considerations then to more specific evaluations as the diet continues to meet nutritional expectations. The following section is a review of common questions to assist in effective comparisons and determinations of pet foods. It is essential to review the information available on a pet food to assess its ability to meet the needs of pets during different stages of life. A review of information available on a pet food label is shown in Fig. 7-5.

Does This Pet Food Produce the Desired Results?

Questions about fecal consistency, quality of product, and physiological response to a diet from previous recommendations should also become part of the information retained at the veterinary clinic regarding diet comparisons that must be answered by assessment of clinical trial and experience. Keeping records of this valuable information is important to be able to draw upon in the future.

Pet foods should also be tested by AAFCO (Association of American Feed Control Officials). AAFCO provides a resource to formulate uniform and equitable regulations and policies. These laws apply to ingredient definitions, labeling, and feeding trials. Diets to be considered for veterinary clinic recommendation should be tested by AAFCO with approved feeding trials to substantiate adequacy in actual application of the diet to a particular species and life stage as it is intended to be fed.

How Do You Choose What Pet Food to Feed?

Decisions on feeding for pets must be based on activity level, breed, age, health status, and reproductive condition (spayed or neutered). Considerations must be made about what will provide the pet with a consistent, high-quality and balanced diet that produces the best results in the pet. Periodically, a diet should be re-evaluated to verify it's appropriateness for the pet and that the right amount is being fed.

Can I Free Feed My Pet?

Allowing pets free access to food at any time increases the incidence of excess caloric intake that leads to obesity. In most situations, free feeding should be discouraged. Free feeding may be acceptable for cats that are able to maintain their weight without obesity, lactating females, and particularly fussy pets. The goal is to maintain optimal weight.

Which is Better to Feed—Canned or Dry?

While canned food has greater palatability, there are some concerns regarding dental health. For that purpose, dry food may be a better choice. Some pets that are finicky may find canned food to their preference over dry food. If

EVALUATING PET FOOD LABELS

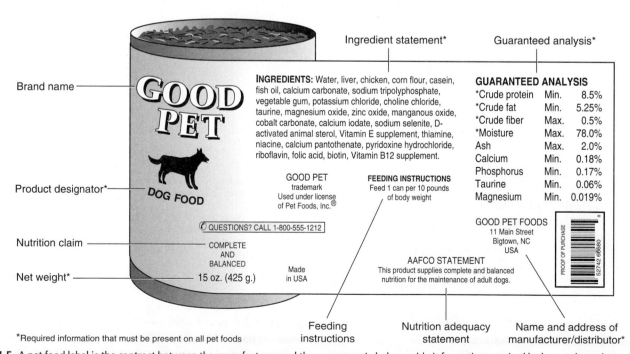

Fig. 7-5 A pet food label is the contract between the manufacturer and the consumer. Labels provide information required by law and may have optional information, such as feeding instructions. *(Courtesy Hill's Pet Nutrition, Inc., Topeka, Kan.)*

caloric intake falls in a pet, increasing palatability can assist in rectifying the situation. It is also important to rule out the presence of disease if a pet's feeding habits change. Palatability of a diet can be enhanced by warming canned food to body temperature or by adding warm water to dry food as well as using a small amount of fat/oil as a top dressing for dogs. Additional palatability factors can be found in Box 7-7.

NUTRITIONAL SUPPORT FOR ILL OR DEBILITATED PATIENTS

Proper nutritional support is an important aspect of therapy for hospitalized patients. Sick or injured patients need good nutritional support to counteract the immunosuppressive effects of sepsis, neoplasia, chemotherapy, anesthesia, and surgery. This support enhances wound healing and minimizes the length of hospitalization without significant weight loss and muscle atrophy. Initiation of nutritional support early in the course of hospitalization is crucial for a successful outcome.

Nutritional status should be assessed when the patient is admitted into the hospital and daily during hospitalization. During the physical examination, the patient's weight is recorded and compared with that of previous visits. A history from the owners regarding type of food, quantity fed, and frequency of feeding is helpful. During hospitalization, the patient is a candidate for nutritional support if the following occurs:

- The patient loses more than 10% of body weight.
- The patient has a decreased appetite or anorexia.
- The patient loses body condition from vomiting, diarrhea, trauma, or wounds.
- The patient has increased needs because of fever, sepsis, wounds, surgery, low serum albumin, organ dysfunction, or chronic disease.

Unfortunately, nutritional support in hospitalized patients is often delayed because the patient is not reassessed daily for nutritional needs, the amount of food a patient consumes is not recorded, the patient is not weighed daily, and dextrose and electrolyte solutions are erroneously thought to provide adequate nutritional support. Most previously healthy dogs can go approximately 1 week without nutritional support and suffer few ill effects. Cats, however, especially overweight cats, can go only a few days without nutritional support before ill effects develop, such as hepatic lipidosis. Nutritional support is often the last consideration when evaluating a patient's daily treatment regimen, until the patient does not recover as quickly as expected. The goal of nutritional support is to provide the patient's nutritional requirements while it is recovering from its disease process and/or anorexia, trauma, or surgery, until the patient is able to eat enough on a regular basis to accommodate any ongoing losses. With nutritional support, patients can gain weight and have an improved response to medical or surgical therapy.

The route of nutritional support administration can be enteral, parenteral, or a combination of both. Enteral feeding may be accomplished with orogastric, nasogastric, nasoesophageal, pharyngostomy, gastrostomy, and jejunostomy tubes. Parenteral nutrition is administered via a catheter placed in the cranial or caudal vena cava. The route selected depends on such factors as function of the gastrointestinal (GI) tract, the disease process, duration of support, equipment and personnel available to provide the necessary support, and cost of the chosen method. Enteral support is chosen most often because it is physiologically sound, easy, relatively free of complications, and inexpensive. If the gastrointestinal tract is functional and the patient can swallow, use as much as possible. Parenteral support should be used if the patient has a medical or surgical condition that prevents ingestion or digestion of nutrients (e.g., vomiting, diarrhea, ileus, pancreatitis, malabsorption, reconstructive surgery, coma), and as adjunctive therapy for patients with organ failure or when malnutrition is severe.

Enteral Nutritional Support

Hand feeding favorite foods and tempting with warm, odoriferous foods in multiple, small meals can be used in conjunction with other methods of nutritional support. Forced feeding can be stressful to the patient and may deliver only a portion of the nutrition required for recovery.

Orogastric intubation is excellent for rapid administration but can cause aspiration and trauma and is very stressful for patients other than neonates. This method is for short-term use only.

Placement of a nasoesophageal or nasogastric tube is an easy, simple, and relatively inexpensive procedure that allows liquid nutritional support for an extended time and can be easily administered by the owner at home for continued convalescence (Box 7-8).

A nasoesophageal or nasogastric tube is placed through the nasal cavity into the distal esophagus or stomach to

---

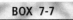

BOX 7-7

Palatability Factors

Texture
Odor
Temperature
Fat/protein levels
Moisture content
Shape of dry food (cats)
Acidity (cats)

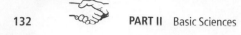

BOX 7-8

Methods of Enteral Feeding

Oral feeding (increased palatability)
Oral feeding (forced feeding)
Orogastric tube feeding
Nasogastric tube feeding
Pharyngostomy tube feeding
Esophagostomy tube feeding
Gastrostomy tube feeding
Jejunostomy tube feeding

---

bypass the oral cavity (Box 7-9). Placement is contraindicated in patients with nasal masses, esophageal disorders (e.g., megaesophagus), or no gag reflex. A nasoesophageal or nasogastric tube can usually be placed without chemical restraint (ideal for animals unable to tolerate general anesthesia). It is tolerated by most patients and used when the animal is anorexic, too stressed for forced feeding, and not

receiving enough nutrition through hand feeding. The tube can remain in place for a week or longer, until the patient's appetite increases or the oral cavity can be used again. Feedings through the tube can start immediately after placement, unlike pharyngostomy or gastrostomy tubes. Have the patient in a sitting position when tube feeding. Common problems with nasoesophageal or nasogastric tubes include epistaxis (nosebleed) when the tube is first placed, accidental placement in the trachea, patient intolerance of the tube, and tube obstruction by medications or diet.

Soft, flexible pediatric feeding tubes, red rubber tubes, and seamless polyurethane tubes, in a variety of lengths and diameters, are used for cats and dogs. Animals weighing less than 5 kg require a 5-French feeding tube, whereas some cats and all dogs weighing 5 to 15 kg can accept an 8-French tube. In larger dogs, the larger-diameter feeding tubes require a guidewire for placement in the esophagus or stomach.

For nasoesophageal placement with the tube tip at the level of the midthoracic esophagus, measure from the tip of the nose to the eighth or ninth rib (Fig. 7-7). For

---

BOX 7-9   *procedure*

Nasoesophageal Tube Placement

1. Restrain the animal in sternal recumbency or sitting, with the head held level or slightly elevated. Anesthetize the nostril with a few drops of topical ophthalmic anesthetic. While waiting for the topical anesthetic to take effect, lubricate the tip of the feeding tube with a water-soluble lubricant or 5% lidocaine jelly.

2. Place the tip of the tube in the nares and direct the tube dorsomedial to the alar fold. After the tip has been inserted 1 or 2 cm into the nostril, direct the tube caudoventrally into the esophagus.

3. When the tube is inserted to the premeasured line, infuse a small amount of sterile saline into the tube. If coughing occurs, the tube is probably in the trachea. Remove and reinsert the tube. If no coughing occurs, aspirate the syringe. If air is removed from the tube, the tube could be in the trachea. If negative pressure is evident, the tube is in the esophagus. If fluid is aspirated, the tube is in the stomach. If there is any question of tube location, make a lateral radiograph to determine placement.

4. Move the proximal end of the tube laterally alongside the nares, place a small strip of elastic tape around the tube, and either suture or glue it alongside the nares. The tube may be sutured without tape using a series of handties around the tube. Move the tube caudally between the eyes (alongside the dorsal nasal midline) and suture or glue (Fig. 7-6). Cap the end of the tube to prevent air from entering.

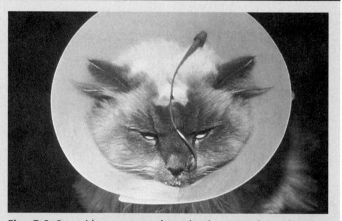

Fig. 7-6 Cat with a nasoesophageal tube sutured in place. An Elizabethan collar has been applied to prevent dislodgment of the tube. *(Courtesy Dr. Nancy Poy, Michigan State University.)*

5. Apply an Elizabethan collar to prevent the patient from removing the feeding tube (see Fig. 7-6). Evaluate the sutures or glue at each feeding to ensure that the tube is stable and not malpositioned.

6. To remove the tube, flush the tube with air to clear fluid out of the tube. Remove the sutures or gently pull the glued tube away from the skin, and pull the tube out of the nose.

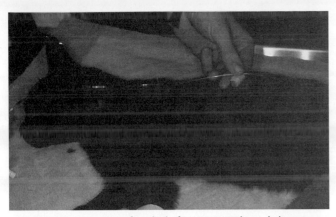

Fig. 7-7 Measurement of a tube before nasoesophageal placement.

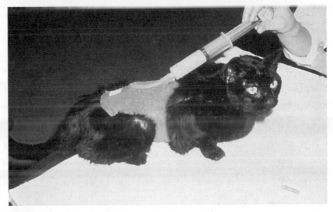

Fig. 7-8 Feeding through a gastrostomy tube. *(Courtesy Dr. Nancy Poy, Michigan State University.)*

nasogastric placement, measure from the tip of the nose to the thirteenth rib to assure safety in its position. Occasionally, tubes placed in the stomach may cause gastroesophageal reflux and irritation, but this is usually not a problem with a small-diameter tube. Mark the premeasured length on the tube with a permanent marker.

For nasoesophageal tube feeding, aspirate the tube before each feeding. If air is aspirated, do not feed. During aspiration, there should be negative pressure on the syringe if the tube is correctly placed. Accidental tracheal intubation can cause aspiration pneumonia. Before each feeding, also assess tube location by injecting 3 ml of sterile water through the tube and listening for coughing or gagging. If this occurs, do not administer the feeding; remove the tube.

A pharyngostomy tube is placed through the wall of the pharynx into the esophagus or stomach, bypassing the oral cavity. Placement requires general anesthesia and surgery. The many possible complications (e.g., esophagitis, pharyngitis, laryngitis, vomiting, regurgitation, aspiration pneumonia) and the difficulty of pharyngostomy tube placement outweigh the benefits.

A jejunostomy tube is a feeding tube surgically placed in the mid- to distal duodenum or proximal jejunum, bypassing the stomach. Continuous feeding of easily digestible diets through the jejunostomy tube requires prolonged hospitalization, without the benefits of home care. This procedure is rarely used because of the cost of placement and maintenance and possible complications.

A gastrostomy tube is placed through the body wall into the lumen of the stomach, bypassing the mouth and esophagus (Fig. 7-8). A gastrostomy tube is used for patients requiring long-term nutritional supplementation because of orofacial neoplasia, surgery or trauma, esophageal disorders, or liver disease. The diet can be easily prepared and administered by the owner, increasing owner compliance. The tube's bulb or mushroom tip helps retain the tube in the desired location. Gastrostomy tubes can be placed with

use of endoscopic equipment (i.e., percutaneous endoscopic gastrostomy) or without endoscopic equipment (i.e., blind percutaneous gastrostomy). Placement requires general anesthesia and trained personnel.

Enteral Nutrition Daily Caloric Requirements

Diet selection is based on caloric density, diameter of the feeding tube, and daily caloric needs of the patient. Each illness is assigned a factor to increase the calculated estimate of the patient's basal energy requirements by 25% to 75% (Figs. 7-9 and 7-10). The volume and consistency of the diet are limited by the size of the animal's stomach and diameter of the feeding tube, but total caloric requirements can usually be delivered when using a calorically dense diet. Stomach volume is approximately 20 ml/kg body weight. Daily water requirement is 12 ml/kg.

Patients with a nasoesophageal or nasogastric tube require a liquid diet (because of small tube diameter). Human enteral feeding products are easily administered through these tubes but are not developed for veterinary patients and may need supplementation with additional nutrients. Hyperosmolar diets can cause diarrhea. Liquid veterinary products, such as CliniCare Canine and CliniCare Feline, are available. Also, canned diets, such as Hill's a/d and Eukanuba Nutritional Recovery Formula, can be delivered through a feeding tube as small as 8-French.

Select the appropriate diet of canned food, and calculate the caloric density (kcal/ml) of the diet based on information on the label or supplied by the manufacturer. The total volume (ml) to be delivered per day is calculated by using the maintenance energy requirement (MER) and caloric density (Box 7-10).

For anorexic patients, after placement of the tube, the volume fed is gradually increased over 3 days, with 5 ml of water administered through the tube every 2 hours for 12 hours. Change to the selected diet, and double the volume

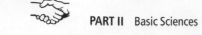

MICHIGAN STATE
U N I V E R S I T Y

Veterinary Teaching Hospital
East Lansing, Michigan 48824-1314

TPN WORKSHEET FOR DOGS

Date:_____

Body weight_____ kg.

1. Basal energy requirement (BER)
   BER = (30 × body weight in kg) + 70 = _____ kcal/day (for animals >2 kg)
   　　　or 70 (body weight in kg)$^{0.75}$　= _____ kcal/day (for animals <2 kg)

2. Maintenance energy requirement (MER)
   - cage rest:　　　　　　　　　　MER = 1.25 × BER
   - post surgery:　　　　　　　　MER = 1.35 × BER
   - major trauma, neoplasia:　　MER = 1.5　× BER
   - sepsis, major burn:　　　　　MER = 1.75 × BER

   MER = _____ × _____ (BER) = _____ Kcal/day (provided as non-protein calories)

3. Protein requirement (renal failure see below)
   - Adult dogs =　　　　　　　　4 gm/100 Kcal/day
   - Dogs with extra protein losses =　6 gm/100 Kcal/day

   _____ (4-6 gm) × _____ (Kcal from step 2) divided by 100 = _____ gm/day

4. Volume of solutions needed****
   - Dextrose 50% = 1.7 Kcal/ml (to provide 50% of Kcal/day from step 2)
     　　　　_____ Kcal/day ÷ 2 = _____ Kcal ÷ 1.7 = _____ ml Dextrose 50%
     (On day 1 use ½ of dextrose increase day 2 if blood glucose <200 mg/dl)
   - Lipid 20% = 2 Kcal/ml (to provide 50% of Kcal/day from step 2)
     　　　　_____ Kcal/day ÷ 2 = _____ Kcal ÷ 2　= _____ ml Lipid 20%
   - Amino Acid 8.5% with electrolytes = 0.085 gm/ml
     　　　　　　　　　　　_____ gm/day ÷ 0.085 = _____ ml A.A. 8.5%
   - Additional fluids (LRS)　　　　　　　　　　　　　= _____ ml LRS
     　　　　　　　　　　　　　　Total Volume　= _____ ml
     　　　　　　　　Rate = total volume ÷ 24　= _____ ml/hr
   - Add multivitamin (MVC) 3 ml/1000 ml total volume　= _____ ml MVC

****Note:　　For volumes >300 ml round off volume to nearest 100 ml
　　　　　　For volumes <300 ml round off volume to nearest 10 ml

Renal Failure Patients:　　1. Use Amino Acid without Electrolytes 2 gm/100 Kcal
　　　　　　　　　　　　　2. Add 20 ml TPN electrolytes II/1000 ml total volume

References:
   - Remillard RL, Thatcher CD: Parenteral nutrition support in the small animal patient. Vet. Clin. North Am. Sm. Animal Pract. 19:1287, 1989.
   - Lippert AC, Armstrong PJ: Parenteral nutrition support. CVT X, 1989, pp 25-30.
   - Lewis LD, Morris ML, Hand MS: Small animal clinical nutrition III, 1990, Ch 5, pp 2-43.
   - Remillard RL, Martin RA: Nutritional support in the surgical patient. Semin. Vet. Surg. 5:197, 1990.

Fig. 7-9 Worksheet used to calculate fluid requirements for total parenteral nutrition in dogs. *(Courtesy Michigan State University Veterinary Teaching Hospital.)*

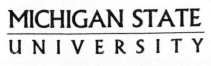

Veterinary Teaching Hospital
East Lansing, Michigan 48824-1314

TPN WORKSHEET FOR CATS

Date:_____

Body weight_____ kg.

1. Basal energy requirement (BER)
   BER = (30 × body weight in kg) + 70 = _____ kcal/day (for cats >2 kg)
   or 70 (body weight in kg)$^{0.75}$ = _____ kcal/day (for cats <2 kg)

2. Maintenance energy requirement (MER)
   - cage rest: MER = 1.25 × BER
   - post surgery: MER = 1.35 × BER
   - major trauma, neoplasia: MER = 1.5 × BER
   - sepsis, major burn: MER = 1.75 × BER

   MER = _____ × _____ (BER) = _____ Kcal/day (protein and non-protein calories)

3. Protein requirement (renal failure see below) 6 gm/100 Kcal/day
   6 gm × _____ (Kcal/day from step 2) divided by 100 = _____ gm/day

4. _____ gm/day of protein × 4 Kcal/gm = _____ Kcal from protein
   MER - Kcal from protein = _____ Kcal to be provided by non-protein (Dextrose & Lipid)

5. Volume of solutions needed****
   - Dextrose 50% = 1.7 Kcal/ml (to provide 50% of non-protein Kcal/day from step 4)

     _____ Kcal/day ÷ 2 = _____ Kcal ÷ 1.7 = _____ ml Dextrose 50%

     (On day 1 use ½ of dextrose increase day 2 if blood glucose <200 mg/dl)
   - Lipid 20% = 2 Kcal/ml (to provide 50% of non-protein Kcal/day from step 4)

     _____ Kcal/day ÷ 2 = _____ Kcal ÷ 2 = _____ ml Lipid 20%
   - Amino Acid 8.5% with electrolytes = 0.085 gm/ml

     _____ gm/day ÷ 0.085 = _____ ml A.A. 8.5%
   - Additional fluids (LRS)   = _____ ml LRS
                                      Total Volume = _____ ml
                          Rate = total volume ÷ 24 = _____ ml/hr
   - Add multivitamin (MVC) 3 ml/1000 ml total volume = _____ ml MVC

****Note: For volumes >300 ml round off volume to nearest 100 ml
             For volumes <300 ml round off volume to nearest 10 ml

Renal Failure Patients: 1. Use Amino Acid without Electrolytes 2 gm/100 Kcal
                           2. Add 20 ml TPN electrolytes II/1000 ml total volume

References:
- Remillard RL, Thatcher CD: Parenteral nutrition support in the small animal patient. Vet. Clin. North Am. Sm. Animal Pract. 19:1287, 1989.
- Lippert AC, Armstrong PJ: Parenteral nutrition support. CVT X, 1989, pp 25-30.
- Lewis LD, Morris ML, Hand MS: Small animal clinical nutrition III, 1990, Ch 5, pp 2-40.
- Remillard RL, Martin RA: Nutritional support in the surgical patient. Semin. Vet. Surg. 5:197, 1990.

Fig. 7-10 Worksheet used to calculate fluid requirements for total parenteral nutrition in cats. *(Courtesy Michigan State University Veterinary Teaching Hospital.)*

BOX 7-10

Enteral Feeding Calculation

Calculate Resting Energy Requirement (RER):

$$RER = 70 \times bw \text{ (body weight in kg)}$$

Calculate Illness/Infection/Injury Energy Requirements (IER):

$$Factor = 1.2 - 1.5$$

Multiply chosen factor by RER to equal IER:
Choose a veterinary-specific critical care formula.
Calculate the volume of diet required, and identify amount of Kcals per ml:

$$IER/Kcals \text{ per ml} = ml \text{ of diet per day}$$

Calculate the number and volume of feedings:

$$ml \text{ of diet per day/number of feedings per day} = ml \text{ diet/feeding}$$

to 10 ml every 2 hours for 12 to 24 hours. Gradually increase the volume to achieve full caloric intake, divided into four to six feedings per day, by the third day. For patients with delayed or inadequate gastric emptying, a meal may need to be skipped, or smaller, more frequent feedings administered if too much food remains in the stomach. If the patient vomits, skip the next scheduled feeding and adjust the amount, rate, and frequency of the feeding.

To prepare the diet using canned food, place one can of food in a blender and add enough water to achieve a consistency that will pass through a large-bore nasogastric tube or a gastrostomy tube. You can also use dry food by allowing the food to soak thoroughly in water before blending. The mixture must be blended well and then strained twice to remove any large chunks that would occlude the feeding tube. All food should be able to pass through a syringe without occluding the tip. For example, one can of Hill's Feline p/d mixed with 340 ml of warm water is of the consistency to pass through the feeding tube; it has a caloric density of 0.8 kcal/ml.

The volume of water added to the canned food when blended is usually adequate for the patient's water requirement. All feedings should be administered slowly, at room temperature. Hill's a/d and Iams Eukanuba Nutritional Recovery Formula can be given straight out of the can through an 8-French feeding tube, at room temperature or slightly warmed, with no premixing with water. The a/d provides 1.2 kcal/ml, and Nutritional Recovery Formula provides 2.1 kcal/ml. If a smaller-diameter tube is used, mixing two 5.5-oz. cans of a/d with 50 ml of water

provides a caloric density of 1.0 kcal/ml. Flush the tube with 5 or 10 ml of water after each feeding to prevent tube occlusion.

Animals with feeding tubes in place should be offered fresh food before each feeding once the oral cavity and esophagus can be used. Most animals begin to eat with the feeding tube still in place. When the animal begins to voluntarily eat at least half of its maintenance energy requirement daily, the amount of food given through the feeding tube can be decreased until the patient is consuming its full caloric intake per os. The change from enteral feedings to the normal diet should be gradual over 3 to 5 days if the patient's normal diet is not used for enteral feedings.

Clients can be instructed on how to feed their animal through the tube at home, if necessary. Ease of administration, minimal maintenance, and owner compliance makes this method of nutritional support a viable alternative for patient care in a nonhospital situation.

Parenteral Nutritional Support

Patients that cannot receive enteral nutrients must be supported by total parenteral nutrition (TPN), which involves intravenous infusion of nutrient solutions. This is a practical alternative for patients that cannot absorb nutrients through the GI tract (e.g., malabsorption), require rest of the GI tract (e.g., vomiting due to severe pancreatitis), cannot swallow (e.g., comatose patients), or are so debilitated that additional nutrition must be administered by another route.

Carbohydrates are administered in the form of dextrose. The most common concentration used is 50% dextrose, which provides 1.7 kcal/ml. Dextrose and lipids each provide 50% of the canine patient's daily MER. Dextrose and lipids are used in a 1:1 ratio to meet the MER (see Figs. 7-9 and 7-10).

Gradual introduction of dextrose is necessary to avoid hyperglycemia. On the first day of TPN, only half of the calculated amount of dextrose is administered. If the patient's urine glucose remains negative and the blood glucose level is below 200 mg/dl, the entire calculated dose of dextrose can be administered on day two. Occasionally, a patient requires addition of insulin to the TPN solution. This should be added immediately before administration of the parenteral nutrition.

Lipids (including essential fatty acids) provide the fat required by the patient. These are available in 10% and 20% solutions, with 20% more commonly used. Made of soybean or safflower oil, egg yolk phospholipids, and glycerol, they provide a concentrated energy source that supplies 50% of the patient's energy requirements. Visually checking the patient's plasma for lipemia on a daily basis can help decrease hyperlipidemia. Patients with hepatic, pancreatic, or endocrine disease may develop hyperlipidemia. For patients with severe hyperlipidemia, decrease the rate of infusion or the concentration of the lipids, or discontinue use of lipids altogether.

Proteins are supplied in the form of crystalline amino acids, made of essential and nonessential amino acids, available in a variety of concentrations, with or without electrolytes. The most common concentration used is 8.5% with electrolytes. The basic solutions of amino acids contain all of the essential amino acids required by dogs and cats, except taurine. If TPN is to be continued for longer than 1 week, supplementation of taurine is essential in cats. For patients with renal or hepatic insufficiency, reduced amounts of amino acids or specially formulated amino acid products should be administered.

Electrolytes can be included in the amino acid solutions. This is usually sufficient to maintain a normal electrolyte balance. Hypokalemia is the most common electrolyte abnormality. For patients with ongoing potassium losses (e.g., vomiting), additional supplementation may be necessary. If the patient is in renal failure, amino acids are administered without electrolytes.

Vitamins are administered as a multivitamin supplement. B complex vitamins should be added daily to the feeding solution. Vitamin K is incompatible with parenteral solutions and should be administered by subcutaneous or intramuscular injection only if parenteral nutrition is continued longer than 1 week.

Trace elements only need to be supplemented if long-term (more than 1 week) parenteral nutritional support is needed. Zinc may need to be supplemented after 1 week in patients with GI disease. Phosphorus may be added for diabetics.

Figs. 7-9 and 7-10 show how to calculate daily TPN feeding requirements for dogs and cats. The total daily fluid volume for maintenance TPN is 30 ml/lb of body weight. If the total volume of TPN is less than the calculated required amount, add an additional amount of balanced electrolyte solution or sterile water to equal the calculated fluid requirements. If the patient is experiencing ongoing fluid losses, a second catheter or an additional lumen on a central catheter can be used to deliver the fluids.

When mixing the appropriate solutions, strict asepsis is essential. Using a laminar flow hood, an automatic mixing pump, or an "all-in-one" bag will help keep contamination to a minimum. Add the dextrose and amino acids before the lipids to prevent lipid destabilization. Add the water or electrolyte solutions next, and any vitamins last.

Parenteral nutrition is administered via a catheter in the cranial or caudal vena cava. A double-lumen catheter is of benefit if additional medication, fluids, blood products, or blood sampling are needed. Administration by a fluid pump is the most accurate method of delivering parenteral nutrition.

Many complications of parenteral nutrition involve problems with the catheter. Sepsis is another complication of parenteral nutrition. Nutrient solutions are an excellent growth medium for bacteria. Contamination of the solutions, lines, or catheters can cause fever, depression, and pain or swelling at the catheter insertion site. Daily patient monitoring can help eliminate or minimize this complication. Administering TPN through a "dedicated" IV line can decrease the likelihood of sepsis. The catheter should be used for parenteral nutrition only, and not for blood sampling, medication administration, or CVP monitoring. New bags of TPN solution should be made daily for the patient and hung for a maximum of 24 hours at room temperature before changing to another bag. All administration lines should be changed every 48 hours when the bag is changed. The catheter bandage should be replaced whenever it is soiled, as well as every 48 hours, when the administration lines are changed.

Gradually tapering off of TPN can prevent hypoglycemia. If TPN must be discontinued abruptly, use a 5% dextrose solution to maintain blood glucose levels. Patients on TPN longer than 1 week may develop intestinal villus atrophy. Partial parenteral nutrition in conjunction with enteral nutrition may be advised when parenteral nutrition is being withdrawn. Care must be taken when changing from one diet to another; the transition should be gradual. Table 7-2 summarizes the nutritional requirements of pets with various diseases.

FEEDING CONSIDERATIONS FOR SMALL MAMMALS

Pet rodents can be fed commercial rodent chows or pellets. "Party mix" diets containing seeds and nuts are not recommended. These are high in fat, and many rodents prefer these to the formulated pellets. Seeds and nuts can be offered as an occasional treat (less than 10% of the daily diet). Fresh, well-cleaned vegetables and occasionally a small amount of fruit can be offered as well. Leafy green vegetables (not lettuce or celery) can be offered, as well as yellow and orange vegetables. The total daily amount of these "people foods" should not make up more than 10% of the diet. The diet should consist of 90% commercial pellets, 5% to 10% vegetables and fruits, and a few seeds or nuts as occasional treats. Hay (alfalfa or clover) may be offered free-choice as a source of fiber.

Unlike most other pets, guinea pigs require a dietary source of vitamin C. They should be fed guinea pig chow (pellets), which is supplemented with vitamin C. However, the shelf-life of vitamin C is about 90 days from the time of milling, not from the time of purchase. Therefore, vitamin C should also be supplied in the drinking water. A simple way to do this is to crush a 200-mg vitamin C tablet into powder. Mix the powder in 1 liter of water. This solution should be made fresh *daily* and used as the pet's drinking water. Fresh green vegetables (broccoli, cabbage, bok choy) can also be used to supply vitamin C.

TABLE 7-2

Summary of Small Animal Clinical Nutrition*

Disease	Objectives	Considerations	Product†	Comments
Allergy, food Dog	Reduce antigen ingestion	Novel highly digestible protein source or protein hydrolysate Reduce total protein content Simplify food Distilled H₂O	Prescription Diet Canine d/d or Canine z/d	8- to 10-week trial period Avoid treats, snacks, access to other food sources, chewable medications, supplements
Cat		Same as dog except Control Mg²⁺ intake Provide taurine Control urine pH	Prescription Diet Feline d/d or Feline z/d	
Anemia	Support RBC production	↑ Iron, cobalt, and copper ↑ B-complex vitamins ↑ Protein	Prescription Diet Canine p/d Feline p/d	
Anorexia	Prevent protein/caloric malnutrition Stimulate appetite	Establish fluid/electrolyte balance Acid-base balance ↑ Protein and fat ↑ Micronutrients	Prescription Diet Feline/Canine a/d Canine p/d Feline p/d	Cat foods are suitable for dogs in acute care settings
Ascites	Reduce fluid retention	Restrict sodium chloride Maintain hydration	Prescription Diet Canine h/d, k/d Feline h/d, k/d	h/d = marked salt restriction k/d = moderate salt restriction
Bone loss and fracture healing	Correct deficiency of energy and protein	↑ Protein ↑ Energy Avoid supplementation	Prescription Diet Canine p/d Feline p/d	Extra dietary calcium does not increase rate of fracture healing
Cancer	Increase longevity and quality of life	↓ Soluble carbohydrate ↑ Fat and n-3 fatty acids ↑ Arginine	Prescription Diet Canine n/d Canine/Feline a/d	Use in conjunction with chemotherapy or other forms of cancer therapy
Colitis	Normalize gastrointestinal motility Rebalance microflora Provide local healing factors	Feed small meals 3-6 times/day Control dietary antigens Vary levels of dietary fiber	Prescription Diet Canine w/d, i/d, d/d Feline w/d, d/d	
Constipation	Normalize gastrointestinal motility Maintain stool water Maintain stool bulk	>10% fiber	Prescription Diet Canine w/d Feline w/d	No table scraps or bones Increase exercise Encourage water intake Cats: keep litter box clean

Mg, Magnesium; *RBC,* red blood cell.

*Nutrients in table are expressed on a dry weight basis.

†Other North American therapeutic brands with wide distribution include CNM (Purina), VMD, Medi-Cal, and IVD Select Care (Heinz), Eukanuba Veterinary Diets (Iams), and Waltham Veterinary Diets (Mars).

Condition	Objective	Dietary modification	Diet	Comments
Copper storage disease	Restrict copper intake	<1.2 mg copper/100 g dry diet	Prescription Diet Canine l/d	No table scraps or treats
Debilitation	Restore tissue, plasma, and nutrients	↑Protein ↑Fat ↑Macronutrients and micronutrients	Prescription Diet Canine/Feline a/d	Assist feed if needed
Developmental orthopedic disease	Reduce rapid growth	↓Fat and energy density ↓Calcium	Prescription Diet Canine p/d Large breed	Avoid calcium-phosphorus supplements
Diabetes mellitus	Even rate of glucose absorption Consistent caloric intake	>10% fiber ↓Soluble carbohydrates	Prescription Diet Canine w/d Feline w/d	Weigh animal frequently and note in medical record
Diarrhea, acute	Normalize gastrointestinal tract motility and secretion	Withhold food for 1-2 days Feed small amounts 3-6 times/day ↓Fiber ↓Sugar ↑Digestibility	Prescription Diet Canine i/d Feline i/d	Electrolyte disturbances and dehydration are common
Eclampsia	Provide Ca/P in correct quantity and ratio prepartum	High digestibility of diet Balanced minerals/vitamins	Prescription Diet Canine p/d Feline p/d	Avoid supplementation
Flatulence	Decrease aerophagia Avoid food fermentation	Avoid milk or milk products Feed small meals 3-6 times/day ↑Caloric density	Prescription Diet Canine i/d Feline i/d	Feed in a flat, open dish Avoid vitamin or fatty acid supplementation Separate competitive eaters
Gastric dilatation/bloat (postoperative)	Prevent gastric distension	Avoid exercise before and after feeding ↑Digestibility of diet Small frequent feedings	Prescription Diet Canine i/d	Diet form or type is *NOT* related to risk of occurrence or recurrence
Heart failure Dogs	Control Na$^+$ retention	↓Na$^+$ intake	Prescription Diet Canine h/d Canine k/d	Prescription Diet h/d has moderate Na$^+$ restriction
Cats		Maintain energy and protein intake ↑B-complex vitamins ↓Na$^+$ intake ↑Taurine Control Mg^{2+} levels	Prescription Diet Feline h/d Feline k/d	Avoid high Na$^+$ treats and water (see Table 14-5)
Hyperlipidemia	Control fat intake	↑Fiber intake ↓Fat intake	Prescription Diet Canine w/d Feline w/d	Common in schnauzers Consider fat in treats, table foods, and supplements
Hyperthyroidism (cats)	Support increased energy need	↑Energy intake ↑Vitamins and minerals ↑Protein	Prescription Diet Feline a/d	Monitor for evidence of concurrent renal disease

Continued

TABLE 7-2

Summary of Small Animal Clinical Nutrition—Cont'd

Disease	Objectives	Considerations	Product[†]	Comments
Liver disease (fat-tolerant)	Reduce protein metabolism Maintain liver glycogen Prevent ammonia toxicity	↑ Digestible energy Protein restriction High biologic value proteins Control Na⁺ intake	Prescription Diet Canine l/d Feline l/d	May feed small meals (4-6 times/day)
Lymphangiectasia	Decrease dietary fat	↓ Intake of long-chain triglycerides Control protein levels Consider medium-chain triglycerides	Prescription Diet Canine w/d or r/d	Medium-chain triglyceride oils and powder can increase caloric density
Obesity	Maintain intake of all nutrients except energy	↓ Energy digestibility Replace digestible calories with indigestible fiber Increase bulk to control hunger Added carnitine	Prescription Diet Canine r/d Feline r/d	Requires professional advice and teamwork with veterinary technician and client
Oral disease: gingivitis (gum inflammation), periodontitis (loss of tooth attachment)	Control accumulation of plaque, stains, and calculus Maintain gingival health	Food that promotes chewing and mechanical cleansing of teeth	Prescription Diet Canine t/d Feline t/d	Many treats make dental claims but are not effective
Pancreatitis, acute (recovery phase)	Control pancreas secretions	↓ Fat ↑ Digestibility Feed small meals 3-6 times/day	Prescription Diet Canine i/d Feline i/d	Frequent, small meals
Pancreatic exocrine insufficiency	Reduce requirements for digestive enzymes	↓ Fiber ↓ Fat Highly digestible carbohydrates ↑ Caloric density	Prescription Diet Canine i/d Feline i/d	Pancreatic enzymes complement highly digestible food
Renal failure	Reduce signs of uremia Slow progression of disease	↓ Protein (↑ biologic value of protein) ↑ Nonprotein calories ↓ Phosphorus and sodium Increase B-complex vitamins	Prescription Diet Canine k/d Canine g/d Canine u/d Prescription Diet Feline k/d Feline g/d	Small meals 4-6 times/day Conversion to a protein-restricted diet may take 7-10 days Water available at all times
Canine urolithiasis (struvite): Treatment	↑ Urine volume ↓ Urine pH Restrict Mg²⁺, NH₄⁺, PO₄	↓ Protein ↓ PO₄, Mg²⁺ ↑ Na⁺ ↓ Urine pH (5.9-6.1)	Prescription Diet Canine s/d	Evaluate and treat urinary tract infection Average duration of stone dissolution is 36 days; follow-up via radiography
Prevention	Maintain physiologic level of urinary solutes and urine pH	Control protein excess ↓ Ca²⁺, P, Ma²⁺ ↓ Sodium mildly ↓ Urine pH (6.2-6.4)	Prescription Diet Canine c/d	Monitor urine sediment for crystalluria and infection

Na, sodium; *P*, phosphorus; *Ca*, calcium.

Condition	Nutritional goals	Prescription Diet	Comments
Canine urolithiasis (ammonium urate): Prevention	↓ Protein ↑ Nonprotein calories ↓ Nucleic acids ↓ Ca^{2+}, P, Mg^{2+}, Na^+ Urine pH (6.7-7.0)	Prescription Diet Canine u/d	Drugs plus diet may be successful treatment Monitor urinary crystalluria Prevention may require long-term drug treatment
Canine urolithiasis (calcium oxalate and cystine): Prevention	↓ Urinary concentration of calcium oxalate or cystine ↓ Protein ↑ Nonprotein calories ↓ Ca^{2+}, P, Na^+, Mg^{2+} ↑ Urine pH (6.1-7.0)	Prescription Diet Canine u/d	Treatment by surgical removal Prevention by dietary management ± drugs
Feline urolithiasis (struvite): Treatment	↑ Urine volume ↓ Urine pH (5.9-6.1) Restrict Mg^{2+}, Ca^{2+}, PO_4 ↑ Caloric density ↓ P and Ca^{2+} Mg^{2+} >20 mg/100 Kcal ↑ Na^+ Urine pH (6.2-6.4)	Prescription Diet Feline s/d	Dissolution is complete 1 month after negative radiographs Recurrence is high if prevention is not implemented
Prevention	Maintain physiologic levels of urinary solutes and urine pH Mg^{2+} >20 mg/100 Kcal (0.1% DMB) ↓ P ↑ Caloric density Urine pH (6.2-6.4)	Prescription Diet Feline c/d-s	In obesity, use calorie-restricted diets that maintain urine pH 6.2-6.4 (Prescription Diet w/d is suggested)
Feline urolithiasis (calcium oxalate): Prevention	↑ Urine volume ↓ Urinary Ca^{2+}, oxalate ↑ Urine pH ↓ Protein ↑ Nonprotein calories ↓ P, Ca^{2+}, Na^+ Mg^{2+} <20 mg/100 Kcal	Prescription Diet Feline c/d-oxl	Monitor urinary crystalluria
Vomiting	Minimize gastric secretion Gastrointestinal rest ↑ Digestibility ↑ Caloric density	Prescription Diet Canine i/d Feline i/d	Frequent, small meals

Ca, Calcium; *DMB*, dry matter basis; *Mg*, magnesium; *Na*, sodium; NH_4, ammonium; *P*, phosphorus; *PO*, phosphate; *RBC*, red blood cells.

Rabbits should be fed mainly free-choice hay. Alfalfa hay can be offered in small amounts, but it is too rich to be the sole source of fiber. Timothy grass or clover hay are better choices. Commercial pelleted feed should be offered each day at no more than ¼ cup per 5 pounds of body weight. The increased fiber helps prevent diarrhea and formation of trichobezoars (hairballs).

Ferrets can be fed commercial kitten food or cat food, or specially formulated ferret diets. As with dogs and cats, periodontal disease is common in ferrets. A dry diet can help reduce tartar accumulation.

FEEDING CONSIDERATIONS FOR REPTILES AND AMPHIBIANS

The subject of feeding reptiles and amphibians is vast and beyond the scope of this chapter. However, it is important to understand the dietary needs of reptiles, especially because improper diet is a common cause of many diseases in pet reptiles. This section discusses the general dietary needs of common pet reptiles and amphibians.

Iguanas

Regardless of what pet store clerks tell clients, iguanas are *herbivorous*. This means that a major portion of the diet must be plant material. There is some controversy among veterinarians as to whether it is acceptable to feed iguanas small amounts of animal protein, such as crickets, moths, or worms. Most veterinarians would probably agree that limiting these animal protein sources to no more than 10% of the diet is safe, although the iguana may not even require these foods (and some iguanas will not eat them).

Most of an iguana's diet should consist of flowers (and leaves), such as roses, hibiscus, carnations, and mums, and green leafy vegetables (not celery and iceberg lettuce, which are low in nutritional value). A small amount of fruits can also be offered. Commercial dog and cat foods are too high in protein and vitamin D and are not recommended. Vegetable and flower "salad" should be chopped into pieces suitable for the iguana's size and offered fresh daily or every other day. A *light* dusting of calcium powder (daily) and vitamin powder (weekly) is often recommended. Fresh water should be available at all times. Metabolic bone disease is common in green iguanas and results from a deficiency of dietary calcium, such as when only lettuce and fruit or lettuce and crickets are fed.

Snakes

Most species of snakes are carnivorous and eat whole prey. Suitable prey items include rats, mice, hamsters, and gerbils. Some species prefer one type of rodent, so it is wise to check reference texts regarding the snake species in ques-

tion. To prevent injury or death of the snake, it is best to feed killed prey, either freshly killed (or stunned) or thawed, frozen prey. If the snake will eat only live prey, the owner *must* observe the snake after feeding it the prey. If the snake has not killed and eaten the prey within 15 minutes, the prey should be removed and the snake fed at a later time.

Box Turtles

Like iguanas, box turtles eat a large amount of plant material; like snakes, they also eat animal protein. As a rule, the diet should consist of about 50% plant material (similar to that for the iguana; hay can also be offered) and 50% animal protein. This can include commercial turtle pellets, tofu, sardines, crickets, or worms. Vitamin A deficiency commonly results when turtles are offered only lettuce and fruit or lettuce and crickets. A proper diet helps prevent this common disorder. As with iguanas, a *light* daily sprinkling of calcium and weekly sprinkling of vitamins can help supplement the diet of box turtles.

Amphibians

Most amphibians are carnivorous as adults. Improper diet, such as a diet consisting of only crickets, can cause nutritional problems, such as metabolic bone disease. An improper diet, such as one consisting entirely of dog or cat food, may cause the opposite problem and lead to hypervitaminosis D or gout. Reference texts should be consulted regarding the proper diet for the species of amphibian in question.

FEEDING CONSIDERATIONS FOR LABORATORY ANIMALS

Animals should be fed a clean, wholesome, and nutritious diet *ad libitum*. It is important to feed a balanced diet, freshly milled, formulated for that particular species. In most instances, the food should be placed in a feeder hung in the animal's cage. This prevents soiling of the food with urine and feces, keeping it dry and clean. If vegetables or fruit are offered to supplement the diet, they should be fresh and washed before feeding them. Any uneaten vegetables or fruits should be removed daily. Animals should have access to fresh water via an automatic watering system or water bottles with sipper tubes.

NUTRITIONAL PECULIARITIES OF LIVESTOCK

Livestock species (cattle, horses, pigs, sheep, goats) require certain essential nutrients to meet metabolic and physiologic needs. Essential nutrients include water, energy, amino acids (proteins), fatty acids, minerals, and vitamins; these are discussed in the first part of this chapter.

There is a unique feature to protein nutrition in ruminants (cattle, sheep, goats). As a result of their pregastric fermentation system, nonprotein nitrogen (e.g., urea), in addition to rumen-degradable dietary protein, can be used by the resident microbes as a nitrogen source of synthesis of microbial proteins. Microbial protein then passes into the abomasum (true stomach) and is digested like any other dietary protein. Microbial protein can account for a significant amount of dietary protein in ruminants.

Dietary fiber is required to maintain adequate gastrointestinal function in herbivores (plant-eating animals) with active microbial fermentation chambers. These include ruminants and hind gut fermenting animals (horses). Therefore, gastrointestinal anatomy has a very critical role in the animal's ability to derive essential nutrients from the feedstuffs available. Domestic livestock extract essential nutrients from plant materials. The plant material consumed by livestock species contains cellulose, hemicellulose, pectin, and lignin compounds that are indigestible by people and carnivorous predators. Microbes within the gut use these plant compounds, and the animal uses the end products of microbial fermentation. Animals have evolved in many ways to take advantage of microbial fermentation in their digestive process.

The alimentary tract includes the mouth and associated structures, esophagus, stomach, small intestine, cecum, and colon (large intestine). The rumen of cattle, sheep, and goats functions as a pregastric fermentation vat (Fig. 7-11). This allows ruminants to efficiently derive nutrients from plant material. In hind gut fermenters, such as horses, a greatly enlarged colon serves as a fermentation vat. These animals can also digest plant material, but not to the same extent as ruminants. As a result of differences in their anatomy, ruminants digest preformed feed material, whereas hind gut herbivores ferment predigested feed material. Pigs are considered omnivores, which means that they can digest materials of both plant and animal origin, although they are primarily fed less bulky plant materials. Pigs have some microbial fermentation capacity in their enlarged, sacculated colon (Fig. 7-11), but not to the extent of hind gut fermenters or ruminants.

Feedstuffs

A *feedstuff* is any dietary component that provides some essential nutrient or serves some other function. Non-nutritive feedstuffs may provide bulk, flavor, odor, or color, or act as an antioxidant to protect other dietary components. More than 2000 different feedstuffs have been fed to domestic livestock throughout the world. The variety of feedstuffs available for use in a given geographic area depends on the crops grown locally. Potential feedstuffs

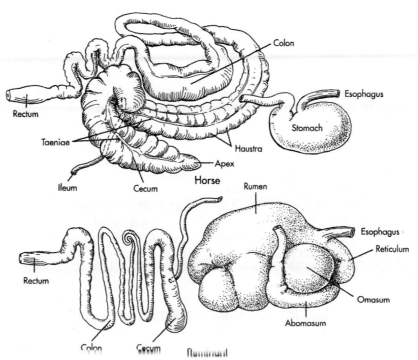

Fig. 7-11 Diagram comparing the gastrointestinal tract of ruminants and horses. (Most of the small intestines omitted for clarity.) (From McBride DF: *Learning Veterinary Terminology*, ed 2, St. Louis, 2002, Elsevier.)

must be matched with the appropriate livestock species, based on nutrient requirements and gastrointestinal tract capabilities. Feedstuffs may be divided into a number of categories, based on their source and nutrient concentration. General categories include forages (roughages), concentrates, by-products, mineral and vitamin supplements, and nonnutritive additives.

Forages are feeds made up of most or all of the plant. Forages generally have large amounts of fiber, low energy density, and high bulk (low weight per unit volume). This is a direct result of the amount of plant cell wall material present. Plant cell walls are composed of cellulose, hemicelluose, lignin, and other compounds. A forager's protein content depends on the type of plant and stage at harvesting. For example, alfalfa hay has much higher protein levels than grass hays at a comparable stage of plant growth. Within plant species, there is an increase in fiber content and a decrease in protein content, energy content, and overall digestibility with advancing maturity of the plant. The decrease in digestibility with maturity is due to increasing *lignin* content of the plant. Lignin is an inert compound that increases rigidity of the plant cell wall. Straw represents the most mature and indigestible form of forages.

Forages fed to livestock belong to either the legume or grass plant families. Legumes commonly used for forage production include alfalfa, red and white clover, bird's foot trefoil, and vetch. Grasses offer more variety for forage production and include bahia grass, bermuda grass, bluegrass, bromegrass, fescue, timothy, orchard grass, reed canary grass, ryegrass, and Sudan grass. Other grass forages that can be used for cereal grain production include corn, wheat, rye, oats, and sorghum. Of these, corn is the most important forage and cereal grain product grown for livestock.

Forage products are harvested and stored for livestock feeding purposes in a number of ways. Livestock may graze grasses, legumes, and other broadleaf vegetation (forbs and browse). Allowing livestock to harvest forage avoids costs incurred in mechanical harvesting and storage. However, forage quality and quantity can be extremely variable, depending on plant maturity and environmental conditions. A more controlled method of grazing called *intensive rotational grazing* is being adopted. In this method, animals are allowed to graze restricted areas of forage for limited periods and are then moved to another area; the forage in the grazed area is allowed to regrow until the animals are returned for grazing. With highly managed rotational grazing, forage quality can be maintained at a very high level.

Forage crops can also be mechanically harvested, stored, and fed using various methods. *Green chop* or *spoilage* represents forage harvested at a given stage of development and fed directly. Green chop contains a high water content (75% to 85%) and available nutrients; however, it must be harvested daily to avoid rapid deterioration with storage. *Ensiling* is a harvesting process by which forage is chopped

and placed into a storage unit (e.g., silo), which excludes oxygen. As the forage ferments, lactic acid is produced and the pH decreases. This effectively "pickles" the forage to a partially fermented state called *silage*. Good-quality silage can be stored indefinitely in upright silos, bunker silos, or plastic bags, the important feature being exclusion of oxygen. Silage has an intermediate water content (55% to 75%) and has the least loss of nutrients from harvesting and storage. Grass, legume, and corn silages are the most common ensiled forages fed to livestock. *Hay* is forage that is cut and allowed to dry before being collected into bales for storage. Hay should have less than 15% water to be stable in storage. Harvesting losses are high in hay making, but storage losses are usually minimal if it is properly dried.

Concentrates are generally low in fiber and high in energy and/or protein. Cereal grains, such as barley, corn, millet, oats, rye, sorghum, and wheat, are the seeds of many of the grass species. Corn is the most common grain fed to livestock and the standard with which others are compared. Cereal grains contain large amounts of energy in the form of starch and are added to diets to increase energy density. Other feed products used as energy concentrates include molasses, root crops (e.g., turnips, beets, carrots), and potatoes. Fats and oils of plant or animal origin contain 2.25 times the energy density of carbohydrates and are also used as energy concentrates.

Concentrate feeds that contain more than 20% crude protein are subclassified as *protein supplements*. Protein supplements may be of plant or animal origin, including marine fish. Plant-based protein products are derived from oilseed crops, such as soybean, canola, cottonseed, sunflower, and peanut seed meals. Of these, soybean meal is by far the most common oilseed meal fed to livestock. Oil from the seeds is harvested for a variety of industrial and nutritional uses; the remaining seed contains more than 40% crude protein. Animal-based protein supplements are derived from rendered animal or fish tissues or from dried-milk products. Animal proteins generally range from more than 50% crude protein to 90% crude protein. As compared with plant-based protein sources, animal protein sources have a better amino acid composition relative to requirements. However, there is much variability in the quality of animal-based products and the way in which they are manufactured.

By-product feeds are residues of the feed-processing industry and span a wide array of feedstuffs. Examples of by-product feeds include sugar beet pulp, bakery waste, blood, bone meal, brewer's grains, tallow, and whey. Many by-product feeds contain substantial amounts of fermentable fiber, energy, and protein.

Mineral and *vitamin supplements* are sources of individual or combination of minerals, with or without vitamins. Fat-soluble vitamins are supplemented primarily in the form of premixes. Fat-soluble vitamins are sensitive to oxidation, sunlight, heat, and fungal growth. Certain water-soluble vitamins may be supplemented in swine and horse diets; they are not routinely supplemented in ruminant diets. Yeast cultures are good sources of B complex vitamins and are commonly added to livestock diets.

Nonnutritive feed additives can include buffers, hormones, binders, and medications. Feed medications may include antibiotics, antifungals, anthelmintics, antiparasitics, and ionophores (antibiotics with growth-promoting effects). Their use is regulated by the Food and Drug Administration in an effort to prevent tissue residues (see Chapters 8 and 9). Nonnutritive additives are used to stimulate animal performance, improve feed efficiency, and improve animal health or metabolic status.

Feed Analysis

Different classes of feedstuffs contribute variable amounts of the essential nutrients (Table 7-3). Even within certain feed groups, such as forages, nutrient composition can vary tremendously. *Feed analysis* is a procedure by which chemical analysis determines the proportion of specific components of a feedstuff. The *proximate analysis* includes determinations of dry matter (DM), crude protein (CP), ether extract (EE, crude fat), crude fiber (CF), and ash. The nonfiber carbohydrate portion of the feed, termed *nitrogen-free extract* (NFE), is determined using the equation NFE 1002 CP2 CF2 EE2 ash. More recently, crude fiber analysis has been replaced with neutral and acid detergent fiber analysis, improving our estimate of cell wall components and their availability. Feed analysis should be routinely completed in any nutritional diagnostic problem.

FEEDING MANAGEMENT

The goal of any livestock feeding management program is to provide sufficient daily amounts of the essential nutrients for optimal (cost-effective) productivity. Because feed costs account for the greatest amount of total production costs in the livestock industry, we must minimize feed costs to ensure profitability. By-product feeds are so widely used when available, because they usually are of lower cost.

Dairy Cattle

Dairy cattle are segregated and housed by production stages and fed according to specific nutrient requirements. Typical feeding groups on a dairy farm include milk-fed calves, growing replacement heifers, nonlactating pregnant cows (dry cows), and lactation groups. Lactation groups are usually based on level of milk production, parity (first lactation vs. older cows), days in milk, or a combination of these factors.

Feeding systems and housing facilities vary among dairy farms, depending on prevailing environmental conditions. Smaller family dairies with fewer than 100 cows generally have individual tie stalls, and cows are fed individually. The amount of forage and concentrates are fed according to production level and body condition score (Table 7-4).

TABLE 7-3

Relative Nutrient Content of Various Feedstuffs for Livestock

			Relative Nutrient Content				
	Protein	Energy	Minerals		Vitamins		Fiber
			Macro	*Micro*	*Fat-Sol.*	*B-Complex*	
Feedstuff Group							
High-quality roughage	++ +	++	++	++	+++	+	+++
Low-quality roughage	+	+	+	+	−	−	+++ +
Cereal grains	++	+++	+	+	+	+	+
Grain millfeeds	++	++	++	++	+	++	++
Fats and oils	−	+ +++	−	−	−	−	−
Molasses	+	+++	++	++	−	+	−
Fermentation products	++ +	++	+	++	−	+++ +	±
Oil seed proteins	++ ++	++ +	++	++	+	++	+
Animal proteins	++ ++	++ +	+ ++	+ ++	++	+++	+

From Church DC: *Livestock feeds and feeding*, ed 3, Englewood Cliffs, NJ, 1991, Prentice-Hall.

+ to ++ ++: low to very high content.

±: may or may not be present in significant amounts.

−: not present.

TABLE 7-4

Body Condition Scoring Classifications for Livestock

Body Condition Scoring Scale*		Generalized Animal Description†
1.0	1	*Emaciated.* All bones obviously protruding; no subcutaneous fat evident
1.5	2	*Very thin.* Bones visible and easily palpated; minimal subcutaneous fat
2.0	3	*Thin.* Thin, flat musculature; prominent ribs, pelvic bones, and spinal processes
2.5	4	*Moderately thin.* Minimal subcutaneous fat; individual ribs not obvious
3.0	5	*Moderate.* Smooth musculature; bones not visible but palpable
3.5	6	*Moderately fleshy.* Fat palpable; soft fat over ribs and covering pelvis
4.0	7	*Fleshy.* Fat visible; ribs barely visible; spinal processes buried in fat
4.5	8	*Fat.* Thick neck; ribs difficult to palpate; rounded appearance to pelvis
5.0	9	*Grossly obese.* Bulging fat all over; patchy fat pads around tailhead

*The body condition scoring scale used depends on the species. Dairy cattle, sheep, pigs, and goats are typically scored on a scale of 1 to 5, whereas beef cattle and horses are scored on a scale of 1 to 9.

†When determining body condition score, evaluate for the presence or absence of fatty tissue over the neck, ribs, spine, and pelvis, independent of animal body weight and frame size.

These farms are predominantly found in the northeastern and midwestern United States as a result of the cold winters. In larger dairies, cows are generally housed in free-stall barns or in open drylots, depending on environmental conditions. Drylots are found primarily in the southern and western United States, whereas free-stall barns are found anywhere in the United States. In larger dairy management systems, cattle are fed in groups at a common feedbunk, rather than individually. Feedbunks may be located within the free-stall facility or along one side of the drylot.

Although feeding management of dairy cattle depends on the type of facility available, there are some options as to how feed is delivered to the animals. Forage (hay, silage) may be fed separately from concentrates in any of the feeding management systems described. Concentrates may be fed separately in the milking parlor or from computerized feeders. Parlor grain feeding and computerized feeding are becoming more common with current interest in pasture-grazing management systems. In large dairies, the most common method of feed delivery is by total mixed ration (TMR). In this system, all individual feed ingredients are mechanically mixed in a feed wagon and presented as a single mixture to the cows. This allows cows to consume the same blend of nutrients in each bite and minimizes selectivity. Some dairies feed what might be termed a partial TMR in that dry hay is fed separate from the rest of the diet.

Beef Cattle

Beef cattle management can be divided into cow-calf and cattle feeding (feedlot) operations. Cow-calf enterprises produce calves that enter the breeding herd or are sent to cattle-feeding operations (feedlots). Forage use is the basis of cow-calf enterprises. Feed costs account for more than 60% of production costs and therefore must be minimized.

Cows are allowed to graze pasture or range land, depending on availability, and then are supplemented with energy, protein, and vitamin-mineral supplements as necessary to meet specific nutritional requirements. Depending on geographic location and season, pasture grazing may be replaced with feeding of dry hay or silage. Supplementation programs depend on prevailing forage quality relative to nutrient requirements of the various production units. Cow-calf operations may have feeding groups for bulls, replacement heifers, growing calves, maintenance, and pregnant or lactating cattle.

Cattle-feeding enterprises involve feeding calves from weaning to slaughter and include backgrounding, stocker, and feedlot systems. In backgrounding and stocker feeding systems, weanling calves are placed on low-cost pasture and supplementation feeding programs to gain weight at a moderate rate and then sold to feedlot operations. The goal of a feedlot enterprise is to maximize rate of gain and feed conversion efficiency for the lowest cost. New arrivals at the feedlot are initially fed a high-forage, low-concentrate diet to acclimate the animal to the operation. The proportion of forage is gradually reduced and concentrate increased to facilitate the desired rate of gain. To minimize feeding costs, a wide variety of by-product feeds and grain products is fed. To ensure animal health with high-grain feeding, ionophores, buffers, and antimicrobial agents are incorporated into the feedlot diet. Generally, the feedlot diet is fed as a TMR similar to the method for dairy cattle.

Nutrition in the Debilitated Calf

Feeding colostrum

Because calves are born essentially *agammaglobulinemic* (without immunoglobulins), provision of colostrum shortly after birth is critically important for the calf to obtain passive maternal antibodies. As a rule of thumb, beef calves should be fed all of the dam's first-milking colostrum as soon as they develop a suckle reflex. If dairy cow colostrum is used, be sure that the colostrum is of sufficient *quality*. The quality of colostrum is a rough measure of the concentration of immunoglobulin. This is most easily determined by use of a *colostrometer*, a simple tool that measures the specific gravity of the colostrum.

Dairy cows produce much more colostrum than beef cows do, but generally the quality and the concentration of immunoglobulin is lower. As a rule of thumb, if calves are provided with dairy cow colostrum, it can be administered orally at 10% of body weight over the first 24 hours of life. Absorption of maternal colostral immunoglobulin by the calf's intestine usually begins to decrease after the first feeding of colostrum or at about 8 hours of age. Therefore, it is important that the first feeding of colostrum is usually of fairly large magnitude. If the calf has a vigorous suckle reflex, allow the calf to nurse all of the dam's colostrum that it will consume. If more colostrum is available, continue to feed it throughout the first 24 hours, offering it at 2-hour intervals and allowing the calf to suckle. If the calf does not have a suckle reflex, continue to offer the colostrum frequently, looking for development of a suckle reflex up to about 6 hours of age. If the calf has not developed a suckle response at that time, intubate the calf and give all of the colostrum from a beef heifer or 5% of the calf's body weight in colostrum from a dairy cow.

For administration of colostrum or milk, allowing the calf to suckle versus intubating is an important question. If the calf has already been nursing the dam and is presented for treatment beyond the first several days of age, it is common for the calf to refuse a rubber nipple feeder. It may be worthwhile to reintroduce the calf to the dam because it may then suckle the dam quite readily. On the other hand, if it is a newborn calf that has not yet suckled the dam, it will usually suckle from a nipple feeder as readily as from the dam's teats.

Development of a suckle reflex is a very important indicator of the calf's status. Calves with a variety of problems, including hypoxemia, hypoglycemia, hypothermia, or acidosis resulting from dystocia, frequently do not develop the reflex until these problems are corrected. Therefore, lack of a suckle reflex is a good indicator of one or more of these problems. In some cases, if these problems are present, the calf may not absorb immunoglobulin, even if colostrum is provided via intubation.

For these reasons, allow the calf to suckle. Development of a suckle reflex usually suggests improvement in an underlying condition. Further, when other problems are present, the calf's gastrointestinal tract may not be fully functional. Therefore, repeated intubation of newborn calves or calves of older ages suffering from similar problems may result in large accumulations of fluid in the forestomachs or abomasum. If you resort to intubation to supply the calf with oral fluids or milk, carefully monitor the calf for fecal production and palpate its abdomen, looking for evidence that the fluid administered is sequestering in the gastrointestinal tract, rather than proceeding on through and being absorbed. If the calf will not suckle and there is evidence that fluid has accumulated in the gastrointestinal tract, continue to offer fluids frequently via nipple feeder but discontinue orogastric intubation.

Stimulation of the calf to develop a suckle reflex is another important function of the dam. Most calves are very responsive to stroking or rubbing along the back, especially near the tailhead. If the calf is not suckling well, such rubbing stimulation can often provide very rewarding results. If the calf has been sleeping or is compromised by one of the aforementioned problems, it may require several minutes before the calf begins to suckle. Therefore, it is worthwhile to repeatedly introduce the nipple into the calf's mouth and try to deliver a small amount of milk before giving up and assuming the calf does not have a suckle reflex.

Feeding milk

Beyond colostral feeding, provision of milk as nutrition is obviously of critical importance. Although dairy calves are often raised with the provision of only 10% of body weight per day as fluid milk, this practice should not be mistakenly construed as providing optimal nutrition. The strategy of providing 10% of body weight per day is geared to enhancing intake of solid feeds so that dairy calves can be weaned at an early age. Most calves, if given the opportunity, freely consume between 20% and 30% of their body weight in milk per day. Although sick calves may not have a very hearty appetite, a recovering calf or premature calf commonly has an exaggerated appetite. For these reasons, provide a calf with up to 3% of its body weight per feeding and offer milk feedings at approximately 2-hour intervals. With this regimen, some calves consume more than 30% of their body weight in milk per day.

Feeding electrolytes

For calves with fluid loss because of neonatal enteritis, oral electrolyte solutions are commonly offered as a means to provide additional fluid therapy. Calves with mild to moderate dehydration may respond adequately with only oral fluid supplementation, whereas calves with severe dehydration require intravenous fluid support. It has been a common practice to withhold milk from calves with enteritis. You do not have to hold to that practice, but rather offer milk via nipple feeder if the calf will accept it. Because milk alone will not provide the electrolytes that have been lost through the gastrointestinal tract, provide oral electrolyte solutions at alternate feedings with the milk. The electrolyte fluids and milk or milk replacer should not be mixed, because this adversely influences normal milk digestion. Offer milk at 2% to 3% of body weight maximum, alternating with oral fluid feedings offered at 5% of body weight per feeding, with the alternate feedings at 2-hour intervals. Many calves refuse the milk feedings but eagerly suckle the electrolyte. With this regimen, even when calves do refuse the milk, they can be provided as much as 30% of body weight per day in additional oral electrolyte fluids.

Horses

Horse feeding management is primarily designed to meet the nutritional requirements of individual horses. Although horses are not ruminants, they require a substantial amount of dietary fiber, in the form of forage, to maintain a healthy digestive tract. Forages fed to horses are primarily hay and pasture. Silage is not commonly fed to horses because of their sensitivity to the molds and mycotoxins potentially found in silage. Many varieties of grasses and legumes can be suitable hay forages for horses. Energy, protein, and mineral-vitamin supplementation depends on forage quality and nutrient requirements of the horse. Corn, barley, and oats are common grain supplements fed to horses for added energy. Recently, fat supplementation has been advocated to provide energy for growing, lactating, and working horses. Such protein sources as linseed, canola, and soybean meal are commonly used. By-products containing fermentable fiber, such as rice bran and beet pulp, are becoming more popular. Many commercial horse feeds are available to horse owners. These range from complete feeds (no supplementation required) to specific vitamin-mineral supplements. Various grain supplements containing energy, protein, minerals, and vitamins are available. These commercial grain supplements may be formulated specifically for growing foals, lactating mares, or geriatric horses, or they may be more generic in purpose. Horse owners should match the concentrate to their forage relative to energy, protein, mineral, and vitamin requirements. A proper horse-feeding program would provide adequate amounts of water and provide sufficient energy to achieve and maintain proper body condition. The diet must then be balanced for protein, minerals, and vitamins according to the National Research Council recommendations. Appropriate dental care and parasite management programs should accompany all horse-feeding systems.

Feeding and watering hospitalized horses

Hospitalized horses often have special dietary needs. Their diseases can often create a catabolic state. The horse may require extra calories to maintain its weight. Horses that can chew and swallow normally should be fed their usual diet if their disease permits. Good-quality alfalfa or grass hay, such as timothy hay, can be fed. Good-quality oat hay is also a suitable feed. Horses with gastrointestinal distur-bances, such as colic or diarrhea, need special consideration. Horses recovering from impactions may need more laxative feeds, such as alfalfa hay, grass pasture, and even bran mashes. Horses with diarrhea or those that have been operated on for colic may benefit from a diet that is not so rich, such as timothy or oat hay. Hay pellets or cubes that contain alfalfa or a mixture of alfalfa and bermuda or oat hay can also be used. If added carbohydrate is needed, a pelleted feed that also contains grains may be fed.

Pelleted feed produces less dust and may be better for horses recovering from respiratory allergies or pneumonia. Horses recovering from gastrointestinal ulceration may also need to be fed a pelleted ration, because the increased fiber and stem in hay may irritate and exacerbate certain kinds of ulcers. Pellets soaked to make gruel can be fed to horses with oral lesions, facial fractures, dental problems, or recurrent episodes of choke. Feed softened in this manner is easier for the animal to chew and swallow. Horses with neuromuscular disorders, such as botulism, may be unable to chew and swallow normally. A pelleted ration that has been soaked may be the only feed the animal can eat.

Fresh water should always be available. Some horses may not know how to use an automatic waterer if it requires the horse to push on a lever to fill the water cup. Water buckets or tubs should always be provided in these cases. Salt may need to be provided topically on the feed or in the form of a salt lick during hot weather, or for horses that have diseases that create a sodium deficiency, such as colitis.

Pigs

Pig feeding management is similar to beef cattle management in that there are breeding-farrowing (reproductive) and growing enterprises. The farrowing unit produces baby pigs as reproductive replacements or to enter the growing unit for feeding to slaughter weight. The pig industry is one of the most intensively managed agricultural enterprises. Current pig production units are moving to total confinement farrow-to-finish operations containing many animals. Within these operations, feeding groups are segregated according to nutrient requirements, with diets for lactating and gestating sows and gilts, boars, nursery pigs, and growing pigs. For the most part, animals in the farrowing unit are housed and fed as individuals to better control body weight and condition. Within the feeding operation, starting with the nursery pigs, all animals are group-housed and fed according to age and moved between groups as an entire unit. As omnivores, pigs have a digestive tract that can accommodate a certain level of dietary fiber. Given the economics of rate of gain from forages versus grains, pig diets consist primarily of concentrates, along with energy, protein, mineral, and vitamin supplements. All feed ingredients are thoroughly mixed and provided as a single diet, like the TMR for cattle. Dietary ingredients depend on the nutritional requirements of the specific group of animals being fed. The classic pig diet consists of corn grain and soybean meal, with a vitamin-mineral pre-mix. Learning more about the specific nutrient requirements of pigs has resulted in more sophisticated diets for pigs. Crystalline amino acids, high-quality animal by-product protein meals, fiber sources, and vitamin-mineral supplements have been incorporated into specific pig diets to improve growth efficiency.

Sheep

Sheep are managed similarly to beef cattle in that there are reproductive and lamb-growing enterprises. Sheep are raised under a wide variety of conditions, ranging from large flocks on western rangelands to small flocks in confinement. The basis of any sheep production system is forage. The advantage of feeding sheep is their ability to selectively graze. This allows sheep to consume a diet of higher nutritional value than the quality of the total forage. A variety of forage types including harvested and stored forages can be used for feeding sheep. As ruminants, sheep can also use a wide variety of by-product feeds efficiently.

For the most part, sheep diets consist of vitamin-mineral supplements added to the base forage. The composition of the vitamin-mineral supplement depends on the forage. Grazing sheep are provided with minerals as a block ("salt lick") or loose from a feeder. Additional energy and protein supplementation may be used for late gestation, lactation, and growing diets. A wide variety of feed sources may be

used, with cost being of primary concern. These supplements may be top-dressed on (spread on top of) the forage or fed by themselves in a feed bunk. Commercial concentrate pellets are also available for ewes and growing lamb diets. Growing lambs may be sent to slaughter directly from grazing high-quality forage or after feeding in a feedlot. Lamb feedlots are similar in organization and feeding practices to beef feedlots. Lambs are acclimated from a high-forage to high-concentrate TMR diet to increase grain and feed efficiency.

Goats

Goats are managed similarly to dairy cattle because of their milk production. However, some breeds of goats are primarily used for mohair (wool) or meat production. Forage is the primary component of goat-feeding programs. Like sheep, goats can selectively graze the more nutritious parts of plants. Goats raised for mohair and meat are managed with grazing or browsing rangeland or pasture and appropriate energy and protein supplementation when necessary. Dairy goats are managed more intensively because of their higher nutritional requirements for milk production.

Dairy goats are usually housed in smaller areas and fed stored forages, such as dry hay. Pasture grazing alone cannot support milk production, so supplements are necessary. The energy and protein feed supplements for goats are similar to those of dairy cattle. Many commercial concentrate products used for horses, sheep, and dairy cattle can also be

---

TABLE 7-5

Nutritional History in Livestock (Specific Information Depends on the Species of Livestock)

General Categories of Information	Specific Information
Identify the people involved	Names and telephone numbers of the owner, herdsman, veterinarian, nutritionist, others
Owner's primary concern	Pertaining to the presenting problem
Historical information about the agribusiness	Ask questions relating to years of ownership, number of hired hands, new animal purchases, acreage, other farms, etc.
Herd information	Function, breeds, average weights, and age distribution of animals on the farm
Production information	Level of performance (milk production, weaning weights, litter size, etc.) in the herd over time; use production record systems if available
Housing facilities	Type of housing, stall surfaces, and bedding used for each group of animals; adequacy of ventilation
Feeding system	Feed storage facilities, feeding system used, feed and water availability, bunk space per animal, number of times fed per day, etc.
Dietary information	Feed ingredients and their nutrient analyses, specific feeds for each feeding group; obtain feed samples if feed analysis or feed tag information is unavailable
Herd disease information	Disease prevalence for pertinent disease problems, animal culling and mortality rates over the past month, 6 months, and year
Reproductive information	Measures of fertility, pregnancy losses, etc.
Preventive medicine practices	Vaccinations, treatments, and dewormings administered and when; ask if routine herd health visits are made by the veterinarian

fed to goats. The amount and nutrient composition of the supplement depend on the nutrient requirements of the animal being fed and on forage quality. Lactating goats require substantial energy supplementation and should be fed the highest-quality forages. Supplements may be top-dressed on forage in a feedbunk or provided in the milking parlor.

CLINICAL NUTRITION

A basic understanding of nutrition can be applied to medical management of livestock. The most important part of clinical nutrition is obtaining an appropriate nutritional history. This is used to determine the potential role of nutrition in a medical problem. Questions one should ask in obtaining a nutritional history are outlined in Table 7-5.

Following the history taking, assess the nutritional status of the animal through physical assessment of the animal and via blood chemistry determinations. Physical assessment of the animal involves obtaining an accurate body weight, height measurement, and body condition score. Body height at the shoulders (withers) can be used to assess frame size and growth. Body weight and height measurements can be compared with those in standardized growth charts to assess growth performance. *Body condition scoring* is a method of subjectively quantifying subcutaneous body fat reserves. Animals are scored on a scale of 1 to 5 or 1 to 9, with the low and high scores representing emaciated and obese animals, respectively (see Table 7-4). Changes in body condition score represent either a positive (increased) or negative (decreased) energy balance. A negative energy balance suggests that the diet contains insufficient energy to meet needs and that body fat reserves are being mobilized.

Beyond this quantitative measure, physical assessment of the animal may include observations of haircoat, hoof quality, hydration status, manure consistency, and attitude. Assess these factors and record them in the animal's records daily for hospitalized patients. Indirect measures of nutritional status may be evaluated through metabolite concentrations in blood.

RECOMMENDED READING

Case LP et al: *Canine and feline nutrition*, ed 2, St Louis, 2000, Mosby.

Cheeke PR: *Applied animal nutrition: feeds and feeding*, New York, 1991, Macmillan.

Church DC: *Livestock feeds and feeding*, ed 3, Englewood Cliffs, NJ, 1991, Prentice-Hall.

Ensminger ME, Olentine CG, Heinemann WW: *Feeds and nutrition*, ed 2, Clovis, Cal, 1990, Ensminger.

Morris ML et al: *Small animal clinical nutrition III*, Topeka, Kan, 1987, Mark Morris.

National Research Council: *Nutrient requirements of beef cattle*, ed 7, Washington, DC, 1996, National Academy Press.

National Research Council: *Nutrient requirements of dairy cattle*, ed 6, Washington, DC, 1988, National Academy Press.

National Research Council: *Nutrient requirements of goats: angora, dairy, and meat goats in temperate and tropical countries*, Washington, DC, 1981, National Academy Press.

National Research Council: *Nutrient requirements of horses*, ed 5, Washington, DC, 1989, National Academy Press.

National Research Council, *Nutrient requirements of sheep*, ed 6, Washington, DC, 1985, National Academy Press.

National Research Council: *Nutrient requirements of swine*, ed 9, Washington, DC, 1988, National Academy Press.

8

Pathology and Response to Disease

Michelle Mayers

Learning Objectives

After reviewing this chapter, the reader should understand the following:

- Ways in which tissues respond to injury
- Phases of inflammation and the cells involved
- Ways in which injured tissues heal
- Ways in which pathogens affect tissues
- Types of immune response

- Physiologic basis for vaccination
- Hypersensitivity reactions
- Ways in which animal disease can affect people
- General principles of epidemiology and their application to public health
- General principles of food hygiene and their application to public health
- Common zoonotic diseases that pose a threat to people
- Ways to control spread of zoonotic diseases

Pathology, simply stated, is the study of disease. Disease is any alteration from the normal state of health. Disease may range from a superficial skin laceration to widely disseminated metastatic neoplasia (malignant tumors spread to many different organs). A *pathologist* is one who studies diseases and often is responsible for accurate diagnosis, as well as determining the cause, or etiology, of those diseases. Pathologists are trained in different areas of expertise, including either anatomic pathology or clinical pathology. A veterinary pathologist is a specialist who, after receiving an advanced degree in veterinary pathology, is employed by veterinary schools, state diagnostic laboratories, or pharmaceutical companies.

The primary responsibility of a veterinary anatomic pathologist is the prosection (dissection) of cadavers (carcasses) presented for *necropsy*, which is analogous to an *autopsy* in humans. During necropsy the pathologist collects tissue sections from lesions, which are grossly observable diseased tissues, and examines them with a microscope. Evaluating tissues with a microscope is called *histopathology*. Histopathology may allow the pathologist an insight into the etiology and prognosis of the disease. The prognosis is the expected outcome of the patient affected by the disease, and is usually stated as good, guarded, or poor. Veterinary anatomic pathologists also evaluate tissues that have been surgically removed by the veterinarian. Thus, these tissues are often referred to as *surgical biopsies*.

Veterinary clinical pathologists evaluate components of the blood as well as bodily fluids such as transudates and exudates. These provide valuable information regarding the causes and prognoses of diseases.

TERMINOLOGY

Pathologists use specific terms to describe the lesions observed at necropsy and with the microscope. Gross lesions are described by stating the location, color, size, texture, and appearance of the altered tissue (Box 8-1). The diagnosis may be a *morphologic* (anatomic) diagnosis or an *etiologic* (cause) diagnosis. The morphologic diagnosis is usually limited to describing the lesion within that organ system. An example of a morphologic diagnosis is "acute necrotizing enteritis," which states that the intestine is inflamed and necrotic and that it occurred very suddenly. The corresponding etiologic diagnosis may be "enteric salmonellosis," which means that the animal had the intestinal form of infection by *Salmonella* bacteria. Other bacterial and viral agents may also cause the lesions described in the morphologic diagnosis, so acute necrotizing enteritis does not always indicate a specific diagnosis of enteric salmonellosis.

Inflammation and Response to Injury

Inflammation is a protective response of the animal's body to fight infection resulting from pathogens (disease-causing

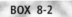

BOX 8-1

Description of Gross Lesions

Location
Color
Size
Texture
Appearance of altered tissue

agents). Pathogens include viruses, bacteria, parasites, fungi, and molds. Pathogens are described in more detail later in the chapter.

Signs of Inflammation

The five cardinal signs of inflammation are *heat, redness, swelling, pain,* and *loss of function* (Box 8-2). These signs result from complex interactions between the cells and fluids in the involved area. Initial *vasodilatation* (dilation of blood vessels) increases the flow of blood to the site of inflammation, resulting in an increase in temperature and redness. The swelling is caused by decreased flow of blood away from the site of inflammation, as well as possible edema, or increased fluid in the tissues. The pain and loss of function (if the inflammation is severe) are the result of pressure on the peripheral nerves at the site of inflammation. Additionally, the immune system and hemostatic (blood clotting) factors may be involved in the inflammatory process, making it a very integrated and complex series of biochemical events.

Cells of the Inflammatory Process

The cells involved in the inflammatory process are the *leukocytes* (white blood cells). Leukocytes include *neutrophils, eosinophils, lymphocytes,* and *monocytes.* Other cells throughout the body (but not within the bloodstream), such as *mast cells* and *macrophages* or *histiocytes,* also play a key role in the inflammatory process.

BOX 8-2

Signs of Inflammation

Heat
Swelling
Pain
Redness
Loss of function

Neutrophils are the first leukocytes participating in the chain of events that occurs during an inflammatory reaction. The cells exit the blood vessels at the site by "squeezing" through the microscopic space between the endothelial cells lining the blood vessels. The primary function of neutrophils in the inflammatory process is *phagocytosis,* or ingestion of pathogens, as well as release of lysosomal enzymes, which destroy the pathogens. Neutrophils are very short-lived; they survive for only 24 to 48 hours once they leave the blood vessels and enter the host tissues.

Eosinophils, so named because they have eosinophilic (pink to reddish-orange) granules, also participate in inflammatory reactions. However, they are more specific than neutrophils and usually are prominent only in inflammation associated with parasitic infestations and allergic reactions. Like neutrophils, eosinophils have two major roles: (1) phagocytosis and (2) lysosomal enzyme release.

A lymphocyte is another type of important leukocyte in the inflammatory process. Like neutrophils, lymphocytes migrate to the tissue site of inflammation, but they have a very different role in the inflammatory process. They are responsible for humoral antibody production and cellular immunity. Lymphocytes can be divided into B-lymphocytes and T-lymphocytes; however, these two groups cannot be distinguished microscopically. B-lymphocytes can be transformed into plasma cells, which produce antibodies. T-lymphocytes are capable of directly killing cells. They also secrete *lymphokines,* chemical substances that allow macrophages to easily phagocytize pathogens.

Monocytes are a stage in the development of tissue macrophages. Once monocytes leave the bloodstream and enter the tissue at the site of the inflammatory process, they become activated macrophages. Macrophages are the workhorses of the inflammatory process; they contain a large number of lysosomal enzymes that kill pathogens. They are also capable of phagocytosis.

Inflammatory Exudates

An *exudate* is the visible product of the inflammatory process. It is usually composed of cellular debris, fluids, and cells that are deposited in tissues as well as on tissue surfaces, such as the serosal, mucosal, and skin surfaces. Exudates may be classified based on their primary constituent, such as *serous, fibrinous, purulent* (or *suppurative*), or others.

A serous exudate consists primarily of fluid with a low protein content. Cutaneous blisters are examples of lesions that contain a serous exudate. A fibrinous exudate is composed chiefly of fibrin, which is derived from a plasma protein, fibrinogen. Fibrinous exudate is observed in traumatic reticulopericarditis ("hardware disease"). This disease can occur when a cow ingests a metallic foreign body (nail or wire) that penetrates the forestomach (reticulum) and subsequently penetrates the diaphragm and pericardium, the membranous sac surrounding the heart. As a result, a large amount of fibrin collects in the pericardial sac. The proper morphologic diagnosis for this lesion is fibrinous pericarditis (Fig. 8-1).

Purulent or suppurative exudates are composed primarily of large numbers of neutrophils and cellular debris. Abscesses contain a purulent or suppurative exudate (Fig. 8-2).

A *hemorrhagic* exudate consists primarily of erythrocytes that have collected in a tissue after disruption of the vascular system. Other less common types of exudate include *mucopurulent* (or *catarrhal*), *eosinophilic*, and *nonsuppurative*. Mucopurulent exudates consist of a mixture of purulent and mucous exudates. They are commonly found in tissues that secrete mucus (i.e., have a mucous membrane), such as the intestinal tract and the respiratory tract. Eosinophilic exudates are composed primarily of eosinophils and are associated with such diseases as salt poisoning of pigs and eosinophilic myositis of dogs. Nonsuppurative exudates are composed primarily of monocytes, such as histiocytes and lymphocytes. The term *nonsuppurative* is usually restricted to exudates in only two anatomic sites: (1) the central nervous system and (2) the integumentary system (skin). Finally, exudates may consist of the combination of the above-mentioned types, such as *fibrinopurulent* or *necrohemorrhagic exudates*.

Vascular Changes Associated With Inflammation

The cellular response associated with inflammation is only a part of the inflammatory process; the blood vessels or vascular system are also involved. Blood vessels are highly dynamic structures that respond rapidly during inflammation. The first response of the blood vessel to vascular injury is dilatation, which means the diameter of the blood vessel increases, allowing more blood to flow into the affected area. This is caused by local release of histamine

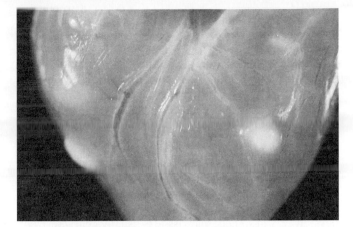

Fig. 8-2 A heart with multiple abscesses.

from mast cells. Next there is increased vascular permeability, which means the blood vessels become slightly "leaky." This is the result of contraction of endothelial cells lining the inside of blood vessels. Increased vascular permeability allows a wide array of proteins to pass through the vessel walls to the site of inflammation. Immediately after vascular permeability increases, the process of exudation allows an influx of leukocytes and red blood cells to the inflammatory site. Congestion of the blood vessels occurs in the next step, which means *stasis* or "sludging" of blood flow in the vessels from fluid loss through exudation.

All of these events work in concert with the cells associated with inflammation such that the host is able to repair the injured site and defend itself against infection. The entire process occurs rapidly, beginning with vascular dilatation, which occurs within minutes of the initial insult, and ending with initiation of congestion within 8 hours of the initial vascular dilatation.

Healing and Repair of Damaged Tissues

The repair process really starts as soon as injury occurs, but healing is the last event to be completed in the inflammatory process. In almost every organ system, the end result of tissue repair is fibrosis or scarring. The exception to this is in the central nervous system, which includes the brain and the spinal cord. Fibrosis does not occur in the central nervous system because it would be detrimental to the functioning of these vital tissues. Repair can take place by first-intention or by second-intention healing.

With first-intention healing of the skin, the edges of the wound surfaces close together with no discernible scarring. Proliferation of fibroblasts and endothelial cells rapidly forms a collagenous matrix. This matrix forms a bridge that brings the edges of the wound together. The last step in this process is re-epithelialization, whereby the wound surface is re-covered with epithelium (cells lining the outer surface of the skin).

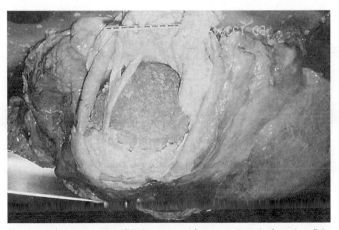

Fig. 8-1 Fibrinous pericarditis in a cow with traumatic reticulopericarditis.

Second-intention healing repairs wounds involving much greater tissue damage. Fibroblasts and endothelial cells proliferate. Unlike first-intention healing, second-intention healing produces granulation tissue. Granulation tissue is a highly vascularized connective tissue that is only produced after extensive tissue damage. Re-epithelialization eventually occurs unless excessive granulation tissue forms, a condition commonly referred to by lay people as "proud flesh." This excessive granulation tissue must be removed before the wound surface can be re-epithelialized.

Fibrosis or scar tissue primarily comprises dense fibrous connective tissue and collagen and contracts when mature. In parenchymatous organ systems, such as the lungs, kidneys, liver, and spleen, scar tissue is usually characterized as a small, irregular focus that has shrunken beneath the capsule of the organ (Fig. 8-3).

PATHOGENS

Pathogens are infectious organisms that can cause disease in a host. Pathogenic agents include parasites, bacteria, fungi, rickettsiae, mycoplasmas, chlamydiae, and viruses. Many of these organisms are very specific in their ability to cause disease in only certain animal species. In most cases, they affect very specific organs or organ systems of the body.

Parasites

Parasites are organisms that have adapted to live within or on a host, deriving all of their nutrients from that host, ideally without killing the host. Chapter 11 contains an extensive discussion of internal and external parasites.

Bacteria

Bacteria make up another group of pathogens that cause disease in animals. Within the infected host, bacteria may be found in the *interstitium* (between cell layers), within inflammatory cells, or on epithelial surfaces. Bacteria are classified as either *gram-positive* or *gram-negative*, depending on their staining characteristics with Gram stain. Gram-positive organisms stain purple, and gram-negative organisms stain red. As a general rule, gram-negative bacteria contain *endotoxins* (substances that cause disease), while gram-positive bacteria contain preformed *exotoxins*. Some bacteria are *pyogenic* and cause the host to produce a purulent (suppurative) exudate (pus). See Chapter 13 for more information.

Animals with bacterial infections are often febrile, lethargic, and anorexic. This is due in part to the associated endotoxins, which stimulate release of an endogenous pyrogen from neutrophils. Endogenous pyrogen is a protein that causes fever and associated lethargy and inappetence. However, this protein aids the animal by increasing the body temperature and allowing neutrophils to be more effective in killing bacteria. Bacterial virulence factors determine the pathogenicity of bacteria. The surface of bacteria comprises such structures as *pili*, *capsules*, and the *cell wall*. These virulence factors allow the bacteria to more easily attach to and colonize tissues and minimize the host immune response. Additionally, bacteria may possess a wide variety of enzymes or proteins, also known as *soluble factors*, which inhibit host functions and provide the bacteria a "foothold" within the host.

Viruses

Viruses are extremely small organisms, ranging from 30 to 450 nm in diameter, which can cause disease in a wide variety of animals. For viruses to cause disease, they must enter the animal's body, bind to the surface of a cell, enter the cell, and destroy it.

Certain viruses are specific for the type of cells they attack. For example, *epitheliotropic* viruses attack epithelial cells, such as respiratory, intestinal, or urinary epithelium. The clinical signs of viral diseases are associated with death of the infected cells. For example, canine distemper virus, a morbillivirus, attaches to and destroys the epithelium of the dog's lungs. Dogs with distemper may develop coughing and respiratory distress because of the effect of viral infection of the lung. The result is interstitial pneumonia caused by the inflammatory infiltrates within the interstitium of the lung. Transmissible gastroenteritis virus of pigs, caused by coronavirus, destroys the gastric and intestinal epithelium of preweanling pigs. A lesion of transmissible gastroenteritis virus is villous atrophy; affected intestinal villi become shortened and blunted and have an atrophic appearance. Clinical signs include vomiting, diarrhea, dehydration, and death (Fig. 8-4).

Viruses classified as *neurotropic* invade and destroy cells of the central nervous system. Examples of disease caused by these viruses include rabies and equine encephalitis.

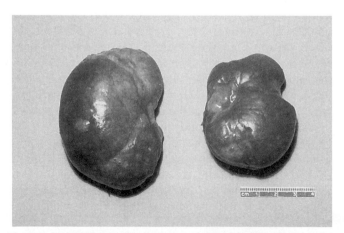

Fig. 8-3 Multiple bands of scar tissue on the outer surface of kidneys in a dog.

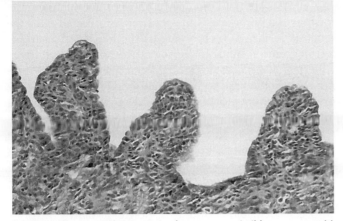

Fig. 8-4 Villous atrophy in a pig due to transmissible gastroenteritis virus. Note the blunt, short villi.

Rabies is caused by a rhabdovirus and has a worldwide distribution. Most cases of rabies are spread by animal bites; the virus is present in the saliva of infected animals. After the virus enters the body, it travels to the central nervous system by way of peripheral nerves. Once it enters the central nervous system, it infects and destroys neurons. Animals infected with this virus develop behavioral changes and sometimes become aggressive, which may result in biting other animals or humans. The lesions of rabies are those of nonsuppurative encephalitis. Diagnosis is dependent on demonstration of characteristic Negri bodies (eosinophilic inclusion bodies) within affected neurons.

As is the case of parasites and bacteria, a large number of viruses can infect animals. A list of some common viruses that cause disease in animals is presented in Table 8-1.

NONPATHOGENS

Disease can also be produced in animals by nonpathogens. Nonpathogenic causes of disease include trauma associated with mechanical, sonic, thermal, and electrical injuries, temperature extremes, and irradiation.

The primary effect of trauma, regardless of the initiating cause, is tissue necrosis and hemorrhage. Trauma is a physical wound or injury. A *wound* is an injury caused by physical means, with disruption of normal structures. An *abrasion* is an injury whereby the epithelium is removed from the tissue surface. A *contusion* is a bruise or injury with no break in the surface of the tissue. A *laceration* is a tear or jagged wound. A *concussion* is a violent shock or jarring of the tissue, a common injury to the brain after blunt trauma to the head. In all of these instances, the inflammatory process occurs as described previously in this chapter, with the exception of destruction and removal of the pathogen.

IMMUNE RESPONSE

The immune system is another inherent protective mechanism of the body. This highly complex and complicated system has many components that, along with the inflammatory process, prevent pathogens from causing disease.

Responses of the immune system can be divided into *humoral immune responses* and *cell-mediated immune responses*. The primary components of the humoral response are antibodies produced by plasma cells or *plasmacytes*, which are transformed *B-lymphocytes*. The other major subset of lymphocytes, referred to as *T-lymphocytes*, plays a major role in the cell-mediated response. B-lymphocytes are distributed throughout the body within the lymph nodes, spleen,

---

TABLE 8-1

Some Viruses That Cause Disease in Animals

Virus Classification	Disease	Host	Lesions
Morbillivirus	Canine distemper	Canidae, mink, raccoon, ferret	Pneumonia, encephalitis
Herpes virus	Pseudorabies	Pig	Abortion, encephalitis
Herpes virus	Infectious laryngotracheitis	Avian	Laryngotracheitis
Adenovirus	Infectious canine hepatitis	Canidae	Acute necrotizing hepatitis
Papillomavirus	Sarcoid	Horse	Sarcoids (neoplasm)
Rhabdovirus	Rabies	Mammals	Fatal encephalomyelitis
Coronavirus	Transmissible gastroenteritis (TGE)	Pig	Enteritis, villous atrophy
Coronavirus	Feline infectious peritonitis (FIP)	Cat	Peritonitis, pleuritis
Alphavirus *(Arbovirus)*	Eastern, western Venezuelan equine encephalitis	Horse	Encephalitis

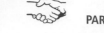

Peyer's patches, and other organs. B-lymphocytes are so named because they were first discovered in the bursa of Fabricius, which is a lymphoid organ of birds. T-lymphocytes are so designated because they arise from the thymus, a lymphoid organ of birds and mammals. All mammals, as well as birds, possess both B-lymphocytes and T-lymphocytes. These lymphocytes cannot be distinguished by their morphology because they look identical under the microscope; however, they can be differentiated by their function. They may also be differentiated by their cell surface markers, which are molecules attached to their surface, necessary for binding with substances such as antigens, antibodies, etc.

Humoral Immunity

Humoral immunity implies that antibodies are produced against a particular pathogen. When the pathogen enters the host's body, it becomes coated with antibody, allowing it to be more easily destroyed by cells involved in the inflammatory process. Antibodies are protein molecules that can attach to the surface of cells and coat pathogens.

Antibodies can be detected in the serum of animals; the study and application of this science is known as *serology*. The principles of serology and immunology are discussed in more detail in Chapter 12. The level of antibodies present in the serum (blood) is reported as an antibody *titer*. Antibody titers represent the reciprocal of the highest dilution of the serum containing antibody that still gives a positive reaction to the serologic test being performed. Although a very high antibody titer to certain pathogens may indicate protection against or immunity to a specific pathogen, it may be very difficult to differentiate between vaccine-induced immunity or natural immunity. This difficulty can be seen with Lyme disease. A special test called a Western Blot must be done to differentiate from vaccine-induced immunity and natural immunity from exposure.

Natural immunity implies that the animal has been exposed to the pathogen by natural means rather than through vaccination. With natural immunity, the animal may have previously become ill from infection with a specific pathogen and may have produced antibodies against the pathogen during the disease.

Antibodies, or *immunoglobulins*, can be classified by their molecular weight into immunoglobulin isotopes, including IgG, IgM, IgA, and IgE. The IgG immunoglobulin is the most common antibody and is found in the highest concentration in the blood. It helps defend tissues by opsonizing or coating the outer surface of pathogens, which allows them to be more easily phagocytized by macrophages.

The IgM immunoglobulin is the second most common antibody in the blood. It is the major immunoglobulin isotype produced in a primary immune response. It is more efficient than IgG in opsonization and neutralization of viruses. The antibody isotype IgA is of primary importance for mucosal immunity. This antibody is secreted onto the mucosal surface of such organs as the lungs and gastrointestinal tract. It binds to pathogens to prevent them from adhering to mucosal surfaces, preventing them from gaining a foothold in the body. The antibody isotype IgE is the primary immunoglobulin associated with Type-1 hypersensitivity reactions, which are discussed later in the chapter. It also plays a role in helminth infestations, along with certain cells from the inflammatory process, including eosinophils.

Cell-Mediated Immunity

The cell-mediated immune response primarily involves T-lymphocytes and macrophages. Much less is known about this type of immunity as compared with humoral immunity. Cell-mediated immunity begins when a T-lymphocyte binds a pathogen to its cell surface. The T-lymphocyte may then present the pathogen to a macrophage, which phagocytizes and kills it, or it may produce specific cytokines, also called *lymphokines*. These lymphokines stimulate macrophages to become more efficient in phagocytosis and pathogen destruction, and recruit more T-lymphocytes to the area.

Response to Vaccination

Animals can be immunized (vaccinated) against a wide variety of diseases, ranging from blackleg in cattle to distemper in dogs. These vaccines are commonly administered by injection. The vaccine often consists of a portion of the pathogen, such as the cell wall of the causative bacterium or a small unit of the virus. After injection, the vaccine does not cause disease but stimulates the cells of the immune system to develop antibodies against that particular pathogen. Upon the next exposure to the pathogen, a vaccinated animal will not become infected because it has been immunized.

Hypersensitivity Reactions

Abnormally severe inflammatory responses mediated by the immune system are called hypersensitivity reactions. These allergic reactions have been classified into four types: Type I (immediate); Type II (cytotoxic); Type III (immune complex); and Type IV (delayed).

Type-I hypersensitivity reactions occur within minutes after exposure to an antigen. An antigen is any foreign substance causing an abnormal immune response upon exposure to that substance. Animals may be exposed to antigens by direct contact, inhalation, ingestion, insect bites or stings, or injection. Examples of antigens include pollen, proteins (e.g., in food, milk, or bacterial cell walls), and plant resins (e.g., in poison ivy or poison oak). Antigens are often referred to as allergens when they evoke an allergic reaction.

Type-I reactions are mediated by IgE on the surface of mast cells located on mucosal surfaces (airways, intestines) and in connective tissues. Upon exposure, the antigen is bound by IgE, causing the mast cells to release granules containing various factors, such as histamine, serotonin, and leukotrienes. These factors cause vasodilation, increased vascular permeability, smooth muscle contraction, and other inflammatory changes.

The severity and manifestation of a Type-I hypersensitivity reaction depend on the location and number of mast cells stimulated as well as the route of exposure and amount of antigen involved. Reactions may be relatively mild, such as *urticaria* (hives) after a bee sting or diarrhea after eating a particular food ingredient. However, Type-I reactions can also be very severe, such as acute anaphylaxis, which is characterized by profound hypotension (low blood pressure), pulmonary edema, and collapse, caused by massive exposure to an antigen.

Type-II hypersensitivity reactions involve destruction of certain cells by neutrophils and macrophages or by activation of *complement*. Complement is a group of enzymes that act in sequential fashion, leading to disruption of tissue or bacterial cell membranes and resulting in the cell's destruction. An adverse reaction to blood transfusion is an example of a Type-II reaction.

Red blood cells contain on their cell surface antigens called *blood group antigens.* Animals of the same species tend to develop antibodies against blood groups other than their own. The red cells function normally, and no immune response results if blood from one animal is transfused to a recipient with the same blood group. However, if blood is transfused into a recipient with a different blood group, the donor's red cells are destroyed by *hemolysis* (rupture) or phagocytosis, or become *agglutinated* (clumped). The first of such incompatible transfusions may be well tolerated. However, the transfusion stimulates production of antibodies, and these antibodies immediately destroy the red cells in a second transfusion.

In Type-III hypersensitivity reactions, antigens and antibodies interact to form immune complexes in various tissues, such as the skin, joints, eyes, lungs, or blood vessel walls. Macrophages gather in these areas to destroy the immune complexes, resulting in inflammation. Examples of Type-III reactions include rheumatoid arthritis and equine viral arteritis.

Type-IV hypersensitivity reactions occur hours after sensitized animals are again exposed to a particular antigen. These delayed hypersensitivity reactions reach their peak at about 24 hours after exposure and are mediated by sensitized T-cells. The tuberculin test used in cattle is a classic example of Type-IV hypersensitivity. A small volume of extract of *Mycobacterium tuberculosis* is injected into the skin of the animal. Normal cattle show no significant response to the injection. Cattle previously exposed to *Mycobacterium tuberculosis*, however, develop a large, warm swelling at the injection site within 12 to 24 hours.

Public health is a community's effort to prevent disease and promote life and health. The effort usually includes sanitation of the environment, control of communicable infections, education of individuals in personal hygiene, and organization of medical and nursing services to ensure proper health care. Veterinary public health plays an important role in protecting and improving human well-being by using veterinary knowledge and skills to preserve the healthy relationship between humans and animals. The veterinary profession's major roles in preventing disease in people are in epidemiology, food hygiene, and zoonotic disease.

EPIDEMIOLOGY

Epidemiology is the study of the occurrences of disease and the risk factors that cause disease in a population. Some texts refer to the study of disease in an animal population as *epizootiology*, but the term *epidemiology* is appropriate for both human and animal populations and is a more widely recognized term. Descriptive epidemiology studies the frequency of disease in a population and describes the type of animals affected and how and when they are affected. In other words, it describes the disease in terms of the animal or people affected and the time and geographic region in which they are affected. This information gives epidemiologists clues about the cause of disease, allows epidemiologists to form hypotheses about the cause, and helps epidemiologists determine the risk that animals or people will become ill. Epidemiologists can then design more elaborate analytic epidemiologic studies to test these hypotheses. Once the cause of the disease and the risk factors that influence the disease are identified, programs for control or prevention of the disease can be implemented. Epidemiologists are essential professionals in veterinary and human public health efforts to study the cause and to initiate the control of disease.

FOOD HYGIENE

The field of food hygiene involves making sure that food is safe and wholesome for human consumption. Proper food hygiene is important in preventing foodborne diseases. Millions of people in the United States become ill with foodborne diseases every year. Primarily, veterinarians are involved in the food hygiene process through inspection and processing of animals for food. Proper inspection and processing are essential in prevention of foodborne diseases that originate from contamination with bacteria at the slaughterhouse. These organisms are the cause of significant disease in people. Some of the most common organ-

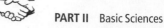
isms involved are *Salmonella* spp., *Campylobacter* spp., and *E. coli* 0157:H7. An *E. coli* outbreak occurred recently in a number of people, particularly children, who ate undercooked hamburgers at a restaurant. *E. coli* 0157:H7 infection causes hemolytic uremia and may result in death. The most common source of Salmonella in the United States is poultry or poultry products, such as eggs. In fact, *Salmonella enteritidis* infection has become a highly reported foodborne disease in the United States and has generated new recommendations for the public in handling raw egg products. Proper cooking and handling of meat can help prevent serious disease. Other foodborne diseases can be caused by contamination of food and improper handling, such as *Staphylococcus* infection, *Clostridium* infection (botulism), and hepatitis.

An important step in food hygiene before an animal reaches the slaughterhouse is prevention of adulterating residues. Residues are hormonal compounds, antibacterials, antimycotics, anthelmintics, antiprotozoals, or pesticides in meat or milk that have accumulated to levels that are above the established safe tolerance levels. The U.S. Department of Agriculture (USDA) monitors foodstuffs for the presence of residues and is responsible for inspection of food. The Environmental Protection Agency (EPA) sets the residue limits for pesticides. The Food and Drug Administration (FDA) sets the limits for drug residues.

How do drugs become residues? Most drug residues are caused by misuse of drugs. Misuse of drugs includes not following label directions, using drugs in unapproved species, and not adhering to withdrawal times. Residues can occur in meat or milk through misuse of drugs in mastitis treatments or with injectable antibiotics. In addition, feed or drinking water can be contaminated with drugs or pesticides.

Residues are important to public health because they can cause toxic or allergic reactions in people. For example, penicillin residues in milk can cause a severe, life-threatening reaction in a person who is allergic to penicillin. Veterinarians and veterinary technicians are responsible for using drugs in food animals according to standard veterinary practice.

ZOONOTIC DISEASES

Zoonoses are the major area of involvement for veterinarians in public health. Zoonoses are diseases that are transmitted between animals and people. Other infectious diseases are common to but not transmitted between animals and people; these can be caused by similar exposures to the same infectious organism. Over 150 zoonoses have been reported. Zoonoses are a significant cause of human disability, hospitalization, death, and high economic cost in the United States and in underdeveloped countries. Table

8-2 lists the causative organism, hosts, and mode of transmission for some common zoonoses.

Primarily, veterinarians are concerned with monitoring and surveillance of zoonoses, evaluating risks to people, and planning and coordinating prevention and control programs with appropriate agencies and individuals. Part of that surveillance is looking for an outbreak or an epidemic of the disease. An epidemic is an increase over the normal expected number of disease cases in a geographic area or over a certain period. An endemic disease is one that has maintained a certain level of disease over time in a given geographic area. For example, rabies is endemic or always present at a certain level in raccoons in the eastern United States. However, in the late 1970s and early 1980s, when rabies began appearing in the mid-Atlantic area, it was considered epidemic. Surveillance of zoonoses or any other disease is dependent on knowledge about the cause of the disease, transmission of the disease, and how the disease is maintained in the population.

DISEASE TRANSMISSION

For an infectious disease to survive in a population, the agent causing the disease must be transmitted. The mode of transmission is an important epidemiologic clue in understanding the disease. It is important for the veterinary profession to be aware of how specific diseases are transmitted so that preventive measures can be taken and the public educated. Reservoirs and hosts of a specific disease are important to identify because these are essential in transmission of a disease and its maintenance in the population. Control programs for a disease are often aimed at the reservoirs or hosts of the disease. For example, spraying programs aimed at controlling mosquito populations are initiated when there is an outbreak of encephalitis.

Reservoirs can be inanimate (e.g., soil) or animate (e.g., animals, people, birds). Reservoirs are essential and necessary for the survival and reproduction of the organism. *Hosts* are living beings that offer an environment for maintenance of the organism, but they are not necessary for the organism's survival. Depending on the disease, the infectious organism may be transmitted through several hosts of different species. This is particularly true of helminth and protozoal diseases. Several hosts or reservoirs are required for the egg to develop to a larva and then to an adult. An infectious disease can be transmitted from the reservoir to a host or from one host to another host.

Direct transmission of disease requires close association or contact between a reservoir of the disease and a susceptible host. Contact with infected skin, mucous membranes, or droplets from an infected human or animal can cause disease. Examples of disease that are transmitted directly are rabies transmitted by a bite, leptospirosis by contact with

TABLE 8-2

The Causative Organisms, Animal Hosts, and Modes of Transmission for Selected Common Zoonoses

	Causative Organisms	Small Animal Hosts	Livestock Hosts	Wildlife Hosts	Modes of Transmission
Viral Diseases					
Rabies	Rhabdovirus	Most	Most	Most	Animal bite
Encephalitis (EEE, WEE)	Togavirus		Horses, poultry	Birds, rodents	Mosquito bite
Lymphocytic choriomeningitis	Arenavirus	Mice			Varied
Contagious ecthyma (orf)	Pox virus	Sometimes dogs	Sheep, goats		Contact
Simian herpes (B virus)	Herpesvirus simiae			Primates	Animal bite, direct contact
Newcastle disease	Paramyxovirus	Domestic birds	Poultry	Wild fowl	Contact, inhalation
Yellow fever	Togavirus			Primates	Mosquito bite
Hantavirus infection	Hantavirus			Rodents	Contact
Rickettsial Diseases					
Q fever	*Coxiella burnetii*		Cattle, sheep, goats	Birds, rabbits, rodents	Inhalation, milk ingestion, contact
Rocky Mountain spotted fever	*Rickettsia rickettsii*	Dogs		Rodents, rabbits	Tick bite
Psittacosis	*Chlamydia psittaci*	Psittacine birds	Turkeys, ducks	Birds	Inhalation
Mycoses					
Ringworm	*Tricophyton* spp., *Microsporum* spp.	Cats, dogs	Cattle, horses, pigs, sheep	Rodents	Contact
Parasitic Diseases					
Trichinosis	*Trichinella spiralis*		Pigs	Rats, bears, carnivores	Ingestion
Scabies	*Sarcoptes scabiei*	Dogs, rodents, cats	Horses	Primates	Contact
Taeniasis, Cysticercosis	*Taenia* spp., *Cysticercus*		Pigs, cattle	Boars	Ingestion
Hydatid disease	*Echinococcus* spp.	Dogs	Herbivores	Wolves	Ingestion
Schistosomiasis	*Schistosoma* spp.	Dogs, cats	Pigs, cattle, horses	Rodents	Contact
Larva migrans	*Toxocara, Ancylostoma, Strongyloides*	Dogs, cats	Pigs, cattle	Raccoons	Ingestion
Bacterial Diseases					
Anthrax	*Bacillus anthracis*	Dogs	Most	Most except primates	Contact
Brucellosis	*Brucella* spp.	Dogs	Cattle, pigs, sheep, goats	All except primates	Contact, inhalation, ingestion
Plague	*Yersinia pestis*	Cats		Rodents, rabbits	Flea bite
Campylobacteriosis	*Campylobacter fetus fetus*	Dogs, cats	Cattle, poultry, sheep, pigs	Rodents, birds	Ingestion, contact
Cat-scratch disease	*Bartonella henselae*	Cats		Cats	Cat bite, scratch
Leptospirosis	*Leptospira* spp.	All, especially dogs	All, especially cattle, pigs	Rats, raccoons	Contact with urine
Salmonellosis	*Salmonella* spp.	All, especially dogs, cats	All, especially pigs, poultry, cattle	Rodents, reptiles	Ingestion
Tuberculosis	*Mycobacteria* spp.	Dogs, cats	Cattle, pigs, goats, sheep, poultry	All except rodents, monkeys	Ingestion, inhalation
Tularemia	*Francisella tularensis*	All	All except horses	Rodents, rabbits	Tick bites, contact with tissue

Continued

TABLE 8-2

The Causative Organisms, Animal Hosts, and Modes of Transmission for Selected Common Zoonoses—Cont'd

	Causative Organisms	Small Animal Hosts	Livestock Hosts	Wildlife Hosts	Modes of Transmission
Erysipelas	*Erysipelothrix rhusiopathiae*		Pigs, sheep, cattle, horses, poultry	Rodents	Contact
Tetanus	*Clostridium tetani*		Horses	Reptiles	Wound
Lyme disease	*Borrelia burgdorferi*	Dogs, cats	Cattle, horses	Deer, birds, rodents	Tick bite
Protozoal Diseases					
Cryptosporidiosis	*Cryptosporidium* spp.	Most	Calves, sheep	Birds	Ingestion
Toxoplasmosis	*Toxoplasma gondii*	Cats, rabbits, guinea pigs	Pigs, sheep, cattle, horses	Cats	Ingestion
Balantidiasis	*Balantidium coli*		Pigs	Rats, primates	Ingestion
Sarcocystosis	*Sarcocystis* spp.	Dogs, cats	Pigs, cattle		Ingestion
Giardiasis	*Giardia lamblia*	Dogs, cats	Pigs, cattle	Beavers, zoo monkeys	Ingestion

contaminated urine, and brucellosis by contact with infected tissues. Another example of direct transmission is through contact with the wool, hair, or hide of an infected animal. Anthrax, although not very common in the United States, is transmitted to people through skin contact with contaminated bone meal from infected cattle or direct contact with infected wool or hair.

Animal bites can be a source of infections, trauma, and even zoonotic disease. Pasteurella is responsible for 50% of dog bite infections and 90% of cat bite infections. Cat bites are 10 times more likely to become infected than dog bites. Mixed infections include *Staphylococcus aureus*, *Staphylococcus epidermidis*, *Streptococcus* spp., *Bacteroides* spp., *Fusobacterium* spp., and other gram-negative bacteria that can cause fever, septicemia, meningitis, endocarditis, and septic arthritis.

Soil or vegetation contaminated with parasites, bacteria, or spores may be another source of direct transmission. *Visceral larva migrans* is transmitted when children eat soil or vegetables that have been contaminated with feces that contain Toxocara (roundworm) eggs. The eggs hatch in the individual's gastrointestinal system and the larvae migrate through the organs. The disease is usually mild and chronic, with eosinophilia, fever, hepatomegaly, and pulmonary signs. If the larvae migrate to the eye, there may be loss of vision or the eye. A similar disease occurs with Ancylostoma (hookworm). The signs of cutaneous larva migrans are those of dermatitis, which is caused by the hookworm larvae migrating in the skin.

Droplet spread is differentiated from airborne transmission by the fact that the droplets travel only a short distance (i.e., a few feet) and involve larger particles that often are removed by mechanisms in the upper respiratory passages.

Psittacosis is an occupational risk at poultry processing plants. People are infected by inhalation of *Chlamydia psittaci* from the droppings or secretions of infected birds. Cage and aviary birds, especially infected large birds that are shipped into pet stores from foreign countries and not properly treated with antibiotics, can also infect people.

Indirect transmission of disease is more complicated and involves intermediaries that carry the agent of disease from one source to another. The intermediary may be airborne; vector-borne (an arthropod); or vehicle-borne through water, food, blood, or an inanimate object. A *vector* is a living organism that transports the infectious agent. A *vehicle* is simply the mode of transmission of an infectious agent from the reservoir to the host. Indirect airborne transmission involves spread of the agent through tiny dust or droplet particles over long distances. Particles smaller than 5 microns in diameter can be inhaled into the alveoli deep within the lungs. *Q fever* is most commonly transmitted by airborne transmission. It is transmitted by inhalation of the rickettsia, *Coxiella burnetii*, in dust from areas that are contaminated by tissue or excreta from infected animals. Airborne particles with the infective organism can travel a long distance, which makes it difficult to locate the source of the infection. Q fever can also be transmitted by direct contact with contaminated wool, other materials, and milk. Infected individuals may have an inapparent infection or they may have chills, headache, weakness, and sweats.

Various types of arthropods may serve as vectors. These may include mosquitoes, ticks, and fleas. Each type of arthropod has its own life cycle that is often reflected by seasonal and geographic patterns in transmission of disease. For example, ticks may have two- or three-host maturation cycles and may take 2 years to complete a life cycle. Arthropods may carry the agent mechanically to a susceptible host, or they may be involved biologically in multiplication of the organism or in a stage of development.

Plague is the best-known vectorborne disease involving the flea as a vector. Plague still occurs in the western United States. The natural reservoir for plague is wild rodents, such as ground squirrels. Infected fleas that spend time on rabbits and especially on domestic cats are a source of infection for people. The most common source of transmission is through the bite of an infected flea. In addition, people can be infected by handling infected tissues during hunting of small ground animals or even by airborne transmission. The mortality (death rate) from untreated plague can be 50%.

Several diseases are transmitted by ticks. Lyme disease *(borreliosis)* is the most commonly reported tickborne disease, but Rocky Mountain spotted fever is the deadlier disease. Other newly discovered diseases in which the role of animals is less clear are *ehrlichiosis* and *babesiosis*. Rocky Mountain spotted fever causes high fever, headache, chills, severe muscle pain, and malaise. In about 50% of patients, a rash occurs on the palms and soles and then spreads to the rest of the body. Mortality is about 15% to 20% if the disease is not treated. Rocky Mountain spotted fever is maintained in nature by ticks, either the dog tick *Dermacentor* or the Lone Star tick *Ambylomma*. People are infected by the tick bite during outdoor activities in tick-infested areas or from contact with ticks on pets. Wearing tick repellents in areas infested with ticks and keeping pet dogs free of ticks prevents tick-transmitted diseases.

Food and water are also vehicles of indirect transmission of disease. Both are sources of bacterial, viral, and parasitic diseases. Foodborne diseases are acquired by consumption of contaminated food or water. Foodborne intoxications are caused by toxins produced by certain bacteria that may contaminate food, such as *Staphylococcus aureus, Clostridium* spp., *and Vibrio* spp. The toxins may be present in the food or may be formed in the intestinal tract after the contaminated food is eaten. Foodborne infections are caused by bacterial or viral organisms that cause infection. These include *Salmonella* spp., *Campylobacter* spp., hepatitis virus, and *Vibrio* spp. The type of organism involved determines the incubation period and how quickly the clinical signs appear. Each organism also causes certain clinical signs, such as diarrhea, vomiting, or nausea. These specific incubation periods and particular clinical signs help epidemiologists determine the organism's identity and source.

Parasitic diseases are also transmitted through food and water. Nematode and trematode infections are most often transmitted either through ingestion of eggs or through ingestion of undercooked meat that contains cysts. Giardia is a protozoan that causes gastrointestinal disease in people; giardiasis can be quite serious in immunosuppressed individuals. Although Giardia is most often transmitted from person to person, it is also a source of waterborne outbreaks when people use mountain streams as community water sources without proper filtration techniques or drink the water during outdoor activities. Beavers and other domestic animals are reservoirs.

Cryptosporidiosis is another disease that can be transmitted by contaminated water and is a serious disease in immunosuppressed individuals. Cattle and other domestic animals are reservoirs. Proper water filtration and treatment are essential in preventing waterborne diseases.

Pasteurization of milk is important to prevent diseases that can be transmitted through milk. Milk can transmit disease directly from animal to animal or from animals to people through ingestion of contaminated milk. Diseases directly transmitted through milk include *brucellosis, Q fever, tuberculosis, toxoplasmosis,* and *listeriosis*. Milk can be contaminated with bacteria, such as *Campylobacter* spp., *Salmonella* spp., and *E. coli,* either from the animal or from the environment. These bacteria can cause disease in people.

MAINTENANCE OF DISEASE

Included in the transmission cycle of disease is maintenance of disease in the human or animal population. There are several ways in which zoonotic diseases are maintained in a population. A direct zoonosis is transmitted by a single vertebrate species. For example, the organism that causes cat-scratch fever is maintained in the feline population. In the eastern United States, rabies virus is maintained in the raccoon and bat population.

A *cyclozoonosis* requires several cycles of disease, usually a parasitic disease, to occur in several different vertebrate species. An example of this is hydatid disease caused by the tapeworm *Echinococcus*. The signs of echinococcosis in infected people depend on the number, size, and location of the cysts of Echinococcus. The primary reservoir of the adult tapeworm is the dog; eggs are produced and are shed in dog feces. The intermediate hosts are cattle, sheep, pigs, and goats. These species eat grasses and plants that are contaminated with feces. The eggs hatch and become larvae in the intermediate hosts, and cysts are formed in their organs. Dogs are reinfected by eating the organs and tissues of dead cattle, sheep, and other infected livestock, and the cycle begins again. People are infected by ingesting tapeworm eggs while handling contaminated materials or soil, or infected dogs.

A *metazoonosis* is maintained by both invertebrate (tick or mosquito) and vertebrate species. An example is *encephalitis*. This viral disease is maintained in the vertebrate population of wild or domestic birds and horses through transmission by a mosquito. People are often infected accidentally.

A *saprozoonosis* depends on an inanimate reservoir to maintain the cycle of infection. Visceral larva migrans, caused by *Toxocara* spp., is considered a saprozoonosis, although the disease also involves vertebrate reservoirs. Soil is essential for transmission of the disease to people and for reinfection of dogs and cats. Infected dogs and cats shed Toxocara eggs in their feces. Humid soil is most favorable for survival of the eggs.

CONTROL OF ZOONOTIC DISEASES

Because of their regular contact with animals, animal tissues, animal environments, and pet owners, veterinarians and veterinary technicians are often the first to notice a zoonotic disease or the potential for one. In fact, animals can act as sentinels for a potential epidemic or outbreak of infection in people. A good example are the arboviral diseases, such as eastern equine encephalitis, western equine encephalitis, California and St. Louis encephalitis, and Japanese encephalitis. Fever and headache characterize mild forms of these diseases; the most serious forms can cause death in people. Mortality depends on the specific type of virus involved. The diseases are transmitted by the bite of an infected mosquito. Mosquitoes acquire the infection from birds, horses, and even pigs (Japanese encephalitis). Eastern equine encephalitis is transmitted among birds; horses and people are uncommon hosts. Both eastern equine encephalitis and western equine encephalitis viruses can cause encephalitis in horses. Venezuelan equine encephalomyelitis rarely causes encephalitis in people but typically causes a flulike viral infection in people. Horses are the reservoir for infection in people. Cases of encephalitis in birds or horses can signal a potential problem for humans; consequently, preventive programs can be implemented before a large outbreak of disease occurs in the human population.

Knowledge of how zoonotic diseases are transmitted and maintained in a population is important for preventing spread of diseases and preventing infection in veterinarians and veterinary technicians. Because of their close working contact with animals, veterinary professionals are at risk of contracting zoonotic diseases. It is important to determine what diseases are most common in certain animal species so that the risk of contracting a particular disease can be estimated. Certain groups of people are more susceptible and suffer more serious effects to zoonotic diseases than others.

Children and the elderly are more susceptible because their immune systems function at a lower level than those of normal healthy adults. AIDS, lupus, and chemotherapeutic medications suppress function of the immune system, making an individual more susceptible to disease. Children are also more likely to put contaminated soil or materials in their mouth. Pregnant women are also highly susceptible. Some diseases, such as *toxoplasmosis*, represent a serious disease threat to newborn infants.

Control of zoonotic diseases is aimed at the reservoir of disease or the intermediaries that transmit the disease. Control measures include spraying for mosquitoes, use of tick repellent, pasteurization of milk, adequate water filtration, and proper cooking and handling of food. Control programs also include treatment of infected animals in the reservoir population and decrease of contact with infected animals in the reservoir to prevent further transmission. Prevention programs require a thorough knowledge of the disease and how it is maintained and transmitted in order to break the cycle of disease in the population or prevent disease transmission. Prevention programs include vaccination of animals in the reservoir population, potential hosts, and people, if vaccines against that disease are available. Prevention of human infection is possible by treatment of infected animals that may transmit the disease to people. For example, treating puppies and kittens for roundworms and hookworms can prevent contamination of soil by feces containing infective eggs. Veterinarians and veterinary technicians can also test animals for infection, such as for tuberculosis and brucellosis.

The content of this chapter does not necessarily reflect the views or policies of the Department of Health and Human Services or the Food and Drug Administration, nor does the mention of trade names, commercial products, or organizations imply endorsement by the U.S. government.

RECOMMENDED READINGS

August JR: Dog and cat bites, *J Am Vet Med Assoc* 193:1394-1398, 1988.

AVMA: *Zoonoses update*, ed 2, American Veterinary Medical Association, 1996.

Benenson AS, ed: *Control of communicable diseases in man*, ed 16, Washington, D.C., 1996, American Public Health Association.

Breitschwerdt EB: Tick-borne zoonoses, *Vet Tech* 11(5):249-251, 1990.

Cheville NF: *Introduction to veterinary pathology*, ed 2, Ames, Iowa, 1999, Iowa State University Press.

Cotran RS, et al: *Robbins' pathologic basis of diseases*, ed 6, Philadelphia, 1999, WB Saunders.

Gershwin LJ, et al: *Immunology and immunopathology of domestic animals*, ed 2, St Louis, 1995, Mosby.

Jubb KVF, et al: *Pathology of domestic animals*, ed 4, San Diego, 1993, Academic Press.

McCapes RH, Osburn BI, Riemann H: Safety of foods of animal origin: responsibilities of veterinary medicine, *J Am Vet Med Assoc* 199:870-874, 1991.

McGavin MD, Carlton WW, Zachary JF: *Thomson's special veterinary pathology*, ed 3, St Louis, 2001, Mosby.

National Association of State Public Health Veterinarians, Inc: Compendium of animal rabies control, *J Am Vet Med Assoc* 208:214-218, 1996.

Tizard IR: *Veterinary immunology: an introduction*, ed 6, Philadelphia, 2000, WB Saunders.

9

Pharmacology and Pharmacy

Katie Samuelsen

Learning Objectives

After reviewing this chapter, the reader should understand the following:

- Various categories of drugs and their clinical uses
- Dosage forms in which drugs are available
- Ways in which drug dosages are calculated

- Routes by which various types of drugs are administered
- Ways in which drugs exert their effect and affect body tissue
- Procedures used to safely store and handle drugs
- Primary drugs affecting various body systems

DRUG NAMES

Drugs are generally referred by three different names. Their *chemical name*, such as D-alpha-amino-p-hydroxybenzyl-penicillin trihydrate, describes the drug's chemical composition. The *nonproprietary name* (sometimes called the *generic name*) is a more concise name given to the specific chemical compound. Examples of nonproprietary names are aspirin, acetaminophen, and amoxicillin. The *proprietary* or *trade name* is a unique drug name given by a manufacturer to its particular brand of drug. Examples of proprietary or trade names include Excedrin™, Tylenol™, and Amoxitabs™. Because the trade name is a proper noun, it is capitalized and the superscript© or™ is added to signify that the trade name is a registered trademark and cannot be legally used by other manufacturers. Because many drug manufacturers produce similar products, a single generic drug can be sold under multiple trade names. For example, the antibiotic amoxicillin is manufactured by several different companies, each of which has its own trade name for amoxicillin (e.g., Amoxi-Tabs, Robamox-V, Amoxil).

When a drug company develops and patents a new drug (not just a new trade name for an old drug, but a new chemical), and obtains FDA approval to sell the new drug, the company has the exclusive rights to manufacture this drug for a number of years. During that time, no other drug manufacturer can produce the same drug. This allows the drug company to recover, at the expense of the consumer, the costs of the research, development, and testing the company has invested to bring the drug to market. After these patent rights expire, other companies can legally produce the drug. These copycat drugs are called *generic equivalents*, because they have properties equivalent to those of the original compound. Generic equivalents are usually sold at a much lower price than the original manufacturer's product, because the generic manufacturer has not had to underwrite development of the original drug.

DOSAGE FORMS

Drugs are also described by their *dosage form*. *Solid* dosage forms include tablets, which are powdered drugs compressed into pills or disks, and capsules, which are powdered drugs enclosed within gelatin capsules. *Enteric-coated* tablets have a special covering that protects the drug from the harsh acidic environment of the stomach and prevents dissolving of the tablet until it enters the intestine.

Suppositories are inserted into the rectum, where they dissolve and release the drug to be absorbed across the membranes of the intestinal wall. Sustained-release forms of oral drugs release small amounts of the drug into the intestinal lumen over an extended time.

The authors acknowledge and appreciate the original contribution of Robert L. (Pete) Bill, whose work has been incorporated into this chapter.

A *solution* is a drug dissolved in a liquid vehicle that does not settle out if left standing. In contrast, a *suspension* contains drug particles that are suspended, but not dissolved, in the liquid vehicle. These drug particles usually settle to the bottom of the container when the container is left standing, so one must shake it back into suspension before administration to ensure consistent dosing. *Syrups*, such as cough syrups, are solutions of drugs with water and sugar (e.g., 85% sucrose). *Elixirs* are solutions of drugs dissolved in sweetened alcohol. Elixirs are used for drugs that do not readily dissolve in water. It is therefore important that you do not dilute an elixir with water, because the water will stratify into a layer separate from the elixir solution.

Tinctures are alcohol solutions meant for *topical application* (applied onto the skin). Topical products are available as liniments, which contain a drug in an oil base that are rubbed into the skin, or lotions, which are drug suspensions or solutions that are dabbed, brushed, or dripped onto the skin without rubbing (e.g., poison ivy medications). *Ointments*, *creams*, and *pastes* are semisolid dosage forms that are applied to the skin (ointments, creams) or given orally (pastes). Ointments and creams are designed to liquefy at body temperatures, whereas pastes tend to keep their semisolid form at body temperature.

Injectables are administered via a needle and syringe. Repository forms of injectable drugs are formulated to prolong absorption of the drug from the site of administration and thus provide a more sustained effective drug concentration in the body. *Implants* are solid dosage forms that are injected or inserted under the skin and dissolve or release a drug over an extended period.

PRESCRIPTIONS AND DISPENSING MEDICATION

Writing Prescriptions

A *prescription* is an order from a licensed veterinarian directing a pharmacist to prepare a drug for use in a client's animal. When writing prescriptions, veterinarians must adhere to the following guidelines:

- Veterinary prescription drugs must be used only by or on the order of a licensed veterinarian.
- A valid veterinarian/client/patient relationship must exist.
- Veterinary prescription drugs must meet proper requirements for labeling.
- Appropriate records of all prescriptions issued must be maintained.
- Veterinary prescription drugs must be appropriately handled and stored for safety and security.

Components of a Prescription

A hypothetical prescription is shown in Fig. 9-1. Fig. 9-2 shows common abbreviations used in prescriptions and their meanings. Valid prescriptions must contain the following items:

- Name, address, and telephone number of the person who wrote the prescription
- Date on which the prescription was written
- Owner's name and address and species of animal (animal's name is optional)
- Rx symbol (abbreviation of *recipe*, Latin for "take thou")
- Drug name, concentration, and number of units to be dispensed
- *Sig* (abbreviation of *signa*, Latin for "write" or "label"), indicating directions for the client in treating the animal
- Signature of the person who wrote the prescription
- Drug Enforcement Administration (DEA) registration number if the drug is a controlled substance

Containers for Dispensing Medication

Many veterinary practices dispense tablets and capsules in plastic containers with a childproof lid. If medication is dispensed in a paper envelope and a child becomes poisoned, the veterinarian could be found negligent in dispensing the medication in a manner that placed the child at risk.

CALCULATING DRUG DOSES

Calculating the dose of drug to be administered involves the following steps:

1. Weigh the animal and convert the weight in pounds to kilograms (if necessary).
2. Depending on how the drug is usually dosed (e.g., mg/kg, U/kg), use the animal's weight to calculate the correct dose (e.g., in mg, ml, units, g).
3. Based on the concentration of the drug (e.g., mg of drug/ml of solution or mg of drug/tablet), determine what volume or number of tablets to administer. Simple algebra helps calculate the amount (dose) of drug to be given (e.g., mg or ml), along with the animal's weight and the recommended drug dosage (e.g., mg/kg). You can also calculate the number of units to give (e.g., tablets or ml) if you know the amount of drug in each unit (e.g., mg/ml or mg/tablet) and the duration of treatment (days). Common metric conversion factors used in calculating drug doses are listed in Fig. 9-3.

Step 1. Set up an equation so that the units (e.g., kg, lb) are the same on the top (numerator) and bottom (denominator) on both sides of the equation. Then solve for x (e.g., kg of body weight). This is shown in Step 1 of Fig. 9-4.

Step 2. Once the animal's weight has been converted to the appropriate units (in this case, kg), determine the amount of drug (dose) to be given. On the left of the equation is the drug dosage (e.g., milligrams of drug/kilogram body weight), and the x you are solving for is the total drug dose (in milligrams). This is shown in Step 2 of Fig. 9-4.

HOMETOWN VETERINARY ASSOCIATES

2000 West Chelsea Ave., Momack, PA
(324) 555-4313

Date: November 22, 1995

Patient: Cricket **Species:** Canine

Owner: Lee Ann Wozniak **Phone:** 555-0127

Address: 929 Christopher Robin Lane, Brookside, PA 13235

℞ Amoxicillin tablets 100mg #30 tabs
Sig: 1 tab q8h POPRN until gone

Robert L. Bill **D.V.M.**

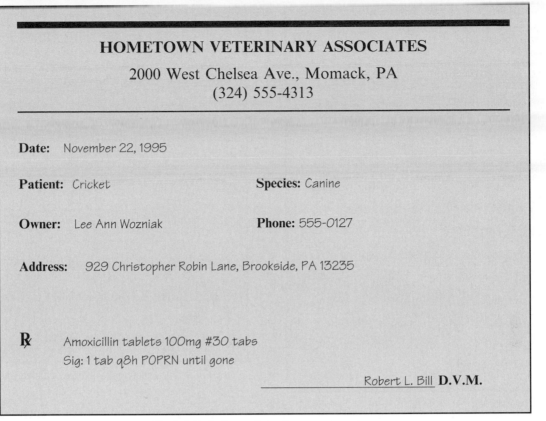

Fig. 9-1 Typical prescription for a veterinary drug.

BID	twice a day	**po**	by mouth
cc	cubic centimeter	**prn**	as needed
disp	dispense	**q**	every
g	gram	**q8h**	every 8 hours
gm	gram	**qd**	every day
gr	grain	**QID**	four times daily
h	hour	**QOD**	every other day
lb	pound	**SID**	once a day
mg	milligram	**stat**	immediately
ml	milliliter	**TID**	three times daily
od	right eye	**tsp**	teaspoon
os	left eye		

Note: SID is rarely used or recognized by pharmacists outside of the veterinary profession

Fig. 9-2 Abbreviations commonly used in prescriptions. *(From Bill RL:* Pharmacology for veterinary technicians, *St Louis, 1993, Mosby.)*

1 kg = 1000g = 100,000 milligrams (mg)

1 kg = 2.2 lb

1 gram = 1 gm = 1000 mg = 0.001 kg

1 gram = 1g = 15.43 grains (gr)

1 grain = 64.8 milligrams (usually rounded to
60 or 65 mg)

1 lb = 0.454 kg = 16 ounces (oz)

1 mg = 0.001 g = 1000 micrograms (μg or mcg)

1 liter (L) = 1000 ml = 10 deciliters (dl)

1 ml = 1 cc = 1000 microliters (μl or mcl)

1 tablespoon (tbsp) = 3 teaspoons (tsp)

1 tsp = 5 ml

1 gallon (gal) = 3.786 L

1 gal = 4 quarts (1qt) 8 pints (pt) = 128 fluid
ounces (fl oz)

1 pt = 2 cups (c) = 16 fl oz = 473 ml

Fig. 9-3 Metric conversion factors. *(From Bill RL:* Pharmacology for veterinary technicians, *ed 2, St Louis, 1997, Mosby.)*

Step 3. After the total dose is determined (in mg or some other measure), calculate the volume (e.g., ml) or number of solid units (tablets, capsules) to be administered using the concentration of drug in the solution

What volume of a drug solution should we give to a 44-lb dog if the recommended dosage is 5 mg/kg and the concentration of the solution is 50 mg/ml?

Step 1: Convert pounds to kilograms.

$$X \text{ kg} = 44 \text{ lb} \times \frac{1 \text{ kg}}{2.2 \text{ lb}} = \frac{44}{2.2} = 20 \text{ kg}$$

Step 2: Calculate the total drug dose.

$$X \text{ mg} = \frac{5 \text{ mg}}{\text{kg}} \times 20 \text{ kg} = 5 \times 20 = 100 \text{ mg}$$

Step 3: Calculate the volume of solution needed.

$$\frac{50 \text{ mg}}{\text{ml}} = \frac{100 \text{ mg}}{X \text{ ml}} = \frac{100 \text{ mg}}{50 \text{ mg/ml}} = 2 \text{ ml}$$

Fig. 9-4 Simple algebraic calculation used to calculate a drug dose.

How many 25-mg tablets should we dispense for a 10-lb cat if the recommended dosage is 5 mg/lb twice daily for 7 days?

Step 1: Calculate the number of tablets needed per dose.

$$10 \text{ lb} \times \frac{5 \text{ mg}}{\text{lb}} = 50 \text{ mg per dose}$$

$$50 \text{ mg} \times \frac{1 \text{ tablet}}{25 \text{ mg}} = 2 \text{ tablets per dose}$$

Step 2: Calculate the number of tablets needed daily.

2 tablet per dose × twice daily = 4 tablets daily

Step 3: Calculate the number of tablets needed for 7 days.

4 tablets daily × 7 days = 28 tablets

Fig. 9-5 Calculating the number of tablets to dispense.

(mg of drug/ml of solution) or in each solid unit (mg of drug/tablet), solving for ml of liquid or number of tablets. This is shown in Step 3 of Fig. 9-4.

When dispensing solid units (tablets, capsules), round to the nearest unit (or half or quarter tablet if the tablet is designed to be broken and greater accuracy is essential). The steps for calculating the total number of solid units required during a course of treatment are detailed in Fig. 9-5. Always check the rounded dosage with the veterinarian as some drugs have a very narrow margin of safety and may need to be rounded *down* versus up.

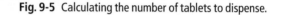

STORING AND HANDLING DRUGS IN THE PHARMACY

Drugs that are improperly stored (e.g., exposed to extreme temperature or light) can degenerate or become inactivated, providing little or no benefit to the animal in which they are used. Drugs still on the pharmacy shelf after the listed expiration date on the container may be less effective. In some cases, such as with tetracycline, these expired drugs can become hazardous to the animal. Store drugs at their optimum temperature to prevent damage. Temperatures used for drug storage, according to label specifications, are as follows:

Cold: not exceeding 8° C (46° F)
Cool: 8° to 15°C (46° to 59° F)
Room temperature: 15° to 30° C (59° to 86° F)
Warm: 30° to 40°C (86° to 104° F)
Excessive heat: greater than 40° C (104° F)

Drugs that are sensitive to light are usually kept in a dark amber container. Tablets and powders tend to be sensitive to moisture, and their containers usually contain silica packets to absorb moisture. Some drugs are destroyed by physical stress, such as vibrations. Insulin is one such drug that can be inactivated by violent shaking of the vial.

STORING AND PRESCRIBING CONTROLLED SUBSTANCES

A *controlled substance* is defined by law as a substance with potential for physical addiction, psychological addiction, and/or abuse. Controlled drugs are sometimes called *schedule* drugs. Controlled substances must be stored securely under lock and key to prevent access by unauthorized personnel. By law, a written record must be kept describing when, for what purpose, and how much of the controlled drug was used. These records must include receipts for purchase or sale of controlled substances and must be maintained for 2 years. Although ketamine is not listed as a controlled drug, its hallucinogenic characteristics increase the potential for abuse; ketamine should therefore be handled as a controlled substance.

Drug manufacturers and distributors are required to identify a controlled substance on its label with a capital *C*, followed by a Roman numeral, which denotes the drug's theoretical potential for abuse.

C-I denotes extreme potential for abuse with no approved medicinal purpose in the United States. These include such drugs as heroin, LSD, and marijuana.

C-II denotes a high potential for abuse. Use may lead to severe physical or psychological dependence. These include such drugs as opium, pentobarbital, and morphine.

C-III denotes some potential for abuse, but less than for C-II drugs. Use may lead to low to moderate physical dependence or high psychological dependence. These include such drugs as morphine derivatives and Fentanyl.

C-IV denotes low potential for abuse. Use may lead to limited physical psychological dependence; includes such drugs as phenobarbital and diazepam (Valium).

C-V also denotes low potential for abuse, but these drugs are subject to state and local regulation (e.g., Robitussin AC).

For veterinarians to legally use, prescribe, or buy a controlled substance from an approved manufacturer or distributor, they must have obtained a certification number from the DEA. This DEA certification number must be included on all prescriptions or any order forms for *Schedule* (controlled) drugs. Even with a valid DEA number, veterinarians cannot prescribe Schedule I (C-I) drugs.

Prescriptions for Schedule II (C-II) drugs, which have the most potential for abuse, must be in written form (many states have special forms for C-II drug prescriptions) and cannot be telephoned to a pharmacist. In the event of an emergency, when the prescription must be ordered by telephone, the verbal prescription must be followed by a written order within 72 hours. Schedule II drug prescriptions may not be refilled; a new prescription must be written for each treatment period.

Handling Toxic Drugs

Veterinary professionals may be exposed to toxic drugs in various ways, including the following:
- Absorption through the skin via spillage from a syringe or vial, or other contact
- Inhalation of aerosolized drug as a needle is withdrawn from a vial that is pressurized by injection of air to facilitate removal of the drug
- Ingestion of food contaminated with drug via aerosolization or direct contact
- Inhalation resulting from crushing or breaking of tablets and subsequent aerosolization of drug powder
- Absorption or inhalation during opening of glass ampules containing antineoplastic agents

The best way to avoid exposure is to educate all involved personnel about safe handling and storage of these drugs. Training may be in-house or formal. Such safety training should be periodically repeated to emphasize the importance of handling precautions and as a refresher for staff members.

THERAPEUTIC RANGE

The concentration of a drug in the body must be such that the detrimental effects are minimized and benefits are maximized. This ideal range of drug concentration is referred to as the *therapeutic range*. If an excessive dose results in accumulation of too much drug in the body, drug concentrations are said to be *toxic*, and signs of toxicity develop. If a small drug dose does not produce drug concentrations within the therapeutic range, drug concentrations are said to be at *subtherapeutic levels*, and the drug's beneficial effect is not achieved.

DOSAGE REGIMEN

There are three components of therapeutic administration of drugs: the *dose*, the *dosage interval*, and the *route of administration*. Altering any of these components can result in drug concentrations that are too high or too low.

A drug's *dose* is the amount of drug administered at one time. For accuracy and clarity in communicating with pharmacists or other veterinary professionals, always state the dose in units of mass (e.g., mg, g, gr). *Do not* state the dose in number of product units (e.g., tablets or capsules) or volume (ml, L), because manufacturers may produce the same

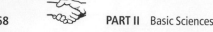

drug in solid dosage forms of various sizes or solutions with various concentrations. For example, writing in an animal's record that the animal received "1 tablet of amoxicillin" is of no value because amoxicillin is available in tablet sizes ranging from 50 mg up to 500 mg. The same is true if you state, "Give 3 ml of xylazine," because 3 ml of a xylazine solution with a concentration of 20 mg/ml contains much less xylazine than 3 ml of a solution with a concentration of 100 mg/ml.

The time between administrations of separate drug doses is referred to as the *dosage interval*. Dosage intervals are often expressed with the Latin abbreviations shown in Fig. 9-2.

The dose and the dosage interval together are often referred to as the *dosage regimen*. The total amount of drug delivered to the animal in 24 hours is the *total daily dose* and is determined by multiplying the dose by the frequency of administration (e.g., 100 mg given 4 times daily results in a total daily dose of 400 mg).

ROUTES OF ADMINISTRATION

The amount of a drug that reaches the target tissues in the body can be significantly altered if the proper route of administration is not used. The route of administration is how the drug enters the body. Drugs given by injection are said to be *parenterally administered*. Drugs given by mouth, or *per os (PO)*, are said to be *orally administered*. If a drug is applied to the surface of the skin, as with lotions and liniments, it is said to be *topically administered*.

Parenteral administration of drugs is further broken down into specific routes. Intravenous (IV) administration involves injecting the drug directly into a vein. Intravenous injections can be given as a single volume at one time, called a *bolus*, or they can be slowly injected or dripped into a vein over several seconds, minutes, or even hours as an intravenous infusion. Drugs that are given over long periods of time ranging from hours to days are termed as being given by *continuous rate infusion (CRI)*. The differences in drug concentrations achieved by these variations of intravenous administration are shown in Fig. 9-6.

Note that *intravenous* injection is not the same as *intra-arterial* injection. Drugs given by intra-arterial injection are injected into an artery (not a vein), quickly producing high concentrations of drug in tissues supplied by that artery. After intravenous injection, blood containing the drug passes to the heart and is mixed and diluted with the remaining blood in circulation before it is delivered to body tissues. Inadvertent injection of drugs intra-arterially (e.g., injection into the carotid artery instead of the jugular vein) delivers a bolus of a drug directly to tissues. These accidental intra-arterial injections can produce severe effects, such as seizures or respiratory arrest. Injection of a drug outside

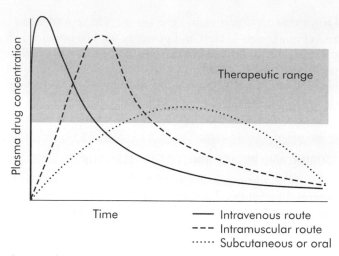

Fig. 9-6 Plasma drug concentrations attained after intravenous, intramuscular, subcutaneous, and oral administration.

of the blood vessel (not within the vessel lumen) is an extravascular or perivascular injection.

Some drugs cause extreme local inflammation and tissue death if accidentally injected extravascularly. *Intramuscular (IM) administration* involves injecting the drug into a muscle mass. *Subcutaneous (SC or SQ) injections* are administered deep to (beneath) the skin, into the subcutis. *Intradermal (ID) injections* are administered within (not beneath) the skin with very small needles. The intradermal route is usually reserved for skin-testing procedures, such as testing for tuberculosis or reaction to allergenic substances. *Intraperitoneal (IP) injections* are administered into the abdominal body cavity and are frequently used when IV or IM injections are not practical (as in some laboratory animals), or large volumes of solution must be administered for rapid absorption.

Movement of Drug Molecules in the Body

Pharmacokinetics describes how drugs move into, through, and out of the body. Knowledge of a drug's pharmacokinetics facilitates understanding of why the drug must be given by different routes or dosage regimens to achieve therapeutic success under different clinical circumstances. Pharmacokinetics involves absorption, distribution, metabolism, and elimination.

Movement of drug molecules from the site of administration into the systemic circulation is called *absorption*. After a drug has been ingested, injected, inhaled, or applied to the skin, it must be absorbed into the blood and travel to the body areas where it will have its intended effect (target tissues). IV injections almost instantaneously achieve their peak concentration (highest level) in the blood (see Fig. 9-6). Drugs given by IM administration take some time to diffuse from the injection site in the muscle, into the systemic circulation. Drugs given by PO administration and

SC injection take longer to be absorbed because they must diffuse farther to reach the systemic circulation (SC injection) or they must pass through several barriers to be absorbed (PO administration). Drugs given IM, SC, or PO attain therapeutic concentrations more slowly than drugs given IV.

Distribution describes movement of a drug from the systemic circulation into tissues. Drugs generally are distributed most rapidly and in greater concentrations to well-*perfused* (rich blood supply) tissues. Examples of well-perfused tissues include active skeletal muscle, the liver, kidney, and brain. In contrast, inactive skeletal muscle and adipose (fat) tissue are relatively poorly perfused, so it takes more time for drugs to be delivered to these tissues. Some drugs bind to proteins in the blood; these protein-bound drug molecules are unable to leave the systemic circulation and so are not distributed to tissues. Thus, a significant portion of a highly protein-bound drug remains in systemic circulation, where these protein-bound drug molecules act as a "reservoir" of additional drug.

Many drugs are altered by the body before being eliminated. This process is referred to as *biotransformation* or *drug metabolism*. The altered drug molecule is referred to as a *metabolite*. The liver is the primary organ involved in drug metabolism or biotransformation. However, other tissues, such as the lung, skin, and intestinal tract, may also biotransform drug molecules. The product of biotransformation (metabolite) is usually readily eliminated by the kidney or liver. Removal of a drug from the body is called *drug elimination* or *excretion*. The two major routes of elimination are via the kidney (into the urine) and via the liver (into the bile and subsequently into the feces). Inhalant anesthetics and other volatile agents are mostly eliminated via the lungs, although some inhalant anesthetics (methoxyflurane and halothane) have some hepatic biotransformation and renal excretion. Drug elimination is greatly affected by dehydration; kidney, liver, or heart disease; age; and a variety of other physiologic and pathologic (disease) conditions.

By law, all drugs approved for use in food animals have mandated withdrawal times. The *withdrawal time* is the period after drug administration during which the animal cannot be sent to market for slaughter, and the eggs or milk must be discarded.

HOW DRUGS EXERT THEIR EFFECT

For cells to respond to a drug molecule, usually the drug must combine with a specific protein molecule on or in the cell, called a *receptor*. A given receptor combines only with the molecule of certain drugs, based upon their shape or molecular makeup.

This concept is illustrated by a key and lock, where the drug is the key and the receptor is the lock into which only the correct key will fit (produce an effect). The effect of the correct drug molecule-receptor combination is some cellular change, such as causing the cell to secrete substances, muscle cells to contract, or neuronal cells to depolarize (fire). Cells do not have receptors for all drugs; only certain cells respond to certain drugs.

DRUGS AFFECTING THE GASTROINTESTINAL TRACT

Drugs or functions related to the stomach are called *gastric*, as in gastric ulcers, gastric blood flow, or gastric emptying. Drugs or functions related to the duodenum, jejunum, or ileum are usually referred to as *enteric*. Drugs and functions related to the colon are termed *colonic*.

Emetics

Emetics are drugs that induce vomiting. The complex process of emesis is controlled by a group of neurons in the medulla of the brain stem, known as the *vomiting center*. Emetics are most often used to induce vomiting in animals that have ingested toxic substances. They should not be used in all cases of poisoning, however, because the risk of aspiration (inhalation) of stomach contents into the lungs may outweigh the benefit of induced vomiting. Also, vomiting should not be induced if a corrosive substance or volatile liquid was ingested.

Apomorphine quickly causes emesis in dogs when given by IV or IM injection, or when an apomorphine tablet is placed in the conjunctival sac of the eye. Apomorphine is a less effective emetic in cats. An effective emetic for cats is the sedative xylazine (Rompun, Anased, and others), which produces emesis within minutes of injection. Syrup of ipecac does not produce vomiting until 10 to 30 minutes after administration. This is because the ipecac must pass from the stomach into the intestine to produce the required local irritation (local effect) and also to be absorbed (central effect on the vomiting center). The 10- to 30-minute lag time between ipecac administration and the onset of vomiting can lead uninformed clients or veterinary professionals to believe the initial dose was ineffective, causing them to administer multiple doses of the drug before vomiting begins. Other local emetics include hydrogen peroxide; a warm, concentrated solution of salt and water; and a solution of powdered mustard and water. These emetics do not work consistently.

Antiemetics

Antiemetics are drugs that prevent or decrease vomiting. Antiemetics should only be used when the vomiting reflex is no longer of benefit to the animal. Phenothiazine tranquilizers, such as acepromazine (PromAce), chlorpromazine (Thorazine), and prochlorperazine (Compazine, Darbazine), are commonly used to combat vomiting caused by motion sickness. The antihistamines dimenhydrinate (Dramamine) and diphenhydramine (Benadryl) are also used occasionally for prevention of motion sickness.

Atropine, aminopentamide (Centrine), and isopropamide (combined with prochlorperazine in Darbazine) are anticholinergic drugs that prevent vomiting by blocking the impulses traveling to the CNS via the vagus nerve and the motor impulses traveling via the vagus nerve to the muscles involved with the vomiting reflex. These drugs are used less commonly due to the availability of other more locally effective drugs.

Metoclopramide (Reglan) is a centrally acting antiemetic that also has local antiemetic activity. Metoclopramide has been useful in otherwise healthy dogs that intermittently vomit small amounts of bile-tinged fluid, usually in the morning. Cisapride (Propulsid) has been used to reduce regurgitation in dogs with megaesophagus (dilated esophagus) and in cats with chronic constipation or cats that frequently vomit hairballs.

Ondansetron (Zofran) is a selective serotonin reuptake inhibitor (also known as a 5-HT3 receptor antagonist). It is unclear as to whether it acts centrally, peripherally, or both because the 5-HT3 receptors for serotonin are located peripherally (the vagus nerve) and centrally (the chemoreceptor trigger zone in the brain). Ondansetron is used when other more widely used antiemetics are not effective due to the expense and the limited experience in veterinary medicine.

Antidiarrheals

Antidiarrheals are drugs used to combat various types of diarrhea. Narcotics commonly used to combat diarrhea include diphenoxylate (Lomotil), paregoric (tincture of opium), and loperamide (Imodium). A disadvantage of narcotics when used as antidiarrheals is that their analgesic effect can mask pain that otherwise could be used to monitor progression or resolution of disease. Another disadvantage is that narcotics can cause excitement in cats ("morphine mania").

The anticholinergics atropine, propantheline bromide, isopropamide (Darbazine), and aminopentamide (Centrine) are used as antispasmodics because they decrease spastic colonic contractions and combat diarrhea associated with these contractions. These drugs are not particularly effective for most small-bowel diarrhea.

Bismuth subsalicylate, the active ingredient in Pepto-Bismol, breaks down in the gut to bismuth carbonate and salicylate. The bismuth tends to coat the intestinal mucosa, perhaps protecting it from enterotoxins, and seems to have some antibacterial activity. The major antisecretory effect, however, is probably from the salicylate (an aspirin-like compound), which decreases inflammation and blocks formation of prostaglandins that would normally stimulate fluid secretion.

Adsorbents and Protectants

Locally irritating substances, such as bacterial endotoxins, can produce acute diarrhea. Any drug that prevents these agents from contacting the intestinal mucosa could theoretically reduce the diarrheal response. That is the underlying principle of adsorbents and protectants. An adsorbent causes another substance to adhere to its outer surface, thus reducing contact of that substance with the intestinal tract wall.

Activated charcoal adsorbs enterotoxins to its surface, preventing them from contacting the bowel wall. The charcoal and the adsorbed enterotoxin then pass out in the feces. Kaolin and pectin (Kaopectate) are often used together for symptomatic relief of vomiting or diarrhea. The kaolin-pectin combination is thought to adsorb enterotoxins. It is questionable as to whether kaolin-pectin has any significant effect in controlling diarrhea in veterinary patients.

Laxatives, Lubricants, and Stool Softeners

Laxatives, cathartics, and purgatives facilitate evacuation of the bowels. Laxatives are considered the most gentle of this class of drugs, whereas cathartics are more marked in their evacuating effect, and purgatives are quite potent in their actions. *Irritant laxatives*, including castor oil and phenolphthalein, work by irritating the bowel, resulting in increased peristaltic motility.

Bulk laxatives are much gentler than irritant laxatives. These drugs osmotically pull water into the bowel lumen or retain water in the feces. Hydrophilic colloids or indigestible fiber (bran, methylcellulose, Metamucil) are not digested or adsorbed to any degree and therefore create an osmotic force to produce their laxative effect. Psyllium is a hydrophilic compound that has gained popularity for its supposed health benefits. Hypertonic salts, such as magnesium (Milk of Magnesia, Epsom salts) and phosphate salts (Fleet Enema), are poorly absorbed and create a strong osmotic force to attract water into the bowel lumen.

Lubricants (mineral oil, cod liver oil, white petrolatum, glycerin) are given to make the stool more "slippery" for easy passage through the bowel. Mineral oil is most commonly used for horses with impactions and is administered by stomach tube. The greatest danger associated with use of this oil is aspiration into the lungs, with subsequent pneumonia. Glycerin is most commonly used as a suppository.

Docusate sodium succinate (Colace) is a stool softener that acts as a "wetting agent" by reducing the surface tension of feces and allowing water to penetrate the dry stool. Docusate sodium succinate and related calcium and phosphate compounds may also stimulate colonic secretions, resulting in increased fluid content of feces.

Lactulose is another laxative that increases osmotic pressure drawing water into the colon and making fecal material contain more liquid. It has an acidifying aspect as well that is used in treatment of hepatic encephalopathy as it traps ammonia in the form of ammonium. It is used most commonly in small animals with chronic constipation problems. The most common danger with the use of Lactulose is excessive fluid loss leading to dehydration. Fluids may be warranted with initial use.

Antacids and Antiulcer Drugs

Antacids reduce acidity of the stomach or rumen. *Nonsystemic antacids*, in liquid or tablet form, are composed of calcium, magnesium, or aluminum, and they directly neutralize acid molecules in the stomach or rumen. Such over-the-counter (OTC) products as Tums and Rolaids are nonsystemic antacids made primarily of calcium. Other nonsystemic antacids include magnesium products (Riopan, Carmilax), aluminum products (Amphojel), and combinations of magnesium and aluminum products (Maalox).

Systemic antacids decrease acid production in the stomach. Systemic antacids include cimetidine (Tagamet), ranitidine (Zantac), and famotidine (Pepcid). Sucralfate (Carafate) is an antiulcer drug used to treat ulcers of the stomach and upper small intestine. The drug has been called a "gastric Band-Aid" because it forms a sticky paste and adheres to the ulcer site, protecting it from the acidic environment of the stomach.

Ruminatorics and Antibloat Medications

Ruminatorics, such as neostigmine (Stiglyn), are drugs used to stimulate an atonic ("limp") rumen. *Antibloat* medications act by reducing numbers of gas-producing rumen microorganisms or by breaking up the bubbles formed in the rumen with frothy bloat. Mineral oil or ordinary household detergents mixed with mineral oil are often used to decrease the viscosity of the rumen contents, decrease the stability of the bubbles, and remove the froth. Some commercial antibloat preparations contain poloxalene. Dioctyl sodium succinate (DSS) also reduces the viscosity of rumen contents, allowing the foam to dissipate.

DRUGS AFFECTING THE CARDIOVASCULAR SYSTEM

Antiarrhythmic Drugs

An *arrhythmia* is any abnormal pattern of electrical activity in the heart. Arrhythmias are divided into two general groups: arrhythmias that result in an increased heart rate (tachycardia) and those that cause a decreased heart rate (bradycardia). Once the type of arrhythmia has been determined, an effective antiarrhythmic drug is used to re-establish a normal conduction sequence *(sinus rhythm)*.

Lidocaine, mexiletine, quinidine, and procainamide reverse arrhythmias primarily by decreasing the rate of movement of sodium into heart cells. Lidocaine, which is also used as a local anesthetic under the name of Xylocaine, is only available in injectable form. Veterinary technicians must realize that lidocaine is packaged in vials with or without epinephrine. Lidocaine with epinephrine is designed for use as a local anesthetic, *not* as an antiarrhythmic drug. Accidental IV injection of lidocaine containing epinephrine in an animal with an arrhythmia could cause death. For this reason, it is important to always check the lidocaine bottle before use in treating arrhythmias to be sure it does not contain epinephrine.

Procainamide and quinidine have been used for supraventricular arrhythmias in horses, but they are not very effective against atrial fibrillation in dogs or cats. Hence, they are more commonly used for their ventricular antiarrhythmic effects. Because quinidine and procainamide are available in oral forms, they are used for long-term maintenance of patients with ventricular arrhythmias.

When stimulated by the sympathetic nervous system or by sympathomimetic drugs (drugs that mimic the effects of the sympathetic nervous system), beta-1 receptors in the heart cause the heart to beat more rapidly and with greater strength. Such beta-1 stimulation can produce arrhythmias. Drugs that block beta receptors are known as beta-blockers. Beta-blockers cause the heart to contract with less force. Propranolol (Inderal) blocks stimulation of beta-1 receptors by epinephrine, norepinephrine, and other beta-stimulating drugs. It decreases the heart rate and prevents tachycardia in response to stress, fear, or excitement. Atenolol (Tenormin) and metoprolol (Lopressor) act similarly to propanolol, but at high doses the beta-1 receptor activity may be lost causing beta-2 blockade. Atenolol and metoprolol are preferred in animals with asthma.

Calcium channel blockers include verapamil and diltiazem. Although calcium channel blockers are not commonly used to treat arrhythmias in veterinary patients, verapamil and diltiazem have been used successfully for treatment of supraventricular tachycardia, atrial fibrillation, and atrial flutter. A more common use of diltiazem is in cats with hypertrophic cardiomyopathy, in which the heart becomes very thickened and enlarged to the point where it cannot contract very efficiently. These drugs combat arrhythmias by blocking calcium channels of cardiac muscle cells, resulting in decreased conduction of depolarization waves and decreased automaticity of parts of the conduction system.

Another calcium channel blocker most commonly used for hypertension in small animals is amlodipine. It acts by dilating the peripheral arteries and thereby reducing afterload. It is eliminated quickly from the system, and hypertension can return rapidly if any doses are missed.

Positive Inotropic Agents

Drugs that increase the strength of contraction of a weakened heart are referred to as *positive inotropic drugs (positive*

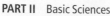
inotropes). Digoxin is the drug of choice for maintaining long-term positive inotropic effects. Digoxin exerts its positive inotropic effect primarily by making more calcium available for the contractile elements within cardiac muscle cells. Digoxin, available as tablets and an elixir, is often used to control supraventricular tachycardia caused by atrial fibrillation. Digoxin has a small *therapeutic index*, meaning that therapeutic concentrations are very close to toxic concentrations. Early signs of digoxin toxicity include anorexia, vomiting, and diarrhea. Owners of animals receiving digoxin should be instructed to watch for these early signs of toxicity and to contact the veterinarian immediately if they should occur.

Dobutamine is also an inotropic agent that is used mostly commonly for short-term management of heart failure and in shock patients when fluid therapy alone is not working. It is used only as a CRI due to its limited availability and quick metabolization by the system. This drug is most commonly used in the ICU setting.

Vasodilators

Vasoconstriction of peripheral blood vessels is a normal physiologic response to the drop in blood pressure caused by congestive heart failure, hemorrhage, and dehydration. Vasodilators open (dilate) constricted vessels, making it easier for the heart to pump blood through these vessels.

Hydralazine is a vasodilator that causes arteriolar smooth muscle to relax, which benefits animals with a poorly functioning left atrioventricular (mitral) valve (mitral insufficiency). Hydralazine allows more blood to flow into the aorta and less to flow back into the left atrium. Although the valve itself remains poorly functional, blood flow through the left heart is improved.

Nitroglycerin relaxes the blood vessels on the venous side of the circulation; it may also help dilate coronary arterioles. The drug is well absorbed through the skin and mucous membranes. In animals, nitroglycerin cream and nitroglycerin in patch form are applied to the skin to improve cardiac output and reduce pulmonary edema and ascites (abdominal fluid accumulation). Nitroglycerin cream is applied every 4 to 6 hours to the hairless inner aspect of the pinna, thorax, or groin. A nitroglycerin patch provides drug diffusion for 24 hours and can be cut into small pieces to adjust the dose for smaller patients.

Nitroprusside acts much like nitroglycerin but is usually found only in the ICU setting due to the necessity to constantly monitor blood pressure and the need to give the drug as a CRI.

Other vasodilators are enalapril (Enacard) and captopril, which block angiotensin-converting enzyme and prevent formation of angiotensin II (potent vasoconstrictor) and aldosterone. For this reason, they are sometimes referred to as *angiotensin-converting enzyme (ACE) inhibitors.* Enalapril and captopril are "balanced" vasodilators that relax the smooth muscles of both arterioles and veins, so they are useful in treating animals with cardiac disease that involves the right and the left ventricle (e.g., severe cardiac valvular disease, cardiomyopathy).

Diuretics

Diuretics are drugs that increase urine formation and promote water loss (diuresis). In animals with congestive heart failure, sodium retention from aldosterone secretion and concomitant retention of water in the blood and body tissue lead to pulmonary edema, ascites, and an increased cardiac workload. Removing water from the body with diuretics reduces these deleterious conditions. Diuretics should be used cautiously in animals with hypovolemia (low blood volume) or hypotension (low blood pressure), because they further decrease the fluid component of blood and reduce blood pressure.

Loop diuretics, such as furosemide (Lasix), produce diuresis by inhibiting sodium resorption from the loop of Henle in nephrons. When sodium resorption is inhibited, osmotic forces are exerted that retain additional water in the urine. In the distal convoluted tubule, potassium is exchanged for sodium so that sodium is still resorbed and conserved by the body to some degree. Because loop diuretics cause potassium to be excreted in the urine, prolonged use of loop diuretics may result in hypokalemia (low blood potassium).

Thiazide diuretics, such as chlorothiazide, are not often used in veterinary medicine because of the safety and effectiveness of furosemide. Thiazides are less potent than loop diuretics because of their site of action in the distal convoluted tubule. Thiazide diuretics can cause loss of potassium, with resultant hypokalemia.

Spironolactone is a diuretic that is a competitive antagonist of aldosterone, the hormone that normally causes sodium resorption from the distal renal tubules and collection ducts. When aldosterone is inhibited, more sodium remains in the lumen of the renal tubules, osmotically retaining water and preventing its resorption. Because sodium is excreted and potassium is conserved in the body, drugs like spironolactone are called *potassium-sparing diuretics.*

Mannitol is a carbohydrate (sugar) used as an *osmotic diuretic.* Mannitol is poorly resorbed from the renal tubule, thus providing a solute that osmotically retains water in the renal tubular lumen. Mannitol is not used in treatment of cardiovascular disease but is used to reduce cerebral edema associated with head trauma and as a diuretic for flushing absorbed toxins from the body.

DRUGS AFFECTING THE RESPIRATORY SYSTEM

Antitussives

Antitussives are drugs that block the cough reflex, which is coordinated by the cough center in the brain stem.

A *productive cough* refers to a cough that produces mucus and other inflammatory products that are coughed up into the oral cavity. A *nonproductive cough* is "dry" and "hacking," and no mucus is coughed up. Antitussives suppress the coughing that normally removes mucus, cellular debris, exudates, and other products that accumulate within the bronchi as a result of infection or inflammation. For this reason, in animals with a very productive cough (much mucus produced), antitussive drugs should be used cautiously and large doses should be avoided. In such situations, suppression of coughing with cough suppressants can result in accumulation of excessive mucus and debris.

Antitussives should be used in animals with a dry, nonproductive cough producing little or no inspissated mucus. Often these coughs keep the animal (and owner) awake, preventing the animal from getting the rest it needs to recover. Antitussives are commonly used in treating uncomplicated tracheobronchitis ("kennel cough") in dogs. This "retching" type of cough is often punctuated by gagging up small amounts of mucus the owner interprets as vomitus. This type of cough is extremely irritating to the upper airway mucosa; such irritation stimulates more coughing, which further irritates the airway. This pattern can continue for weeks if the cough is not treated.

Butorphanol (Torbutrol) is a centrally acting opioid cough suppressant that, unlike most other opioid cough suppressants, is not classified as a controlled substance in most states. In antitussive doses, butorphanol causes little sedation, as compared with stronger opioid drugs.

Hydrocodone (Hycodan) is a C-III narcotic available only by prescription from a veterinarian with a DEA clearance for writing C-III prescriptions. Sedation is often noted in treated animals, and long-term administration can result in constipation.

Codeine is a relatively weak opioid/narcotic that is a component of many cough suppressant preparations. Most products containing codeine are prescription preparations with a C-V controlled substance rating. The sedative effect of codeine is similar to that of hydrocodone, and use of the compound can become habit forming.

Dextromethorphan is a common ingredient in OTC nonprescription cough, flu, and cold preparations. Its actions are similar to those of the more potent narcotic antitussives, but it is not a controlled substance. Dextromethorphan is generally not as effective in controlling coughs in veterinary patients as butorphanol or other prescription antitussives; however, owners often initially use human cold products containing dextromethorphan to curtail coughing in their pets. Although dextromethorphan in OTC products is fairly harmless, the other compounds in cold or flu preparations can cause significant harm to animals (e.g., acetaminophen can be very toxic in cats); therefore, it is unwise to recommend that pet owners use OTC products to control coughing in their animals.

Mucolytics, Expectorants, and Decongestants

Mucolytic agents are designed to break up ("lyse") mucus and reduce the viscosity of mucus so that the cilia can move it out of the respiratory tract. Acetylcysteine (Mucomyst) is a mucolytic agent that decreases the viscosity of mucus. Acetylcysteine may be administered by nebulization (inhalation of a fine mist containing the drug) or given PO (although the taste is awful and must be masked with flavoring agents, or it must be administered by feeding tube). Nebulized saline and other fluids are used to increase the fluid content of respiratory mucus in the lower airways. Acetylcysteine is also used as the treatment for acetaminophen toxicity in cats.

Expectorants are compounds that also increase the fluidity of mucus in the respiratory tract by generating liquid secretions by respiratory tract cells. Guaifenesin (glycerol guaiacolate) and saline expectorants (ammonium chloride, potassium iodide, sodium citrate) are given PO. The volatile oils, such as terpin hydrate, eucalyptus oil, and pine oil, directly stimulate respiratory secretions when their vapors are inhaled.

Many OTC human cold preparations that contain expectorants also contain *decongestants*, such as phenylephrine or phenylpropanolamine, for relief of nasal congestion. Decongestants reduce congestion (vascular engorgement) of the mucous membranes.

Bronchodilators

Bronchoconstriction is caused by contraction of smooth muscles surrounding the small terminal bronchioles deep within the respiratory tree. Drugs that inhibit bronchoconstriction are called *bronchodilators*. Terbutaline and albuterol are available in an oral dosage form and as an inhaler. The methylxanthines include such bronchodilators as theophylline and aminophylline. The difference between theophylline and aminophylline is that aminophylline is approximately 80% theophylline and 20% ethylenediamine salt. Because 100 mg of aminophylline contains only 80 mg of active theophylline, the dose of theophylline must be adjusted if the animal is switched to aminophylline or vice versa based upon the amount of active ingredient (theophylline) in the compound.

DRUGS AFFECTING THE ENDOCRINE SYSTEM

Drugs Used to Treat Hypothyroidism

Drugs used to treat hypothyroidism (insufficiency of thyroid hormone) include levothyroxine (T_4) and synthetic liothyronine (T_3). Supplementing a hypothyroid animal with levothyroxine (T_4) provides the various organs and tissues with the appropriate amount of thyroid hormone, as each organ or tissue converts T_4 to T_3. With T_3 supplementation, the local tissue regulation of thyroid hormone conversion is bypassed.

Another advantage of synthetic levothyroxine is its ability to trigger the natural negative-feedback mechanism, thus emulating the normal regulatory mechanism for thyroid hormone production. Levothyroxine (e.g., Synthroid, Soloxine) is usually the drug of choice for treating hypothyroidism. Also, T_3 products (e.g., Cytomel) are generally more expensive than T_4 products and must be administered three times daily, rather than once daily.

Drugs Used to Treat Hyperthyroidism

Hyperthyroidism is an increase in thyroid hormone production. It is most common in cats and is associated with a hormone-secreting thyroid tumor. Hyperthyroidism is treated by surgical removal of the thyroid gland, with drugs that decrease thyroid hormone production, or drugs that destroy the thyroid tissue (antithyroid drugs).

Methimazole (Tapazole) and propylthiouracil have been used to control hyperthyroidism in cats by blocking the thyroid tumor's ability to produce T_3 and T_4. Of the two drugs, methimazole causes fewer complications and is preferred over propylthiouracil for decreasing thyroid hormone production. Methimazole can be compounded for topical application (onto the ear pinna) as well.

Radioactive iodine (I-131) is an alternative to oral treatment of hyperthyroidism. The radioactive iodine is injected IV. The iodine, a normal component of thyroid hormone, is taken up and concentrated by the active thyroid tumor cells, which are then destroyed by the radioactivity.

Endocrine Pancreatic Drugs

Insulin is responsible for movement of glucose from the blood into tissue cells. Lack of insulin results in diabetes mellitus, a condition characterized by high blood glucose levels (hyperglycemia) and passage of glucose in the urine (glucosuria). Blood glucose levels can be controlled by one or two *SC insulin* injections a day. The insulins of choice for maintaining diabetic dogs are *NPH insulin* and *lente insulin*, which are of intermediate duration. Diabetic cats sometimes require the longer-acting *ultralente insulin*, which is administered once or twice daily. Regular insulin is not commonly used to maintain diabetic cats or dogs because its short duration of activity requires multiple doses during a 24-hour period. However, because regular insulin is the only type that can be given IV, it is used initially to stabilize the glucose concentrations of animals with severe, uncontrolled diabetes or diabetic ketoacidosis.

Glipizide is a tablet used in treating diabetes for owners that are unwilling or unable to give the insulin via injection to cats. Glipizide has fallen out of favor with most veterinarians, as it does not usually regulate the diabetes well enough.

Drugs Used to Treat Hypoadrenocorticism

Hypoadrenocorticism (Addison's disease) is characterized by a lack of glucocorticoid and/or mineralocorticoid secretion from the adrenal cortex. It can result from the gland itself or from a hormone (ACTH) that aids in telling the gland to secrete the corticoids. Hypoadrenocorticism is treated with corticoids supplementation. Mineralocorticoid supplementation is achieved with desoxycorticosterone pivalate (DOCP), or fludrocortisone acetate. Desoxycorticosterone is a long-acting mineralocorticoid that requires functioning kidneys to work properly. It is used only in dogs and as an injection once every 23 to 25 days. Desoxycorticosterone may require the use of concurrent glucocorticoids. Fludrocortisone has both mineral and glucocorticoid activity and is used in both dogs and cats. It is used daily by oral administration. Since fludrocortisone has some glucocorticoid activity, additional supplementation may not be necessary.

Glucocorticoid supplementation is achieved using any number of glucocorticoid agents including betamethasone, dexamethasone, fludrocortisone, flumethasone, hydrocortisone, methylprednisolone, prednisolone, prednisone, or triamicinolone. The glucocorticoids vary in duration of effectiveness, which is usually the determining factor for the choice of drug used.

Drugs Used to Treat Hyperadrenocorticism

Hyperadrenocorticism (Cushing's disease) is characterized by excess glucocorticoids in the system. This can be due to bilateral adrenocortical hyperplasia (caused by a pituitary microadenoma), functional adrenal tumors (benign or cancerous), or by excessive or prolonged administration of oral, parenteral, or topical corticosteroids (termed *iatrogenic hyperadrenocorticism*).

Treatment of hyperadrenocorticism is based on suppressing the adrenal gland, by discontinuing the corticosteriod use, or by surgically removing the adrenal gland. Mitotane (o.p'-DDD, lysodren) causes selective necrosis of two sections of the adrenal gland decreasing the release of corticosteriods. It is administered daily at first and eventually is tapered to twice-weekly dosing. Ketoconazole reversibly inhibits the development of corticosteroids by twice-daily administration. All forms of treatment can lead to hypoadrenocorticism.

DRUGS AFFECTING REPRODUCTION

Hormone drugs, either natural or synthetic, are used in food animals and horses to synchronize estrous cycles, terminate pregnancies, and induce ovulation. In dogs and cats, they are used primarily to prevent pregnancy or alter the state of the uterus. Gonadotropin-releasing hormone (GnRH) drugs (e.g., Cystorelin) stimulate release of luteinizing hormone (LH) and/or follicle-stimulating hormone (FSH) from the pituitary gland, causing the ovary to develop follicles. The FSH and LH produced by the pituitary gland are also called *gonadotropins*. In addition to pituitary gonadotropins, some species produce chorionic gonadotropins from the placenta. These can be used as drugs and include human chorionic gonadotropin (HCG), a hormone produced by pregnant women, and equine chorionic gonadotropin (ECG), formerly known as pregnant mare serum gonadotropin (PMSG). These drugs are sometimes used in food animals to induce superovulation (release of ova from multiple follicles) and occasionally in dogs and cats to induce estrus.

Estrogens, such as estradiol cypionate, have been used to induce estrus in anestrual mares. Their most common use in small animals is to prevent pregnancy after "mismating."

Progestins are reproductive hormones that are similar to progesterone. Progestins can prevent an animal from coming into full estrus. The progestins used in veterinary medicine include altrenogest (Regu-Mate) and norgestomet.

In livestock breeding systems, the estrous cycles of females can be synchronized so that many animals can be artificially inseminated at the same time. Injecting cows with prostaglandins during diestrus lyses the corpus luteum, causing return to estrus within two to five days. Prostaglandin drugs used include *dinoprost tromethamine* (Lutalyse), *cloprostenol* (Estrumate), *fluprostenol* (Equimate), and *fenprostalene* (Bovilene).

Because equine breed registries encourage birth of foals as soon as possible after January 1, veterinarians are often asked to help mares conceive during spring. To stimulate more predictable ovulation during this period of transitional estrus, progesterone or a progestin is given for 10 to 14 days to mimic diestrus. Drug use is then halted to mimic lysis of the corpus luteum. Such hormonal therapy is often coupled with exposing the mares to artificial lighting to artificially lengthen the photoperiod. This causes the mare to cycle as though it were summer.

Pregnancy can be prevented (contraception) by suppressing the estrous cycle or by preventing implantation of the fertilized ova in the uterine wall. Megestrol acetate (Ovaban) is an oral progestin used for contraception in female dogs and cats. Megestrol use increases the risk of cystic hyperplasia of the endometrium, endometritis, or pyometra. Prolonged use of megestrol can result in mammary hyperplasia (proliferation of mammary tissue). Mibolerone (Cheque Drops) is another contraceptive used in female dogs. Because mibolerone is a testosterone analog (similar structure), it produces effects similar to those of high levels of testosterone, including increased production of anal sac secretions, masculinization of developing female fetuses, and increased vulvar discharge. Estradiol cypionate (ECP) is an injectable estrogen used after mismating in dogs. Estrogens prevent pregnancy by increasing the number and thickness of folds within the oviducts, preventing passage of the ova to the uterus. Because there are safer alternatives to estradiol therapy, such as ovariohysterectomy (spaying), many theriogenologists (specialists in animal reproduction) do not recommend use of estradiol in dogs.

Prostaglandin administration causes lysis of the corpus luteum, resulting in a decrease in progesterone levels and subsequent fetal death. Fluprostenol (Equimate) and dinoprost tromethamine (Lutalyse) are both approved for termination of pregnancy in mares. Prostaglandins are only effective in cows if given before the fourth month of pregnancy. Corticosteroids (e.g., dexamethasone) may induce abortion in mares or cows by mimicking the elevated levels of cortisol that occur at the beginning of normal parturition.

Oxytocin is commonly used to increase uterine contractions in animals with dystocia (difficult birth) related to a weakened or fatigued uterus. Anabolic steroids, such as testosterone and progesterone, have been used to increase the weight and conditioning of feedlot cattle. Progestins (e.g., megestrol acetate) have been used to modify behavior in cats.

DRUGS AFFECTING THE NERVOUS SYSTEM

Anesthetics

Barbiturates are frequently used to produce short-term anesthesia, induce general anesthesia, control seizures, and euthanize animals. Thiobarbiturates contain a sulfur molecule on the barbituric acid molecule; oxybarbiturates contain an oxygen molecule. Thiamylal and thiopental are thiobarbiturates; methohexital, pentobarbital, and phenobarbital are oxybarbiturates. Thiobarbiturates have a more rapid onset but shorter duration of action than oxybarbiturates.

Propofol is usually injected as an IV bolus and provides rapid injection of anesthesia and a short period of unconsciousness. It is relatively expensive and may cause pain when injected IV.

Ketamine and tiletamine are short-acting injectable anesthetics that produce a rather unique form of anesthesia in which the animal feels dissociated (apart) from its body. Retention of laryngeal, pharyngeal, and corneal reflexes, lack of muscular relaxation (often rigidity), and an increased heart rate characterize this dissociative effect. The lack of muscular relaxation makes ketamine unsuitable as a sole anesthetic agent for major surgery. Ketamine and tiletamine produce good somatic (peripheral tissue) analgesia (pain relief) and are suitable for superficial surgery; however, they are much less effective in blocking visceral (internal organ) pain and should not be used alone as anesthesia for internal procedures. Tiletamine is included with zolazepam, a benzodiazepine tranquilizer, in a product marketed as Telazol. Zolazepam reduces some of the CNS excitation and side effects produced by tiletamine.

Nitrous oxide, also referred to as "laughing gas," is very safe when used properly and has much weaker analgesic qualities than other inhalant anesthetics. The major role of nitrous oxide is to decrease the amount of the more potent inhalant anesthetics needed to achieve a surgical plane of anesthesia.

Methoxyflurane (Metofane, Penthrane) is an inhalant anesthetic characterized by good muscle relaxation, a relatively slow rate of anesthetic induction (as compared with halothane and isoflurane), and a prolonged recovery period. Unlike halothane and isoflurane, methoxyflurane does not require a precision vaporizer for administration. Like methoxyflurane, halothane (Fluothane) is a nonflammable, nonirritating inhalant anesthetic that can be used in all species. Anesthesia is induced much more rapidly with halothane than with methoxyflurane. Because of its chemical and physical properties, halothane should be administered with a precision vaporizer.

Isoflurane (Forane, Aerrane) is an inhalant anesthetic that has gained popularity in veterinary practice because of its rapid, smooth induction of anesthesia and short recovery period. Other inhalant agents with similar properties of isoflurane include enflurane (Ethrane), desflurane (Suprane), and sevoflurane (Ultane). Chapter 19 contains detailed information on anesthetic agents.

Tranquilizers and Sedatives

Acepromazine maleate is a phenothiazine tranquilizer that reduces anxiety and produces a mentally relaxed state. It is often used to calm animals for physical examination or transport. Unlike xylazine or detomidine, phenothiazine tranquilizers have no analgesic effect (do not relieve pain).

Droperidol is a butyrophenone with much more potent sedative effects than most phenothiazine tranquilizers. Droperidol has been combined with fentanyl, a strong narcotic analgesic with emetic activity, and marketed as a neuroleptanalgesic product called Innovar-Vet.

Diazepam (Valium), zolazepam (contained in Telazol), midazolam (Versed), and clonazepam (Klonopin) are benzodiazepine tranquilizers often used with other agents as part of a preanesthetic protocol for their calming and muscle relaxing effect.

Xylazine (Rompun, Anased), medetomidine (Domitor), and detomidine (Dormosedan) produce a calming effect and somewhat decrease an animal's ability to respond to stimuli. These drugs also have some analgesic activity. A disadvantage of xylazine is that sedative doses produce vomiting in about 90% of cats and 50% of dogs.

Analgesics

Analgesics are drugs that reduce the perception of pain without loss of other sensations. Oxymorphone (Numorphan) is commonly used for preanesthesia and anesthesia. Butorphanol (Torbutrol, Torbugesic) is used for cough control and GI-related pain in small animals and for reducing colic pain in horses. Fentanyl has an analgesic effect 250 times greater than that of morphine. Meperidine (Demerol) is a fairly weak analgesic/sedative and is often injected SC to restrain cats. Pentazocine (Talwin) is a weak analgesic used in horses with colic and dogs recovering from painful surgery. Buprenorphine (Buprenex) is commonly combined with sedatives or tranquilizers (acepromazine, xylazine, detomidine). It is also used alone in dogs and cats as an analgesic, both for its potency (30 times the analgesic potency of morphine) and its long duration of analgesia (6 to 8 hours). Etorphine (M-99) is an extremely potent narcotic (1000 times the analgesic potency of morphine) used to sedate and capture wildlife or zoo animals. Butorphanol, pentazocine, and buprenorphine are sometimes used to partially reverse some of the respiratory depression and sedation caused by stronger narcotic agents. Nalorphine is another reversal agent.

Neuroleptanalgesia refers to a state of CNS depression (sedation or tranquilization) and analgesia induced by a combination of a sedative (e.g., xylazine) or tranquilizer (e.g., acepromazine), and an analgesic (oxymorphone). Phenothiazine tranquilizers or butyrophenone tranquilizers (droperidol) calm the animal and also decrease or block the emetic (vomiting) side effect of a narcotic analgesic.

Anticonvulsants

Seizures are periods of altered brain function characterized by loss of consciousness, altered muscle tone or movement, altered sensations, or other neurologic changes. Drugs used to control seizures are called *anticonvulsants*. Phenobarbital is the drug of choice for long-term control of seizures in dogs and cats. This barbiturate is inexpensive and, because of its long half-life, may be given orally once or twice a day. The dose of phenobarbital is often measured in grains (1 grain = approximately 60 mg). Although primidone has some anticonvulsant activity, most of its efficacy is attributable to phenobarbital, produced by metabolism of primidone.

Phenytoin (Dilantin) is a human anticonvulsant that was once popular for use in treating epilepsy in animals. The major disadvantage of phenytoin is that it is difficult to maintain therapeutic plasma concentrations in dogs. Diazepam (Valium) is the drug of choice for emergency treatment of convulsing animals. Diazepam is very effective when given IV, but it is poorly effective when given PO and is absorbed irregularly if injected SC or IM. Clonazepam (Klonopin) is occasionally used with phenobarbital in animals in which plasma concentrations of barbiturate are in the therapeutic range, but the seizures are not adequately controlled.

Potassium Bromide (KBr) is also used alone or in conjunction with phenobarbital to control seizures. The exact mechanism in not fully understood, but it is thought that it has generalized depressant effects on neuronal excitability and activity. The bromide also competes for chloride transport raising the seizure threshold. The main disadvantage of bromides is the long half-life and consequent necessity to take it for at least one month before seeing therapeutic effects. Bromides are commonly used in dogs but not in cats.

Central Nervous System Stimulants

Central nervous system (CNS) stimulants are primarily used to stimulate respiration in anesthetized animals or to reverse CNS depression caused by anesthetic or sedative agents. The active ingredient in chocolate is theobromine. A dosage as low as 90 mg/kg (41 mg/lb) can produce toxicity in dogs. For a 10-lb dog, it would take two or three chocolate bars to produce serious toxicity. Fortunately, ingestion of that much chocolate by such a small dog would likely produce vomiting, thus decreasing the amount of theobromine absorbed.

Doxapram (Dopram) is a CNS stimulant that increases respiration in animals with apnea (cessation of breathing) or bradypnea (slow breathing). Doxapram is most often used in animals that have received large amounts of these respiratory depressant drugs. Yohimbine, tolazoline, and atipamezole increase respiration through reversal of CNS depression caused by such drugs as xylazine, detomidine, and medetomidine.

ANTIMICROBIALS

Antimicrobials are drugs that kill or inhibit the growth of microorganisms or "microbes," such as bacteria, protozoa, viruses, or fungi. The term *antibiotic* is often used interchangeably with the term *antimicrobial*. An antimicrobial can be classified by the type of microorganism against which it is effective and whether the antimicrobial kills the microorganism or prevents the microorganism from replicating and proliferating.

The suffix *-cidal* generally describes drugs that kill the microorganism (e.g., bactericidal). The suffix *-static* usually describes drugs that inhibit replication but generally do not kill the microorganism outright (e.g., fungistatic). Examples include the following:
- *bactericidal:* kills bacteria
- *bacteriostatic:* inhibits bacterial replication
- *virucidal:* kills viruses
- *protozoistatic:* inhibits protozoal replication
- *fungicidal:* kills fungi

Antimicrobials work by different mechanisms to kill or inhibit bacteria and other microorganisms. Antimicrobials generally exert their effects on the cell wall, cell membrane, ribosomes, critical enzymes or metabolites, or nucleic acids of microorganisms.

Some microorganisms have developed the ability to survive in the presence of antimicrobial drugs. This ability to survive is referred to as *resistance*. Bacteria may become resistant to certain drugs because of genetic changes inherited from previous generations of bacteria, or they may acquire resistance by spontaneous mutations of chromosomes.

A *residue* is an accumulation of a drug or chemical or its metabolites in animal tissues or food products, resulting from drug administration to an animal or contamination of food products. Use of drugs in animals intended for food (meat, egg, milk, etc.) must be stopped a specific number of days (the withdrawal period) before the animal is slaughtered or the food products are to be marketed as food for people. *Most antimicrobial residues in food are not degraded by cooking or pasteurization.*

Penicillins

Penicillins are bactericidal and can usually be recognized by their *-cillin* suffix on the drug name. The most frequently used penicillins in veterinary medicine include the following: the natural penicillins, penicillin G and penicillin V; the broad-spectrum aminopenicillins, ampicillin, amoxicillin, and hetacillin; the penicillinase-resistant penicillins, cloxacillin, dicloxacillin, and oxacillin; and the extended-spectrum penicillins, carbenicillin, ticarcillin, piperacillin, and others. Penicillins are generally effective against gram-positive bacteria and varying types of gram-negative bacteria. Penicillins are generally well absorbed from injection sites and the GI tract. A penicillin that should not be given PO is penicillin G. Penicillin G is inactivated by gastric acid and so is used only in injectable form.

Amoxicillin/Clavulanic acid (Clavamox) is another bactericidal aminopenicillin with beta-lactamase inhibitor, which expands its spectrum of coverage. It is most commonly used in dogs and cats for urinary tract, soft tissue, and skin infections by susceptible organisms.

Cephalosporins

Cephalosporins are bactericidal beta-lactam antimicrobials with a *ceph-* or *cef-* prefix in the drug name. Cephalosporins are classified by generations, according to when they were first developed. *First-generation cephalosporins* are primarily effective against gram-positive bacteria (*Streptococcus, Staphylococcus*). They are less effective against gram-negative bacteria than the *second-* or *third-generation cephalosporins*. Veterinary products include cefadroxil (first-generation, Cefa-Tabs), cefazolin (first-generation, Kefzol, Ancef, Zolicef, and cefazolin sodium), cephapirin (first-generation, Cefa-Lak and Cefa-Dri intramammary infusions), and ceftiofur (third-generation, Naxcel injectable). Human products used in veterinary medicine include cefixime (third-generation, Suprax), cefoperazone (third-generation, Cefobid), cefpodoxime proxetil (third-generation, Vantin), cefotetan disodium (second- or third-generation, Cefotan), cephalothin (first-generation, Keflin), ceftriaxone (third-generation, Rocephin), cephalexin (first-generation, Keflex), cefoxitin (second-generation, Mefoxin), and cefotaxime (third-generation, Claforan). First-generation cephalosporins are well absorbed from the GI tract.

Bacitracins

Bacitracins are a group of polypeptide antibiotics, of which bacitracin A is the major component. Bacitracin is a common ingredient in topical antibiotic creams or ointments. It is often combined with polymyxin B and neomycin to provide a broad spectrum of antibacterial activity.

Aminoglycosides

Aminoglycosides used in veterinary medicine include gentamicin, amikacin, neomycin, streptomycin, dihydrostreptomycin, apramycin, kanamycin, and tobramycin. With the exception of amikacin, most aminoglycosides can be recognized by the -*micin* or -*mycin* suffix in the nonproprietary name. Aminoglycosides are bactericidal and are quite effective against many aerobic bacteria (bacteria that require oxygen to live), but are not effective against most anaerobic bacteria (those that do not require oxygen). Aminoglycosides are potentially nephrotoxic (toxic to the kidney) and ototoxic (toxic to the inner ear), even at "normal" dosages.

Fluoroquinolones

Fluoroquinolones (quinolones) are bactericidal antimicrobials used commonly for their effectiveness against a variety of pathogens. Quinolones are not effective against anaerobes. Enrofloxacin (Baytril) is approved for use in dogs, cats, cattle, horses, ferrets, reptiles, birds, and rodents. It has also been used extra-label (in unapproved ways) to treat neonatal diseases in swine. Ciprofloxacin (Cipro) is similar to enrofloxacin and mostly used when larger dosages are necessary. Orbifloxacin (Orbax) is also similar to enrofloxacin and is approved for use in dogs and cats against susceptible infections. Difloxacin (Dicural) and marbofloxacin (Zeniquin) are approved for use against suspectible infections in dogs only. Sarafloxacin (Saraflox) was the first quinolone approved for use in food animals (poultry only). The quinolones are effective against common gram-negative and gram-positive bacteria found in skin, respiratory, and urinary infections. Quinolones can cause arthopathies in immature, growing animals and therefore should not be used in these animals.

Tetracyclines

Tetracyclines are bacteriostatic drugs with a nonproprietary name ending in -*cycline*. They work most effectively against mycoplasma, spirochetes (including lymes), chlamydia, and rickettsia. The gram-positive organisms they have been effective against in the past are becoming more resistant. Tetracycline and oxytetracycline have similar spectra of antibacterial activity and actions in the body. The newer and more lipophilic doxycycline and minocycline are human drugs that are being used more frequently in animals (unapproved use) because of their longer half-life (increased duration of activity), broader spectrum of antibacterial action, and better penetration of tissues than the older tetracyclines. After oral administration, doxycycline and minocycline are absorbed better than oxytetracycline or tetracycline. Oxytetracycline is the most commonly used injectable tetracycline because of its good absorption from IM injection sites. Chlortetracycline is used as a food or water treatment or as an ophthalmic agent.

Sulfonamides and Potentiated Sulfonamides

Because sulfonamides ("sulfa drugs") have been in use for many years, many strains of bacteria have become resistant to them. To increase the efficacy of sulfonamides and convert them from bacteriostatic to bactericidal drugs, they are sometimes combined with other compounds, such as trimethoprim and ormetoprim, to *potentiate* (increase) their antibacterial effects. Some of the more common sulfonamides used in veterinary medicine include sulfadimethoxine (combined with ormetoprim in Primor), sulfadiazine (combined with trimethoprim in Tribrissen), sulfamethoxazole (combined with trimethoprim in Septra), sulfachlorpyridazine (used in livestock and poultry), and sulfasalazine (used for its antiinflammatory effect in inflammatory bowel disease). Potentiated sulfas used in veterinary medicine have a fairly broad spectrum of antibacterial activity, including many gram-positive organisms (e.g., *Streptococcus*, *Staphylococcus*, *Nocardia*). Although sulfas and potentiated sulfas are not very effective against gram-negative organisms, they are the drugs of choice for treating some protozoal infections, including *Coccidia* and *Toxoplasma*.

Lincosamides

Lincosamide antibiotics, including linocomycin and clindamycin (Antirobe), can be bacteriostatic or bactericidal, depending on the concentrations attained at the site of infection. The lincosamides are generally effective against many gram-positive aerobic cocci. Lincomycin is approved for use in a variety of species (dogs, cats, swine, poultry), but clindamycin is approved only for use in dogs, cats, and ferrets. Pirlimycin is approved for use only in cattle and Tilmicosin for cattle and poultry.

Macrolides

The macrolide antibiotics erythromycin, azithromycin, and tylosin (Tylan) are approved for use in a variety of companion animals and food animals, including dogs, cats, swine, sheep, cattle, and poultry. Although tylosin is approved for use in dogs and cats, its primary use is in livestock. Both drugs are bacteriostatic and share similar spectra of antibacterial activity and bacterial cross resistance. *Tilmicosin* (Micotil) is a macrolide approved for SC administration for treatment of bovine respiratory diseases.

Metronidazole

Metronidazole (Flagyl) is a bactericidal antimicrobial that is also effective against protozoa that cause intestinal disease, such as *Giardia* (giardiasis), *Entamoeba histolytica* (amebiasis), *Trichomonas* (trichomoniasis), and *Balantidium coli* (balantidiasis).

Nitrofurans

The nitrofurans are a large group of antimicrobials, of which nitrofurantoin (Furadantin) is most commonly used in veterinary medicine. Nitrofurantoin is bacteriostatic or bactericidal, depending on concentrations attained at the site of infection. Because about half of the drug administered is secreted into the renal tubule, it is used to treat infections of the lower urinary tract (bladder, urethra) in dogs, cats, and occasionally horses.

Chloramphenicol and Fluorfenicol

Chloramphenicol is an antimicrobial that is bacteriostatic at low concentrations but may become bactericidal when used at higher dosages. Chloramphenicol has produced fatal aplastic anemia in humans. For this reason, *chloramphenicol is totally banned from any use in food animals.* Fluorfenicol is a new drug similar to chloramphenicol but without the risk of aplastic anemia. It is approved for treatment of respiratory disease in cattle.

Rifampin

Rifampin is a bactericidal or bacteriostatic antimicrobial belonging to the rifamycins. It is primarily used with or without erythromycin for treatment of *Rhodococcus equi* infections in young foals, and sometimes in conjunction with antifungal agents for treatment of aspergillosis or histoplasmosis in dogs and cats.

ANTIFUNGALS

Amphotericin B and Nystatin

Amphotericin B is an antifungal that is administered IV for treatment of deep or systemic mycotic infections. Nystatin, because of its toxicity to tissues, is used only to treat *Candida* infections (candidiasis) on the skin, mucous membranes (e.g., mouth, vagina), and lining of the intestinal tract in dogs, cats, and birds.

Flucytosine

Flucytosine is an antifungal agent used mostly against *Cryptococcus* and *Candida*. It is often used in conjunction with amphotericin B as resistance is quite common when used alone.

Fluconazole, Ketoconazole, and Itraconazole

Fluconazole, ketoconazole, and itraconazole are imidazole antifungals with fewer side effects than amphotericin B. Of the imidazoles, fluconazole has the least side effects and is apparently safe for use in multiple species.

Griseofulvin

Griseofulvin is a fungistatic drug used primarily to treat infections with *Trichophyton*, *Microsporum*, and *Epidermophyton* dermatophytes (superficial fungi) in dogs, cats, and horses. These fungi usually infect the skin, hair, nails, and claws, causing the condition known as *ringworm*. Griseofulvin is available as a veterinary product (Fulvicin) for oral use as a powder (for horses) or tablets.

DISINFECTANTS AND ANTISEPTICS

Disinfection is the destruction of pathogenic microorganisms or their toxins. *Antiseptics* are chemical agents that kill or prevent the growth of microorganisms on living tissues. *Disinfectants* are chemical agents that kill or prevent growth of microorganisms on inanimate objects (surgical equipment, floors, tabletops). Antiseptics and disinfectants may also be described as *sanitizers* or *sterilizers*. Sanitizers are chemical agents that reduce the number of microorganisms to a "safe" level, without completely eliminating all microorganisms. Sterilizers are chemicals or other agents that completely destroy all microorganisms. As with antimicrobials, it is important to know against what organisms the antiseptic or disinfectant is effective (Table 9-1).

Phenols

Phenols are used as scrub soaps and surface disinfectants. Phenols are also the main disinfecting agents found in many household disinfectants (Lysol, pine oil, and similar cleansers). They are very effective against gram-positive bacteria but generally not effective against gram-negative bacteria, viruses, fungi, or spores. Hexachlorophene is a phenolic surgical scrub that has decreased in popularity because of its suspected neurotoxicity (damage to the nervous system) and teratogenic effects (birth defects) in pregnant nurses who performed hexachlorophene scrubs on a regular basis.

Alcohols

Alcohols, such as ethyl alcohol or isopropyl alcohol, are among the most common antiseptics applied to skin. Solutions of 70% alcohol are used to disinfect surgical sites, injection sites, and rectal thermometers. Nonenveloped viruses are not susceptible to the virucidal effects of alcohol.

TABLE 9-1

Relative Efficacy of Disinfectants and Antiseptics*

	Chlorhexidine	Quaternary Ammonium Compounds	Alcohol	Iodophor	Chlorine	Phenols
Bactericidal	3+†	2+	2+	3+	2+	2+
Lipid-enveloped virucidal	3+	2+	2+	2+	3+	1+
Nonenveloped virucidal	2+	1+	(–)‡	2+	3+	(–)
Sporicidal	(–)	(–)	(–)	1+	1+	(–)
Effective in presence of soap	1+	(–)	2+	2+	2+	2+
Effective in hard water	1+	1+	1+	2+	2+	1+
Effective in organic material	3+	1+	1+	(–)	(–)	(–)

* Ratings are relative indicators, and the effectiveness is dependent upon concentration of compound used.
† The higher the positive number, the greater the efficacy.
‡ Hyphens (–) indicate lack of efficacy.

Alcohol is also ineffective against bacterial spores and must remain in contact with the site for several seconds to be effective against bacteria (several minutes for fungi). Therefore, a cursory swipe with an alcohol-soaked swab on an animal's skin, especially if the skin is encrusted with dirt or feces, does little to disinfect an injection site.

Quaternary Ammonium Compounds

Quaternary ammonium compounds are used to disinfect the surface of inanimate objects. One of the most commonly used quaternary ammonium compounds in veterinary medicine is benzalkonium chloride. Quaternary ammonium compounds are effective against a wide variety of gram-negative and gram-positive bacteria, but they are ineffective against bacterial spores and have poor efficacy against fungi. Although quaternary ammonium compounds can destroy enveloped viruses, they are ineffective against nonenveloped viruses, such as parvovirus. They act rapidly at a site of application and are not normally irritating to the skin or corrosive to metals.

Chlorine Compounds

Chlorine compounds, such as sodium hypochlorite (Clorox, household bleach), can kill enveloped and nonenveloped viruses and are the disinfectant of choice against parvovirus. Chlorines are also effective against fungi, algae, and vegetative forms of bacteria. Like many other disinfectants, chlorine is not effective against bacterial spores.

Iodophors

Iodophors are used as topical antiseptics before surgical procedures or for disinfection of tissue. An iodophor is a combination of iodine and a carrier molecule that releases the iodine over time, prolonging the antimicrobial activity. The most common iodophor is iodine combined with polyvinylpyrrolidone, more commonly known as *povidone-iodine*. Iodophors are bactericidal, virucidal, protozoicidal, and fungicidal.

Biguanides

Chlorhexidine, a biguanide antiseptic, is commonly used to clean cages and to treat various superficial infections in animals. Its wide variety of uses is likely related to its low tissue irritation and its virucidal, bactericidal (both gram-positive and gram-negative), and fungicidal activity. Because chlorhexidine binds to the outer surface of the skin, it is thought to have some residual activity for up to 24 hours if left in contact with the site.

ANTIPARASITICS

Anthelmintic is a general term used to describe compounds that kill various types of internal parasites (helminths or "worms"). A *vermicide* is an anthelmintic that kills the worm, as opposed to a *vermifuge*, which only paralyzes the worm and often results in passage of live worms in the stool. Antinematodal compounds are used to treat infections with nematodes (roundworms). Nematodes include hookworms, ascarids, whipworms, and strongyles. Anticestodal compounds are used to treat infections with cestodes (tapeworms or segmented flatworms). Antitrematodal compounds are used to treat infection with trematodes (flukes or unsegmented flatworms), including *Paragonimus*, *Fasciola*, and *Dicrocoelium*. Antiprotozoal compounds are used to treat infection with protozoa (single-celled organisms), including *Coccidia*, *Giardia*, and *Toxoplasma*. Coccidiostats are drugs that inhibit the growth of coccidia specifically.

Internal Antiparasitics

Piperazine, a vermicide and vermifuge, is the active ingredient in most of the "once-a-month" dewormers sold in grocery stores and pet shops. Piperazine is very safe but is only effective against ascarids. The benzimidazoles include fenbendazole (Panacur), mebendazole (Telmin, Telmintic), thiabendazole (Equizole, Tresaderm Otic), oxibendazole (Anthelcide EQ, Filaribits-Plus), albendazole, oxfendazole, and cambendazole.

Organophosphates are used as internal antiparasitics (Task, Combot), as well as external antiparasitics to combat fleas, ticks, and flies. The organophosphates most commonly used internally are dichlorvos and trichlorfon. Ivermectin (Ivomec, Eqvalan, Heartgard-30) is an avermectin widely used in almost every species treated by veterinarians. Ivermectin can produce adverse reactions in Collies and Collie cross-breeds. Anticestodals used in animals include praziquantel (Droncit) and epsiprantel (Cestex).

Anthelmintics containing pyrantel (Strongid, Nemex, Banminth, Imathal) safely remove a variety of nematodes in domestic species. They are marketed as pyrantel pamoate and a more water-soluble salt, pyrantel tartrate. Morantel tartrate (Nematel) is very similar to pyrantel and has similar uses. Febantel is marketed in a palatable paste formulation for horses or in combination with the anticestodal drug praziquantel (Vercom) for dogs and cats or with the organophosphate trichlorfon (Combotel) for horses.

For years, thiacetarsamide sodium (Caparsolate) had been the only drug approved for treatment of adult heartworms; thiacetarsamide is given by IV injection. In 1996, melarsomine dihydrochloride (Immiticide) was approved as an adulticide; it is given by IM injection. After adulticide treatment, a microfilaricide can be administered to eliminate circulating heartworm microfilariae. Ivermectin (e.g., 1% Ivomec injectable, approved for use in livestock) is the microfilaricide of choice. Milbemycin oxime (Interceptor), a drug very similar to ivermectin, is also used as a microfilaricide. After microfilariae have been cleared from the blood, the animal can begin receiving heartworm preventive to prevent reinfection. Diethylcarbamazine (DEC), marketed as Caricide, Nemacide, and Filarbits, is given daily during seasons when an animal could be bitten by a mosquito and for 2 months thereafter. Because they must be given only once a month, ivermectin (Heartgard-30) and milbemycin (Interceptor) have captured a significant percentage of the heartworm preventive market. Ivermectin is also available as a heartworm preventive for cats (Heartgard-30 for Cats).

Antiprotozoals are most commonly used against coccidia, *Giardia*, and other protozoa. They include sulfonamide antimicrobials, such as sulfadimethoxine (Albon, Bactrovet), metronidazole, and amprolium (Corid).

External Antiparasitics

Chlorinated hydrocarbons constitute one of the oldest group of the synthetic insecticides. The only chlorinated hydrocarbon currently used in veterinary medicine is lindane, which is incorporated in some dog shampoos. Lindane is easily absorbed through the skin and can produce harmful side effects if absorbed in sufficient quantities.

Organophosphates and carbamates are usually grouped together because of their similar mechanism of action, effects on insects, and toxic effects. Unlike the chlorinated hydrocarbons, organophosphates and carbamates decompose readily in the environment and do not pose a significant threat to wildlife. Included in this group are chlorpyrifos, carbaryl (Sevin), and propoxur (Baygon).

Pyrethrins and pyrethroids (synthetic pyrethrins) constitute the largest group of insecticides marketed for use against external parasites and as common household insect sprays. They are generally quite safe. Pyrethrins and pyrethroids produce a quick "knockdown" effect, but the immobilized flies or fleas may recover after several minutes. Pyrethroids include resmethrin, allethrin, permethrin, tetramethrin, bioallethrin, and fenvalerate.

Amitraz is a diamide insecticide that was one of the first effective agents available for treatment of demodectic mange in dogs. Since its introduction, amitraz has been incorporated into other insecticidal products. Amitraz is toxic to cats and rabbits, so it should not be used in those species. The liquid form, available as a dip or sponge-on bath product (Mitaban), is used to treat demodectic mange in dogs. Amitraz is also available as Preventic, a tick collar for dogs, and as Taktic, a liquid topical or a collar for use in cattle.

Imidacloprid (Advantage) is a chloronicotinyl nitroguanidine insecticide used topically to kill adult fleas on dogs and cats. Imidacloprid is applied to the back of the neck in cats or between the shoulder blades in dogs (and over the rump area of large dogs), and kills adult fleas upon contact. Fipronil (Frontline and Top Spot), and selamectin (Revolution) are once-a-month flea spray and topical applications that resemble ivermectin in their insecticidal activity.

Rotenone (Derris Powder) is a natural insecticide derived from derris root. It may be included with other insecticides in dips, pour-ons, and powders. D-limonene, derived from citrus peels, purportedly has some slight insecticidal activity. When included in insecticidal products, it imparts a pleasant citrus smell to the haircoat. Sulfur is sometimes included in "tar and sulfur" shampoos to help reduce skin scaling and to treat sarcoptic mange. These products are usually recognized by their strong sulfur odor. Insect growth regulators are compounds that affect immature stages of insects and prevent maturation to adults. They are insecticidal without toxic effects in mammals. Methoprene (Siphotrol, Ovitrol) and fenoxycarb (Basus, Ectogard, and others) were some of the first insect growth regulators incorporated into topical products or flea collars. These compounds are distributed over the animal's skin. Female fleas absorb the drug, and it is incorporated into the flea eggs. The drug-impregnated eggs hatch and the larvae do not mature to adult fleas. Lufenuron (Program) is an insect development inhibitor given once a month as a tablet for dogs and cats and as an oral liquid for cats.

Lufenuron interferes with development of the insect's chitin, which is essential for proper egg formation and development of the larval exoskeleton. If flea larvae survive within the egg despite a defective shell, they will be unable to hatch. Because lufenuron is orally ingested and distributed throughout the animal's tissue fluids, a flea must bite the animal to be exposed to the drug.

Insect repellents are used to repel insects and keep them off of animals. Butoxypolypropylene glycol (Butox PPG) has been incorporated into flea and tick spray products for use in dogs and cats. It is also used in equine fly repellents.

Diethyltoluamide (DEET) is a common ingredient in repellent products formulated for use in people.

ANTIINFLAMMATORIES

Drugs that relieve pain or discomfort by blocking or reducing the inflammatory process are called *antiinflammatories*. There are two general classes of antiinflammatories: *steroidal antiinflammatory drugs* (glucocorticoids) and *nonsteroidal antiinflammatory drugs (NSAIDs)*. Most of these drugs relieve pain indirectly by decreasing inflammation; however, some also have direct analgesic (pain-relieving) activity.

Glucocorticoids

When veterinarians use the terms *cortisone* or *corticosteroid*, they are usually referring to glucocorticoids. A glucocorticoid that exerts an antiinflammatory effect for less than 12 hours, such as hydrocortisone, is considered a *short-acting glucocorticoid*. Many glucocorticoids used in veterinary medicine are classified as *intermediate-acting glucocorticoids*, with activity for 12 to 36 hours. These include prednisone, prednisolone, triamcinolone (e.g., Vetalog), methylprednisolone, and isoflupredone. *Long-acting glucocorticoids*, such as dexamethasone, betamethasone, and flumethasone, exert their effects for more than 48 hours.

Glucocorticoids are generally available in three liquid forms: aqueous solutions, alcohol solutions, and suspensions. Glucocorticoids in aqueous (water) solution are usually combined with a salt to make them soluble in water. Dexamethasone sodium phosphate (Azium SP) and prednisolone sodium succinate (Solu-Delta-Cortef) are aqueous solutions of glucocorticoids. The advantage of aqueous forms is that they can be given in large doses IV with less risk than alcohol solutions and suspensions (suspensions should never be given IV). The aqueous forms are often used in emergency situations (shock, CNS trauma) because they can be delivered IV in large amounts and have a fairly rapid onset of activity. If the label of a vial of dexamethasone specifies the active ingredient as dexamethasone, without mention of sodium phosphate, it is likely an alcohol solution. Suspensions of glucocorticoids contain the drug particles suspended in the liquid vehicle. Suspensions are characterized by their opaque appearance (after shaking), the need for shaking the vial before use, and the terms *acetate, diacetate, pivalate, acetonide,* or *valerate* appended to the glucocorticoid name. When injected into the body, the drug crystals dissolve over several days, releasing small amounts of glucocorticoid each day and providing prolonged action. Topical preparations of glucocorticoid suspensions using the acetate ester are used in topical ophthalmic medications. Oral tablets are available for prednisone and prednisolone.

Overuse of glucocorticoid drugs can produce Cushing's syndrome. The signs of Cushing's syndrome are related to the effects of glucocorticoids and include alopecia (hair loss), muscle wasting, pot-bellied appearance, slow healing of wounds, polyuria, polydipsia, and polyphagia. Physical changes (alopecia, muscle wasting) do not become apparent until the animal has been treated for weeks.

Nonsteroidal Antiinflammatory Drugs

The advantage of nonsteroidal antiinflammatory drugs (NSAIDs) over glucocorticoids centers around the many side effects of glucocorticoids as compared with the few adverse effects associated with NSAIDs. NSAIDs decrease protective prostaglandins in the stomach and kidney. In large doses or in sensitive animals, NSAIDs can produce gastric ulcerations or decreased blood flow to the kidneys.

Phenylbutazone is given PO or IV to horses for relief of musculoskeletal inflammation. Aspirin (acetylsalicylic acid) is a fairly safe NSAID in most animal species. Like other NSAIDs, aspirin is metabolized by the liver. Aspirin is metabolized much more slowly in cats than in other species. Aspirin has a half-life of 1.5 hours in people, approximately 8 hours in dogs, and 30 hours in cats. Thus, as with many other drugs, the aspirin dosage for cats is lower than dosages used in other species and usually consists of one "baby aspirin" tablet (81 mg) every two or three days. If used prudently, however, aspirin is one of the safest and most effective NSAIDs for cats.

Ibuprofen, ketoprofen, and naproxen are available as OTC medications (ibuprofen is marketed as Advil, naproxen is marketed as Aleve, ketoprofen is marketed as Orudis). Naproxen is marketed as the veterinary product Naprosyn. A ketoprofen product, Ketofen, is approved for use in horses. Flunixin meglumine (Banamine) is also is a potent analgesic used primarily in equine medicine for treatment of colic; dogs are very sensitive to the GI side effects of flunixin. Carprofen (Rimadyl) is a new veterinary NSAID that decreases prostaglandins associated with

Inflammation but does not significantly reduce the protective prostaglandins of the stomach and kidneys.

Meclofenamic acid (Arquel) is commonly administered to horses as granules mixed in the feed. Dimethyl sulfoxide (DMSO) is used topically and parenterally, primarily in horses. DMSO is also a component of some otic (ear) preparations used in dogs and cats. Orgotein (superoxide dismutase) is most commonly used to treat horses with joint and vertebral disease.

Other Antiinflammatories

Although acetaminophen is not an antiinflammatory drug, it is included here because its analgesic and antipyretic (fever-reducing) properties often cause it to be grouped with NSAIDs. Acetaminophen (e.g., Tylenol) does not cause the GI upset, ulcers, or interference with platelet clumping associated with NSAIDs. Unfortunately, the metabolites of acetaminophen can have other severe side effects, especially in cats. A single "extra-strength" acetaminophen tablet (500 mg) can kill an average-sized cat. In dogs, a higher dosage (above 150 mg/kg) is required before signs of hepatic necrosis, weight loss, and icterus (jaundice) become evident.

Phenacetin is a compound found in many "cold preparations." This drug is metabolized to acetaminophen and thus can produce acetaminophen toxicity in susceptible species and individual animals. Gold salts, such as aurothioglucose, have been used to treat severe immune-mediated skin problems, such as the various forms of pemphigus. The antiinflammatory activity of dipyrone is weak compared with its analgesic properties and its ability to decrease fever.

RECOMMENDED READING

Adams HR: *Veterinary pharmacology and therapeutics*, ed 7, Ames, Iowa, 1995, Iowa State University Press.

Allen DG: *Handbook of veterinary drugs*, Philadelphia, 1993, JB Lippincott.

Bill RL: *Pharmacology for veterinary technicians*, ed 2, St Louis, 1997, Mosby.

Gilman AG, et al: *Goodman and Gilman's The pharmacological basis of therapeutics*, ed 7, New York, 1985, MacMillan.

Mosby's Drug Consult, St Louis, 2004, Mosby.

Plumb DC: *Veterinary drug handbook*, ed 4, Ames, Iowa, 2002, Iowa State University Press.

Veterinary Pharmaceuticals and Biologicals 1997/1998, ed 10, Lenexa, Kans, 1997, Veterinary Medicine Publishing.

Wanamaker BP, Pettes CL: *Applied pharmacology for the veterinary technician*, ed 2, St Louis, 2000, WB Saunders.

10

Behavior

Stuart L. Porter

Learning Objectives

After reviewing this chapter, the reader should understand the following:
- The value of taking a proactive approach toward the behavior of patients
- Where behavior comes from and how it develops
- Role of veterinary professionals in helping clients prevent behavior problems
- Role of veterinary professionals in managing behavior problems
- Appropriate procedure for referring clients to professionals to resolve behavior problems

Most experts agree that behavior problems are common and a leading cause of death in dogs and cats. Usually the "problem" is normal dog and cat behavior that the owner finds inappropriate and then makes worse in attempts to correct it (Fig. 10-1). This often starts early with housebreaking and continues with attention-getting behaviors, destruction, barking, and aggression. Often these owners don't know where to go for advice, and it is here that the veterinary practice can provide an important service to its clients and their pets. However, veterinarians have not been very involved in animal behavioral issues, possibly because so few veterinary schools have behaviorists on the faculty. Certainly there are now many books and continuing education programs on this topic, which would allow someone to become educated as to the depth of the problem. There is even a new Society of Veterinary Behavior Technicians for those interested in learning more about this field.

WHAT IS BEHAVIOR, AND WHERE DOES IT COME FROM?

Behavior is any act done by an animal. An animal does not exhibit a behavioral act without a reason, although the reason may not be obvious to humans. For any behavior to occur, there must be a *stimulus*, some internal or external change that exceeds a threshold causing stimulation of the nervous and/or endocrine systems. This receptor and cellular stimulation and integration of information requires a number of chemical messengers in the animal's body including epinephrine, acetylcholine, dopamine, serotonin, and many others (probably many not yet described). Some problem behaviors are due to increased or decreased amounts of these neurotransmitters. This has resulted in the development of animal psychopharmacology.

Any animal's behavior results from a combination of genetic inheritance from an animal's sire and dam and what the animal learns as it develops. In human behavior, scientists are still debating which is most important in behavioral development, nature or nurture. Many behavioral scientists believe that behavior is approximately 33% genetics and 66% environment in origin. The most important time period for behavior development in dogs and cats is from 4 to 16 weeks. At this young age, the animals learn about its environments, how to interact with others, and what not to fear. What occurs during this habituation or socialization period can affect the animal for the rest of its life. For example, fearful events during this period can result in an animal developing a lifelong phobia (Fig. 10-2). While veterinary professionals have little effect on genetics (other than to recommend that an animal not be bred), they can play an important role by educating clients about the correct way to raise and interact with their pets. Of course, it is important to remember that diseases also play a role in animal behavior problems such as in hypothyroidism in dogs, hyperthyroidism in cats, and cognitive dysfunction in older

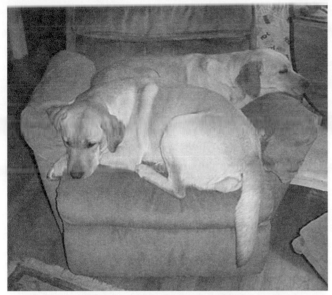

Fig. 10-1 Owners need to decide whether a particular behavior is a problem, because the animal rarely recognizes it as such. For example, barking may be a desirable behavior for one owner, but a problem for another.

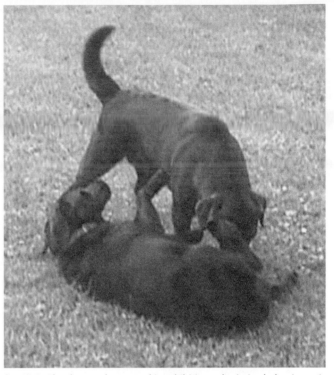

Fig. 10-3 The dog on the ground is exhibiting submissive behavior to its sibling. It is important for owners to recognize and respect the canine hierarchy in the home, or interdog aggression may result.

animals. Sometimes aggression or even housesoiling may be due to a medical problem.

Animals also need to learn how to interact with one another. Many households have more than one dog or cat and often have both. Introducing young animals is usually easier than introducing adults. Being social animals, dogs have a hierarchy or pecking order that determines which one gets first access to coveted resources such as food, toys, owners, and resting spots (Fig. 10-3). Sometimes interdog aggression develops when owners interfere with this hierarchy by allowing the subordinate animal to be petted or fed first.

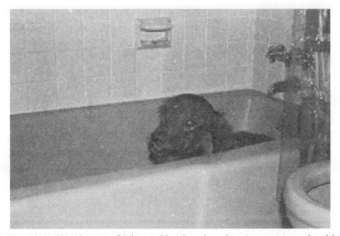

Fig. 10-2 This dog was frightened by thunder when it was 10 weeks old and became afraid of thunder and then loud noises for the next 14 years. For years, it exhibited destructive behavior trying to escape the noise. The dog finally found refuge in the bathtub.

PREVENTING BEHAVIOR PROBLEMS IN COMPANION ANIMALS

Most behavior problems are easier to prevent than to correct. Aggression is the most common problem for which owners seek guidance, but many pet owners are annoyed when their animals damage household belongings and exhibit housesoiling behavior. Techniques based on scientifically valid ethologic and learning principles minimize such behaviors. However, much of the information in popular literature to which owners have easy access does not always meet these criteria. Thus, technicians can be an important source of scientifically accurate information on preventing behavior problems.

Housetraining

Housetraining is one of the most important and first behaviors that young pets are expected to learn. Many owners use outdated methods to housetrain their pets. These methods often interfere with success or damage the relationship with a pet. Problems related to housetraining may result in the animal being turned loose, isolated in a yard or tied, or given away. Dogs and cats can be encouraged to eliminate reliably in locations that are acceptable to their human owners. Cats, as well as pigs and rabbits, learn to use litter boxes. Other species of domestic companion animals are either caged or kept outside because their elimination behavior is not restricted to specific locations.

Dogs

People have probably been training dogs not to eliminate in the house for almost as long as dogs have been domesticated. You might assume that thousands of years of practice have resulted in good housetraining techniques. Surprisingly, this is not the case.

Housebreaking requires that the dog be taken out frequently, especially when it wakes up, after it eats, and whenever it appears to be sniffing around the house. When a puppy cannot be monitored, it should be confined to a crate (Figs. 10-4 and 10-5). Most "accidents" occur when the puppy is left alone. There are different types of crates, including collapsible ones, and those made of wire, plastic, and wood (fabric ones do not work well for young puppies). Training with a crate is also useful for preventing destructive behaviors such as chewing. The use of the crate should not be excessive, because 8-week-old puppies cannot hold their bowels longer than 4 to 6 hours. Dogs will soil in the crate if they cannot get out when they need to eliminate or

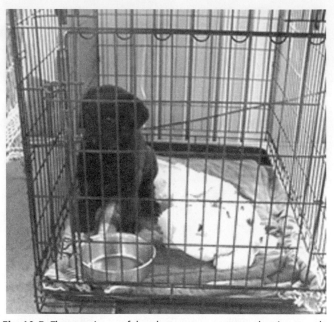

Fig. 10-5 The crate is a useful tool to manage a puppy when it cannot be supervised in the home. This helps with housebreaking as well as preventing destructive behavior.

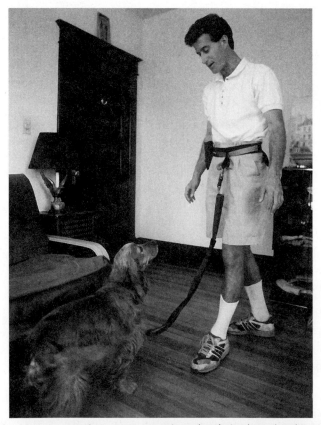

Fig. 10-4 A convenient way to supervise a dog during housebreaking is to keep the dog with you at all times by tying a leash to your belt or by using a Hands-Away Leash Belt. *(Photo courtesy Woof Whirled, Boulder, CO.)*

if the crate is too large. While it is desirable to purchase a crate suitable to hold a full-grown dog, it may be necessary to use plywood or cardboard to subdivide it when the puppy is small.

Owners must be made aware of several important points when housetraining their dog. First, a dog's confinement to a crate must not exceed the time the animal can control its bladder and bowels. For young puppies, this can be as little as 1 hour, or sometimes as much as 2 or 3 hours at a time. In addition, many puppies need to eliminate at least once during the night.

Second, the dog must be actively taught, by reinforcing correct behavior, the desired location for elimination. Owners should reward elimination outside with verbal praise and petting, and possibly a special tidbit. The timing of this reward, however, is critical. Research in animal learning suggests that a delay of longer than 0.5 seconds between the behavior and the subsequent reinforcement significantly decreases the effectiveness of the reinforcement. Thus, if the owner waits by the door to reinforce the puppy as it returns from eliminating in the yard, the behavior that has been reinforced is returning to the house. In these cases, owners often complain that all the puppy does when taken outside is to stand by the door. This should come as no surprise because standing by the door is what the puppy has inadvertently been rewarded for doing. To reinforce the elimination behavior, the owner must go outside with the puppy and provide reinforcement immediately following elimination at the location where it occurs.

Finally, use of physical punishment in housetraining is never appropriate. Interactive punishment that involves the owner (even if delivered at the time of housesoiling) may cause the dog to become reluctant to eliminate in the owner's presence at other times or may even result in the dog becoming afraid of the owner. This interferes with the owner's attempts to appropriately reinforce elimination outside. Remote punishment, such as a loud noise or other startling but harmless stimuli, should be sufficient to temporarily interrupt the behavior. The dog can then be taken outside in a positive, nonthreatening manner and rewarded if it eliminates.

In an ideal housetraining program, the dog's environment and behavior should be so well managed that correct behavior is reinforced with 100% consistency, and opportunities for inappropriate behavior never occur. In reality, this ideal is seldom met, but if owners are made aware of it through your educational efforts, it may give them a much more accurate perspective on the time and effort required for housetraining.

Educating owners about housetraining dogs should be much more detailed than simply telling them to "get a crate and put the dog in it when you can't watch him." Handouts on this important process should also be provided.

Cats

One of the reasons people choose cats as pets instead of dogs is because they can be readily trained to use a litter box for elimination and do not need to be walked. The process of encouraging cats to consistently use litter boxes is based on different developmental events than is housetraining dogs. It is normal instinctual behavior for kittens and cats to use a substrate for elimination. Kittens do not need to observe the queen eliminating or have the owner demonstrate part of the process by raking the cat's paws in the litter. Providing a clean, easily accessible litter box with an acceptable substrate is sufficient. However, the accessibility of the litter box and suitability of the substrate must be examined from the kitten's or cat's perspective. The major complaint owners have is that their cats stop or inconsistently use the litter box and choose to eliminate somewhere else in the house. If this problem is not corrected, these cats may be confined to the outdoors or given away. Since there are many reasons for a cat to stop using its litter box, a detailed history is needed to determine the cause.

Because kittens are physically and behaviorally immature, a litter box should be within easy access at all times. This may mean providing several litter boxes at strategic locations in the house or initially limiting the cat's access to only portions of the house. The litter box should be easily accessible but also should afford some privacy. High-traffic areas are not a good choice, but neither is locating the box in a basement with a cold cement floor. Close proximity to appliances that make unexpected, startling noises, such as the washer, furnace, or hot water heater, should also be avoided.

One study found that cats seem to prefer the softer texture of fine-grained substrates (Fig. 10-6). Thus, a cat is less likely to develop an aversion to a clumping litter comprising very small particles. However, cats develop idiosyncratic preferences for substrates and locations for elimination for reasons that are not well understood. These changing preferences are often the basis of many inappropriate elimination problems in cats. Sometimes these preferences can be influenced by the condition of the litter material. Cats may avoid litter that is consistently dirty, too deep, or scented. One study found that cats with elimination problems were more likely to have scented than unscented litter as compared with cats without such problems.

Owners are sometimes under the impression that the more litter they put in the box, the less often they need to clean it. General guidelines are to keep the litter depth at no more than 2 inches, remove feces and urine clumps daily, and change the litter frequently enough to prevent odors from developing and to ensure that the majority of the litter is always dry (Fig. 10-7).

Another consideration influencing the cat's perception of litter box accessibility is the presence of other cats in the household. A litter box may be temporarily unavailable because another cat is either using it or "guarding" it. Thus, advise owners to provide at least as many litter boxes as there are cats, and to keep the boxes in different locations so that a single cat cannot block another cat's access to the litter box area. In addition, the litter box location should allow the cat using it to be aware of the presence of other cats in order to prevent any surprise attacks that may occur during elimination. The owner must also understand that if the cat learns to associate the litter box with punishment such as catching it in order to administer medication, it may stop using it.

PREVENTING DESTRUCTIVE BEHAVIOR BY CATS

Probably more owners recognize the need to provide their cats with litter boxes than to provide scratching posts. Because cats scratch for a variety of reasons, cats may want to scratch in different locations for different reasons. One of the most important motivations for cats scratching objects with their front claws is territorial marking. Scratching leaves a visual as well as an olfactory mark that serves as an indication of the cat's presence. In addition to marking, scratching also serves to stretch the muscles and tendons of the legs and remove the worn outer sheaths from the claws. It may also be used as a greeting or play behavior.

Scratching objects should be provided in locations in which the behavior is likely to be triggered. Even if the cat scratches objects when allowed outdoors, it still should have access to an acceptable object indoors. Merely provid-

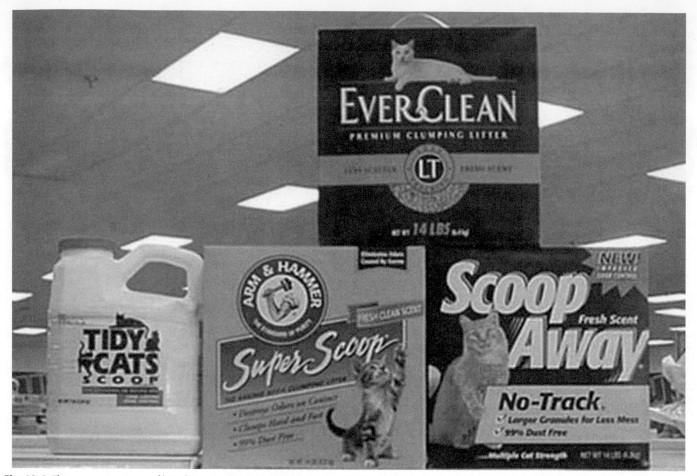

Fig. 10-6 There are many types of kitty litters on the market, and cats do exhibit preferences for particular types. Switching litter brands may trigger a cat to stop using the litter box.

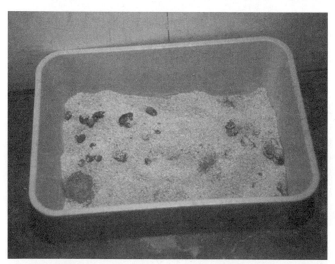

Fig. 10-7 Cats are fastidious, and one reason they stop using the litter box is that it is too dirty for them. Litter boxes should be cleaned daily, and there should be at least one litter box per cat in the household.

ing a scratching object does not guarantee the cat will use it preferentially to carpet, drapes, or furniture. The scratching objects must match the cat's preferences for desirable locations, and with regard to height, orientation, and texture (Fig. 10-8).

If a new cat is encouraged to use its own scratching post, it may avoid exercising its claws on furniture or drapes. Owners must understand that they should discourage cats from clawing their possessions. They can do this by distracting the cat caught in the act or preventing its access to the items. Unfortunately, many clients merely resort to having the cat declawed as a preventive measure or solution to the problem behavior.

Height

Many scratching posts available commercially do not permit the cat to reach vertically to its full height to scratch, as many cats like to do. Also they aren't sturdy enough to support the cat's weight and readily fall over, frightening

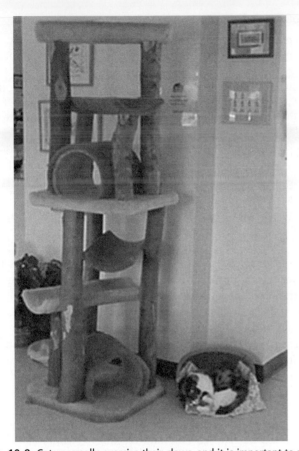

Fig. 10-8 Cats normally exercise their claws, and it is important to provide them with scratching posts that are large and sturdy enough to support their weight. The scratching posts must also be located in appropriate places in the home.

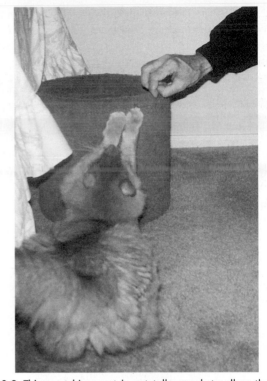

Fig. 10-9 This scratching post is not tall enough to allow the cat to stretch to its full height while using it. This may result in the cat finding more suitable objects to use, such as the couch or the curtains.

the cat. For larger cats using relatively short posts, this means they are scratching almost with their abdomen on the floor (Fig. 10-9). It may be a good idea to talk to owners about the desirability of taller, or even floor-to-ceiling scratching poles. If the back of the couch allows the cat to reach to its full height to scratch but the scratching post does not, it is easy to guess which surface the cat will prefer.

Orientation

Not all cats scratch vertically all of the time. Some cats may prefer to stretch their legs out in front and rake backward in a horizontal motion. If this is the case, the cat may be more likely to use a flat, horizontal object (Fig. 10-10) than a vertical post. Some cats may use both, depending on where, when, and why they scratch. One unusual cat was reported to only scratch upside down by pulling herself along on her back as she scratched the underside of the couch.

Texture

This may be the most frequently overlooked aspect of providing an acceptable scratching object. As with other aspects of the behavioral pattern of scratching, cats vary in

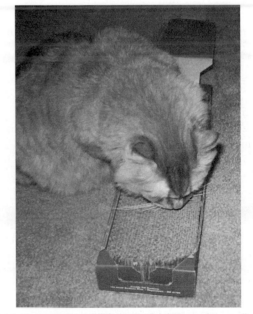

Fig. 10-10 Horizontal scratching objects such as this cardboard pad scented with catnip may be preferred over vertical objects.

textures they prefer. Cats that like to rake their claws in long, vertical motions may be more likely to use an object with a texture that permits this. If the cat scratches vertically and the texture is not conducive to those motions, the cat may not use the object. Other cats use more of a "picking" motion and may prefer items covered with sisal, wrapped horizontally. It has been proposed that an object that has been scratched repeatedly, with the result that the covering is somewhat shredded and holds the cat's scent, will be preferred over a new, unused object. This suggests that owners should not replace well-worn scratching posts, even if they appear unsightly.

The scratching object should be placed in a location where the cat is likely to be motivated to scratch, or adjacent to an unacceptable item the cat is already using. To encourage the cat to use the desirable object, it can be scented with catnip or a commercial pheromone (Feliway™, Abbott), or a toy can be attached to the top to entice the cat to reach high up the post. Raking the cat's feet up and down the post is not necessary and may actually have adverse effects. The most reliable way to discourage scratching of inappropriate objects is to first provide an appropriate substitute and then change the texture of the "off-limit" items. Owners can change the texture by covering it with plastic, sandpaper, or another covering with an unpleasant (from the cat's perspective) texture.

PREVENTING DESTRUCTIVE BEHAVIOR BY DOGS

Destructive behavior is a classification of behavior based more on the owner's view of the result (destruction) than on the actual behavior that caused it. Digging, chewing, tearing, scratching, moving objects from one place to another, and removing the contents from the trash are all considered destructive behavior and are self-rewarding.

Dogs show these behaviors for a variety of reasons. Destructive behavior that is the symptomatic manifestation of other problems, such as separation anxiety or noise phobias, can be treated but may not be prevented. In these cases, the underlying problem must be resolved, rather than trying to treat the symptom. However, destructive behavior that occurs as the result of a normal developmental process, such as teething, play, and investigative behavior, can often be prevented or at least minimized.

Dogs vary in their need for physical activity and play. Some dogs are content to lead relatively inactive lives, whereas others seem to be on the move constantly. Just as with cats' scratching, the goal in minimizing problem destructive behavior due to teething, play, and investigative behavior is not to eliminate the behavior, but to direct it toward acceptable objects by making acceptable toys more attractive than household items. This needs to be done on a consistent basis, or some items may be destroyed.

Appealing Toys

Dogs should be exposed to suitable toys when they are young. The attractiveness of acceptable toys can be maximized by first rewarding the dog every time it plays with them. Toys should also elicit the play patterns that the dog is likely to exhibit. For example, dogs that like to shake toys may be more satisfied with one made of lambskin than with a tennis ball. Toys should be available for chewing and tearing, as well as for carrying and chasing, if the dog displays both patterns of play behavior. It may be helpful to establish a toy rotation so that different toys are available each day to make them more appealing.

If the dog is caught chewing an unacceptable item, the item should be taken away and replaced with one that is acceptable (Figs. 10-11 and 10-12). To decrease the dog's interest in household items, even when the owner is not present, attempts can be made to lessen their appeal. Commercial products, such as Bitter Apple, are available to give objects a bad taste. Motion detectors or Snappy Trainers (modified mousetraps that do not harm the animal) can discourage animals from bothering specific items or areas, or items can be "booby-trapped" in other creative ways. Remind owners of the advisability of "dog-proofing" the house just as they would for a young child.

Dogs that insist on digging outside can be provided with their own area in which to do so. This area should consist of loose soil or sand to facilitate digging. Owners can shallowly bury enticing items in this area to attract the dog.

PREVENTING AGGRESSIVE BEHAVIOR PROBLEMS

Aggressive behavior is normal behavior for most species of animals, including companion animals. *Aggression*, defined as behavior that is intended to harm another individual, is only one aspect of *agonistic* behavior. Agonistic behaviors are behaviors that animals show in situations involving social conflict. Submission, avoidance, escaping, offensive and defensive threats, and offensive and defensive aggression are all part of the agonistic behavior system. There are many different types of aggression displayed by dogs and cats. Aggression may be directed against people, family members or strangers, children, or other dogs and species. Different types of aggression include dominant, fearful, territorial, maternal, intermale, interfemale, predatory, play-related, redirected, and others. It is important to determine which type is present in order to treat it. The most common complaint from dog owners is aggression toward people, while the most common complaint from cat owners is aggression toward other cats. Because the factors that determine when and where an animal will display aggressive or threatening behavior are not fully understood, it is unlikely that preventing problems will be a simple process.

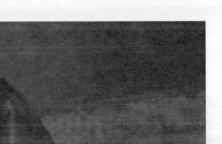

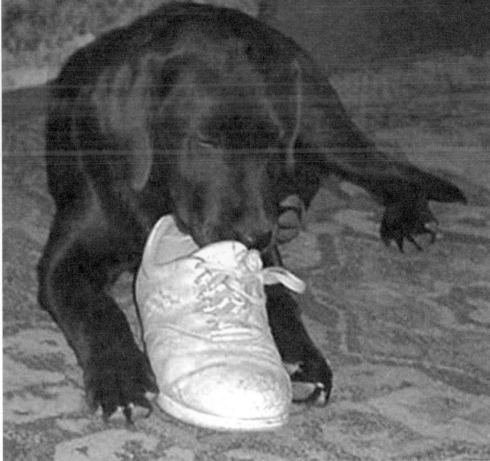

Fig. 10-11 Chewing is normal dog behavior and needs to be directed to acceptable objects. Owners should remove their things from the dog's mouth and replace them with the dog's own toys. A dog cannot tell the difference between an old shoe and a new one.

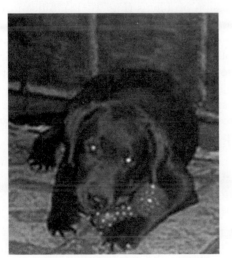

Fig. 10-12 This puppy didn't even notice that a different item had been placed in its mouth. It is best to introduce puppies to suitable toys when they are young and encourage them to play with the toys.

Aggression directed at children is considered the number-one public health problem in children, as more than 60% of victims are between 5 and 14 years of age. Dogs need to be socialized to children when they are young, and children need to be taught how to behave around dogs, particularly strange ones. Parents also often worry about dog aggression toward infants. This aggression is actually a form of predatory behavior. It is important to advise new parents about how to introduce their new baby to their dog (Fig. 10-13).

Puppy Tests

One way to prevent aggression problems in animals would be to select pets that are unlikely to develop such problems. Popular literature describes of a variety of "puppy tests" that supposedly predict a puppy's likelihood for dominant behavior or aggression problems as an adult. This information can be used to suggest behavioral tendencies and to

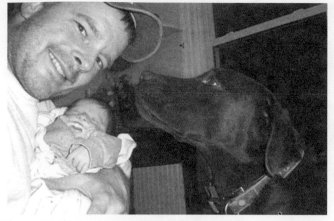

Fig. 10-13 This parent is supervising the introduction of his new infant son to his 2-year-old dog. Isolating the dog from his new baby may result in problems. There are brochures available that instruct owners how to prepare their dog for a new baby.

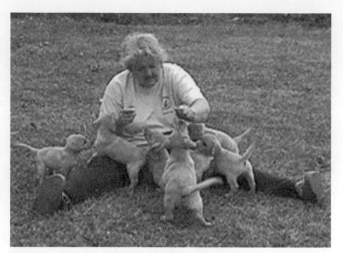

Fig. 10-14 Puppy training should start at an early age. These 5-week-old puppies are being clicker-trained by a breeder.

match puppies and new owners. A submissive owner and a dominant puppy are a bad match, which can result in aggression problems. No such selection tests have been devised for cats or other species of companion animals. At Cornell University, scientists are developing a "kitten personality test" based on expectations of the pet as an adult.

Dominance Exercises

Several authors have suggested that puppies should be restrained in a variety of subordinate positions on a regular basis, and any struggling should be firmly reprimanded. These exercises supposedly teach the puppy to be subordinate and prevent biting, especially aggression that is directed toward children. It is important that the puppy understand that it is subordinate to people. These exercises in addition to basic obedience training help accomplish this goal. Training should start as soon as the puppy enters its new home before it is old enough to attend classes. Some breeders actually begin training once the pups are mobile (Fig. 10-14).

Castration

Castrating male animals clearly reduces some forms of aggressive behavior in many species, including dogs, cats, and horses. Postpubertal castration seems to be as effective as prepubertal. Reports on dog bite statistics show that male dogs are more often involved in serious attacks, and the majority of these dogs are not castrated. Therefore, selection of female animals as pets may reduce problems with aggressive behavior. All dogs should be castrated unless they are purebreds that are to be used in a breeding program. In addition to aggression, castration prevents other potential problems such as roaming, urine marking, and prostate problems.

Socialization

Many species of mammals and birds have sensitive periods of development of normal species-typical social behavior. This sensitive period in dogs has been well studied, and to a lesser degree in cats and horses. The sensitive socialization period usually occurs fairly early in life. For example, in dogs it is from 4 to 16 weeks of age and in cats from 2 to 12 weeks.

Companion animals must have a variety of pleasant experiences with different types of people, other animals, and environments during these sensitive periods so that they are able to accept humans as their social peers later in life. Poorly socialized animals are typically fearful of people or may attach strongly to one or two individuals but are unable to generalize this acceptance to unfamiliar individuals. This fear of people can sometimes develop into defensive aggression problems (Fig. 10-15). Since many young animals are seen in the veterinary hospital, it is important that these experiences be pleasant to avoid fear and aggression problems (Fig. 10-16). Veterinary technicians should encourage dog owners to enroll puppies in puppy classes and to expose both puppies and kittens to a variety of gentle handling and play sessions with people outside the family. A procedure for developing good social relationships between people and horses has also been used.

PROVIDING PROBLEM PREVENTION SERVICES

Knowing what to tell clients to prevent problems is a separate issue from finding sufficient time to do so. It may not be realistic to expect the veterinary professional to do so during a 15-minute office visit when the time is allocated to addressing the presenting medical concern, or in a brief telephone call while greeting clients at the front desk or

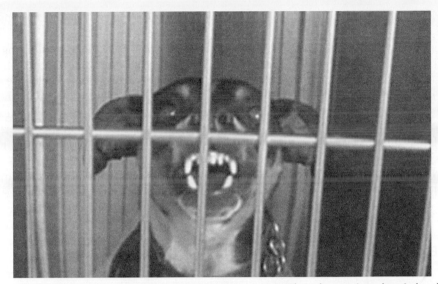

Fig. 10-15 Aggression is a common owner complaint. Sometimes the aggression occurs only in the veterinary hospital and is related to fear. Veterinary health professionals should strive to prevent this from occurring and attempt to find ways to alleviate this behavior in hospitalized animals.

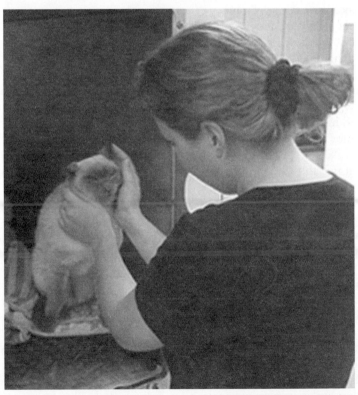

Fig. 10-16 Cats are often poorly socialized. It is worth our time to make them feel comfortable in the veterinary clinic to help prevent aggression and stress-related behaviors.

searching for a client record. Veterinarians and technicians must purposely decide how the valuable information regarding problem prevention can be disseminated. One obvious way is to make it a policy to schedule extra time for appointments involving new animal examination and to

charge accordingly. These are often new puppy and kitten appointments, but not always. The fee structure for new animal appointments can include an extra 15 to 20 minutes of staff time, even if the problem prevention discussion takes place separately from the medication examination and vaccination time. Talking to clients about these issues is preferable to relying on videos and written materials alone. However, written materials can be of value because they reinforce what was said and allow clients to read them as often as needed and at their convenience. It can also be argued that the expenses for the time required for problem prevention, even if not charged directly as a fee, may be recouped indirectly. Problem prevention sessions can improve the chances that the animal will remain in the home and thus continue being a patient. Also, the owner's perception of the clinic is enhanced, making word-of-mouth referral of new clients more likely.

PROVIDING PROBLEM RESOLUTION SERVICES

Problem resolution is almost always a more complex process than is problem prevention. It requires first arriving at a behavioral diagnosis for the type of problem. The presenting complaint, whether it be excessive barking, housesoiling, or aggression, can be thought of as behavioral signs similar to medical signs, such as vomiting, limping, or a poor hair coat. Each of these signs can potentially be related to a variety of problems. In the case of behavior problems, medical conditions that may account for the behavioral signs should first be evaluated. This is especially important with aggression and housesoiling. Once this is done, arriving at a behavioral diagnosis requires obtaining a complete behavioral history and ideally observing the animal and its environment. For some types of problems, such as feline elimination problems, seeing the animal in its home environment may make it possible to identify physical features of the environment that are contributing to the problem. Behavioral diagnosis can sometimes require several hours to interview the owner and observe the animal. In some cases, the owner may need to return home and maintain a log or even videotape the behavior.

Once the type of problem has been narrowed down to one or a few possibilities, a behavior modification plan must be devised. The type of problem dictates the specific procedures used. Time is required to explain these procedures to the owner, provide written handouts, demonstrate them if necessary, and have the owner practice them, if appropriate. Once treatment begins, the case must be followed up with either additional in-home or clinic visits or regularly scheduled telephone calls. These follow-up contacts may be relatively brief (sometimes less than 15 minutes) or longer in more complex cases.

A number of pharmaceuticals are used to treat animal behavior problems such as aggression, housesoiling, and various phobias. Currently there are only two drugs approved by the FDA to treat behavior problems. They are Clomicalm® (clomipramine, Novartis) for separation anxiety and Anipryl® (selegiline, Pfizer) for canine cognitive dysfunction. However, there are many different human tranquilizers and antianxiety drugs that have shown some promise as an adjunct in treating problem behaviors. Clients need to be aware of the limitations of these products in behavioral therapy, including the fact that the problem may return when the drug therapy is stopped, the dosages may need to be adjusted to see the desired effect, and side effects may occur. Some form of behavior modification is needed to accompany drug therapy to increase the chances of a successful resolution of the problem. The goal is to ultimately wean the animal from the drugs and for the problem to be corrected.

The process of problem resolution cannot be collapsed into "25 words or less" solutions. This oversimplified approach to problem solving trivializes the importance of the problem and omits the scientific knowledge required to successfully modify behavior. Because technicians often have the opportunity to solve behavior problems but may not have the time or expertise to do so, it is important to be aware of the veterinary practice's policies regarding referrals and to become proficient in referring cases to behavior specialists.

REFERRING CASES TO BEHAVIOR SPECIALISTS

Before referral of an animal to a behavior specialist, evaluate medical conditions that could contribute to the problem behavior. Behavior referrals should be based on the same model of professionalism as are medical case referrals. This includes determining the qualifications of the referral resource, learning the preferred method of referral, facilitating contact between client and specialist, and informing the client of what type of services to expect from the referral.

Evaluating Referral Resources

Many types of professionals offer to assist pet owners with animal behavior problems. These can range from self-taught dog trainers to academically trained, degreed, and certified behavior specialists. Veterinarians who meet the established criteria may become board certified by the American College of Veterinary Behavior and are considered behavior specialists. The Animal Behavior Society, the largest organization in North America dedicated to the study of animal behavior, offers two levels of certification to individuals holding a master's or doctoral degree in the behavioral sciences and who meet educational, experiential, and ethical criteria. Although veterinary behaviorists can be board certified, and applied behaviorists can be certified by the Animal Behavior Society, anyone, regardless of academic training, can legally use the professional title of animal behaviorist.

The National Association of Dog Obedience Instructors (NADOI) and the Association of Pet Dog Trainers (APDT) are two professional organizations that dog trainers can join. NADOI membership is open only to trainers who meet the organization's qualifications. APDT, which recently developed its own certification program, encourages and promotes use of positive reinforcement in training, but its membership is open to anyone who trains dogs.

It is the referring professional's responsibility to evaluate the credentials, knowledge, competence, and philosophies of individuals considered as potential referral resources for the clinic. This is because certification does not guarantee competence, and professionally trained and some qualified people may not be certified. This may include interviewing these individuals and also observing their classes and/or behavior consulting sessions. Gathering information about the individuals from others who offer behavioral assistance can be a valuable service the technician can perform for the clinic.

When choosing a referral resource for behavior cases, technicians should be aware that obedience or command training does not resolve behavior problems. Teaching a dog *sit*, *down*, and/or *stay* does not address aggression, separation anxiety problems, housesoiling problems, or other types of problems unrelated to obedience performance. However, obedience classes can be a useful tool in helping dog owners exert better verbal control over their dogs and establish a more consistent relationship. You may want to identify referral resources for dog obedience classes as well as for behavior counseling for whatever species of animal the clinic provides medical care. You may need to select several individuals. Certified behavior specialists consult only on those species with which they have experience. Thus, a behaviorist may work with cats and dogs but not birds or horses. Every veterinary hospital should refer all of their puppy owners to an obedience trainer. Some practices offer obedience classes in the hospitals, which may even be taught by staff members.

Making the Referral

Handle behavior referral cases as you would medical referrals. When referring a client to a veterinary medical specialist, such as a cardiologist or oncologist, a veterinary professional probably would not instruct the client to call the specialist for "tips" or "advice." Unfortunately, all too often this is the way clients are referred to behavior specialists. Find out whether the behavior specialist prefers the initial contact to be from the client or from the veterinary medical professional. If contact from the veterinary professional is preferred, be prepared to provide a pertinent medical and behavioral history during the initial conversation.

Give the client a reasonable set of expectations about the referral. Discuss information about the fee structure, where the consultation will take place, how to schedule the appointment, and the amount of time required. You can also encourage the client to seek behavioral help without giving false expectations. Although most animal behavior problems can benefit from professional assistance, not all problems can be completely and permanently resolved.

Dealing with behavior referrals in a professional manner may help clients to view the behavior consulting process as a legitimate aspect of health care and overcome some of their embarrassment about seeking "psychological help" for their pets. It may also help them to better understand why behavior specialists charge fees for professional services, just as veterinarians do. The veterinary clinic can facilitate referrals by having business cards, brochures, and other information about the behavior specialist available to give to clients at the clinic.

RECOMMENDED READING
Beaver BV: *Feline behavior: a guide for veterinarians*, ed 2, Philadelphia, 2003, WB Saunders.

Beaver BV: *Canine behavior: a guide for veterinarians*, Philadelphia, 1999, WB Saunders.

Beaver BV: *The veterinarian's encyclopedia of animal behavior*, Ames, 1994, Iowa State University Press.

Bergnman A: Ain't misbehavin': feline play aggression, *Vet Tech:* May 2001.

Borchelt PL: Cat elimination behavior problems: advances in companion animal behavior, *Vet Clin North Am, Small Anim Pract:* 21(2):257-264, 1991.

Campbell WE: *Behavior problems in dogs*, ed 2, St Louis, 1992, Mosby.

Fraser AF: *The behaviour of the horse*, Wallingford, UK, 1992, CAB International.

Hart BL, Hart LA: *Canine and feline behavioral therapy*, Philadelphia, 1985, Lea & Febiger.

Hofmeister E: Once bitten, twice shy: handling hospitalized canine patients, *Vet Tech* 2(26):June, 2001.

Houpt KA: *Domestic animal behavior for veterinarians and animal scientists*, ed 3, Ames, Iowa, 1998, Iowa State University Press.

Karsh EB, Turner DC: The human-cat relationship. In Turner DC, Bateson P, eds: *The domestic cat: the biology of its behaviour*, New York, 1988, Cambridge University Press.

McCobb EC, Brown E, Damiani, K, et al: Thunderstorm phobia in dogs: an internet survey of 69 cases, JAAHA 37, 2001.

McMillan FD: Effects of human contact on animal health and well being, *J Am Vet Med Assoc* 215(11):1592-1598, 1999.

Miller RM: Imprint training the newborn foal, *Large Animal Vet* 44(4):21, 1989.

Mills D, Nankervis K: *Equine behavior: principles and practice*, Oxford, UK, 1999, Blackwell Science.

Overall, K: *Clinical behavioral medicine for small animals*, St Louis, 1997, Mosby.

Overall K, Love M: Dog bites to humans—demography, epidemiology, injury, and risk, *J Am Vet Med Assoc* 218(12):June, 2001.

Patronek G, Dodman N: Attitudes, procedures, and delivery of behavior services by veterinarians in small animal practice, *J Am Vet Med Assoc* 215(11):June, 1999.

Riegger MH, Guntzelman J: Prevention and amelioration of stress and consequences of interaction between children and dogs, *J Am Vet Med Assoc* 196(11):1781-1785, 1990.

Serpell J, ed: *The domestic dog: its evolution, behaviour and interactions with people*, New York, 1995, Cambridge University Press.

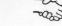

Voith VL, Borchelt PL, eds: *Readings in companion animal behavior,* Trenton, N.J., 1996, Veterinary Learning Systems.

Volhard J, Bartlett M: *What all good dogs should know: the sensible way to train,* New York, 1991, Howell Book House.

Wright JC: Canine aggression toward people: bite scenarios and prevention. Advances in Companion Animal Behavior: *Vet Clin North Am Small Anim Pract* 21(2):299-314, 1991.

BEHAVIOR ORGANIZATIONS

American College of Veterinary Behaviorists www.avma.org
American Veterinary Animal Behavior Society www.avma.org/avsab/profile.html
Animal Behavior Society www.animalbehavior.org
Society of Veterinary Behavior Technicians www.svbt.org

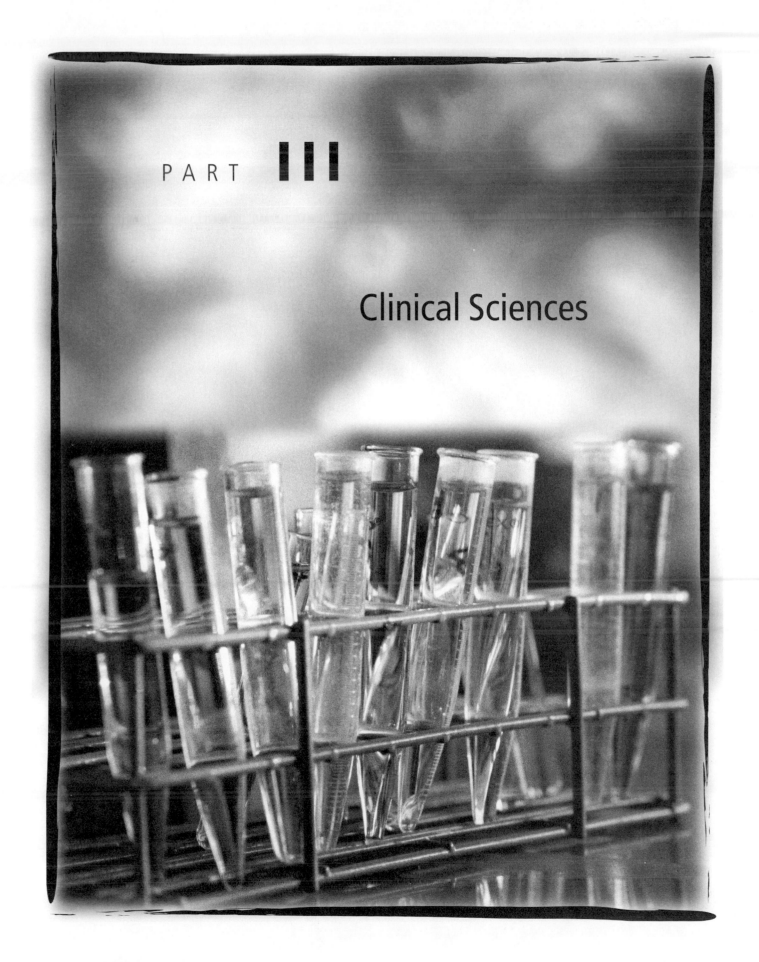

PART **III**

Clinical Sciences

11

Hematology and Hemostasis

Margi Sirois

Learning Objectives

After reviewing this chapter, the reader should understand the following:

- Methods used to collect blood samples for laboratory examination
- Ways in which diagnostic samples are prepared for laboratory examination
- Hematologic examinations commonly performed on blood
- Methods used to maintain accuracy of laboratory test results
- Methods for evaluation of hemostasis in domestic animals

Hematologic examination, or the analysis of blood, is a very powerful diagnostic tool. Veterinary technicians provide a valuable service by acquiring the skills necessary to perform this analysis. Only through practice and attention to detail can the veterinary technician develop the confidence and proficiency to perform these procedures.

Hematologic procedures include collecting and handling blood samples, performing a CBC, assisting with bone marrow examination, and helping with routine blood coagulation tests. The recent focus on economic health of the veterinary clinic has also provided an opportunity for veterinary technicians to perform additional diagnostic testing, improve overall animal care, and provide an additional source of revenue for the clinic.

LABORATORY INSTRUMENTATION AND EQUIPMENT

A variety of types of equipment are needed for the in-house hematology laboratory. One of the most important items is the microscope. Ideally, each practice laboratory will have at least two microscopes. One should be designated solely for use with blood films and cytology preparations. The other can be used for examination of parasitology and urine specimens. This will help to maintain the microscopes in the best working order since the corrosive fluids sometimes used in parasitology testing can damage the microscope. Examination of blood films requires a high-quality binocu-

lar microscope, preferably with planachromatic (flat-field) lenses and a focusable substage condenser (Fig. 11-1). Centrifuges are also required for clinical testing. The centrifuge is used to prepare blood samples for chemical testing and for completion of the packed cell volume test that is part of the complete blood count (CBC). There are thousands of types of centrifuges available for the clinic laboratory. Several centrifuges are now available that allow the use of small volumes of sample. Other equipment and supplies that may be needed for the veterinary practice laboratory include:

- Refractometer
- Pipettes
- Differential cell counter
- Hand tally counter
- Automated or manual cell-counting equipment
- Water bath or heat block

LABORATORY SAFETY

The veterinary practice laboratory has the potential to be a safety hazard if specific policies and procedures are not in place to ensure safe working conditions. A sample laboratory safety policy can be found in Box 11-1. For example, individuals that wear contact lenses should be required to remove them when working in the laboratory. Contact lenses block fluids used to flush the eyes in an emergency,

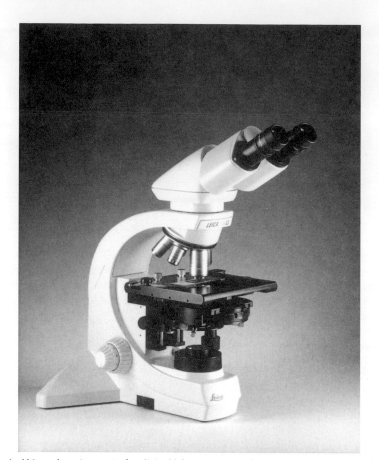

Fig. 11-1 Typical binocular microscope for clinical laboratory procedures. *(Courtesy of Leica Microsystems Inc. Bannockburn, IL)*

and most individuals are too disoriented to be capable of removing them during an emergency. Assuring that all chemicals are stored properly and that the laboratory has adequate ventilation can minimize chemical hazard from volatile fumes. Specific recommendations for chemical safety are contained in the material safety data sheet (MSDS) provided by each chemical manufacturer. MSDSs contain storage concerns, requirements for personal protective equipment use, and emergency procedures that may be needed. All personnel in the clinic must be made aware of the hazards associated with working in the veterinary practice laboratory and the procedures to be used in emergencies. Even when the clinic has an appropriate written safety policy, safety concerns may arise unless the policies are followed and enforced by everyone in the clinic. There are also laws that require specific safety procedures. Additional safety concerns also relate to quality control. In particular, proper maintenance of equipment is essential. Some laboratory equipment can be hazardous if not properly maintained (e.g., centrifuges). This maintenance requirement affects the operation of the equipment and the accuracy of results obtained from its use.

QUALITY CONTROL

Veterinarians expect veterinary technicians to present them with dependable analytic results. Through a well-planned and carefully controlled quality-control program, veterinary technicians can provide veterinarians with accurate laboratory results. *Quality control* (also called *quality assurance*) is a series of steps and procedures to ensure that the analytic results from a laboratory represent the state of the animal from which a sample was taken. If these *in vitro* results are to be of any value to a veterinarian, they must match as closely as possible the *in vivo* values of the animal at the time the sample was obtained.

Unlike human medical office laboratories, there are no laws that require quality control and proficiency programs for veterinary practice laboratories. However, without an appropriate quality control program, the *accuracy* and *precision* of test results cannot be assured. Accuracy refers to how closely the test result is to the actual patient value. Precision refers to the reproducibility of a test result. Inaccurate test results can lead a veterinarian to make an incorrect diagnosis.

BOX 11-1

Laboratory Safety Policy

The safety procedures contained in this document are designed to minimize any potential source of injury to employees of this facility. All employees are required to adhere to these policies to ensure a safe workplace for everyone.

The clinical lab is equipped with the following safety equipment: fume hood, eye wash station, electrical surge and drop-out extension, first aid kit, pipettors, chemical spill cleanup kit, fire extinguisher, and fire blanket.

All employees are required to familiarize themselves with these devices and be able to use and operate them effectively.

General Rules

1. Smoking, eating, or drinking is prohibited in the lab.
2. No foods or beverages may be stored in the lab refrigerator or general lab area.
3. Lab coats must be worn at all times.
4. Long hair must be confined while in the lab.
5. Shoes must be worn in the lab; open-toe or canvas shoes are prohibited.
6. No pipetting of materials by mouth!
7. All employees are responsible for safe and proper operation of equipment. Read the operator's manual and be familiar with the operation of any instrument before attempting its use.

Lab Housekeeping

1. All glassware must be washed immediately after use. Cracked or chipped glassware must be discarded at once.
2. All work surfaces must be cleaned with a 10% bleach solution at the end of the work period.

3. Lab work areas must be kept clear of personal belongings.
4. Employees must wash hands thoroughly before leaving the lab.

Reagents

1. Fume hood must be used for dispensing reagents with potentially hazardous fumes.
2. All reagents will be stored properly in designated areas.
3. Carrying reagents must be done cautiously, using unbreakable containers whenever possible.
4. All reagent, stock, and dispensing containers MUST be labeled with identity, date, and initials of individual preparing reagent and MUST contain proper hazard warning labels.

Biologicals

1. All biologicals (blood, urine, body fluid, control materials) must be treated as potentially infectious.
2. Disposable latex gloves MUST be worn at all times when handling or transporting biological materials.
3. Spilled biological material must be cleaned up with 10% bleach solution.

Disposal

1. Reagents suitable for sewage disposal should be poured into running water in the sink.
2. Hazardous reagents will be disposed of in proper central waste containers.
3. All reagent bottles must be thoroughly rinsed before disposal.
4. Biological materials and their containers should be disposed of in biohazard bags.

From Sirois M: *Veterinary clinical laboratory procedures*, St Louis, 1995, Mosby.

Based on inaccurate test results, the veterinarian may prescribe medications that are contraindicated or may withhold medications that are essential for recovery. There are a few tests performed in the laboratory that may have a relatively low precision rating simply as a function of the test methodology. For example, manual cell counts have one of the lowest accuracy ratings since there are numerous components of the test that could be faulty. For that reason, it is often necessary to repeat the procedure and then calculate a mathematical average of the two test results to report as the patient value. Any test with a low precision rating should be repeated and the results averaged to improve accuracy.

Other factors that affect accuracy and precision include test selection, test conditions, sample quality, technician skill, electrical surges, and equipment maintenance.

Test Selection and Test Conditions

Test selection refers to the principle of the test method. Many of the tests used in veterinary laboratories were adapted from human medical laboratory tests. Since the veterinary clinic often sees a diversity of species with very different physiologic parameters, some of these tests may not provide an accurate representation of patient health status. For example, some tests for amylase may be invalid when used with canine samples. This is often due to limitations in the linearity of a test. That is, the test may not be capable of measuring in a range likely to be found in a given species. Additionally, the clinical significance of test results may vary among different species. In addition to assuring that the test method is appropriate, tests should be chosen based on their accuracy. Regardless of the method used,

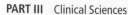
care must be taken to follow the analytical procedure exactly. Any deviation can seriously affect accuracy of results. Some tests can be carried out only under specific conditions of temperature or pH. These tests will be highly inaccurate with even slight variations in test conditions.

Sample Quality

Sample quality also greatly affects quality of test results. In veterinary medicine, this can be a significant concern. Samples that are lipemic, icteric, or hemolyzed require special handling before use with most clinical analyzers. Collection of blood samples from properly fasted animals using appropriate techniques and equipment will minimize this significant source of error.

Technician Skill

Human error is perhaps the most difficult testing parameter to control. Personnel responsible for performance of clinical testing must be appropriately trained in test principles and procedures. Even the use of the wrong type of pipetting device can seriously affect test accuracy. Mechanisms should be in place to provide for the continual education of all clinical laboratory personnel.

Electrical Power Surges

Although not an obvious source of error, electrical power surges and dropouts can significantly alter equipment function. Repeated surges shorten the life of light sources in microscopes and spectrophotometric equipment. Changes in the intensity of the light source yield inaccurate test results. All electrical equipment should be connected to a device designed to protect it from surges and electrical dropout.

Equipment Maintenance

Maintenance of equipment must also be included in quality control programs. A regular, written schedule of equipment maintenance is vital to ensure their proper operation. This will allow changes in equipment function to be detected before obvious errors begin to occur. Always follow manufacturer recommendations for routine maintenance of instruments and equipment.

The accuracy of clinical instruments must also be verified on a regular basis by analyzing control materials. Control material contains specific concentrations of blood constituents. Busy practice laboratories should run controls on a daily basis. The equipment manufacturer provides recommendations regarding the frequency of control material analysis. The control is analyzed as if it were a patient sample. The control is designed to function the same as a patient sample would under the same conditions. Control results should be charted and analyzed regularly to help identify any changes in performance of the equipment. Standards are not acceptable as substitutes for controls.

Standards are nonbiological substances used to calibrate equipment.

Record Keeping

The results of assays of control samples should be recorded, graphed, and kept in a permanent file (Fig. 11-2). If the results of a control assay do not fall within the acceptable range, the sample should be reassayed. If the results are not within the acceptable range for the second assay, the instrument and the technician's technique must be evaluated. When the control sample values continually fall outside the acceptable range, there has been a shift of the mean itself and a systematic error is involved. Graphing the control results enables laboratory personnel to detect changes or trends in assay results. Fig. 11-2 shows an example of a control serum graph used in a clinical laboratory that assays control serum once a day.

Some manufacturers provide a quality-control service in which test samples are sent to many clinical laboratories for assay each month. The results from all the laboratories are collected and compared. From these results, the manufacturer can identify laboratories with accuracy problems.

SAMPLE COLLECTION

As mentioned previously, sample quality has a significant impact on test accuracy. Careful attention to collection procedures will minimize these problems. When preparing to collect blood, the technician should first determine what specific test procedures will be needed. This will determine, in part, the equipment and supplies needed and the choice of a particular blood vessel from which to collect the sample. Unless the purpose of the test is to monitor therapy, always collect the blood sample before any treatment is given. It is important to remember that treatments, such as fluid therapy, may affect results. Certain test methods cannot be accurately performed once the patient has received certain pharmaceutical therapies. *Fasted* samples, or samples from an animal that has not eaten for some time, are ideal. *Postprandial* samples, or samples collected after the animal has eaten, may produce many erroneous results. Increased amounts of lipid *(lipemia)* may also be present in postprandial blood samples. Lipemia also increases the likelihood of hemolysis in the sample, and further complicates analyses.

Improper handling of blood may render a blood sample unusable for analysis or result in inaccurate results. The methods and sites of blood collection depend on the species, the amount of blood needed, and personal preference.

Venous blood is frequently used in hematologic tests and is easily accessible in most species. The cephalic vein is the preferred site in dogs and cats. The saphenous vein (lateral in the dog, medial in the cat) is a reasonable substitute,

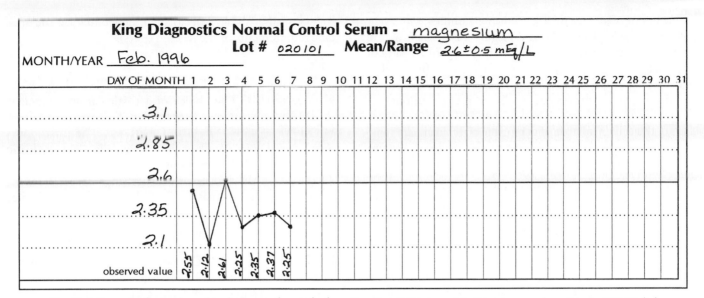

Fig. 11-2 Example of a graph used to chart normal control values. *(From Sirois M:* Veterinary clinical laboratory procedures, *St Louis, 1995, Mosby.)*

especially in fractious cats. Jugular venipuncture is an efficient way to collect a large volume of blood. It is the preferred site in large domestic animals (Table 11-1). The wing vein is the preferred site in birds. If only a small amount of blood is needed, you may clip a nail and draw blood into a microhematocrit tube by capillary action. Vasoconstriction related to the stress of restraint may restrict blood flow after nail clipping. If this happens, it is best to let the bird calm down and try to collect again later, rather than keep clipping more nails.

TABLE 11-1

Commonly Used Blood Collection Sites

Canine	Cephalic vein
	Jugular vein
	Saphenous vein
Feline	Cephalic vein
	Jugular vein
Equine	Jugular vein
Bovine	Caudal vein
	Mammary vein
	Jugular vein
Avian	Wing vein
	Toenail clip
Rabbit	Ear vein
	Toenail clip
Rodents	Tail vein
	Cardiac puncture

From Sirois M: *Veterinary Clinical Laboratory Procedures*, St. Louis, 1995, Mosby.

The ear vein in rabbits works well for blood collection. The tail vein, infraorbital sinus, and cardiac puncture can be used in laboratory animals if the animals are anesthetized.

Ideally, you should clip the collection site to remove hair. Then clean the site with alcohol or another suitable antiseptic and allow it to dry before proceeding with the venipuncture.

Take care not to stress the animal during blood collection. Use only the amount of restraint necessary to immobilize the animal. Excitement and stress can cause splenic contraction, which can alter the results of tests performed on red blood cells (RBCs). Results of several white blood cell (WBC) tests are also affected.

Collection Equipment

A variety of collection equipment is available for use with veterinary patients. Blood may be collected in a syringe or specialized vacuum device, such as the Vacutainer system (Becton-Dickinson, Rutherford, N.J.). When the needle/syringe method is used, the needle chosen should always be the largest one that the animal can comfortably accommodate. For most small animals, 20- to 25-gauge needles work well. In large animals, 16- to 20-gauge needles are routinely used. The syringe chosen should be one that is closest to the required sample volume. Use of a larger syringe could collapse the patient's vein. Using a large syringe with a small-bore needle can result in hemolysis (rupture of red blood cells) when the syringe plunger is pulled back with great speed and force. Remove the needle before expelling the blood into the collection tube. *Erythrocytes* (red blood cells, or RBCs) may *hemolyze* (rupture) if forced back through the needle.

Vacutainers are useful for multiple samples and when blood can be collected from a larger vessel, such as the cephalic or jugular vein. The Vacutainer system consists of a special needle, a needle holder, and vacuum-filled tubes that may be empty (clot tubes) or may contain a premeasured amount of anticoagulant. Draw a fixed amount of blood into the tube, based on tube size and amount of vacuum in the tube. Collapse of veins, especially in smaller animals, may occur because of excessive negative pressure exerted by the vacuum. Using small vacuum tubes may remedy this problem.

Fill collection tubes with the proper amount of blood, regardless of the method used to collect the sample. Unless otherwise directed, fill the tube about ⅔ to ¾ full. This ensures a proper blood-to-anticoagulant ratio. Mix the blood adequately by inverting the tube *gently* for 10 to 20 seconds after transferring the blood. It is important always to try for a precise venipuncture to prevent formation of blood clots in the sample because of contamination with tissue fluids aspirated after multiple attempts at venipuncture. Serious errors may result if a sample is not labeled immediately after it has been collected. Label the tube with the date and time of collection, owner's name, patient's name, and patient's clinic identification number. If submitted to a laboratory, include with the sample a request form that includes all necessary sample identification and a clear indication of which tests are requested.

Sample Type

Whole blood

Whole blood is composed of cellular elements (*erythrocytes, leukocytes,* and *platelets*), and a fluid called *plasma.* To collect a whole blood sample, place the appropriate amount of blood into a container with the proper *anticoagulant* (discussed later) and gently mix the sample by inverting the tube multiple times. Whole blood may be refrigerated if analysis is to be delayed, but it should never be frozen unless the plasma has been separated from the cellular elements. If the blood has been refrigerated, warm the sample to room temperature and mix gently before analysis.

Plasma

To obtain a plasma sample, collect the appropriate amount of blood in a container with the proper anticoagulant and gently mix well. Centrifuge the closed container for 10 minutes at 2000 to 3000 rpm to separate the fluid from the cells. After the sample is centrifuged, remove the plasma from the cells, being careful not to contaminate the plasma with any pelleted cells, and transfer the plasma into another appropriately labeled container. Separate plasma from the cellular elements as soon as possible after collection to minimize any artifactual changes. Plasma can be refrigerated or frozen until analysis is performed, depending on the specific requirements of the desired test(s).

Anticoagulants

Anticoagulants are used when whole blood or plasma samples are needed. The choice of a particular anticoagulant should be based on the tests needed. Some anticoagulants can interfere with certain test methods. The most commonly used anticoagulant is ethylenediaminetetraacetic acid (EDTA). EDTA functions as an anticoagulant by binding calcium, which is necessary for clotting to occur. It is preferred for routine hematologic studies because it preserves cell morphology better than other anticoagulants. Even if collected in an EDTA tube, blood should be analyzed as quickly as possible, preferably within 2 hours after collection. Blood preserved in EDTA stays fresh for several hours or even overnight if stored in a refrigerator at 4° C. However, morphologic changes in the cells, such as cytoplasmic vacuolation, irregular cell membranes, and *crenation* (shrinkage of RBCs), may occur in stored samples. This can make interpretation of observations difficult and result in inaccuracies.

It is for this reason that blood smears are best made immediately with fresh blood or within 1 hour after collection in an EDTA tube. If there is any delay in examining the blood, it is important to gently remix the blood by inverting it several times before making a blood smear. Crenation may occur if the tubes are not sufficiently filled, causing a relative excess of EDTA in the sample. Tubes that contain EDTA have a lavender or purple rubber stopper.

Heparin functions as an anticoagulant by activation of antithrombin III, which prevents conversion of prothrombin to thrombin. Heparin is not a permanent anticoagulant; it inhibits coagulation for only 8 to 12 hours. Tubes containing heparin (green-top tubes) may be used if blood smears are made immediately and tests run on whole blood are done promptly, because heparin may cause cells to clump and stain poorly. Heparin tubes may be a good choice for storing small blood samples from birds, because you can use the whole blood for hematologic tests and then collect plasma after spinning the sample.

Sodium citrate (blue-top tubes) anticoagulant is used for coagulation tests. However, it is generally not suitable for routine hematologic studies because it can cause distortion in cell morphology.

FORMATION AND FUNCTIONS OF BLOOD AND BLOOD CELLS

Blood is composed of plasma and cells. Blood plasma is more than 90% water. The remainder of plasma consists of proteins, hormones, vitamins, and similar substances. The cells contained in plasma make up about 45% of the total blood volume and include *erythrocytes* (red blood cells), *leukocytes* (white blood cells), and *platelets*.

The formation of blood cells is called *hematopoiesis*. In the adult animal, blood cell formation occurs in the bone marrow. In the prenatal animal, blood cell formation occurs in multiple organ sites such as the liver and spleen. Other organs play a role in blood cell formation, both in the adult and prenatal animal.

Erythropoiesis

The formation of erythrocytes is called *erythropoiesis*. This process is stimulated by the hormone erythropoietin. Cells in the kidney monitor the oxygen levels in tissues and stimulate the release of the hormone in response to tissue hypoxia. Erythropoietin stimulates the erythrocyte stem cell, the *hemocytoblast* (located in the bone marrow), to differentiate into a *rubriblast*. Mitosis of erythrocyte precursor cells continues in the bone marrow as the cells continue to mature. Once the cell reaches the reticulocyte stage, it may be released from the bone marrow into peripheral circulation. Reticulocytes can continue their maturation in circulation. Younger cells within the maturation series are not capable of further development once released from the bone marrow.

Hemoglobin Synthesis

Hemoglobin is a protein that comprises approximately 30% of the volume of an erythrocyte. The remainder of the cell consists of about 65% water and 5% organelles, enzymes, and salts. Hemoglobin functions to bind oxygen and thus allow the erythrocyte to carry oxygen to the body tissues. It also binds carbon dioxide and removes it from the tissues. Hemoglobin formation begins during the rubricyte stage of erythrocyte maturation and ends during the metarubricyte stage. Since mature erythrocytes do not contain a nucleus, they cannot synthesize cellular enzymes. Cellular enzymes needed to provide energy to the cell are synthesized as the cell matures in the bone marrow. This limitation in the amount of available enzymes is responsible for the relatively short life span of an erythrocyte. This life span is variable among different species (Table 11-2).

An increase in the numbers of circulating erythrocytes is termed *polycythemia*. Polycythemia may be pathologic, physiologic, or apparent. Apparent polycythemias are seen in dehydrated patients. Physiologic polycythemia results when an animal is stressed during blood collection. Stress causes splenic contraction and releases vast numbers of red blood cells into circulation.

Anemia refers to a decrease in the oxygen-carrying ability of the blood. This may be due to decreased production of erythrocytes, increased destruction of erythrocytes, or decrease in hemoglobin concentration of the erythrocytes. Hemoglobin testing, packed cell volume (PCV), and RBC indices are used to differentiate the specific cause of anemia. Evaluation of erythrocyte morphology on the differential blood film also provides diagnostic information useful in classification of anemia.

TABLE 11-2

Erythrocyte Life Span

Species	Life Span (days)
Bovine (adult)	160
(3 mos)	55
Equine	140-150
Porcine	62
Canine	107-115
Feline	68
Ovine	70-153
Caprine	125

From Sirois M: *Veterinary Clinical Laboratory Procedures*, St Louis, 1995, Mosby.

Leukopoiesis

The formation of white blood cells (leukocytes) is called *leukopoiesis*. Leukocyte maturation occurs primarily in the bone marrow, although other organs are also involved. Leukocytes are classified as either granulocytes or agranulocytes, and the formation and maturation of these two groups of leukocytes differs considerably. Leukocytes perform their function within the tissues and not in the blood. Therefore, most leukocytes remain in circulation only a few hours. Some leukocytes continue maturation once in tissue spaces. The granulocytes, neutrophils, eosinophils, and basophils develop from a stem cell known as a *myeloblast*. Maturation then proceeds through a *promyelocyte*, *myelocyte* (Plate 21 in color insert), *metemyelocyte* (Plate 22), band, and segmented stage. Production of specific granules occurs during the myelocyte stage. In most veterinary species, the band and segmented stages are commonly found in peripheral circulation.

Agranulocytes, lymphocytes, and monocytes have diverse patterns of development and maturation. The monocyte seen in peripheral circulation is one stage in the development of the tissue macrophage. Monocytes, therefore, do not perform their functions in circulation. Lymphocytes show extreme diversity in maturation, function, and appearance. Their primary functions relate to production of antibody and regulation of the immune system.

An increase in the numbers of circulating leukocytes is termed *leukocytosis*. Leukocytosis is often the result of viral or bacterial inflammation. *Leukopenia* is the term used to describe a decrease in circulating leukocytes.

Hematopoietic tumors (neoplasia of blood forming tissues) are common in domestic animals. These disorders are broadly classified as either *lymphoproliferative* or *myeloprolif-*

erative, depending on the type of cell or cells from which the tumor originates. Lymphoproliferative disorders originate from lymphocytes or plasma cells (a tissue cell of lymphoid origin). Myeloproliferative disorders arise from nonlymphoid cells that originate in the bone marrow. Neoplasms of red blood cell and megakaryocyte origin are also included in this group. These tumors are called *leukemias* if the neoplastic cells originate in the bone marrow.

Hematopoietic disorders are often diagnosed by finding specific early stages (blast forms) of cell types in peripheral blood and/or bone marrow. Lymphoblastic leukemia may be diagnosed by finding lymphoblasts in the blood and/or some marrow. If neoplastic cells are found in the peripheral blood, the term *leukemic blood profile* is often used.

COMPLETE BLOOD COUNT

The CBC is a cost-effective way to obtain valuable hematologic information on a patient. With practice and attention to detail, you can perform a CBC quickly, easily, and accurately in any veterinary hospital. CBCs are indicated for diagnostic evaluation of disease states, well-animal screening (e.g., geriatric), and as a screening tool prior to surgery. A CBC includes total erythrocyte and leukocyte counts, packed cell volume, hemoglobin concentration, and RBC indices. Additional tests that should be included at the time of the CBC are measurement of total solids and platelet count.

The CBC can be performed manually or with automated analyzers. A variety of methods are available for both methods. Automated analyzers can provide accurate and cost-effective results. However, care should be taken in choosing the most appropriate instrument for your clinic. Hematology analyzers for veterinary use employ impedance methods, buffy coat analysis, or laser methods when evaluating a sample. Each method has specific advantages

and disadvantages. Regardless of which analyzer you use, an understanding of the test principles used with your analyzer is essential. Knowing the limitations of the analytical system enhances the validity of your test results. Regular quality control is also essential for assuring the accuracy of your test results.

Cell Counts

Counting of erythrocytes and leukocytes is a routine part of the CBC. Cell counts can be performed using manual or automated methods. The total white blood cell (*leukocyte*, WBC) count is one of the most useful values determined in a CBC. Total red blood cell (erythrocyte, RBC) and platelet (thrombocyte) counts, although more difficult and less accurate, may also be performed manually with a hemacytometer or through automated methods. Manual cell count methods usually utilize the Unopette system (Fig. 11-3; Becton-Dickinson, Rutherford, N.J.). This system includes a pipette that holds a predetermined amount of blood and a reservoir that contains a diluting and lysing agent (Box 11-2).

The most commonly used WBC counting Unopette system uses a 20-μl (microliter) pipette and 3% acetic acid as a diluent (Box 11-3). The RBC counting system (Box 11-4) uses a 10-μl sample pipette and 0.85% saline as a diluent (the RBCs are not lysed in this count). Unopette systems contain a premeasured volume of diluent and provide a specific dilution ratio. Once filled with the appropriate volume of blood and mixed, a small amount of the blood-diluent mixture is placed on a hemocytometer. The hemocytometer contains an optical quality cover glass and measured grid that contains a specific volume.

Hemacytometers are counting chambers used to determine the number of cells per microliter (μl, mm^3) of blood. Several models are available, but the most common type used has two identical sets of fine grids of parallel and perpendicular etched lines called *Neubauer rulings* (Fig. 11-6). Each grid is divided into nine large squares. The

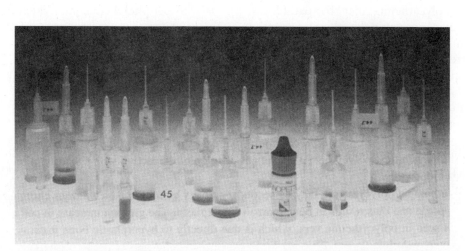

Fig. 11-3 Unopette blood dilution system. *(Courtesy Becton-Dickinson VACUTAINER Systems.)*

BOX 11-2

Blood Counts With the Unopette System and Hemacytometer

1. After thoroughly mixing anticoagulated blood, fill the Unopette pipette with blood by capillary action. Carefully wipe excess sample from the outside of the pipette.
2. Transfer the blood into the reservoir containing the diluting agent. Be careful not to lose any of the sample during this step. See the Unopette package insert for more detailed instructions. Thoroughly mix the sample and the diluting agent.
3. After letting the sample stand for an appropriate time (to lyse RBCs, if needed), mix the sample to resuspend the cells so that a consistent sample can be delivered to the hemacytometer. Make sure the hemacytometer and its special coverslip are clean and free of dirt and fingerprints. Clean them with lens cleaner and paper.
4. After squeezing 3 to 4 drops of sample and discarding, immediately charge (fill) each side of the hemacytometer at the etched groove. Do not overfill or underfill the counting chamber. This can cause uneven distribution of cells throughout the Neubauer ruling and contributes to an inaccurate count.
5. Place the hemacytometer on the microscope stage. Lower the condenser of the microscope to increase contrast so that the cells are easier to see.
6. Count all of the cells in the appropriate squares. Cells that touch the lines between two squares are considered as within that square if they touch the top or the left-center lines (Fig. 11-4). Cells that touch the bottom or right lines

are not counted with that square. Squares from each side (grid) of the hemacytometer are counted, and these counts are averaged. This value is then used to calculate the count for each cell type being evaluated.

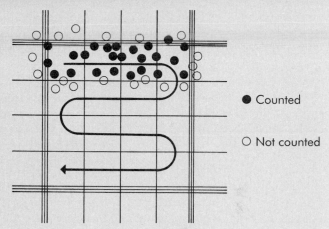

● Counted

○ Not counted

Fig. 11-4 Each area of the hemacytometer is scanned in a systematic pattern after counting blood cells. In this diagram, the solid spheres represent cells already counted, whereas the open spheres represent cells not yet counted. Count the cells that touch the top and left-center lines of an individual square. Do not count cells touching the bottom and right lines of a square.

BOX 11-3

Total WBC Count Procedure

1. Fill the appropriate 20-μl Unopette pipette with blood, and wipe off the excess.
2. Transfer the blood to 3% acetic acid diluent (lysing agent). Make sure all blood is transferred into the diluent by squeezing the plastic reservoir a few times. Mix the vial by inversion. The diluted sample is stable for 3 hours.
3. Let the sample stand for at least 10 minutes to allow RBCs to hemolyze.
4. Mix the sample by inversion, discard the first 3 to 4 drops, and charge (fill) the hemacytometer. Let the cells settle for about 1 minute.
5. Under 100× magnification, count the WBCs in the nine large squares of the Neubauer grid (Fig. 11-5). Count each side separately and average these counts. The counts for the two sides should be within 10% of each other. If not, clean the hemacytometer and do the count again. With practice, you can do this consistently. White blood cells appear as dark dots of varying shapes. These are the nuclei of WBCs. Be careful not to count dust particles or other contaminant debris.
6. Once you have this average count, add 10% and multiply by 100 (or multiply by 110%). This gives you the number of WBCs/μl of blood. For example, if the average count of both sides of the hemacytometer is 80, add 10% of 80 (8) to that. Report this value to the clinician.

$$88 \times 100 = 8,800 \text{ WBCs}/\mu\text{l of blood}$$

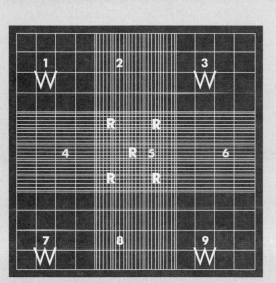

Fig. 11-5 Neubauer rulings and hemacytometer. Each *W* indicates a zone counted for the total WBC count. Each *R* indicates a square counted for the total RBC count when using a standard dilution.

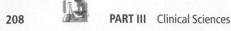

BOX 11-4

procedure

Total RBC Count Procedure

1. Fill the appropriate 10-μl Unopette pipette with blood, and wipe off the excess.
2. Transfer the blood from the pipette to the reservoir containing 0.85% saline, and mix by inversion. The diluted sample is stable for 6 hours.
3. Discard the first 3 to 4 drops of sample and immediately charge (fill) each side of the hemacytometer as in the procedure for total WBC count.
4. Under 400× magnification, count the RBCs in the four corner squares and the one center square within the large center square of the grid (Fig. 11-5). Count each side, and

average these counts. Erythrocytes tend to be packed tightly and are harder to count than leukocytes. It is difficult to achieve agreement within 10% of the counts for the two sides. Therefore, it is usually considered adequate if agreement is within 20%.
5. Add four zeros to the value counted in the five smaller squares on the grid. For example, if the average RBC count is 550, adding four zeros to that value would yield an RBC count of 5,500,000 RBCs/μl of blood. Another way of reporting this is $5.5 \times 10^6/\mu$l.

4 corner squares are divided into 16 smaller squares and the center square is divided into 400 tiny squares (25 groups of 16 each). The area of each grid (Neubauer ruling) is designed to hold a precise amount of sample (0.9 μl). Knowing the number of cells in set parts of the grid and the amount of sample in that area is the basis for calculating the number of cells per microliter of blood. Mechanical counters are available to manually keep track of the number of each cell type observed.

Red blood cell counts may also be estimated by dividing the packed cell volume by 6. For example, if the PCV is 36, the estimated RBC count is 36/6 = 6 million RBCs/μl.

The Unopette system also provides a method for manually counting platelets. The procedure is similar to counting WBCs. A 20-μl pipette is used with 1% ammonium oxalate as a diluent. The ammonium oxalate hemolyzes the RBCs but preserves the WBCs and platelets. The WBCs and platelets can be counted at the same time by this method. The platelets are counted at 400× magnification in the 25 small squares located in the large center square of the grid. The number of platelets counted is then multiplied by 1000 to calculate the number of platelets per μl of blood. Counting platelets is especially difficult because of their small size and tendency to clump together. Platelets are counted after the WBCs, because it takes about 10 minutes for the platelets to settle within the hemacytometer counting chamber. Platelet counts can be roughly estimated while viewing a blood smear with a microscope (see the "Platelet Counting Methods" section).

Automated analyzers used for counting blood cells are present in many veterinary clinics. Automated analysis of hematologic samples has become more common in recent years. Several veterinary analyzers are currently available. CBCs performed in this manner may be cost-effective if several CBCs are done each day. Advantages of automation include speed, accuracy, and consistent results.

Disadvantages of certain analyzers include the need for regular maintenance and quality control. Automated hematologic examination only partially replaces a manual CBC. The veterinary technician still must perform several aspects of the CBC, usually the differential count and total protein concentration. Each instrument has a specific protocol for use; therefore, the technician should study the operator's manual or contact the manufacturer before using the equipment. Following is a brief description of the types of automation used in veterinary practice.

Impedance counters

Impedance counters can rapidly and efficiently count RBCs, WBCs, and platelets. They are based on the idea of counting particles (cells) as they flow past a detection device. The analyzers are designed to count all particles of a specific size that pass through an aperture. The analyzer must be set to the sizes of the blood cells seen in the species being evaluated. A blood sample is placed in an electrolyte solution and then drawn through the aperture (Fig. 11-6). As cells pass through the aperture, a specific amount of the electrolyte solution is displaced. The analyzer counts each of these displacements as a cell. Some units also determine hemoglobin concentration and the red cell indices. These counters have computer-based settings for species and type of cells being counted. Because the RBCs and WBCs of animal species vary greatly in size, the instrument is calibrated and set for the proper species. Platelet clumps, especially seen in cats, can be erroneously counted as leukocytes by cell counters. Examine a blood smear if you suspect this. Proper sample collection and handling usually alleviates this problem.

Qualitative buffy coat system

Buffy coat analyzers provide an estimate of the cell count rather than a true count. This estimate is then used to calculate other hematologic parameters, such as PCV and

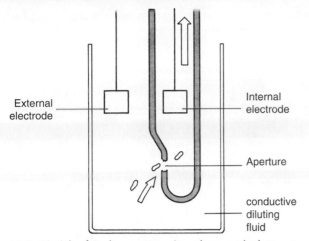

Fig. 11-6 Principle of Coulter counter—impedance method. *(From Powers LW:* Diagnostic hematology, *St Louis, 1989, Mosby.)*

hemoglobin concentration. Qualitative buffy coat (QBC) analysis is based on measurement of a centrifuged, stained, and expanded buffy coat by a computerized automatic microhematocrit reader. The QBC Vet Autoread (Idexx Laboratories) uses a specialized microhematocrit tube that is coated with stain. The tube is filled with EDTA anticoagulated blood and then centrifuged. The centrifuged blood separates into layers based on density of the cells. RBCs are found at the bottom of the tube, as in the manual microhematocrit method. The buffy coat is expanded into several layers and is divided into a granulocyte (combined neutrophil, eosinophil, basophil) layer, an agranulocyte (combined lymphocyte/monocyte) layer, and a platelet layer. If many reticulocytes or nucleated red blood cells (NRBCs) are present, these may form a layer at the top of the RBC column (below the buffy coat). The tube is then placed in an optical scanning device, which measures the degree of stain fluorescence in each cell layer. The analyzer prints out a report with 12 different hematologic values and a graph illustrating cell numbers and fluorescence for each cell layer. These values include hematocrit, hemoglobin, mean corpuscular hemoglobin concentration (MCHC), total WBC count, granulocyte count (percentage and absolute count), eosinophil count (absolute count, dogs only), lymphocyte/monocyte count (percentage and absolute count), platelet count, and reticulocyte/NRBC count (if present). The QBC Vet Autoread performs only a partial CBC and cannot replace blood smear evaluation. It is especially important to examine the blood smear if findings are abnormal. Total protein concentration can be measured on plasma separated in the specialized tube.

Laser flow cytometry

Laser-based analyzers are the most accurate of the hematology analyzers. A focused laser beam is used, and the rela-

tive size and density of the cells differentiates the various cell types. This method also allows for an accurate differential blood cell analysis and a reticulocyte count. Rapid test performance and built-in quality control procedures are characteristic of laser-based analyzers. These analyzers tend to be quite expensive and are not yet in common use in veterinary practice.

Hemoglobin Testing, PCV, and RBC Indices

A variety of methods are used to measure hemoglobin concentration. These require that the red blood cells be lysed to release the hemoglobin from the cells. Once that step is accomplished, the hemoglobin measurement may employ a color-matching method or a photometric method. Color-matching methods tend to be the least accurate analyses. A color standard is used to compare the color of the lysed blood sample and equate it to a specific hemoglobin concentration. Automated and semiautomated methods are available that utilize this technology. Photometric analysis of hemoglobin concentration is more accurate than color-matching methods. The photometric technique requires mixing the lysed blood sample with a specific reagent and measuring the resulting colored-complex with a photometer. The light absorbance of the colored complex equates to a specific hemoglobin concentration. Unlike color-matching methods, photometric methods are capable of measuring all forms of hemoglobin. Most color-matching methods only provide the concentration of oxyhemoglobin.

The PCV is another vital part of the CBC. The PCV, also known as the hematocrit (Hct), is an expression of the percentage of whole blood occupied by RBCs. PCV can be performed with either a macrohematocrit or microhematocrit technique. The microhematocrit method, abbreviated mHct, is the most commonly performed PCV test in veterinary practice (Box 11-5). A blood-filled capillary tube is centrifuged for 2 to 5 minutes, depending on the type of centrifuge. The blood separates into a plasma layer, a white buffy coat composed of WBCs and platelets, and a layer of packed red cells (Fig. 11-8). Measuring the RBC layer in the capillary tube determines the PCV. The precision of a PCV is approximately 1%, making it a very accurate test.

A low PCV may indicate anemia. There are many causes of anemia, including blood loss, neoplasia, parasitism, and chronic infection. An increased PCV also has several possible causes, including dehydration and splenic contraction in an excited animal.

PCV values may be erroneously high because of clots in the sample, failure to adequately mix the EDTA and blood, and insufficient centrifugation time.

PCV values may be erroneously low if the microhematocrit tube contains excessive plasma because of inadequate mixing of the sample. Sample dilution because of low blood-to-anticoagulant ratio may also cause a spurious decrease in PCV.

BOX 11-5 *procedure*

Microhematocrit Procedure

1. Fill two microhematocrit tubes about three fourths full with whole blood. Wipe the excess blood from the outside of the tube. Use plain (anticoagulant-free) microhematocrit tubes with anticoagulated blood. Use heparinized tubes when collecting blood from a venipuncture site.
2. Push sealing clay into one end of each microhematocrit tube. Rotate each tube as it is pressed into the clay to ensure a tight seal.
3. Put the tubes in a microhematocrit centrifuge, with the clay seal to the *outside*. Centrifuge for 2 to 5 minutes, depending on the model of the centrifuge used.
4. Determine the PCV for each tube by measuring the length of the column of RBCs using a microhematocrit tube reader. Average the two readings. A popular tube reader is a plastic sheet known as a Critocap chart (Sherwood Medical, St Louis, MO). Place the centrifuged tube perpendicular to the chart lines with the clay/RBC interface on the zero line. Slide the tube along the chart until the 100% line intersects the plasma/air interface in the center of the meniscus. Read the PCV (percentage) directly from the chart at the RBC/buffy coat interface (Fig. 11-7).

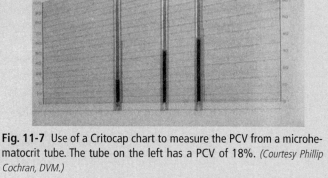

DIRECTIONS FOR USE:
Place the centrifuged Micro-Hematocrit Tube vertically on the chart with the bottom edge of the CRITOCAP just touching the red line below the "0" percent line. The bottom of the column of blood should then be at the "0" percent line. Slide the tube along the chart until the meniscus of the plasma intersects the "100" percent line. The height of the packed red cell column is then read directly as percent cell volume.

Fig. 11-7 Use of a Critocap chart to measure the PCV from a microhematocrit tube. The tube on the left has a PCV of 18%. *(Courtesy Phillip Cochran, DVM.)*

After determining the PCV, evaluate the plasma for turbidity and color (Box 11-6). An icteric, or yellow, plasma layer may occur with liver disease or hemolytic anemia. Normal adult ruminants and horses may have yellow plasma resulting from carotenes in the blood. A hemolytic, or red, sample can occur from improper sample collection and handling or with hemolytic anemia. Sometimes the buffy coat is red-tinged, especially in very sick animals or if there is an increased number of immature RBCs in the circulation. Lipemic plasma appears cloudy (turbid) and white, indicating excessive lipids in the blood. This can occur if blood was collected from an animal that was not fasted, or it may be pathologic.

Icterus, hemolysis, and lipemia may be quantified as slight, moderate, or marked. The width of the buffy coat should be assessed. With experience, you may be able to generally assess the WBC count from buffy coat width, if the total WBC count is very high or low. This is not an accurate method, but can signal the technician to be on the lookout for an abnormal WBC count.

Microfilariae in heartworm-positive dogs are also observable at the buffy coat/plasma interface. The interface should be examined with a microscope at low power (100× magnification). The wiggling movement of the microfilariae displaces the plasma.

In certain situations, it may be valuable to microscopically examine the buffy coat for infectious agents and cell types, including cancer cells. This may be done using the *macrohematocrit*, or *Wintrobe*, method. This requires a larger hematocrit tube and 1 ml of blood. The main purpose of this method is to locate cells present in very low numbers in the buffy coat. After centrifugation, make a smear of the buffy coat. Air-dry the smear and send it to a commercial laboratory for analysis. The slide may also be stained and examined for neoplastic cells or infectious agents.

Total Plasma Protein Determination

The serum or plasma total protein level can be rapidly and reliably measured using a handheld refractometer (Box 11-7). Several types of refractometers are available. Those encountered in practice have built-in scales that you can view by looking through a viewfinder at one end of the refractometer. Most refractometers have a scale to measure both protein and specific gravity. The protein value is read directly from the scale in g/dl. Calibration of the refractometer should be verified periodically as part of routine quality control procedures. This involves taking a reading on distilled water at an ambient temperature of 21° to 29° C (70° to 85° F). The reading should be at 1.000 on the urine

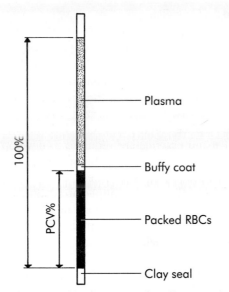

Fig. 11-8 Separated layers in a centrifuged hematocrit tube.

Visual Assessment of Plasma Turbidity and Color

Normal:	Clear and colorless to light straw yellow
Icterus:	Clear and yellow
Hemolysis:	Clear and red
Lipemia:	Turbid and white

specific gravity scale. If it is not, adjust the reading by turning the zero-set screw on the instrument. Refer to the manufacturer's manual for details.

Accurate plasma protein determination is difficult in lipemic samples, because the turbidity produces an indistinct line of demarcation on the scale. Hemoglobinemia caused by hemolysis can falsely increase plasma protein values because of the presence of the heme portion of hemoglobin. The yellow color of an icteric sample does not interfere with refractometry.

Normal plasma protein values vary from 6 g/dl to 8 g/dl. Common causes of increased plasma protein levels include dehydration and increased production of globulins associated with inflammation. Plasma protein values decrease with overhydration, renal disease, gastrointestinal losses, and reduced protein production by a diseased liver.

Erythrocyte Indices

Erythrocyte indices are calculated values that utilize the cell count, hemoglobin measurement, and PCV. The RBC

procedure

Plasma Protein Determination

1. After centrifuging a filled microhematocrit tube, carefully break the tube just above the buffy coat/plasma interface.
2. Transfer plasma to the refractometer by allowing the sample to fill the space between the cover plate and glass surface by capillary action. You need only a very small amount of the sample. Use a syringe and needle to force the plasma onto the surface of an open refractometer. Do not tap the sample out of the tube, because this can scratch the surface of the refractometer.
3. Hold the refractometer horizontally, allowing the overhead light to reach the top of the instrument.
4. Look through the viewfinder and focus the scale by turning the eyepiece.
5. Read the protein value in g/dl at the interface of the light and shaded area (Fig. 11-9). Record the *v* value. Readings may vary slightly when different people read values on a refractometer. This results from a slight variation in an individual's perception of where the shaded line is read.
6. Clean the instrument with water and a soft, lint-free cloth or lens paper.

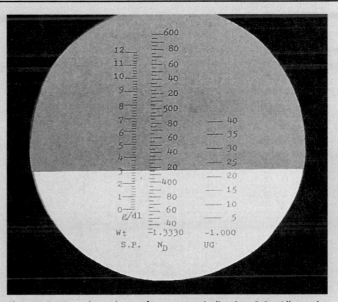

Fig. 11-9 View through a refractometer indicating 3.0 g/dl on the serum protein (S.P.) scale. *(Courtesy Phillip Cochran, DVM.)*

indices include the mean corpuscular volume (MCV), mean corpuscular hemoglobin (MCH), and mean corpuscular hemoglobin concentration (MCHC). The term *corpuscular* is an old term used to describe red blood cells. These measurements provide data on the overall size of the red blood cells as well as the relative amount of hemoglobin within the individual red blood cells. The equations used to calculate the RBC indices are in Table 11-3.

Of the three RBC indices, the MCHC is considered the most accurate since the tests used to calculate the ration (PCV and HB) are more accurate than cell counts. RBC indices should be confirmed by evaluating the morphology of the erythrocytes on the differential blood film.

DIFFERENTIAL BLOOD FILM

Although most veterinary hematology analyzers provide at least a partial differential white blood cell count, a blood film must still be prepared and evaluated. There are a large number of abnormalities that are not routinely reported by automated analyzers. These include:

- Nucleated red blood cells
- "Mega-platelets"
- Heinz bodies
- Bacteria
- Lymphoblasts
- Basophils
- Neoplastic cells
- Cellular inclusions (e.g., parasites, viral materials)
- Toxic granulation
- Platelet clumps
- Polychromasia
- Target cells
- Hemoparasites
- Left shift
- Hypersegmentation

Evaluating the Blood Film

The CBC must include a differential blood film that enumerates various types of white blood cells present and also describes morphology of both red and white blood cells. A platelet estimate is also performed on the differential blood film. In addition to reporting the morphologic changes, a rating system is used to characterize the relative numbers of abnormal cells seen on the differential blood film.

Patience and practice are required to develop the skills necessary to make and interpret blood films. Only one drop of blood is needed to make a smear. It is best to use blood from the tip of the needle immediately after the blood is collected. This prevents development of artifacts related to the presence of anticoagulant. If you cannot make a smear immediately, make the smear as soon as possible after collection.

The two methods of preparing blood smears are the wedge (glass slide) method and the coverslip method. Always use precleaned, glass microscope slides and coverslips. It is important to hold slides by their edges to avoid smudging with grease or fingerprints.

The wedge method is the most common type of smear used for routine hematology (Fig. 11-10). The coverslip method is often preferred for avian blood smears because it renders a thinner film, which facilitates cell identification. It is also less traumatic on fragile avian blood cells.

Coverslip smears are made by putting one drop of blood in the center of a clean, square coverslip (see Fig. 11-10). Place a second coverslip diagonally on top of the first, causing the blood to spread evenly between the two surfaces. Then pull the coverslips apart in a single smooth motion before the blood has completely spread. Wave the smears in the air to promote drying and stain them in a similar manner as described in Box 11-8 for making wedge smears.

Improper technique and inappropriate staining can result in inferior or useless blood smears. Jerky movements

TABLE 11-3

Equations Used to Calculate RBC Indices

Parameter	Equation	Units
MCV	$\dfrac{PCV \times 10}{RBC\ count}$	Femtoliter
MCH	$\dfrac{Hb \times 10}{RBC\ count}$	Picogram
MCHC	$\dfrac{Hb \times 100}{PCV}$	Percent

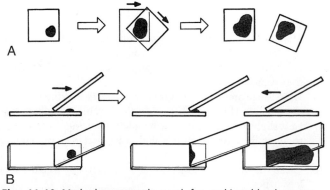

Fig. 11-10 Methods commonly used for making blood smears. **A,** Coverslip method, **B,** Wedge method. *(From Powers LW:* Diagnostic hematology, *St Louis, 1989, Mosby.)*

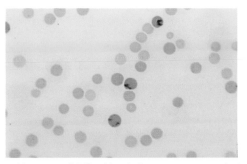

PLATE 1 In this smear of feline blood, three aggregate reticulocytes are evident in the center. Also present throughout the smear are punctate reticulocytes (brilliant cresyl blue). *(Courtesy of Dr. Mary Anna Thrall.)*

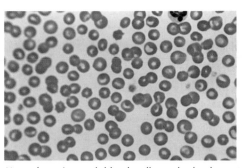

PLATE 2 Normal canine red blood cells and platelets. *(Courtesy of Dr. E. Lassen.)*

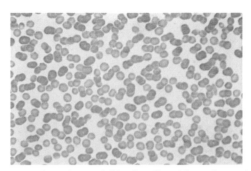

PLATE 3 Normal equine red blood cells with rouleaux formation. *(Courtesy of Dr. E. Lassen.)*

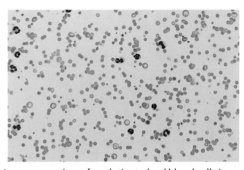

PLATE 4 Low-power view of agglutinated red blood cells in a smear from a dog with immune-mediated hemolytic anemia. *(Courtesy of Dr. Mary Anna Thrall.)*

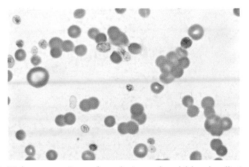

PLATE 5 High-power view of agglutinated red blood cells in a smear from a dog with immune-mediated hemolytic anemia. *(Courtesy of Dr. Mary Anna Thrall.)*

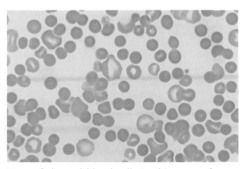

PLATE 6 Most of the red blood cells in this smear from a dog with immune-mediated hemolytic anemia are spherocytes, lacking central pallor. *(Courtesy of Dr. Mary Anna Thrall.)*

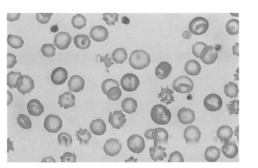

PLATE 7 The large, bluish-staining red cells in this smear of canine blood are polychromatophils. Also present are leptocytes (folded cells and target cells) and acanthocytes (spur cells). *(Courtesy of Dr. Mary Anna Thrall.)*

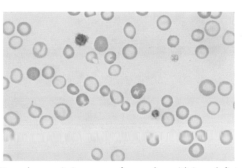

PLATE 8 Hypochromasia in a smear from a dog with iron deficiency. Note the increased central pallor. Several polychromatophils are also present. *(Courtesy of Dr. Mary Anna Thrall.)*

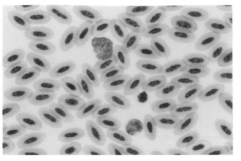

PLATE 25 Heterophil *(top center)* in an avian blood smear. Also present are a thrombocyte *(center)* and a lymphocyte *(bottom center)*. *(Courtesy of Dr. Mary Anna Thrall.)*

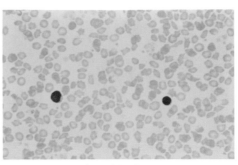

PLATE 26 Lymphocytes in a feline blood smear. *(Courtesy of Dr. E. Lassen.)*

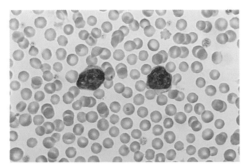

PLATE 27 Large lymphocytes *(center)* with nucleolar rings in a bovine blood smear. *(Courtesy of Dr. Mary Anna Thrall.)*

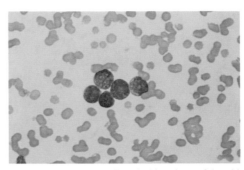

PLATE 28 Atypical lymphocytes (lymphoblasts) in a feline blood smear. *(Courtesy of Dr. E. Lassen.)*

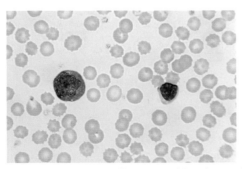

PLATE 29 Reactive lymphocyte *(left)* and normal lymphocyte *(right)* in a canine blood smear. *(Courtesy of Dr. Mary Anna Thrall.)*

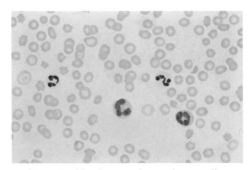

PLATE 30 In this canine blood smear, the two larger cells are monocytes; the smaller cells are segmented neutrophils. *(Courtesy of Dr. E. Lassen.)*

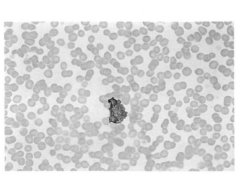

PLATE 31 Eosinophil in an equine blood smear. *(Courtesy of Dr. E. Lassen.)*

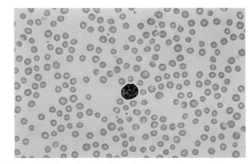

PLATE 32 Basophil in a bovine blood smear. *(Courtesy of Dr. E. Lassen.)*

BOX 11-8 *procedure*

Making a Wedge Smear

1. Place a small drop of blood at the end of a clean glass slide using a microhematocrit tube or the end of a wooden applicator stick. Place this slide on a flat surface or suspend in midair between the thumb and forefinger.
2. Hold a second slide (the spreader slide) at a 30-degree angle and pull back into contact with the drop of blood, spreading blood along the edge of the spreader slide. Push the spreader slide forward in a rapid, steady, even motion to produce a blood film that is thick at one end and tapers to a thin, feathered edge at the other (Fig. 11-11). The blood film should cover about three-quarters of the length of the slide.
3. Air-dry the smear by waving the slide in the air. This fixes the cells to the slide so that they are not dislodged during staining.
4. Label the slide at the thick end of the smear. If the slide has a frosted edge, this may be written on.
5. After drying, stain the smear with Wright's stain or a Romanowsky-type stain, available in commercial kits (e.g., Wright's Dip Stat3; Medi-Chem, Santa Monica, CA). These kits contain an alcohol fixative, a methylene blue mixture to stain cell nuclei and certain organelles bluish-purple, and eosin to stain hemoglobin and some WBC granules reddish-orange. Follow the directions packaged with the staining kit. Smears typically must be immersed in each solution for 5 to 10 seconds (5 to 10 dips).
6. After staining, rinse the slide with distilled water. Allow the slide to dry upright with the feathered edge pointed upward. This allows the water to drip off the slide away from the smear.

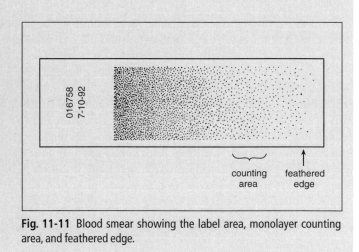

Fig. 11-11 Blood smear showing the label area, monolayer counting area, and feathered edge.

and dirty slides may cause streaks on the film. Using too little or too much blood results in improper smear length. Clots in the blood can cause small holes in the smear and an uneven feathered edge. If the blood is anemic (decreased PCV), increase the spreader slide angle to about 45 degrees. Conversely, the angle should be decreased to about 20 degrees if the blood is concentrated (increased PCV). Increasing the spreader slide angle makes a thicker smear, whereas decreasing it makes a thinner smear.

Table 11-4 lists problems related to staining. Cells appear dark if overstained, whereas extensive rinsing may cause them to look faded. Changing stains regularly is necessary for consistent results and preventing stain precipitation on the film. Refractile artifacts on RBCs are another common problem. These are usually caused by moisture in the fixative solution. Take care not to confuse these artifacts with cellular abnormalities.

Examining the Blood Smear

Place the slide on the microscope stage and examine the blood smear in a systematic manner. It is important to examine slides the same way each time to avoid making mistakes in counting cells or missing important observations (Fig. 11-12). Scan the smear at low power (100× magnification) to assess overall cell numbers and distribution. With practice, you can quickly estimate the total WBC count as either too high or low. Platelet clumps (*aggregates*) and blood parasites (*microfilariae*) are sometimes found at the feathered edge; note these.

A *monolayer* (single layer of blood cells) is located adjacent to the feathered edge. The cells should have even distribution and minimal overlapping. It is here, using the oil-immersion objective (1000× magnification), that the differential WBC count takes place. The differential count is performed in the smear monolayer using oil-immersion (1000×) magnification. There are 100 WBCs counted, identified, and recorded during this count. Because 100 WBCs are counted, the number of each WBC type observed is recorded as a percentage. This is called the *relative WBC count*. Various counting devices are available to aid the differential WBC count. Once the relative percentages of each cell type have been determined, the absolute value of each cell type must be calculated. This is accomplished by multiplying the total white blood cell count by the percentage of each cell type.

Total WBC count = 6000/μl, with 80% neutrophils observed

6000 × 80% = 4800 neutrophils/μl of blood

TABLE 11-4

Some Possible Solutions to Problems Seen with Common Romanowsky-Type Stains

Problem	Solution
Excessive Blue Staining (RBCs May be Blue-green)	
Prolonged stain contact	Decrease staining time
Inadequate wash	Wash longer
Specimen too thick	Make thinner smears, if possible
Stain, diluent, buffer, or wash water too alkaline	Check with pH paper and correct pH
Exposure to formalin vapors	Store and ship cytologic preps separate from formalin containers
Wet fixation in ethanol or formalin	Air dry smears before fixation
Delayed fixation	Fix smears sooner, if possible
Surface of the slide was alkaline	Use new slides
Excessive Pink Staining	
Insufficient staining time	Increase staining time
Prolonged washing	Decrease duration of wash
Stain or diluent too acidic	Check with pH paper and correct pH; fresh methanol may be needed
Excessive time in red stain solution	Decrease time in red stain solution
Inadequate time in blue stain solution	Increase time in blue stain solution
Mounting coverslip before preparation is dry	Allow preparation to dry completely before mounting coverslip
Weak Staining	
Insufficient contact with one or more of the stain solutions	Increase staining time
Fatigued (old) stains	Change stains
Another slide covered specimen during staining	Keep slides separate
Uneven Staining	
Variation of pH in different areas of slide surface (may be due to slide surface being touched or slide being poorly cleaned)	Use new slides, and avoid touching their surfaces before and after preparation
Water allowed to stand on some areas of the slide after staining and washing	Tilt slides close to vertical to drain water from the surface or dry with a fan
Inadequate mixing of stain and buffer	Mix stain and buffer thoroughly
Precipitate on Preparation	
Inadequate stain filtration	Filter or change the stain(s)
Inadequate washing of slide after staining	Rinse slides well after staining
Dirty slides used	Use clean new slides
Stain solution dries during staining	Use sufficient stain, and do not leave it on slide too long
Miscellaneous	
Overstained preparations	Destain with 95% methanol and restain; Diff-Quik-stained smears may have to be destained in the red Diff-Quik stain solution to remove the blue color; however, this damages the red stain solution
Refractile artifact on RBC with Diff-Quik stain (usually due to moisture in fixative)	Change the fixative

From Cowell RL, Tyler RD, Meinkoth JH: *Diagnostic cytology and hematology of the dog and cat*, ed 2, St Louis, 1999, Mosby.

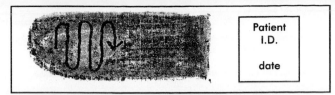

Fig. 11-12 Scanning pattern used for performing a differential WBC count. *(From Sirois M: Veterinary clinical laboratory procedures, St Louis, 1995, Mosby.)*

The morphology of RBCs and WBCs is then assessed and recorded. The presence of any abnormal cells or toxic changes should be semiquantified (Table 11-5). A platelet estimate is also performed (see "Platelet Counting Methods" section).

ERYTHROCYTE MORPHOLOGY

Normal erythrocyte morphology varies greatly among different species (Table 11-6). Unlike the RBCs of mammals, avian RBCs are nucleated. Veterinary technicians should be able to identify normal as well as abnormal RBC morphology. Morphology is evaluated using the oil-immersion objective (1000× magnification) in the monolayer portion of the smear.

Changes in the appearance of erythrocytes occur in a variety of conditions. In general, these changes fall into one or more of the following categories: (1) changes in size, (2) changes in shape, (3) changes in color, (4) changes in cell behavior, and (5) appearance of inclusions. The following sections describe the terms used to describe variations in erythrocytes on the blood film.

Morphologic Variation in Size

Anisocytosis

Anisocytosis is a condition in which the size of the RBCs varies. It is seen in splenic or liver disorders and is a sign of regeneration of anemia

Macrocytes

Macrocytes are RBCs that are larger than normal. This variation represents immature cells. *Macrocytosis* appears as reticulocytes with an NMB stain.

Microcytes

Microcytes are RBCs that are smaller than normal. This variation is often seen in iron deficiency.

Morphologic Variation in Shape

Normocytes

Normocytes in canine appear as biconcave disks. In feline, this variation appears as round cells.

TABLE 11-5

Semiquantitative Evaluation of Erythrocyte Morphology Based on Average Number of Abnormal Cells Per Oil-immersion (1000×) Field

	1+	2+	3+	4+
Anisocytosis				
Dog	7-15	16-20	21-29	>29
Cat	5-8	9-15	16-20	>20
Cow	10-20	21-30	31-40	>40
Horse	1-3	4-6	7-10	>10
Polychromasia				
Dog	2-7	8-14	15-29	>29
Cat	1-2	3-8	9-15	>15
Cow	2-5	6-10	11-20	>20
Horse	Rarely observed			
Hypochromasia				
All species	1-10	11-50	51-200	>200
Poikilocytosis				
All species	3-10	11-50	51-200	>200
Leptocytes (Target and Folded Cells)				
All species	3-5	6-15	16-30	>30
Spherocytes				
Dogs only	5-10	11-50	51-150	>150
Echinocytes, Heinz Bodies (and Eccentrocytes)				
All species	5-10	11-100	101-250	>250
Acanthocytes, Schistocytes, and Stomatocytes				
All species	1-2	3-8	9-20	>20

Modified from Weiss DJ: Uniform evaluation and semiquantitative reporting of hematologic data in veterinary laboratories, *Vet Clin Pathol* 13(2):27, 1984.

Poikilocytes

Poikilocyte is a generic name for any abnormally shaped cell. The specific abnormality should be further characterized as appropriate.

Schistocytes

Schistocytes or *schizocytes* are fragmented RBCs. This variation is caused by vascular trauma. Schistocyte is seen in disseminated intravascular coagulation (DIC), neoplasia, and other disorders (Plate 13).

Acanthocytes

Acanthocytes are long, irregular projections from the surface of an RBC (Plate 7).

TABLE 11-6

Characteristics of Normal Red Blood Cells in Animals

Species	Diameter	Rouleux	Central Pallor	Anisocytosis	Poikilocytes	Basophilic Strippling in Regenerative Response	Reticulocytes (Normal PCV)
Dogs	7.0 μ	+	++++	—	—	—	±1.0%
Pigs	6.0 μ	++	±	+	++++	—	±1.0%
Cats	5.8 μ	++	+	±	—	±	±0.5%
Horses	5.7 μ	+++	±	±	—	—	0% (will not increase in response to anemia)
Cattle	5.5 μ	—	+	++	—	+++	0% (will increase in response to anemia)
Sheep	4.5 μ	±	+	+	—	+++	0% (will increase)
Goats	3.2 μ	—	—	±	++ (in young)	++	0% (will increase)

Number of plus (+) signs indicates degree of characteristic; number of minus (–) signs indicates degree of absence of characteristic.

Echinocytes

Echinocytes are characterized by the scalloped border (regular projections) from the surface of the RBC (Plate 12).

Spherocytes

Spherocytes are small dense RBCs with no area of central pallor (Plate 6).

Stomatocytes

Stomatocytes are RBCs with a slitlike center opening. This variation is seen in regeneration.

Leptocytes

Leptocytes are RBCs with an increase in membrane surface relative to cell volume. This variation appears as target cells, or codocytes (Plate 13).

Morphologic Variation in Color

Polychromasia

Polychromasia is characterized by cells that exhibit a bluish tint.

Hypochromasia

Hypochromasia is characterized by cells with an increase in the area of central pallor (Plate 8).

Hyperchromic cells

Hyperchromic or *Hyperchromatophilic* cells appear darker than normal. These are often microcytic spherocytes.

Variation in Cell Behavior

Rouleux

Rouleux cells appear to be stacked on top of one another. These cells are normal in equine blood. This variation is

seen as an artifact if a sample is held too long before making the blood film (Plate 3).

Autoagglutination

Autoagglutination is characterized by three-dimensional clumps of cells. This variation is seen in immune-mediated hemolytic anemia (Plates 4 and 5).

Other Abnormalities

Basophilic stippling

Basophilic stippling is characterized by bluish granular bodies on the surface of an RBC. This abnormality is seen in regenerative anemia in ruminants, and is diagnostic for lead poisoning in small animals (Plate 10).

Heinz bodies

Heinz bodies are round structures within the RBC representing denatured hemoglobin (Plate 11). A small number may be normally present in feline. This abnormality may be caused by onion toxicity, Tylenol toxicity, etc.

Howell-Jolly bodies

Howell-Jolly bodies are basophilic nuclear remnants in the RBC. This abnormality is common in feline regenerative anemias (Plate 10).

Nucleated RBCs

Nucleated RBCs are seen in regenerative anemias, lead poisoning, extramedullary hematopoiesis, and bone marrow disease (Plate 9). If 5 in 100 or more WBCs are found, a corrected total WBC count should be calculated. The corrected total WBC count is necessary because total WBC counts performed on hemacytometers and some automatic cell counters include all nucleated cells, including RBCs.

The equation used to calculate a corrected total WBC count is as follows:

$$\text{Corrected total WBC count} = \frac{\text{Total WBCs} \times 100}{100 + \text{NRBCs}/100 \text{ WBCs}}$$

For example, if the total WBC count is 9000/μl and 6 NRBCs are observed per 100 WBCs, the corrected WBC count is 9000/μl 100/100 6 8490/μl. Note that the corrected total WBC count is always *lower* than the original WBC count. The corrected total WBC count is then used to calculate the absolute count for each type of WBC.

Parasites

Hemobartonella felis

Hemobartonella felis (Plate 14) is a common parasite of feline RBCs. Any anemic cat should be tested for this parasite. The organisms are very small, round, or rod-shaped structures that stain darkly with Wright's or Romanowsky-type stain. They are often found as single organisms or pairs on the periphery of an RBC. They may also appear as chains or rings on an RBC. Because these parasites appear in the peripheral blood in cycles, the blood may need to be examined several times over 3 to 5 days before the infection can be ruled out. Do not confuse this parasite with stain precipitate or Howell-Jolly bodies. Some clinicians prefer to stain with new methylene blue, make a routine smear, and counterstain with a Romanowsky-type stain as for a reticulocyte preparation. This technique may aid in diagnosing other small blood parasites. This disease is commonly known as *feline infectious anemia (FIA)* or *hemobartonellosis*.

Hemobartonella canis

Hemobartonella canis is a rare blood parasite found in dogs. It is observed in immunosuppressed or splenectomized dogs. This parasite resembles its feline counterpart.

Eperythrozoon

Eperythrozoon occurs in cattle, sheep, and swine and appears similar to *Hemobartonella*. Coccal, rod, and ring forms are found on the RBC surface. The ring form is the most common.

Cytauxzoon felis

Cytauxzoon felis is a very rare parasite found in cats. An irregular ring form occurs within RBCs. Macrophages in the bone marrow may also contain the organism.

Anaplasma marginale

Anaplasma marginale (Plate 15) is a blood parasite of cattle and wild ruminants. It can appear as a small, dark-staining spherical body at the margin of RBCs. This organism must not be confused with Howell-Jolly bodies. Early in the disease, the parasite affects a large number of RBCs. Later, severe anemia develops and a smaller number of RBCs are affected. Howell-Jolly bodies usually are not observed in a large number of cells.

Babesia

Babesia (Plate 16) is a blood parasite found in many species. The parasites appear as large, round, oval, or teardrop-shaped bodies. They can occur singly, in pairs, or in multiples of two. Infected RBCs are often seen at the feathered edge of a blood film.

Dirofilaria immitis

Microfilariae of *Dirofilaria immitis*, the heartworm of dogs, can sometimes be found near the feathered edge of a smear. A microfilaria is about the width of an RBC.

LEUKOCYTE MORPHOLOGY

Morphologic Variation in Leukocytes

Segmented neutrophils

Segmented neutrophils, also known as *segs* or *polymorphonuclear* (PMN) cells (Plate 18) are mature WBCs that function mainly as phagocytes and are involved in inflammation. They have an irregular, lobulated nucleus that is dark and dense. Their cytoplasm is usually colorless to pale pink in most species. Bovine neutrophils have pink to orange cytoplasm. The cytoplasm may contain very fine, diffuse, dark granules. They are the most common type of WBC found in most species.

Heterophils

Heterophils (Plate 25) are the functional equivalent of neutrophils in rabbits, rodents, birds, reptiles, and amphibians. They have a segmented nucleus and variably sized red-brown granules. In most birds, the granules are oval- or needle-shaped. Heterophils may exhibit cytoplasmic basophilia and vacuolization as toxic changes.

Blood cells from exotic species

Blood cells from exotic species can be difficult to classify and identify as abnormal. Lymphocytes have a round to slightly indented nucleus that almost completely fills the cell. The cytoplasm is light blue and may contain a few purple granules, especially in ruminants. Lymphocytes vary in size. Small lymphocytes are mature and have a thin rim of cytoplasm (Plate 26). Large lymphocytes (less mature) have larger nuclei and abundant cytoplasm. Lymphocytes are the predominant WBC type in ruminants (Plate 27). Some bovine lymphocytes may be quite large, with nuclei that contain nucleolar rings, causing the lymphocytes to resemble neoplastic lymphoblasts (atypical lymphocytes).

Monocytes

Monocytes (Plate 30) are very large WBCs with diffuse, less dense nuclear chromatin. The nucleus may vary in shape, including oval, kidney bean, bilobed, trilobed, and horseshoe shapes. The cytoplasm of monocytes is blue-gray and abundant. Vacuoles and/or fine granules may be present. Monocytes may be difficult to distinguish from toxic band neutrophils or earlier stages. Identifying an obvious band and noting its color is helpful. The cytoplasm of monocytes is usually darker than that of bands. The cell in question is most likely a monocyte if a left shift is not present.

Eosinophils

Eosinophils (Plate 31) have a lobulated nucleus and red-orange (eosinophilic) granules in their cytoplasm. Canine eosinophils contain round granules that vary greatly in size. They usually stain the same color as RBCs. The eosinophils of sighthounds (e.g., Greyhounds) may be difficult to identify because a colorless area often replaces the granules. Feline eosinophils contain numerous, small, rod-shaped granules. Eosinophilic granules in horses are very large and round, and stain bright orange. The granules in swine and ruminants are uniformly small and round, and they stain pinkish-red. Increased eosinophil numbers (*eosinophilia*) may occur with parasitic disease or allergies.

Basophils

Basophils (Plate 32) have a lobulated nucleus and numerous dark purple (basophilic) granules in the cytoplasm. Canine basophils have few basophilic granules. Feline basophils have many round granules that stain mauve (grayish-purple). Equine and ruminant basophils are usually packed with granules and stain dark blue. Basophil numbers are often increased in allergies and some metabolic disorders.

Variations in Leukocyte Morphology

Changes in the appearance of leukocytes generally occur as a result of disease processes that affect the appearance and/or function of the cell. These changes can also occur as normal reactions to a disease process and may be nonpathological. Leukocyte changes may affect the cell nucleus, cytoplasm, or both. Additional abnormalities include the appearance of juvenile cells and parasites. The following sections contain terms used to describe variations in leukocytes on the blood film.

Hypersegmentation

Hypersegmentation is characterized by a neutrophil nucleus with five or more lobes. This variation is associated with a variety of conditions including chronic infection, pernicious anemia, and steroid use (Plate 24). These are old neutrophils with a prolonged time in circulation. Neutrophils normally do not age in peripheral blood, but corticosteroid administration, hyperadrenocorticism, or chronic inflammation may keep the cells in peripheral blood for extended periods. Increased number of old neutrophils is called a *right shift.*

Karyohexis/Karyolysis/Pyknosis

Karyohexis/karyolysis/pyknosis describes a nucleus that is condensed, lysed, or damaged. In WBCs in peripheral circulation, this is an artifact caused by the use of inappropriate anticoagulants.

Döhle's bodies

Döhle's bodies are coarse, irregular, gray to blue cytoplasmic inclusions representing ribosomal material. This variation is common in feline and may be seen with chronic bacterial infection and some viral diseases (Plate 22). They often are seen in pairs near the periphery of the cell. When alone, they represent a mild toxic change. Feline neutrophils appear to easily form Döhle's bodies.

Vacuolization

Vacuolization is one of several toxic changes seen in both lymphocytes and neutrophils. This variation is associated with septicemia. It is also produced as an artifact if a sample is held for extended time in anticoagulant (Plate 23). Vacuolization of the cytoplasm (Plate 23), ranging from a few vacuoles to many and causing a foamy appearance, is another toxic change in neutrophils. Vacuolization is recorded as moderate to severe, depending on the number and size of vacuoles observed.

Toxic granulation

Toxic granulation is the appearance of numerous large granules that range in color from dark purple/red to black. This variation is seen in most infectious diseases. Toxic granulation may be described by number (few, moderate, many) or severity (slight, moderate, marked), as indicated in Table 11-7. The overall toxicity is based on the most severe change observed. Toxic granulation is a moderate to severe toxic change. It is particularly evident in equine blood. The granules are purplish-blue and stain quite prominently.

Parasites

A number of parasites, including *Ehrlichia* and *Histoplasma* may be seen within leukocytes. Usually, these organisms are small in number so are best demonstrated with a buffy coat smear. *Erlichia* (Plate 17) is an intracellular parasite of lymphocytes, monocytes, and neutrophils. The organism appears as small clusters in the cytoplasm. Infected animals are usually anemic, neutropenic, and thrombocytopenic. Examination of buffy coat smears may aid in diagnosis.

TABLE 11-7

Semiquantitative Evaluation of Toxic Changes in Neutrophils by Amount

Number of Cells With Toxic Change	Percentage (%)*
Few	5-10
Moderate	11-30
Many	>30
Observed Change	Severity of toxic change
Döhle bodies	Slight
Cytoplasmic basophilia	Slight to marked, depending on intensity
Cytoplasmic vacuolization (Foamy cytoplasm)	Moderate to marked, depending on amount
Indistinct nuclear membrane	Marked
Severe cell degeneration	

*If toxic changes occur in less than 5% of neutrophils, they are not reported.

Juvenile forms

The presence of immature WBCs in circulation is seen in a variety of conditions that result in increased bone marrow activity. In most species, small numbers of band neutrophils may normally be seen in peripheral circulation. The appearance of increased numbers of band cells and/or more immature forms of any of the leukocytes is referred to as a *left shift*. Band neutrophils (Plates 18 and 19) are immature neutrophils with a horseshoe- or S-shaped nucleus. The nucleus may have indentations up to 50% of its width, and that neutrophil may still be classified as a band cell. The nucleus of band cells is smooth and is often lighter in color than that of segmented neutrophils.

Metamyelocytes

Metamyelocytes (Plate 20) and *myelocytes* (Plate 21) are even earlier stages of neutrophils and are found in the bone marrow. They are not usually found in peripheral blood unless severe inflammation or infection is present. If there is any doubt about the identification of a neutrophil stage, always classify it as the more mature cell.

Reactive lymphocytes

Reactive lymphocytes are cells with dark blue cytoplasm and a darker nucleus. They are seen in chronic infection (Plate 29). Reactive lymphocytes (immunocytes) are lymphocytes with a very dense, eccentric, irregular nucleus. Their cytoplasm typically stains intensely royal blue and may have a pale Golgi zone (Plate 29). Reactive lymphocytes may be observed during periods of antigenic stimulation. They are occasionally present in normal animals; report them as a

morphologic change only if more than 5% of lymphocytes are of this type. Reactive and atypical lymphocytes are counted along with the other lymphocytes in the differential count. They may be quantified as *few*—5% to 10% of lymphocytes, *moderate*—11% to 30%, and *many*—more than 30%.

Atypical lymphocytes

Atypical lymphocytes show a variety of changes including eosinophilic cytoplasm and changes in nuclear texture and shape. They exhibit a wide variety of morphologic differences from large to classic small lymphocytes. These variances include divided nuclei and nucleoli. A nucleolus is a round, light-blue structure within the nucleus. A few of these lymphocytes with nucleoli may be seen in sick animals. Another atypical lymphocyte is the *lymphoblast*. Lymphoblasts (Plate 28) are large, immature lymphocytes that contain a nucleolus. Large numbers of circulating lymphoblasts suggest a neoplastic disease of lymphocytes (lymphoproliferative disorders). Extreme lymphocytosis (more than 20,000/μl) may be present in these cases (Plate 28).

Basket cell

Basket cell is a common term used to describe degenerative WBCs that have ruptured. They are also referred to as *smudge cells*. These may be an artifact if blood is held too long before making the smear. Basket cells are also associated with leukemia. They appear as pale-staining, amorphous bodies of stain. A few smudge cells may be expected, but large numbers may indicate excessive cell fragility, which is common in very sick animals.

PLATELETS

Platelets are sometimes referred to as *thrombocytes*. In mammals, they are derived from the bone marrow cell called a *megakaryocyte*. Mammalian platelets are fragments of the cytoplasm of this bone marrow cell. In other animal species, the platelets are actual cells with a different bone marrow precursor. Platelets function to provide an initiating coagulation factor. They are also capable of plugging small ruptures in small blood vessels.

Platelet Counting Methods

A platelet estimate is performed by counting the number of platelets seen on the differential blood film as averaged over ten oil-immersion fields. The presence of an average of 7 to 21 platelets is reported as "adequate." To get an indirect measure of platelet number, count the number of platelets seen per 100 white blood cells on the differential blood film. This number is then used to calculate the platelet estimate using the following equation:

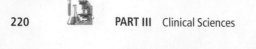

$$\frac{thrombocytes}{100\ leukocytes} \times \frac{total\ WBC\ count}{\mu l} = thrombocytes/\mu l$$

Platelets can also be evaluated with manual methods (Unopette 5855) and with some automated analyzers. Manual methods involve the use of a Unopette and a hemocytometer. The number of platelets is calculated with the same equation used for cell counts. Automated analyzers may also provide a platelet count. Morphologic changes in platelets include *aggregation* and *giant platelets*. These abnormalities will not be evident with automated analyzers and must therefore be detected using the differential blood film.

Reticulocyte counts

The presence of increased numbers of basophilic macrocytic cells on a differential blood film usually indicates an increase in the number of circulating reticulocytes. Although reticulocytes are capable of completing maturation in the peripheral blood, their oxygen-carrying capacity is less than a mature erythrocyte. An increase in the number of circulating reticulocytes is an indication of regenerative anemia. Reticulocyte counts can be performed using a blood film stained with a vital stain such as new methylene blue. Vital stain allows for visualization of the intracellular structures found in reticulocytes, specifically iron not yet incorporated into hemoglobin as well as fragments of cellular organelles. Reticulocytes are immature RBCs that contain ribonucleic acid (RNA) that is lost as the cell matures. Reticulocyte numbers increase when the bone marrow is responding to an anemic state. When reticulocytes are stained with a vital stain, such as new methylene blue, their RNA is visible as blue granules or aggregates. These cells correspond to the larger, blue-gray polychromatic RBCs seen in Wright's-stained smears.

Cats have two types of reticulocytes. The aggregate type is similar to those found in other species and is the type that is counted in all species (Plate 1). The punctate type has a few small, blue-stained granules (not aggregates). This type of reticulocyte may compose up to 10% of RBCs in healthy animals. Their numbers are increased in regenerative anemia, but only the aggregate type is counted.

Reticulocytes do not occur in horses, even with regenerative anemia. They are not found in healthy ruminants but do increase in responding anemias. Reticulocytes are common in healthy suckling pigs. Less than 1% of the RBCs in adult pigs are reticulocytes; reticulocyte numbers increase in regenerative anemias of pigs.

To make a blood smear to examine for reticulocytes, mix a few drops of blood with an equal amount of new methylene blue stain in a test tube and allow it to stand for at least 10 minutes. Make a wedge-type smear with the mixture and allow it to air-dry. Many clinicians like to counterstain this slide with Wright's or Romanowsky-type stain because the RBCs stain reddish and the aggregate granules stain a prominent blue, making the reticulocytes easier to count. Counting the reticulocytes allows the clinician to evaluate the degree of bone marrow response in anemia.

Count the reticulocytes using the oil-immersion objective (1000× magnification). Count the number of aggregate reticulocytes among an estimated 1000 RBCs. The observed percentage can easily be calculated by dividing by 10 the number of reticulocytes counted per 1000 RBCs. Correct this percentage for the degree of anemia present by multiplying it by the patient's PCV and dividing by the normal mean PCV (45% in the dog, 37% in the cat). A corrected reticulocyte percentage above 1% in dogs and above 0.4% in cats indicates a regenerative response to anemia. For example, a dog has a PCV of 21%, with 20% reticulocytes.

$$\begin{array}{c}observed\ \%\\reticulocytes\end{array} \times \frac{patient's\ PCV}{normal\ mean\ PCV} = Corrected\ \%\ reticulocytes$$

$$20\% \times \frac{21\%}{45\%} = 9\%$$

If a total RBC count has been performed, you can calculate an absolute reticulocyte count by multiplying the observed reticulocyte percentage by the RBC count. This gives the number of reticulocytes per microliter (μl) of blood. In most animals (except horses), an absolute reticulocyte count above 60,000/μl indicates a regenerative response to anemia.

Miscellaneous Hematologic Tests

Erythrocyte sedimentation rate (ESR) and erythrocyte fragility testing are occasionally performed in veterinary medicine. The ESR is a measure of the rate that red blood cells fall in their own plasma under controlled conditions. This rate is affected by a number of factors including membrane defects. Since the total number of RBCs affects the ESR, the observed ESR must be corrected for the PCV. This is accomplished by subtracting the observed ESR from the ESR that would be expected from a normal animal of the same species (Table 11-8). For example, a canine with a PCV of 45% would be expected to have an ESR of 5 mm. If the observed ESR is 12 mm, the corrected ESR would be reported as +7 mm.

Erythrocyte fragility testing provides an evaluation of the relative resistance of the RBC to lysis. The procedure uses a set of Unopettes with varying saline concentrations. The blood sample is incubated in these Unopettes. Lysis of cells will occur and create a color change in the liquid. This color change is then measured photometrically and a percent lysis in each solution is calculated.

TABLE 11-8

Erythrocyte Sedimentation Rate Anticipated Values

PVC%	Canine/feline (at 1 hour)	Equine (at 20 min)
10	79	86
15	64	80
20	49	70
25	36	60
30	26	47
35	16	28
40	10	11
45	5	2
50	0	0

BONE MARROW EXAMINATION

Veterinary technicians may assist the veterinarian in examination of bone marrow. This procedure is indicated when there is evidence that the bone marrow is not responding appropriately or when certain types of neoplasia are suspected. Specific indications include unexplained nonregenerative anemia, leukopenia, thrombocytopenia, and pancytopenia (decreased numbers of all cell lines). Bone marrow evaluation is also used to confirm certain infections (e.g., ehrlichiosis) and diagnose hematopoietic neoplasms (e.g., lymphoproliferative disorders).

In small animals, bone marrow is aspirated under general anesthesia or using local anesthesia. Local anesthesia is preferred for large animals. It is crucial to follow aseptic technique throughout the procedure. The proximal end of the femur, the craniolateral portion of the humerus, and the iliac crest are common sites of bone marrow aspiration in dogs and cats. The sternum, ribs, and iliac crest are often used in large animals. Special bone marrow needles are preferred, although an 18-gauge needle may be used in cats with thin bones. Bone marrow needles have a stylet to prevent occlusion of the needle with bone and surrounding tissue as it is inserted into the marrow cavity. A syringe is used to aspirate a few drops of bone marrow, filling the hub of the needle and perhaps the distal part of the syringe. The needle is removed from the bone and the contents immediately used to make slides. Alternatively, the marrow may be mixed with EDTA so smears can be made a short time later.

Marrow smears are prepared in a similar manner to peripheral blood. Bone marrow is thicker than blood and should contain particles or spicules. Blood contamination can be minimized by vertically positioning the slide to drain off excess blood before making the smear. The smear is air-dried and stained as described previously. You may then examine smears or send them to a commercial laboratory for analysis.

If you examine the stained smears, do so at low-power (100×) magnification for overall cellularity and mega-karyocyte (thrombocyte precursor cell) number. Cellularity is normal if the particles are composed of about 50% nucleated cells and 50% fat (Fig. 11-13). Describe the marrow as *hypercellular* or *hypocellular*, based on the proportion of cells present. There should be 2 to 3 megakaryocytes per low-power field.

At higher magnification, examine erythroid (red) and myeloid (white) cells. Rubricytes and metarubricytes should make up 90% of the nucleated erythroid cells. Metamyelocytes, bands, and segmented myeloid cells should make up 90% of the myeloid cells. Determine the ratio of myeloid to erythroid cells (M:E ratio) by counting 500 nucleated cells and classifying them as erythroid or myeloid. Normal M:E ratios should be between 0.75:1.0 and 2.0:1.0. Neoplasia is a possibility if all the cells look alike. Bone marrow status should never be evaluated without the results of a concurrent peripheral hemogram. If his-

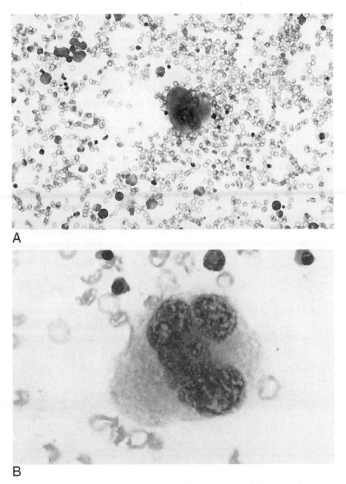

A

B

Fig. 11-13 A, Bone marrow smear from a normal dog, with megakaryocyte at center. **B,** High-power view of a megakaryocyte. *(Courtesy Dr. Mary Anna Thrall.)*

tologic examination of marrow is required, a special biopsy needle is used to obtain a larger core sample for analysis.

HEMOSTASIS

Hemostasis refers to the ability of the body systems to maintain the integrity of the blood and blood vessels. Hemostasis is a complex interaction between blood vessel walls, platelets, and coagulation factors. The result of this interaction is formation of a blood clot (hemostatic plug) made up of platelets and fibrin. Fibrin is the end product of a complex series of chemical steps known as the *coagulation cascade*. Activation of either the intrinsic or the extrinsic coagulation pathway may trigger this cascade. The intrinsic pathway is essential for clot formation and occurs in the blood vessels. Tissue damage (such as needle puncture of a vessel wall) initiates the extrinsic pathway, which enhances coagulation. These separate pathways lead to a common

pathway where the final reaction involves fibrinogen conversion to fibrin. The hemostatic plug (clot) eventually degrades as tissue heals. Fig. 11-14 provides an overview of hemostasis.

Coagulation of blood proceeds through a mechanical phase and a chemical phase. The mechanical phase, also known as *primary hemostasis*, is initiated when a blood vessel is ruptured or torn. The exposed blood vessel subendothelium is charged surface. Platelets are immediately attracted to this surface. As platelets congregate at this site, they undergo morphologic and physiologic changes. These changes cause the platelets to adhere to each other as well as the blood vessel. This also causes platelets to release the initiating factor in the chemical phase of hemostasis. The chemical phase is generally divided into a secondary and tertiary phase and is referred to as the coagulation cascade. A number of coagulation factors are involved. Table 11-9 lists the coagulation factors and their common synonyms. Each factor participates in a chemical reaction that serves to

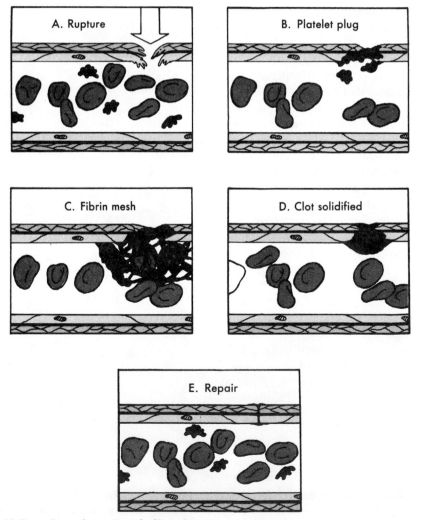

Fig. 11-14 Formation and retraction of a fibrin clot. *(From Powers LW:* Diagnostic hematology, *St Louis, 1989, Mosby.)*

TABLE 11-9

Blood Coagulation Factors

Designation	Synonym
Factor I	Fibrinogen
Factor II	Prothrombin
Factor III	Tissue thromboplastin
Factor IV	Calcium
Factor V	Proaccelerin
Factor VII	Proconvertin
Factor VIII	Anithemophilic factor
Factor IX	Christmas factor, Plasma thromboplastin
Factor X	Stuart-Prower factor
Factor XI	Plasma thromboplastin antecedent
Factor XII	Hageman factor
Factor XIII	Fibrin-stabilizing factor

initiate the next reaction in the pathway. The end result of the coagulation cascade is the formation of a mesh of fibrin strands that forms the clot. Fig. 11-15 shows the chemical phase of the coagulation pathways.

Hemostatic Defects

Most bleeding disorders found in veterinary species are secondary to some other disease process. Primary coagulation disorders are more rare and are usually the result of an inherited defect in production of coagulation factors. Disorders in concentration or function of coagulation factors are the least common cause of bleeding problems in veterinary species. The most common inherited disorder of domestic animals is von Willebrands disease. The disease results when production of von Willebrands factor is decreased or deficient. The disease occurs with relative frequency in Doberman dogs and has been reported in other

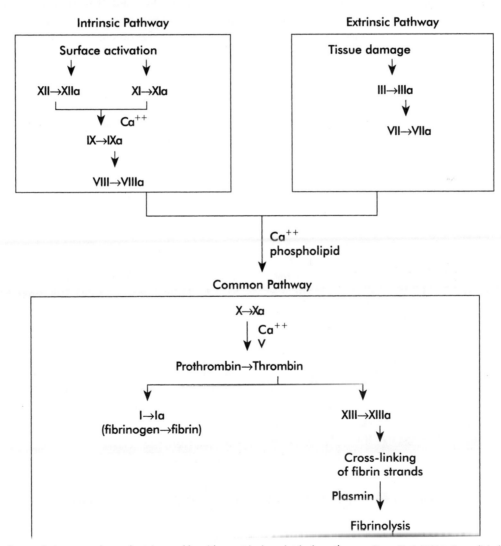

Fig. 11-15 The blood coagulation cascade can be triggered by either extrinsic or intrinsic pathways. *(From Sirois M:* Veterinary clinical laboratory procedures, *St Louis, 1995, Mosby.)*

canine breeds as well as rabbits and swine. Three distinct forms of the disease have been identified based on their patterns of inheritance. Primary coagulation disorders are rare in cats.

Secondary coagulation disorders can result from decreased production or increased destruction of platelets as well as nutritional deficiencies, liver disease, and ingestion of certain medications or toxic substances. Thrombocytopenia refers to a decreased number of platelets and is the most common bleeding disorder of hemostasis in veterinary patients. This can occur as a result of bone marrow depression that reduces the production of platelets, or autoimmune disease that increases the rate of platelet destruction. A large number of infectious agents, such as *Ehrlichia*, *Dirofilaria*, and parvovirus, can also affect thrombocyte production and destruction. Since the liver is the site of production of most coagulation factors, any condition that affects liver function can result in a coagulation disorder. Ingestion of toxic substances such as warfarin can also create bleeding disorders. Warfarin is a common component of rodenticides and acts to inhibit vitamin K function. Since vitamin K is required for synthesis of coagulation factors II, VII, IX, and X, this can create a deficiency in several necessary components of the coagulation cascade. Ingestion of medications such as aspirin can also cause bleeding disorders.

Disseminated Intravascular Coagulation

Although not a disease entity on its own, DIC is associated with many pathologic conditions. DIC is often seen in trauma cases as well as a large number of infectious diseases. A large number of events can trigger DIC. The resulting hemostatic disorder may manifest as systemic hemorrhage or microvascular thrombosis. Since the triggering event and the resulting disorder are diverse, the laboratory findings are highly variable. Most patients with DIC have alterations in three or more coagulation tests, including prolonged partial thromboplastin time (APTT) and elevated fibrinogen, as well as significant thrombocytopenia.

Clinical presentation of patients with bleeding disorders include *petechia* (pinpoint hemorrhage), *ecchymoses* (superficial hemorrhage of about 1 cm in diameter), *purpura* (bruising), *epistaxis* (bleeding from the nares), and prolonged bleeding following trauma or surgery. Patients may also have bleeding into joint cavities, or into the urinary bladder, evidenced as *hematuria*, or digestive tract, evidenced as *melena*.

Assessment of Coagulation and Hemostasis

Coagulation tests may be appropriate if a bleeding disorder is suspected or as part of a presurgical screening protocol. Coagulation tests are designed to evaluate specific portions of the hemostatic mechanisms. Some tests measure just the mechanical phase of hemostasis. Others can measure specific parts of the chemical phase. All patients should be evaluated for coagulation defects prior to undergoing surgery. Most coagulation tests can be completed with minimal time and equipment and are relatively inexpensive. Platelet counts described earlier are part of all coagulation profiles. Samples for coagulation testing are plasma collected into an appropriate anticoagulant. Tests to determine the concentration and/or function of specific coagulation factors are not routinely performed in veterinary practice.

ACTIVATED CLOTTING TIME

This test can evaluate every clinically significant clotting factor except Factor VII. The test utilizes a preincubated Vacutainer tube that contains a diatomaceous earth material. Venipuncture is performed, and 2 ml of blood is collected directly into the tube. A timer is started as soon as the blood enters the tube. The tube is mixed once by gentle inversion and placed in a 37° incubator or water bath. The tube is observed at 60 seconds and then at 5 second intervals for presence of a clot. Increases in activated clotting time are not usually seen unless one of the coagulation factors is reduced to 5% of normal.

BUCCAL MUCOSAL BLEEDING TIME

This is a primary assay for the detection of abnormalities in platelet function. The test requires a Simplate I or II spring-loaded lancet, blotting paper or #1 Whatman filter paper, a stopwatch, and a tourniquet. The patient should be anesthetized and placed in lateral recumbency. A strip of gauze is used to tie the upper lip back in order to expose the mucosal surface and to act as a tourniquet (Fig. 11-16). A 1-mm-deep incision is made using the Simplate device. Standard blotting paper or #1 Whatman filter paper is used to blot the incision site. This is performed by lightly touching the paper to the drop of blood, allowing it to absorb. Blotting is repeated every five seconds until bleeding has stopped. A prolonged bleeding time occurs with most platelet dysfunction syndromes. It will also be prolonged in thrombocytopenia so a platelet count must also be performed.

FIBRINOGEN DETERMINATION

Fibrinogen is a protein produced by the liver and is involved in blood coagulation. Fibrinogen synthesis increases when inflammation is present. This is especially apparent in large animals, making fibrinogen a useful indicator of inflammation in large animals. Automated analysis of fibrinogen is complicated and not routinely available for

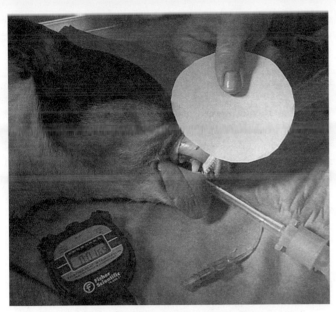

Fig. 11-16 Bleeding time. *(Photo courtesy Barry Mitxner, DVM.)*

use on in-house laboratory analyzers. One manual method that may be used for fibrinogen determination involves the use of two hematocrit tubes. The tubes are centrifuged as for a PCV, and the total solids on one tube is determined with a refractometer. The second tube is then incubated at 58° C for 3 minutes. The second tube is recentrifuged, and the total solids are measured. This test is based on the idea that fibrinogen becomes denatured and precipitates out of plasma heated to 56° to 58° C. This test is rapid and provides a reasonable approximation of plasma fibrinogen levels. Because only a small amount of fibrinogen is normally present in serum, it is more reliable to detect increased levels than decreased levels in plasma. Fibrinogen is then calculated using the following equation (Box 11-9).

$$\text{TS mg/dl}_{(\text{nonincubated})} - \text{TS mg/dl}_{(\text{incubated})} = \text{fibrinogen mg/dl}$$

Normal plasma fibrinogen concentrations are 100 to 700 mg/dl, depending on the species. Severe inflammation cause increases above this value. This test is usually reserved for large animals because increases are a consistent finding in these species.

PROTHROMBIN TIME TEST

The prothrombin time (PT) test is usually performed with automated analyzers (Fig. 11-17). This test evaluates the extrinsic coagulation pathway. Most analyzers require a citrated plasma sample to which tissue thromboplastin reagent is added. A reagent designed to recalcify the sample is then added. Under normal conditions, a clot should form within 6 to 20 seconds. Some automated analyzers are available that can utilize whole-blood samples and provide a rapid and accurate Prothrombin time test.

ACTIVATED PARTIAL THROMBOPLASTIN TIME TEST

The activated APTT test requires an automated coagulation analyzer. The test evaluates the intrinsic pathway and common pathways. Older instruments used for these tests were generally not practical for use in veterinary clinics. Several reagents were required, and the tests were difficult to perform accurately. New analyzers for APTT testing are now available that can utilize whole-blood or plasma samples (collected in citrate anticoagulant tubes) and have no requirement for external reagent. The tests are simple, rapid, and provide an accurate evaluation of APTT. APTT increases can occur when any of the coagulation factors are reduced to 30% of normal.

PIVKA TEST

PIVKA is an acronym that refers to *Proteins induced (or invoked) by vitamin K absence*. Recall that vitamin K is required to activate coagulation factors II, VII, IX, and X.

BOX 11-9 *procedure*

Plasma Fibrinogen Procedure

1. Measure the plasma protein concentration on one of two centrifuged microhematocrit tubes.
2. Insert the remaining tube into a warm-water bath or an incubated sand-filled heat block at 56° to 58° C. Make sure the entire plasma column is immersed in the water or sand.
3. Heat the tube for at least 3 minutes. Remove the tube and examine the plasma layer for turbidity.
4. Recentrifuge to concentrate the fibrinogen in the top portion of the buffy coat.
5. Carefully break the tube at the plasma/fibrinogen interface and measure the plasma protein concentration. Subtract the second value from the first. The difference is the fibrinogen concentration. This value is measured as g/dl but may also be reported as mg/dl. (To convert from g/dl to mg/dl, move the decimal point three places to the right.)

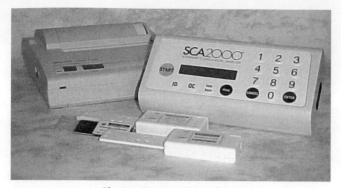

Fig. 11-17 SCA2000 analyzer.

When vitamin K is deficient, the concentration of the precursor proteins of those coagulation factors build up and can be detected by the PIVKA. The test can be used to differentiate rodenticide toxicity from primary hemophilia when ACT is prolonged. It is more sensitive than PT when there is a depletion of these factors. The APTT test usually does not prolong until 48 hours after exposure. The PIVKA test usually becomes prolonged within 6 hours following ingestion of an anticoagulant rodenticide.

FIBRIN DEGRADATION PRODUCTS AND D-DIMER TESTS

These tests are important in evaluating thrombus formation and detecting the presence of DIC. Fibrin Degradation Products (FDPs) are formed when the protein plasmin acts on fibrin or fibrinogen to dissolve a clot. The clot is broken down into several fragments, some of which can be detected with the FDP test. An increase in the presence of FDPs indicates active fibrinolysis. This is a common finding in DIC.

The FDP test requires some special instrumentation but is rapid and easy to perform. D-dimers are a type of FDP resulting from the degradation of cross-linked fibrin strands in the clot. The concentration of D-dimers increases in DIC, as well as thrombosis, liver failure, trauma, and hemangiosarcomas. Several rapid in-house test kits are now available for detecting canine D-dimers. The kits differ significantly in test principle. They may be based on immunochromatography, latex agglutination, or immunoturbidometric analysis.

RECOMMENDED READING

Benjamin MM: *Outline of Veterinary Clinical Pathology*, ed 3, Ames, Iowa, 1981, Iowa State University.

Coles EH: *Veterinary Clinical Pathology*, ed 4, Philadelphia, 1986, Lea & Febiger.

Colville J: The veterinary practice laboratory. In Hendrix CM: *Laboratory procedures for veterinary technicians*, ed 4, St Louis, 2002, Mosby.

VanSteenhouse, JL: *Clinical pathology*. In McCurnin D and Bassert J: *Clinical textbook for veterinary technicians*, ed 5, Philadelphia, 2002, WB Saunders.

Sirois M: *Veterinary Clinical Laboratory Procedures*, St Louis, 1995, Mosby.

Sodikoff CH: *Laboratory Profiles of Small Animal Disease*, ed 3, St Louis, 2001, Mosby.

12

Clinical Chemistry and Serology

Margi Sirois

Learning Objectives

After reviewing this chapter, the reader should understand the following:
- Methods used to collect samples of blood for laboratory examination
- Ways in which diagnostic samples are prepared for laboratory examination
- Biochemical assays commonly performed on blood
- Assays commonly performed to assess organ function
- Immunologic and serologic tests commonly used in veterinary practice
- Methods used to maintain accuracy of laboratory test results

Laboratory analysis of blood biochemical constituents is performed for a variety of reasons. A blood sample may be collected from a patient as part of a general wellness screening process, to confirm or rule out a specific disease, as part of management of a clinical case to evaluate the status of a previously diagnosed condition, or as part of emergency medical therapy. Biochemistry profiles, or groups of tests, are routinely performed using serum as the preferred sample type, although heparinized plasma may also be used. Determinations of levels of the various chemical constituents in blood can provide valuable diagnostic information. The chemicals being assayed are usually enzymes associated with particular organ functions or metabolites and metabolic by-products that are processed by certain organs. Serologic testing usually refers to immunodiagnostic testing. These tests are generally performed on the same type of sample as the blood chemistry profile.

SAMPLE COLLECTION

Unless the purpose of the test is to monitor therapy, always collect the blood sample before any treatment is given. Administration of certain medications and treatments often affects results of biochemical testing. Preprandial samples, or samples from an animal that has not eaten for 12 hours, are ideal. Postprandial samples, or samples collected after an animal has eaten, may produce erroneous results. For example, after meals, the blood glucose concentration frequently increases. Also, an increased BUN concentration may be present if the meal was high in protein. Increased amounts of lipid (lipemia) may also be present in postprandial blood samples.

Blood Collection

Regardless of the method of blood collection, it is vital that the sample be labeled immediately after it has been collected. The tube should be labeled with the date and time of collection, the owner's name, the patient's name, and the patient's clinic identification number. If submitted to a laboratory, include with the sample a request form that includes all necessary sample identification and a clear indication of which tests are requested.

Make venipuncture with the least tissue injury possible to minimize contamination with tissue fluid and to minimize hemolysis. Use of a vacuum tube (Vacutainer, Becton-Dickinson, Rutherford, N.J.) or syringe is determined by the size of the animal (and vein) and the quantity of sample desired. All blood samples collected in a tube containing anticoagulant should be gently inverted several times immediately after collection to distribute the anticoagulant. If a Vacutainer is used, fill the tube to capacity to ensure the proper blood-to-anticoagulant ratio. If a syringe and needle are used, remove the needle from the syringe before transferring the blood to the vial, because forcing blood through the needle may result in hemolysis.

Small animals

In adult dogs and cats, the jugular vein is the preferred site for collection of blood samples. It is relatively easy to locate, and the size of the vein allows adequate quantities of blood to be collected. Alternate sites include the cephalic and saphenous veins in dogs, and the cephalic and femoral veins in cats. Vacutainers may be used with large dogs, but in very small animals the vacuum in the tube can collapse the vein. Blood samples from small animals are routinely collected with a calibrated syringe and a needle of appropriate size. If the needle bore is too small or too large, it may cause disruption of erythrocytes (hemolysis). Needles of 20 to 25 gauge work well for collection of samples from dogs and cats.

Large animals

The jugular vein is a suitable site for collection of blood samples in most large animals. In adult cattle, the subcutaneous abdominal (milk) vein and coccygeal (tail) vein are alternate sites. Alternate sites for sample collection from horses include the cephalic, lateral thoracic, and saphenous veins. Vacutainers work well, but needles and calibrated syringes can also be used. Needle gauges range from 16 to 20, with lengths of 1.5 to 2 inches; 20-gauge needles of 1.5 to 4 inches are used to obtain samples from the cranial vena cava of pigs. Because the blood of goats is easily hemolysed if collected with a Vacutainer, a syringe and a 20-gauge needle are recommended for collection of caprine blood samples.

SAMPLE TYPE

Whole Blood

Whole blood is composed of cellular elements (erythrocytes, leukocytes, platelets) and a fluid called *plasma*. Collect the whole-blood sample by placing the proper amount of blood into a container containing the appropriate anticoagulant and then gently mixing the sample by inverting the tube multiple times. Whole blood may be refrigerated if analysis is to be delayed, but it should never be frozen. If the blood has been refrigerated, warm the sample to room temperature and gently mix before analysis. Few blood chemistry or serology tests are capable of utilizing whole-blood samples. Plasma or serum samples are more commonly used.

Plasma

To obtain a plasma sample, collect the appropriate amount of blood in a container with the proper anticoagulant and gently mix well. Centrifuge the closed container for 10 minutes at 2000 to 3000 rpm to separate the fluid from the cells. After the sample is centrifuged, remove the plasma from the cells, being careful not to contaminate the plasma with any of the pelleted cells, and transfer the plasma into another appropriately labeled container. Separate plasma from the cellular elements as soon as possible after collection to minimize any artifactual changes. Plasma can be refrigerated or frozen until analysis is performed, depending on the specific requirements of the desired test(s).

Plasma collected in tubes containing heparin as the anticoagulant (sodium heparin, potassium heparin, ammonium heparin, or lithium heparin) can be used for most assays included on a routine biochemical profile. However, do not use potassium heparin if electrolyte levels are being measured, because artifactual increases of potassium concentrations can occur. Heparin functions as an anticoagulant by activation of antithrombin III, which prevents conversion of prothrombin to thrombin. Heparin is not a permanent anticoagulant; it inhibits coagulation for only 8 to 12 hours. When biochemical analysis must be performed quickly, as in an emergency situation, collection of a blood sample with a heparin anticoagulant is indicated. The plasma can be harvested immediately after collection and centrifugation, rather than the time delay (necessary for the blood to clot and the clot to retract) required to harvest a serum sample.

Plasma collected in tubes containing ethylenediaminetetraacetic acid (EDTA) as the anticoagulant (which is routinely used for complete blood counts) should not be used for serum biochemical analysis, because spurious values for electrolytes, trace elements, and many serum enzymes will result. EDTA functions as an anticoagulant by binding calcium, which is necessary for clotting to occur. Because EDTA binds calcium, any test procedure that requires calcium cannot be performed on samples collected in EDTA. All other anticoagulants, such as potassium oxalate and sodium citrate, also function by binding calcium, and therefore should not be used to collect plasma for biochemical analysis.

Serum

Serum is plasma that has had the coagulation proteins, such as fibrinogen, removed during the clotting process. A serum sample is obtained by placing blood in a container with no additives and allowing it to clot at room temperature. Once sufficient time has passed for the clot to form (usually 30 minutes), the closed container is then centrifuged at 2000 to 3000 rpm for 10 minutes, and the serum is harvested. Centrifugation for longer periods can result in hemolysis.

If the serum is not separated from the clot, numerous artifactual changes can result in erroneous laboratory values. An artifactual decrease in glucose concentration can occur due to glucose metabolism by blood cells. Release of inorganic phosphorus from high-energy phosphate bonds results in artifactual increases in serum phosphorus concentrations. Leakage of potassium from red blood cells (RBCs) occurs in large animal species and in some small animal species, resulting in erroneously high potassium concentrations. Artifactual increases of serum enzymes such as aspartate aminotransferase (AST) and alanine aminotransferase (ALT) may also occur.

Once harvested, the serum may be refrigerated or frozen. Freezing may affect some test results, so check the test protocol prior to freezing the sample.

Blood can also be collected in serum tubes containing a gel substance that, during centrifugation, moves into a position between the clot and the serum. Using this type of serum tube, called a *serum separator tube*, does not necessarily prevent artifactual changes. The benefit of a serum separator tube is that the gel substance facilitates removal of serum without accidental aspiration of clot elements, which would contaminate the serum sample.

All of the above-mentioned artifactual changes can occur without the problems of hemolysis or lipemia being present. Hemolysis can result from difficult blood collection, mixing too vigorously after sample collection, forcing the sample through a needle when transferring it to a tube, or freezing a whole-blood sample. The syringe must be completely dry before it is used, because water in the syringe can cause hemolysis. Also, it is beneficial to remove the needle from the syringe before transferring the blood into a tube. Cells can be ruptured when blood is forced through the needle. To reduce the chance of hemolysis occurring when transferring blood to a tube, expel the blood slowly from the syringe without causing bubbles to form. Hemolysis may cause errors in testing resulting from direct interference, dilution, and/or release of substances found in high concentrations within erythrocytes.

Hemolysis may not be apparent until after a blood sample has been centrifuged. A trained observer can detect visibly hemolytic serum (slight pink discoloration) at hemoglobin concentrations as low as 20 mg/dl. Mild to moderate hemolysis has minimal effect on most routine serum chemistry assays, but bilirubin and ALT levels are often increased. Also, lipase activity is inhibited by hemolysis, resulting in falsely decreased values. If marked hemolysis is present, the results of most assays are likely to be affected, resulting in inaccurate values.

Lipemia also affects the results of serum biochemical assays, resulting in erroneous values. *Lipemia* describes the milky appearance of serum or plasma resulting from increased concentrations of triglyceride-containing lipoproteins. Transient lipemia is common approximately 4 to 6 hours after a meal. Ideally, collect blood samples from an animal that has been fasted for at least 12 hours. This should eliminate any lipemia resulting from ingestion of food. Water need not be withheld. Lipemia can cause erroneous results for all routine clinical chemistries. Light scattering is the most common source of error in testing of lipemic samples. Light scattering may result in falsely

increased or decreased values, depending on whether lipemia in the sample results in an increase or decrease in light absorbance measured by the spectrophotometer.

Endpoint enzymatic assays are generally more severely affected by lipemia than are kinetic enzymatic assays. However, results are invalid in markedly lipemic samples and should be interpreted with caution even in mildly lipemic samples. Lipemia can result in falsely decreased values of electrolytes if a flame photometer is used to measure the electrolytes. If an ion-specific electrode is used to determine electrolyte concentrations, lipemia does not affect results (see "Electrolytes" section).

LABORATORY SELECTION

There are several choices of where to obtain clinical chemistry results. Veterinary reference laboratories, human hospitals, or in-clinic chemistry machines are the most common choices. There are advantages and disadvantages to each choice. Price, service, and quality are the main variables to consider.

The main benefit to choosing a veterinary reference laboratory is that the staff members should be familiar with and should have established reference ranges (normal values) for domestic species with the equipment used in that particular laboratory. Some laboratories may have reference ranges for certain exotic animal species, as well. In addition to providing chemistry profiles, these laboratories may also offer endocrine testing, microbiology, cytology, and histopathology services. Using a single laboratory for all services can be very convenient. Also, many of these laboratories offer consultations with specialists, such as internists, clinical pathologists, or anatomic pathologists. These laboratories are generally available only in larger cities. Some reference laboratories may have arrangements with an overnight mailing service so that results are available the next day. Most of these laboratories provide results via telephone or fax, in addition to mailing a printed copy of the results. One disadvantage is that quality assurance standards have not been established for veterinary laboratories, in contrast to the standards that have been established for human laboratories.

Laboratories in human hospitals provide an alternative for obtaining clinical chemistry results. Unlike veterinary reference laboratories, these laboratories must adhere to rigorous quality control standards, and the testing methods are of high quality. Human hospital laboratories are not likely to have established reference ranges for animal species. The cost of having animal samples analyzed at a human hospital may be quite reasonable because of the high volume of human samples assayed. Most of the assays included in routine chemistry profiles performed at human hospital laboratories are valid for animal species.

It is important not to assume, however, that every assay is valid. Certain reagents that human hospitals use in their testing methods may not provide accurate or reliable results for animal species. If the validity of any assay is in question, check to confirm the proper testing protocol for that assay and possibly for the animal species. Keep in mind that technicians at human hospitals may not be aware of which procedures are valid for veterinary species.

Certain tests can be performed using commercially available dry chemistry strips. Some examples include blood urea nitrogen (Azostix, Bayer, Elkhart, Ind.) and blood glucose (Chemstrip bG, Boehringer Mannheim, Indianapolis, Ind.).

LABORATORY EQUIPMENT

Chemistry machines designed for in-clinic use are increasing in quality and becoming more affordable and easier to use. A great advantage of in-clinic chemistry analyzers is that the results can be obtained very quickly. Also, performing these tests in-clinic can be a source of profit. Factors to consider are the initial cost of the machine, cost of the reagents, anticipated use of the machine, and amount of maintenance the machine requires. Quality control procedures are essential for any test that is performed on an in-clinic basis. The machine must be kept calibrated, and regular control samples that contain known quantities of a substance or substances must be assayed. If these are not done, the potential for erroneous results is great.

FEATURES AND BENEFITS OF COMMON ANALYZER TYPES

Most in-clinic automated blood chemistry analyzers employ photometric principles. Photometry involves the addition of a reagent to a serum or plasma sample that creates a color change in the system. The degree of color change is then measured with a spectrophotometer (Fig. 12-1). The primary difference between the various photometric analyzers lies in the format of the tests. Several important questions must be answered when determining which type of analyzer to purchase for in-house testing. These include the intended purpose of the testing (i.e., presurgical versus tracking disease progress), anticipated test volume, and ease of operation and maintenance. Methods for ensuring quality of results should also be evaluated when choosing an analyzer. Costs associated with various analyzers also vary a great deal. When determining costs, be sure to include technician time to prep and run samples and instrument prep and maintenance time along with the actual costs per test or profile.

Analyzers utilizing "dry" systems include those with reagent-impregnated slides, pads, or cartridges (Fig. 12-2). Most of these utilize reflectance assays (rather then the absorbance assay of a traditional photometric analyzer). Dry systems tend to have comparatively higher costs associated with them than other analyzer types. Most are not configured for veterinary species and have fairly high incidences of sample rejection with compromised samples or samples from large animals. However, they have the benefit of not requiring reagent handling, and performance of single tests is relatively simple. Running profiles on these types of systems tends to be more time-consuming than most other analyzer types.

Liquid systems include those that utilize lyophilized reagent or those that provide prepared liquid reagent. The most common type of lyophilized reagent systems for veterinary clinical practice use rotor technology. The rotors consist of individual cuvettes (optical quality reagent wells) to which sample is added. These systems tend to be quite accurate, although some are not configured for veterinary species. They are usually cost-effective for profiles but are generally incapable of running single tests. Other liquid systems in common use include those with unitized reagent cuvettes and those with bulk reagent. The unitized systems have the advantage of not requiring reagent handling but tend to be the most expensive of all the liquid reagent

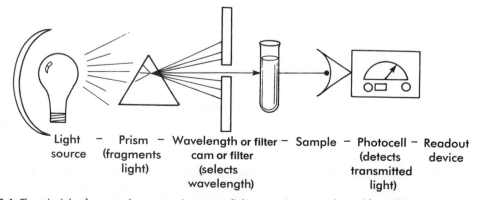

Fig. 12-1 The principle of spectrophotometry. A tungsten light source is commonly used for visible wavelengths.

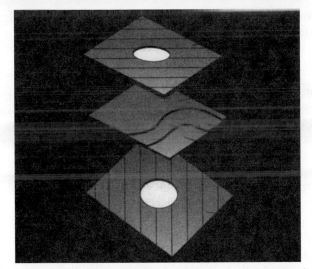

Fig. 12-2 An exploded view of a "dry" reagent clinical chemistry slide. Reagents are located on the central pad of the slide and sample is added to this area. *(Photo courtesy Eastman Kodak Company. KODAK is a trademark.)*

TABLE 12-1

Effects of Sample Compromise

Sample Characteristic	Effect	Result
Lipemia	Light scattering	↑
	Volume displacement	↓
	Hemolysis	↑↓*
Hemolysis/blood substitutes	Release of analytes	↑
	Release of enzymes	↑↓*
	Reaction inhibition	↓
	Increased OD (absorbance)	↑
	Release of water	↓
Icterus	Spectral interference	↑
	Chemical interaction	↑
Hyperproteinemia	Hyperviscosity	↓
	Analyte binding	↑↓*
	Volume displacement	↓
Medications	Reaction interference	↑↓*

*Variable effect depending on analyte and test method.

systems. It is also time-consuming to run profiles with these systems, but single testing is simple. Bulk reagent systems may supply reagent either in concentrated form that must be diluted or in working strength. Working strength reagent systems do not usually require any special reagent handling. These analyzers are the most versatile in that they can perform either profiling or single testing with relative ease. Most require little prep time. However, some have extensive maintenance time, in particular with calibration of test parameters.

Samples that are compromised by hemolysis, icterus, or lipemia may yield inaccurate results with many of the automated analyzers (Table 12-1). Most automated blood chemistry analyzers work by passing light in the ultraviolet or visible range of the spectrum through the sample-reagent complex and measuring the amount of light transmitted. Hemolysis, icterus, and lipemia affect the amount of light transmitted through the complex. Newer chemistry methods that utilize infrared wavelengths have minimized these problems.

Types of Photometric Testing

Most photometric analyzers utilize endpoint readings. The analyzer then uses either a one-point calibration or an internal standard curve (Fig. 12-3) to calculate the patient results. Some assays utilize kinetic methods rather than endpoint. These are primarily used for enzyme assays or when the reagent is enzyme-based. Kinetic reactions measure changes in color development over specific periods of time. Fixed-time reactions are similar to kinetic except that the color development is not linear at any prolonged point throughout the reaction. These tests utilize

readings at two points during the reaction taken at the times when the reaction is closest to linear.

HEPATOBILIARY FUNCTION TESTING

Hepatic cells exhibit extreme diversity of function and are capable of regeneration if damaged. As a result, there are over 100 types of tests to evaluate liver function. In most cases, evaluation of several liver function tests is required to evaluate the overall status of the liver. Liver cells also compartmentalize the work, so damage to one zone of the liver

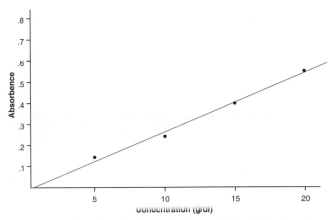

Fig. 12-3 Completed standard curve for hemoglobin plotting absorbance vs. concentration.

may not affect all liver functions. Liver function tests are usually done with serial determinations. Usually, liver disease is greatly progressed before clinical signs appear. Liver function tests are designed to measure substances that are produced by the liver (primarily proteins), modified by the liver (e.g., bilirubin), or released when hepatocytes are damaged (primarily liver enzymes).

The most common type of tests for hepatobiliary disease is the *leakage enzyme tests*, which includes ALT, AST, glutamate dehydrogenase (GD), and sorbitol dehydrogenase (SD) tests. The *cholestatic tests* include the alkaline phosphatase (ALP) and gamma glutamyl transferase (GGT) tests. Other general tests of liver function include total bilirubin, direct bilirubin, indirect bilirubin, bile acids, ammonia, albumin, globulin, and cholesterol.

Following liver parenchymal damage, ALT increases, followed by AST. AST returns to normal more rapidly than ALT, provided there is no subsequent muscle tissue damage. Chronic or ongoing liver damage is likely if ALT and AST both remain elevated.

SD and GD indicate acute damage, but these tend to return to normal within a day or two. SD can be used to determine if an AST increase is due to liver or muscle damage. Cholestatis can result from impaired bile flow or can be drug-induced. ALP and GGT are normally present in very low concentrations in serum.

Impaired bile flow stimulates production of ALP. This may also be linked to retention of bile acids. Increased ALP may also be caused by excessive glucocorticoid concentration or administration of anticonvulsants or megestrol acetate.

Protein

In the small veterinary practice, total protein is usually measured with a refractometer. This instrument gives a measurement of the refractive index of a substance and is a function of the total amount of material dissolved in the plasma. Proteins represent the primary solid component in plasma or serum. Total plasma protein measurements include fibrinogen values. Total serum protein concentrations include all plasma proteins except fibrinogen and certain other coagulation proteins, which have been removed during the coagulation process. The majority of serum proteins are produced by hepatocytes. Most chemical analyses to measure total protein utilize the biuret method, which involves the addition of reagent that acts on molecules with multiple peptide bonds. Precipitation (trichloroacetic acid) and dye-binding (Coomassie blue) methods have been used to measure the low levels of protein found in such fluids as cerebrospinal fluid and urine.

Serum protein levels are affected by the rate of protein synthesis in the liver, the rate of protein catabolism in the animal, hydration status, and alterations in distribution of proteins in the body. Dehydrated animals usually have elevated total protein values; overhydrated animals usually

have decreased total protein values. Other conditions in which total protein concentrations may be helpful include coagulation (clotting) abnormalities, hepatic disease, renal disease, weight loss, diarrhea, edema, and ascites.

Marked hemolysis falsely increases total protein values. Do not use lipemic samples, especially if the refractometric method is used. Moderate icterus has no effect on the refractometric method. Heat, ultraviolet light, surfactant detergents, and chemicals can break down proteins, leading to artificially low results.

Albumin

Albumin is one of the most important proteins in plasma or serum. It makes up approximately 35% to 50% of the total serum protein concentration. Albumin is synthesized by the liver. Severe hepatic insufficiency is a cause of decreased albumin levels. Albumin levels are also influenced by dietary intake, renal disease, and intestinal protein absorption. Albumin functions as a transport and binding protein of the blood and is responsible for maintaining osmotic pressure of plasma.

The most commonly performed test for albumin is the dye-binding assay. The test involves conjugation of albumin to a biological dye (usually bromcresol green) at a specific pH. This test is affected by certain anticoagulants, so plasma samples are not usually used for albumin testing. Hemolysis may increase the apparent albumin level if the bromcresol green method (commonly used in veterinary laboratories) is used. Methods of measurement used in some human laboratories (those that use bromcresol purple) can be unreliable. Check the test protocol for the method used. Keep the sample covered to prevent dehydration, which can falsely elevate protein levels.

Globulin

Globulins are a complex group of proteins that include all of the proteins (plasma or serum) other than albumin and coagulation proteins. The globulins are separated into three major classes by electrophoresis: alpha, beta, and gamma globulins. Most alpha and beta globulins are synthesized by the liver. The proteins in these groups include complement, transferrin, ferritin, other acute-phase proteins of inflammation, and lipoproteins. The gamma globulins (immunoglobulins) are synthesized by plasma cells and are responsible for the body's immunity provided by antibodies. Immunoglobulins identified in animals include IgG, IgD, IgE, IgA, and IgM.

Direct measurement of globulin is not usually performed. Globulin concentration is calculated by subtracting the albumin concentration from the total serum protein.

Albumin-to-globulin ratio

The albumin:globulin (A:G) ratio may be reported on chemistry profiles. The normal A:G ratio is approximately

0.5 to 1.5 across species. An increased A:G ratio may occur with any condition that increases albumin (e.g., dehydration) and/or decreases globulin. A decreased A:G ratio may occur with any condition that decreases albumin and/or increases globulin (e.g., inflammation). Although A:G ratios are frequently reported, they are of little significance without knowledge of the absolute total protein, albumin, and globulin values.

Fibrinogen

Fibrinogen is synthesized by hepatocytes. It is one of the factors necessary for clot formation and is the precursor of fibrin, which is the insoluble protein of blood clots. Clot formation is impaired when fibrinogen concentrations are decreased. Because fibrinogen is removed from plasma when a blood clot forms, no fibrinogen is present in serum. Acute inflammation or tissue damage can elevate fibrinogen levels.

Fibrinogen concentration can be determined with automated analyzers or estimated as described in Chapter 11.

Bilirubin

Bilirubin is an insoluble molecule derived from the breakdown of hemoglobin in the spleen. The molecule is bound to albumin and transported to the liver. The hepatic cells metabolize and conjugate the bilirubin to the molecule bilirubin glucuronide. This molecule is then secreted from the hepatocytes and becomes a component of bile. Bacteria within the gastrointestinal system act on the bilirubin glucuronide and produce a group of compounds collectively referred to as urobilinogen. Urobilinogen is broken down to urobilin before being excreted in feces. Bilirubin glu-

curonide and urobilinogen may also be absorbed directly into the blood and excreted via the kidneys (Fig. 12-4).

Measurements of the circulating levels of these various populations of bilirubin can help to pinpoint the cause of jaundice. Differences in the relative solubility of each of these molecules allow them to be quantified individually. In most animals, the prehepatic (bound to albumin) bilirubin composes about two thirds of the total bilirubin in serum. Alterations in the ratios of the various bilirubin compounds help determine whether liver damage is present or other conditions (e.g., bile duct obstruction) are contributing to disease. Both unconjugated and conjugated bilirubin are found in plasma (and serum). Assays can directly measure total bilirubin (conjugated plus unconjugated) and conjugated bilirubin. Conjugated bilirubin is also referred to as *direct bilirubin*, because test methods directly measure the amount of conjugated bilirubin in the sample. Unconjugated bilirubin is also referred to as *indirect bilirubin*, because it reacts with test substrates only after addition of alcohol (indirect reacting). Measuring the color produced before addition of alcohol gives the concentration of conjugated bilirubin (direct reacting); measuring the color after addition of alcohol gives the concentration of total bilirubin. The concentration of unconjugated (indirect) bilirubin is determined by subtracting the conjugated (direct) bilirubin concentration from the total bilirubin concentration.

Bilirubin is assayed to determine the cause of jaundice (icterus), to evaluate liver function, and to check the patency of bile ducts. Blood levels of conjugated bilirubin are elevated with hepatocellular damage or bile duct injury and/or obstruction. Excessive erythrocyte destruc-

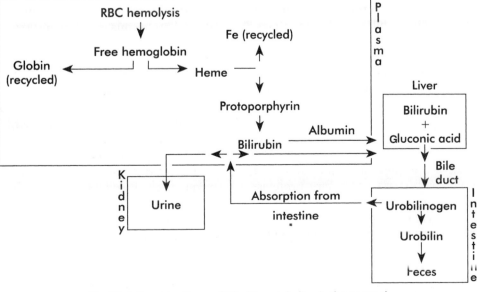

Fig. 12-4 Normal pathway of bilirubin metabolism in the mammal.

tion often results in production of more unconjugated bilirubin than the liver can clear. Initially, the elevated bilirubin levels in the blood are primarily composed of unconjugated bilirubin; however, with time, more and more conjugated bilirubin appears.

Bile acids

Bile acids are produced from cholesterol in the liver and serve many functions, including aiding in fat absorption and modulating cholesterol levels. The gallbladder stores bile acids, and they are then released into the intestinal tract. Most bile acids are actively resorbed in the ileum and carried to the liver where they are reconjugated and excreted as part of the enterohepatic circulation of bile acids (Fig. 12-5). This recirculation functions to conserve bile acids and is so efficient that the entire pool of bile acids is generally recirculated three to five times after every meal, with only small amounts being lost in the feces or bypassing the liver into the systemic circulation. Because of this, blood levels of bile acids in normal animals are very low, especially in fasted animals. When functional hepatic mass is reduced, extraction of bile acids from blood is affected. Measurement of bile acid concentration is, therefore, a good indicator of hepatobiliary function. In general, elevated bile acid concentrations are not specific for the type of underlying disease. Increased bile acid concentrations can also result from extrahepatic diseases (e.g., hyperadrenocorticism) that secondarily affect the liver. In small animals, measurement of bile acids in paired (fasting and 2-hour postprandial) samples is often useful in increasing the overall test sensitivity. Cholestasis causes backup of bile acids into blood (along with conjugated bilirubin). Other variables independent of hepatobiliary function affect bile acid concentrations including decreased gastrointestinal transit time or spontaneous gallbladder contraction. Prolonged fasting, intestinal malabsorption, or increased intestinal transit time through the bowel (e.g., diarrhea) can lower bile acid concentrations. In horses, increased bile acid concentrations result from hepatobiliary disease or decreased feed intake. Most horses with hepatobiliary disease have markedly increased bile acid concentrations. The normal bovine has extremely variable serum bile acids concentration, making the test ineffective in detection of disease.

Ammonia

Ammonia is produced in the intestine (primarily in the colon) from the action of bacteria on dietary proteins. Ammonia is absorbed in the intestine and carried in the portal vein to the liver, where it is effectively cleared from the circulation. The hepatocytes convert ammonia to urea via the urea cycle. Much like bile acids, blood ammonia levels are increased with reduced hepatic mass and abnormalities in portal circulation. Ammonia levels have been measured in cases of suspected hepatic encephalopathy.

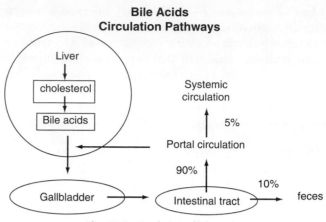

Fig. 12-5 Circulation of bile acids.

Samples for ammonia determination are not stable and must be stored on ice immediately after collection, centrifuged in a refrigerated centrifuge, separated from the RBCs, and assayed as soon as possible (preferably within 15 minutes). Sample collection must be as smooth as possible, because occlusion of a vein for prolonged periods results in ammonia accumulation.

Cholesterol

Cholesterol is produced in almost every cell in the body and is especially abundant in hepatocytes, adrenal cortex, ovaries, testes, and intestinal epithelium. The liver is the primary site of synthesis in most animals. Cholesterol levels are frequently elevated in animals with hypothyroidism, although other conditions may also result in increased cholesterol levels. These include hyperadrenocorticism, diabetes mellitus, and nephrotic syndrome. Dietary causes of hypercholesterolemia are rare but may include very-high-fat diets or postprandial lipemia. (*Note:* Cholesterol alone does not cause the grossly lipemic plasma seen after eating. This lipemia is due to the presence of triglycerides.)

Enzyme Analyses

Enzymes are specialized proteins that catalyze various chemical reactions. Most enzymes work intracellularly at a very specific pH. Enzymes are usually not present in high concentrations in serum. Increased concentrations of enzymes in serum often indicate cellular damage. Enzyme assays usually involve measurement of the outcome of enzyme activity rather than specific measurement of the enzyme itself. Enzymes related to liver function in most mammals include the phosphatases, transaminases, and dehydrogenases.

Phosphatases

Blood contains two major groups of phosphatases. They are the alkaline phosphatases (ALPs) and the acid phosphatases (ACPs). Determinations of ACP levels are not commonly done, but may help in diagnosis of certain types of hemolytic anemia. ALPs are isoenzymes with multiple organ sources, including the liver, kidney, bone, and intestine. The extent of the increase aids in determining whether the patient has intrahepatic damage or extrahepatic damage. The half-lives of intestinal and renal isoenzymes are extremely short (minutes), as compared with the half-lives of hepatic enzymes (hours to days). Because of this, the intestinal and renal isoenzymes of ALP are not usually found in serum (or plasma) in high concentrations. Special analytic methods in commercial or research laboratories can be used to determine which isoenzyme is increased. Increases in circulating levels of ALPs are almost always due to liver damage.

ALP is most often used to detect cholestasis in dogs and cats. Production of ALP is induced by increased pressure within the biliary system during any form of cholestasis. The cholestasis may be intrahepatic because of tumors, swelling, inflammation, or anything blocking bile flow, or it may be extrahepatic because of bile duct obstruction. ALP is a sensitive indicator of cholestasis in dogs and cats, but it is not useful in large animals because of the wide variation of ALP concentrations found in normal large animal species.

In dogs, certain drugs induce ALP synthesis. The magnitude of increase may be great. The most commonly used drugs that induce ALP synthesis are glucocorticoids, such as prednisone or cortisone. Exogenously administered or endogenous (due to hyperadrenocorticism) glucocorticoids stimulate this effect. It occurs through induction of a unique isoenzyme of ALP. Anticonvulsants, such as phenobarbital, primidone, and diphenylhydantoin, also induce synthesis of ALP (hepatic isoenzyme). These increases in ALP are due to drug induction and do not necessarily indicate liver disease.

ALP levels can be increased in young growing animals because of bone remodeling and increases in the bone isoenzyme. Other causes of increased osteoblastic activity, such as primary hyperparathyroidism, fracture healing, and neoplasia, can also result in increased serum ALP activity. Placental ALP is present in mares and queens during pregnancy.

Transferases

This group of enzymes is found primarily in tissues that have high rates of protein metabolism, especially kidney, liver, and muscle. In veterinary medicine, the transferases of clinical significance are GGT, ALT, and AST. In dogs and cats, damage to hepatocytes results in release of large amounts of ALT. In other species, ALT levels have little clinical significance. AST assays are used primarily to evaluate the extent of skeletal muscle damage in the equine and may also be used to evaluate cardiac muscle damage in some species.

Gamma glutamyltransferase. GGT is similar to ALP in that it is bound to microsomal membranes within the cell. Serum levels of GGT are increased when the cell is stimulated to increase synthesis. GGT is present in most cells but is found in high concentration in liver, pancreatic, and renal tubular cells. GGT from renal tubular cells is released into the urine during renal tubular damage, not into the blood. Pancreatic GGT is apparently secreted into the intestines and also does not cause elevated serum concentrations. Therefore, serum GGT is considered a liver-specific enzyme. As with ALP, the major inducer of hepatic GGT is cholestasis. This occurs in all species. GGT is an excellent indicator of cholestasis in horses, ruminants, and swine. GGT can also be used in dogs and cats, although it offers no advantage over ALP for these species.

Alanine aminotransferase. ALT is formerly known as serum glutamate pyruvate transaminase (SGPT). This enzyme is considered a liver-specific enzyme and a good indicator of hepatocellular damage in dogs, cats, and primates because the primary/major source of serum ALT is the hepatocyte. It is not useful in large animal species, such as horses, cattle, sheep, and pigs, because the hepatocytes of these species contain insignificant amounts of ALT.

Aspartate aminotransferase. AST is formerly known as serum glutamate oxaloacetate transaminase (SGOT). Hepatocytes are one source of serum AST, but there are other sources. Both skeletal and cardiac muscle contain significant amounts of AST. Other sources include erythrocytes, kidneys, and pancreas. Increased levels of AST indicate liver or muscle damage. It is important to remember that AST is not considered a liver-specific enzyme.

Dehydrogenases

This group of enzymes functions in cellular metabolism and include the lactate dehydrogenases (LD) and the sorbitol dehydrogenases (SD). Any disease characterized by membrane defect will result in release of LD into surrounding tissue. SD is present in a variety of organs, but in most species it has the greatest concentrations in the liver. SD is the preferred assay to evaluate equine liver function.

Lactate dehydrogenase. Lactate dehydrogenase (LD) values are frequently included in biochemistry profiles. This enzyme is not considered organ-specific, because it has many sources and the concentrations in each tissue are not high enough to result in significant elevations. LD is found in the liver, skeletal muscle, cardiac muscle, kidney, leukocytes, erythrocytes, and skin.

Sorbitol dehydrogenase. Sorbitol dehydrogenase (SD) is found in high concentrations in hepatocytes of all species, including large animals, and is considered a liver-specific enzyme. SD is unstable, and serum activity decreases rapidly. Samples should be analyzed within 12 hours of collection.

Glutamate dehydrogenase. GD is highly concentrated in the liver of cattle and sheep, as well as in the liver of other species. Increased serum values of GD indicate hepatic necrosis. GD is considered a liver-specific enzyme.

Other enzymes

Other enzymes can leak from damaged or dead liver cells. However, no standard methodology has been developed for laboratory testing, and enzymes are not routinely measured. Following are enzymes that are occasionally assayed.

Arginase. Arginase is present in significant concentrations in the liver of mammals. Studies evaluating arginase levels in dogs, cats, horses, sheep, and pigs have been published. It is considered a liver-specific enzyme, and increased serum values indicate hepatic necrosis.

Ornithine carbamoyltransferase. Similar to GD, ornithine carbamoyltransferase (OCT) is a liver-specific enzyme that indicates liver necrosis. Studies have been conducted on cattle, swine, and dogs.

Kidney Function Testing

The kidneys have an important role in the homeostatic mechanisms of the body. They function to maintain the volume and composition of extracellular fluid and are involved in excretion of metabolic waste products and other chemicals. The functional unit of the kidney is the *nephron*, which consists of a network of capillaries (the glomerulus) and tubules that are lined with epithelial cells. Nearly all blood constituents pass through the glomerulus and enter the tubules. In a normally functioning nephron, about 80% of the water and all of the amino acids and glucose that enter the tubules are either reabsorbed or actively transported back into circulation. Ions (primarily sodium, chloride, and bicarbonate) are also selectively reabsorbed. Any constituent not reabsorbed or transported back into circulation is excreted in the urine.

Kidney damage may result in an inability of the glomerulus to retain cells and proteins, or impair the resorptive capability of the tubules. The primary chemical tests of kidney function are urea nitrogen and creatinine.

Urea nitrogen

Urea nitrogen (BUN) is the principal product of protein catabolism. Normally, all urea passes through the glomerulus and about half is reabsorbed by passive diffusion.

Azotemia (increase in urea nitrogen levels) can occur when blood flow through the kidneys alters the glomerular filtration rate, or when the urinary tract is obstructed. Dehydration will also result in azotemia since urea must be excreted in a large amount of water. Differences in rates of protein catabolism between male and female animals, young and adult animals, different species, and nutritional status will also affect blood urea nitrogen (BUN) levels.

The majority of tests for urea nitrogen are photometric analyses.

Creatinine

Serum creatinine is produced from metabolic breakdown of phosphocreatine in muscle tissue. The day-to-day rate of creatinine production is relatively constant in any animal and is dependent on muscle mass. Creatinine is also primarily cleared by the kidney. Glomerular filtration is the primary mode of elimination. Creatinine is minimally resorbed by the tubules, so it is not influenced by the rate of urine flow, as is BUN.

Creatinine is used to evaluate renal function based on the ability of the glomeruli to filter creatinine from the blood and eliminate it in urine. Like BUN, if serum creatinine values are increased because of decreased renal function, this indicates that approximately 75% of the nephrons are nonfunctional.

Creatinine testing is often done in conjunction with urea nitrogen testing. An alteration in the ratio of the concentrations of these two components is a more significant indicator of renal disease than individual measurements of either component. There are a number of photometric procedures available for serum creatinine testing.

Uric acid

Uric acid is an end product of catabolism of nucleic acids. It is the primary end product of nitrogen metabolism in avian species, and is actively secreted by the renal tubules. Measurement of plasma or serum uric acid is therefore preferred over urea levels as an indicator of kidney function in birds. In most animals, uric acid is bound to albumin, passes through the glomerulus, and then is reabsorbed. It is usually converted to allantion and excreted in the urine. In Dalmatian dogs, the liver is unable to convert uric acid, so these animals excrete uric acid rather than allantion. This also predisposes the breed to urate urolithiasis. Photometric analysis of uric acid is a complex procedure not commonly performed in veterinary clinical practice. However, newer methods of chemical analysis using liquid stable reagents can allow for uric acid testing in the veterinary practice laboratory. In birds, increases in uric acid concentration can be an artifact seen when samples are collected from a toenail that has fecal urate contamination.

Pancreatic Function Testing

The pancreas functions as both an endocrine and exocrine organ. Endocrine functions include the production of the hormones insulin and glucagon. Exocrine activities of the pancreas involve the production of digestive enzymes (Table 12-2). Trauma to pancreatic tissue is often associated with pancreatic duct inflammation that results in a backup of digestive enzymes into peripheral circulation.

TABLE 12-2

Major Pancreatic Enzymes

Enzyme	Digestive Activity
Amylase	Carbohydrates
Lipase	Lipids
Nucleases	Nucleic acids
Chymotrypsinogen	Protein
Trypsinogen	Protein

Amylase

Amylase is produced in a variety of tissues, including the salivary glands, small intestine, and pancreas and functions in the breakdown of starch to glucose. The majority of amylase test methods are photometric assays that utilize starch as a substrate in the test system. Serial determinations of amylase in conjunction with lipase provide the best indication of pancreatic function.

Nearly all serum lipase is derived from the pancreas. Excess lipase is easily filtered through the kidneys, so lipase levels tend to remain normal in early stages of pancreatic disease. Gradual increases are seen as disease progresses. With chronic, progressive pancreatic disease, damaged pancreatic cells are replaced with connective tissue that cannot produce enzyme. As this occurs, amylase and lipase levels both decrease. Tests for serum lipase involve a substrate such as oil with the resulting products measured photometrically.

The sources of amylase activity are the pancreas, small intestine, and liver. Amylase functions in the breakdown of starches and glycogen in sugars to form such sugars as maltose and residual glucose. Increased levels of amylase can occur with acute pancreatitis, flareups of chronic pancreatitis, and obstruction of the pancreatic ducts.

Nonpancreatic disease may also increase serum amylase levels. Most commonly, amylase levels are elevated with renal disease. Renal disease can cause amylase levels that are approximately 2.5 times the upper limit of normal. Increased amylase levels have also been reported with certain liver and intestinal diseases (intestinal obstructions).

Amylase levels can be determined by two methods: *amyloclastic or saccharogenic.* Amyloclastic methods measure the rate of disappearance of starch and should be used for canine serum. Saccharogenic methods, which measure the rate of appearance of reducing sugars and are valid for humans, give falsely elevated results in canine samples because of other enzymes found in canine serum.

Lipase

Lipase functions to break down the long-chain fatty acids of lipids. In experimental pancreatitis, lipase levels rise rapidly and are elevated for more than a week. Clinical cases are not as consistent, and not all animals with pancreatitis have elevated lipase levels. Some studies suggest that lipase is more valuable than amylase because it is more consistently elevated.

Lipase activity may also be elevated by nonpancreatic factors, such as chronic renal failure, exploratory surgery, and corticosteroid use.

Test methods for determining lipase activity are usually based on hydrolysis of an olive oil emulsion into its constituent fatty acids. The quantity of NaOH required to neutralize the fatty acids provides a measure of lipase activity.

Glucose

A small portion of the pancreas is involved in the production of insulin. Insulin is required to facilitate the uptake of glucose by body cells. Blood glucose measurements provide an indicator of the status of pancreatic endocrine activity. However, these can be affected by a variety of factors, including diet and stress. The blood glucose level reflects the net balance between glucose production (dietary intake, conversion from other carbohydrates) and glucose utilization (energy expended, conversion to other products). It also reflects the balance between blood insulin and glucagon levels.

Glucose utilization depends on the amount of insulin and glucagon being produced by the pancreas. As the blood insulin level increases, so does the rate of glucose utilization, resulting in decreased blood glucose levels. Glucagon acts as a stabilizer to prevent blood glucose levels from becoming too low. As the insulin level decreases, so does glucose utilization, resulting in increased blood glucose concentration. Although excess serum glucose can result from a variety of disease conditions, the highest blood glucose values are seen in diabetes mellitus. This condition results from either decreased or defective production of insulin. Without sufficient insulin, the body cells are unable to take up glucose. Although the nephron normally resorbs blood glucose from the filtrate, excess glucose cannot be effectively resorbed by the nephron. This results in glycosuria (glucose in the urine). Glycosuria alters the solute concentration of the filtrate and causes an increased loss of electrolytes and nitrogen into the urine.

A variety of photometric test methods are available to evaluate blood glucose. Dedicated instruments for blood glucose testing are also readily available. Most of these were initially designed for use in human medicine to allow diabetic patients to monitor their own blood glucose levels. It is vital that the blood serum or plasma be removed from contact with the erythrocytes immediately after blood collection. If the sample is left in contact with the erythrocytes, the blood glucose levels will drop up to 10% per hour at room temperature. Erythrocytes use glucose for energy. In a blood sample, erythrocytes may decrease the glucose level

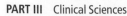

enough to give false-normal results if the original sample had an elevated glucose level. If the sample originally had a normal glucose level, a falsely low level may result. If the blood sample cannot be centrifuged and the serum or plasma is not separated from the erythrocytes, collect the sample in a sodium fluoride tube. This anticoagulant tube contains potassium oxalate. The sodium fluoride inhibits utilization of glucose by erythrocytes and therefore stabilizes glucose levels in the sample. Glucose levels remain stable for 12 hours at room temperature and for 48 hours if the sample is refrigerated. Fill this tube at least halfway with blood; otherwise the fluoride concentration may be high enough to interfere with glucose analysis.

Refrigeration slows glucose utilization by erythrocytes. Because eating raises the blood glucose level and fasting decreases it, a 12-hour fast is recommended when possible for all animals, except for mature ruminants, before the blood sample is collected.

Fructosamine

Fructosamine is a more specific indicator of pancreatic endocrine activity than glucose. Fructosamine is a glycosylated serum protein. The reaction between glucose and the protein is irreversible. It therefore provides an indication of the average glucose levels over the life span of the protein (approximately 1 to 3 weeks).

Traditional test methods for fructosamine were complicated and difficult to perform in-house. New technology now makes these methods practical for in-house testing.

β-Hydroxybutyrate

When cells cannot utilize glucose for energy, other metabolic pathways are activated. Although the same pathways are used in normal metabolism, cells of the diabetic patient overutilize these pathways. This leads to the buildup of abnormal levels of metabolic by-products, such as ketones. Ketones cause decreased body pH and affect all metabolic systems. This condition is known as *ketoacidosis*. The primary ketone produced in ketoacidosis is β-hydroxybutyrate (βHB). Test kits are now available that allow this testing to be performed in-house.

Creatine kinase

Creatine kinase (CK), also referred to as *creatine phosphokinase (CPK)*, is a cytoplasmic enzyme that appears in the serum in increased concentrations after cellular injury. This enzyme consists of three isoenzymes: CK_1, CK_2, and CK_3. CK_1 is found in neurologic tissue, cerebrospinal fluid, and viscera. This isoenzyme is not present in serum and/or plasma. CK_2 is found mainly in cardiac muscle. CK_3 is found in skeletal and cardiac muscle. The last two isoenzymes are present in serum and/or plasma. Therefore, changes in CK concentrations are specific for muscle (skeletal and cardiac) injury or necrosis.

CK is a very sensitive enzyme, and serum levels can be dramatically increased after relatively minor insults to muscle. Intramuscular injections are enough to raise CK levels several times above the normal range. Other causes of muscle damage include the following:

- Inflammatory myopathies from infectious causes (e.g., *Clostridium*) or noninfectious causes (e.g., immune-mediated, eosinophilic)
- Traumatic myopathies (e.g., accidental, postoperative, downer animals, CNS diseases, seizures)
- Degenerative myopathies (e.g., muscular dystrophy, myotonia, hyperadrenocorticism, hypothyroidism, equine rhabdomyolysis, transport myopathy, malignant hyperthermia, capture myopathy)
- Nutritional myopathies (e.g., vitamin E/selenium deficiency)
- Ischemic myopathies (e.g., bacteria endocarditis, heartworm disease, thrombosis)

Aspartate aminotransferase

AST is a cytoplasmic enzyme found in most tissues, but is in highest concentrations in the liver and muscle. Increased serum AST levels are due to hepatic injury (as previously discussed), muscle cell injury, or hemolysis. Elevations of AST along with elevations of CK suggest muscle damage. Elevations in AST with normal CK levels suggest hepatocellular injury or prior muscle injury in which the CK level has returned to normal.

Lactate dehydrogenase

Like CK, lactate dehydrogenase (LD) is a serum enzyme with many isoenzymes. Different amounts of isoenzymes are present in different tissues. Almost all tissues have LD, although liver, muscle, and erythrocytes are the major sources of increased blood LD levels. As compared with CK, the magnitude of LD rise is less dramatic following muscle injury.

Electrolytes

Electrolytes are minerals that exist as positively charged or negatively charged particles in an aqueous solution. Positively charged particles are called *cations*, and negatively charged particles are called *anions*. These particles play essential roles in processes that are vital to normal physiologic function and life. They function primarily in regulation of acid/base and osmotic balance of the body. There are two commonly used methods of measuring electrolytes: *flame photometry* and *ion-specific electrodes*. Flame photometry has been the standard for many years and is still used in some laboratories. This method measures concentrations of electrolytes relative to the entire plasma volume. Ion-specific electrodes, which more recently have achieved wider use, measure the concentration of electrolytes relative to the amount of plasma water. Automated ion specific instruments are readily available and reasonably priced, so many veterinary practices now have the ability to perform electrolyte testing. Plasma is approximately 93% water, with the remaining percentage composed of lipids and proteins; electrolytes are distributed only in the water phase. Samples that are hyperlipemic or hyperproteinemic may demonstrate reduction in electrolyte activity due to displacement of plasma water by lipids or proteins.

Some of the functions of electrolytes include maintenance of water balance and fluid osmotic pressure, normal conduction of nervous impulses, normal contraction of muscles, and maintenance and regulation of body fluid pH. Electrolytes also function as vital cofactors in many enzymatically mediated metabolic reactions.

The electrolytes that are most commonly measured are sodium, potassium, chloride, calcium, inorganic phosphorus, and magnesium. Electrolytes can be measured using serum or heparinized plasma. It is important to remember that different salts of heparin are available: sodium heparin, potassium heparin, ammonium heparin, and lithium heparin. When selecting an anticoagulant, do not choose a form of heparin that contains the substance that is being measured.

Sodium

Sodium (Na) is the major cation of plasma and interstitial fluid. Plasma and interstitial fluid make up what is known as *extracellular fluid*. Sodium plays an important role in maintaining extracellular fluid and vascular volume, because it is the most important contributor to effective osmolality. *Effective osmolality* is a term used to describe the number of particles that cannot easily cross cellular membranes (impermeant particles) in a solution. Effective osmolality is the major factor in determining fluid shifts between intracellular and extracellular fluid. *Hyponatremia* (decreased sodium) causes hypoosmolality and movement of fluid from the vascular space to the intracellular space. This causes vascular hypovolemia and may result in cellular swelling. *Hypernatremia* (increased sodium) results in hyperosmolality and movement of intracellular water into the extracellular space, leading to cellular dehydration.

Potassium

Potassium (K) is the major intracellular cation. Because potassium is found predominantly intracellularly, the measure of plasma potassium concentration is not necessarily a good indicator of total body potassium. Potassium distribution across the cell membrane is important in normal function of cardiac and neuromuscular tissues. *Hypokalemia* (decreased potassium) decreases cell excitability, causing weakness and paralysis. *Hyperkalemia* (increased potassium) increases cell excitability; the most serious manifestation is abnormal cardiac rhythm.

Using potassium heparin as the anticoagulant may result in falsely elevated values. Hemolysis may falsely elevate the results in large animal species (cattle, horses, pigs, some species of sheep) because intraerythrocytic potassium concentrations are higher than potassium concentrations in plasma (or serum). This is not true for cats and most species of dogs. Mild hemolysis in cats and dogs does not affect plasma or serum potassium concentration. One notable exception is the Akita. This breed of dog has high intraerythrocytic potassium concentrations. Platelets and leukocytes have enough intracellular potassium to affect plasma potassium levels only if they are present in markedly increased numbers and the plasma is not separated from the clot quickly.

Chloride

Chloride (Cl) is the predominant extracellular anion and is an important component of serum osmolality. It also helps to maintain electroneutrality (equal number of positive and negative charges) for all of the sodium present.

An increase in chloride is termed *hyperchloremia;* a decrease is termed *hypochloremia*.

Calcium

Approximately 99% of calcium (Ca) in the body is found in bones. Only a small percentage of calcium is present in extracellular fluid (including blood), but its presence is essential. Calcium ions are required for preservation of skeletal structure, muscle contraction, blood coagulation, activation of several enzymes, transmission of nerve impulses, and decreasing cell membrane and capillary permeability. Calcium in whole blood is found primarily in plasma (or serum), as erythrocytes contain very little calcium.

An increase in calcium is termed *hypercalcemia;* a decrease is termed *hypocalcemia*. Although not a specific indicator of pancreatic function, serum calcium levels are often altered as a result of the acidosis found in many diabetic patients. In normal animals, calcium levels remain fairly constant. Assays for total serum calcium employ photometric methods. Do not use EDTA or oxalate anticoagulants when collecting samples for calcium analysis, because they bind calcium and therefore make it unavailable for assay. Hemolysis may result in a slight decrease because of dilution with erythrocytic fluid.

Inorganic phosphorus

More than 80% of the phosphorus (P) in the body is found in bones, with less than 20% in extracellular fluids. These extracellular phosphorus ions play an important role in carbohydrate metabolism as metabolic intermediates and high-energy phosphate bonds. Phosphorus is also a component of nucleic acids, phospholipids, nucleotides, and body fluid buffers. Most of the phosphorus in whole blood is found within erythrocytes as organic phosphorus (phosphoric esters). The phosphorus in plasma and serum is inorganic, and it is usually measured in the laboratory.

An increase in phosphorus is termed *hyperphosphatemia;* a decrease is termed *hypophosphatemia.*

Magnesium

Magnesium (Mg) is the fourth most common cation in the body and the second most common intracellular cation. Magnesium is found in all body tissues, although approximately 60% is found in bones. It is an activator (catalyst) for many biological enzymes, and the actions of magnesium extend to all major anabolic and catabolic processes. Magnesium balance is primarily affected by absorption from the gastrointestinal tract and excretion by the kidney. Clinical disorders related to magnesium deficiency are primarily seen in cattle and sheep, although disorders of magnesium metabolism have been reported in cats, horses, and goats.

An increase in magnesium is termed *hypermagnesemia;* a decrease is termed *hypomagnesemia.*

BASIC PRINCIPLES OF IMMUNOLOGY

The term *immune system* refers to a variety of cells, tissues, organs, and organ systems that are involved in the body's defense mechanisms. Some components are present and active in the body at all times. Others are created or activated in response to a foreign substance. Immunity can generally be divided into two types: *passive* and *active.* Passive immunity includes maternal antibodies from colostrum and physicochemical barriers, such as the skin and mucous membranes. Active immunity is developed or acquired and is classified as *humoral* or *cell-mediated* immunity.

Humoral immunity is mediated by production of unique proteins *(antibodies),* which are responsible for specific recognition and elimination of antigens. Foreign substances that are capable of generating a response from the immune system are referred to as *antigens.* Antigens include bacteria, viruses, parasites, or even the body's own tissues. Specific substances on the surface of the antigen are responsible for the recognition of an antigen by the body's immune system. These substances are usually proteins and act as "markers" for the immune system. Recognition of these markers often results in the formation of antibody by the immune system. When antibodies are produced, the immune system retains a memory of the antigen and can respond more quickly to future attacks by the same antigen.

Cell-mediated immunity is dependent on cells, in particular lymphocytes. Like antibodies, these lymphocytes recognize specific antigens, such as those of fungi, parasites, intracellular bacteria, or tumor cells, and help remove them from the animal by lysing the infected/cancerous cell or organism (Table 12-3).

Components of the immune system that are present continuously include the skin, mucous membranes, and certain body fluids and cells. These components are collectively referred to as the *natural defenses* and provide physical and/or chemical barriers to invasion by antigens. The natural defenses generally act in the same manner regardless of which specific antigen is encountered. For example, hydrochloric acid in the stomach or lysozymes in saliva both are capable of destroying bacterial antigens. The action of the hydrochloric acid and lysozymes is similar regardless of the specific bacteria present. Similarly, intact skin acts as a physical barrier to prevent antigens from entering the body.

Components of the immune system that are involved in reacting to specific antigens include several types of white blood cells and a number of biochemicals. These components are collectively referred to as the *adaptive defenses.* The biochemicals are primarily enzyme systems that function in the formation of antibodies. The major enzyme system is known as the *complement system.* The complement system represents a series of enzymes that must react in a stepwise fashion in order to function. The completion of each step results in generation of additional compounds whose end result will be neutralization or lysis of the

TABLE 12-3

Humoral Immune Response vs. Cell-mediated Immune Response

	Humoral Immune Response	Cell-mediated Immune Response
Cell type involved	B lymphocyte that transforms into a plasma cell after antigenic stimulation	T lymphocyte that transforms into a cytotoxic T cell, helper T cell, or suppressor T cell after antigenic stimulation
Substance produced	Immunoglobulins (antibodies)	Lymphokines
Cellular mobility	B lymphocytes and plasma cells stay in lymphoid tissue; antibodies are released into plasma	T lymphocytes can enter circulation and travel to the site where an antigen entered the body

antigen. Additional biochemicals are involved in the formation of specific antibodies.

Role of White Blood Cells in Immunity

Each of the white blood cells (leukocytes) has a specific role within the immune system. Most mammals have two types of white blood cells: *granulocytes* and *agranulocytes*.

Granulocytes

Granulocytes play a role in both the natural defenses and the adaptive defenses. Both eosinophils and basophils are involved in the inflammatory response generated when an antigen invades the body. Eosinophils and basophils release specific chemicals to help activate other aspects of the immune system. Neutrophils also play a major role in the immune response. The respiratory, digestive, and urinary systems contain groups of neutrophils, referred to as *resident neutrophils*, which act as scavengers and function to phagocytize foreign substances. Phagocytosis literally means "cell eating." The neutrophils release chemicals that damage the foreign agent and then engulf the antigen. This phagocytic activity is part of the natural defenses. When these defenses are incapable of fully neutralizing the antigen, the neutrophils become active within the adaptive defenses. Specific neutrophils function in the adaptive defenses by "processing" the antigen and "presenting" it to a cell that is capable of triggering the cascade of reactions that result in antibody formation. Antigen processing is a complex process that results in exposure of the surface marker protein on the antigen. This allows for recognition of the antigen as a foreign substance. The neutrophil then interacts with another cell that will respond by triggering additional parts of the adaptive defenses.

Agranulocytes

Monocytes and lymphocytes each have unique roles within the immune system. Monocytes act in a manner similar to phagocytic neutrophils. They are often referred to as *tissue macrophages* and are capable of phagocytosis, and antigen processing and presentation. Lymphocytes are the primary cellular components of the antibody-producing systems. Specific subpopulations or subgroups of lymphocytes each play a specific role in this process. These subgroups are referred to as T-lymphocytes and B-lymphocytes. Although there are no apparent differences in appearance of the cells in different subgroups, they are biochemically and functionally diverse groups that are derived and matured in different ways and in different locations in the body.

T-lymphocytes are involved in assisting in full activation of B-lymphocytes (although B-lymphocytes can be activated without this interaction). B-lymphocytes are responsible for creation and secretion of antibody that is specific for a certain antigen. The process is triggered when an antigen-presenting cell (e.g., macrophage or neutrophil) presents an antigen to a B-lymphocyte. That specific B-lymphocyte then is sensitized to that particular antigen and begins to synthesize and release antibody. B-lymphocytes have an additional capability of memory. As B-lymphocytes are maturing, they develop with the capability of producing antibody against a specific antigen that has been presented to them during their maturation. When an antigen that has been previously encountered by a B-lymphocyte is encountered again, the B-lymphocyte is able to respond more quickly and begin producing antibody almost immediately. The production of specific antibody is referred to as *humoral immunity* since the antibody is secreted into the body fluids, or humors. T-lymphocytes, in addition to their role in the activation of B-lymphocytes, are also capable of direct attack on antigens. This is referred to a *cellular immunity*.

Antibodies

The production of a specific antibody is a critical part of the immune system response. Antibodies are protein molecules produced by a certain subgroup of B-lymphocytes when they are presented with a substance that is recognized as foreign (the antigen).

Antibodies are also referred to as *immunoglobulins* and are present in several forms in the body. Each type is responsible for a specific activity within the immune system. The five types of antibodies are referred to with the abbreviation Ig (for immunoglobulin) followed by a letter that designates the type of antibody (Fig. 12-6). The five types of antibodies found in most mammalian organisms are IgG, IgM, IgA, IgD, and IgE.

Each antibody is produced at a specific time in the immune system response. Some are also produced when certain types of antigens are involved (e.g., parasites). Over the past two decades, in-house diagnostic testing has taken an increasing role in small animal veterinary clinics. Where once we had limited ability to perform accurate testing in-house for common canine and feline diseases, we now have the ability to perform nearly all essential testing in-house. This is particularly true of immunological testing for viral and parasitic diseases. These tests are referred to as *immunoassays*. An immunoassay is any test that uses interactions between antibody and antigen to produce a result.

In general, these tests are very easy to perform, take minimal time, and are relatively inexpensive. However, a few in-house immunoassays have developed reputations for unusually high levels of false-positive or false-negative results. In nearly all cases, the incidence of false results is due to errors by the operator in performing the test.

The antigens are usually present in the blood, so the sample used for immunoassays is often a blood sample. Depending on the test being used, the sample may be whole, anticoagulated blood, serum, or plasma. A few immunoassays may use urine, feces, or saliva as the sample.

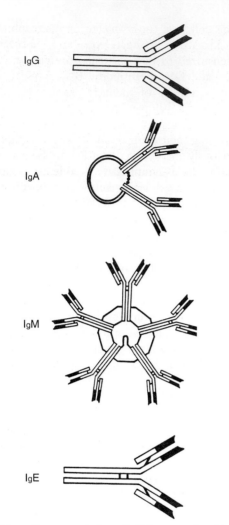

IgG

IgA

IgM

IgE

Fig. 12-6 Schematic representation of IgM (pentamer) and IgG and IgE (monomers) and IgA (dimer). *(From Gershwin:* Immunology and immunopathology of domestic animals, *ed 2, St Louis, 1995, Mosby.)*

With a few exceptions, in-house immunologic test kits utilize enzyme-linked immunosorbent assay (ELISA) or immunochromatography (ICT) assay methods. It is vital that veterinary technicians understand the principles of these in-house immunologic tests to avoid false results.

TYPES OF IMMUNOLOGIC TESTS

Dysfunction of the immune system can lead to an overactive immune system that produces immune-mediated disease, or an underactive immune system that produces immunodeficiency disorders. These disorders can involve any component of the immune system (passive, humoral, or cell-mediated). In addition, the cellular components of the immune system can undergo neoplastic transformation, resulting in lymphoma or plasma-cell tumor. Serologic testing is based on the ability to detect antibody-antigen

interactions. Immunoassays most often contain monoclonal antibodies to an antigen or part of an antigen, such as a viral capsule or a surface protein of a parasite. The tests, therefore, detect that portion of the antigen for which the test kit manufacturer has created a specific antibody. There are a few tests that detect circulating antibody, rather than antigen, but these are only used when the antigen is not readily available for testing. Serologic tests formerly required a reference laboratory; however, many kits are now available for in-house testing for a variety of infectious agents (Table 11-13). Many kits are based on ELISA technology and may detect either antigens (organism) or antibodies (humoral immune response), depending on the kit.

Enzyme-Linked Immunosorbent Assay

ELISA tests are the most common types of immunologic tests performed in veterinary clinics. Every ELISA test has the same basic components:

- solid phase
- conjugate
- chromogen

The solid phase may be a microwell, wand, flow-through membrane, or chromatographic strip. Conjugate reagents are imbedded on the solid phase and usually consist of monoclonal antibodies bound to an enzyme. The chromogen is a photosensitive reagent that produces a color change in the test system. Adding patient sample to the solid phase is the first step in the test. The sample is allowed to incubate. If specific antigen is present in the sample, it will bind to the antibody on the test surface. After the appropriate incubation time, the patient sample is washed away. If antigen has bound to the solid phase, it will not be washed away. Chromogen is then added that can react with the bound enzyme-antigen-antibody complex, if present, and produce a color change in the test system (Fig. 12-7).

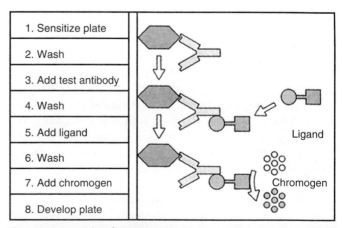

| 1. Sensitize plate |
| 2. Wash |
| 3. Add test antibody |
| 4. Wash |
| 5. Add ligand |
| 6. Wash |
| 7. Add chromogen |
| 8. Develop plate |

Ligand

Chromogen

Fig. 12-7 Principle of ELISA reaction. *(From Roitt I, Brostoff J, Male D:* Immunology, *ed 3, London, 1993, Mosby.)*

Immunochromatography

The ICT assay is similar to the ELISA method except that gold staining is used to replace the chromagen. This format has become more common in veterinary practice in recent years. In ICT test formats, also known as *lateral flow assays*, the conjugate is an antibody bound to colloidal gold or latex, instead of an enzyme. The solid phase of an ICT test is a chromatographic strip. Most ICT tests require a flow solution, usually a buffered saline, to aid in the movement of the sample across the chromatographic strip. Some ICT tests do not require flow solution since the sample volume is large enough to flow onto the solid phase without additional steps. The ICT method does not use temperature-sensitive enzymes, so the test kit can be kept at room temperature.

Chromatographic strips have been used for many years in reference laboratories in the performance of certain serum chemistry assays. The ICT test is performed by adding patient sample to the absorptive pad on the solid phase. The absorptive pad functions to absorb the sample and filter out solid substances, such as blood cells. The conjugate is released as the sample flows onto the solid phase. The sample and conjugate then pass across two test areas. The first test area, known as the patient line, contains antibodies to the antigen being tested for. If the antigen is present in the sample, they will bind to the antibodies on the patient line. When that occurs, conjugate also reacts and produces a color change on the patient line. The sample and conjugate continue to flow to the second test area. The second area is a control line that contains antibodies to the conjugate. A color change is produced on this line and indicates that the test is functioning correctly

Agglutination Test

Agglutination tests are used for detection of antibodies to large particulate antigens. The test requires adding a specific antigen to the test sample. If the sample contains the antibody for that antigen, agglutination (clumping) occurs.

In some agglutination tests, the antigen may be coated with latex beads to induce agglutination reactions. Agglutination tests are usually performed on a slide. Latex agglutination is commonly used to diagnose brucellosis in dogs. Latex particles are coated with *Brucella* antigen. Serum from the patient is added to these particles. If the animal's serum contains antibodies to *Brucella*, they form complexes with the latex particles, causing agglutination (Fig. 12-8). The serum can further be manipulated to detect separate classes (IgG versus IgM) of antibody. Other kits using this methodology include tests for organisms that cause mastitis and for canine rheumatoid factor.

Precipitation Tests

There are three major types of precipitation tests: immunodiffusion, radioimmunodiffusion, and immunoelectrophoresis.

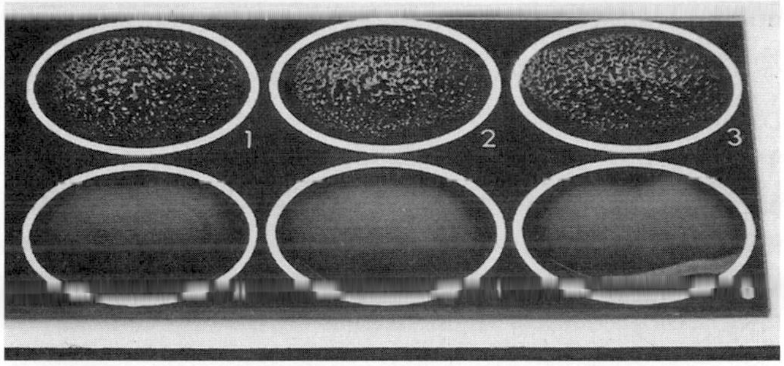

Fig. 12-8 Clumped latex particles representing antigen-antibody complexes. Samples 1, 2, and 3 indicate a positive reaction. Samples 4, 5, and 6, showing no clumping, indicate a negative reaction. *(Canine RF Test; courtesy Synbiotics.)*

Immunodiffusion

The immunodiffusion method is used to test for equine infectious anemia. This is commonly referred to as the Coggin's test. The test requires an agar plate with wells cut into it. The wells contain patient sample, a positive control, and negative control. If specific antibody is present in the sample, precipitate forms where the diffusing antigen (positive control) and antibody meet (Fig. 12-9).

Radioimmunoassay

The radioimmunoassay is usually performed in research laboratories rather than clinical practice. The principle is similar to ELISA except that a radioisotope is used in place of the conjugate. This procedure can detect either antigen or antibody. The amount of radiation detected equates to a volume of antigen or antibody present in the sample.

Immunoelectrophoresis

Fluorescent antibody tests are often used to verify diagnoses. The test is designed to detect antibody and requires a fluorescent labeled antiantibody. There are two types of

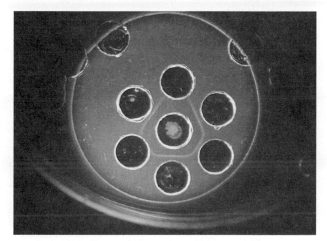

Fig. 12-9 Agar plate showing lines of precipitation. No lines of precipitation are evident near negative patient wells. *(EIA Immunodiffusion; courtesy Synbiotics.)*

fluorescent antibody tests: the *direct method* and the *indirect method*.

Coombs' Test

The Coombs' test is used to detect auto-antibodies (antibodies to one's own tissues). The test detects immunoglobulin (IgG or IgM) or complement (C3) bound to the surface of RBCs. There are two types of Coombs tests. The indirect Coombs detects circulating autoantibodies. The direct Coombs test is used for diagnosis of hemolytic disease. In the direct Coombs test, RBCs from the patient are incubated with a species-specific antiglobulin reagent. The sample is then evaluated for agglutination (irregular clumps of 3 to 5 or more RBCs). Agglutination occurs if the erythrocytes have enough antibody or complement on their surface to allow cross-linking between the cells (Fig. 12-10). Although the Coombs test is fairly simple to perform, the expense of stocking the species-specific Coombs reagent for only occasional tests makes it impractical to run in-house. The tests are usually sent to an outside reference laboratory.

Antinuclear Antibody Test

The antinuclear antibody (ANA) test is an example of an indirect fluorescent antibody (IFA) test (Fig. 12-11). This test is used to rule out the diagnosis of systemic lupus erythrematosus, a systemic autoimmune disorder. The patient's serum is serially diluted, and the dilutions are added to slides coated with cells, such as mouse liver or tissue-culture cell lines. If the patient's serum contains antinuclear antibodies, these bind to the cells on the slides. The slides are washed to remove unbound antibody and are then further treated with species-specific antiglobulin, which is fluorescein-labeled. The fluorescein-labeled antibodies bind to antibody from the patient's serum that is now bound to the cells. The slides are then evaluated using a fluorescence microscope. A positive result is determined to the highest dilution, which is reported as a *titer*. Results from different laboratories should not be compared, as there may be variation in reagents used and the interpretation of fluorescence by different technicians.

The ANA test takes some expertise to run and requires specific reagents and special instrumentation and is thus not practical to run in-house. The ANA test requires a

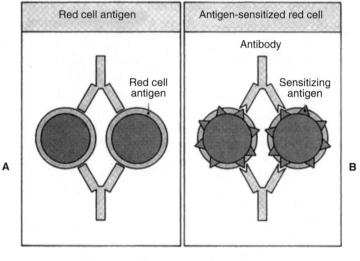

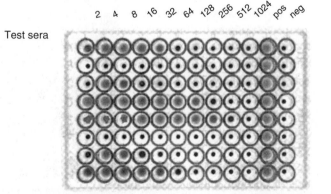

Fig. 12-10 Principles of the Coombs reaction. **A,** Direct Coombs test. **B,** Indirect Coombs test. *(From Roitt I, Brostoff J, Male D:* Immunology, *ed 3, London, 1993, Mosby.)*

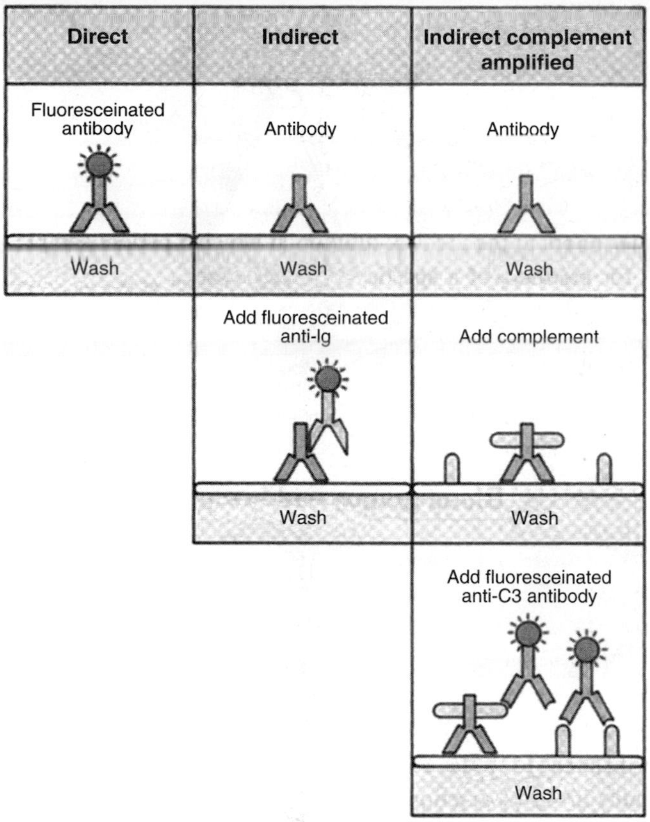

Direct	Indirect	Indirect complement amplified
Fluoresceinated antibody	Antibody	Antibody
Wash	Wash	Wash
	Add fluoresceinated anti-Ig	Add complement
	Wash	Wash
		Add fluoresceinated anti-C3 antibody
		Wash

Fig. 12-11 Fluorescent antibody technique. *(From Roitt I, Brostoff J, Male D: Immunology, ed 3, London, 1993, Mosby.)*

serum sample that may be kept refrigerated if the test is to be done soon or frozen if there will be a delay in testing.

Serum Protein Electrophoresis

Serum protein electrophoresis is occasionally done to help assess the cause of severe hyperproteinemia, in particular, hypergammaglobulinemia. The test requires approximately 0.5 ml of serum, which may be refrigerated or frozen. The serum is placed on a gel preparation and subjected to an electrical current. The size and charge of the various proteins (albumin, globulins) determine how far they migrate across the gel. These bands are then visualized by applying a protein-binding dye. The density of these bands (assessed by a densitometer) corresponds to the amount of protein present. A very sharp, dense band in the beta- or gammaglobulin region is called a *monoclonal spike*, typically associated with a lymphoid or plasma-cell tumor. On the other hand, a wide band in this region is associated with a polyclonal gammopathy, typically caused by chronic antigenic stimulation, such as feline infectious peritonitis or some types of chronic liver disease.

Antibody Titers

Results of some antibody tests may be reported as *positive* or *negative*. In other words, the test indicates the presence or absence of antibody to the particular infectious agent in the patient's serum. Results of other antibody tests may be reported as antibody *titers*, or levels. The patient's serum is serially diluted to different concentrations, such as 1:10, 1:40, and 1:160, meaning 1 part serum in 9 parts saline, 1 part serum in 39 parts saline, and 1 part serum in 159 parts saline, respectively. A test to detect antibodies (e.g., hemagglutination test, complement-fixation test, or IFA test) is done on each of these dilutions, and the greatest dilution that tests positive is reported. For example, if 1:10 and 1:40 are positive and 1:160 is negative, the titer is reported as 1:40. If none of the dilutions is positive, the titer may be reported as negative or the test may be repeated at lesser dilutions, such as 1:2, 1:4, or 1:8. A higher titer (positive at greater dilutions) indicates that more antibody is present. More antibody is present in a sample with a titer of 1:160 than in a sample with a titer of 1:40.

Note that antibody titers are conventionally expressed in terms of dilution. It is important to note that when measuring titers of antibodies to infectious agents, they are typically measured in two samples collected over a 2- to 4-week period to assess for a fourfold increase in antibody titer. An antibody titer in a single sample may indicate only that the animal has been previously exposed to an infectious agent; the animal may not currently have an active infection. A rising titer in two or more samples indicates an active infection. Usually it is best to run both titers at the same time to minimize the error in measuring antibody at two different times. This requires that the first sample is drawn, separated, frozen, and stored in such a way that it can be easily retrieved when the second sample is collected.

COMMON ERRORS AND ARTIFACTS

In spite of what may seem like very simplistic technology, the proper performance of the tests is vital to ensuring accurate results. Each test method mentioned has specific advantages and limitations. However, if the test is not performed correctly, a number of other factors can produce false-positive or false-negative results. A false-positive result is a positive test result on a sample from a patient that is in fact negative for the antigen. A false-negative result is a negative test result on a sample from a patient that is in fact positive for the antigen. Many immunoassays incorporate controls that help determine the accuracy of the test results. A visible positive control indicates that the test kit is functional. The most common causes of false results are poor sample quality, inadequate washing (ELISA tests), improper incubation, cross-reacting proteins, or expired or improperly stored kits.

Although it is uncommon, a test may produce false results when the patient sample contains very high levels of antigen and/or antibody. A patient can be exhibiting a very strong immune response and be producing high levels of antibody. It is possible for these antibodies to bind all the antigen in the sample so that none is available for binding to the solid phase.

Sample Quality

Manufacturers of immunoassays usually provide very specific information on the type of sample required for proper test performance. In most cases, the use of hemolyzed or lipemic samples will lead to ambiguous or erroneous test results. Hemolysis and lipemia can interfere with the absorption and flow of sample on an ICT test and can create background color on both ICT and ELISA tests that complicate interpretation of results.

Washing

Each of the common in-house test methods (ELISA and ICT) function on the premise that conjugate binds to the antigen from the patient sample that has bound to the antibody of the solid phase. At that point in the test, nothing short of a major chemical reaction can break the bond between the antigen-antibody complex.

This is a critical feature of an ELISA test since the next step in the test is usually the wash step. The purpose of the wash step is to remove any unbound sample and conjugate. If any unbound conjugate remains after the wash step, it will react with the chromogen and produce a false-positive result (Fig. 12-12). It is impossible to overwash an ELISA test system. However, underwashing is the most common cause of false-positive results. In addition to the positive control mentioned above, ELISA tests also contain negative controls. No color in the negative control indicates that the wash step was adequate and no known cross-reacting substances are present. A few test kits state that the positive control should merely be of greater color intensity than the negative control. However, any color development in the negative control indicates that the washing step may have been inadequate. Some ELISA tests have the wash step built into the system. The SNAP test is an example of this type of test (Fig. 12-13). The SNAP test is a membrane-ELISA test that contains wash solution within the test unit. The wash solution is released when the test is "snapped." This minimizes the possibility of false-positive results from inadequate washing of the test system.

Incubation

Test incubation times are established to give optimum accuracy. Not waiting the full time may decrease the sensitivity of the test (i.e., the ability to detect positives) and lead to false-negative results. Overincubation may lead to false-positive results. The final incubation period is particularly important. It is possible that very small amounts of chromagen may remain after the wash step. The conjugate can continue to react with the chromagen and generate color

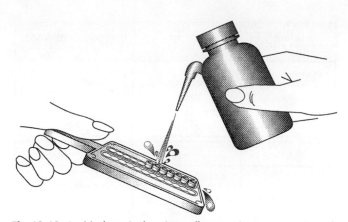

Fig. 12-12 A critical step in the microwell enzyme immunoassay is washing away the unbound enzyme-labeled antibodies. *(Pet Check heartworm antigen test kit; courtesy IDEXX Laboratories.)*

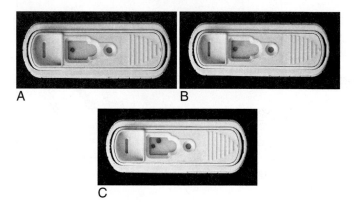

Fig. 12-13 Enzyme immunoassay for heartworm antigen (Snap whole blood heartworm antigen test, IDEXX). **A,** Negative reaction. **B,** Weak positive reaction. **C,** Strong positive reaction. *(Courtesy IDEXX Laboratories.)*

after the normal incubation period. A test that is negative at the end of the incubation period and then appears positive even a few minutes later is still considered a negative test result.

Storage

The enzyme-conjugate reagent used in ELISA tests requires refrigeration. Improper storage of the kit (i.e., storage at room temperature) can inactivate the reagent and lead to false-negative results. However, it is crucial that the ELISA kit be warmed to room temperature prior to use. The reaction between the enzyme-conjugate and the chromagen is temperature-dependent. When the enzyme-conjugate is at a lower then normal temperature, the reaction with the chromagen will be delayed and the incubation period will not be sufficient to detect a positive result.

CHOOSING A TEST KIT

There are numerous parameters to consider when choosing a diagnostic test kit. Cost is often a primary factor.

Microwell ELISA tests tend to be less expensive and more accurate than other ELISA methods. Membrane ELISA tests are more expensive but somewhat easier to carry out. Test accuracy should also be a primary concern when choosing a test kit. No test is 100% accurate. The test manufacturer provides data on *sensitivity* and *specificity* of the test. Sensitivity refers to the ability of the test to yield positive results on a sample that is in fact positive. Specificity refers to the ability to yield negative results on a sample that is in fact negative. *Predictive value* is a term used to describe the percentage of false-positive and false-negative results that are obtained with a particular test. Predictive value is a function of both test sensitivity and specificity as well as the prevalence of the antigen in the test population. For example, most heartworm antigen tests kits are approximately 95% sensitive and 99% specific. If the prevalence of heartworm disease in dogs is 1% (i.e., 1 in 100 dogs has the antigen), the test is likely to detect the 1 animal in 100 that has the antigen. However, since the specificity is 99%, there is a chance that 1 in 100 animals tested will yield a false-positive result. When the disease prevalence is higher, say 5%, the same test sensitivity and specificity will most likely detect all 5 positive patients in 100. However, the 99% specificity still will likely yield 1 in 100 false-positive results. That is, for every 100 patients tested, 6 positive results will likely be obtained. There will be 5 true positives and 1 false positive. Therefore, as the prevalence of a specific antigen in the population increases, the incidence of false-positive results decreases.

TEST SIGNIFICANCE

The results of immunoassays are only one part of the information the veterinarian considers when making a diagnosis. Physical examination results, patient history, and test results are all part of the diagnostic process. The veterinary technician must be able to provide accurate and reliable test results to aid the veterinarian in determining the diagnosis and prognosis for the patient.

For many years, the only means available for completing immunologic examination in animals was to submit samples to referral and reference laboratories. This often delayed the diagnosis and treatment of the patient. The ready availability of accurate, reliable in-house immunoassays has greatly improved service to our clients and patients.

RECOMMENDED READING

Coles EH: *Veterinary clinical pathology*, ed 4, Philadelphia, 1986, WB Saunders.

Hendrix CM: *Laboratory procedures for veterinary technicians*, ed 4, St Louis, 2002, Mosby.

Sirois M: *Veterinary clinical laboratory procedures*, St Louis, 1995, Mosby.

Sodikoff CH: *Laboratory profiles of small animal disease*, ed 3, St Louis, 2001, Mosby.

13

Microbiology, Cytology, and Urinalysis

Elaine Anthony and Margi Sirois

Learning Objectives

After reviewing this chapter, the reader should understand the following:

- Methods used to collect samples of body tissues and fluids for laboratory examination
- Methods used to prepare diagnostic samples for laboratory examination
- Microbiologic tests commonly performed to identify bacterial, fungal, and viral pathogens

- Procedures used in cytologic examination of body tissues and fluids
- Tests commonly performed in analyzing urine specimens
- Techniques of sample collection and processing for cytology and microbiology samples
- Identification of common normal cells in cytology samples
- Identification of common abnormal cells in cytology samples
- Methods for differentiation of inflammatory and neoplastic cytology samples

MICROBIOLOGY

The term *microbiology* refers to the study of microbes, specifically bacteria. Bacteria are small prokaryotic cells that are anuclear and have few cellular organelles. Microbiologic evaluations of tissues and body fluids can be used to determine the presence of specific disease-causing organisms and to aid in managing patient therapy. Samples for microbiologic evaluation can be collected quickly by various methods, including swabbing, scraping, and aspiration. The specific techniques utilized depend on the type of lesion and its location on the animal's body. Careful attention to aseptic technique is critical to achieving diagnostic quality results.

Characteristics of Bacteria

Bacteria are variable in size, ranging from 0.2 to 2.0 μm. They can be classified into one of four general categories and can take a variety of arrangements (Fig. 13-1). Although most cellular organelles are absent, bacteria contain cell walls, plasma membranes, and ribosomes. Some contain capsules and flagella, and can develop endospores. These characteristics are often used in the differentiation of specific bacterial pathogens.

Most bacteria are chemoheterotrophic. That is, they obtain nutrients from nonliving components of their environment. Growth factors such as vitamins, amino acids, and nucleotides, are also essential. Oxygen and temperature requirements vary among different species (Box 13-1). The majority of species require a pH in the range of 6.5 to 7.5. Bacteria reproduce primarily by binary fission, and their numbers grow exponentially until essential nutrients are depleted, toxic waste products accumulate, and/or space becomes limiting. Generation time refers to the time required for bacterial populations to double and is variable with different species and under different environmental conditions (Fig. 13-2).

MYCOLOGY

The study of fungi is referred to as *mycology*. Fungi are groups of organisms that are characterized by vegetative structures known as *hyphae*. Hyphae can grow into matted structures known as *mycelia*. Fungi contain eukaryotic cells with cell walls composed of chitin. The organisms are heterotrophic and may be parasitic or saprophytic. Fungi can be differentiated based on the structure of the hyphae and on the presence of spores. Different groups of fungi produce different types of spores. A variety of fungal organisms can affect veterinary species and cause superficial mycosis or deep mycosis. Table 13-1 summarizes fungal pathogens of veterinary importance, species affected, resultant diseases or lesions, and specimens required for diagnosis.

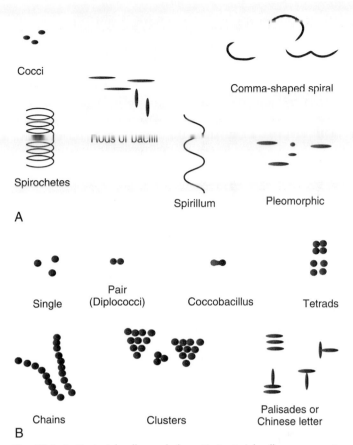

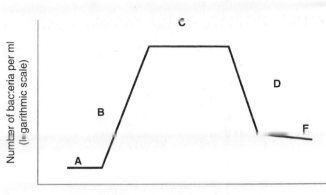

Fig. 13-2 Bacterial growth curve. **A,** Lag phase (phase of cell enlargement). **B,** log phase (exponential growth phase). **C,** maximum growth phase (stationary phase). **D,** logarithmic decline phase (death phase). **E,** dormant phase (endospores survive).

Fig. 13-1 A, Bacterial cell morphology. **B,** Bacterial cell arrangement. *(From Hendrix CM: Laboratory procedures for veterinary technicians, ed 4, St Louis, 2002, Mosby.)*

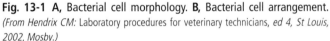

MATERIALS NEEDED FOR THE IN-HOUSE MICROBIOLOGY LAB

A review of scientific or veterinary supply catalogs will yield hundreds of products used in microbiology and cytology

testing. The average small animal practice in-house laboratory requires just a few of these. A high-quality binocular microscope is an essential piece of equipment. Microbiology equipment requirements include a small incubator, autoclave, and a refrigerator for storage of supplies. Consumable supplies needed are those required for sample collection and preparation as well as culture media and stains for microbiology specimens. The specific choice of collection method depends on the location of the lesion on the animal's body as well as the specific type of testing desired. Samples that are to be immediately processed can usually be collected using sterile cotton swabs. However, this is the least suitable method of collection since contamination risk is high and cotton can inhibit microbial growth. Oxygen can also be trapped in the fibers, making recovery of anaerobic bacteria less likely. Should delays in processing the sample be expected, a rayon swab in transport media (e.g., Culturette) must be used to preserve the quality of the sample. Aspirated samples and tissue samples can be collected in a fashion similar to that described later in this chapter for cytology samples.

The following guidelines should be kept in mind for proper specimen collection and handling:

- *Collect the specimen aseptically.* Specimen contamination is the most common cause of diagnostic failure. The importance of aseptic collection of microbiologic specimens cannot be overemphasized. Collect samples as soon as possible following the onset of clinical signs.
- *Collect tissue samples that are at least 5 to 15 cm² (block or wedge-shaped).* This will allow for processing the sample with a variety of methods if needed.
- *Keep multiple specimens separate from each other to avoid cross-contamination.* This is essential for intestinal specimens because of the normal flora found there. In addition, samples that contain formalin should be stored and/or shipped to outside laboratories in containers that

---

BOX 13-1

Temperature and Oxygen Requirements of Bacteria

Optimum Temperature
- Psychrophiles: 0°–30° C
- Mesophiles: 20°–40° C
- Thermophiles: 40°–80° C

Oxygen Requirements
- Aerobes require oxygen
- Anaerobes require absence of oxygen
- Facultative can grow under a variety of conditions
- Microaerophilic prefer reduced oxygen tension
- Capnophilic require high levels of carbon dioxide

TABLE 13-1

Summary of Pathogenic Fungi, Species Affected, Disease or Lesions Caused, and Specimens for Diagnosis

Organism	Species Affected	Disease or Lesion	Specimens
Microsporum		Ringworm	Fresh plucked hair and skin scrapings from edges of lesions; send to laboratory in paper envelopes
M. canis	Dogs, cats		
M. distortum	Dogs, cats, horses, pigs		
M. gallinae (T. gallinae)	Chickens, turkeys ("white comb")		
M. gypseum	Horses, cats, dogs, other species		
M. nanum	Pigs		
M. persicolor	Voles, bats, dogs		
Trichophyton			
T. equinum	Horses, donkeys		
T. erinacei	Hedgehogs, dogs, people		
T. mentagrophytes	Most animal species		
T. rubrum	Primarily people, but also dogs, cats		
T. simii	Poultry, monkeys		
T. verrucosum	Primarily cattle		
Candida albicans Some other *Candida* spp. (such as *C. tropicalis*) can cause lesions	Chickens, turkeys, other birds	Infection of mouth, crop, esophagus	Fresh affected tissue or scrapings from affected tissue
	Dogs	Mycotic stomatitis	Fixed affected tissue
	Cats	Enteritis of kittens	
	Calves, foals	Infections of oral and intestinal mucosae	
	Cattle	Mastitis	Most common after extensive antibiotic therapy
	Horses	Genital infections—both sexes	
	Pigs	Infection of esophagus and stomach	
Malassezia pachydermatis	Dogs	Chronic otitis externa	Fresh ear swabs
Cryptococcus neoformans (worldwide distribution)	People, dogs, cats (infection frequently affects nervous systems)	Subacute or chronic affected tissue	Fresh nasal discharge, milk
	Cattle	Sporadic cases of mastitis	Fixed affected tissue, brain, lung
Coccidioides immitis (SW USA and South America; occurs in soil)	People, horses, cattle, sheep, dogs, cats, captive feral animals	Disease characterized by granulomas, often in bronchial and mediastinal lymph nodes and lungs; can cause lesions in brain, liver, spleen, kidneys	Fresh and fixed lesions and affected tissue
Histoplasma capsulatum (NE, central, and S central USA; occurs in soil)	People, dogs, cats, sheep, pigs, horses	Disease that generally affects reticuloendothelial system; dogs, cats: ulcerations of intestinal canal; enlargement of liver, spleen, lymph nodes; TB-like lesions	Fresh and fixed lesions or affected tissue

Organism	Host species	Disease/characteristics	Specimen
Histoplasma farciminosum (Mediterranean, Asia, Africa, and part of Russia)	Horses, mules, donkeys	Epizootic lymphangitis, African farcy, or Japanese glanders	Fresh pus and discharges from lesions
Blastomyces dermatitidis (USA, Canada, and Africa; occurs in soil)	People, dogs, cats, sea lions	Granulomatous lesions in lungs and/or skin and subcutis	Fresh and fixed lesions and affected tissue
Sporothrix schenckii	People, horses, dogs, pigs, cattle, fowl, rodents	Subcutaneous nodules or granulomas that eventually discharge pus; can include involvement of bones and visceral organs	Fresh and fixed pus, granulomas
Rhinosporidium seeberi (not yet cultured in vitro)	Horses, dogs, cattle, people	Characterized by polyps on the nasal and ocular mucous membranes	Fresh nasal discharge and polyps; fixed polyps
Aspergillus A. fumigatus main pathogen; potentially pathogenic *A. flavus* *A. nidulans* *A. niger*	Many animal species and birds	Fowl: air sac infection; diffuse and nodular forms in lungs; "brooder pneumonia" in chicks and poults; cattle: occasional mycotic abortion and mastitis; horses: guttural pouch mycosis; dog: infection of nasal chambers	Fresh deep scrapings or affected tissue Abortions: see text
A. flavus *A. parasiticus* *A. ochraceus*	Ducklings, domestic birds, pigs, dogs	Aflatoxicosis; affects liver and sometimes kidneys	Suspect food product
A. clavatus	Pigs	Hemorrhagic disease; profuse hemorrhage in many tissues, jaundice, and liver lesions	
	Cattle	Trembling syndrome: *A. flavus* and *A. fumigatus* toxins; abortion; toxins of *A. ochraceus* cause fetal death; hyperkeratosis lesions on muzzle and mouth from *A. clavatus* toxins	
Petriellidium boydii (*Allescheria boydii*)	Cattle	Abortion, mastitis	Fresh milk, uterine discharges, affected tissue
	Equidae	Abortion, metritis, infertility	
	People, other animals	Mycetoma; progressive disease of subcutis	Fixed affected tissue

From Hendrix CM: *Laboratory Procedures for veterinary technicians*, ed 4, St Louis, 2002, Mosby.

are separate from prepared slides and nonformalinized specimens. Formalin fumes can render samples unsatisfactory for further analysis.

- *Label the specimen container, especially if a zoonotic condition is suspected,* such as anthrax, rabies, leptospirosis, brucellosis, or equine encephalitis. Tissues from animals with suspected zoonoses should be submitted in a sealed, leakproof, unbreakable container.

- *Keep the specimen cool during transport.* Any sample that can be frozen should be frozen (especially in summer). Swabs must be sent in transport medium. Bacteriologic, virologic, and *Mycoplasma* tests require separate swabs for each. Samples for anaerobic culture must be submitted cool or frozen.

- *If shipping involves dry ice, seal the container or swab to prevent entry of CO_2 into the container.* Carbon dioxide released by dry ice may kill bacteria and viruses.

- *Swabs placed in viral transport medium cannot be used for bacterial culture.* Use duplicate bacterial transport medium.

- *If using an outside referral laboratory, send the specimen to the diagnostic laboratory by the fastest possible means.* If the sample will be arriving during a weekend, inform the laboratory ahead of time so that arrangements can be made for pickup.

- *Discuss the results with the veterinarian promptly,* in a clear, concise manner. Failure to do so reflects adversely on both the veterinarian and the laboratory.

Fig. 13-3 shows the typical sequence of procedures used in processing microbiologic specimens.

Sample Processing Materials

Preparation of samples for microbiology requires some unique supplies. Glass slides and cover slips are needed when performing Gram stain procedures, and they can be of average quality. Inoculating loops or wires for transfer of specimens to culture media are also needed. A propane (Bunsen) burner or alcohol lamp is required to sterilize the inoculating loops and to flame the mouth of culture tubes before inoculation. When anaerobic or microaerophilic microbes are suspected pathogens, a candle jar or anaerobe jar (Gas Pak) will be required to provide the appropriate environment for microbial growth.

Culture Media

Culture media are available in dozens of formulations. General-purpose nutrient media provides basic requirements for bacterial growth. Selective media contain additives that allow certain microorganisms to grow while inhibiting the growth of others. Enriched media also promote growth of certain microbes by providing specific growth factors for bacteria with strict nutrient requirements. These types of bacteria are referred to as *fastidious.* Differential media contain additives that detect certain bio-

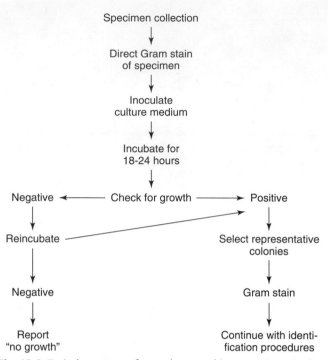

Fig. 13-3 Typical sequence of procedures used in processing microbiologic specimens. *(From Hendrix CM:* Laboratory procedures for veterinary technicians, *ed 4, St Louis, 2002, Mosby.)*

chemical reactions of the bacteria. Media is also available that incorporate characteristics of more then one type. Most small-animal practice microbiology laboratories will require just a few of these. Media are also supplied as either solid forms on culture plates or in tubes, liquid form in tubes, or in dehydrated form. Dehydrated media are the least expensive. However, they require additional preparation time and must be autoclaved before use. This may not be financially justifiable unless the practice is performing very large numbers of microbiology tests.

In veterinary practice, the most commonly used solid media in culture plates are Mueller-Hinton, Trypticase soy agar with 5% sheep blood (commonly called blood agar), and MacConkey or Eosin-Methylene Blue (EMB). Mueller-Hinton is the recommended media for culture and sensitivity testing. MacConkey and EMB are both selective media that support the growth of gram-negative bacteria and incorporate an additional indicator to allow differentiation among gram-negative enteric bacteria based on their ability to ferment lactose. Blood agar is an enriched general-purpose media that allows differentiation among specific hemolytic organisms. The degree to which the organisms hemolyze the cells of the media aids in identification of pathogenic bacteria. The type of hemolysis present on a blood agar is classified as alpha (α), beta (β), or gamma (γ). Beta hemolysis is complete destruction of the red blood cells and will alter the color of the media from bright red to clear. Pathogenic bacteria exhibit beta hemolysis. Alpha hemolysis is partial destruction of the red blood cells. The media around the bacterial colony will appear green. Gamma hemolysis produces no change in the color of the media. These are nonhemolytic species.

Solid media in culture tubes are used primarily for growth of fungi and yeasts. Additional media available in this form include those used for biochemical testing of microbes. The most common types of slant media tubes are Sabaroud Dextrose or Bismuth-Glucose-Glycine Yeast (commonly referred to as "biggy"). The media is usually solidified into a slant-top configuration. Either type is suitable for growth of dermatophytes and is usually described as dermatophyte test media (DTM) regardless of which specific media is present. Fungal cultures of solid tissue samples may require the use of a 20% potassium hydroxide reagent for preparation of the sample.

A variety of companies produce culture plates that incorporate several different media within individual compartments on a culture plate. Items such as the Bullseye® Veterinary Plate and the Bacti-Vet® Culture System provide five different types of media that can simultaneously select and differentiate microbes as well as provide antibiotic sensitivity data.

Broth media in tubes is necessary for blood cultures and is also available in forms to provide differentiation of gram-negative enteric bacteria. Thioglycollate broth is a general-purpose media that can be used for urine cultures. Specific blood culture tubes are available as evacuated tubes used for blood collection. These contain both anticoagulant and culture media.

Bacteria may often be partially differentiated based on their growth patterns on agar plates. Evaluation of colony characteristics should include form, elevation, margin, texture, and pigmentation (Fig. 13-4). The specific configuration a bacterial colony makes depends on the type of culture media used as well as environmental conditions.

Stains

Gram stain is an essential component of the microbiology lab. These are available in kit form or can be purchased as individual solutions. For differentiation of certain types of bacteria, a variety of other stains are also available. *Acid-fast* stains are useful in the identification of *Mycobacteria*. These involve the addition of an agent such as DMSO before addition of the primary stain. The agent allows the stain to penetrate the stain-resistant cells of *Mycobacterium*. The subsequent addition of acid alcohol or dilute alcohol removes the stain. If the stain is not removed, the organism is said to be *acid-fast*. The Ziehl-Nelson technique is a modification of this procedure.

Flagella stains, capsule stains, endospore stains, and fluorescent stains are also available but have limited application in the average veterinary microbiology lab. Fluorescent stains tend to be quite expensive and are used primarily for the identification of *Legionella* and *Pseudomonas*. Flagella stain usually contains crystal violet and is used to detect and characterize bacterial motility. These tend to be somewhat expensive for the small veterinary practice laboratory. Other methods that can be used to test motility include the hanging drop preparation and the use of motility test media. Capsule stains are used for detection of pathogenic bacteria. All bacteria that contain capsules are pathogenic. However, not all pathogenic bacteria contain capsules. Capsule stains often require the use of bright-field phase contrast microscopy. Endospore stains are used to detect the presence, location, and shape of spores. These characteristics can aid in differentiation of bacteria. Spores may be centrally located, terminal, or subterminal (Fig. 13-5). Endospore staining is performed on older cultures (>48 hours) since spore formation occurs during the log decline phase. The procedure involves addition of malachite green to the specimen on the slide and then heating the slide. The slide is washed and counterstained with safranin or basic fuscin. Spores appear dark blue/green with the remainder of the bacterial cell pink or red. Spores may also be found free from cells. Simple stains, such as crystal violet or methylene blue, are usually used for yeasts.

Lactophenol cotton blue stain is often needed to prepare fungal culture samples for analysis and can also be used for cellophane tape preparations of external lesions.

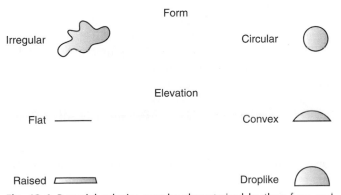

Fig. 13-4 Bacterial colonies may be characterized by their form and elevation. *(From Hendrix CM: Laboratory procedures for veterinary technicians, ed 4, St Louis, 2002, Mosby.)*

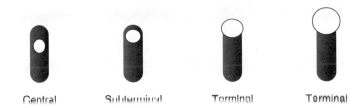

Fig. 13-5 Bacterial endospores. *(From Hendrix CM: Laboratory procedures for veterinary technicians, ed 4, St Louis, 2002, Mosby.)*

Additional Materials

Antimicrobial sensitivity disks are necessary when performing a culture and sensitivity. The specific types of antimicrobial disks purchased depend on the suspected pathogens. Antimicrobial disks are available in a variety of concentrations. These allow more specific determination of therapeutic levels needed once the antimicrobial is chosen. A 3% potassium hydroxide solution (used to perform the catalase test) should be available for clarification of results when gram staining yields ambiguous or variable answers. Concave slides are useful to prepare *hanging drop* slides for determination of bacterial motility.

Inoculating Culture Media

Aseptic technique is crucial to achieving diagnostic quality results in microbiology. Culture media and processing supplies must be sterile. There are several methods for inoculation of culture media depending on the characteristics of the sample and the type of testing needed. Since many samples contain multiple types of bacteria, the majority of bacterial tests involve an initial step designed to isolate the bacterium of interest. Before inoculating the culture plate, an inoculation loop or wire is passed through a flame and briefly cooled. The loop or wire is lightly touched to the sample and then streaked onto a culture plate using the quadrant method (Fig. 13-6). If the sample was collected using a sterile swab, the swab can be used directly on the culture plate. The procedure for inoculating agar slants requires a sterile wire. The slant is generally divided into a butt portion, and slant surface. The media can be inoculated either on the butt only, the slant only, or both (Fig. 13-7). Motility test media is prepared as an agar slant. Broth media, such as blood culture tubes, are inoculated in a manner similar to that used for agar slants.

Incubating Bacterial Cultures

The optimum time and temperature for growth of bacterial cultures depends on the type of media being used, the bacterial species' generation time, and preferred temperature

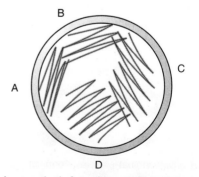

Fig. 13-6 Quadrant method of streaking a culture plate. *(From Hendrix CM: Laboratory procedures for veterinary technicians, ed 4, St Louis, 2002, Mosby.)*

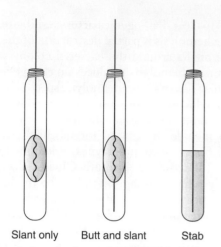

Slant only   Butt and slant   Stab

Fig. 13-7 Inoculation of culture tubes with an inoculating wire. *(From Hendrix CM: Laboratory procedures for veterinary technicians, ed 4, St Louis, 2002, Mosby.)*

characteristics of the bacterial species. Most pathogenic bacteria are incubated at 37° C. Some incubators also contain mechanisms to read and record the biochemical reactions.

Incubators should contain thermostatic controls (temperature and preferably humidity). Some have oxygen and carbon dioxide controls as well.

Biochemical Test Materials

Biochemical tests are often necessary to differentiate specific types of microbes. Fig. 13-8 provides an example of how biochemical testing and other criteria are used for primary identification of bacteria. Biochemical testing may involve the use of specific liquid reagents or use media that contain the necessary reagents. The most commonly performed tests in the small veterinary practice laboratory are the oxidase test and catalase tests. Reagents to perform these tests are quite inexpensive and readily available. Some are available in a slide form that contains the necessary reagent impregnated in a pad on the slide. Coagulase testing may sometimes be required and can be performed as either a slide or tube test. Coagulase reagent tends to be relatively expensive.

Enterotubes® are a type of commercially available microbiology test kit that incorporates multiple types of media designed to provide differentiation of enteric bacteria based on their biochemical reactions on the media. These tend to be relatively expensive and may not be financially justified unless large numbers of microbiology tests are performed on a variety of species. Individual culture media tubes can be purchased that provide many of the same test results as Enterotubes®. These may decrease the overall cost of testing when only a few biochemical tests are needed. The most commonly used biochemical tests that utilize differential media are the Sulfide-Indole-Motility

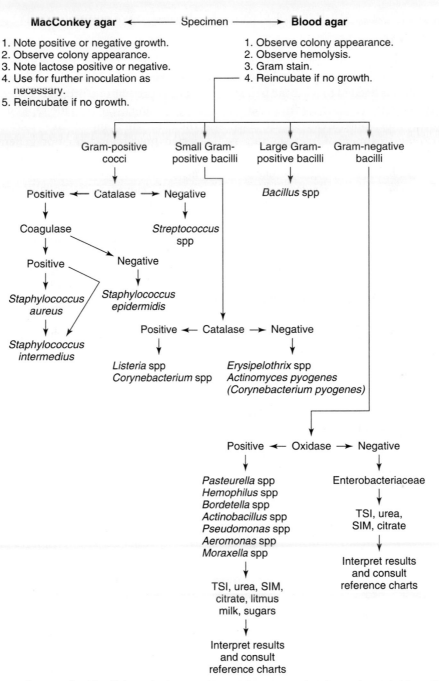

Fig. 13-8 Flowchart of procedures used to identify bacteria. *(From Hendrix CM: Laboratory procedures for veterinary technicians, ed 4, St Louis, 2002, Mosby.)*

(SIM) media, Simmons' Citrate Media, and Triple Sugar-Iron media. These are all solid media prepared in tubes with slanted surface agar. SIM testing requires the addition of Kovac's reagent following incubation of the sample.

IMMUNOLOGIC TESTING

Since microbes contain compounds that can serve as antigens, immunologic tests can sometimes be used for determi-

nation of the presence or absence of specific microbes. The majority of these types of tests require specialized and expensive equipment and reagent that may not be financially justifiable for the small veterinary practice. Immunologic tests utilizing the enzyme-linked-immunosorbent reaction are available for detection of *Brucella* antibodies and are also available for some species of *Salmonella*, and *Staphylococcus*.

Table 13-1 summarizes bacterial pathogens of veterinary importance, species affected, resultant diseases or lesions, and specimens required for diagnosis.

ANTIMICROBIAL SENSITIVITY TESTING

Bacterial samples isolated from patient samples are often processed with the antimicrobial sensitivity test. This test indicates which antimicrobial is needed to treat the patient and at which concentrations it should be administered. The test must be performed on a pure, fresh culture taken before the initiation of any treatment. Gram staining is used to determine which antimicrobial discs to use. The most common method for performing antimicrobial sensitivity testing is the *agar diffusion method*. The test uses paper discs impregnated with antimicrobials that are placed on the surface of the bacterial culture (usually a freshly-inoculated Mueller-Hinton agar plate) and allowed to incubate. After the incubation period, usually 18 to 24 hours, the plate is examined for bacterial growth. If the bacterium is sensitive to a particular antimicrobial, a zone around the paper disc will be evident. The diameter of the zone is then measured and interpreted using a standardized comparative chart. A similar method can be used to determine the minimum inhibitory concentration (MIC) of an antimicrobial. This is the smallest concentration of the specific antimicrobial that can inhibit the growth of a given bacteria. Paper discs with varying concentrations of the chosen antimicrobial are placed on a freshly inoculated culture plate and incubated. Measuring the zones of inhibition around each of these discs will aid in choosing an appropriate concentration of medication to be given to the patient.

QUALITY CONTROL CONCERNS

An effective quality control program is vital to achieving accurate and reliable results in any laboratory. Samples for microbiologic analysis are greatly affected by inappropriate or improperly performed collection methods. Careful attention to aseptic technique is critical. The timing of sample collection and processing must also be considered. Samples that are collected after medical treatment has begun or that are held long periods of time before processing will yield unreliable results. Staining supplies and reagents must be stored and used correctly for maintenance of the integrity of these items. In addition to maintaining the sterility of collection and processing supplies, equipment used in the microbiology laboratory requires regular verification of performance. This includes verification of temperatures in autoclaves and incubators. Such routine quality control must be performed on a regular schedule and the results recorded so that equipment malfunctions can be detected early.

CYTOLOGY

The primary goal of the cytology evaluation is differentiation of inflammation and neoplasia. The types and numbers of cells present in a properly collected and prepared cytology specimen can provide rapid diagnostic information to the clinician. Samples for cytology evaluation can be collected quickly and do not generally require specialized materials or equipment for proper evaluation. With careful attention to appropriate collection, preparation, and staining technique, a high-quality cytology sample can be obtained. Such samples yield valuable results for the clinician and often preclude the need for more invasive procedures to determine diagnosis, treatment, and prognosis for a patient.

Several different preparations are often made from each sample. This allows for additional diagnostic testing without additional collection. Samples may be processed as impression smears, squash or modified squash preparations, line smears, starfish smears, or simple smears. The exact type of preparation depends on the characteristics of the sample. Some samples may also require concentration by centrifugation. Fluid samples usually require anticoagulant and/or preservatives. A variety of staining techniques is also available for cytology specimens. Some samples will require processing with more than one staining procedure.

Collected and processed correctly, a cytology specimen is characterized as inflammatory, neoplastic, or mixed. The specimen is then described according to the presence of specific cell types. Neoplastic cells are further evaluated for malignant changes. Inflammatory processes are characterized as either *suppurative*, *pyogranulomatous*, or *eosinophilic* when specific cell types and numbers of cells are evident on the cytology preparation. In general, samples that are inflammatory are characterized by a predominance of neutrophils and macrophages (tissue monocytes). Neoplastic processes are characterized by large numbers of tissue cells. There may be a combination of cell types present. This may indicate a neoplastic disease with secondary inflammation. Box 13-2 contains a list of commonly used supplies for cytology sample collection.

COLLECTION AND PREPARATION OF SAMPLES FROM TISSUES AND MASSES

Impression Smears

Impression smears (Box 13-3) are prepared from active lesions on an animal's body or from tissues removed during surgical procedures. For impression smears from active lesions, an initial impression is made before cleaning the

Basic Equipment Used for Cytologic Examination

- Binocular microscope (Nikon, Olympus, American Optical, Swift)
- Immersion oil
- 20- or 22-gauge, 1.5-inch needles
- 6- and 12-ml syringes
- Glass slides and cover slips
- Stains: Diff-Quik (Scientific Products), Hema-Quik (Curtis Matheson Scientific), Quik Stain II (Scientific Products) new methylene blue, gram stain
- Coplin staining jars
- Specimen tubes: red-top tubes contain no anticoagulant; lavender-top tubes contain EDTA as anticoagulant
- Forceps, scalpel blades
- Refractometer
- Hemacytometer

BOX 13-3 *procedure*

Preparing Impression Smears

Materials
- Scalpel
- Forceps
- Paper towels and/or gauze sponges
- Glass slides

Procedure
1. Section the tissue to expose a fresh surface.
2. Hold the tissue fragment with forceps.
3. Blot excess fluid on a paper towel or gauze sponge until the tissue is nearly dry.
4. Gently touch the tissue to the surface of a slide repeatedly down the length of the slide. Reblot as needed.
5. Allow the slide to air dry.

lesion or initiating treatment. Additional smears are prepared after cleaning the lesion. To prepare the smear, gently touch a clean glass slide to several areas of the lesion. Although this type of sample can be prepared quickly and easily, it tends to yield the fewest number of cells and can also be contaminated by bacteria that may be present due to secondary bacterial infection. Impression smears of tissue samples are made in a similar manner except that a fresh section of the tissue is made and then the tissue is blotted to remove excess blood and tissue fluid. These excess fluids may prevent tissue cells from adhering to the slide.

Scrapings

Scrapings can be prepared from either external lesions or from tissues removed during surgical procedures. This type of sample yields a greater number of cells than impression smears. To prepare a scraping, the lesion or tissue must be cleaned and blotted dry. If using tissue samples, a fresh section is cut before obtaining the sample. A dull scalpel blade is held at a 90° angle to the lesion or tissue and is gently pulled across the surface. A squash prep is then prepared from the material on the edge of the scalpel blade. The sample can also be smeared across a slide directly from the scalpel blade.

Swabbings

Swab smears can provide valuable diagnostic information for certain types of specimens. This type of sample preparation is most useful for fistulated lesions or collections from the vaginal canal. A sterile cotton swab is moistened with 0.9% saline and lightly swabbed along the surface of the tissue. Then the swab is gently rolled across the surface of a clean glass slide.

Fine-Needle Aspiration

A fine-needle aspiration collection can often provide a great amount of information to the clinician and may preclude the need for biopsy of lesions of internal organs. This type of sample preparation may also be preferred for collection of samples from superficial lesions since bacterial contamination can be kept to a minimum (Box 13-4). Equipment needed for fine-needle aspiration includes a 3- to 20-ml syringe and a 21- to 25-gauge needle. Samples collected from softer tissue require smaller syringes and needles. Firmer tissues require larger syringes and large bore needles. Collection of samples from solid masses is

BOX 13-4 *procedure*

Fine-Needle Aspiration

Materials
- 21- or 25-gauge, 1.5-inch needles
- 3- to 30-ml syringes
- Glass slides

Procedure
1. Clean the site.
2. Immobilize the mass or lymph node with one hand.
3. Insert the needle into the mass and redirect through the mass several times while aspirating to collect cells.
4. Release pressure from the syringe plunger before removing the needle from the mass.
5. Prepare squash or push smears immediately.

performed by inserting the needle into the tissue and pulling the plunger about three-fourths of the way out of the barrel. This exerts a negative pressure on the tissue and draws material into the needle. Samples should be collected from several areas of the tissue by releasing the pressure on the syringe and redirecting the needle into another location. An alternative method, known as a *nonaspirate procedure*, can be used to collect samples from masses. To perform this procedure, attach a 22-gauge needle to a 10-ml syringe that has been prefilled with air (Fig. 13-9). Introduce the needle into the mass, and move the needle rapidly back and forth through the mass. Shearing and capillary action force cells into the needle. Once removed from the mass, the material is expelled onto a clean glass slide by rapidly pressing the plunger of the syringe.

Preparation Techniques for Solid Samples

Samples collected from organs and masses can be prepared in several ways. Regardless of preparation method chosen, the smear must be made quickly to avoid deterioration of the sample. Several smears should be made and rapidly air-dried.

Squash technique

This method has been widely used for many years for preparation of cytology specimens (Box 13-5). The technique is similar to that employed for preparation of avian blood smears. A small amount of sample is placed on a clean glass slide or cover slip. A second slide or cover slip is placed on top at a 90° angle to the first. The second slide is then gently pulled away from the first (Fig. 13-10).

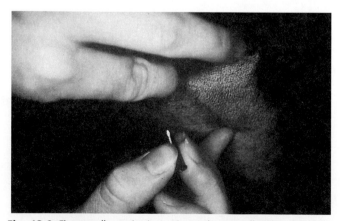

Fig. 13-9 Fine-needle aspiration using only a needle. The cutaneous and/or subcutaneous mass is usually immobilized using one hand. In this case, the mass is so large both hands are needed. The hair has been clipped to better visualize the area. After redirecting the needle through the mass, the needle is removed from the mass, then attached to a syringe with the plunger withdrawn in preparation for making a squash smear. *(Photo courtesy Dr. Anthony Carr, University of Wisconsin, Madison).*

BOX 13-5

Preparing Squash Smears

Materials
- Glass slides

Procedure
1. Place one drop of aspirated material on one end of a slide.
2. Allow material to spread by capillary action
3. Place a second slide gently on top of and parallel or at a right angle to the first.
4. Pull the second slide across the surface of the first slide using a smooth motion
5. Allow the slides to air-dry.

Modified squash technique

This technique can be useful for samples that are highly viscous or very fragile. The technique involves placing a small amount of sample near the middle of a clean glass slide. A second slide is placed on top at a right angle. The top slide is then rotated 45° and then removed (Fig. 13-11).

Combination method

This technique involves placing a small amount of sample near the middle of a clean glass slide. The edge of a second slide is then placed on top and at a right angle to the first so that it covers about one-third of the specimen. The second slide is then gently slid across the specimen, leaving the middle one-third portion of the specimen untouched. The final one-third portion of the specimen is then smeared in a manner similar to that used for preparation of a routine blood smear, with somewhat less pressure applied to the smear (Fig. 13-12).

COLLECTION AND PREPARATION OF FLUID SAMPLES

Removal of fluid from the abdominal, thoracic, and pericardial cavities can be accomplished in a manner similar to that for fine-needle aspiration of tissue samples (Box 13-6). Aspirated fluid samples should be well mixed with an appropriate anticoagulant (e.g., EDTA) and the specimen prepared as quickly as possible to prevent cellular deterioration. Slides can be prepared directly from the nonconcentrated fluid or from concentrated sediment following centrifugation of the sample.

Transtracheal and Bronchial Washes

Evaluation of mucus secretions from the trachea, bronchi, and bronchioles can aid in differential diagnosis of

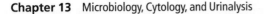

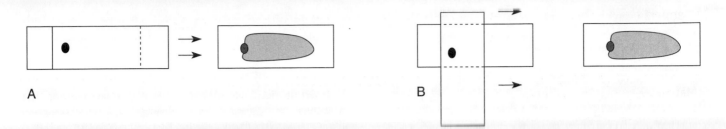

Fig. 13-10 Squash smear. The second slide may be placed in a parallel, **A,** or perpendicular, **B,** orientation. Care should be taken not to push forcefully on the two slides, because most of the cells would be ruptured.

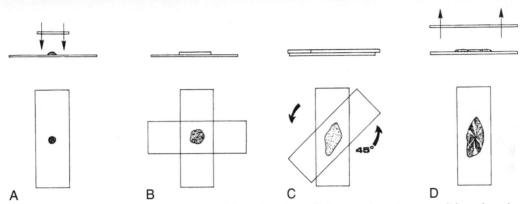

Fig. 13-11 A modification of the squash preparation. **A,** A portion of the aspirate is expelled onto a glass microscope slide, and another slide is placed over the sample. **B,** This causes the sample to spread. If necessary, gentle digital pressure can be applied to the top slide to spread the sample more. Care must be taken not to use excessive pressure and cause cell rupture. **C,** The top slide is rotated about 45° and lifted directly upward, producing a spread preparation with subtle ridges and valleys of cells, **D.** *(From Cowell R, Tyler R, Meinkoth J:* Diagnostic cytology and hematology of the dog and cat, *ed 2, St Louis, 2002, Mosby.)*

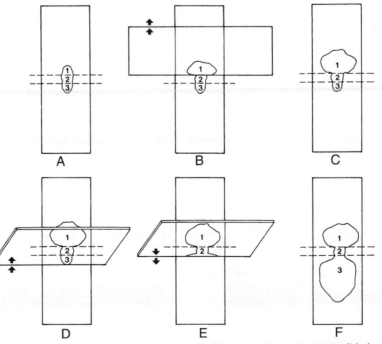

Fig. 13-12 Combination cytologic preparation. **A,** A portion of the aspirate is expelled onto a glass microscope slide (prep slide). **B,** Another glass slide is placed over about one third of the preparation. If additional spreading of the aspirate is needed, gentle digital pressure can be used. Excessive pressure should be avoided. The spreader slide is smoothly slid forward. **C,** This makes a squash prep of about one third of the aspirate *(area 1).* The spreader slide also contains a squash prep *(not depicted).* Next, the edge of a tilted glass slide (second spreader slide) is slid backward from the end opposite the squash prep until it contacts about one third of the expelled aspirate, **D** and **E.** Then the second spreader slide is slid rapidly and smoothly forward. **F,** This produces an area *(3)* that is spread with mechanical forces like those of a blood smear preparation. The middle area *(2)* is left untouched and contains a high concentration of cells. *(From Cowell R, Tyler R, Meinkoth J:* Diagnostic cytology and hematology of the dog and cat, *ed 2, St Louis, 2002, Mosby.)*

BOX 13-6

Abdominocentesis and Thoracentesis

Materials

- Surgical prep materials
- Local anesthetic
- 18- or 20-gauge, over-the-needle catheter or needles (cats, dogs)
- 2- or 3-inch teat cannula, bitch catheter, 18-gauge, 1½-inch needle (cattle, horses)
- 6- to 12-ml syringe
- Red-top and lavender-top tubes
- 3-way stopcock (thoracentesis)
- Sterile IV extension tubing (horses)

Procedure

1. Anesthetize or tranquilize the animal as necessary.
2. Surgically prepare the site (thorax: cranial rib ventral to the fluid line; abdomen: ventral midline). Local anesthetic may be used to infiltrate the site of the catheter, needle, or cannula insertion.
3. Insert the needle or catheter in the appropriate location. If using a needle, use care to avoid lacerating internal organs. Attach the needle or catheter to a three-way stopcock or syringe when entering the thoracic cavity to avoid causing pneumothorax.
4. Use a three-way stopcock between the catheter and syringe if you are collecting multiple syringefuls from thoracic cavity. IV extension tubing is also helpful, particularly when draining large volumes of thoracic fluid from a horse. Collect samples in a red-top and lavender-top tube if the sample is very bloody.
5. Note the volume of fluid removed.
6. Place a small amount of fluid in a sterile tube.
7. Place a small amount of fluid in EDTA.
8. Note gross appearance of fluid.
9. Prepare slides from the fluid samples. Allow the slides to air-dry.
10. Perform a cell count. Assess SG (protein content) using a refractometer

---

inflammation, neoplasia, mycosis, and bacterial and protozoal diseases. There are various techniques for collecting these samples, such as the percutaneous (jugular catheter) and endotracheal tube methods (Box 13-7). Both methods involve infusion of saline into the trachea. Fluid is collected either by aspirating the fluid or waiting for the animal to cough. It is important to collect all fluid coughed up by the animal, even if it requires that the sample be collected in a nonsterile fashion (e.g., from the bottom of the cage floor). Specimens collected in this manner should be noted as such before performing any testing.

Concentration techniques

Fluid samples may be centrifuged in order to concentrate the solid material before preparing smears. The technique is similar to that used for preparation of urine sediment for microscopic analysis. The anticoagulated fluid is placed in a standard clinical centrifuge and spun for five minutes at 1000 to 2000 rpm (165 to 400 G). The supernatant is poured off, leaving a few drops in the tube. The sediment is then gently resuspended in the remaining supernatant. A few drops of this concentrate are then used to prepare several smears. Ideally, several preparations should be made utilizing several different techniques.

Slide preparation

The squash technique described previously may be used for fluid samples, particularly ones that are highly viscous or contain a large amount of particulate material. Wedge films

(blood smear) are usually suitable for fluid samples (Fig. 13-13). An alternative technique, the line smear, will also provide excellent specimens.

Line smear

This technique is primarily utilized when fluid samples cannot be concentrated or when the amount of sediment is very small. A small drop of the sample is placed near the end of a clean glass slide, and a second slide used to spread the specimen in a manner similar to that used for preparation of a peripheral blood film. When the smear covers approximately three-fourths of the slide, the second slide is abruptly lifted off the first. This produces a smear with a thick edge, rather than a feathered edge (Fig. 13-14). The thick edge should contain a line of concentrated sediment from the sample.

Starfish smear

Although used infrequently, this technique can be utilized for sample preparation from both solid masses and viscous fluid aspirates. The aspirate is gently spread onto the slide by dragging the point of the needle across the slide in several directions (Fig. 13-15). This technique is probably the least damaging to the cells but often results in cells that are surrounded by large volumes of tissue fluid.

Staining of Cytology Specimens

A variety of stains can be used for cytological examination. The most commonly used stains in veterinary practice

BOX 13-7

Tracheal Wash and Bronchoalveolar Lavage

Materials

- Surgical prep materials
- Local anesthetic
- 18-gauge jugular catheter
- Sterile polyethylene tubing and trocar (horses)
- Sterile scalpel blade
- 20- to 30-ml syringe
- Sterile buffered saline
- Endotracheal tube

Procedure

1. A standing animal is preferred; sedation may be necessary. If an endotracheal tube is used, general anesthesia is necessary.
2. The transtracheal approach requires surgical preparation over the cricothyroid area.
3. Infiltrate a local anesthetic agent over the cricothyroid membrane and skin (dogs, cats) or over the tracheal rings (horses, cattle).
4. Make a stab incision with the scalpel blade in the anesthetized area.
5. Insert the catheter (or trocar) into the trachea and direct toward the tracheal bifurcation.
6. Attach a saline-filled syringe (approximately 10 ml for small dogs and cats, 20 ml for large dogs, 30 ml for large animals) and flush into the trachea. An animal that is not anesthetized typically coughs.
7. Bronchoalveolar lavages are done with an endoscope or through an endotracheal tube. Move the catheter or endoscope as far down the trachea as possible (until wedged in a bronchus) before infusing the fluid and aspirating.
8. Aspirate fluid into the syringe by pulling back on the plunger while gently pulling the catheter back and forth within the trachea. Only a portion of the fluid will be recovered.
9. Note volume of fluid recovered. Collect additional fluid if animal coughs after procedure and note this as a nonsterile collection.
10. Place a small amount of fluid in a sterile tube for culture and sensitivity testing.

---

are Romanowsky-type stains. Although there is some variation in staining patterns of cells when using different Romanowsky-type stains, these rarely complicate evaluation once the cytologist becomes familiar with the staining pattern of the particular stain used.

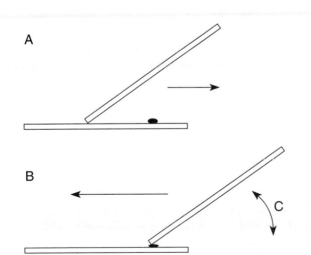

Fig. 13-13 Wedge film. **A,** The upper slide is slowly drawn back into the drop of fluid. The fluid is allowed to spread along the edge of the slide until it nearly reaches the edges. **B,** The slide is then pushed along the surface of the first slide to make the smear. **C,** The length of the smear can be varied by altering the pushing speed, changing the amount of fluid on the slide, or changing the angle of the top slide.

In general, stains should be applied according to the recommendations of the manufacturer. In some cases, the density or thickness of the tissue may require alteration in that technique. Denser, thicker preparations tend to require longer amounts of time in order to stain structures correctly, usually, twice the time required for staining of blood films.

Examination of Cytology Specimens

The primary goal of the initial cytology evaluation is differentiation of inflammation and neoplasia. In general, samples that are inflammatory are characterized by a predominance of neutrophils and macrophages or eosinophils. Neoplastic processes are characterized by large numbers of tissue cells. There may be a combination of cell types present. This mixed cell population often indicates neoplastic disease with secondary inflammation.

The initial evaluation of the cytology preparation should be performed on low magnification (100×) to determine if all areas are adequately stained and to detect any localized areas of increased cellularity. Large objects such as parasites, crystals, and fungal hyphae will normally also be evident on the low-power examination. This initial evaluation should be used to characterize the cellularity and composition of the sample by recording the types of cells present and relative numbers of each type. A high-power (450× to 1000×) should then be performed to evaluate and compare

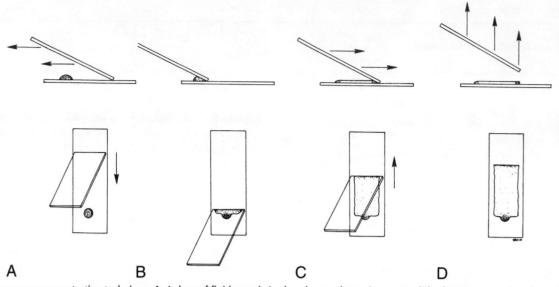

Fig. 13-14 Line smear concentration technique. **A,** A drop of fluid sample is placed onto glass microscope slide close to one end, and another slide is slid backward to contact the front of the drop. **B,** When the drop is contacted, it rapidly spreads along the juncture between the two slides. **C,** The spreader slide is then smoothly and rapidly slid forward. **D,** After the spreader slide has been advanced about two thirds to three fourths of the distance required to make a smear with a feathered edge, the spreader slide is raised directly upward. This produces a smear with a line of concentrated cells at its end, instead of a feathered edge. *(From Cowell R, Tyler R, Meinkoth J:* Diagnostic cytology and hematology of the dog and cat, *ed 2, St Louis, 2002, Mosby.)*

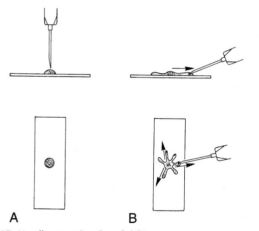

Fig. 13-15 Needle spread or "starfish" preparation. **A,** A portion of the aspirate is expelled onto a glass microscope slide. **B,** The tip of a needle is placed in the aspirate and moved peripherally, pulling a trail of the sample with it. This procedure is repeated in several directions, resulting in a preparation with multiple projections. *(From Cowell R, Tyler R, Meinkoth J:* Diagnostic cytology and hematology of the dog and cat, *ed 2, St Louis, 2002, Mosby.)*

individual cells and further characterize the types of cells present. A systematic approach is vital to achieving high-quality results. Fig. 13-16 contains a sample flowchart for use in evaluating cytology specimens.

Terminology

Consistent terminology must be used when describing cell types. Specific details on the morphology of each cell type will also assist the clinician in making the diagnosis. Neutrophils and macrophages should be evaluated for

presence of vacuoles or phagocytized material. Neutrophils should be evaluated for the presence of degenerative changes, such as pyknosis, karyorrhexis, and karryolysis. Squamous epithelial cells should be characterized as *cornified* or *noncornified*. Neoplastic cells should be evaluated for malignant changes in the cell nucleus, such as mitotic figures, multiple nucleoli, and basophilic cytoplasm.

Fluid samples should also be evaluated for gross appearance, total protein, and total cell count. The total nucleated cell count (TNCC) and total protein values for the sample will allow it to be classified as *transudate, modified transudate,* or *exudate* (Box 13-8). Transudate samples are noninflammatory, appear clear or colorless, and have TNCC less than 500/microliter and total protein less than 2.5 g/dl. Modified transudates are noninflammatory and represent fluids that are passively leaked into tissues with a cell count between 500 and 800/microliter and total protein between 2.5 and 5.0 g/dl. Exudates are characterized by increased cellularity of greater than 3000/microliter and total protein greater than 3.0 g/dl. This higher cell count and protein value is usually indicative of inflammation. Exudates must be evaluated for the presence of intracellular bacteria and then further classified as septic or nonseptic.

Cytology samples can be classified into one of five general categories:
1. Inflammation
2. Cyst formation
3. Hemorrhagic lesions
4. Neoplasia
5. Mixed cell population

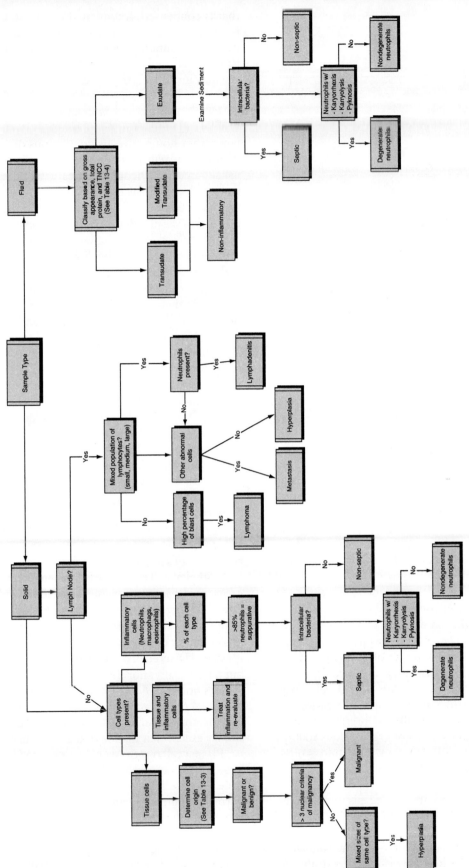

Fig. 13-16 Flowchart for use in evaluating cytology specimens.

BOX 13-8

Classifying Fluid Samples

1. Note volume removed from cavity
2. Save a small amount of fluid in EDTA
3. Save a small amount of fluid in a sterile tube
4. Complete gross examination
5. Perform TNCC and Total Protein Evaluations
6. Classify fluid as transudate, modified transudate, or exudate

	Transudate	Modified Transudate	Exudate
Protein	< 2.5 g/dl	2.5–5.0 g/dl	> 3.0 g/dl
Appearance	Clear, colorless	slightly turbid, white	turbid, pink
Cellularity	< 500/μl	500–800/μl	> 3000/μl

It is usually not necessary to collect cytology samples from hemorrhagic lesions or cysts. In most cases, the veterinary technician will be responsible for making the initial determination to classify a lesion as inflammatory, neoplastic, or mixed.

Inflammation

Inflammation is a normal physiologic response to tissue damage or invasion by microorganisms. This damage releases substances that have a chemotactic effect on certain white blood cells. These chemotactic factors, therefore, are involved in attracting white blood cells to the site of inflammation. The first white blood cells to arrive are the neutrophils. Neutrophils phagocytize dead tissue and microorganisms. The process of phagocytosis creates pH changes both within the neutrophils and in the site. As the pH changes, neutrophils become unable to phagocytize any further and the cells quickly die. At this point, macrophages move in to the site and pick up the phagocytic activity. Cytology samples from inflammatory sites are therefore characterized by the presence of white blood cells, particularly neutrophils and/or macrophages. Occasionally, eosinophils or lymphocytes may also be present. In fluid samples, total nucleated cell counts of greater then 5000/μl is a common finding with inflammation. The fluid is often turbid and may be white or pale yellow. Total protein is often greater than 3 g/dl.

Once designated as inflammatory, the cells must also be evaluated for evidence of degeneration and presence of microorganisms. Nuclear changes that may be found in inflammatory cells (e.g., neutrophils) include *karyolysis*, *karyorrhexis*, and *pyknosis*. These terms describe a nucleus that is condensed, fragmented, or lysed. Cells should also be evaluated for the presence of bacteria. Inflammatory cells that contain phagocytized bacteria or fungal organisms are referred to as *septic*. Additional phagocytized material may include erythrocytes or parasites.

Neoplasia

Unlike inflammation, neoplastic specimens normally contain rather homogeneous populations of a single cell type. Although mixed cell populations are sometimes seen, these usually involve a neoplastic area with a concurrent inflammation. Neoplasia is indicated when the cells present are of the same tissue origin. Once identified as neoplastic, the technician should identify the tissue origin and evaluate the cells for presence of malignant characteristics.

Neoplasia must first be differentiated as either benign or malignant. Benign neoplasia is represented by hyperplasia with no criteria of malignancy present in the cells. Although there may be some minor morphologic variations, the cells are of the same type and are relatively uniform in appearance. Cells that display at least three abnormal nuclear configurations are identified as malignant. Nuclear criteria of malignancy can include any of the abnormalities listed in Table 13-2.

In general, if three or more nuclear criteria of malignancy are present, the specimen is identified as malignant. Exceptions to this general rule would be indicated if inflammation is also present or only a few cells display malignant characteristics.

Specimens that have been classified as malignant should be further evaluated to determine the cell type involved. The basic tumor categories seen in mammals include *epithelial* cell tumors, *mesenchymal* cell tumors, and *discrete round* cell tumors. Table 13-3 summarizes the overall characteristics of samples from each cell type.

Epithelial cell tumors are also referred to as *carcinoma* or *adenocarcinoma*. The samples tend to be highly cellular and often exfoliate in clumps or sheets. Mesenchymal cell tumors are also referred to as *sarcoma* and are usually less cellular. The cells tend to exfoliate singly or in wispy spindles. Discrete round cell tumors exfoliate very well but are usually not in clumps or clusters. Round cell tumors include *histiocytoma, lymphoma, mast cell tumors, plasma cell tumors, transmissible venereal tumors,* and *melanoma*. Histiocytoma and transmissible venereal tumors appear similar except that histiocytoma is not usually highly cellular. Plasma cell tumors can be recognized by the presence of large numbers of cells with a prominent perinuclear clear zone. Mast cells can be recognized by their prominent dark purple granules. Melanoma is characterized by cells with prominent dark black granules.

Examination of lymph node tissue is perhaps one of the most complex of cytology evaluations. Normal lymph nodes usually have a mixture of small, intermediate, and

TABLE 13-2

Easily Recognized General and Nuclear Criteria of Malignancy

Criteria	Description	Schematic Representation
General criteria		
Anisocytosis and macrocytosis	Variation in cell size, with some cells ≥1.5 times larger than normal.	
Hypercellularity	Increased cell exfoliation due to decreased cell adherence.	Not depicted
Pleomorphism (except in lymphoid tissue)	Variable size and shape in cells of the same type.	
Nuclear criteria		
Macrokaryosis	Increased nuclear size. Cells with nuclei larger than 10μ in diameter suggest malignancy.	RBC
Increased nucleus:cytoplasm ratio (N:C)	Normal nonlymphoid cells usually have a N:C of 1:3 to 1:8, depending on the tissue. Increased ratios (1:2, 1:1, etc) suggest malignancy.	See "macrokaryosis"
Anisokaryosis	Variation in nuclear size. This is especially important if the nuclei of multinucleated cells vary in size.	
Multinucleation	Multiple nucleation in a cell. This is especially important if the nuclei vary in size.	
Increased mitotic figures	Mitosis is rare in normal tissue.	normal abnormal
Abnormal mitosis	Improper alignment of chromosomes.	See "increased mitotic figures"
Coarse chromatin pattern	The chromatin pattern is coarser than normal. It may appear ropy or cord-like.	
Nuclear molding	Deformation of nuclei by other nuclei within the same cell or adjacent cells.	
Macronucleoli	Nucleoli are increased in size. Nucleoli ≥5μ strongly suggest malignancy. For reference, RBCs are 5-6μ in the cat and 7-8μ in the dog.	RBC
Angular nucleoli	Nucleoli are fusiform or have other angular shapes, instead of their normal round to slightly oval shape.	
Anisonucleoliosis	Variation in nucleolar shape or size (especially important if the variation is within the same nucleus).	See "angular nucleoli"

From Cowell RL, Tyler RD, Meinkoth JH: *Diagnostic cytology and hematology of the dog* and *cat*, ed 2, St Louis, 1999, Mosby.

Continued

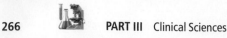

TABLE 13-3

General Appearance of the 3 Basic Tumor Categories

Tumor Type	General Cell Size	General Cell Shape	Schematic Representation	Cellularity of Aspirates	Clumps or Clusters Common
Epithelial	Large	Round to caudate		Usually high	Yes
Mesenchymal (spindle cell)	Small to medium	Spindle to stellate		Usually low	No
			Mast cell Lymphosarcoma		
Discrete round cell	Small to medium	Round	Transmissible veneral tumor Histocytoma	Usually high	No

From Cowell RL, Tyler RD, Meinkoth JH: *Diagnostic cytology and hematology of the dog and cat*, ed 2, St Louis, 1999, Mosby.

large lymphocytes in relatively even percentages. Lymph nodes may show evidence of inflammation (lymphadenitis), hyperplasia (benign neoplasia), mixed (both inflammatory and neoplastic cells present), neoplasia (lymph node cells with abnormal nuclear features), and metastasis (neoplastic cells from other body tissues that spread to lymph nodes). Each of these has specific cell types associated with the abnormality.

Vaginal Cytology

Cytologic evaluation of vaginal tissues is used to determine the stage of estrous in the dog and cat, and as an aid in timing of mating or artificial insemination. Samples are collected with the animal in a standing position with the tail elevated. The external genitalia should be cleaned and rinsed. A lubricated vaginal speculum is inserted into the vagina, followed by a sterile moistened swab. The swab is gently rolled against the vaginal wall and then prepared for evaluation. Two preparations should be made by gently rolling the swab onto two clean glass slides. Approximately ⅔ of each slide should contain material from the vaginal wall. The slides must be air-dried before staining. Any stain

appropriate for general staining of blood films is adequate for vaginal cytology preparations. The slide is initially examined on low power, and quality of preparation is determined. High power can then be used to determine the presence of specific cell types. The cells seen in vaginal cytology samples include epithelial cells (intermediate, large, and cornified), blood cells, and bacteria. Some references may use the terms *parabasal* (for the youngest epithelial cells), *small intermediate* and *large intermediate*. Cornified cells are also referred to as superficial cells and further characterized as either *anuclear* or *pyknotic* (Fig. 13-17). Interpretation of results of vaginal cytology is combined with recent behavioral history and clinical signs in determining estrous stage.

Semen Evaluation

Evaluation of semen is commonly performed when preparing for artificial insemination to determine quality and quantity of sperm present in a sample. Methods used for collection of semen vary with different species. A "teaser" female may be used, and techniques include massage, electro ejaculation, and use of an artificial vagina. Once collected, samples must be protected from rapid changes in

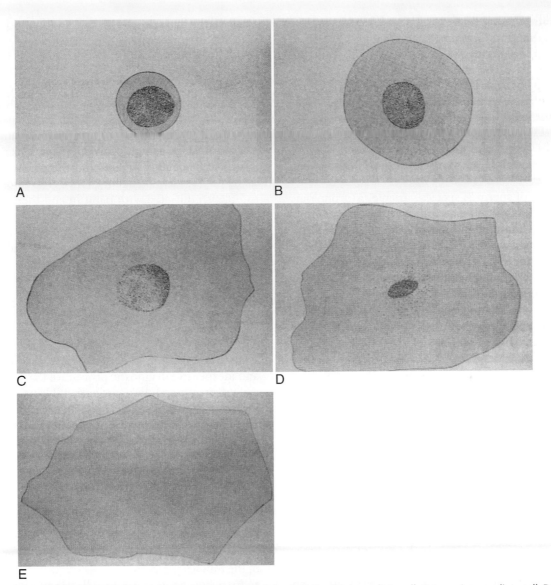

Fig. 13-17 Diagrams of cells from the canine vagina. **A,** Parabasal epithelial cell. **B,** Small intermediate cell. **C,** Large intermediate cell. **D,** Superficial cell with pyknotic nucleus. **E,** An anuclear superficial cell. *(Courtesy Kal Kan Forum.)*

temperature and pH and must not contact water, disinfectants, or other chemicals. All equipment and supplies used to collect, store, or process samples must be clean, dry, free of detergent residue, and warmed to 37° C before use. Tests used to evaluate semen include volume, gross appearance, wave motion, motility, concentration of sperm, live-to-dead sperm ratio, morphology, and determination of the presence of foreign cells and other materials.

Semen volume demonstrates significant species variation and is also affected by method of collection. The largest volumes are obtained with electro ejaculation combined with the use of a teaser female. Volume is evaluated with the use of a volumetric flask. Gross appearance involves evaluation of degree of opacity. This is considered to be a rough indication of sperm concentration and is usually recorded as creamy, thick, opaque, or milky.

Sperm motility can be assessed with either the wave motion tests or progressive motility tests. Wave motion is a subjective assessment based on the amount of activity seen when observing a drop of semen at 40× magnification. If distinct, vigorous swirling activity is seen, the sample is rated as very good (VG). Moderate, slow swirling is rated as good (G). Barely discernible swirling is rated fair (F). Lack of obvious swirling activity is rated poor (P). Progressive motility testing requires dilution of 1 drop of semen in 1 drop of isotonic saline. The sample is examined at 100× magnification for rate of motility and relative percent of motile sperm.

Concentration of sperm is determined by diluting the sample with saline and formalin. A blood dilution pipette is used to dilute the sample, and a hemacytometer is used to count and calculate the numbers of sperm present. The live-to-dead sperm ratio requires a small drop of warmed eosin/nigrosin stain added to a drop of sperm on a glass slide. The slide is air dried and examined under high power. Live sperm resist staining and appear pale/clear against a background of stain. Dead sperm stain pink/red. Two hundred sperm are counted and the ratio of live to dead sperm is recorded.

Morphology of sperm is species variable. Morphologic examination is used to detect the presence of abnormal sperm. Abnormalities may be seen in the head (bicephaly, microcephaly, pyriform, etc.) or tail (coiled, double, etc.) of the sperm (see Fig. 6-11). One hundred sperm are counted, and the number of abnormal sperm seen is expressed as a percentage. Other components that may be seen in semen include blood cells, epithelial cells, and other contaminants from the prepuce.

Histology

Many samples collected for cytology analysis will also require histologic evaluation. Histology samples are usually collected by biopsy and require special preparation in order to preserve the cells for detailed evaluation. The steps required for preparation of permanent histology samples are listed in Box 13-9. Fixation of tissues is a critical first step. The fixative must rapidly denature cellular proteins to avoid autolysis of the sample. Fixatives are chosen based on their speed and penetrating ability. They must not excessively harden or soften tissues and ideally, be nontoxic to the user and inexpensive. Common fixatives include acetic acid, isopropyl or isobutyl alcohol, chromic acid, and formalin. The size of the tissue sample also affects rate of fixation. Samples must be sectioned so that the fixative can penetrate the entire tissue within 24 to 48 hours. For large tissue samples, several cuts should be made into the tissue

to allow the fixative to penetrate rapidly. Most fixatives are capable of penetrating approximately 2 to 4 mm per 24 hours. The amount of solution needed is generally 10 to 20 times the volume of the sample. Once adequately fixed, the sample can be transferred into a smaller container.

Dehydration and washing of the tissue usually involves transferring the sample into increasingly greater concentrations of isopropyl over a 24- to 30-hour time period. The sample is then cleared (alcohol removed) using one of several clearing agents. Xylene, toluene, and/or benzene may all be used as clearing agents. Once cleared of alcohols, the sample is infiltrated with paraffin and then imbedded in a block of paraffin. The paraffin block is sectioned, and the sections are mounted on glass slides. Stains are then added and the tissue examined microscopically. Slides can be permanently maintained by adding a cover slip with mounting media.

URINALYSIS

Complete examination of urine is a relatively simple, rapid, and inexpensive diagnostic procedure that can provide crucial information to the veterinarian. Urinalysis is a valuable diagnostic procedure for evaluating patients. Abnormalities in the urine may reflect a variety of disease processes involving several different organs. The basic equipment needed to perform a urinalysis is minimal and readily available in most veterinary clinics.

Sample Collection

Collect urine samples in clean glass or plastic containers. Sterile containers are not necessary unless you are performing a urine culture. Urine samples are collected using one of the following methods.

- Free-flow or clean catch: collecting a specimen as the animal urinates.
- Expressing the bladder: manual compression of the bladder using gentle, steady pressure applied through the abdominal wall.
- Catheterization: placing a urinary catheter through the urethra into the bladder.
- Cystocentesis: inserting a needle into the bladder through the ventral abdominal wall.

Bladder expression and cystocentesis require the bladder to be full enough to palpate and hold in position. Cystocentesis and catheterization require sterile collection equipment and aseptic technique. Only specimens collected by cystocentesis or catheterization are suitable for urine culture. Cystocentesis and catheterization are also performed to relieve bladder distention in animals unable to urinate. Manual compression cannot be performed on an obstructed animal because this could rupture the bladder. Bladder expression, catheterization, and cystocentesis all

---

BOX 13-9

Preparation of Samples for Histopathology

- Tissue fixation
- Dehydration and washing
- Clearing
- Paraffin infiltration
- Sectioning
- Mounting
- Permanent cover slip

cause some degree of trauma. It is not unusual to find some red blood cells on microscopic examination of the urine. A first-morning urine sample is the preferred specimen because this sample is the most concentrated. The first few drops should be discarded since there is a high incidence of contamination by the debris normally present at the urethral opening in the first few drops. In females, the first drops of urine may also be contaminated with material from the genital tract, such as blood from an intact bitch in proestrus.

Because physical, chemical, and microscopic characteristics of a urine specimen begin to change as soon as urine is voided, urine specimens should be analyzed immediately after collection. Samples left at room temperature for an hour or more will have increases in pH, turbidity, and bacteria and decreases in glucose, bilirubin, and ketones. If specimens are left at room temperature for longer than one hour, cells and casts may also disintegrate, especially in dilute alkaline urine, or urine color may change because of oxidation or reduction of metabolites. If analysis cannot be done immediately, refrigeration will minimize deterioration of the specimen. The specimen should be brought to room temperature before testing. Chemical preservatives can also be added to urine. However, preservatives usually act as antimicrobial agents, so chemically preserved urine cannot be used for culture and may interfere with biochemical testing.

THE COMPLETE URINALYSIS

A complete urinalysis has the following four parts:
1. Gross examination
2. Specific gravity
3. Biochemical analysis
4. Sediment examination

A systematic approach is vital to achieving high-quality, reproducible results. The gross examination includes an evaluation of color, clarity, odor, and volume. Normal canine and feline urine is light amber-colored, clear, and has a characteristic odor. Normal urine output for canine and feline patients is 10 to 20 cc per pound in a 24-hour period. Common changes found during gross examination of the urine sample are summarized in Table 13-4.

Specific Gravity

Specific gravity (SG) is a measure of the ratio of a volume of urine to the weight of the same volume of distilled water at a constant temperature. SG is an indicator of the concentration of dissolved materials in the urine and provides an indication of kidney function. Alteration in the concentrating ability of the kidneys is an early indicator of renal tubular damage. The preferred method for determining SG is with the use of a refractometer. SG indicator pads on urinalysis dipstick tests may be unreliable in veterinary species. SG can be measured before or after centrifugation,

TABLE 13-4

Gross Examination of Urine

Quality	Shows Evidence of
Changes in Color	
Colorless	Dilute urine with low SG; often seen in conjunction with polyuria
Deep amber	Highly concentrated urine (low SG); associated with oliguria
White	Associated with presence of leukocytes
Red to red/brown	Usually indicates presence of RBCs and/or hemoglobin
Changes in Turbidity	
Cloudy	Usually indicates presence of cells (e.g., WBCs, epithelial cells, bacteria)
Milky	Usually indicates presence of fatty material
Changes in Odor	
Sweet	Usually indicates presence of ketones
Pungent	Associated with presence of bacteria
Changes in Volume	
Polyuria	Increase in volume of urine voided in a 24-hour period
Oliquria	Decrease in volume of urine voided in a 24-hour period
Anuria	Absence of urine voiding

as long as the procedure is always performed consistently in the clinic. All individuals performing the test should perform it in the same manner on the same type of sample.

Biochemical Testing

Chemical evaluation of urine is used to detect substances that may have passed into the urine as a result of damage to the nephron or overproduction of specific analytes. The majority of in-house urinalysis chemical tests utilize the dipstick format. Dipsticks can be used to perform individual tests or multiple tests. Each reagent pad on the dipstick contains reagent for one specific chemical test. The reagent pad changes color during the reaction, and the color is visually compared to a color chart. Before using the dipstick, always note the expiration date and general condition of strips. Containers of dipsticks should be stored at room temperature with the lid tightly capped. Avoid placing containers or color charts in direct sunlight. Always use well-mixed, room temperature urine samples and perform chemical testing before adding any chemical preservatives. Read the instructions carefully, and evaluate color changes at the correct time interval. Since dipsticks are not configured for veterinary species, some tests (i.e., SG, nitrite, leukocytes) may be unreliable with some species.

Protein

Protein is normally present in very low quantities in the urine (at or below the limit of sensitivity of the urine reagent strips). Physiologic (nonpathologic) proteinuria can occur with fever or strenuous exercise that results in increased permeability of the glomeruli to plasma proteins. Postrenal proteinuria is the result of serum proteins being added from hemorrhage or inflammation in the lower urinary tract (bladder) or genital tract. Renal proteinuria is fairly common and may be due to glomerular damage.

Glucose

Glucose is normally not present in the urine in quantities detectable on dipsticks. The presence of glucose in the urine is called *glucosuria* or *glycosuria*. Glucosuria occurs with any condition that causes the blood glucose level to exceed the renal threshold for resorption. Diabetes mellitus is a common cause of glucosuria resulting from excessive blood glucose concentrations.

Ketones

Ketonuria can occur with diabetes mellitus in small animals, during lactation in cows, and during pregnancy in cows and ewes. It also occurs with high-fat diets, starvation, fasting, anorexia, and impaired liver function.

pH

The pH is an indication of the hydrogen ion (H^+) concentration, and it is a measure of the degree of acidity or alkalinity of urine. A pH greater than 7.0 is alkaline; a pH less than 7.0 is acidic. High-protein diets produce a lower urine pH, whereas vegetable diets result in high urine pH. Carnivores typically have acidic urine, whereas herbivores have alkaline urine. Nursing herbivores have acidic urine from consumption of milk.

Bilirubin

Normal dogs occasionally have small amounts of bilirubin in their urine. Any bilirubinuria is abnormal in other species. Bilirubinuria can be seen with a number of diseases, including hemolytic diseases, hepatic insufficiency, and diseases that cause obstruction of bile flow.

Occult blood

The occult blood reagent detects both myoglobin and hemoglobin in urine. The hemoglobin may be free hemoglobin (*hemoglobinuria*) or within intact erythrocytes (*hematuria*). Hematuria is detected by a positive occult blood test, along with observation of intact red blood cells on urine sediment examination. Cloudy urine that appears red, brown, or wine-colored denotes the presence of moderate to large amounts of blood. Similar colors, but with a transparent appearance, that remain after centrifugation indicate hemoglobinuria. Hemoglobinuria is usually due to intravascular hemolysis. Myoglobin is a protein found in muscle. Myoglobinuria is usually seen in horses with rhabdomyolysis. A positive occult blood reading is most commonly associated with hematuria, rather than with hemoglobinuria.

Microscopic Examination of Urine Sediment

The primary purpose of microscopic examination of urine is to determine the presence of abnormal formed elements (i.e., cells, casts, crystals) in the sample. Such abnormalities may be present even in samples that are otherwise normal. The microscopic examination can be partly standardized with the use of specific urine sediment evaluation preparation and counting chambers. The examination requires 5 to 10 ml of fresh urine. The sample should be centrifuged at low speed for about 5 minutes and then the supernatant poured off, leaving about 1 ml of supernatant with the sediment. The remaining sediment is resuspended in the supernatant and mixed gently. A drop of this suspension is then placed on a microscope slide, a cover slip is added, and the specimen is examined microscopically. Although stain may be added to the sample, this often creates artifacts and can add bacteria to the sample. When stain is needed to classify cell types, they should be added after the initial evaluation of the specimen.

The specimen should first be scanned with a low-power lens. Large formed elements (e.g., casts) are evident at lower magnifications. A minimum of 10 microscopic fields with a high-power lens should be observed. The results of the microscopic examination are reported as the number of elements seen per low-power field (LPF) or high-power field (HPF). Report cells and bacteria in numbers/HPF and casts in numbers/LPF. Box 13-10 contains a summary of the steps required to perform a complete urinalysis.

Elements in Urinary Sediment

Urinary sediment may contain a variety of cells, casts, crystals, and miscellaneous components such as parasites. The presence of specific formed elements usually provides detailed diagnostic information to the clinician.

Cells

Erythrocytes and leukocytes. The presence of intact erythrocytes (RBCs) (hematuria) in urine may indicate bleeding within the urogenital tract (Fig. 13-18). Up to five RBCs per high-power field is considered normal. RBCs are smaller than leukocytes (WBCs) or epithelial cells; they are round and slightly refractile and lack internal structure (Fig. 13-19).

In concentrated urine, the RBCs crenate (shrivel); in dilute urine they swell and lyse, and appear as colorless rings (ghost cells) that vary in size and shape.

Up to five WBCs per high-power field can be found in the urine sediment of normal animals (Fig. 13-20). Greater than 5 WBC/HPF can indicate inflammation. These cells are round and granular, larger than RBCs, and smaller than epithelial cells. They degenerate in old urine and may lyse in hypotonic or alkaline urine.

Epithelial cells. Unless the sample was collected by cystocentesis, squamous epithelial cells are a common finding in urine samples (Fig. 13-21). They are the largest of the three types of epithelial cells found in urine samples. The cells are thin and flat with angular borders and large nuclei. The cells originate in the distal urethra, vagina, vulva, or prepuce. The presence of squamous cells is usually

not significant. Transitional epithelial cells originate in the bladder, ureters, renal pelvis, and proximal urethra. They are usually round, but can be oval or caudate. The nucleus is dense and round.

Transitional epithelial cells may occur in clumps, especially if the urine was collected by catheterization. Sheets of transitional cells in a free-flow sample may reflect transitional cell carcinoma. The morphology of these cells requires close examination for changes suggestive of malignancy. An increase in the number of transitional cells of normal appearance suggests inflammation. Renal epithelial cells are the smallest epithelial cells seen in urine. They originate in the renal tubules, and their presence may represent tubular degeneration. They are small, round, and slightly larger than WBCs.

Casts

Urinary casts are cylindrical structures formed from a matrix of protein secreted by the renal tubules. They form in the loop of Henle and distal tubules of the kidney (Fig. 13-22). The cast takes on the shape of the tubule. Any component in the urine can be incorporated into the cast, such as cells or bacteria. Cast types include hyaline casts, cellular casts, granular casts, and waxy casts, depending on the material trapped in the protein matrix at the time of formation and the age of the casts. Therefore, the presence of a specific type may aid in identification of the location of damage within the nephron. Casts dissolve in alkaline urine, so identification and quantification is best done with fresh urine samples. Although a few casts may be seen in normal urine, the presence of casts in urine samples usually indicates tubular damage. The formation of casts requires slow-moving filtrate. Casts are fragile structures that are easily destroyed with improper preparation of sample.

BOX 13-10　　　　　　　　　　　　　　　　　　　　　　　　　　*procedure*

Microscopic Examination of Urine Sediment

1. Place a small drop of suspended urine sediment on a glass slide and cover with a 22- × 22-mm coverslip.
2. Place the slide on the microscope and swing the 10X lens into place.
3. Reduce the light intensity and lower the substage condenser.
4. Focus on the material on the slide.
5. Scan the slide and identify larger elements, such as casts and crystals. Both the center and edges of the slide should be examined.
6. Swing the 40X lens into place and readjust the light, if necessary.
7. Identify formed elements, including RBCs, WBCs, epithelial cells (and their type), casts, crystals, and bacteria.

8. Evaluate the sediment as follows:
   - Crystals and casts—numbers per low-power field (LPF)
   - Cells (and sometimes casts and crystals)—numbers per high-power field (HPF)
   - Bacteria and sperm

Rare	=	Only 2 or 3 seen on scanning several HPF
1+	=	Less than 1/HPF
2+	=	1-5/HPF
3+	=	6-20/HPF
4+	=	Greater than 20/HPF

9. Record the results.

From Pratt PW: Laboratory procedures for veterinary technicians, ed 3, St Louis, 1997, Mosby.

Red blood cells

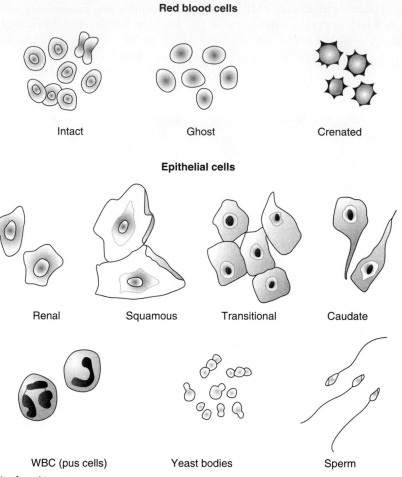

Intact   Ghost   Crenated

Epithelial cells

Renal   Squamous   Transitional   Caudate

WBC (pus cells)   Yeast bodies   Sperm

Fig. 13-18 Cell types that may be found in urine. *(From Cowell R, Tyler R, Meinkoth J: Diagnostic cytology and hematology of the dog and cat, ed 2, St Louis, 2002, Mosby.)*

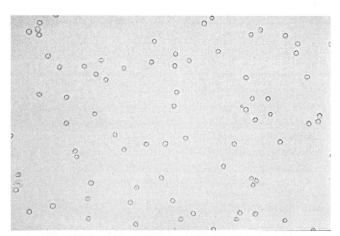

Fig. 13-19 RBCs in urine sediment. Although cells are similar in size, some have irregular borders because they are crenated as a result of increased urine osmolarity (unstained, original magnification 400×). *(From Cowell R, Tyler R, Meinkoth J: Diagnostic cytology and hematology of the dog and cat, ed 2, St Louis, 2002, Mosby.)*

Hyaline casts are colorless and translucent (Fig. 13-23). Cellular casts contain specific recognizable cells (WBCs, RBCs, epithelial cells). Granular casts are formed when cellular casts degenerate. Granular casts should be described as either coarse or fine. The presence of granular casts usually indicates severe kidney damage. Waxy casts (Fig. 13-24) are wide and smooth, with sharp margins and blunt ends. Fatty casts contain high amounts of lipid material incorporated into the protein matrix of the cast.

Crystals

The presence of crystals in the urine is called *crystalluria* (Fig. 13-25). Crystals are common in urine sediment, but only a few types are significant. Formation of crystals is dependent on the amount of the substance in the urine and the solubility of the particular crystal type. The pH and SG of the urine affects the formation of crystals. Crystals found in acidic urine include: calcium oxalate, amorphous urates,

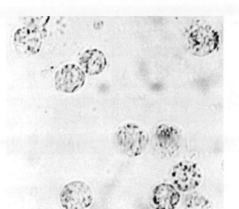

Fig. 13-20 White blood cells in canine urine. (500×) *(From Cowell R, Tyler R, Meinkoth J: Diagnostic cytology and hematology of the dog and cat, ed 2, St Louis, 2002, Mosby.)*

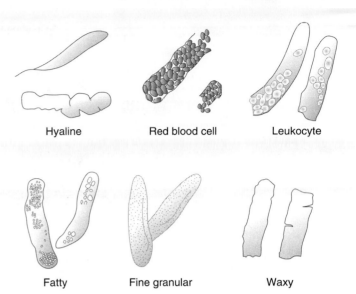

Hyaline Red blood cell Leukocyte

Fatty Fine granular Waxy

Fig. 13-22 Various types of casts that may be found in urine. *(From Cowell R, Tyler R, Meinkoth J: Diagnostic cytology and hematology of the dog and cat, ed 2, St Louis, 2002, Mosby.)*

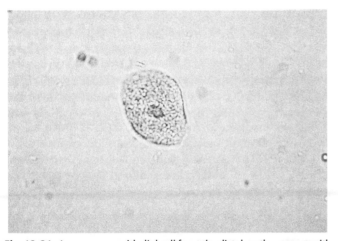

Fig. 13-21 A squamous epithelial cell from the distal uretha as seen with reduced illumination and bright field microscopy. *(From Cowell R, Tyler R, Meinkoth J: Diagnostic cytology and hematology of the dog and cat, ed 2, St Louis, 2002, Mosby.)*

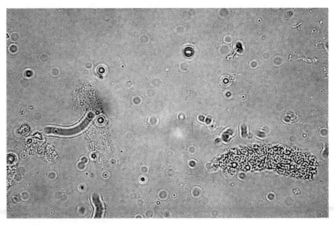

Fig. 13-23 Hyaline and granular casts. Bright-field microscopy. *(From Cowell R, Tyler R, Meinkoth J: Diagnostic cytology and hematology of the dog and cat, ed 2, St Louis, 2002, Mosby.)*

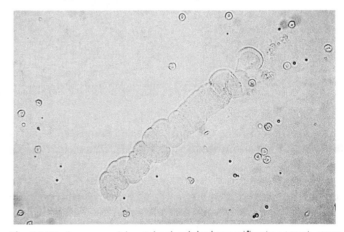

Fig. 13-24 A waxy cast (unstained, original magnification 280×). *(From Cowell R, Tyler R, Meinkoth J: Diagnostic cytology and hematology of the dog and cat, ed 2, St Louis, 2002, Mosby.)*

sodium urates, uric acid, calcium sulfates, and cystine. Alkaline urine may contain amorphous phosphates or struvite crystals.

Struvite crystals have a characteristic "coffin lid" appearance. This type of crystal, sometimes referred to as *triple phosphate*, is a common finding in urolithiasis in dogs and cats but may also be seen in urine samples from normal patients. Amorphous phosphate crystals appear as a

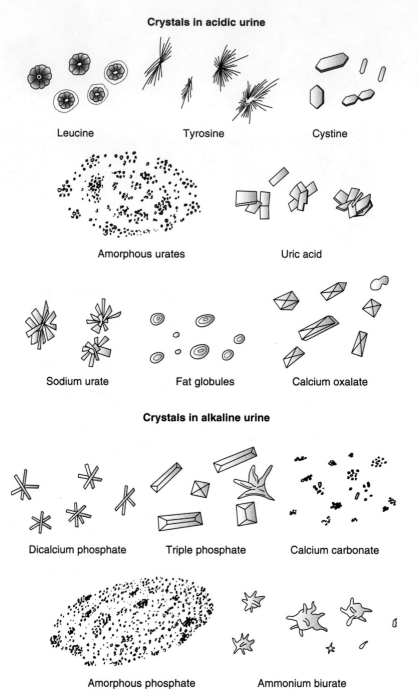

Fig. 13-25 Various types of crystals that may be found in urine. *(From Hendrix CM: Laboratory procedures for veterinary technicians, ed 4, St Louis, 2002, Mosby.)*

granular precipitate. Calcium oxalate crystals and stones are also found in normal urine and are common in urine from older dogs and cats.

Calcium carbonate crystals are commonly found in the urine of normal horses and cattle. These crystals resemble colorless "dumbbells" and can be seen in neutral or alkaline urine. Amorphous urate crystals, seen in acidic urine, resemble amorphous phosphates (a granular precipitate), but amorphous phosphates are seen in alkaline urine.

Calcium oxalate dihydrate crystals can be found in the urine of normal animals. They are seen in acidic, neutral, or alkaline urine, and appear as small squares or "envelopes" containing an *x*. These crystals can be associated with oxalate ingestion in large animals and ethylene glycol (antifreeze) poisoning in small animals. Calcium oxalate monohydrate crystals are most commonly associated with ethylene glycol poisoning but can also be seen in animals with calcium oxalate urolithiasis. Uric acid crystals can be seen in alkaline urine and are associated with a metabolic defect (most common in Dalmatians) and formation of uroliths.

Ammonium biurate (also known as ammonium urate) crystals are found commonly in Dalmatians and with presence of certain liver diseases. These crystals are round and brownish, with long thorny apple-shaped spicules and are not present in the urine of normal animals; they are seen in the urine of animals with liver disease or portosystemic shunts. Monohydrate calcium oxalate crystals are seen in ethylene glycol toxicity. Cystine, leucine, and tyrosine are pathological crystals that may be found in urine samples. Cystine crystals appear as flat, hexagonal (six-sided) plates and are associated with congenital defects in cystine metabolism and are common in certain canine breeds (e.g., Newfoundland). Leucine and tyrosine crystals often occur together and are present in acute liver disease.

Bacteria

Bacteria may be present as the result of infection or contamination. Normal urine is free of bacteria but may be contaminated by bacteria from the distal urethra and genital tract. Urine obtained by cystocentesis is the preferred sample for evaluation of bacteria because contamination is avoided. Bacteria numbers are reported as few, moderate, or many. Because bacteria often proliferate in urine that has been left standing for some time, it is important to examine a fresh sample.

Miscellaneous

Parasites and/or their ova may be seen in urine sediment. *Capillaria plica* (Fig. 13-26), *Dichtopyma renale*, and some liver flukes may be present. Additional organisms such as mites are seen as contaminants when samples are collected improperly. Fungal organisms, microfilaria of *D. immitis*, and sperm may also be seen.

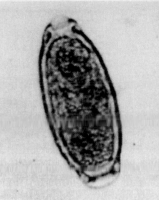

Fig. 13-26 An egg of *Capillaria plica*, the bladder worm of dogs (400×). *(From Hendrix CM: Laboratory procedures for veterinary technicians, ed 4, St Louis, 2002, Mosby.)*

RECOMMENDED READING

Baker R, Lumsden J: *Color atlas of cytology of the dog and cat*, St Louis, 2000, Mosby.

Coles EH: *Veterinary clinical pathology*, ed 4, Philadelphia, 1986, Saunders.

Cowell R, Tyler R, Meinkoth J: *Diagnostic cytology and hematology of the dog and cat*, ed 2, St Louis, 2002, Mosby.

Dow SW, Jones RL, and Rosychuk RA: Bacteriologic specimens: selection, collection, and transport for optimum results. In *Veterinary laboratory medicine in practice*, Trenton, N.J., 1997, Veterinary Learning Systems.

Graff L: *A handbook of routine urinalysis*, Philadelphia, 1992, Lippincott Williams & Wilkins.

Hendrix CM: *Laboratory procedures for veterinary technicians*, ed 4, St Louis, 2002, Mosby.

Meyer DJ: The management of cytology specimens. In *Veterinary laboratory medicine in practice*, Trenton, N.J., 1997, Veterinary Learning Systems.

Raskin R, Meyer DJ: *Atlas of canine and feline cytology*, Philadelphia, 2001, Saunders.

14

Veterinary Parasitology

Margi Sirois

Learning Objectives
After reviewing this chapter, the reader should understand the following:

- Common internal parasites of domestic animals
- Common external parasites of domestic animals
- Procedures used to diagnose parasites

PARASITOLOGY

Parasitology is the study of organisms that live *in* (internal parasites, *endoparasites*) or *on* (external parasites, *ectoparasites*) another organism, the *host*, from which they derive their nourishment. Parasitism is a type of symbiotic relationship. *Symbiosis* involves two organisms living together and can be of three types:

- Commensalism: one organism benefits, the other is unaffected
- Mutualism: both organisms benefit
- Parasitism: one organism benefits, the other is harmed

The organism that the parasite lives in or on is called its host. The host may be a definitive host, sheltering the sexual, adult stages of the parasite, or an intermediate host, harboring asexual (immature) or larval stages of the parasite. There are also *paratenic* hosts or *transport* hosts for some parasites, in which the parasite survives without multiplying or developing. Parasite life cycles can be simple with direct transmission, or complex and involve one or more vectors. A vector can be mechanical or biological. Mechanical vectors transmit the parasite but the parasite does not develop in the vector. Biological vectors serve as intermediate hosts for the parasite. The term *life cycle* refers to maturation of a parasite through various developmental stages in one or more hosts. For a parasite to survive, it must have a dependable means of transfer from one host to another and the ability to develop and reproduce in the host, ideally without producing serious harm to the host. This requires the following:

- Mode of entry into a host (infective stage)
- Availability of a susceptible host (definitive host)
- Accommodating location and environment in the host for maturation and reproduction (gastrointestinal, respiratory, circulatory, urinary, or reproductive system)
- Mode of exit from the host (feces, sputum, blood, urine, smegma), with dispersal into an ecologically suitable environment for development and survival.

For parasites that have one or more intermediate hosts, the definitive host is the one in which sexual maturity takes place.

Parasites have a wide distribution within host animals. They can have a negative impact in a number of ways, including the following:

- Injury on entry (e.g., creeping eruption)
- Injury by migration (e.g., Sarcoptes)
- Injury by residence (e.g., heartworms)
- Chemical and/or physiological injury (e.g., digestive disturbances)
- Injury due to host reaction (e.g., hypersensitivity, scar tissue)

CLASSIFICATION OF PARASITES

Parasites of domestic animals are found in the Kingdom Protista and the Kingdom Animalia and in a large number of phyla in those kingdoms.

Kingdom Protista, Subkingdom Protozoa

There are about 65,000 known protozoans in a wide variety of habitats. Only a small percentage of protozoans are parasitic. Protozoa are single-celled organisms with one or more membrane-bound nuclei containing DNA and specialized cytoplasmic organelles. Parasitic protozoa can be found in three primary phyla: (1) Sarcomastigophora; (2) Apicomplexa; and (3) Ciliophora. The life cycles of protozoa can be simple or complex. Reproduction may be asexual (binary fission, schizogony, budding) or sexual (syngamy, conjugation). With certain groups of protozoa, reproductive stages are useful in identification. The *trophozoite* (also known as vegetative form) is that stage of the protozoal life cycle that is capable of feeding, movement, and reproduction (Fig. 14-1).

Organelles for locomotion consist of *flagella* (long whiplike structures), *cilia* (short flagella usually arranged in rows or tufts), *pseudopodia* (temporary extensions and retractions of the body wall), and *undulatory ridges* (small snakelike waves that form in the cell membrane and move posteriorly). Locomotor organelles and modifications of them are frequently used to help identify the type of protozoa recovered from animals. The trophozoite is often too fragile to survive transfer to a new host and generally is not infective. Transmission to a host often occurs when the protozoan is in the cyst stage. Most metabolic functions are suspended when the parasite is encysted. The cyst wall prevents desiccation. The cyst stage occurs under certain conditions that include:

- Lack of nutrients
- Low oxygen tension
- Lack of water
- Low pH
- Accumulation of waste
- Overcrowding

Phylum sarcomastigophora (Sarcodina)

This phylum includes the amoebas and flagellates. There are about 44,000 known species in this phylum, but only about 2300 are parasitic. Genera of veterinary importance in this phylum include:

- *Trypanosoma*
- *Leishmania*
- *Giardia* (see Fig. 14-1)
- *Trichomonas*
- *Histomonas*
- *Entamoeba*

Phylum apicomplexa

These are the sporozoans. There are about 4600 species and all are parasitic. Sporozoans are unique in that all their life cycle stages are haploid except for the zygote. Sporozoal parasites are found within the host cells and commonly occur in the intestinal tract cells and blood cells. *Oocyst* is the name given to the cyst stage of this group of intestinal protozoa. The genera of veterinary importance include the following intracellular parasites:

- *Eimeria* (Fig. 14-2)
- *Isospora* (Fig. 14-3)
- *Cryptosporidium* (Fig. 14-4)
- *Klossiella*
- *Toxoplasma* (Fig. 14-5)
- *Sarcocystis*
- *Plasmodium*
- *Babesia* (Fig. 14-6)

Phylum ciliophora

There are about 7200 species in the phylum Ciliophora, of which about 2200 are parasitic. Only one genera, *Balantidium*, is of veterinary significance.

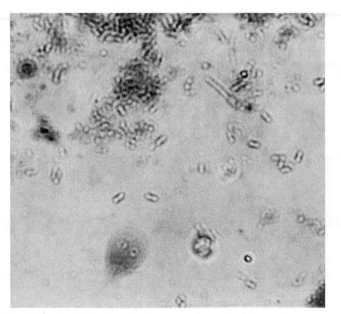

Fig. 14-1 *Giardia* trophozoite (Romanowsky-stained impressions smear of duodenum).

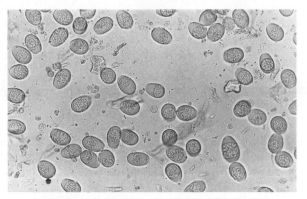

Fig. 14-2 *Eimeria* spp. oocysts (fecal flotation).

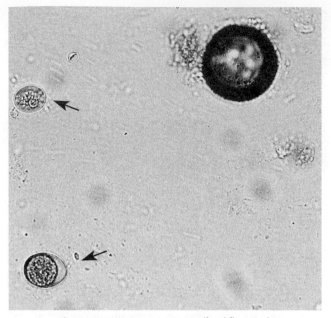

Fig. 14-3 *Isospora* spp. oocysts (fecal flotation).

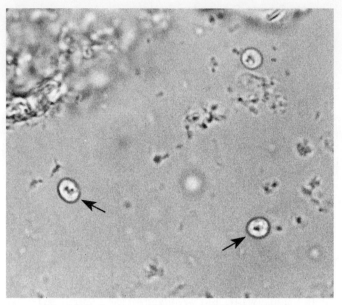

Fig. 14-4 *Cryptosporidium m* oocysts (fecal flotation).

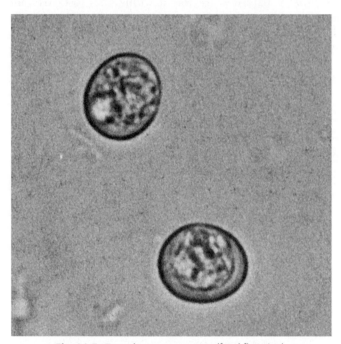

Fig. 14-5 *Toxoplasma* spp. oocysts (fecal flotation).

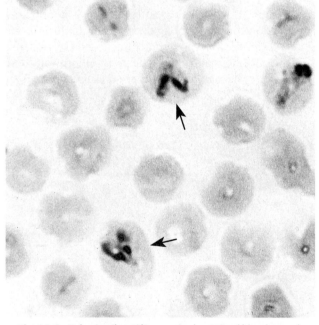

Fig. 14-6 *Babesia gibsoni* (Romanowsky-stained blood smear).

Kingdom Animalia

Three of the phyla in this kingdom contain hundreds of species that are of veterinary significance. These include (1) Platyhelminthes: the flatworms; (2) Nematoda: the roundworms; and (3) Arthropoda: ticks, mice, and lice. The phylum Acanthocephala contains just a few species of veterinary significance.

Phylum platyhelminthes

Organisms in the phylum Platyhelminthes are commonly called flatworms because of the dorsoventral flattening of their body tissues. The two groups of veterinary importance are the cestodes (tapeworms) and trematodes (flukes).

Cestodes. Two major groups of tapeworms are important in veterinary medicine. The first group is composed of the cyclophyllidean tapeworms, which typically have one intermediate host (such as *Dipylidium caninum*, *Taenia* spp., *Echinococcus* spp., *Moniezia* spp.) (Figs. 14-7 and 14-8). The second group is composed of the pseudophyllidean tapeworms, which have two intermediate hosts (such as *Diphyllobothrium latum*). Typically the larval stages of cestodes in domestic animals are more harmful (pathogenic) than the adult stages in the intestinal tract. However, the adult stages are the source of eggs, especially for cestodes, which can use people as an intermediate host and pose a risk to human health (zoonotic).

Cestodes are multicellular organisms that lack a body cavity. Their organs are embedded in loose cellular tissue (*parenchyma*). The body of tapeworms is long and dorsoventrally flattened, and consists of three regions. The head (*scolex*) is modified into an attachment organ and bears two to four muscular suckers, or *bothria*. The suckers may

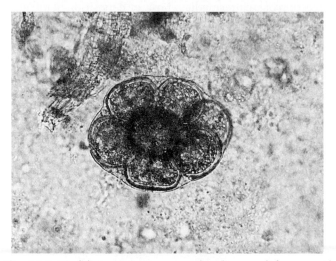

Fig. 14-7 *Dipylidium caninum* egg packet (recovered from gravid proglottid).

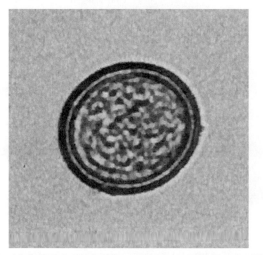

Fig. 14-8 *Taenia* spp. egg (recovered from gravid proglottid).

be armed with hooks. There may also be a snout (*rostellum*) on the head, which can be fixed or retractable. The rostellum can also be armed with hooks. Caudal to the head is a short neck of undifferentiated tissue, followed by the body (*strobila*). The body is composed of segments (*proglottids*) in different stages of maturity. Those near the neck are immature, followed by sexually mature proglottids, and terminating with gravid segments containing eggs. Gravid proglottids break off and pass out of the body of the definitive host in the feces. New proglottids are continually formed from the undifferentiated tissue of the neck. Cestodes lack a digestive tract, and nutrients are absorbed directly through the body wall. The most prominent organs in cestodes are the organs of the reproductive system. Both male and female reproductive organs occur in an individual tapeworm. Cestodes also have a nervous system and an excretory system.

The cestode egg contains a fully developed embryo, which has six hooks in three pairs (*hexacanth embryo* or *oncosphere*), or a zygote that develops into a ciliated embryo (*coracidium*). The life cycle of tapeworms is always indirect and involves one or two intermediate hosts. The intermediate hosts may be arthropods, fish, or mammals. Domestic animals can be definitive hosts and/or intermediate hosts for tapeworms. The larval stages of some tapeworms found in domestic animals are called *bladder worms* because they resemble fluid-filled sacks with one or multiple scoleces. When ingested by a definitive host, the bladder worms are released from the tissue of the intermediate host and develop into adult tapeworms within the digestive tract of the definitive host. Some cestodes have larval forms that are solid bodies (*procercoid*, *plerocercoid*, *and tetrathyridium*). Domestic animals become infected with the larval stages of tapeworms by ingestion of the cestode egg or procercoid.

Trematodes. The trematodes (flukes) are flatworms that, like cestodes, lack a body cavity. They are unsegmented and leaflike. The organs are embedded in loose tissue (parenchyma), and they also possess two muscular attachment organs or suckers. One sucker, the anterior sucker, is located at the mouth. The other sucker, the ventral sucker or *acetabulum*, is located on the ventral surface of the worm near the middle of the body or at the caudal end. There are three main groups of trematodes, but only the *digenetic* trematodes are parasites of domestic animals.

Digenetic trematodes have an outer body wall or cuticle. They have a simple digestive tract consisting of a mouth, pharynx, esophagus, and an intestine that divides into two blind sacs (ceca). The main organs visible in trematodes are the reproductive organs. Most trematodes have both male and female reproductive organs in the same individual, but a few have separate sexes (e.g., *Schistosoma*). A nervous system and an excretory system are also present.

The life cycle of digenetic trematodes is complicated. They pass through several different larval stages (miracidium,

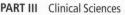

sporocyst, redia, cercaria, and metacercaria) and typically require one or more intermediate hosts, one of which is nearly always a mollusk (snail, slug). Multiplication takes place in both the definitive (sexual) and intermediate (asexual) hosts. The eggs of digenetic trematodes are capped (operculated), and they contain a ciliated embryo called a miracidium. Through penetration or ingestion, the miracidium enters a suitable snail and develops through several stages that eventually give rise to a motile, tailed stage referred to as a cercaria. Cercariae are released from the snail and swim actively. Sometimes, depending on the species of fluke, the cercariae encyst on vegetation. This encysted stage, the metacercaria, is infective for the definitive host. In other species, the cercaria may penetrate the skin of the definitive host or encyst in another intermediate host. Examples of digenetic trematodes of domestic animals are *Fasciola hepatica* (Fig. 14-9), *Heterobilharzia americana, Paramphistomum cervi, Nanophyetus salmincola* (Fig. 14-10), and *Paragonimus kellicotti.*

Phylum nematoda

Organisms in the phylum Nematoda are commonly called roundworms because of their cylindrical body shape.

Nematodes are multicellular, and possess a body wall composed of an external, acellular, protective layer called the *cuticle;* a cellular layer beneath the cuticle called the *hypodermis;* and a layer of longitudinal, somatic muscles that function in locomotion. The digestive tract and reproductive organs of roundworms are tubular and are suspended in the body cavity *(pseudocoelom).* The digestive tract is a straight tube that runs the length of the body from the mouth to the caudal end (anus). The sexes for most nematodes are separate. The reproductive organs are also tubular but typically are longer than the body and coil around the intestinal tract of the worm. Nematodes have a nervous system and an excretory system, but no respiratory system.

The life cycle of nematodes follows a standard pattern consisting of several developmental stages: the egg, four larval stages that are also wormlike in appearance, and sexually mature adults. The infective stage may be an egg containing a larva, a free-living larva, or a larva within an intermediate host or transport host. A life cycle is considered *direct* if no intermediate host is necessary for development to the infective stage. If an intermediate host is required for development to the infective stage, the life cycle is considered *indirect.* Transmission to a new definitive host (host harboring sexually mature adults) can occur through ingestion, skin penetration of infective larvae, ingestion of an intermediate host, or deposition of infective larvae into or on the skin by an intermediate host.

Once a nematode gains entry into a new host, development to the adult stages may occur in the area of their final location or may occur after extensive migration through the body of the definitive host. The diagnostic stages of parasitic nematodes are typically found in feces, blood, sputum, or urine. Most parasitic nematodes are found in the intestinal tracts of their respective definitive hosts, but some are found in the lungs, kidney, urinary bladder, or heart.

The following 11 taxonomic superfamilies of nematodes are significant in veterinary medicine:

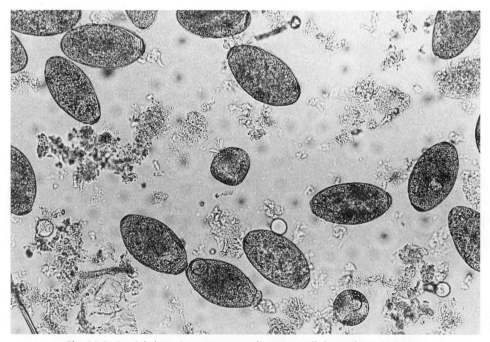

Fig. 14-9 *Fasciola hepatica* eggs surrounding a centrally located *Moniezia* egg.

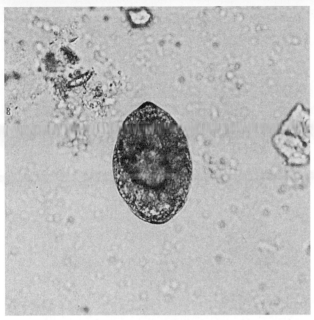

Fig. 14-10 *Nanophyetus salmincola* eggs (sedimentation).

1. Ascaridoidea (Figs. 14-11 to 14-14) (*Toxocara* spp., *Toxascaris* spp., *Ascaris* spp., *Parascaris equorum*, *Toxocara vitulorum*)
2. Strongyloidea (Fig. 14-15) (*Strongylus* spp., *Ancylostoma* spp., *Bunostomum* spp., *Uncinaria* spp., *Syngamus* spp., *Oesophagostomum* spp.)
3. Trichostrongyloidea (*Haemonchus* spp., *Ostertagia* spp., *Trichostrongylus* spp., *Cooperia* spp., *Nematodirus* spp., *Ollulanus tricuspis*, *Dictyocaulus* spp.)

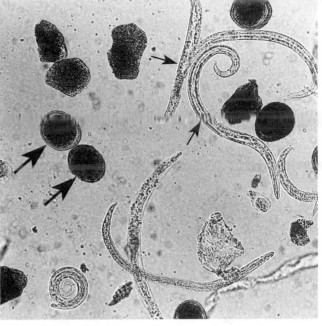

Fig. 14-12 *Toxocara cati* eggs (*large arrows*) and *Aelurostrongylus abstrusus* larvae (*small arrows*) (fecal flotation).

4. Metastrongylidae (*Metastrongylus* spp., *Protostrongylus* spp., *Muellerius capillaris*, *Filaroides* spp., *Aelurostrongylus abstrusus*)
5. Oxyuroidea (Fig. 14-16) (*Oxyuris equi*, *Skrjabinema ovis*)
6. Trichuroidea (Figs. 14-17 and 14-18) (*Trichuris* spp., *Capillaria* spp., *Trichinella spiralis*, *Ancylostoma*)

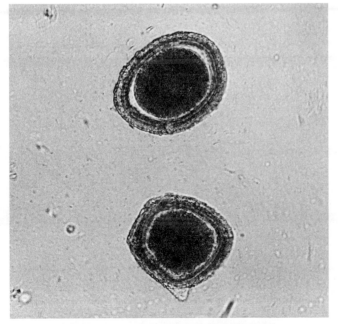

Fig. 14-11 *Toxocara canis* eggs (fecal flotation).

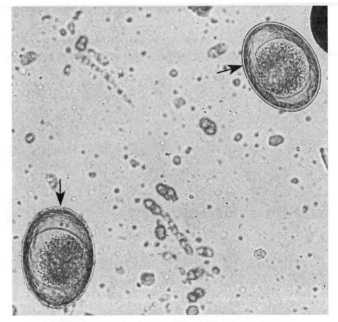

Fig. 14-13 *Toxascaris leonina* eggs (fecal flotation).

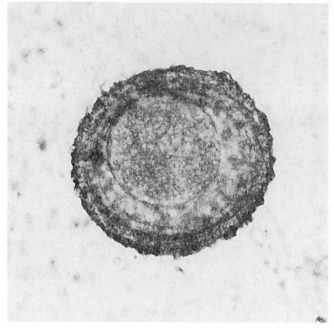

Fig. 14-14 *Parascaris equorum* egg (fecal flotation).

7. Filaroidea (Figs. 14-19 and 14-20) (*Dirofilaria immitis, Dipetalonema reconditum, Onchocerca* spp., *Setaria* spp.)
8. Rhabditoidea (*Strongyloides* spp.)
9. Spiruroidea (*Habronema* spp., *Thelazia* spp., *Spirocerca lupi, Ascarops strongylina, Physaloptera* spp.)
10. Dracunculoidea (*Dracunculus* spp.)
11. Dioctophymoidea (*Dioctophyma renale*)

Phylum acanthocephala

Acanthocephalans are commonly referred to as "thorny-headed worms." This group of intestinal parasites is rarely encountered, but occasionally they are found in pigs and dogs. They are wormlike in appearance after fixation, and have a spiny, protrusible snout *(proboscis)*. They have a body

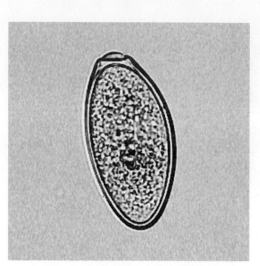

Fig. 14-16 *Oxyuris equi* egg (fecal flotation).

cavity and lack a digestive tract; the sexes are separate. The life cycle of acanthocephalans is complex and involves an intermediate host, usually a crustacean or an insect. Mature adults produce eggs that are shed through the feces of the definitive host. The eggs contain an embryo, the *acanthor,* which is surrounded by three to four envelopes. This gives the eggs a layered appearance, which is useful for identification. When an aquatic crustacean or insect ingests the eggs, continuous development through two stages occurs to produce the infective stage *(cystacanth)*. Infection of the definitive host occurs by ingestion of the intermediate host. The main acanthocephalan of concern is *Macracanthorhynchus hirudinaceus* (Fig. 14-21), which is found in the

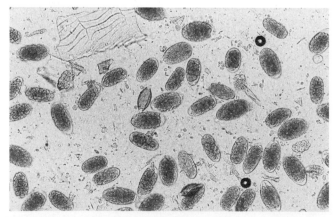

Fig. 14-15 Strongyle eggs surrounding a centrally located *Trichuris* egg (fecal flotation).

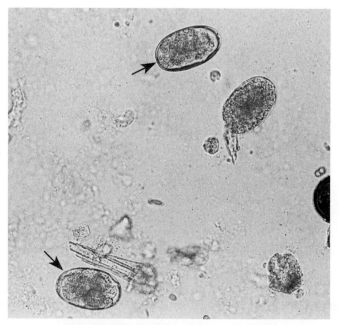

Fig. 14-17 *Ancylostoma caninum* eggs *(arrows)*.

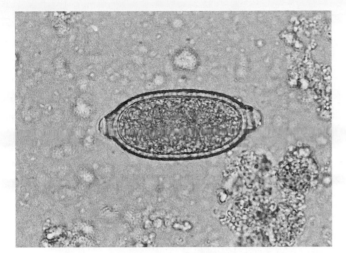

Fig. 14-18 *Capillaria aerophilous* egg (fecal flotation).

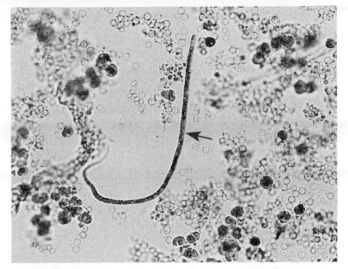

Fig. 14-20 *Dipetalonema reconditum* microfilaria (modified Knott's).

small intestines of pigs. *Oncicola canis* is an acanthocephalan found in dogs. Other hosts for acanthocephalans are aquatic birds, fish, amphibians, and monkeys.

Phylum arthropoda

Organisms in the phylum arthropoda are characterized by the presence of jointed legs. They have a chitinous exoskeleton composed of segments. In the more advanced groups, some segments have fused together to form body parts, such as a head, thorax, and abdomen. Arthropods have a true body cavity *(coelom)*, a circulatory system, a digestive system, a respiratory system, an excretory system, a nervous system, and a reproductive system. The sexes are separate, and reproduction is by means of eggs. Only certain groups of arthropods are parasitic. Members of other groups may act as intermediate host for the other parasites previously discussed. When a parasite resides on the surface of its host, it is called an *ectoparasite*. Most ectoparasites are either *insects* (fleas, lice, flies) or *arachnids* (ticks, mites).

The following general characteristics differentiate the two major classes of arthropods of veterinary importance: Insects have three pairs of legs, three distinct body regions (head, thorax, and abdomen), and a single pair of antennae. Arachnids (adults) have four pairs of legs, a body divided

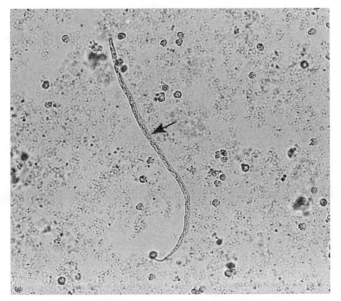

Fig. 14-19 *Dirofilaria immitis* microfilaria (modified Knott's).

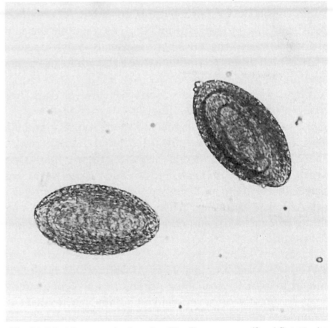

Fig. 14-21 *Macracanthorhynchus hirudinaceus* eggs (fecal flotation).

into two regions (cephalothorax, abdomen), and no antennae. Pentastomids (tongue worms) are another group of parasitic arthropods rarely encountered in the respiratory passages of vertebrates. They resemble worms rather than arthropods in the adult stage. Adults have two pairs of curved, retractile hooklets near the mouth. Immature stages are mitelike, with two or three pairs of legs.

The mouth parts of insects vary in structure, depending on feeding habits, with adaptations for chewing-biting, sponging, or piercing-sucking. The thorax may have one or two pairs of functional wings, in addition to the three pairs of jointed legs. The sexes are separate, and reproduction results in production of eggs or larvae. Development often involves three or more larval stages called *instars*, followed by formation of a pupa and a change in form or transformation (complete metamorphosis) to the adult stage. In other insects, development occurs from the egg through several immature stages *(nymphs)*, which resemble the adult in form but are smaller (incomplete metamorphosis). Fleas and flies demonstrate complete metamorphosis, and lice demonstrate incomplete metamorphosis. Insects may produce harm to their definitive host as adults and/or larvae.

The arachnids include ticks, mites, spiders, and scorpions. Ticks and mites are the more important groups of arachnids in veterinary medicine, although some spiders and scorpions can harm domestic animals by way of toxic venoms. Arachnids are generally small, often microscopic. Their mouth parts are borne on a structure called the *basis capituli* and consist of a pair of mobile digits adapted for cutting *(chelicerae)* and a pair of sensory structures *(palps)*. The *hypostome* is a structure with recurved teeth that maintains attachment to the host and bears a groove that permits the flow of arthropod saliva and host blood or lymph. Life cycle stages consist of egg, larva, nymph, and adult. There can be more than one nymphal instar. Nymphs resemble the adult in form but are smaller. There is usually only one larval stage, which differs from the nymphs and adults in size and has only three pairs of legs.

Fleas. Fleas are blood-sucking parasites of dogs, cats, rodents, birds, and people. They are vectors of several diseases, such as bubonic plague and tularemia. Cat and dog fleas, *Ctenocephalides felis* (Fig. 14-22) and *C. canis*, respectively, can act as intermediate hosts for the common tapeworm, *Dipylidium caninum*. Heavy infestations with fleas, especially in young animals, produce anemia. Flea saliva is antigenic and irritating, causing intense *pruritus* (itching) and hypersensitivity, known as *flea-bite dermatitis* or *miliary dermatitis*.

Fleas are laterally compressed, wingless insects with legs adapted for jumping. They move rapidly on the host and from host to host. Flea infestations are encountered most frequently on dogs and cats. They can be detected around the tailhead, on the ventral abdomen, and under the chin.

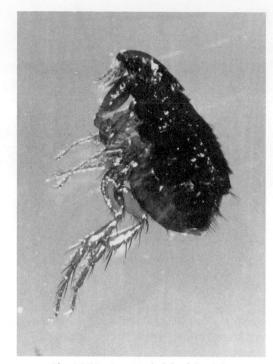

Fig. 14-22 *Ctenocephalides felis* adult.

Fleas demonstrate complete metamorphosis. Eggs deposited on the host fall off and develop to larvae in the environment. The larvae (Fig. 14-23) can occasionally be found in the animal's bedding, on furniture, or in cracks and crevices of the animal's environment. The larvae are maggotlike, with a head capsule and bristles. Flea larvae feed on

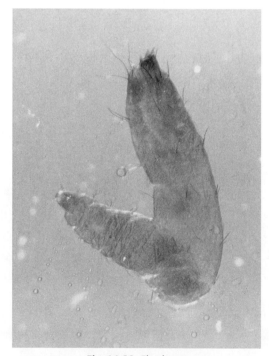

Fig. 14-23 Flea larva.

organic debris, including the excrement of adult fleas. Flea droppings are reddish brown, comma-shaped casts of dehydrated blood. Flea droppings in the animal's haircoat indicate flea infestation.

Specific identification of fleas requires the expertise of an entomologist. Other fleas of veterinary importance are *Pulex irritans, Xenopsylla cheopis, Tunga penetrans, Ceratophyllus gallinae,* and *Echidnophaga gallinacea.* Fleas have preferred hosts, but they attack any source of blood if the preferred host is not available. Adult fleas can also survive for extended periods off the host and can heavily infest premises.

Lice. Lice are dorsoventrally flattened, wingless insects with clawed appendages for clasping to the host's hairs. Lice are separated into two Orders, based on whether their mouth parts are modified for chewing (*Mallophaga,* Fig. 14-24) or sucking (*Anoplura,* Fig. 14-25). Sucking lice feed on blood and move slowly on the host. They have a long, narrow head. Biting lice feed on epithelial debris and can move rapidly over the host. They have a broad, rounded head. Lice are host-specific, remain in close association with the host, and have preferred locations on the host. Lice glue their eggs or *nits* (Fig. 14-26) to the hairs or feathers of the host. Transmission is usually by direct contact but can occur through equipment contaminated with eggs, nymphs, or adults.

Louse infestations (*pediculosis*) tend to be more severe in young, old, or poorly nourished animals, especially in overcrowded conditions and during the colder months. Sucking lice produce anemia, whereas biting lice are irritating and disturbing to the animal. Common biting lice of domestic animals include *Trichodectes canis* (dog), *Damalinia equi* (horse), *D. bovis* (cow), *D. ovis* (sheep), *D. caprae* (goat), and *Felicola subrostratus* (cat). Common sucking lice of domestic animals include *Linognathus* setosus (dog), *Haematopinus asini* (horse), *Haematopinus vituli, Haematopinus eurysternus, Solenopotes capillatus, Haematopinus quadripertusus* (cow), *Linognathus ovillus, Linognathus pedalis* (sheep), and

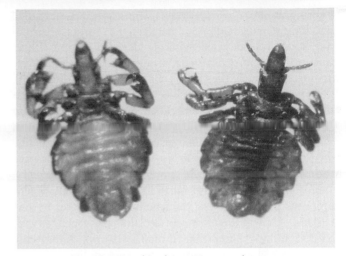

Fig. 14-25 Sucking louse, *Haematopinus* spp.

Haematopinus suis (pig). Identification of lice beyond their Order is difficult, but not usually necessary.

Flies. Flies are a diverse group of insects that undergo complete metamorphosis. They have one pair of wings, which may be scaled or membranous, and a pair of balancing structures called halters. The mouth parts may be adapted for sponging or piercing-sucking. Flies produce harm by inflicting painful bites, blood sucking, producing hypersensitive reactions, depositing eggs in sores, migration of larval stages through tissues of the host with escape through holes in the skin (warbles), causing annoyance, and acting as vectors and intermediate hosts to other pathogenic agents.

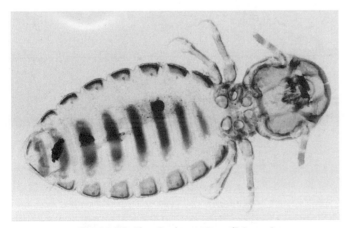

Fig. 14-24 Chewing louse, *Damalinia equi.*

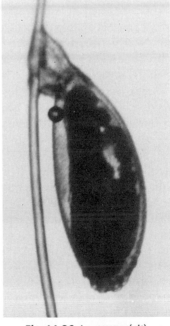

Fig. 14-26 Louse egg (nit).

Biting midges ("no-see-ums"), *Culicoides* spp., are small flies. The females are blood suckers that inflict a painful bite. Some species cause allergic dermatitis, and others transmit helminths, protozoa, and viruses. Blackflies (buffalo gnats) are small flies with a characteristic humped back. They produce similar harm as no-see-ums and in great numbers can exsanguinate a host. Sandflies (*Phlebotomus* species) are mothlike flies, known primarily for their role in the transmission of leishmaniasis and viral diseases. The females suck blood. Mosquitoes are a large and important group of flies known for the annoying bites of the females, which suck blood, and also for their role in transmission of numerous protozoal, viral, and nematode diseases to animals and people. Horseflies and deerflies are large flies with serrated mouth parts that inflict a painful bite. Only females suck blood. They are serious pests of livestock, can transmit filarial nematodes, and act as mechanical vectors of bacterial, viral, and rickettsial disease agents.

Muscid flies include the house fly, face fly, horn fly, and stable fly. The house fly and face fly do not suck blood, but are annoyances because they are attracted to excrement and secretions. Both act as intermediate hosts for spirurid parasites (*Habronema* spp., *Thelazia* spp.) and can mechanically transmit bacteria. The horn fly and the stable fly inflict painful bites and suck blood. Horn flies spend most of their life on the host (cattle). Stable flies feed intermittently and rest on fences and in barns. The stable fly can spread bacterial and viral diseases to cattle and horses and is an intermediate host for the stomach worm of horses (*Habronema*).

Blowflies, flesh flies, and screwworm flies are larger flies with bright coloration. The adults do not suck blood but deposit their eggs in decaying organic matter, septic wounds, or living flesh. The larvae of *Callitroga hominovorax* and *Wohlfahrtia opaca* are the only primary invaders of living tissue in North America. Other members are attracted to septic wounds and are known as secondary invaders. Botflies (*Gastrophilus* spp., *Hypoderma* spp., *Cuterebra* spp., *Oestrus ovis*) are beelike flies, the adults of which do not feed. The adult flies glue their eggs to the hairs of the host or deposit them at the entrance of animal burrows. The larvae (Fig. 14-27) hatch and penetrate the skin of the host. Some migrate extensively through the host's body, and others develop locally. They produce large pockets in the subcutaneous tissues of the host with airholes in the skin, and are known as *warbles*. Hippoboscids or sheep keds (*Melophagus ovinus*) are dorsoventrally flattened, wingless flies that resemble ticks. They suck blood and spend their entire life on the host (sheep). They cause pruritus and damage the wool.

Ticks. Ticks are blood-sucking arachnids. They are dorsoventrally flattened in the unengorged state. There are two types of ticks: hard ticks (*Ixodidae*, Fig. 14-28) and soft ticks (*Argasidae*, Fig. 14-29).

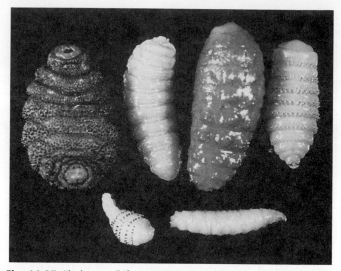

Fig. 14-27 Fly larvae *(left to right, top row)*, *Cuterebra* spp., *Oestrus ovis*, *Hypoderma* spp., *Gastrophilus* spp.; *(left to right, bottom row)*: *Dermatobia hominis*, *Callitroga* spp.).

Hard ticks are important vectors of protozoal, bacterial, viral, and rickettsial diseases. The saliva of female ticks of some species is toxic and produces flaccid, ascending paralysis in animals and people *(tick paralysis)*. The adults, larvae, and nymphs attach to the host and feed on blood. Eggs are deposited in the environment. Hard ticks are dorsoventrally flattened, with well-defined lateral margins in the unengorged state. They have a hard, chitinous covering *(scutum)* on the dorsal surface of the body. Hard ticks may have grooves, margins, and notches *(festoons)*, which are useful for identification purposes. They may attach to and feed on one to three different hosts during a life cycle and are referred to as *one-host*, *two-host*, or *three-host ticks*.

Important hard ticks in North America include *Rhipicephalus sanguineus*, *Dermacentor variabilis*, *Dermacentor*

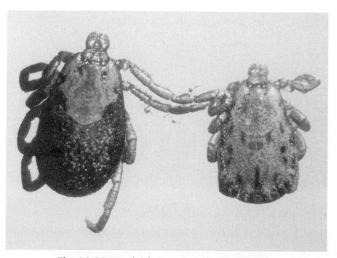

Fig. 14-28 Hard tick, *Dermacentor occidentalis*.

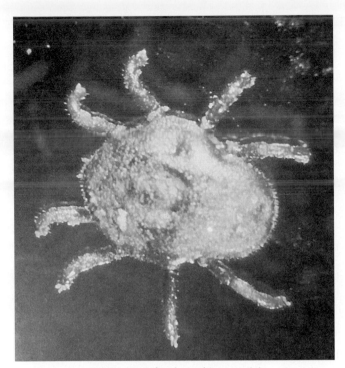

Fig. 14-29 Soft tick, *Otobius megnini*.

andersoni, *Dermacentor occidentalis*, *Dermacentor albipictus*, *Ixodes scapularis*, *Ixodes cookei*, *Ixodes pacificus*, *Amblyomma americanum*, *Amblyomma maculatum*, *Haemaphysalis leporispalustris*, and *Boophilus annulatus*. *R. sanguineus* is unusual in that it can become established in indoor dwellings and kennels.

Soft ticks lack a scutum, and their mouth parts are not visible from the dorsal surface. The lateral edges of the body are rounded. The females feed often, and eggs are laid off the host. Soft ticks are more resistant to desiccation than hard ticks, and they can live for several years in arid conditions. There are three genera of veterinary importance: *Argas* spp., *Otobius megnini*, and *Ornithodoros* spp.

Argas spp. are ectoparasites of birds. The larvae, nymphs, and adults live in cracks and crevices of poultry houses and feed at night about once a month. They cause restlessness, loss of productivity, and severe anemia. They also serve as a vector for bacterial and rickettsial diseases of birds. *O. megnini*, the spinose ear tick, occurs on housed stock, dogs, and even people. Only the larval and nymphal stages are parasitic. They live in the external ear canal and suck blood, causing inflammation and production of a waxy exudate. *Ornithodoros* spp. live in sandy soils, in primitive housing, or in shady areas around trees. This genus is probably more important on people and rodents than on domestic animals, but *Ornithodoros coriaceus* is known to transmit the agent of foothill abortion in California.

Mites. Mites are arachnids that occur as parasitic and free-living forms, some of which act as intermediate hosts for cestodes. Most parasitic mites are obligate parasites, which spend their entire life cycle on the host and produce the dermatologic condition referred to as *mange*. A few species found on birds and rodents live off the host and visit the host only to obtain a blood meal (*Dermanyssus gallinae*, *Ornithonyssus bacoti*). Most mite infestations are transmitted through direct contact with an infested animal. Burrowing mite infestations are diagnosed with deep skin scrapings at the periphery of lesions.

Mites can be divided into two main groups: burrowing mites and nonburrowing mites. Another group of mites is parasitic only as larvae, the trombiculid mites or "chiggers." The burrowing mites include: *Sarcoptes scabiei* (Fig. 14-30), *Notoedres cati* (Fig. 14-31), and *Knemidokoptes* spp. These mites tunnel into the superficial layers of the epidermis and feed on tissue fluids. Infestations begin as localized areas of inflammation and hair loss, but they spread rapidly to become generalized. Females deposit their eggs in the tunnels. Mating occurs on the surface of the skin. Sarcoptic mange caused by *S. scabiei* can affect most animal species, including people, but it is most commonly seen on dogs and pigs. It is characterized by loss of hair and intense pruritus. Each animal species has its own variety of *S. scabiei*, and cross-transmission does not occur. However, temporary infestation may take place without colonization of the skin. Notodectic mange (caused by *Notoedres*) is more restricted in host range and occurs in cats and occasionally rabbits. *Knemidokoptic mange* (caused by *Knemidokoptes*) affects birds.

Demodex spp. (Fig. 14-32) are also burrowing mites that live in the hair follicles and sebaceous glands of the skin. They are considered part of the normal skin fauna of most mammals. Demodectic mange is most common in dogs and can be localized or generalized. Immunodeficiency, both

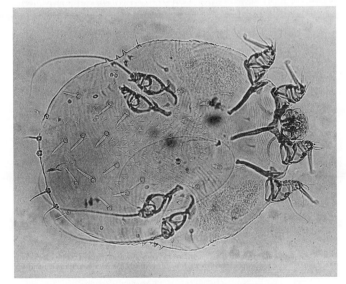

Fig. 14-30 *Sarcoptes scabiei* (skin scraping).

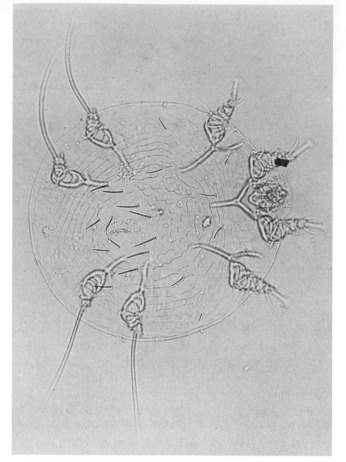

Fig. 14-31   *Notoedres cati* (skin scraping).

spp. (Fig. 14-33), *Chorioptes* spp. (Fig. 14-34), *Otodectes cynotis* (Fig. 14-35), *Psorergates ovis,* and *Cheyletiella* spp. (Fig. 14-36) are examples of nonburrowing mites. Psoroptic mange is important in sheep. The mites are active in the superficial keratinized layer of the skin but also pierce the skin with their mouth parts. Vesicles develop, with crusting and intense pruritus. Chorioptic mange is less severe and tends to remain localized. *Chorioptes bovis* is the more important species and a common parasite of cattle.

Cheyletiella and *Otodectes* are parasites of dogs and cats. *Cheyletiella* produces a mild condition referred to as "walking dandruff." *Otodectes cynotis* lives in the external ear canal of dogs and cats. A brownish, waxy exudate accumulates, with crust formation, ulceration, and secondary bacterial infections. Infested animals scratch frequently at the ears and shake their head. Head shaking can result in rupture of blood vessels and hematomas of the pinna. The mites can be found in the waxy exudate and crust within the ear canal.

DIAGNOSTIC TECHNIQUES IN PARASITOLOGY

Parasites may be located in the oral cavity, esophagus, stomach, small and large intestines, internal organs, and skin of animals. Diagnostic stages can be found in sputum, feces, blood, urine, secretions of the reproductive organs, and epidermal layers of the skin. Samples collected for examination should be as fresh as possible and examined as soon as possible, preferably within the first 24 hours after

genetic and induced by the mites, is necessary for an infestation to become clinically apparent. The disease is characterized by loss of hair, thickening of the skin, and pustule formation. Pruritus is not a manifestation of this type of mange. Deep skin scrapings are used to recover the cigar-shaped mites for diagnosis.

Nonburrowing mites live on the surface of the skin and feed on keratinized scale, hair, and tissue fluids. *Psoroptes*

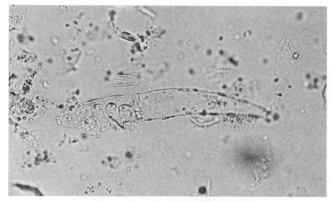

Fig. 14-32   *Demodex canis* (skin scraping).

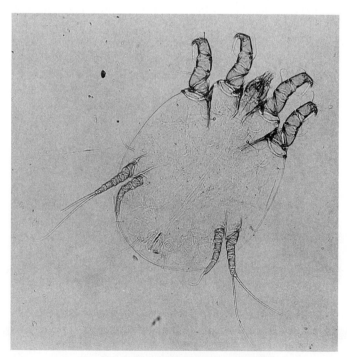

Fig. 14-33   *Psoroptes ovis* (skin scraping).

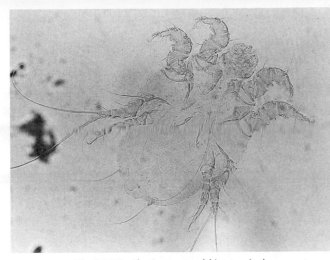

Fig. 14-34 *Chorioptes* spp. (skin scraping).

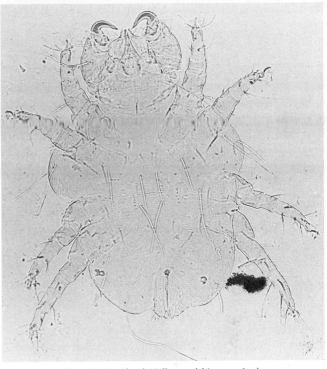

Fig. 14-36 *Cheyletiella* spp. (skin scraping).

collection. Clients can collect samples and store them in any clean, sealable container, or collection can occur at the clinic. Refrigeration or fixation may be necessary if prompt examination is not possible. A sample of 5 to 50 g (the size of a pecan or walnut) may be needed, depending on which procedures are necessary. Pooled samples from a herd or kennel can be used, but generally it is better to examine several samples from individual animals.

It is vital to take proper precautions when working with samples to prevent contamination of the work environment and to ensure personal health when handling agents transmissible to people. Wear gloves and/or wash your hands frequently with warm water and soap. Clean and disinfect work areas after examinations. Also, clean equipment frequently.

Maintenance of good records is important. Label samples with the client's name, date of collection, species of host, and identification of the animal. Records should include identification information, procedures performed, and the results. An adequate history, including clinical signs, duration of signs, medications given, environment, vaccinations, stocking density, and number of animals affected, should accompany the sample.

Parasitologic examination begins with gross examination of the sample, noting consistency, color, presence of blood, mucus, odor, adult parasites, or foreign bodies such as string. Normal feces should be formed yet soft. Diarrhea or constipation can occur with parasitic infections. Most secretions are clear and moderately cellular. A yellowish discoloration with excessive mucus could signal infection. Blood in a sample can be fresh and bright red or partially digested (hemolyzed), appearing dark reddish brown to black and tarry. Excessive mucus in a sample generally indicates irritation to a mucosal membrane, with proliferation of mucus-producing cells. This is common in parasitic infections of the respiratory system and lower digestive tract. Adult parasites, such as roundworms and tapeworm proglottids, can be found in vomitus or feces, and can be identified.

Microscopic examination of samples is the most reliable method for detection of parasitic infections. A binocular microscope with 10×, 40×, and 100× objectives is needed. A stereo microscope is also helpful for identifying gross parasites. A calibrated ocular micrometer may be necessary to determine sizes and specific differentiation of some

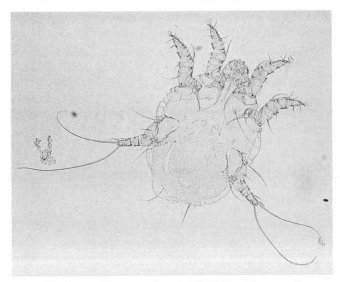

Fig. 14-35 *Otodectes cynotis* (swab of external ear canal).

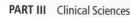
parasitic stages, such as microfilariae. Samples are generally mounted on a glass slide in a fluid medium with a cover slip on top. The sample should be thoroughly and systematically viewed, beginning at one corner of the cover slip and ending at the opposite end using the 10× objective. Parasite stages usually are in the same plane of focus as air bubbles or the edge of the cover slip. Any materials or objects observed can be viewed and verified with more powerful objectives. A good working knowledge of the parts of the binocular microscope and adjustments to produce Kohler illumination is essential for parasitology examinations.

Parasitology testing is one of the most common activities of the practicing veterinary technician. This section provides an overview of sample collection and handling as well as principles and general procedures for the most common parasitology tests performed.

Sample Collection and Handling

Fecal samples

For tests to be valid, the fecal sample must be fresh and stored properly if testing is to be delayed. With small animals, it is common to provide the client with a collection container. Instruct the client to witness the animal defecating and collect the sample immediately. Samples can also be collected directly from the rectum using a fecal loop. The sample should be refrigerated until it is to be examined. Large animal specimens are often collected directly from the rectum. Herd animal samples are normally collected as pooled samples. Several samples are taken from the area where the animals are confined.

Blood samples

The specific collection procedure varies somewhat depending on the tests to be performed. Whole blood in EDTA or serum may be required. Standard collection methods for these sample types will yield appropriate samples for parasitologic testing.

Miscellaneous samples

Skin scrapings, cellophane tape collections, transtracheal washes, urine sample collections, and swabbings are all performed in parasitology. Standard protocols for these collections will yield appropriate samples. Some of these methods are described later in more detail.

Evaluation of Fecal Specimens

Depending on clinical signs and patient history, it is likely that specific parasite infestations may be suspected. This information helps to guide the choice of test to be performed. All parasitology samples should undergo gross evaluation for the presence of abnormalities such as blood, mucus, and parasites that are large enough to see with the unaided eye (e.g., tapeworm segments). Additional tests can then be performed.

Direct smear

Fecal direct smears are the simplest of the evaluation procedures. Feces, sputum, urine, smegma, and blood can be observed with the technique described in Box 14-1. It requires a minimum amount of equipment and materials and is a rapid scan for parasite stages. The procedure involves placing a small amount of feces on a clean glass slide and examining it microscopically for the presence of eggs and larvae. This method will also allow visualization of the trophozoite stages of protozoal parasites, such as *Giardia*.

Unfortunately, a direct smear alone is not an adequate examination for parasites, because only a small quantity of sample is examined and parasitic infections can be missed. However, it should be incorporated as a routine part of any parasitology examination.

Fecal flotation

Flotation methods are based on differences in the specific gravity of life cycle stages of parasites found in feces and fecal debris. Simple fecal flotation is an example of a flotation method (Box 14-2). Specific gravity refers to the weight of an object compared with the weight of an equal volume of distilled water, and is a function of the total amount of dissolved material in the solution. Most parasite eggs have a specific gravity between 1.10 and 1.20 g/ml.

BOX 14-1 *procedure*

Direct Smear of Feces

Materials
- 75 glass microscope slides (25-mm)
- Glass cover slips (22-mm² #1)
- Wooden applicator sticks
- Water or saline

Procedure

1. Dip the applicator stick into the feces (only a small amount should adhere to the stick).
2. Place a drop of saline on a slide.
3. Mix the feces with the saline to produce a homogeneous emulsion that is clear enough to read newsprint through it. (A common mistake is to make the smear too thick.)
4. Place the cover slip over the emulsion.
5. Examine the slide at 100× and 400× magnification for eggs, cysts, trophozoites, and larvae.

Optional: To demonstrate diagnostic features of protozoa, add a drop of Lugol's iodine:

1. To make a 5% Lugol's stock solution, add 5 g iodine crystals to 10 g potassium iodide/100 ml distilled water.
2. Store solution in an amber bottle away from light.
3. Dilute 1 part 5% Lugol's stock solution to 5 parts distilled water to make a staining solution.

BOX 14-2 *procedure*

Simple Fecal Flotation

Materials

- 75 glass microscope slides (25-mm)
- Glass cover slips (22-mm #1)
- Wooden tongue depressors
- Waxed paper cups (90–150 ml)
- Cheesecloth or 10 cm gauze squares or metal screen tea strainer
- Shell vial, (1.25–2.0 cm or 5.0–7.5 cm); or 15-ml conical centrifuge tube
- Saturated salt or sugar flotation solution

Procedure

1. Place approximately 2–5 g of feces in the paper cup.
2. Add 30 ml of flotation solution.
3. Using the tongue depressor, mix the feces to produce an evenly suspended emulsion.
4. If using cheesecloth, bend the sides of the cup to form a spout and cover the top with the cheesecloth squares while pouring the suspension from the shell vial. If using a metal strainer, pour the suspension through the metal strainer into another cup and fill the shell vial with the filtered solution.
5. Fill the shell vial to form a convex dome (meniscus) at the rim. *Do not overfill the vial.* Fresh solution can be used to form this dome.
6. Place a cover slip on top of the filled shell vial.
7. Allow the cover slip to remain undisturbed for 10 to 20 minutes.
8. Pick the cover slip straight up and place it on a glass slide, fluid side down.
9. Systematically examine the surface under the cover slip at 100× magnification.

Flotation solutions are formulated with a specific gravity that is higher than that of common parasite ova. Therefore, the ova float to the surface of the solution. Saturated solutions of sugar and various salts are used as flotation solutions and have a specific gravity ranging between 1.18 and 1.40. Fecal debris and eggs with a specific gravity greater than that of the flotation solution do not float. Fluke eggs are generally heavier than the specific gravity of most routinely used flotation solutions, with a few exceptions (*Paragonimus*, *Nanophyetus*), and are not usually recovered using this technique. Nematode larvae can be recovered but frequently are distorted from crenation, making identification difficult. If the specific gravity of the flotation solution is too high, a plug of fecal debris floats and traps parasite stages in it, obscuring them from view.

Commonly used flotation solutions are sugar, sodium chloride, sodium nitrate, magnesium sulfate, and zinc sulfate. Each solution has advantages and disadvantages, including cost, availability, efficiency, shelf life, crystallization, corrosion of equipment, and ease of use. Selection is often determined by the type of practice and common parasites encountered in the area. Some companies (Synbiotics Corporation, San Diego, Calif.) have packaged flotation kits (Ovassay Plus®) using prepared solutions of sodium nitrate or zinc sulfate, disposable plastic vials, and strainers. They are convenient but more expensive. Supplies to conduct simple flotations can be acquired through suppliers of scientific equipment and chemicals (e.g., Scientific Products, McGaw Park, Ill.). Formulas for making flotation solutions are shown in Box 14-3.

The specific gravity of flotation solutions can be checked using a hydrometer and adjusted by adding more salts or more water to the solution. Leaving extra crystals of salt on the bottom of the solution ensures that the solution is saturated.

Centrifugal flotation

This procedure is similar in principle to the flotation procedure except that once the sample and solution are mixed, the specimen is strained (to remove excess debris). Add a coverslip and centrifuge the specimen at 400 to 650 G for 5 minutes. Centrifugal force holds the coverslips in place during spinning, provided the tubes are balanced. A bacteriology loop is then used to remove a drop of liquid from the surface of the tube, and the drop is examined microscopically. Centrifugal flotation is more sensitive than simple flotation. It recovers more eggs and cysts in a sample in less time (Box 14-4). However, it requires access to a tabletop centrifuge with a head for rotation buckets. Fixed-angle heads do not work for this procedure as described. They can be adapted for this procedure by not filling the tubes and omitting the coverslip during centrifugation.

Fecal sedimentation

The sedimentation procedure is used when suspected parasites produce ova too large to be recovered with standard flotation (i.e., fluke ova). The fecal sample is mixed in a small volume of water and strained into a centrifuge tube. The sample can be centrifuged at 400 G for 5 minutes or allowed to remain undisturbed for 20 to 30 minutes. The supernatant is poured off, and a pipette is used to remove a drop of the sediment. A drop from the upper, middle, and lower portions of the sediment is removed. These drops are then examined microscopically.

BOX 14-3

Formulas for Making Flotation Solutions

Sugar Solution (specific gravity 1.275):

- 454 g granulated sugar
- 355 ml water
- 1 g crystalline phenol/100 ml solution

Heat the water and add the sugar. Continue heating until all sugar is dissolved. Add the phenol as a preservative. Sugar is thick and viscous, and eggs take longer to float. It is also sticky and attracts ants and flies. However, it is readily available, inexpensive, and efficient. Slides can also be stored for a longer time in sugar. Some protozoan cysts collapse rapidly in sugar. It is a recommended flotation solution for recovery of *Cryptosporidium* oocysts.

Sodium Chloride Solution (specific gravity 1.20):

- 360 g sodium chloride (better to use crude salt than refined salt)
- 1000 ml water

Heat the water and add the salt. An excess of crystals in the container ensures a saturated solution. Brine solution is inexpensive and clean to use. It crystallizes rapidly, collapses some protozoan cysts and nematode larvae, and fails to float some heavier nematode eggs. It is also corrosive.

Sodium Nitrate Solution (specific gravity 1.39):

- 850 g sodium nitrate
- 1000 ml water

Add the sodium nitrate to the water and allow the solution to sit overnight at room temperature, stirring often. The water may also be heated before adding the salt. This solution is very efficient at floating eggs, even heavier eggs, such as ascarid eggs, trichurid eggs, and some fluke eggs. It tends to form air bubbles and floats more fecal debris. It also crystallizes rapidly and is more expensive.

Magnesium Sulfate Solution (specific gravity 1.285):

- 920 g magnesium sulfate
- 1000 ml water

Add the magnesium sulfate to the water and allow the solution to sit overnight at room temperature, stirring often. Magnesium sulfate is economical, accessible, and more efficient than sodium chloride at floating some of the heavier eggs. It also crystallizes fairly rapidly.

Zinc Sulfate Solution (specific gravity 1.18):

- 336 g zinc sulfate
- 1000 ml water

Add the zinc sulfate to the water and allow the solution to sit overnight at room temperature, stirring often. Zinc sulfate solution floats protozoan cysts and nematode larvae without distorting them.

BOX 14-4

procedure

Centrifugal Flotation

Materials

- Glass microscope slides (25-mm)
- Glass cover slips (22-mm^2 #1)
- Waxed paper cups
- Cheesecloth or 10 cm gauze squares, or metal screen tea strainer
- Funnell Conical centrifuge tubes (15-ml)
- Test tube rack
- Flotation solution
- Centrifuge with rotating buckets
- Wooden tongue depressors
- Balance scale

Procedure

1. Prepare a fecal emulsion using 2–5 g of feces and 30 ml of flotation solution.
2. Strain the emulsion through the cheesecloth or tea strainer into the centrifuge tube. (Suspending a funnel over the tube facilitates filling the tube.)
3. Fill the tube to create a positive meniscus with flotation solution.
4. Place a cover slip on top of the tube.
5. Create a balance tube of equal weight, containing another sample or water.
6. Place the tubes in the centrifuge buckets, and weigh them on a balance. You may add water to the buckets to make them equal weights.
7. Centrifuge the tubes for 5 minutes at 400–650 gravities (approximately 1500 rpm).
8. Remove the cover slips from the tubes by lifting straight up, and place them on a slide.
9. Systematically examine the slides at 100× magnification.

Sedimentation concentrates parasite stages as well as fecal debris (Box 14-5). Because of the debris, parasite stages may be obscured from view; this technique is also more laborious. Sedimentation is used primarily when fluke infections are suspected. Most fluke eggs do not float, or they are distorted by flotation solutions with a higher specific gravity, making it difficult to recognize them. A few drops of liquid detergent can be added to the water as a surfactant to help remove excess fats and debris from the sample.

Cellophane tape preparation

This method is often used to recover ova of *Oxyuris* (pinworms). It can also aid in identification of tapeworms. A piece of cellophane tape is wrapped around a tongue depressor with the adhesive side out. The animal's tail is raised and the tongue depressor firmly pressed against the anus. The tape is then removed and applied to a glass slide that has a small amount of water on it and then examined microscopically (Box 14-6). Pinworms can be found in primates, horses, and ruminants. The adult female worms migrate out of the anus and deposit their eggs on the skin around the anus (perianal region). The activity of the female worms is

---

BOX 14-5

procedure

Fecal Sedimentation

Materials

- Waxed paper cups (90–150 ml)
- Wooden tongue depressors
- Cheesecloth or 10 cm gauze squares, or metal screen tea strainer
- Funnell Conical centrifuge tubes (50-ml)
- Disposable pipettes (2-ml)
- Glass microscope slides (25-mm)
- Glass cover slips (22-mm^2 #1)

Procedure

1. Mix 2–5 g of feces in a cup with 30 ml of water.
2. Strain the fecal suspension through the cheesecloth or tea strainer into a 50-ml conical centrifuge tube. (Suspending a funnel over the tube facilitates filling the tube.)
3. Wash the sample with water until the tube is filled.
4. Allow the tube to sit undisturbed for 15 to 30 minutes.
5. Decant the supernatant off, and resuspend the sediment in water.
6. Repeat steps 4 and 5 two more times.
7. Decant the supernatant without disturbing the sediment.
8. Using a pipette, mix the sediment and transfer an aliquot to a slide.
9. Place a cover slip over the sediment, and systematically examine the slide with 100× magnification.
10. Repeat steps 8 and 9 until all sediment has been examined.

BOX 14-6

procedure

Cellophane Tape Preparation

Materials

- Transparent adhesive tape
- Wooden tongue depressors
- Glass microscope slides (25-mm)

Procedure

1. Place adhesive tape in a loop around one end of the tongue depressor, with the adhesive side facing out.
2. Press the tape firmly against the skin around the anus.
3. Place a drop of water on the slide. Undo the loop of tape and stick the tape to the slide, allowing the water to spread out under the tape.
4. Examine the taped area of the slide microscopically for the presence of pinworm eggs.

---

irritating and produces itching. Pinworm eggs are not consistently found on fecal flotations and are suspected when animals rub their tails on objects, resulting in loss of hair. *Oxyuris equi*, the pinworm of horses, can be a problem. Pinworm species of domestic animals are not transmissible to people. People can be infected with *Enterobius vermicularis* through direct contact with another infected person or premises contaminated with *Enterobius* eggs. Frequently, infected people are misinformed and believe that their infections came directly from their animals.

Baermann technique

The Baermann technique is sometimes used to recover larvae from fecal samples. The procedure requires construction of a Baermann apparatus that consists of a large funnel supported in a ring stand. A piece of rubber tubing is attached to the end of the funnel and placed in a collection tube. The fecal sample is placed in the funnel on top of a piece of metal screen. Warm water or warmed physiologic saline is passed through the sample. The larvae are stimulated to move by the warm water and then sink to the bottom of the apparatus. A drop of the material in the collection container is examined microscopically for presence of larvae. The Baermann technique is used to recover nematode larvae from feces, fecal culture, soil, herbage, and animal tissues (Box 14-7). The warm water stimulates larvae to migrate out of the sample and relax. They then sink to the bottom of the apparatus, where they can be collected relatively free of debris. Free-living larvae must be distinguished from parasitic ones, especially if the sample is collected off the ground, from soil, or from herbage. This may require the expertise of an experienced helminthologist. Preserve samples by adding 5% to 10% formalin to the

BOX 14-7   *procedure*

Baermann Technique

Materials

- Baermann apparatus (ring stand, ring, funnel, rubber tubing, clamp, wire screen)
- Cheesecloth or Kimwipes
- Disposable pipettes
- Centrifuge tubes (15-ml) or Petri dishes
- Pinch clamps

Procedure

1. Construct a Baermann apparatus by fastening the ring to the ring stand. Attach 3 to 4 inches of rubber tubing to the narrow portion of the funnel. Ensure that there is a good seal (tubing can be glued on). Place the funnel in the ring. Place the wire screen in the top portion of the funnel to support the feces. Put several layers of cheesecloth or Kimwipes over the wire screen. Place the pinch clamps at the end of the rubber tubing and check, using water, to ensure a tight seal. Put 30 to 50 g of feces on top of the Kimwipes and fill the funnel with warm water (not hot) to a level above the fecal sample. (An alternative method, which is more practical in a practice setting, is to use long-stem, plastic champagne glasses with hollow stems. The feces are wrapped in several layers of Kimwipes, similar to a tea bag. The fecal pouch is then set in the glass. Fill the glass with warm water to a level above the fecal sample.)

2. Allow the apparatus to remain undisturbed for a minimum of 1 hour up to 24 hours.
3. Collect the fluid in the rubber tubing (stem of the glass) and transfer to a Petri dish or centrifuge tube.
4. Examine the Petri dish for larvae using a stereo microscope, or centrifuge the solution to pellet the larvae. Remove the supernatant from the centrifuge tube and place the pellet on a microscope slide.
5. Examine the slide for larvae and identify them. The slide can be passed over the flame of a Bunsen burner several times to kill the larvae in an extended position before identification.

---

pellet for submission to an expert. Kill free-living larvae by adding 1% hydrochloric acid to the pellet, and examine the preparation without heat fixation. Unfortunately, identification of motile larvae is more difficult.

The Baermann technique is routinely performed on feces of domestic animals when lungworm infections (*Dicytocaulus, Aelurostrongylus, Filaroides, Crenosoma, Muellerius, Protostrongylus*) are suspected. Ideally, samples should be fresh and collected rectally. In dogs and cats, a Baermann technique should be conducted when *Strongyloides* spp. infections are suspected. If the sample is not fresh, a fecal culture may be needed to distinguish first-stage hookworm larvae from first-stage larvae of *Strongyloides*. The third-stage filariform larva of *Strongyloides* is diagnostic and characterized by an esophagus that is half the length of the larva and a forked (bipartite) tail. Care should be taken when handling *Strongyloides* fecal cultures because of the zoonotic potential.

Miscellaneous fecal examinations

Some parasites produce intestinal bleeding. This bleeding may be evident as frank blood in the fecal sample or as darkened feces. Some intestinal bleeding can only be identified with chemical testing. This is referred to as fecal occult blood testing. Several types of kits are available for this procedure. They primarily act to identify the presence of hemoglobin in the sample.

Examination of vomitus may also aid in diagnosis of parasitism. Some parasites (e.g., *Toxacara canis*) are often present in vomitus of infected patients.

Fecal culture is used to differentiate parasites whose eggs or larvae are not easily distinguished by examination of a fresh fecal sample (Box 14-8). Trichostrongyle eggs in ruminant feces are indistinguishable from strongyle eggs. Small strongyle eggs in a horse sample cannot be distinguished from large strongyle eggs. First-stage hookworm larvae in a dog or cat sample and some free-living nematode larvae in soil or on grass cannot be easily distinguished from first-stage *Strongyloides* larvae. After fecal culture, the third-stage larvae of many of these parasites can be identified to genus level. Because the life cycles, pathogenicity, and epidemiology of some species may differ, identification may be necessary for proper treatment and control. Identification may require the help of an experienced helminthologist.

An additional type of fecal flotation test is the modified McMaster technique. This technique provides an estimate of the number of eggs or oocysts per gram of feces, primarily with livestock species and horses (Box 14-9). Originally it was adapted from a technique used in people infected with hookworms to estimate the worm population in the host. However, it is impossible to calculate the actual worm population in a host, especially in livestock and horses, because many factors influence egg production, and the number of eggs produced varies with the species and number of worms present.

Typically, livestock and horses are infected with several species of worms at one time, and some species are more prolific and pathogenic than others. Also, lesions often result from damage produced by immature stages of the parasites. In ruminants, the parasites of interest are coccidia

BOX 14-8 *procedure*

Fecal Culture

Materials

- Glass jar with tight-fitting lid
- Charcoal or vermiculite
- Wooden tongue depressors

Procedure

1. Moisten 50 g of charcoal or vermiculite with water. The charcoal or vermiculite should be damp but not wet.
2. Using the tongue depressor, mix an equal amount of feces with the moistened substrate.
3. Place the fecal mixture in a glass jar, and seal with the jar lid.
4. Place the jar in indirect light at room temperature for up to 7 days.
5. Check the jar periodically to ensure that the contents remain moist. A spray bottle of water can be used to moisten the fecal mixture if it becomes too dry. Be sure not to saturate the material.
6. Do a Baermann technique on the fecal culture at 48-hour intervals to recover developing stages. Some larvae migrate up the wall of the jar and congregate in condensation droplets. These can be collected by flushing the sides of the jar with water and collecting the excess fluid in a centrifuge tube or Petri dish.
7. Identify the larvae recovered.

and trichostrongyles. In horses, the parasites of interest are large and small strongyles. Both trichostrongyles and strongyles infect ruminants and horses. The eggs of trichostrongyles and strongyles cannot be readily distinguished from one another and are referred to as strongyle eggs (see Fig. 14-15). Nevertheless, counts in excess of 1000 are considered indicative of heavy infections, whereas those greater than 500 indicate moderate infections. A low egg count can indicate a low level of infection, or severe infections in which the parasites are just becoming mature. Egg counts must always be interpreted in view of the clinical signs observed, age, sex and nutritional level of the animals, and stocking density of a herd or flock.

More recently, egg counts have been used in epidemiologic investigations and herd health management programs as predictors of peak pasture contamination and transmission potential for different geographic regions and individual farms. This information is applied toward prevention programs involving strategic use of broad-spectrum anthelmintics and pasture rotation schemes aimed at reducing the infective levels of pastures and exposure rates. When herd studies are conducted, individual samples are taken from at least 10% of the herd. Egg counts are also used to monitor development of resistance to anthelminthics. Egg counts are done before treatment and again three weeks following treatment to determine the effectiveness of the anthelminthic used and development of resistance in a given worm population.

BOX 14-9 *procedure*

Modified McMaster Quantitative Egg Counting Technique

Materials

- McMaster slides (Olympic Equine Products, 5003 228th Avenue S, Issaquah, Wash., 98027)
- Waxed paper cups (90 to 150 ml) or beakers
- Graduated cylinder
- Balance scale
- Saturated sodium chloride solution
- Wooden tongue depressors
- Disposable pipettes
- Rotary stirrer (optional)

Procedure

1. Using the scale, weigh 5 g of feces into a cup.
2. Add a small amount of the flotation solution to the cup.
3. Mix the feces and flotation solution together thoroughly with a tongue depressor to make an even suspension.
4. Add sufficient flotation solution to bring the total volume to 75 ml.
5. Turn the rotary stirrer on, and place the cup containing the fecal suspension in it. If a rotary stirrer is not available, the fecal suspension can be mixed with a tongue depressor.
6. Using a pipette, withdraw a portion of the mixing suspension and fill the chambers of the McMaster slide.
7. Allow the slide to sit undisturbed for 10 minutes.
8. Using the 10× objective, focus on the grid etched in the McMaster slide. Count all eggs or oocysts seen in the six columns of the etched square, keeping a separate count for each species of parasite seen.
9. Multiply the numbers counted by the appropriate dilution factor (dependent on the number of squares counted), and record the results as eggs per gram (epg) of feces. The volume under the etched area is 0.15 ml. If 5 g per 75 ml total volume equals 1 g per 15 ml total volume, then 0.01 g is contained in 0.15 ml. Therefore, if one chamber is counted, multiply by 100. If two chambers are counted, multiply by 50 to arrive at the total epg.

Evaluation of Blood Samples

Examination of blood samples may reveal adult parasites and/or their various life cycle stages either free in the blood or intracellularly. A variety of methods can be used for this determination. Thin or thick blood smears are prepared in the same way that smears for a WBC differential count are prepared. (Preparation of smears for a WBC differential count is described in Chapter 11.) Most parasites are carried with the laminar flow to the feathered edge of the slide. Parasites may be located between cells, on the surface of cells, or in the cytoplasm of cells. Thin blood films are most effectively used to study the morphology of protozoan and rickettsial parasites. If parasitemia is low, infections can be missed. A thick blood film or a buffy coat smear is more effective because it concentrates a larger volume of cells (Box 14-10).

The buffy coat smear is a concentration technique for detection of protozoa and rickettsiae in white blood cells. A microhematocrit tube is centrifuged as for a PCV determination. Microfilariae and some protozoa may also be found at the top of the plasma column. The technique is quick but can not be used to differentiate *D. immitis* from *D. reconditum*

Direct drop

This is the simplest of the blood evaluations, although it is also the least accurate due to the small sample size. A drop of anticoagulated whole blood is examined microscopically. The movement of parasites that are extracellular can be detected with this method.

Filter test

The filter technique is a method designed to concentrate microfilariae in blood (Box 14-11). The principles applied are similar to those of the modified Knott's test, except that the blood is passed through a Millipore filter, which collects the microfilariae. Commercial kits use a detergent lysing solution and a different stain. This procedure is quicker and easier than the modified Knott's test, but the differential characteristics of the microfilariae are not as obvious. Identification using the characteristics listed in Table 14-1 is not possible with commercial kits, because the characteristics of the microfilariae are based on fixation with 2% formalin.

Modified Knott's test

This method is used to concentrate microfilaria and can help in differentiation of *Dirofilaria* from *Dipetalonema*. The procedure requires a mixture of blood and formalin in a centrifuge tube. The mixture is incubated at room temperature for 1 to 2 minutes and then centrifuged for 5 minutes. The supernatant is poured off, and a drop of methylene blue is added to the sediment in the tube. A drop of this mixture is transferred to a glass slide for microscopic evaluation. The modified Knott's technique is a rapid method for detection of microfilariae (heartworm larvae) in the blood (Box 14-12). It is used primarily for differentiating *Dirofilaria immitis* and *Dipetalonema reconditum* infections in dogs. The technique concentrates microfilariae while fixing them and lyses red blood cells. When preparing the 2% formalin solution, it is important to remember that 37% formaldehyde is equivalent to 100% formalin. It is also important to use water, not physiologic saline, to prepare this solution because physiologic saline does not lyse red blood cells. For accurate differentiation of the microfilariae, the microscope must have a calibrated ocular micrometer. Table 14-1 lists the characteristics used to distinguish microfilariae. Figs. 14-19 and 14-20 show these microfilariae.

BOX 14-10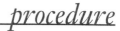

Buffy Coat Smear

Materials

- Hematocrit tubes
- Sealant
- Hematocrit centrifuge
- Glass microscope slides (25-mm)
- Glass cover slips (22-mm^2 #1)
- File
- Permount

Procedure

1. Fill the hematocrit tube with the blood sample, and plug one end with sealant.
2. Centrifuge for 5 minutes.
3. The buffy coat is located in the middle of the centrifuged sample, between the red blood cells and the plasma.
4. Use the file to etch the glass below the buffy coat. Snap the tube by applying pressure opposite the etched spot.
5. Take the end of the tube containing the buffy coat and plasma, and tap the buffy coat onto a glass slide with a small amount of plasma. If too much plasma is released, use a clean Kimwipe to wipe away excess.
6. Apply a clean slide over the buffy coat, and rapidly pull the two slides across each other in opposite directions.
7. Allow the slides to air-dry, and stain with Romanowsky stain.
8. After staining, apply mounting medium and a cover slip.
9. Examine the slides microscopically at 400× and 1000× magnification.

BOX 14-11

procedure

Millipore Filtration Procedure

Materials

- 5-μ Millipore filters
- Millipore filter holders
- 2.5% methylene blue stain
- 2% formalin
- Glass microscope slides (25-mm)
- Glass cover slips (22-mm² #1)
- 12-ml disposable syringes

Procedure

1. Assemble the filter holder with a Millipore filter.
2. Place 1 ml of blood in the syringe.
3. Add 9 ml of 2% formalin to the blood in the syringe, and insert the plunger.
4. Connect the syringe to the filter apparatus, and slowly apply pressure to the syringe plunger.
5. Remove the syringe and fill it with tap water. Allow a few milliliters of air to remain in the syringe. Flush the water through the filter apparatus.
6. Remove the filter from the filter holder, and place top-side-up on a glass slide.
7. Place a drop of the methylene blue stain on the filter, and add a cover slip.
8. Examine the slide microscopically at 100× magnification for microfilariae.

BOX 14-12

procedure

Modified Knott's Technique

Materials

- Blood collection materials
- 15-ml conical centrifuge tubes
- 2% formalin (2 ml 37% formaldehyde/98 ml water)
- 2.5% methylene blue (2.5 g methylene blue/100 ml water)
- Tabletop centrifuge
- Glass microscope slides (25-mm)
- Glass coverslips (22-mm² #1)
- Pipettes

Procedure

1. Mix 1 ml of blood with 9 ml of 2% formalin in a centrifuge tube. Agitate the tube and mix well.
2. Centrifuge the tube at 1500 rpm for 5 minutes.
3. Pour off the supernatant, and add 1 to 2 drops of methylene blue stain to the pellet at the bottom of the tube.
4. Using a pipette, mix the stain and sediment, and transfer the mixture to a glass slide.
5. Apply a coverslip, and examine the sediment microscopically for microfilariae at 100× and 400× magnification.

Immunologic tests

A variety of tests are available to identify antigen and/or antibody to specific parasites. The majority of tests are based on the enzyme-linked immunosorbent assay (ELISA) principle. The tests are highly accurate and precise and can detect occult infections. Canine heartworm infections and *Toxoplasma* infections are routinely diagnosed with these methods. In the ELISA, monoclonal antibodies are used to detect antigens of adult heartworms in the serum or plasma of dogs. These procedures are rapid and easy to perform They are also more sensitive and specific than microfilariae detection methods. The American Heartworm Society currently recommends using antigen-detection methods for routine screening. Antigen-detection methods are preferred to microfilariae concentration methods in cats because such aberrant hosts circulate microfilariae only for a very short time. However, antigen levels in the blood of infected cats may also be too low to detect. Other methods, such as radiography, may be employed to make a diagnosis in cats.

Approximately 25% of heartworm-infected dogs have occult infections. Occult infections are characterized by a lack of circulating microfilaria and occur if the infection is not yet patent, if the population of adult heartworms consists of only one sex, and if immune reactions of the host to microfilariae eliminate this stage from the bloodstream. Occult infections can also occur if animals infected with

The most accurate differentiating characteristics are body width, body length, and shape of the cranial end. The other characteristics are not consistent. The modified Knott's technique cannot detect occult heartworm infections.

TABLE 14-1

Differential Characteristics of *Dirofilaria immitis* and *Dipetalonema reconditum* Microfilariae

Characteristic	Dirofilaria immitis	Dipetalonema reconditum
Body shape	Usually straight	Usually curved
Body width	5–7.5 μ	4.5-5.5 μ
Body length	295-325 μ	250-288 μ
Cranial end	Tapered	Blunt
Caudal end	Straight	Curved or hooked
Numbers	Numerous	Sparse
Movement	Undulating	Progressive

adult heartworms are given heartworm preventive medications of the ivermectin group. These interfere with oogenesis and sterilize the worms.

Miscellaneous parasitologic evaluations

Cellophane tape preparations (previously described) can be used to recover external parasites that live primarily on the surface of the skin (i.e. mites, lice, fleas). Parasites that live in hair follicles or burrows are usually diagnosed with skin scraping using standard procedures.

Samples may be collected from the ear or the respiratory or genital tracts with cotton swabs. These can be examined microscopically using standard preparations as for cytology samples. Transtracheal/bronchial washes can also be used to recover parasites of the respiratory system. Parasites of the urinary system are usually recovered using standard urine sediment examination techniques. (These procedures are described in more detail in Chapter 13.)

Impression smears can be used for diagnosis of intracellular parasites (Box 14-13). They can be useful for diagnosis of parasitic, neoplastic, and fungal diseases antemortem and postmortem. Frequently, protozoal organisms produce systemic disease and are located in the reticuloendothelial cells of lymph nodes, liver, lung, bone marrow, spleen, brain, kidneys, or muscles. Also, the liver, lung, lymph nodes, bone marrow, and spleen filter out damaged and abnormal cells of the blood, collecting parasitized cells. Toxoplasmosis, leishmaniasis, ehrlichiosis, and babesiosis are examples of parasitic diseases that can be diagnosed using this technique.

Skin scrapings are used as a diagnostic tool for dermatologic conditions, especially mange in domestic animals (Box 14-14). Because some mange mites dwell in burrows and hair follicles deep in the epidermis, superficial scrapings are not productive. Other mites live in the more superficial layers of the skin and produce crusty or scaly lesions; deep scrapings are not required to diagnose these infestations. Sometimes the thick crusts interfere with seeing the mites. Soaking the crust in a 10% potassium hydroxide solution helps to dissolve the keratinized skin and releases the mites. Mite infestations usually localize in specific locations (ear margin, tail head) initially, depending on the species of mite involved. Later they may become generalized and more difficult to diagnose. *Sarcoptes* (see Fig. 14-30) and *Cheyletiella* mites can be transmitted to people and produce pruritic reactions requiring attention. Specific identification of mites can be accomplished with the aid of taxonomic keys.

Cheyletiella infestation can be diagnosed by combing the coat of infested animals over a piece of black paper and observing the paper for "moving dandruff" (see Fig. 14-36). *Otodectes cynotis* (ear mite, see Fig. 14-35) infestations of the external ear canal can be diagnosed by otoscopic examination or by taking a swab of the dark waxy debris found in the ear and microscopically examining it in mineral oil.

BOX 14-13   *procedure*

Impression Smear

Materials

- Paper towels
- Glass microscope slides (25-mm)
- Glass coverslips (22-mm^2 #1)
- Romanowsky stain
- Scalpel blade or single-edged razor blade
- Forceps

Procedure

1. With tissue from necropsy or a lesion on an animal, either make a fresh cut of the tissue or remove any crust or scabs over the lesion.
2. Lightly blot the tissue or lesion with a clean paper towel.
3. Press the fresh edge of the tissue or lesion to a glass slide.
4. Stain the slide, and examine it microscopically for parasites at 400× and 1000× magnification.

BOX 14-14   *procedure*

Skin Scrapings

Materials

- Glass microscope slides (25-mm)
- Glass coverslips (22-mm^2 #1)
- Scalpel blades (#10)
- 10% potassium hydroxide solution (10 g potassium hydroxide/100 ml water)

Procedure

1. With one hand, pinch the skin at the periphery of the lesion.
2. Apply a small amount of mineral oil to the area of skin to be scraped and a drop of oil to the center of a glass slide.
3. With the scalpel blade held between the thumb and index finger, scrape the skin until serum and a small amount of blood ooze from the area. Hold the blade perpendicular to the skin so as not to cut the skin.
4. Transfer the hair and epithelial debris from the blade to the oil on the slide.
5. Place a coverslip over the slide, and examine microscopically at 100× and 400× magnification.

BOX 14-15

procedure

Tritrichomonas Foetus Culture

Materials

- Lactated Ringer's solution or phosphate buffered saline
- Pipettes
- Disposable gloves
- Diamond's culture medium or In Pouch TF

Procedure

1. Wear gloves to prevent contamination of the sample to be collected.
2. Perform a preputial wash of the bull or collection of vaginal, cervical, or uterine secretions of the cow, using the Ringer's or saline solution.
3. Transfer the sample immediately to a clean tube, and allow the sample to settle.
4. Inoculate the Diamond's culture medium or In Pouch TF with 1 to 2 ml of the sediment.
5. Inoculate the medium at 37° C
6. Examine the medium within the first 48 hours microscopically for growth of trichomonads. Allow the medium to incubate for 5 days, and re-examine periodically for organisms.
7. If trichomonads are cultured, transfer 3 to 5 drops of the lower (deeper) portion of the medium containing the organisms to a new tube or pouch of culture medium. Repeat the process of incubation and observation for growth.
8. Withdraw a small amount of a positive culture with a pipette, and transfer to a slide to observe motility and morphology microscopically (0.5% formalin can be used to kill the flagellates for viewing with a phase microscope).

Tritrichomonas foetus is a flagellated protozoan parasite of the reproductive tract of cattle that causes early-term abortions and repeat breeding (Box 14-15). Bulls remain permanently infected and must be identified and slaughtered to prevent spread of this organism. The organism can be found in fluid from the abomasum of aborted fetuses, uterine discharges, and vaginal and preputial washes. However, the numbers present are usually low and culture of these materials facilitates diagnosis. Occasionally, intestinal flagellates can contaminate a sample. These must be differentiated from *T. foetus*, which has three cranial flagella and one caudal flagellum attached to an undulating membrane. Isolates of *T. foetus* can be propagated through several passages of culture medium, whereas intestinal flagellates usually cannot. Materials may also be collected and shipped to diagnostic facilities for culture and identification. In Pouch TF (Biomed Diagnostics, San Jose, Calif.) is an excellent transport medium.

Total worm burden estimates provide the most accurate information regarding whether pathogenic levels of parasites are present in an animal or herd (Box 14-16). This technique is used most frequently in grazing animals, but can be used in small animal practices as well. It is frequently employed in scientific studies investigating the epidemiology of parasitic helminths and in drug efficacy studies.

Specific identification of gross parasites recovered from domestic animals is beyond the scope of this book and often requires the expertise of experienced helminthologists, protozoologists, and entomologists. Government, academic, and private diagnostic laboratories often provide these services. However well-preserved specimens must be provided (Box 14-17). Usually both male and female parasites are needed, and numerous samples of the parasite must be examined for appropriate identification. An adequate history is also needed, including host, location in the host, geographic location of the host, travel history, age, sex, nutritional level, clinical signs, and treatments. Specific diagnostic procedures requested should be denoted. Telephoning the laboratory before shipment is helpful to find out how the laboratory handles requests, and the cost, time required, and procedures for specimen processing. Telephone numbers of government and university facilities are listed in the directory of the American Veterinary Medical Association.

Figs. 14-1 to 14-36 show common internal parasites of domestic animals. Tables 14-2 (pp. 301-304) and 14-3 (p. 305) list diagnostic characteristics of internal parasites of domestic animals. Table 14-4 (p. 306) lists some zoonotic internal parasites.

BOX 14-16 *procedure*

Total Worm Counts of the Digestive Tract

Materials

- 6 buckets (12-L capacity)
- String
- Scissors
- Dissection pans
- Stereo microscope
- Petri dishes
- Fine-tipped forceps
- Graduated cylinders (1000–2000 ml)
- Paddle
- Jar of known volume (50–100 ml)
- 37% formaldehyde solution

Procedure

1. At necropsy, detach the digestive tract from the mesenteric attachments. Straighten the tract segments, and remove any adhering mesentery.
2. Using double ligatures, tie off each segment of the digestive tract (stomach, small intestines, large intestines). Cut between the ligatures and separate the segments, placing each segment into a separate bucket.
3. Open the segments into the buckets while flushing the mucosal surface with a gentle stream of water. Rub the surface vigorously to detach adhering debris and worms. Place each washed segment of gut into a separate bucket, submerge in water, and allow it to soak for several hours or overnight.
4. Fill the buckets containing the gut contents with an equal volume of water, and allow the contents to sediment (15 to 30 minutes).
5. Pour off the supernatant (liquid top portion) slowly. Resuspend the sediment again, and allow the contents to settle.
6. Repeat steps 4 and 5 until the top liquid becomes clear.
7. Measure the total volume of each bucket with the graduated cylinders, and return the contents to the buckets.
8. Using a jar of known volume, withdraw 3 volumes (aliquots) of the gut contents while agitating the contents of the bucket with a paddle. Transfer the aliquots to the dissection pans or containers. Concentrated iodine solution may be added to the pans to help visualize worms grossly, or a small amount of the aliquot can be transferred to a Petri dish and examined using a stereo microscope until all the sediment in the aliquot has been examined. Nematodes recovered should be removed with forceps and preserved for identification. Most nematodes in the large intestine can be seen without the aide of a microscope.
9. Identify the parasites, and make separate counts for each species recovered.
10. Determine the dilution factor by dividing the volume of the aliquot into the total volume of the gut contents. The total worm burden can be calculated by multiplying the dilution factor times the average number of the parasites recovered in each of the aliquots for each segment of gut. An alternative approach is to add sufficient formaldehyde to each aliquot to approximate a 10% solution of formalin and submit the aliquots to a reference laboratory for counting and identification. When using this approach, specify the volume of the aliquots and the total volumes for each segment of intestinal tract.
11. Contents from each washed segment of the gut can be processed in a similar manner and examined for larval stages, which tend to migrate out into the warm water.

BOX 14-17 *procedure*

Preservation and Shipment of Parasites

Materials

- 70% ethyl alcohol, 10% formalin, 5% glycerin alcohol, polyvinyl alcohol
- Glass or polypropylene screw-cap specimen containers
- Paraffin
- Labels
- Styrofoam or heavy cardboard mailing containers

Procedure

1. Briefly wash worms recovered from the digestive tract or internal organs to remove adhering debris.
2. Roundworms, tapeworms, and flukes should be placed in a refrigerator for several hours to relax them for identification later.
3. After relaxation, roundworms can be stored in glycerine alcohol or 7% to 10% formalin. Tapeworms and flukes are best preserved in 70% ethanol because they require staining for identification. Most ectoparasites can be transferred directly to 70% ethanol. Fecal samples that are to be shipped should be mixed with 10% formalin (1 part feces to 3 volumes of formalin). If intestinal protozoan trophozoites are present in the feces, feces should also be preserved in polyvinyl alcohol for staining and identification.
4. Place specimens in screw-cap vials, and seal with paraffin.
5. Label vials with the date of collection, preservative used, practitioner's name, client's name, species of animal, animal's identification number or name, geographic location, and location of parasite in the host.
6. Package vials in containers so that they do not break during shipment.
7. Accompany the specimen with a cover letter giving a brief clinical history of the animal and diagnostic tests required.

TABLE 14-2

Diagnostic Characteristics of Internal Parasites of Domestic Animals

Parasite	Location	Prepatent Period	Diagnostic Stage	Test
Dogs				
Toxocara canis (see Fig. 14-11)	Small intestine	3-5 weeks	Dark brown, thick-walled, pitted egg, single-celled zygote 90-75 μ	Fecal Flotation
Ancylostoma caninum (see Fig. 14-17)	Small intestine	2-3 weeks	Clear, smooth, thin-walled hookworm egg; 8-16-cell morula zygote; 55-65 × 27-43 μ	Fecal Flotation
Uncinaria stenocephala	Small intestine	2 weeks	Hookworm egg; 63-93 × 32-55 μ	Fecal Flotation
Trichuris vulpis	Large intestine	3 months	Smooth, amber, thick-walled, barrel-shaped egg with bipolar plugs; single-celled zygote; 72-90 × 32-40 μ	Fecal Flotation
Filaroïdes spp.	Lungs	5-10 weeks	L1 with S-shaped tail lacking a dorsal spine; esophagus ⅓ length of body; 230-266 μ long	Fecal Flotation, Baermann
Crenosoma spp.	Lungs	19-21 days	L1 with a straight, pointed tail; esophagus ⅓ length of body; 265-330 μ long	Baermann
Spirocerca lupi	Esophagus	5-6 months	Clear, smooth, thick-walled, paper-clip-shaped, larvated egg; 30-37 × 11-15 μ	Flotation
Dirofilaria immitis (see Fig. 14-19)	Heart	6-8 months	Microfilaria (L1) lacks an esophagus	Modified Knott's millipore filtration, ELISA, antigen test
Dipetalonema reconditum (see Fig. 14-20)	Subcutaneous tissue	9 weeks	Microfilaria	Modified Knott's millipore filtration
Dioctophyma renale	Kidney	5 months	Dark brown, thick-walled, barrel-shaped egg with a pitted shell and an operculum at each pole; single-celled zygote; 71-84 × 46-52 μ	Sedimentation of urine
Dracunculus insignis	Subcutaneous tissue	309-410 days	Comma-shaped larva with an esophagus and a straight tail; 500-750 μ long	Direct smear of fluid in blister
Cats				
Toxocara cati (see Fig. 14-12)	Small intestine	8 weeks	Dark brown, thick-walled, pitted egg; single-celled zygote; 65-75 μ	Fecal Flotation
Ancylostoma	Small intestine	3 weeks	Hookworm egg; 55-76 × 34-45 μ	Fecal Flotation
Aelurostrongylus abstrusus (see Fig. 14-12)	Bronchioles alveoli	4-6 weeks	L1 with S-shaped tail and a dorsal spine; 360 μ long; esophagus ¼ length of body	Baermann
Platynosomum fastosum	Liver	8-12 weeks	Dark amber, oval, operculated egg containing a miracidium; 34-50 × 20-35 μ	Sedimentation of feces
Toxoplasma gondii (see Fig. 14-5)	Small intestine	1-3 weeks	Clear, smooth, thin-walled spherical oocyst; single-celled zygote; 8-10 μ	Fecal Flotation
Dogs and Cats				
Toxascaris leonina (see Fig. 14-13)	Small intestine	11 weeks	Clear, smooth, thick-walled eggshell with wavy internal membrane; single-celled zygote; does not completely fill egg; 75 × 85 μ	Fecal Flotation
Ancylostoma braziliense	Small intestine	3 weeks	Hookworm egg; 75-95 × 41-45 μ	Fecal Flotation
Uncinaria stenocephala	Small intestine	15 days	Hookworm egg; 63-93 × 32-55 μ	Fecal Flotation
Capillaria aerophilus (see Fig. 14-18)	Trachea Bronchi	6 weeks	Rough, granular, thick-walled, barrel-shaped, straw-colored egg with asymmetric bipolar plugs; single-celled zygote; 58-79 × 29-40 μ	Fecal Flotation
Capillaria plica	Urinary bladder	60 days	Rough, striated, thick-walled, barrel-shaped, amber-colored egg with asymmetric bipolar plugs; single-celled zygote; 60-68 × 24-30 μ	Sedimentation of urine

Continued

TABLE 14-2

Diagnostic Characteristics of Internal Parasites of Domestic Animals—Cont'd

Parasite	Location	Prepatent Period	Diagnostic Stage	Test
Dogs and Cats—Cont'd				
Strongyloides stercoralis	Small intestine	8-14 days	L1 with a rhabditiform esophagus and a straight pointed tail; L3 with a filariform esophagus and a bipartite tail	Baermann fecal culture
Physaloptera spp.	Stomach	56-83 days	Smooth, clear, thick-walled, larvated egg 45-53 × 29-42 μ	Fecal flotation
Dipylidium caninum (see Fig. 14-7)	Small intestine	3 weeks	Proglottid with bilateral genital pores; eggs containing six-hooked hexacanth embryos in packets; 35-60 μ	ID proglottids fecal flotation
Taenia spp. (see Fig. 14-8)	Small intestine	2 months	Dark brown, thick, radially striated eggshell; six-hooked hexacanth embryo; 32-37 μ; rectangular proglottids with unilateral genital pore	ID proglottid
Echinococcus spp.	Small intestine	47 days	Similar to *Taenia* eggs	Fecal flotation
Mesocestoides spp.	Small intestine	16-20 days	Smooth, thin egg capsule containing six-hooked hexacanth embryo; 20-25 μ; globular proglottid with parauterine body	Fecal flotation ID proglottid
Spirometra mansonoides	Small intestine	10-30 days	Unembryonated, thin-walled, smooth, amber-colored operculated egg; 70 × 45 μ	Fecal flotation
Paragonimus kellicotti	Lung	1 month	Smooth, golden brown, urn-shaped, operculated egg; 75-118 × 42-67 μ	Sedimentation of urine
Nanophyetus salmincola (see Fig. 14-10)	Small intestine	1 week	Rough, brown, operculated egg; 52-82 × 32-56 μ	Sedimentation of feces
Isospora spp. (see Fig. 14-3)	Small intestine	4-12 days	Clear, spherical to ellipsoid thin-walled oocyst, size varies with species	Fecal flotation
Sarcocystis spp.	Small intestine	7-33 days	Thin-walled oocyst with 2 sporocyst containing 4 sporozoites each or sporocyst; size varies with species	Fecal flotation
Horse				
Parascaris equorum (see Fig. 14-14)	Small intestine	10 weeks	Rough, brown, thick-walled, spherical egg single-celled zygote; 90-100 μ	Fecal flotation
Eimeria leukarti	Small intestine	15-33 days	Dark brown, piriform, thick-walled oocyst 70-90 × 49-69 μ	Fecal flotation
Cyathostoma (small strongyles)	Large intestine	2-3 months	Smooth, thin-walled, clear strongyle egg zygote 8- to 16-cell morula; size varies with species	Fecal flotation
Strongylus spp. (large strongyles)	Large intestine	6-12 months	Strongyle egg	Fecal flotation
Oxyuris equi (see Fig. 14-16)	Large intestine	5 months	Clear, smooth, thin-walled egg with one side flattened; operculated; 90 × 42 μ	Cellophane tape preparation
Anoplocephala spp.	Small and large intestines	1-2 months	Clear, thick-walled, square eggs with a pear-shaped (piriform) apparatus containing a hexacanth embryo	Fecal flotation
Trichostrongylus axei	Stomach	25 days	Strongyle egg	Fecal flotation
Dictyocaulus arnfieldi	Lung	2-4 months	L1 with dark, granular intestines; esophagus ⅓ length of larva; tapered tail	Fecal flotation Baermann
Habronema and *Draschia* spp.	Stomach	2 months	Thin-walled, larvated egg (rarely seen)	ID adults at necropsy
Strongyloides westeri	Small intestine	8-14 days	Smooth, thin-walled, larvated egg; 40-50 × 32-40 μ	Fecal flotation
Onchocerca spp.	Ligaments of legs and neck	1 year	Unsheathed microfilaria in the skin of ventral midline; 200-370 μ long	Skin biopsy
Setaria equina	Peritoneal cavity		Sheathed microfilaria in the blood; 190-256 μ long	Blood smear ID adults at necropsy

Continued

	Location	Prepatent	Description	Diagnostic test
Gasterophilus spp. (see Fig. 14-27)	Stomach		2.5 cm, robust grub with rows of spines and straight spiracular slits (breathing tubes)	ID 3rd instar at necropsy
Cattle, Sheep, Goats				
Trichostrongyles Haemonchus, Ostertagia, Cooperia, Trichostrongylus (see Fig. 14-15)	Abomasum, small intestine	15-28 days	Strongyle egg	Fecal flotation
Dictyocaulus spp.	Lungs	3-4 weeks	L1 with dark granular intestines; esophagus ⅓ length of larva; straight pointed tail; 550-580 μ long	Baermann
Strongyloides spp.	Small intestine	3-4 weeks	Thin-walled egg with parallel sides; 40-60 × 20-25 μ	Fecal flotation
Oesophagostomum spp.	Large intestine	45 days	Strongyle egg	Fecal flotation
Skrjabinema spp.	Large intestine	25 days	Clear, smooth, thin-walled egg with one side flattened; single-celled zygote	Fecal flotation
Eimeria spp. (see Fig 14-2)	Small and large intestines	10-30 days	Smooth or rough, thin-walled, clear to yellowish brown oocysts; single-celled zygote; size varies with species	Fecal flotation
Moniezia spp. (see Fig. 14-9)	Small intestine	6 weeks	Thick-walled, clear, triangular to square egg with a piriform apparatus containing a hexacanth embryo	Fecal flotation
Thysanosoma actinoides	Bile ducts		Thin-walled egg with hexacanth embryos; 21-45 μ	Fecal flotation
Fasciola hepatica (see Fig. 14-9)	Liver	10-12 weeks	Dark amber, oval, operculated egg; 130-150×63-90 μ	Sedimentation of feces
Dicrocoelium dendriticum	Liver	10-12 weeks	Dark brown, operculated egg; 36-45 × 22-30 μ	Sedimentation of feces
Paramphistomum spp.	Rumen	7-10 weeks	Light greenish, oval, operculated egg; 114-176×73-100 μ	Sedimentation of feces
Bunostomum spp.	Small intestine	2-3 weeks	Strongyle egg	Fecal flotation
Chabertia ovina	Large intestine	47-63 days	Strongyle egg	Fecal flotation
Toxocara vitulorum	Small intestine	3 weeks	Thick-walled, pitted eggshell; single-celled zygote; 90-100 μ	Fecal flotation
Setaria labiatopapillosa	Peritoneal cavity		Sheathed microfilaria in the blood; 240-260 μ	Blood smears; adults at necropsy
Trichuris spp. (see Fig. 14-15)	Large intestine	2-3 months	Dark, brownish, thick-walled, smooth egg with symmetric bipolar plugs; single-celled zygote; size varies with species	Fecal flotation
Capillaria spp.	Small intestine		Brownish, thick-walled striated egg with asymmetric bipolar plugs; single-celled zygote, 45-52 × 21-30 μ	Fecal flotation
Cattle				
Onchocerca spp. nuchae	Ligamentum	1 year	Unsheathed microfilaria in the skin of ventral midline; 170-265 μ	Skin biopsy
Stephanofilaria stilesi	Skin along ventral midline		Microfilaria in the skin along ventral midline; 45-60μ	Skin biopsy
Cryptosporidium muris	Abomasum	4-10 days	Clear, smooth, thin-walled oocyst containing 4 sporozoites; 5 × 7 μ	Fecal flotation
Sheep				
Elaeophora schneideri	Arteries	4-5 months	Microfilaria in skin of the poll; 207 ×13 μ	Skin biopsy
Protostrongylus rufescens	Lungs	30-37 days	L1 with a straight, pointed tail 48 × 56 μ long without a dorsal spine; 340-400 × 19-20 μ	Baermann
Mullerius spp.	Lungs	6 weeks	L1 are 300-320 × 14-15 μ with S-shaped tail bearing a dorsal spine	Baermann
Pigs				
Eimeria spp.	Small intestine	4-10 days	Smooth or rough, thin-walled oocyst; single-celled zygote; size varies with species	Fecal flotation

TABLE 14-2

Diagnostic Characteristics of Internal Parasites of Domestic Animals—Cont'd

Parasite	Location	Prepatent Period	Diagnostic Stage	Test
Pigs—Cont'd				
Isospora suis	Small intestine	5 days	Smooth, clear, thin-walled oocyst; single-celled zygote; $17-25 \times 16-21$ μ	Fecal flotation
Balantidium coli	Large intestine		Thin-walled, greenish cyst with hyaline cytoplasm; $40-60$ μ; trophozoite with rows of cilia $30-150 \times 25-120$ μ	Fecal flotation Direct smear
Ascaris suum	Small intestine	7-9 weeks	Brownish yellow, thick-walled, mammillated egg; single-celled zygote; $50-80 \times 40-60$ μ	Fecal flotation
Strongyloides ransomi	Small intestine	3-7 days	Smooth, thin-walled, larvated egg with parallel sides; $45-55 \times 26-35$ μ	Fecal flotation
Oesophagostomum spp.	Large intestine	32-42 days	Strongyle egg	Fecal flotation
Stephanurus dentatus	Kidney	3-4 months	Strongyle egg	Sedimentation of urine
Hyostrongylus rubidus	Stomach	15-21 days	Strongyle egg	Fecal flotation
Metastrongylus spp.	Lungs	24 days	Rough, clear, thick-walled, larvated egg with a corrugated surface; $45-57 \times 38-41$ μ	Fecal flotation
Ascarops strongylina	Stomach	6 weeks	Oblong, clear, smooth, thick-walled, larvated egg; $34-40 \times 18-22$ μ	Fecal flotation
Physocephalus sexalatus	Stomach	6 weeks	Clear, smooth, thick-walled, larvated egg; $31-45 \times 12-26$ μ	Fecal flotation
Trichuris suis	Large intestine	2-3 months	Brownish yellow, smooth, thick-walled egg with symmetric bipolar plugs; single-celled zygote; $50-56 \times 21-25$ μ	Fecal flotation
Trichinella spiralis	Small intestine	2-6 days	L3 encysted in striated muscles; esophagus composed of stichocytes (single cells stacked on top of one another); cysts are $400-600 \times 250$ μ	Squash preparation of muscle
Macracanthorhynchus hirudinaceus (see Fig. 14-21)	Small intestine	2-3 months	Dark brown, thick-walled egg with 3 membranes; zygote an acanthor with anterior hooks; $67-110 \times 40-65$ μ	Fecal flotation
Dogs, Cats, Cattle, Horses, Sheep, Goats, Pigs				
Thelazia californiensis	Eye and tear duct	3-6 weeks	Adult worm in conjunctival sac	ID adult
Giardia spp. (see Fig. 14-1)	Small intestine	7-10 days	Smooth, clear, thin-walled cyst with 2-4 nuclei; $4-10 \times 8-16$ μ; Piriform, bilaterally symmetric greenish trophozoite with 2 nuclei and 4 pair of flagella; $9-20 \times 5-15$ μ	Fecal flotation Direct smear
Trichomonads	Digestive tract		Spindle-shaped to piriform trophozoite with 3-5 anterior flagella, an undulating membrane and 1 posterior flagellum	Direct smear
Cryptosporidium spp. (see Fig. 14-4)	Small and large intestines	4-10 days	Clear, thin-walled, spherical oocyst containing 4 sporozoites; 5×5 μ	Fecal flotation

TABLE 14-3

Diagnostic Characteristics of Blood Parasites of Domestic Animals

Parasite	Definitive Host	Location	Prepatent Period	Diagnostic Stage	Diagnostic Test
Babesia spp. (see Fig. 1-16)	People, dogs, cattle, horses	Blood (erythrocytes)	10-21 days	Paired piriform (tear-shaped) merozoites in erythrocytes	Romanowsky-stained blood film, indirect fluorescent antibody test
Trypanosoma spp.	People, dogs, cats, cattle, sheep, horses	Blood and lymph, heart, striated muscle, reticuloendothelial muscle	Acute and chronic disease	Trypanosome form, spindle-shaped flagellate with undulating membrane, central nucleus and kinetoplast, found in blood Amastigore form, intracellular spherical bodies with single nucleus and rod-shaped kinetoplast, found in myocardium, striated muscle cells, and macrophages	Blood smears, xenodiagnosis ('clean vector allowed to feed on suspect patient and organism isolated from the vector), biopsy, animal inoculation, serology
Leishmania donovam	People, dogs	Intracellular in cytoplasm of macrophages of reticuloendothelial system	Several months up to a year	Amastigore form, oval, single nucleus, with a rod-shaped kinetoplast, in clusters within the cytoplasm of macrophages	Impression smears and biopsy of skin, lymph nodes and bone marrow

TABLE 14-4

Zoonotic Internal Parasites

Parasite	Host	Reservoir	Infective Stage	Condition
Toxocara spp.	Dogs, cats	Dogs, cats	Egg with L2	Visceral larva migrans
Anoylostoma spp.	Dogs, cats	Dogs, cats	L3	Cutaneous larva migrans
Uncinaria stenocephala	Dogs, cats	Dogs, cats	L3	Cutaneous larva migrans
Toxoplasma gondit	Cats	Cats, raw meat	Sporulated oocyst, bradyzoite, tachyzoite	Toxoplasmosis
Strongyloides stercoralis	Dogs, cats, people	People, dogs, cats	L3	Strongyloidiasis
Dipylidium caninum	Dogs, cats, people	Flea	Cysticercoid	Cestodiasis
Taenia saginata	People	Bovine muscle	Cysticercus	Cestodiasis
Taenia solium	People	Porcine muscle	Cysticercus	Cestodiasis
	People	People	Egg	Cysticercosis
Echinococcus granidosus	Dogs	Dogs	Egg	Hydatidosis
Echinococcus multilocularis	Dogs, cats	Dogs, cats	Egg	Hydatidosis
Spironietra mansonoides	Dogs, cats	Unknown	Procercoid in arthropod	Sparganosis
Sarcocystis spp.	People	Cattle, pigs	Sarcocyst in muscle	Sarcocystiasis
	Dogs, cats	Dogs, cats	Oocyst	Sarcosporidiosis
Cryptosporidium patvum	Mammals	Mammals	Oocyst	Cryptosporidiosis
Balantidium coli	People, pigs	People, pigs	Cyst, trophozoite	Balantidiasis
Ascaris suum	Pigs	Pigs	Egg with L2	Visceral larva migrans
Trichinella spiralis	Mammals	Porcine and bear muscle	Encysted L3	Trichinellosis
Thelagia spp.	Mammals	Flies	L3	Verminous conjunctivitis
Giardro duodenalis	Mammals	Mammals	Cyst	Giardiasis
Babesia microti	Rodents, people	Hard ticks	Sporozoite	Babesiosis
Trypanosoma	Mammals	Reduvirds	Trypanosomal form in kissing bug	Chagas' disease
Leishinania donovani	Mammals	Phlebotomine flies	Leptomonad form in sandfly	Leishmaniasis

RECOMMENDED READING

Bowman DD: *Georgi's parasitology for veterinarians*, ed 7, Philadelphia, 1999, WB Saunders.

Hendrix CM: *Diagnostic veterinary parasitology*, ed 2, St Louis, 1998, Mosby.

Hendrix CM: *Laboratory procedures for veterinary technicians*, ed 4, St Louis, 2002, Mosby.

Sloss MW, Kemp RL, and Zajac AM: *Veterinary clinical parasitology*, ed 6, Ames, Iowa, 1994, Iowa State University Press.

15

Preventive Medicine

Michael D. Cross and Margi Sirois

Learning Objectives
After reviewing this chapter, the reader should understand the following:
- General principles underlying disease prevention
- Features of appropriate housing and nutrition for animals
- Ways in which animals can be identified
- Types and schedules of vaccinations for domestic animal species
- Principles of sanitation used in disease prevention
- Factors that predispose to disease
- General principles of incorporating a wellness program into a veterinary facility

Veterinary preventive medicine is the science of preventing disease in animals. The three major components of a preventive medicine program include *husbandry*, *vaccination or prevention through medication*, and *sanitation*. Husbandry involves the housing, diet, and environment of animals. Vaccination involves the use of vaccines or bacterins to prevent such diseases as rabies or equine encephalomyelitis; medication can be given regularly to prevent heartworms. Sanitation focuses on cleanliness and the use of disinfectants to prevent infection or disease transmission. All three components are interrelated; disease is prevented only by attention to all components. For example, poor husbandry practices cannot be accommodated by overvaccination and rigorous sanitation. Failure to properly vaccinate an animal may well result in disease, even if the husbandry is top-notch, and the sanitation is impeccable. Poor sanitation frequently results in animal and human disease.

The goal of any preventive medicine program is the lowest possible incidence of disease in animals under the care of the veterinary practice. In general, the number of client visits to the hospital or the number of farm visits reflects the efficacy of the preventive medicine program. The mutual goal of veterinary professionals and animal owners should be to preserve animal health using preventive practices.

The authors acknowledge and appreciate the original contribution of R.E. Banks, whose work has been incorporated into this chapter.

Such efforts save money that otherwise would be spent for treatment of disease. Preventive medicine also prolongs the life span, improves the well being of animals, and fosters a good client-veterinarian relationship.

Unfortunately, some clients cannot see the benefit of spending a few dollars for preventive care, such as for vaccination. These clients then complain about the large sums of money they must spend to correct problems that could have been avoided through preventive methods. The challenge for veterinary technicians is to empathize and work with these clients for the benefit of the patient. By educating animal owners on the benefits of proper preventive medicine, you will be given the opportunity to provide the best veterinary care possible.

Tables 15-1 to 15-6 present preventive medicine programs recommended for various species.

HUSBANDRY

Temperature, Light, and Ventilation

For small animals, such as dogs, cats, birds, and small mammals, the ambient (room) temperature should ideally be 65° to 84° F (18° to 29° C). Birds, very young pets, old pets, and those with a sparse haircoat should be maintained at the higher end of this temperature range. Those that are well furred or overweight should be kept at the lower end of this range.

TABLE 15-1

Preventive Medicine Programs Generally Recommended for Dogs

6 to 8 Weeks	10 to 12 Weeks	16 Weeks or Older	Annual Visits
General physical examination	General physical examination	General physical examination	General physical examination
Fecal examination	Fecal examination; treat if required	Fecal examination; treat if required	Fecal examination; treat if required
Vaccinate for distemper, parainfluenza, adenovirus infection, leptospirosis, parvovirus infection, coronavirus infection	Vaccinate for distemper, parainfluenza, adenovirus infection, leptospirosis, parvovirus infection, coronavirus infection	Vaccinate for distemper, parainfluenza, adenovirus infection, leptospirosis, parvovirus infection, coronavirus infection, rabies, possibly borreliosis and tracheobronchitis	Vaccinate for distemper, parainfluenza, adenovirus infection, leptospirosis, parvovirus infection, coronavirus infection, rabies, possibly borreliosis and tracheobronchitis
Begin client education:	Continue client education:	Continue client education:	Continue client education:
Cage/pen care	Ask about cage/pen care	Confirm cage/pen care	Confirm cage/pen care
Exercise/sleep	Check on nutrition	Check on nutrition	Check on nutrition
Nutrition	Discuss grooming practices	Discuss grooming practices	Discuss grooming practices
Grooming	Begin heartworm preventive therapy	Adjust heartworm therapy	Adjust heartworm therapy
Heartworms	Recheck for parasites; treat as needed	Confirm that training is working	Confirm that training is working
Viral diseases	Confirm that training is working	Schedule neutering	Schedule neutering
Parasites	Suggest neutering if not breeding		
Behavior			

TABLE 15-2

Preventive Medicine Programs Generally Recommended for Cats

8 to 10 Weeks	12 to 14 Weeks	Annual Visits

General physical examination
Fecal examination; treat if required
Vaccinate for feline leukemia virus infection, panleukopenia, rhinotracheitis, calicivirus infection, chlamydial pneumonitis
Begin client education:
  Exercise/sleep
  Nutrition
  Grooming
  Play
  Viral diseases
  Parasites
  Behavior
	General physical examination
	Fecal examination; treat if required
	Vaccinate for feline leukemia virus infection, panleukopenia, rhinotracheitis, calicivirus infection, chlamydial pneumonitis, rabies
	Continue client education:
	  Exercise/sleep
	  Nutrition
		General physical examination
		Fecal examination; treat if required
		Vaccinate for feline leukemia virus infection, panleukopenia, rhinotracheitis, calicivirus infection, chlamydial pneumonitis
		Continue client education:
		  Exercise/sleep
		  Nutrition
		  Grooming
		  Viral diseases
		  Parasites
		  Behavior

TABLE 15-3

Preventive Medicine Programs Generally Recommended for Horses

Foals and Weanlings	Yearlings and Adults
Physical examination at time of vaccination Deworm every 2 months (rotate products) Trim feet as needed Vaccinate for tetanus, EEE, WEE, VEE, equine influenza, rhinopneumonitis Discuss feeding regimen Discuss exercise program Monitor body condition	Physical examination at time of vaccination Deworm at least every 2 months (rotate products) Check teeth and float as needed Trim feet as needed Vaccinate for tetanus, EEE, WEE, VEE, equine influenza, rhinopneumonitis Review stall cleaning schedule Discuss feeding regimen Discuss exercise program Monitor body condition

TABLE 15-4

Preventive Medicine Programs Generally Recommended for Cattle

Neonatal Period	1 to 3 Months	5 to 6 Months	Annually
Physical examination Vaccinate for bovine rotavirus and coronavirus infection (if necessary) Review stall-cleaning schedule Monitor body condition	Physical examination Deworm (rotate products) Vaccinate for clostridial diseases Review stall-cleaning schedule Discuss feeding regimen Monitor body condition	Physical examination Deworm (rotate products) Vaccination for clostridial diseases, infectious bovine rhinotracheitis, parainfluenza-3, bovine virus diarrhea Review stall-cleaning schedule Discuss feeding regimen Monitor body condition	Physical examination Deworm (rotate products) Vaccinate for infectious bovine rhinotracheitis, parainfluenza-3, bovine virus diarrhea Review stall-cleaning schedule Discuss feeding regimen Monitor body condition

TABLE 15-5

Preventive Medicine Programs Generally Recommended for Pigs

Neonatal Period	1 to 3 Weeks	4 to 5 Weeks	8 to 10 Weeks	Annually
Physical examination	Physical examination	Physical examination	Physical Examination	Deworm (rotate products)
Dock tails	Vaccinate for transmissible	Vaccinate for atrophic	Treat for ectoparasites	Check for ectoparasites
Castrate (if necessary)	gastroenteritis, atrophic	rhinitis, erysipelas,	Deworm	Physical examination
Clip needle teeth	rhinitis, porcine parvovirus	*Haemophilus* infection,	Discuss feeding regimen	Vaccinate as necessary
Iron dextran injection	infection	swine dysentery	Monitor body condition	Review stall-cleaning schedule
Identify with ear	Monitor body condition	Review stall-cleaning		Discuss feeding regimen
notching	Review stall-cleaning	schedule		Monitor body condition
	schedule	Monitor body condition		

TABLE 15-6

Preventive Medicine Programs Generally Recommended for Goats, Sheep, and Llamas

Neonatal Period	1 to 3 Months	5 to 6 Months	Annually
Physical examination	Physical examination	Deworm (rotate products)	Physical examination
Vaccinate for clostridial	Deworm (rotate products)	Physical examination	Deworm (rotate products)
diseases, tetanus	Vaccinate for clostridial diseases	Review stall-cleaning schedule	Vaccinate as needed
Review stall-cleaning schedule	Review stall-cleaning schedule	Discuss feeding regimen	Review stall-cleaning schedule
Monitor body condition	Discuss feeding regimen	Monitor body condition	Discuss feeding regimen
	Monitor body condition		Monitor body condition

Livestock can survive extremes in outdoor temperatures if sheltered from precipitation and wind. In a barn or stable, good ventilation is more important than ambient temperature. Smaller animals of any species generally require warmer temperatures, whereas larger animals, with their greater body mass, generally require cooler temperatures.

Light sufficient for humans is adequate for most animals. Excessive light can cause eye problems in albino rats. Too little light makes sanitation difficult. Rodents do well in low-light environments. Breeding stock may require adjustment of the photoperiod (periods of daylight and darkness) to maximize breeding potential. Most rodents are best housed with 14 hours of light and 10 hours of darkness. Stallions have improved breeding behavior with long light cycles. All species do better when there is a definite difference between day and night. Animals should never be kept in direct sunlight without access to shade, as they may become sunburned and overheated. Such environmental stress can also predispose to disease.

Ventilation is extremely important in maintaining good health. Inadequate air exchange in an enclosure increases urine odors, ammonia levels, and numbers of airborne bacteria and viruses. Such conditions irritate the respiratory tract and predispose to respiratory disease. Drafty conditions or excessive ventilation can be dangerous. Excessive cool airflow can cause chilling. In a low-humidity environment, as with air conditioning, high airflow can dehydrate an animal. Small pets caged indoors must be kept away from air conditioning drafts or heater vents. It is usually best to place a cage along an interior wall away from ventilation or heating ducts.

Housing

An important aspect of husbandry is housing, such as in cages, pens, or stalls. It is important to keep in mind the following considerations. Housing should:
- Prevent contamination of the animal with feces or urine
- Provide for the psychosocial comfort of companion animals
- Be appropriate for the species
- Be structurally sound
- Be free of dangerous surfaces
- Be constructed so that the animal cannot escape and vermin are not allowed access
- Be easy for the owner to clean

Housed animals should be dry, clean, and protected from environmental extremes. Walls and roofing should be sufficient to protect animals from the sun, wind, rain, and snow. Rabbits held in outdoor hutches can become sunburned. Horses can develop conjunctivitis from wind-driven dust. Pens and corrals must be free of exposed nails, sharp metal edges, or other dangerous features. Attention should be paid to escape-proofing cages. Rodents can squeeze through 1-inch openings; many other small pets learn to flip the latch on their cage door.

Accommodation must also be made for species-specific behavior. For example, pigs should have access to dirt lots for rooting and mud wallowing. Rodents need sufficient bedding for burrowing. Cats need scratching posts. Chinchillas require dust baths.

A major failure of many animal enclosures is that they do not allow sufficient room for normal movement or even postural changes. Cages, pens, and stalls that are too small increase the risk of disease and may predispose to abnormal behavior, such as pacing or excessive barking. Pets may be kept in close confinement for short periods, such as a dog kept for a few hours in a portable kennel or carrier; however, such enclosures should have sufficient room for normal postural movements and stretching. A useful rule of thumb for holding enclosures is a minimum of 10 times the body size of the animal. This recommendation assumes the animal will be given opportunity to exercise routinely outside of the primary enclosure. Also, housing too many animals in a single primary enclosure of insufficient size can create problems. A high concentration of animals in a primary enclosure, whether hamsters or ponies, dramatically increases the risk of stress, aggression, and disease transmission.

Animals of different species should be housed separately, or, in some cases, at least in separate rooms. Do not house natural predators and prey animals in the same room, such as cats with mice or birds, as this leads to stress and possible attack. Also, there are medical reasons for housing different species separately. A disease considered inconsequential in one species can be deadly in another species. For example, healthy rabbits may carry *Bordetella* and *Pasteurella* bacteria, but these agents can quickly kill guinea pigs.

Enclosures should be cleaned and sanitized frequently, from once per day to once per week. Few pet owners clean cages or pens of their pets too often. For large animals, stalls or stanchion areas should be "mucked" daily and new straw or other bedding should be spread. Barn gutters and pens should be shoveled or cleared of manure with a tractor as needed and periodically hosed down. Small cages can be sanitized by hand or even in a dishwasher. Generally speaking, any good dishwashing detergent will effectively clean holding areas. Additional sanitation can be obtained with a dilute solution of laundry bleach, using 1 part bleach to 20 parts of water. All surfaces should be rinsed thoroughly after cleaning and disinfecting. Wet items should be left to dry completely before returning the animal to the cage.

Nutrition

Animals must have free access to fresh potable water. Water in containers should be changed sufficiently to prevent accumulation of slime, algae, or dirt. Bowls should be kept clean and sanitized in a dishwasher (180° F) at least once per month. Water troughs for livestock should be periodically emptied and sanitized. Automatic watering devices must be kept clean and free of ice. Water containers should be sufficient for the number of animals in an enclosure.

Animals should be fed a wholesome, palatable diet on a regular schedule and in sufficient quantity. Feeding devices must be designed to prevent contamination by wastes. Usually this is accomplished with an appropriately sized feeder, positioned off of the floor, in close proximity to the water source. As with water containers, feeding devices should be sanitized routinely—at least monthly or more often as needed.

Clients should be encouraged to purchase good-quality feedstuffs and refrain from feeding outdated or off-brand diets. In general, commercial diets more than 3 months old should not be fed as a sole food source, because certain nutrients deteriorate with long storage. Clients should be cautioned not to buy feeds that show large amounts of oil uptake by the bag or box. Such products have likely been held for considerable time in a warehouse that was warm enough to cause oil to bleed out of the feed.

The diet fed should be formulated for that species. Cats should not be fed food formulated for dogs. Rat rations are of little value for rabbits, dogs, or cats. Guinea pigs require vitamin C in their diet. Rat or mouse diets can produce disease in guinea pigs. Pig rations, with their high carbohydrate component, can cause bloat in horses. Rabbit rations can cause metabolic disease in sheep. Feeding an improperly formulated diet produces nutritional deficiencies, excesses, or imbalances that can predispose to bacterial infections or metabolic disease. Chapter 7 contains detailed information on nutrition.

Animal Identification

An often overlooked aspect of preventive medicine is animal identification. The method of identification depends on the species. For pets allowed outdoors, an implanted microchip or a tattoo is preferred to a collar with a nametag. Collars may be removed or fall off, and tags may be lost. Permanent identification ensures that a lost pet can be identified for return to its owner.

VACCINATION OR USE OF PREVENTIVE MEDICATION

Certain diseases are readily prevented by vaccination. Domestic animals should be routinely vaccinated against prevalent diseases. Such serious diseases as parvovirus infection and distemper in dogs, panleukopenia and feline leukemia virus infection in cats, and equine encephalomyelitis and tetanus in horses can be prevented by vaccination. In some cases, vaccination is beneficial to humans as well as animals. For example, animals at risk of developing rabies from the bite of rabid animals should receive regular rabies prophylaxis.

Most small mammals kept as pets (rodents and rabbits) are not routinely vaccinated because of the relatively small risk of contracting certain diseases for which vaccines are available for the species. Mice can contract rabies, but pet mice housed in a cage in a home are unlikely to encounter a rabid animal. Vaccination recommendations for some species are changing (Table 15-7). In years past, rabies vaccination was not considered necessary for pet ferrets; with the improved rabies vaccines now available, ferret vaccination is considered appropriate.

The decision whether or not to vaccinate an animal is influenced by the risk of contracting the disease, the effects of the disease, and the benefits and cost of vaccination. Vaccination may not be warranted if the disease is unlikely to develop or causes only mild illness. For example, veterinarians do not routinely vaccinate dogs or cats against tetanus because they are unlikely to contract the disease; however, horses are vaccinated against tetanus because they are more likely to develop it. Vaccination against a very rare disease may not be necessary. However, vaccination is worthwhile if contraction of the disease poses a substantial threat to human and animal health, such as with rabies. Vaccination also benefits the offspring of vaccinated females, through transfer of maternal immunity in the mother's colostrum.

The attitude toward vaccination also varies with circumstances. Kennel and cattery owners, breeding farm managers, and ranchers are very concerned with diseases that could sweep through the animal population, with devastating economic effects. Although tracheobronchitis ("kennel cough") is a fairly mild upper respiratory infection of dogs, it could cause great harm in the form of bad public relations if it infected dogs in a boarding facility. An individual owner of a dog, however, would not be overly concerned with kennel cough in his or her pet.

A growing number of practitioners are concerned about the apparent association between vaccines and a particular type of cancer (sarcoma) at the injection site. The American Association of Feline Practitioners currently recommends using different vaccines at different locations on the body.

Animal vaccines are available in many combinations. For example, Duramune PC (Fort Dodge) is a canine vaccine against parvovirus and coronavirus. Duramune DA2PPv protects against five viruses, including parvovirus, but not coronavirus. Duramune DA2PP-CvK/LCI and Vanguard 5/CV-L (Pfizer) protect against six viruses and

two kinds of bacteria. Currently, 8 Duramune and 13 Vanguard products are available in the United States for vaccination of dogs. A similarly wide variety of vaccine products is also available for cats, horses, cattle, pigs, and other species.

Vaccination

Vaccination of dogs

The following vaccines are available for dogs:

- Rabies
- Distemper
- Parvovirus
- Coronavirus
- Canine adenovirus (CAV-1 or CAV-2)
- *Bordetella bronchiseptica*
- Parainfluenza
- Leptospirosis
- Borreliosis

Puppies are usually immunized with one to three doses in the first few months of life and then annually as adults (see Table 15-1).

Vaccination of cats

The following vaccines are available for cats:

- Rabies
- Panleukopenia (feline distemper)
- Chlamydial pneumonitis
- Feline leukemia virus
- Rhinotracheitis
- Calicivirus
- Feline infectious peritonitis
- Feline immunodeficiency virus
- Ringworm

Most cats begin receiving vaccines as kittens, usually around 6 weeks of age. Kittens require boosters after an original series of vaccines. Adult cats may require annual boosters against each of these diseases (see Table 15-2).

Vaccination of horses

The following vaccines are available for horses:

- Rabies
- Encephalomyelitis (Eastern and Western)
- Tetanus
- Influenza
- Equine Herpesvirus 1 and 4
- Potomac horse fever
- Strangles
- Rotavirus
- Botulism
- Anthrax

Most horses begin receiving vaccines as foals. Horses of unknown vaccination status should receive an initial series of vaccines, which is repeated in 4 weeks for maximal antibody production. Adult horses generally require annual boosters against each of these diseases (see Table 15-3).

Vaccination of cattle

The following vaccines are available for cattle:
- Rabies
- Trichomoniasis
- Brucellosis
- IBR
- BVD
- Parainfluenza-3
- Campylobacteriosis
- Leptospirosis
- Rotavirus
- Coronavirus
- *E. coli*
- Clostridial diseases
- Anthrax
- Anaplasmosis

Most cattle begin receiving vaccines as calves, with booster doses after 6 months of age. Cattle of unknown vaccination status should receive an initial series of vaccines, which is repeated in 4 weeks for maximal antibody production. Adult cattle generally require annual boosters against each of these diseases (see Table 15-4).

Vaccination of pigs

The following vaccines are available for pigs:
- Rabies
- Leptospirosis
- Parvovirus
- TGE
- Rotavirus
- Clostridial diseases
- *E. coli*
- *Bordetella bronchiseptica*
- *Pasteurella*
- *Actinobacillus*
- *Mycoplasma*
- PRRS
- Erysipelas
- Pseudorabies
- *Streptococcus*
- Encephalomyocarditis

Most swine begin receiving vaccines as piglets. Pigs of unknown vaccination status should receive an initial series of vaccines, which is repeated in 4 weeks for maximal antibody production. Adult pigs generally require annual boosters against each of these diseases (see Table 15-5).

Vaccination of goats

The following vaccines are available for goats:
- Rabies
- Clostridial diseases
- Tetanus
- Contagious ecthyma
- Anthrax
- Leptospirosis
- Caseous lymphadenitis
- *E. coli*

Most goats begin receiving vaccines as kids, usually around 4 to 6 weeks of age. Kids require boosters after an original series of vaccines. Adult goats require annual boosters against each of these diseases (see Table 15-6).

Vaccination of sheep

The following vaccines are available for sheep:
- Clostridial diseases
- Tetanus
- Vibriosis
- Footrot
- Bluetongue
- Contagious ecthyma
- *E. coli*
- Caseous lymphadenitis

Most lambs begin receiving vaccines at 4 to 6 weeks of age. Lambs require boosters after an original series of vaccines. Adult sheep need annual boosters against each of these diseases (see Table 15-6).

Vaccination of llamas

The following vaccines are available for llamas:
- Rabies
- Clostridial diseases
- Anthrax
- Brucellosis
- Leptospirosis

Most crias (immature llamas) begin receiving vaccines before 4 weeks of age. Crias require boosters after an original series of vaccines. Adult llamas require annual boosters against each of these diseases (see Table 15-6).

Use of Preventive Medication

Certain diseases can be prevented by regular administration of preventive medication. This is best exemplified by use of ivermectin, milbemycin, or diethylcarbamazine to prevent heartworm infection in dogs, or use of ivermectin, lufenuron, or pyrantel to control internal and external parasites in dogs.

SANITATION

The third aspect of the preventive medicine triad is sanitation. A good preventive medicine program involves the judicious use of selected sanitizing and disinfecting agents. Gross accumulations of dirt and organic matter must be removed by cleaning before application of disinfectants. The ideal sanitizing agent has the following characteristics: broad spectrum of antimicrobial activity; no odor; rapid microbicidal effect; no tissue toxicity; no corrosive action; no inactivation by urine or other organic matter; ability to be used at normal environmental temperatures; reasonably priced; readily obtainable; and easily applied. Because no single disinfectant meets all of these criteria, selection is based on the specific needs of the client's preventive medicine program.

Hypochlorites, such as in laundry bleach, are inexpensive, widely available, and effective, and have a wide spectrum of antimicrobial activity. They are most effective in acidic solutions but less effective in the presence of organic matter or detergent residues. These agents can also damage fabrics and may be corrosive to metal. A solution of 30 ml of standard laundry bleach in 1 L of water (1 oz per quart) is an effective sanitizing agent. However, it degrades quickly and a fresh batch should be made daily.

Quaternary ammonium compounds have very low toxicity to most animals, are convenient to use, and have no apparent taste or offensive odor. They are most effective against gram-positive bacteria but less effective against gram-negative bacteria. They have limited efficacy in the presence of organic matter, detergent residues, or in an acidic environment. These agents are useful for sanitation of feed and water containers. All equipment and surfaces disinfected with quaternary ammonium products should be well rinsed because the residues can cause toxicity.

Phenols are good disinfecting products and effectively kill vegetative forms of both gram-negative and gram-positive bacteria. The exception is *Pseudomonas*, which can be a major contaminant in certain animal environments. (Acidification of drinking water can prevent *Pseudomonas* contamination of water for rodents, the animals most commonly affected.) Phenols are recognized by their pine or cedar smell. Phenols are toxic to some species (e.g., cats) and so should not be used to clean feed or water containers. These agents are good for sanitizing the surfaces of pens and cages. Their strong odor, however, can mask the odor of accumulated urine or feces.

Alcohol, such as ethyl alcohol, is a poor disinfectant. To serve as an effective disinfectant, alcohol must remain in contact with the site for 15 to 20 minutes. Because it evaporates long before this, alcohol is not a good choice for most applications. Alcohol is a good solvent and helps to physically remove microorganisms when accumulated materials are wiped away.

Other agents are also used to disinfect the environment of animals (e.g., lye, formaldehyde gas, 10% ammonia), but these usually require specialized application not readily available to most animal owners. Chapter 9 contains additional information on disinfectants and antiseptics.

A practical way to assess sanitation is to avoid use of highly scented products, such as cedar shavings, pine-scented cleaners, or perfumes, on animals or in their surroundings. Although deodorants make the animal or its enclosure smell good, they also mask odors that can be associated with poor sanitation.

FACTORS PREDISPOSING TO DISEASE

Some factors that predispose to disease can be controlled, but others cannot. Although some factors are beyond our control, we can often establish conditions so that even uncontrollable factors have only minimal impact on our animals. Animals are predisposed to disease by genetic, dietary, environmental, and metabolic factors.

Genetic Factors

Genetic factors are largely beyond our control, although they can be reduced to some extent by selective breeding. These include such things as predispositions by gender, inherited mutations, immunodeficiencies, and the effect of inbreeding. Most male tricolored cats are sterile, whereas tricolored female cats are usually fertile. Inherited malocclusions can interfere with chewing. Immunodeficiencies may be noted by an increased incidence of infections. Inbreeding can lead to physical abnormalities or diminished mental (intellectual) capacities.

Dietary Factors

Dietary factors are generally controllable. Animal owners determine most aspects of an animal's diet, such as feed type, quality, amount, and regimen. A high-quality balanced ration is of little value if the feeder is inaccessible. This is occasionally seen with young bunnies, which are too short to reach the feeder. Limited feeding can prevent obesity but can lead to malnutrition if not applied properly. A diet formulated for one type or age of animals may not be healthful for another group of the same species. For example, hard pellets may not be chewable by aged animals. The diet must change as the needs of the animal change.

Environmental Factors

Environmental factors also require consideration in the preventive health plan. Climatic extremes or sudden climatic changes can clearly cause distress or even death. Although we cannot change the weather, we can adjust the animal's housing to reduce environmental stress. Additional bedding improves the insulation around animals housed in extremely cold conditions. Overhead cover is needed to prevent sunburn and heat prostration and shield animals from precipitation.

Inadequate ventilation increases the incidence of respiratory diseases through increased ammonia levels and large numbers of microorganisms in the air. Inadequate ventilation also impairs cooling in animals that use respiration to regulate body temperature (e.g., dogs) and prevents radiation of body heat (e.g., heat loss from the ears of rab-hits). Inadequate ventilation inhibits the drying of bedding, favoring proliferation of bacteria or parasites. At the other end of the spectrum, excessive ventilation is also stressful. Drafts or excessive ventilation can cause chilling, dehydration, or inflamed ocular tissues.

The level of ventilation should be appropriate for the animal, rather than for the animal owner. We must take the time to experience the same conditions that the animal is experiencing. We must evaluate airflow not at the 5-foot level, but at the 5-inch level. A draft along the floor could lead to respiratory disease in a small mammal but may not be evident to the animal owner. A 2 hour period of sunshine directly on a hamster each day could dehydrate the pet, while the owner remains unaware of it. Inadvertent spraying of perfume or other aerosols near a fish tank could kill the fish. If the air in a poorly ventilated barn or stable causes discomfort in farm personnel, such as burning eyes or a sore throat, it is also causing discomfort in the animals.

Metabolic Factors

Metabolic factors also must be considered in preventive health programs. Factors beyond our control include the age of the animal and reproductive status; concurrent disease; and nonspecific stressors. Young, old, pregnant, and lactating animals have different physiologic needs than other animals. These needs may require alteration of the animal's diet and housing.

A common metabolic problem that influences the health of many companion animals, and that can be effectively managed by the animal owner, is obesity from overfeeding and lack of exercise. We often focus on the animal's age group and manage health problems as they relate to age; however, a more effective preventive approach is to address factors under the client's control. Veterinary professionals should discuss proper nutrition and exercise programs with clients so that their animals can benefit from that knowledge.

Wellness Programs

There is no doubt that preventative medicine—specifically the use of vaccines—has been responsible for saving the lives of countless animals during the past few decades. For years the veterinary community has relied on the annual booster vaccination as a means of encouraging yearly visits to the veterinarian. Due to recent controversies surrounding the use of vaccines and client knowledge of these issues, the veterinary community is trying to shift emphasis from yearly booster vaccines to health and wellness examinations.

Because companion animals mature at approximately seven times the rate of humans, annual wellness examinations are essential to ensure their health and to diagnose developing diseases in their early stages (Tables 15-8 and 15-9).

Implementing a wellness program

Creating a wellness program for patients should begin with client education. Veterinary technicians should look for ways to maximize opportunities to educate clients on wellness. Written materials with specific wellness goals can be reviewed with each client. Use an age equivalence chart to help clients understand that a year in the life of a dog or cat can be as much as 20% of its life expectancy! Many clinics have special testing programs for senior pets. However, even healthy young adult pets should be evaluated for early detection and prevention of disease. Once the client agrees to the wellness examination, be sure to provide a written "report card" of the examination, and take time to explain recommendations to the client.

What to include

Wellness programs vary at different veterinary facilities and at different ages and life stages of pets. In general, a complete physical examination should be performed annually. Blood test results, antibody titers, parasite testing, urinalysis, nutritional assessment, behavioral evaluations, and assessment of the pet's home environment may be included. Patients that are considered geriatric (usually older than 7 years) may also need electrocardiographic, radiographic, and other tests for common problems of senior pets.

The in-house laboratory

Although the wellness test profiles can be sent to outside laboratories, providing these services in-house improves service by sparing the client the several hours-to-overnight wait for test results. In addition, the treatment benefit of rapid test turnaround time is one of the goals of a successful wellness program. In-house laboratory testing is also a source of additional revenue for the clinic. Many of the basic supplies needed for in-house testing already are present in most veterinary clinics. Clinics that do not currently perform in-house laboratory services may have additional equipment and supply needs. Box 15-1 (see table2.doc) lists some commonly used supplies for in-house laboratory testing.

During the past two decades, in-house laboratory equipment has become increasingly user-friendly and cost-effective. Laboratory equipment for in-house wellness testing requires a blood chemistry analyzer, hematology analyzer, and supplies for urinalysis and coagulation profiles. Table 15-10 provides an overview of some of the common in-house analyzers marketed to veterinary facilities. Some of these analyzers are also capable of performing electrolyte testing, although most patients will not require those tests. Most of these analyzers are similar in their degree of accuracy. The veterinary staff should determine cost per test based on anticipated test volume. Additional costs include supplies and technician time to prepare and run samples, as

TABLE 15-7

Recommended Guidelines for Vaccination of Cats

Antigen	Vaccine Type	Recommendation for Initial Vaccination Series			Comments
		<12 Weeks Old When First Examined	≥12 Weeks Old When First Examined	Booster Vaccination Interval	
Feline parvovirus[†]	MLV vaccine	Vaccinate at initial visit and every 3 to 4 weeks until ≥12 weeks old	Vaccinate at initial visit (only 1 dose is needed)	1 year after initial vaccination series, then at 3-year intervals	Highly recommended for all cats; vaccine is not for use in pregnant queens or kittens that are 4 weeks old or immunocompromised
	Killed-virus vaccine	Vaccinate at initial visit and every 3 to 4 weeks until ≥12 weeks old	Vaccinate at initial visit and again 3 to 4 weeks later	1 year after initial vaccination series, then at 3-year intervals	Highly recommended for all cats
Feline herpesvirus –1[§] and feline calicivirus	MLV vaccine	Vaccinate at initial visit and every 3 to 4 weeks until ≥12 weeks old	Vaccinate at initial visit (only 1 dose is needed)	1 year after initial vaccination series, then at 3-year intervals[||]	Highly recommended for all cats
	Killed-virus vaccine	Vaccinate at initial visit and every 3 to 4 weeks until ≥12 weeks old	Vaccinate at initial visit and again 3 to 4 weeks later	1 year after initial vaccination series, then at 3-year intervals[||]	Highly recommended for all cats
Rabies virus	Killed-virus vaccine	Not eligible for vaccination	Vaccinate at initial visit (only 1 dose is needed)	1 year after initial vaccination series, then at 3-year intervals[¶]	Highly recommended for all cats
Chlamydia psittaci	Avirulent live vaccine	Vaccinate at initial visit (only 1 dose is needed)	Vaccinate at initial visit (only 1 dose is needed)	1 year after initial vaccination series, then at 3-year intervals	Recommended for cats at high risk of exposure
	Killed vaccine	Vaccinate at initial visit and again 3 to 4 weeks later	Vaccinate at initial visit and again 3 to 4 weeks later	1 year after initial vaccination series, then at 3-year intervals	Recommended for cats at high risk of exposure
Feline infectious peritonitis virus	MLV vaccine	Not recommended[‡]	Vaccinate at initial visit and again 3 to 4 weeks later (first dose should not be given before 16 weeks of age)	1 year after initial vaccination series, then at 3-year intervals	Can be considered for cats at risk of exposure to cats known or suspected to have been exposed to feline coronavirus
FeLV	Killed-virus vaccine	Vaccinate at initial visit and again 3 to 4 weeks later (first dose should be given at ≥8 weeks of age, second dose at ≥12 weeks of age)	Vaccinate at initial visit and again 3 to 4 weeks later	1 year after initial vaccination series, then annually	Recommended for use in cats at high risk of exposure[#]
Microsporum canis**	Killed vaccine	Not recommended	Prevention: vaccinate at initial visit, second dose 2 weeks later, third dose 3 weeks after second dose Treatment: third dose is at veterinarian's discretion	Guidelines not available	Not recommended for routine use; insufficient data to evaluate efficacy in prevention or treatment of disease

From Thomas E, et al: *AAFP/AFM vaccination guidelines.* JAVMA 212:227-241, 1998. *MLV,* Modified-live virus.

*American Association of Feline Practitioners and Academy of Feline Medicine's Advisory Panel on Feline Vaccines recommended guideline for vaccination of cats.

[†]Cause of feline panleukopenia.

[‡]Vaccination of kittens between 4 and 6 weeks old that are in environments where they are at high risk of exposure (e.g., catteries and shelters) and orphan kittens may be indicated.

[§]Cause of feline viral rhinotracheitis.

Booster vaccination interval may be decreased depending on risk of exposure. Cats at high risk of exposure, such as those entering boarding facilities, may benefit from more frequent vaccination.

[||]Duration of immunity beyond 1 year has been evaluated by determining antibody titers, not results of challenge.

[¶]Vaccination interval must comply with local statutes.

[#]Outdoor cats, indoor-outdoor cats, stray cats, feral cats, cats in open, multiple-cat households, cats in FeLV-positive households, and cats in households with unknown FeLV status.

**Cause of dermatophytosis (ringworm).

TABLE 15-8

Age Equivalents for Dogs

Comparative Age in Human Years			
Dog's Age	0-20 lbs	21-50 lbs	51-90 lbs	>90 lbs
5 years	36	37	40	42
6 years	40	42	45	49
7 years	44	47	50	56
10 years	56	60	66	78
12 years	64	69	77	93
15 years	76	83	93	115
20 years	96	105	120	

Adapted from *senior@seven* wellness exam brochures. Antech Diagnostics.

TABLE 15-9

Age Equivalents for Cats

Cat's Age	Comparative Age in Human Years
1	15
2	24
5	36
7	45
12	64
15	76
18	88
21	100

Adapted from *senior@seven* wellness exam brochures. Antech Diagnostics.

BOX 15-1

In-House Laboratory Supplies*

General Supplies

Binocular microscopes
Glass slides and coverslips
Lens tissue
Immersion oil
Lab Timer and stopwatch
Disposable pipettes
Test tube rack
Refractometer
OSHA supplies
  labels, manuals
  personal protective equipment
Blood collection supplies

Hematology Supplies

Microhematocrit centrifuge
Microhematocrit tubes and sealant
Microhematocrit card reader
Differential stain
New Methylene Blue stain
Multi-place tally counter
Staining jars
Hematology analyzer supplies
  sample cups/dilution vials
  dilution fluids
  quality control material
  hemoglobin lysing reagent

Clinical Chemistry Supplies

Chemistry analyzer and supplies
Clinical centrifuge and centrifuge tubes
Sample/dilution cups
Quality control material

Urinalysis Supplies

Urine collection containers
Conical centrifuge tubes
Variable speed clinical centrifuge
E.R.D. Screen Test kit
Quality control material

Coagulation Testing Supplies

Unopette (white blood cell count/platelet)
Hemacytometer and coverglass
Hand tally counter
Bleeding time lancets
Blotting paper
Automated coagulation analyzer and supplies or ACT tubes and
  heat block

Parasitology and Immunodiagnostic supplies

Fecal sample collection supplies
Fecal flotation solution
Heartworm antigen test kits
Antibody test kits

*This list is not meant to be an all-inclusive presentation of supplies needed. The most commonly used equipment and supplies needed for an in-house laboratory performing wellness exams is included.

TABLE 15-10

In-House Analyzers

	In-House Chemistry Analyzers	
	Characteristics	*Manufacturer*
Analyst	Rotor technology	Hemagen Diagnostics
	Profiles or miniprofiles	www.hemagen.com
	Semiautomated dilution	
Irma	Cartridge technology	Diametrics Medical, Inc.
	Portable	www.diametrics.com
	Miniprofiles	
	Limited chemistry menu	
	Includes electrolytes	
VetTest	Slide technology	Idexx Laboratories
	Single tests or profiles	www.idexx.com
Hematology Analyzers		
COULTER A^cT	Impedance counter	Beckman Coulter
	Includes WBC histogram	www.beckmancoulter.com
	Automated quality control	
QBC	Buffy coat technology	Idexx Laboratories
	Estimated cell counts	www.idexx.com
	Partial differential	
Lasercyte	Laser flow cytometry	Idexx Laboratories
	Cell counts	www.idexx.com
	Differential white blood cell count	
	Reticulocyte counts	
Miscellaneous Equipment		
SCA-2000	Performs ACT, APTT, and PT tests	Synbiotics Corp.
	Automated, portable	www.synbiotics.com
Easy Vet	Electrolyte	Medica Corp.
		www.medicacorp.com

well as time required for routine maintenance, calibration, and quality control.

Physical examination

A complete systems examination should be performed on all pets. The pet's weight and overall nutritional status should be evaluated. A complete behavioral history and assessment of the environment in which the pet lives should also be performed. These data will help to determine whether the patient is at any risk of exposure to specific diseases. There are several approaches to performing the physical examination. Box 15-2 (see table4.doc) provides a systematic method of physical examination. Remember that "normal" can vary among species and even among individuals at different times. Appropriate words to use for finding no abnormalities are "characteristic" or "adequate." Each of the systems has a minimum number of parameters that you can and should be evaluating.

Every attempt should be made to show the client the thoroughness and importance of the physical examination. The client should see the veterinarian and/or veterinary technician use the tools that they'd expect to see in their own physician's office (e.g., stethoscope, otoscope, ophthalmoscope). This adds value to the client's perception of the physical examination.

Blood tests

Depending on the age and life stage of the patient, a complete blood count (CBC) and chemistry panel should be performed. These tests can detect literally hundreds of internal diseases, such as diabetes, liver diseases, and kidney diseases. The CBC includes tests that can identify the presence of anemia and can aid in evaluating the pet's nutritional status. The CBC includes red and white blood cell counts, hemoglobin concentration, packed cell volume, and differential blood film examination. All adult

BOX 15-2

Systematic Method of Physical Examination

- Record TPR
- Evaluate and record animal's general condition [(i.e., disposition, activity level, overall body condition, etc.)
- Evaluate and record condition of each body system:
  - Integument: note overall condition of hair coat, presence or absence of alopecia, parasites, lumps, wounds, rashes, etc, note hydration status with skin turgor test.
  - Respiratory: evaluate respiratory rate and rhythm; record presence or absence of rales, ronchi, crepitus, dyspnea, nasal discharge, etc.
  - Cardiovascular: evaluate cardiac rate and rhythm; CRT, presence or absence of pulse: deficit, etc.
  - Gastrointestinal: Record presence/absence of diarrhea, vomiting (note character, if present). Palpate abdomen and record presence or absence of tenderness, impaction, etc.
  - Genitourinary: Palpate kidneys, bladder. Note presence of characteristic urine volume; note any blood, etc., in urine. [In male, check for presence/absence of testicles in scrotum;

penile discharge. In female, record evidence of pregnancy, lactation, vaginal discharge (note character, if present).
  - Musculoskeletal: evaluate presence/absence of swelling (particularly in joints); manipulate limbs; record any abnormal gait, limping, guarding, tenderness; note overall musculature.
  - Nervous: Record presence/absence of head tilt, tremors, etc. Evaluate pupillary light reflexes. Evaluate and record triceps, patellar, and gastrocnemius reflexes.
  - Eyes: evaluate and record, presence/absence of abrasions, ulcers, discharge (note character, if present).
  - Ears: evaluate and record presence/absence of tenderness, parasites, odor, ulcers, discharge (note character, if present).
  - Mucosa: note color of mucous membranes, evaluate odor of mouth, evaluate periodontal tissues.
  - Lymphatic: palpate peripheral lymph nodes, evaluate characteristic size/location of lymph nodes.

patients younger than 7 years should have at least one baseline CBC chemistry panel. It is common for patients to have one or more laboratory values that are outside of accepted "normal" ranges. Normal values are a guideline only. It may be that a particular patient normally has a value that is somewhat beyond the normal range. This may be perfectly acceptable for that patient. If a patient becomes ill and the veterinarian has no baseline data, it is difficult to determine whether an abnormal result is due to the illness or is an idiosyncrasy of the patient. Other tests may be included because of the pet's potential risk. For example, patients that are obese may need thyroid evaluations. Antibody titers for common diseases may also be needed. Many veterinarians are now recommending this as an alternative to routine annual vaccination. Annual vaccinations are a source of much controversy because of the risks that may be associated with vaccine use. Reactions to vaccine administration ranging from localized swelling to anaphylaxis and sarcoma have been reported. Optimal vaccination intervals have not been established for most vaccines, and it seems likely that the vaccinations currently in use provide long-term immunity. However, some patients that are at risk for contracting common diseases may still need vaccination. In particular, pets that are exposed to other dogs or cats on a routine basis or are ill with some other disease (e.g., feline leukemia virus [FELV]) may still need routine vaccinations. An antibody titer can help to determine whether a patient is likely to need booster vaccinations. Pets that are older than 7 years and those with chronic ill-

nesses such as Cushing's disease and diabetes should have more detailed wellness examinations

Coagulation profile

Veterinary patients can be affected by a number of genetic and acquired diseases of the coagulation mechanisms. There are several simple and inexpensive evaluations that can identify these defects. All patients should have a coagulation profile before any surgery to identify any potential bleeding problems. Patients with chronic disease, especially those with poor nutrition, should also be evaluated. Some coagulation abnormalities may be subclinical—that is, the patient does not always have visible signs or symptoms of disease. When these patients have surgery or are involved in traumatic events, bleeding problems become evident and are much more difficult to manage. A platelet count, bleeding time, and activated clotting time test should be performed at least once on all adult patients. Other coagulation tests that may be included in wellness examinations include prothrombin time and activated partial thromboplastin time. Both of these tests require special instrumentation but can be performed easily in-house.

Parasite examinations

Wellness examinations should include a fecal direct smear, fecal flotation, and serum tests for heartworm antigen. The differential blood film can be used to detect other parasites such as *Ehrlichia*, *Haemobartonella*, and *Babesia*. The fecal direct smear is useful for detecting protozoal parasites such as *Giardia*. Fecal flotation can detect the presence of common parasites such as *Toxocara canis, Trichuris vulpis*, and *Ancylostoma caninum*.

Urinalysis

Evaluation of the overall health and function of the urinary system is arguably one of the most valuable sets of tests that can be performed. The kidneys perform many functions in maintaining the health of the patient. Changes in urine chemistry and the presence of certain types of cells and crystals in the urine can provide a great deal of information on the patient's overall health status. Renal disease is a leading cause of mortality in small animals. Early detection can halt or slow progression of a disease. In addition to the CBC and chemistry panel, senior pets should also be tested for microalbuminuria to detect early changes in kidney function. The presence of any protein in urine indicates alteration in glomerular filtration. The microalbuminuria (E.R.D. Screen,© Heska) test acts to detect the protein, albumin in the urine. Since the test is more sensitive to urine protein, it provides for detection of changes in the glomerulus before a reduction in kidney function occurs.

Radiography and electrocardiography

Although not required for every pet, chest radiographs and an electrocardiograph should be performed on all senior pets. Heart disease is extremely common in these patients. Patients that have had prior treatment for heartworm infection and those with chronic illnesses or chronic coughing should also be screened for cardiac health. Early detection of cardiac disease can greatly improve patient prognosis. Many cardiac and respiratory diseases can be successfully treated in their early stages. However, in late-stage disease, tissue damage is often too great for treatment to be effective.

Miscellaneous tests

Keratoconjunctivitis sicca is the most common cause of blindness in dogs. The Schirmer tear test can identify the presence of this condition. Certain dog breeds, such as cocker spaniels, Lhasa apsos, and Shih Tzus, are especially prone to this condition. Glaucoma is the second-most common cause of blindness in dogs and cats. Glaucoma screening can be accomplished with a tonometer or by ocular ultrasound.

RECOMMENDED READING

Birchard SJ, Sherding RG: *Saunders manual of small animal practice*, ed 2, Philadelphia, 2000, WB Saunders.

Bonagura JD: *Kirk's current veterinary therapy XII, small animal practice*, Philadelphia, 1995, WB Saunders.

Harkness JE, Wagner JE: *The biology and medicine of rabbits and rodents*, ed 4, Baltimore, 1995, Williams & Wilkins.

Smith B: *Large animal internal medicine*, ed 3, St Louis, 2002, Mosby.

Veterinary pharmaceuticals and biologicals, ed 10, Lenexa, Kan, 1997, Veterinary Medicine Publishing.

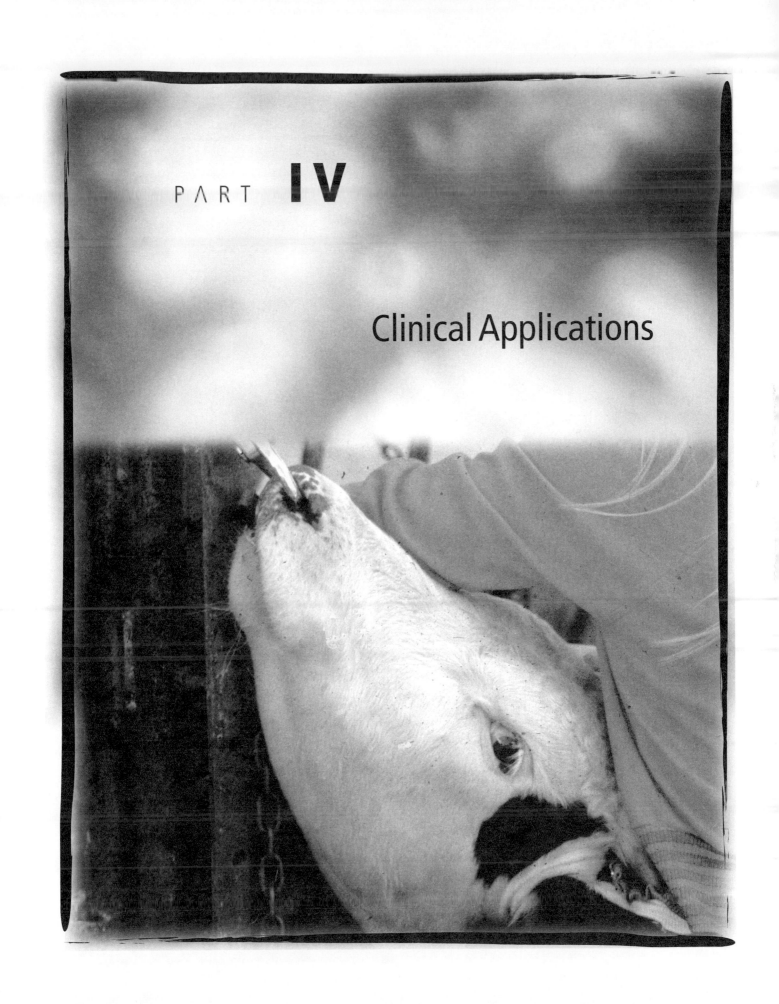

PART **IV**

Clinical Applications

16

Physical Restraint

Teresa Sonsthagen

Learning Objectives

After reviewing this chapter, the reader should understand the following:

- Psychological principles underlying physical restraint techniques
- Safety precautions taken before and during physical restraint
- Methods used to restrain dogs, cats, small mammals, birds, horses, cattle, goats, sheep and pigs
- Typical behavior responses of animals to physical restraint
- Correct use of mechanical devices for physical restraint

RESTRAINT AND HANDLING OF DOGS

Canine Behavior

Dogs exhibit a number of personalities that are important to note before attempting to restrain them. The majority of dogs are happy to be with people and enjoy interacting with others. These dogs rarely bite but can retaliate if they are pushed too hard or are cornered. The second most common personality is the nervous or fearful dog. They exhibit a fearful expression by having ears drawn down and back, showing white around the pupils of their eyes, and cowering away from others. If these dogs are cornered or feel threatened, they often bite. The third personality type is the aggressive dog. Aggressive dog body language is head lowered between the shoulders, a level stare, tail straight out, and they may or may not grimace or growl. These dogs will take offense at improper body language such as a direct look into their eyes and a frontal approach. Aggressive dogs and nervous/fearful dogs should be handled with the thought that they will bite, and appropriate steps such as muzzles and sedation should be considered before working with these dogs. Regardless of the personality, never expose your face to an unfamiliar dog, do approach with your body turned slightly, and avoid a direct stare into their eyes. An extended hand should have the fingers curled in with the palm up.

Danger Potential

A dog's main means of defense is to run and if cornered will fight. This is called the "flight or fight" response, and all animals exhibit this behavior. They are equipped with formidable teeth that are designed to crush and tear. Regardless of personality, if a dog is curling its lips, showing its teeth, growling, or raising its hackles, it is imperative to control its muzzle to avoid being bitten.

A lesser weapon is a dog's toenails. They rarely cause severe injuries but can inflict painful scratches that can become infected.

Mechanical Devices

Leash

The rope leash is a standard tool used for restraining dogs. It can be made of a rolled or flat nylon rope with a handle at one end and a slip ring to form a sliding loop at the other. The loop is easy to keep open and can be flipped over the head and/or body of a dog to bring it out of a cage or run. It is easy to remove by allowing the loop to loosen and the dog to slip its head out. It fits easily into a pocket and can be used on cats just as effectively as dogs.

Gauntlet

These commercially made leather gloves include a band of leather that extends to protect the forearm as well as the hands. Even though they are made of thick leather, most dogs, cats, and birds can pinch or actually bite through the leather. However, it slows them down enough that you can usually escape the worst of it. The best way to use them is to place one partially on your nondominant hand and wave it in front of the animal as a distraction. The animal will usually bite onto the empty fingers while you reach in and scruff or leash it with the other hand. If you do restrain an animal with the gloves on, be careful not to exert too much pressure because the gloves reduce your tactile feeling. Usually once the animal is out of the kennel, it is placed on a table. Then either another person can get a good hold on the animal, or you can wrap your hand and arm around the dog's neck or head, get rid of the gloves, and restrain the animal with your bare hands. If this is not possible because the animal is too aggressive, then keep the gloves on and monitor that the animal isn't turning blue from the pressure you are exerting!

Muzzle

Many commercially manufactured muzzles are available and should be fitted to the dog by the owner. Before coming to the clinic, the client should muzzle an aggressive or nervous dog. A muzzle can also be made with a length of roll gauze, a nylon sock or a length of rope. Using a 4-foot-long piece of gauze, make a loop by tying an overhand knot that is not tightened down. Have the dog either restrained by the scruff of the neck or by a capture pole. Stand slightly to the left or right of the dog's head, just out of its reach, and slide the loop around the dog's muzzle. Quickly tighten the muzzle over the nose by pulling on the ends of the knot, and then tie another overhand knot under the dog's chin (Fig. 16-1). Move in closer, and pass ends behind the ears using a

bowknot. Keep scissors close by in case the muzzle must be quickly cut off. To remove the muzzle, untie the bowknot and gently pull the ends back and forth and forward. Often the dog will help with a paw. Be careful that the dog doesn't bite as the muzzle is removed; have people cleared out or have the head restrained carefully. Also note that this muzzle is only used for short-term procedures, because the dog cannot pant and will overheat if the muzzle is left on for extended periods.

Catchpole

Many types of catchpoles are available commercially. A catchpole is used to move an aggressive or fearful dog to or from a run or cage. The rigid pole separates the restrainer and dog, and a quick-release handle is used to prevent strangulation. The loop at the end of the pole is placed around the dog's neck and tightened. This allows the restrainer to move the dog in and out of a run or cage (Fig. 16-2). Care should be taken not to choke the dog, but the loop has to be tight enough so that its head doesn't slip out. Often another person can approach the rear of the dog and administer a sedative or vaccination without fear of being bitten.

Voice

Dogs and horses especially respond to voice commands and tones. It can be a very useful tool to comfort and soothe or to direct an animal to obey. When using it to direct an animal, make the tone of your voice deep and commanding. Avoid the uplift inflection of a question. For example a sit command is given as a command not a question! Almost all animals will respond to a soothing croon or "shushing" noise as a distraction. So don't be afraid of sounding silly when comforting an animal!

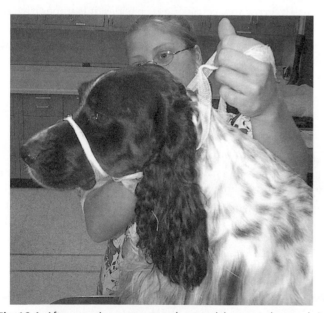

Fig. 16-1 After wrapping a gauze muzzle around the snout, the muzzle is tied behind the head.

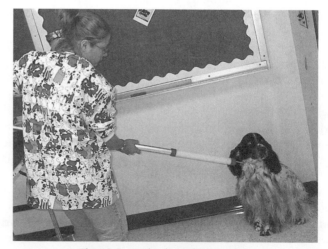

Fig. 16-2 Catchpole applied to a dog.

Restraint Techniques

Removing dogs from cages or runs

Make certain that all escape routes are closed, because many dogs bolt out of a cage or run if given the opportunity. To prevent this, the handler should block the run door with a knee or forearm in the cage door opening.

Nonaggressive nonfearful dogs. Small dogs can usually be grasped gently by the scruff or under the chin and then lifted out of the cage with one hand around and under the dog's thorax. Snug its body close to yours, or place a leash around its neck and place the dog on the floor. Medium-sized to large dogs are usually led out with a leash if in a floor-level cage. Never pull a dog out of a cage allowing it to "jump" to the floor. Most are not ready for the jump, and the height of the cage can cause injury to legs and joints as well as to the neck if it is jerked.

Fearful and aggressive dogs. It takes practice and sensibility to remove fearful or aggressive dogs safely from cages or runs. Ideally, dogs that are likely to bite should be muzzled, sedated, or both before they are placed in a cage or run. If this is not possible, proceed with caution. Do not corner the dog by stepping into the run or leaning into a cage. Calmly encourage the dog verbally with praise, and flip a leash over the dog's head if possible, then walk it out of the run or floor-level cage. If it is a small dog, capture it with a leash as previously described. Once captured, pull it to the edge of the cage, retaining a steady pressure on the neck with the leash, reach in with a gloved hand and grasp a hindquarter, quickly lowering it to the ground. Do not pull the dog out and let it drop to the floor. You can cause severe injury to the legs, joints, back, and neck. It is a good idea to wear gauntlets when attempting this technique.

An alternative with a dog in a run or floor-level cage is to narrowly open the door, stepping behind the door allowing the dog to exit the run. As the dog's head comes through the doorway, quickly flip a leash over its head and move out with it. Most dogs actually calm down once they are "out of its territory" and will come along willingly. Remain on guard, as these animals can turn nasty without much notice.

If a dog is attacking the leash or the front of the kennel, the use of a capture pole is warranted, regardless of whether the dog is small, medium, or large.

Lifting a dog

Small dogs are held draped over a forearm with the other hand holding onto the head just below the mandible. Medium-sized dogs are held around the neck with one arm and around the rear end with the other. Carry both sizes close to your body until it can be placed in a kennel or on an exam table. Large dogs should be lifted by two people, one with an arm around the neck and thorax, the other with an arm around the abdomen and around the rear quarters. A count or signal should be given to lift in concert. Most large dogs get quite nervous on a table; procedures should be done on the floor if possible. If this is not possible, be sure you have enough people to hold the dog securely on the table.

Standing restraint

This technique is used for such procedures as physical exams, anal sac expression, rectal temperature, and obtaining vaginal smears. Place one arm around the dog's neck or muzzle and the other around the abdomen, and hug it close to your body (Fig. 16-3). If the dog is very large, you may have to have another person help as described for lifting a large dog. A gentle hold and some soothing words are often all that is necessary to keep the dog still. Be ready to strengthen your grip if the dog starts to struggle or tries to bite.

Crowding

This technique may be used with very large dogs. Place the dog in a sitting position close to a corner of the room. Gently slide the dog's rear into the corner so it cannot back away. Then straddle the dog and restrain the head with both hands, gripping the mandibles, or kneel to the side and wrap an arm around the neck and steady the front legs with the other hand. Do not make it appear that you are cornering the dog; otherwise it may become frightened and retaliate.

Sitting or sternal recumbency

This technique is usually used on the examination table, and sometimes on the floor with large dogs. This technique is useful for blood collection from the cephalic or jugular vein, intravenous injection, nail trimming, oral and ophthalmic exam or medication, and some radiographs.

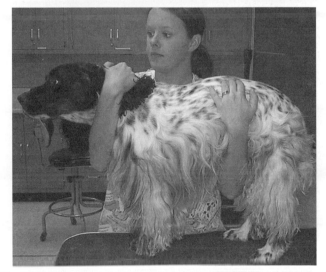

Fig. 16-3 Holding a dog in standing position. One arm is placed in front of the chest, and the other supports the abdomen to prevent sitting.

For restraint in the sitting position, ask or place the dog in a sitting position. Then place one arm around the dog's neck or hold onto the muzzle and put the other arm around the rear of the dog. This will prevent it from biting and from backing away. Pull the dog close to your body to provide added security. If you need to abduct one of the dog's forelegs for venipuncture, move the arm that normally holds onto the rear across the shoulders and grasp the leg opposite from your body (Fig. 16-4). Hold the leg by placing the elbow into the palm of that hand and push the leg forward. To occlude the vein, place your thumb on top of the leg, squeeze, and rotate laterally. This occludes the vein and rolls it dorsally for easier access.

One difficulty with this hold is keeping the dog from scratching you with its front paws. So instead of holding on to the rear, move your arm into the same position as you would for a venipuncture procedure, except you will grasp both legs, with a finger in between the legs, just above the carpals. Lean your body onto the dog's body to keep it from backing up. This will keep the dog from scratching you or the person doing the procedure.

For restraint in sternal recumbency, say "down" or gently pull the front legs out until the dog rests on its sternum. Then hold the neck or muzzle as described above, and use your free hand to either steady the rear or hold the foreleg out for venipuncture. Also, lean some of your body weight

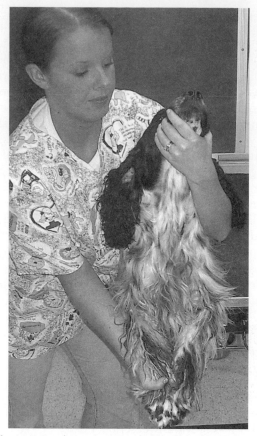

Fig. 16-5 Jugular venipuncture hold in sternal recumbency.

on top of the dog to keep it in the down position. This technique can also be used for jugular venipuncture. One hand reaches over the shoulders under the chin and wraps around the muzzle, raising the head to expose the neck. The other hand grasps both front legs and stretches them over the edge of the table (Fig. 16-5). If you put a finger between the legs and grasp around the carpal area, it will allow you to hold on better. Again, lean your body on top of the dog. This is a very uncomfortable position for you and the dog. Do not apply this hold until the phlebotomist is ready to go!

Lateral recumbency

This technique is usually used on the examination table but also can be used on the floor. It is useful for urinary catheterization, radiographs, suture removal, ECGs, access to the lateral saphenous vein, and other short procedures. Place the dog on its left or right side. Hold the legs touching the table (left legs in left recumbency, right legs in right recumbency), lifting them slightly. Put one wrist or arm across the dog's neck and the other across the flank. This prevents the dog from getting up (Fig. 16-6). If you need one hand free, the only hand available is the hand holding the rear legs. Keeping hold of both front legs, lift so that the dog's weight is shifted onto its shoulder, then you can

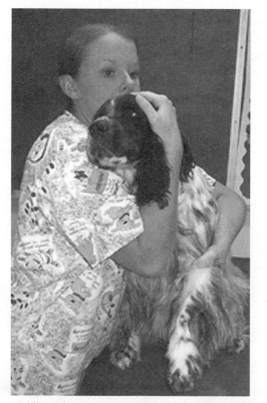

Fig. 16-4 Holding a dog in sitting position with the front leg extended for a cephalic venipuncture.

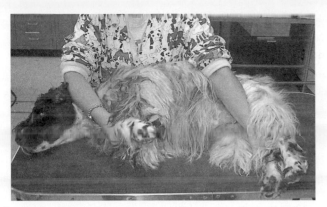

Fig. 16-6 Holding a dog in lateral recumbency. One arm is placed across the dog's neck, and the other is placed across the dog's abdomen. The feet closer to the table are held to prevent rising.

release the rear legs. Maintain pressure on the dog's neck with your forearm. A dog cannot get up without first putting its front legs out in front of it, so if you keep it off-balance by lifting on the front legs, you can free your other hand to assist in the procedure.

Dorsal recumbency

This technique is used for procedures such as radiography, cystocentesis, and blood collection from the jugular vein. It sometimes requires two persons, depending on how squirmy the dog is and how wide! Place the dog in lateral recumbency, then roll it onto its back. If it is a very deep-chested dog, a V-trough or foam wedges may be necessary to keep the dog from rolling. The forepaws are stretched cranially, and back paws are stretched caudally, exposing the thorax and abdomen.

Snubbing

This method can be used to administer an IM injection if you are alone, and it can be used to prevent an aggressive dog from getting too close to the restrainer. In one variation, one end of the leash is run through an eyebolt anchored in a wall. The leash is then pulled, snugly forcing the dog's head up to the eyebolt and tied with a quick-release knot. In another variation, one end of the leash is run through the crack of a door near the hinges or the bars on a low cage. The leash is then pulled so the restrainer is on one side of the door and the dog on the other, again tying with a quick-release knot. This allows another technician to vaccinate or give an injection to the dog.

RESTRAINT AND HANDLING OF CATS

Feline Behavior

There are two things you need to keep in mind before restraining a cat. It establishes its territory very quickly, and

the *minimum* amount of restraint is vital to a successful procedure. If the cat begins to struggle and vigorously resist physical restraint, release it and consider use of chemical restraint after it has calmed. Rough handling, extreme physical restraint, and a hot temper are counterproductive and have no place in restraint of cats. Also keep in mind that it is usually a good idea to make friends before placing a cat in any restraint hold. Relax the cat by petting it, speaking to it gently, and finding its favorite "itchy" spot.

Danger Potential

Cats will also try to get away from a scary or painful procedure; most of the time a cat will try to scare you off by batting at you with its front feet and/or hissing. If you are "foolish" enough to keep coming, then they will resort to bringing out some formidable weapons. Their canines are sharp but small in diameter, and if bitten, the result is a deep puncture wound that often becomes infected. They can also defend themselves with very sharp claws. Hanging onto a cat is very difficult, because they are agile and strong enough to bring into use all four feet and their teeth in defense. Remember, the idea is to not push a cat into fighting "for its life."

Mechanical Devices

Towel and blanket

A large beach towel or small blanket is one of the best tools to keep around to assist in restraining a cat. Either can be used to wrap the cat's body snugly, thus controlling the feet and body. There are two techniques that can be used to wrap a cat. The first is easy to explain if you think of a taco. Drape a towel over the cat so the middle of the towel is directly over the cat's back. Then quickly sweep the sides of the towel together and lay the cat on its side. Continue to wrap the two ends of the towel completely and snugly around the cat. This completely encircles the legs but allows access to the head and rear. The other technique is similar but is wrapped more like a burrito. The towel is placed flat on the table, and the cat is placed at about one third of the way from one end of the towel. Taking the short end or the end closest to the cat, wrap it very snugly around its body. Once that is in place, quickly fold one side over the cat's rear, and wrap the long end around and around its body. This covers everything but the head (Fig. 16-7). Both methods are useful if you have to give an oral or ophthalmic medication by yourself, or can be used for a jugular or cephalic venipuncture. Most cats submit to procedures when wrapped up, and so it is less traumatic for the cat.

Cat restraint bags

Cat restraint bags or cat bags work similar to towels and blankets. They are made of canvas or heavy nylon and have zippered or Velcro closures, with holes in various areas for

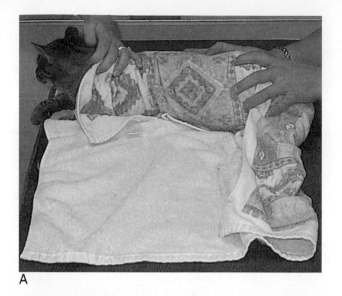

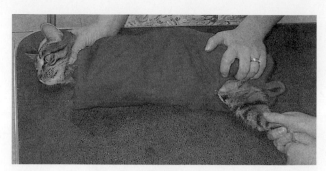

Fig. 16-8 A cat in a restraint bag, with the rear leg protruding for femoral venipuncture.

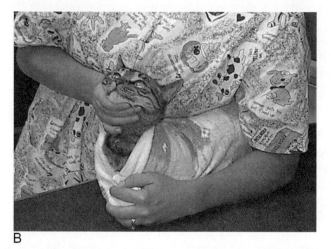

Fig. 16-7 A, Cat wrapped in the first third of a towel. **B,** Cat wrapped completely in the towel

limb exposure. They are available in a variety of sizes, because one size does not fit all! To insert a cat into a cat bag, you must have it laid out and open wide. Place the cat in the middle of the bag and quickly wrap the neck strap around the neck, fastening it snugly, but not so much that it occludes the airway. Then with a hand on its back or over its shoulders and hip, have another person zip the zipper, being careful not to zip hair or skin (Fig. 16-8). Legs can be brought through zippered openings for injections or venipunctures.

Never leave a cat on a tabletop in a cat bag, as it can still roll over and can fall off the table. To remove the cat, unzip the zipper either all of the way or partially and then loosen the neck strap. Most cats will walk straight out. However if the cat is terribly upset, be ready to pull your hands back fast when loosening the neck strap!

Muzzle

Commercial muzzles are available for cats. Most are designed to cover the cat's eyes but leave a fairly small hole for breathing. It seems this often upsets the cat even more. If a situation calls for a muzzle, perhaps sedation would be a better alternative.

Gauntlet

Refer to the dog restraint section; these gauntlets are used in the same manner. The only difference is that you may use them more for cats than dogs.

Distraction Techniques

Cats and horses both respond well to being distracted by the infliction of "mild" pain. The following are some distraction techniques that seem to work well with cats.

Caveman pets

Caveman pets are heavy, but gentle, pats or rubbing on the head. They can be rapid or slow and steady or somewhere in between. The idea is to get the cat to concentrate on what you are doing and ignore the procedure being performed. Varying the pressure and stroke is usually more successful than a continuous pattern. Some people will tap a cat's nose with their finger. This is *not* recommended, as the cat may not be able to resist biting such a tempting target.

Puffs of air

Blowing or puffing air into a cat's face is another way to redirect its interest. Again, vary the speed and force of the puff, and you will get better results.

Rubber band around the base of the ears

Placing a small rubber band around the base of the ears can distract some cats. The trick is to get it low down on the base of the ears. The cat will crouch down and really focus its attention toward its ears. But you have to be quick, and it usually doesn't work well for semipainful procedures.

Restraint Techniques

Removal from a carrier

Be sure all routes of escape are closed before restraining. Most cats will not willingly walk out of a carrier on our time frame. So it is a good idea to open the carrier door as soon as the client is escorted into the exam room. While you are talking to the client, the cat may decide to walk out and explore. If not, you can assess the temperament of the cat and if friendly reach in, gently grasp the scruff, and bring it forward until you can get a hand around its midsection. Most cats don't object to this; however most clients do not understand this and may feel you are hurting their cat. Always explain that scruffing is a natural hold for them since that is how their mother carried them.

If the cat resists, elevate the rear of the carrier and force the cat to slide out. Don't raise it so high that the cat drops from the carrier. If you are not successful, you can dismantle most carriers quickly. This is much safer than reaching into their territory and trying to grab them!

Removal from a cage

If the cat is friendly, reach in across its shoulders, grasp the front feet, quickly lift it out of the cage, and snug its body against yours. Your elbow can gently pin the cat's body against yours, thereby controlling the back legs. Cradle the chin, or encircle the neck with the other hand (Fig. 16-9).

If the cat is upset, you can try a number of things. A large beach towel or small blanket thrown over the cat and then scooped up works well to get them out of the cage. Once they are out of "their territory," they usually calm down and allow you to work with them. It is still recommended that you wear gauntlets while getting them out of the cage. You can also try lassoing them with a rope leash; however, you usually end up getting the leash around their chest, which isn't all that bad. If that does occur, you can pull them to the front of the cage and with a gloved hand reach in for a back leg and quickly transport them to an exam table. If the cat is terribly upset, there are a number of devices designed to trap and/or pin a cat to the floor of a cage or inside a device so a sedative can be administered.

Sitting or sternal recumbency

This procedure can be used for physical exams, oral and ophthalmic exams and medications, and cephalic or jugular venipuncture. For a routine physical examination, have the cat sit and place one hand in front of its chest and have the other steady its back. Gently talk and stroke the animal as it is being examined. When it is time to examine the head or do more invasive procedures, encircle the neck holding the mandibles with one hand; with the other hand reach across the back and grasp the front feet. Snug the cat up against your body. If necessary, lean a bit over the cat to keep its back legs in place (Fig. 16-10). A very gentle grip is a must to keep the cat from getting worried and causing it to struggle. If the procedure is almost done and the cat starts to struggle, it is a simple matter of tightening your grip and hanging on until the procedure is done. If at all possible don't let go! However, if you are losing your grip and the cat is trying to bite and/or scratch, alert the person doing the procedure and when they have stepped away, let go! This works well with most cats, and most cats don't object unless they are being held too tight.

If the procedure is a cephalic venipuncture, you can hold the cat in the same manner as described for the dog. Some people are dexterous enough to tuck the other foot between their little finger and ring finger and hang onto it so the cat can't reach up and scratch.

The jugular venipuncture hold is also similar to the way you hold dogs. However a cat's neck is a lot shorter, which results in having to hold onto the head and mandibles, usually with just a few fingers, as you stretch it up. It can be quite difficult to keep the cat's head under control; however, there is one method of adding support to the hold. As you stretch the head up, jut your chin out and place it

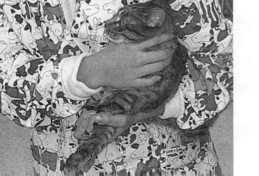

Fig. 16-9 Cat being held or carried.

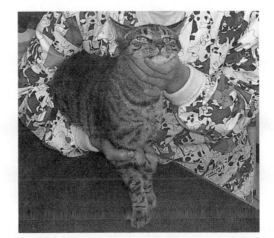

Fig. 16-10 Table hold used for examination or venipuncture of a cat.

against the top of the cat's head. This sounds dangerous, but it really does give you added stability, and you can quickly move out of the way if the cat starts to escape. Again it bears repeating: do this hold in a *very* gentle manner. Most students learning to restrain cats grip the cat too tightly right from the start. This will cause the cat to resist almost immediately, and it hasn't even been poked yet! Hold them gently, talk to them, and only tighten as necessary! Another mistake that students make is putting the cat into a hold before their classmate is ready to do the procedure. Don't start until you are sure the cover is loose on the needle, the cotton ball has alcohol on it, and the student knows where she is going to put the needle!

Fetal hold or "scruffing"

This technique is useful for giving subcutaneous or intramuscular injections, or rectal thermometer. As the cat sits, grasp the scruff of the neck gathering as much of the skin as possible in one hand. Lift the cat slightly off the table and grasp both back legs with the other hand. Stretch the cat's back against the forearm holding the scruff (Fig. 16-11). If the cat is stretched out fully, a reflex causes the cat's tail to curl ventrally toward its abdomen and the legs tend to be relaxed. The person doing the intramuscular injection can either take the top back leg or take both back legs, which then allows the restrainer to grasp the front legs.

Small cats can be lifted off the table, and a back leg can be moved up toward the neck and be hooked by the thumb of the hand holding the scruff. This presents the biceps femoris muscle into which an intramuscular injection can be given by the restrainer with the other hand (Fig. 16-12). *Do not* use this on cats over 7 pounds, because it can cause a lot of damage to tissues and vertebrae! Another precaution when using this technique is to have the injection ready to go and the cotton ball full of alcohol before placing the cat into position. The cat shouldn't be held in this position longer than 5 to 6 seconds; otherwise even a small cat can suffer some injury. But it is a real timesaver if you are alone and an injection needs to be given.

Lateral recumbency

Cats can be restrained in lateral recumbency just as you would for a dog. However, they are very agile and can often maneuver their heads around and bite! This should be

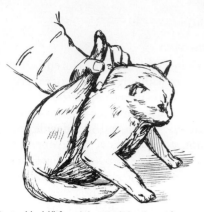

Fig. 16-12 "Pretzel hold" for giving IM injections alone. *(From Sonsthagen T: Restraint of domestic animals, St Louis, 1991, Mosby.)*

reserved for very placid cats and very noninvasive procedures. If you need them in lateral recumbency for a femoral venipuncture, placing them in a cat bag is the safest way to accomplish the task.

Dorsal recumbency

This technique is used for blood collection from the jugular vein, radiography, and cystocentesis. It sometimes requires two persons. However, with practice one person can usually do the hold alone. Scruff the cat, grasp the rear legs with the other hand, and roll it on its back. Coming from the rear with the other hand, palm up, gather the back legs and then the front legs in between the fingers on that hand. Try to grasp the back legs above the hocks and the front legs above the carpals. This gives you more purchase on the legs. The head continues to be scruffed, or you can switch your hold so that you are hanging onto the mandibles from the back of the head (Fig. 16-13). The phlebotomist can hold off the jugular vein with one hand and insert the needle with the other. Often it is easier to insert the needle pointing toward the chest versus the traditional insertion point. If the proce-

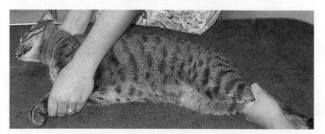

Fig. 16-11 Scruffing combined with holding a cat in lateral recumbency.

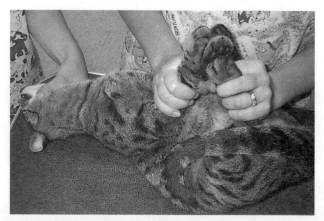

Fig. 16-13 Holding a cat in dorsal recumbency for jugular venipuncture or cystocentesis.

dure is for a radiograph or cystocentesis, you will most likely need two people.

RESTRAINT AND HANDLING OF SMALL MAMMALS

If small mammals (rabbits, gerbils, guinea pigs, rats, mice, ferrets) are restrained correctly, the chances of being bitten are minimal. Many of these "pocket pets" are frequently played with by children and do not resent being handled. If, however, the restrainer is fearful and mishandles the animal, it may become fearful as well.

Danger Potential

Again flight is the main means of defense, and if these little critters cannot get away they will use very sharp incisors to give you a good bite as well as using their toenails for scratching.

Mechanical Devices

A rabbit restraint box is used to securely hold a rabbit for venipuncture or injection using the ear veins. There is a head gate that allows you to adjust it firmly around the neck, and there is a back panel that is used to squeeze the rabbit forward. This prevents the rabbit from hopping and possibly causing a fractured spine.

Mouse and rat restraint chambers are plastic holders that allow you access to the head, tail, and body. The only difficulty is getting them into it! They grab onto the edges of the chamber with their front feet as they are lowered into it and stop their forward motion! You often have to twirl them around by the tail to make them dizzy enough to miss the edges! Once you get the hang of getting them into the chamber, it can prevent a lot of bites.

Restraint Techniques

There are three basic restraint techniques that can be used on these small mammals. They are described here, and under the specific species there is information if the technique needs to be modified.

Capture

There are three ways to capture small mammals. The first method is scooping them up with both hands. Quickly and without hesitation, cup your hands with palms pointing down and cover their bodies; then bring your hands together under the animal and scoop the critter up. The second method is to grasp the tail. Quickly raise it out of the cage and place it on a grate or near an edge, gently pull back on the tail. The animal will hang onto the bars or edge while you scruff them. The third method is to quickly reach in and grasp the animal over the shoulders and wrap your fingers around and under the neck. Lift the body out of the cage and support the rear end with the other hand.

Restraint

The most common method to securely hold them is by the scruff of the neck. Procedures such as gastric lavage and injections other than venipunctures can be accomplished using this procedure. The key to a good hold is to be sure you get all of the skin on the back of the neck. Otherwise the rodent will be able to turn its head and bite. Scruffing is accomplished by placing the animal on a grated surface, poising your index finger and thumb over the neck region, gently pushing down and grasping the skin at the same time. The downward pressure keeps the animal from scooting away. Once you have the animal scruffed, a tail or back leg can be restrained by pinning it to your palm with your little finger (Fig. 16-14).

HAMSTERS, MICE, GERBILS, GUINEA PIGS, AND RATS

Hamsters are nocturnal rodents that tend to be grumpy when handled in the daylight hours. It is always a good idea to knock on their cage to wake them up and give them a moment to get their eyes open before reaching in to capture them. Another thing to avoid doing with hamsters is poking your finger through their cage bars. Most will oblige and give you a good solid bite. Hamsters can be scooped and they can be scruffed. Hamsters have huge pouches on either side of their head and necks. When scruffing a hamster, be sure you have all of the skin!

Fig. 16-14 Scruffing a gerbil.

Mice are captured by grasping the tail. Once caught, you have to move fast or twirl them around by the tail because many are able to climb up their tails and bite. Once captured, place them on a grate or close to the edge of the table so they can grasp it with their front feet. While they have a grasp on the edge of the table or grate, gently pull the tail back toward you. Use your nondominant hand to quickly scruff them. Transfer the tail to that hand by pinning the tail or back leg to your palm with your little finger. This allows a free hand for injections or gavaging.

Gerbils are great jumpers and hard to catch if they are loose on the floor. They are prone to epileptic-like seizures that can occur if startled or handled too harshly. Because a gerbil has a long tail, some people try to use it to capture the animal. Because they are so quick, you usually end up grasping the end of the tail as they run by. When grasping just the tip of the tail, it is possible for the entire tip to come off in your fingers, leaving a few vertebrae and a very sore gerbil! It is better to use the scoop method to capture them and then scruff them if an invasive procedure needs to be done.

Guinea pigs are one of the easiest animals to restrain, because they rarely bite, do not move as quickly as smaller rodents, and tend to remain very still when frightened. Capture the guinea pig by scooping it up with both hands under the thorax. Then transfer one hand to support the hindquarters. They can also be scruffed, set up on their rear, laid on their backs in the crook of your arm, or wrapped in a towel for various procedures.

Rats enjoy attention and generally do not require much more restraint than distraction and simple holding. However, for examinations you hold them as described for the guinea pig. Rats can be wrapped in a towel, allowing the tail to be exposed for venipuncture. They can also be scruffed.

RABBITS

Rabbits can be difficult to restrain; they tend to be nervous and fragile. Rabbits have been known to struggle and kick violently, breaking their own spines.

Danger Potential

Rabbits will bite, but it is their toenails that can inflict painful injuries. When very frightened, rabbits emit high-pitched screams.

Restraint Techniques

Picking up a rabbit

Place one hand over the rabbit's shoulders, grasping as much skin as you can get. Then grasp the hind feet with the other hand. As you lift, face the rabbit away from you to prevent scratching and gently curl the rabbit's body inward (Fig. 16-15). Once out of the cage, tuck the rabbit's head into the crook of your arm and hold the back feet with the opposite hand (Fig. 16-16). Covering their head calms them, and they will "ride" in your arms quite comfortably. Do not use the ears or scruff to lift an adult rabbit. Using the scruff for handling damages the subcutaneous tissues; this is painful and can devalue the animal. Young rabbits can be scruffed for a very short time, although a better method is to pick them up like a ferret or guinea pig. Placing a rabbit back into a cage requires you to set it down and continue to hold it for a second. The rabbit will give a little jump and then walk out of your hold. If you let go as you set it down, it may jump forward and either bang into the cage wall or out the door!

Sternal recumbency

Rabbits can be restrained in sternal recumbency for most procedures. Pad an exam table with a towel or nonslip mat, place the rabbit on the mat, and encircle the rabbit's body with your forearms, holding the head with one hand and the front legs with the other. Examination and medication applications can be performed using this technique.

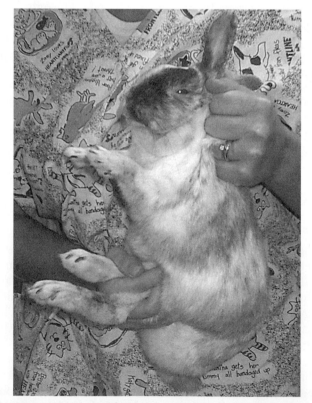

Fig. 16-15 Rabbit being lifted from a cage. Note how the body is curled inward.

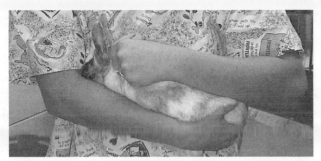

Fig. 16-16 Rabbit being carried with its head in the crook of the elbow.

Wrapping

Like cats, rabbits can be wrapped up in towels for venipunctures. When using this method, watch that the rabbit does not overheat.

Dorsal recumbency

Place a thick towel on the table, and place the rabbit on the towel. Lay the rabbit in lateral recumbency as you would for a dog or cat. Gently roll the rabbit over on its back. Transfer one hand to the head, and gently flex the neck back until the rabbit goes limp. Maintain the position with the head, and add a gentle rub on its stomach. This works for radiographs or examinations of the stomach; it does not work for a painful procedure.

FERRETS

Ferrets are rather easygoing animals that sleep a lot. They may "hiss" as a warning sign, but they usually do not bite unless distressed. Ferrets can easily become hyperthermic. Panting is an indication of overheating; these animals must be quickly cooled.

Danger Potential

When a ferret bites, it sometimes will not let go. If it bites and remains attached, put the ferret under running water. This is the best way to get the ferret to release its grip.

Restraint Techniques

Picking up a ferret

Never pick up a ferret by the tail or neck. Use the same method as for a rat or guinea pig. As it is picked up, move slowly and turn it to face you. Always talk to the ferret to reassure it.

Distraction

Place a dab of liquid treat on the ferret's stomach for non-painful procedures, such as nail trimming, physical examination, vaccination, auscultation, or rectal temperature. The ferret will be engrossed in cleaning it off.

Scruffing

Scruffing can be applied for restraint during procedures that require no movement, such as radiography or cystocentesis. As with cats, grasp the loose skin around the shoulders and neck. Support the back with your other hand, and keep the rear legs off the table. The ferret will often relax and not struggle. This method is recommended for dental examinations, vaccinations, rectal temperature, and other injection. Do not use scruffing for oral drug administration, because the ferret cannot swallow when held by the scruff.

Wrapping

Towels can be used to wrap a ferret for short procedures. If the ferret struggles and begins to pant, this indicates overheating. If this occurs, quickly unwrap the animal.

Venipuncture

If the animal is not going to be anesthetized, you will need two handlers. One will control the front legs and stretch the neck forward; the other will control the rear legs. The ferret can be held in dorsal recumbency or, like other animals, with its front legs stretched over the edge of a table. If the ferret struggles violently, it should be anesthetized.

RESTRAINT AND HANDLING OF BIRDS

Birds can be a challenge to restrain; large parrots may be the most difficult. Restraint of tiny, fragile songbirds and finches requires very careful planning and execution as well. Before applying restraint, carefully check to be sure that all potential escape routes are closed.

Danger Potential

The main defense of birds is flight and biting. The larger parrots can inflict injury to hands with their claws and beak. Medium- to small-sized birds can also draw blood but seldom cause serious injuries.

Restraint Techniques for Large Birds

Removal from a cage

Many birds are territorial and possessive; do not attempt to remove a bird from an owner's arm or shoulder or from its cage with a bare hand. Gently place a wooden dowel (rod or perch) against the bird's legs and ask it to step up. Most birds will hop onto the dowel, which allows you to place them into a more restrictive hold when necessary. Another method is to have the client place the bird on the floor. When the bird is on the floor, it feels vulnerable and is more agreeable to being picked up. Again, offer it the dowel to step on. Do not use your hands to capture birds. Once it is on the dowel, a towel can be used to cover the bird and place it in a more restrictive hold, or you can use gauntlets.

Mechanical Devices

Gauntlet

The same leather gloves used on dogs and cats can be used to capture and hold large birds. Again, you have to be very aware of your grip, as the gloves decrease your tactile sensitivity. Many technicians will capture the bird with gloves on. Then, with help, they will remove the gloves before proceeding with the procedure. This can be tricky, but it gives you a better sense of touch. Some do not recommend using gloves, as they can cause fear and spread disease. However, a large bird can badly mangle a finger or inflict extensive wounds!

First place a thick, folded towel on the exam table. The towel pads the shoulder joints and body of the bird. Then, with the bird standing on the dowel, reach behind the bird's head and wrap your fingers around the head with the thumb and index finger placed around the neck close under the lower beak. Be careful not to twist the neck or occlude breathing by compressing the trachea or thorax. Quickly move your other hand down the bird's back and grasp the wing tips, tail, and feet with the other hand. Stretch the bird a bit, and lean it away from you so its back is almost parallel to the floor. Place the bird on the towel, have someone hold the head through the towel as you get rid of your glove, then repeat for the feet (Fig. 16-17). Holding the bird in this manner allows the bird to breathe freely, and allows the veterinarian to trim toenails, beak, and wing feathers or perform a thorough examination and venipuncture.

Towel

With the bird on the floor or on the dowel, hold the towel over your hand. Coming from behind the bird, quickly grasp the bird in the same manner as described above. The towel can be totally or partially removed to perform medical procedures.

Avian restraint board

The bird is laid in dorsal recumbency with its head placed in an adjustable gate. A gentle hand on either side of the bird will prevent the wings from flapping. Most birds settle down when placed in this device, and the technician doesn't have the worry of injuring the bird with a tight hold or being injured by the bird if it gets loose!

Restraint Techniques for Small to Medium Birds

Most are unaccustomed to being handled and are best caught in a semi-illuminated room. If the bird escapes, a net with a long handle works best for capture. Avoid stressful stimuli, such as barking dogs, loud music, and hurried activity, if possible.

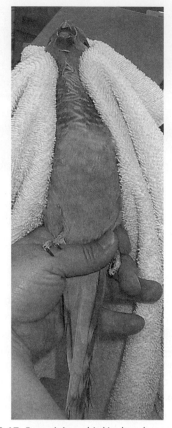

Fig. 16-17 Restraining a bird in dorsal recumbency.

Small birds can be held in one hand for examination. A soft cloth can be used to seize the bird in the cage. Coming from behind the bird, center the cloth around the bird's body. Gently wrap your index finger around the neck with a thumb under the lower beak, or gently squeeze the head between thumb and index finger. The little finger can be used as a "perch" for the bird to grip, or you can hold its feet down by pinning them to the palm of your hand. The restrainer must always be careful not to compress the thorax and abdomen. Restriction of breathing or rupture of air sacks can occur if pressure is applied to these areas. Procedures such as nail, beak, and wing trimming and jugular venipuncture can be done with one person holding the bird.

RESTRAINT AND HANDLING OF HORSES

Equine Behavior

Horses are herd animals that develop strong social relationships. If separated from its herd mates, a horse can become nervous, agitated, distracted, and uncooperative. The horse uses numerous vocal sounds and a variety of body language to communicate with offspring, to indicate social position in the herd, and to signal fear and nervousness. Horses have well-developed senses to detect possible threats.

Horses have keen binocular, stereoscopic vision. Their eyes are situated on the sides of their heads (as in most prey animals) to see in two directions at once. However they have small "blind spots" directly behind them and a short distance laterally from their rear flanks (Fig. 16-18). Although this is very advantageous for horses, it also makes them shy from objects located in their "blind spot." The horse's depth perception is good if it is using both eyes, meaning it has to look directly at the object such as a jump or a hole in the ground. Horses can distinguish the colors yellow, red, and green but have trouble with blue and purple.

Horses have excellent hearing and can recognize each other's calls from great distances. By watching a horse's ears, you can locate the origin of sounds. Although most domestic horses are accustomed to certain amounts of noise, sudden loud sounds can startle a horse into flight.

The sense of touch is well developed in the horse. Horses are very sensitive on the body surface, especially under the belly and in the flank area.

If a horse cannot run away from a threatening situation, it will resort to jumping, kicking, bucking, rearing, and biting. Although unprovoked aggression is rare in horses, defensive biting and kicking are relatively common.

Body Language

A horse's temperament and intentions are often signaled by its "body language."

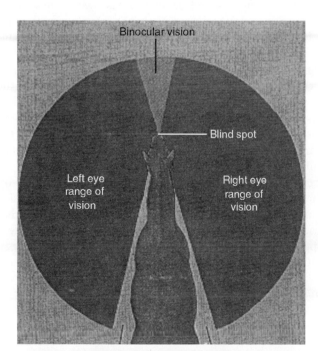

Fig. 16-18 Horse vision areas.

Ears

Pinned-back ears indicate aggression or, if working, thinking hard! Forward-pointing ears indicate listening or attentiveness. One ear pointed forward and the other pointed backward indicates listening in two directions. Drooping or relaxed ears can indicate a sleeping, tired, or unwell horse.

Mouth

An open mouth with teeth exposed may signal attack. Lifting of the upper lip to expose the gums, with teeth together, is the *Flehmen response*, a type of sexual behavior in males. A tightly clamped mouth with a grimace can indicate pain.

Head

A lowered head and pinned-back ears are threatening gestures, as in a mare protecting its foal. An elevated head with eyes widely opened and ears moving in all directions signals attention and/or fright.

Feet

Pawing at the ground indicates impatience. Lifting of a rear foot with slight kicking motion indicates a possible defensive kick. Elevation of both front feet off of the ground signals the intent to rear defensively.

Tail

Tucking of the tail tight against the hindquarters signals fear or pain. Swishing or circling the tail signals agitation.

Danger Potential

The main defense of horses is accurate kicking with the rear feet. The safe zones for passing behind a horse are either 10 to 12 feet away or in direct contact with the rear of the horse. Most horses have a range of 6 to 8 feet, with the apex of the kick being the most deadly. You can be kicked when in close contact with the horse, but it doesn't have the power of the full leg.

Front legs can be used to paw at you or to come down on you from rearing up, or both! That is why it is so important not to stand directly in front of a horse at any time!

Horses have very strong jaws. If a horse does not want to let go, it is nearly impossible to remove yourself from its jaws. A horse can lift an adult off the ground and shake it like a rag doll. A horse can cause horrible bruising and dislocations by biting and shaking. Most horses don't bite, but those that bite or try to bite should be disciplined. If a horse tries to bite, a sharp rap to the muzzle is a must to get them to stop. Once they start biting, it is very hard to get them to stop.

Mechanical Devices

Halter

A halter is the main tool of restraint used on horses. Check your halter and lead rope for worn spots that could tear if the horse bolts. Make sure the lead rope is attached to the center ring at the bottom of the halter and that it is at least 6 feet long. Hold the halter open; if it is tangled, untangle it so that a smooth application of the halter can be accomplished. If the equipment checks out, proceed to halter the horse.

Hold the end of the lead rope and the neck strap of the halter in your left hand. Reach over the neck of the horse, and pass that hand to the end of the lead rope. Tie the lead rope around the horse's neck using a simple overhand knot. This convinces most horses into believing they've been caught. It also gives you something to grasp if the horse decides to move off. Reach back over the neck close to the pole and grasp the long end of the neck strap. Allow the halter to fall open. Pull the nose band over the bridge of the nose, then buckle the neck strap. The halter should fit snugly with two fingers easily slipping under the nose band. Untie the lead rope from around the neck, and loosely loop so that it can be grasped in the left hand. Position the right hand approximately 6 inches from where it is connected to the halter. Stand to the side and slightly ahead of the front feet, facing the same direction as the horse.

Twitch

A twitch is a mechanical device that is attached to a horse's upper lip to distract its attention from a procedure being performed elsewhere on its body. It can be a flat chain that is wound around the lip or a clamp that is closed and tightened over the lip. The horse is haltered and held with the right hand, with the left hand reaching through the opening in the twitch. Standing to the side of the horse's head, grasp as much of the upper lip as possible, curling the lips in to protect the mucous membranes. Slide the twitch around the bunched lip with your right hand, and tighten (Fig. 16-19). If the twitch has been applied properly, the horse should begin to look drowsy. Slightly loosening and tightening the chain twitch or gently squeezing and releasing the clamp twitch will keep the horse focused on the twitch. After the twitch has been released, gently massage the lip.

Chain shank

This is actually more of a discipline technique than a form of restraint. Think of it as a choker collar for horses. It involves the use of a flat chain that is attached to a leather or rope lead. The chain shank is run from one side ring of the halter, over the nose, under the upper lip or inside the mouth, and connected to the other side ring. When the horse misbehaves, the shank is popped or tightened. This immediately disciplines the horse and often results in getting it to lower its head. Quickly loosen the tightened shank and comfort the horse if it settles down.

Some people will put the shank beneath the horse's chin. But when popped or tightened, it causes the horse to throw its head up. The higher the head is, the less control you

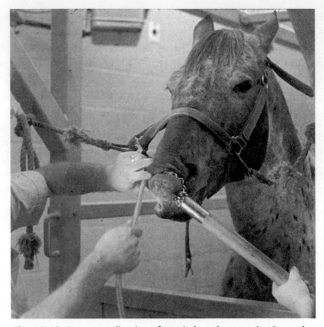

Fig. 16-19 Proper application of a twitch and cross-tying in stocks.

have over the horse. Only an experienced person should use the chain shank, as it can cause a great deal of harm both physically and psychologically. By watching and speaking with an experienced person, you will be able to learn this useful technique.

Stocks

Stocks are the ideal piece of equipment for procedures such as floating teeth, eye treatments, cleaning superficial wounds, changing head bandages, nasogastric intubation, and rectum or uterine examinations. Stocks usually have solid panels on the sides and a gate on either end. The panels are often removable or repositionable to allow access to legs and feet.

To place a horse into a stock, lead the horse up to the stock, allow the horse to go into the stock, and walk outside, passing the rope around the posts. Close the tail and head gates as the horse reaches the front of the stocks. Tie the horse's head with a halter tie. Adjust any parts, such as side rails, as necessary to accommodate the horse. You can cross-tie the head for added security. Take the lead rope off the bottom center ring of the halter, and place it on the side ring of the halter, tying it to the post. Then add another lead rope to the opposite side ring on the halter, and tie it opposite of the first lead rope. You can cross-tie horses without being in stocks as well. However, remember that a horse can still paw at you with its front legs, swing its body, and kick with its back legs!

Distraction Techniques

Distraction techniques are most useful for examinations, suture removal, injections, radiography, hoof work, and oral administration of paste dewormers. The person holding the halter usually applies the distraction techniques. If the horse is really uncooperative, a second person may be called upon to help.

Skin twitch

A horse's sensitivity to touch is used to distract its attention away from other procedures. The restrainer stands on the same side as the person performing the procedure. Grasp a handful of loose skin on the lateral aspect of the neck or shoulder. Roll the skin under and give it a little shake or jiggle. If a second helper is available, have the person use both hands. After release, scratch and pet the area. This is useful for all injections or venipunctures.

Eyelid press

With the halter in place, reach up and give the base of the ears a nice scratch. Then gently move your cupped hand down and cover the eye closest to you. Exert a mild pressure or move your hand in a circular motion very gently. Talk to the horse while you have the eye covered. It will focus on you and ignore most other procedures.

Ear hold

Grasp the very base of the ear, and gently move it in a small circular pattern. Do not bend it over or be too vigorous with the movements. This may cause excessive pain, and the horse may become head shy. You can also tie a light rope around the ear. Fold the edges in, and tie it closed with a piece of baling twine or cotton rope. Again it causes the horse to focus on the ear and not what is going on elsewhere. Once the procedure is finished, release the ear and give a good scratch all over so the horse knows that every time you reach for an ear it is not going to be painful!

Blindfolding

Horses often become docile when blindfolded with a soft towel, jacket, or other large piece of clean cloth. Halter the horse; do not tie it. Standing on the same side as the person performing the procedure, slip the cloth underneath the halter and over the eyes, and secure it. Make sure the horse cannot see around the blindfold. If you do this, talk to the horse continually and move slowly; the horse will depend entirely on you to keep it safe.

Restraint Techniques

Horses are prey animals and therefore have a strong flight or fight response to danger. To restrain a horse, the handler must first convince the horse that it is not being threatened, then win its trust and therefore its cooperation.

Approaching a horse

If possible, try to approach a horse from the left or "near" side. Most horses are trained to be bridled, saddled, and mounted from the left side, so they are accustomed to people working from that side. Call out its name and wait for it to look at you. Approach, gently pat it lower down on the neck, and wait for it to smell you. At that time you can offer it a treat such as grain or an apple or carrot. Then you can proceed to halter or bridle it. If possible, do not approach the horse from the rear. If it is in a stall, it is best to persuade the horse to turn until its head is facing you. Call out to it and offer a treat. If it won't face you, carefully move into the stall paying close attention to the animal's body language. If a rear foot is cocked into the kicking position, try to approach on the other side of the horse. Move close in so that your body is in close contact to its body. This minimizes the strength of a kick if it is coming. Continue to move up to the front of the horse and halter it.

Leading a horse

Never wrap the lead rope around your hand. This is extremely dangerous because of the possibility of injury if the horse bolts. The rope will tighten down around your hand, and you will be dragged with the horse. Loosely loop the lead rope, then grasp it in the middle; it should look like you have a handful of "eights."

Standing on the left side of the horse, give the lead rope a forward tug and ask the horse to move out. This can be a clicking sound made with your mouth or "giddy-up." Watch the front feet so they don't step on you, and watch where the horse is looking and listening. Be very alert to things that may frighten or startle the horse.

If the horse tries to pull ahead, pull back on the lead rope and say, "whoa." Sometimes you may have to jerk the lead rope sharply to get the horse to pay attention to you. If the horse refuses to be led, turn its head toward the right and push on its neck. This forces the horse to move its front feet and usually will get it to move off. Keep the horse's head level with your eye or lower. If the head is allowed to go above your shoulders, it is almost impossible to control the horse if it should bolt. If the horse is startled, the long lead rope allows you to move away from the horse out of danger yet maintain some control! Talk to the horse, and try to work your way back to the original position. Some technicians will use an even longer lead rope, allow the horse to settle down on its own, and then regain control.

If the horse is being uncooperative, it is important to discipline it immediately. Jerking its head away so it cannot be haltered or jerking the lead rope from your hand and running are tricks horses can learn and remember. Every time a horse gets loose by being bad-tempered, it learns the behavior sooner and can sometimes become even more bad-tempered. Not allowing the horse to act this way teaches it to behave and listen to you. This can be accomplished with sharp tugs on the halter with a command to whoa or stop. Sometimes you will have to use a chain shank to really get its attention. If the horse tries to bite, it should be rapped on the muzzle immediately and told to stop it.

Tying a horse

Because a horse tends to frighten easily, never tie it to anything that could be torn loose and dragged behind it. Always tie the lead rope with a quick-release knot around a vertical post or pole. The rope should be at least wither height, with approximately 2½ feet of slack in the lead rope. More slack than this may allow the horse to put its foot over the rope and become entangled. Never pass under the neck of a tied horse to get to its other side. Many people have been injured because a horse was frightened and jumped forward.

Halter tie

The halter tie is a quick-release knot. The knot releases easily when you pull on the free end of the lead rope. The proper type of lead rope is also important; heavy braided, round cotton is the best.

Using a stout post or another appropriate hitching post, place the free end of the rope behind the post. Bring the free end around, and make a loop over the long end (the part attached to the horse) (Fig. 16-20, *A*). Make another loop with the free end. From underneath, push this loop up and through the first loop (Fig. 16-20, *B* and *C*). This traps the long end of the rope and forms a quick-release knot. Test the knot by pulling the free end of the rope (Fig. 16-20, *D*). The knot should release easily. Some horses have learned to pull on the free end of the rope, thus freeing themselves. To thwart them, stick the end of the rope into the loop formed in the knot. Do not tighten the rope. Just leave it hanging loosely. The horse will pull on the end of the rope but will not release or tighten the knot.

Picking up feet

Have someone hold onto the horse on the same side you are on. If the horse decides to bolt, it will then go in the oppo-site direction from you and your helper. To prepare to lift either foot, face toward the rear of the horse with a hand placed firmly on the horse so it knows you are there. Front feet are picked up by first placing your hand at the top of the leg near the shoulder. Firmly run your hand down the front of the leg until you reach the fetlock joint. With one hand on the front of the joint, reach around opposite of you and grasp the back of the joint (Fig. 16-21). Lean against the horse, lift on the joint, and say "up" or "give me your foot." The other hand can grasp the front of the hoof and tip the foot in a flexed position. If the horse begins to resist, flex the foreleg a bit more. Place the hoof between your legs and above your knees. This allows both hands to be free for cleaning, bandaging, or checking for soft spots. When you are finished, hang onto the hoof until your leg is out of the way and then set the foot down. Do not let it drop, as it can startle the horse and cause it to jump.

Rear feet are picked up by first placing your hand at the top of the rump and firmly sliding it down on the inside of the leg until you get to the fetlock joint. Lean into the horse, pull up on the fetlock joint, give the "up" command, and start to walk forward. This brings the leg out to the rear of the horse (Fig. 16-22). Keeping the foot extended prevents the horse from gathering a lot of power in which to kick. It can still kick out but without the force of coming from the ground. Once the foot is extended, rest the hoof on *top* of your thigh. Do not place it between your legs like the front foot! If the horse pulls back, hook your elbow around the hock and take another step forward.

The person restraining the head can aid this process by performing distraction techniques, talking to the horse, and watching it for signs that it is going to move or jump.

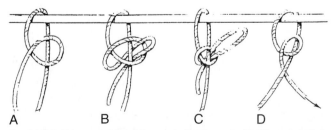

Fig. 16-20 Tying a quick-release or halter knot. **A,** The free end of the rope is run behind the post. **B** and **C,** Another loop is made with the free end and is pushed from underneath up and through the first loop. The long end of the rope is pulled to complete the knot. **D,** The knot can be released quickly by pulling on the free end of the rope. *(From Sonsthagen T:* Restraint of domestic animals, *St Louis, 1991, Mosby.)*

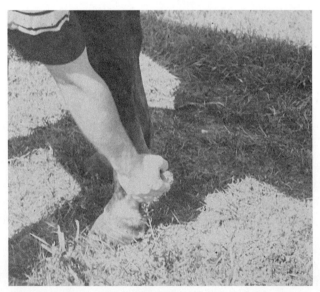

Fig. 16-21 Hand on the fetlock joint just before picking up the leg.

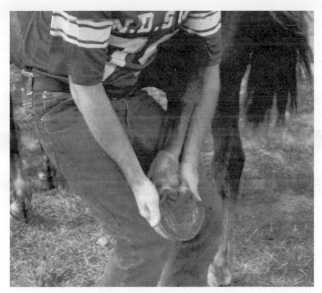

Fig. 16-22 Holding the rear leg to inspect the foot.

Tying a leg

This technique has a very powerful psychological effect on a horse. By taking away its ability to flee, the horse must rely on you to be its protector. The first time this procedure is done, a horse may panic and hop around. Eventually, the horse will relax and allow you to work with it.

The technique involves tying up one front leg in a flexed position. The horse should not be tied to an inanimate object because it may struggle and injure itself. Have someone hold the head while you tie up the leg. Pick the front leg up as you would for any other procedure, but instead of placing the leg between your knees fold it so the leg is in a flexed position. Using a soft cotton rope or a leather strap with a buckle, wrap it around the leg several times and secure with either two half hitches or by buckling the strap (Fig. 16-23). Release the leg and step away from the horse. Once the horse has accepted its fate, you can perform radi-

ographs, bandaging, or other fairly noninvasive procedures. This is not recommended for painful procedures, because the next time to you try to pick up one of its legs, the horse may remember the procedure and react violently.

Tail tie

When tying up its tail, a horse cannot swish it or tuck it under. Procedures such as rectal palpation, Caslick's surgery, and artificial insemination can be performed on the hindquarters. Grasp the tail in one hand, and form a bend in the hair just distal to the last coccygeal vertebra. Then bring the loose end of a heavy braided cotton rope through the loop from the bottom (Fig. 16-24). Wrap the rope around the horse's tail, then bring the end under the rope. Pull up on the short end and down on the long end. Grasp the long end, and tie it to the front leg with a quick-release half hitch.

Restraining foals

Newborn foals can be restrained by placing one arm in front of the foal's chest and the other behind the foal's hindquarters. The foal can also be backed into the corner of a stall and gently held in position with an arm placed in front of the chest. Foals are always kept in mother viewing because both foal and mother will do most anything to be reunited.

Once the foal is up and moving around, a small halter can be fitted to the head. A loop is made in a lariat and placed over the foal's rump. A tug on the lead rope with the appropriate command and a tug on the lariat are usually all that is needed to get the foal to move forward. Praise is appropriate when the foal is walking along with no tugs on the lariat.

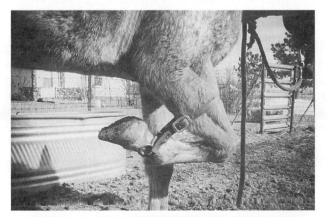

Fig. 16-23 Hobble strap applied to the front leg of a horse.

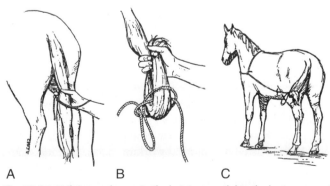

Fig. 16-24 Tail tie on a horse. **A,** The hair just caudal to the last coccygeal vertebra is bent to form a bite. **B,** The rope is brought up from the bottom and through the bite. **C,** The end is passed around the tail and back under the rope coming from the bottom of the bite. **D,** The long end of the rope can be tied around the horse's neck. (*From Sonsthagen T:* Restraint of domestic animals, *St Louis, 1991, Mosby.*)

RESTRAINT AND HANDLING OF CATTLE

Bovine Behavior

Rough or inappropriate handling of cattle can reduce conception rates, the immune response, and rumen function. Understanding cattle behavior will help you predict how they are likely to respond to handling and can facilitate handling, reduce stress on the animal, and improve handler and animal safety.

Remember too that dairy cows are very used to having humans around and do not need a lot of physical manipulation to get them to go where you want. They are often treated either in their stanchions or haltered and tied to a post. Dairy bulls can be very unpredictable in their behavior and should not be handled by a novice. Beef cattle of both sexes can be very shy of humans and should be handled via the use of alleyways and chutes.

Danger Potential

The most common means of defense for cattle are kicking and butting. When cattle kick, it is usually with one leg at a time. Their kick is an arch starting forward, moving off to the side then straight back. Some cattle will kick straight out, but that is usually not the case. Also note that they are very accurate!

Cattle will slam into you with their heads, and once you are on the ground or against a wall or fence they will continue to hold you there. Some will even grind you into the ground. If that should happen, try to curl up and protect your head as much as possible and lie still. Most cattle will back off if you stop moving, but be aware that if you move and they are still watching you they will come back and attack again. This usually occurs when a cow has a calf at her side, although bulls have been known to do this as well. They are very protective of their young and will defend them aggressively no matter how tame they are. Many people have lost their lives while working on a calf and not paying attention to where its mother was.

Mechanical Devices

Squeeze chute

The squeeze chute is a restraint device used almost exclusively on beef cattle. Nearly all medical procedures can be facilitated by use of a properly constructed chute. A chute usually has three mechanical working parts: the head gate, tailgate, and squeeze. An animal is run into a chute by means of an alley. Once the cow enters the chute, the following three things should occur: the head gate closes securely behind the head; the tailgate closes at the same time so another cow doesn't run in behind the captured cow; and the captured cow refrains from backing out of the head gate and to the alley. Adjust the squeeze snugly, but

not so tightly against the cow's sides that it impedes breathing. Cows will usually settle if they feel they are confined in this way. The head gate is closed tight enough so that the animal cannot put a foot through, but not so tight as to clamp the cow's neck to occlude the airway. The side panels can be opened to allow access to the cow's side or feet. The tailgate acts as a barrier between you and the cow's rear legs. The head gate allows you to approach the cow to apply a halter or nose tongs or to administer oral medications.

Be aware that a cow can still stretch its neck quite a way out and can move it from side to side. The danger is being butted with the head, which is usually not fatal, unless there is direct contact to your head! If the head needs to be controlled, a halter should be applied.

Halter

The halter used on cattle is usually a rope halter that can be adjusted to fit any sized cow or bull. Two things to remember when applying a halter: the part that tightens when the lead is pulled goes around the nose and the lead comes off the left side of the cow's head. Before applying the halter, be sure the head stall is large enough to go behind the ears, but not so large that you have to make major adjustments while standing close to the cow's head. Most people will slip the nose band on first, then the headstall behind the ears. Pulling the lead will cause the halter to tighten up, and the cow's head can be tied to the side of the chute. Make sure that you adjust the side straps so they are not resting over the eyes. Halter and tying the head to the chute allows jugular venipuncture or injections, ear tag placement, and ophthalmic procedures to be performed.

Nose tongs

Nose tongs are attached to the nasal septum and are used to hold the head still. These pincerlike instruments should be checked for smoothness of the balls used inside the nose so they don't cause scrapes or cuts. Checked the nose tongs to ensure that the balls are not too close together. This can cut off circulation on the septum. Once applied, nose tongs can be secured to the chute. They should be used only for 20 to 30 minutes at a time (Fig. 16-25).

Stanchions

A stanchion usually consists of a head gate without sidebars to restrict lateral movement. Dairy cattle are often placed in stanchions and are comfortable being worked on in them. The handler must be aware that even though the head is secured, the cattle can kick and pin you between their bodies!

Electric prod

Battery-powered prods are sometimes used to deliver a shock to the hindquarters. These instruments should be used sparingly and only on the most stubborn of cattle. Keep the prod directly behind the animal; prodding on the

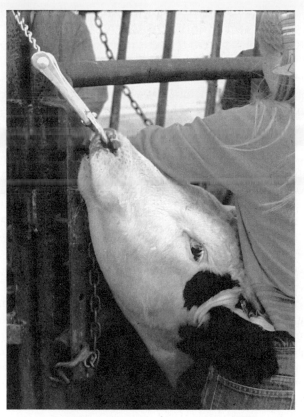

Fig. 16-25 Proper use of a nose tong or lead.

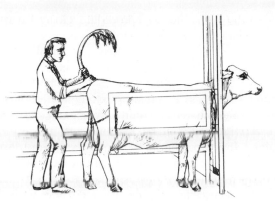

Fig. 16-26 Applying a tail jack to a cow in a stanchion. (*From Sonsthagen T: Restraint of domestic animals, St Louis, 1991, Mosby.*)

top line confuses the cow because in its mind it cannot go down!

Whips

Whips are also used sparingly to make cattle move. If used, they should be flicked at the heels or hindquarters to make the cow move forward. You can also use a whip to make yourself "bigger." This can help when guarding an opening or walking behind them to move them forward.

Hobbles

Hobbles are usually used on dairy cattle that have tendency to kick the milkers. Hobbles can be either a metal clip that is placed on each hock or a padded strap that is buckled around the lower leg. With both types, it is important to keep the cow's legs squared under her. If the back legs are brought in too close, she could lose her balance and fall.

Tilt table

Cattle, especially bulls, often need their feet trimmed. This can be done in a chute, but it is easier to do on a tilt table. Lead the animal or use an alley to put the animal near the table in its vertical upright position. Then sedate the animal and strap it to the table. Tilt the animal so is in lateral recumbency. This allows access to all four feet at a height that is comfortable to work at.

Restraint Techniques

Approaching and moving

Cattle have the same wide-angle vision that horses do. This can be used to the handler's advantage when getting them to move in the correct direction. Standing in their field of vision and giving them some stimulus such as a word or a flick of a whip or strap will cause the cattle to move out. Be aware that cattle will kick if pushed too hard or frightened. They seldom kick straight out, having an arch from front to back. This is important to remember because you can get kicked standing to the side of a cow as well as behind!

Cattle also have a natural tendency to move in a circle. If pushed too hard, they will start to circle and continue until the pressure is eased off. Allow them time to check out new places, and keep noise such as shouts and whistles to a minimum when working with cattle. Solid walls in alleyways that curve are the ideal when cattle are to be moved.

Tail jacking

Tail jacking is lifting the base of the tail straight up (Fig. 16-26). It is used to relax the hindquarters for rectal palpation and tail bleeding. It is not used to make a cow move forward, which is more of a side-twisting motion and should not be done with a lot of force, as it can fracture the vertebrae in the tail. With both techniques, you must be prepared for the cow to kick.

RESTRAINT AND HANDLING OF GOATS

Caprine Behavior

Goats are gregarious, ruminant animals. Although they are herd animals, they do not move together as easily as sheep. Also, goats become very vocal when separated from herd mates. It is usually easier for all involved if a companion goat is kept near the patient during a procedure. Goats that are used to being handled are docile and enjoy attention and petting.

Goats cannot be treated like sheep or controlled by force. They are much more agile and resistant to restraint. Although goats can withstand more stress than sheep, rough handling is unnecessary. Goats also tolerate heat fairly well. Goats become agitated and tend to struggle against restraint after a certain point. When handling goats, it is best to keep untrained dogs away, because goats make a game of attacking a dog. Although goats do not bite or kick, they do rear and charge humans and dogs, especially to defend their kids. Goats are also excellent escape artists and have been known to unlatch gates, climb, and jump over 6 feet.

Restraint Techniques

Catching and holding

When you work with a herd of goats, the ideal restraint is to use a small pen. Lure them into the pen with grain or some other treat. Chasing goats rarely works, as they scatter to the four winds!

Goats can be crowded into a pen, and then an individual goat can be caught and moved out to a work area. You can catch a goat by placing an arm around its neck and the other hand on its tail, much like a foal, then direct its movements with forward or backward pressure. Goats that are handled frequently may have a collar that can be used to lead it to the work area. If the goats are in a panic and you cannot get an arm around the neck, grasp a front leg and hold it off the ground. Most goats will stop and allow you to encircle them with your arms or place a collar or halter on them. Some may throw themselves to the ground and cause a ruckus. Be careful not to wrench the leg if this happens.

Once caught, place the goat's rear end in a corner to prevent it from backing up, and press its body against a wall to prevent lateral movement. Hands can be wrapped around either side of the face to lift the head for medications or jugular venipuncture. Small goats can actually be handled much like a dog; they can be put in lateral recumbency and can be straddled.

Halter

A halter can be used on a goat. It is similar to a horse halter but cut to size. The flat chain collar or a leather collar is most often seen. Goats that are milked or shown can usually be led easily. A goat will stand quietly for short periods if tied securely to an object using a collar or halter and lead. These techniques can be used for such procedures as hoof trimming, vaccination, and blood collection.

Stanchion

Dairy goats that are accustomed to a stanchion can easily be restrained for most procedures in this manner. Grain can be fed as a distraction.

RESTRAINT AND HANDLING OF SHEEP

Ovine Behavior

Sheep depend on their speed and flocking instinct as defense against predators. If we keep that in mind, we can minimize the amount of handling that causes sheep a lot of stress. Sheep become hyperthermic easily because of their wool and normally high body temperature (103° F). Use caution when working with sheep in ambient temperatures above 50° F and high humidity. Working in the early part of the morning with good ventilation is a must to keep sheep from overheating.

Sheep have a frail skeletal system and can be injured easily if they are chased into fences. Rough handling can break their back and legs. Never grab sheep by the wool; it is easily pulled out and the skin tears easily, causing bruising. It also devalues the carcass and pelt.

Although uncommon, at times a sheep may charge and butt a person. Ewes protecting lambs and other adult sheep sometimes charge dogs. Usually sheep that are behaving defensively face the assumed "predator" and stamp their feet. Sheep can bound over obstacles or people when feeling threatened. However, they are not good jumpers and usually catch you mid chest!

Restraint Techniques

Catching and holding

One of the easy things about sheep is that once one goes they all go! This can work very well if they are going in the direction you want them to, but not if they are escaping! Sheep should be moved as a group into a small containment pen. This can be accomplished with portable 4-foot-by-4-foot wooden panel or gate. Once they are in the pen, you can single out the sheep that needs treatment.

To capture a single sheep, place one hand around the tail and the other under the jaw. A forward or backward pressure with your hands will direct the sheep. Be careful not to choke the sheep by placing your hand on the throat. Or use a shepherd's crook to catch a sheep by the hock then hold it as mentioned previously. Move the sheep out to a work area, but not out of sight from the other sheep. This will keep the sheep calmer.

Jugular venipuncture, oral medications, and physical exams can be accomplished using the same technique as described for a goat.

Setting up

Sheep are often set on their hindquarters for shearing and other procedures, such as hoof trimming and subcutaneous injections. The restrainer stands with his or her legs against the sheep's shoulder and flank. The sheep's head is pushed laterally to its shoulder (Fig. 16-27). After a few moments,

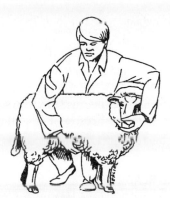

Fig. 16-27 Correct placement of the hands in preparation for setting a sheep up on its rump. (*From Sonsthagen T:* Restraint of domestic animals, *St Louis, 1991, Mosby.*)

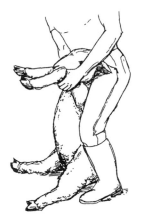

Fig. 16-28 Setting a sheep up on its rump. (*From Sonsthagen T:* Restraint of domestic animals, *St Louis, 1991, Mosby.*)

the sheep will begin to slowly sag. At this point, the restrainer lifts up on the flank, steps back with the leg closest to the flank, pivots on the other leg to throw the sheep off center, and sets the sheep on its rump (Fig. 16-28). Rock the sheep back so that it is resting on the top of the pelvis versus directly on the rear. This keeps the sheep off balance, and it will cease to struggle. Rest the back between your legs, freeing both hands for other work.

Halter

If a sheep restraint table is not available, a sheep halter can be applied after a sheep is caught. Take care not to occlude the nostrils with the nose band. Show sheep are trained to be led using a halter, whereas others must be coaxed and pushed from behind.

RESTRAINT AND HANDLING OF PIGS

Porcine Behavior

Pigs are not herd animals, but they tend to follow other pigs. When one pig becomes distressed and screams, the others may react as a group and panic. Pigs are extremely protective of their young and will come running if a piglet lets out a cry.

Pigs can become hyperthermic if chased or roughly handled in hot weather. Overheated pigs must be cooled immediately or they are likely to die of heat stroke.

Danger Potential

The main defensive weapons of pigs are their teeth. They can tear flesh easily and have very strong jaws; the tusks of boars can be very dangerous. Enter all adult swine enclosures with caution and be prepared to exit quickly. Sows are very dangerous with piglets at their side; a handler should never get into the same pen with a sow and piglets.

Restraint Techniques

Driving and catching

Pigs can be difficult to drive in an open pen. Solid-paneled hurdles work well to move pigs, as well as pieces of PVC piping or a cane. Pigs stop when confronted with a solid barrier, which is what the hurdles do, and the pigs will move along when tapped on the rear quarters. Pigs should be driven into a small pen with solid walls at least as high as the pig's shoulder. They can be separated from the group again using the hurdles and pipe or cane.

Directing a single pig

When moving a single pig, walk behind it with a hurdle in front of you. Use a cane or stick to direct the pig by tapping it on the flank to move it forward or on the shoulder to move it right or left. If it turns and moves toward you, set the edge of the hurdle on the ground and tilt it forward. This prevents the pig from getting its snout under it and lifting, allowing it access to or through your legs.

Hog snare

A hog snare is used for restraining pigs for venipunctures or other injections. The snare is usually a metal pipe with a cable loop on one end. The free end of the cable runs through the hollow pipe, so the size of the loop can be controlled. Hold the loop in front of the pig; most will investigate it in case it is something to eat. When the pig mouths the loop, quickly move the loop into the mouth and over the snout and tighten the loop. Two things happen. The pig will lean back from the snare and emit a loud scream, which it will keep up until released, so it is advisable to wear ear protection when capturing pigs with a snare. When releasing the snare, do it quickly and step out of the way. Excessive tightening can injure the pig's snout. A snare should be in place for a maximum of 20 to 30 minutes. A rope can be used in place of the pipe and cable snare. If using a snare on a boar with tusks, it is important to get the snare behind the tusks. However, this creates a possible hazard if the snare gets hung up on the tusks as it is removed. The pig is strong enough to jerk the snare from your hands and then swing it around. If the snare hits you or becomes airborne, someone is going to get hurt! Be advised that once a pig has experienced a snare, it is difficult to capture them again.

Restraining piglets

Baby pigs weighing less than 30 pounds are captured by grasping a back leg and holding the pig upside down until it can be held on your forearm close to your body or placed in a holding pen. If removing piglets from a sow, do it quickly and move to a different room to do the procedure so that you do not agitate the sow. Piglets can be restrained by holding both hind legs or placing them in a V-trough for such procedures as castration, ear notching, and cutting needle teeth. Piglets weighing more than 30 pounds can be held the same way, but it may take two people to hold them upside down by their hind legs.

Restraining potbellied pigs

Potbellied pigs are usually kept as pets and have a docile temperament; however, some potbellied pigs may show aggression. Small pet pigs tend to squirm, jump, and climb on whomever is trying to restrain them. Ear protection is important for the handler because they can squeal as loud as a full-sized pig. Chemical restraint is sometimes the best choice.

RECOMMENDED READING

Fowler F: *Restraint and handling of domestic and wild animals*, ed 2, Ames, Iowa, 1995, Iowa State University Press.

McBane S and Douglas-Cooper H: *Horse facts*, Dorset Press, New York, 1990.

Sonsthagen T: *Restraint of domestic animals*, Mosby, St Louis, 1991.

Tully T and Mitchell M: *A technician's guide to exotic animal care*, AAHA Press, Lakewood, CO, 2001.

17

Patient History and Physical Examination

Michelle Mayers

Learning Objectives

After reviewing this chapter, the reader should understand the following:
- Importance of clear communication with the client
- Components of the patient's history
- Appropriate ways to elicit information from the client
- Approaches used for physical examination
- Components of a physical examination
- Ways to assess patients in emergency situations

A patient's history and physical examination are the foundations on which sound medical and nursing interventions are based. Animal patients cannot verbally communicate the ailments or discomforts caused by disease. Therefore, pay meticulous attention to the observations and concerns voiced by the client, who provides information from which you may formulate the patient's history. Astute observation from both the veterinarian and the nursing staff is crucial when performing the physical examination.

TECHNICIAN-CLIENT INTERACTION

Communicating With Clients

Communication is the key to successful history taking. The interviewer must be able to ask questions that are easily understood and are geared toward the animal's owner. If necessary, slang words describing certain conditions may be used to facilitate communication and avoid misunderstanding.

The interview is most successfully conducted when the technician is professional but cheerful, friendly, and genuinely concerned about the patient (Fig. 17-1). A dry,

The authors acknowledge and appreciate the original contributions of A.M. Rivera and P. J. Gaveras, whose work has been incorporated into this chapter.

inquisitional approach, consisting of rapid-fire questions, is typically less effective in unearthing important details of the history.

The best clinical interview focuses on the patient. When speaking with the client, determine the primary medical problem (presenting or chief complaint) as well as the way the animal is manifesting the illness. An important interviewing technique employs reflective listening methods that incorporate active listening, infrequent interruption, limited speaking, and asking for clarification when needed. Interrupting an animal owner may disrupt his or her train of thought and prevent the client from reporting important facts.

Allow the client to control the interview, at least in part. Once the client has reported the facts, repeat important information, indicating that you have heard him or her and understand the concern. If the history given is vague, use direct questioning. Asking "how, "where," and "when" is generally more effective than asking "why." The technician's appearance influences the success of the interview. Neatness counts. An untidy interviewer wearing a soiled smock will be viewed as unprofessional, careless, or incompetent. Some clients may view a sloppy appearance as a sign of not caring, and as such will taint their expectations and impressions of the entire veterinary team.

The rule of five vowels is useful in conducting an interview. This rule states that a good interview contains elements of Audition, Evaluation, Inquiry, Observation, and

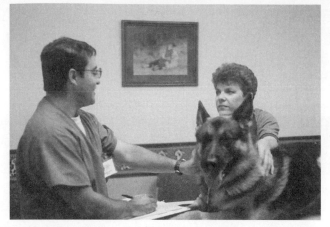

Fig. 17-1 The interview should be conducted in a professional yet friendly manner, while displaying genuine concern for the patient and client. The appearance, attire, and attitude of the veterinary staff set the tone of the visit and convey an impression of the quality of veterinary services being rendered.

Understanding. Audition means listening carefully to the client's story. Evaluation refers to the sorting of data to determine which is important and which is irrelevant. With inquiry, the interviewer probes into the significant areas requiring more clarification. Observation refers to the importance of nonverbal communication, body language, and facial expressions, regardless of what is said. Understanding the client's concerns and apprehensions enables the interviewer to play a more emphatic role.

The physical setting of an interview can enhance or hinder it. Ideally, the interview should take place in a quiet, properly lighted room or with lighting adjusted to produce optimal illumination, although this is not always possible in field situations. Make the client feel as comfortable as possible. If feasible, you and the client should be seated on an even level, allowing for direct eye contact. Maintain a distance of 3 to 4 feet between you and the client. Distances greater than 5 feet are impersonal, whereas distances less than 3 feet intrude on the client's comfort zone. Sit in a relaxed position, and avoid crossing your arms across your chest, because this body language projects an attitude of superiority and may interfere with communication. A key to successful history taking is to put the client at ease.

Obtaining a thorough history by a medical interview depends on the technical knowledge and communication skills of the interviewer. The interview should be flexible and spontaneous, not interrogative. The major goal of the interview is to sort through the reported signs associated with the illness to better understand the pathophysiology of the disease in question. Although the novice may have limited knowledge of the signs associated with various diseases, with experience and education, one can learn to recognize the history and signs as they relate to various injuries and illnesses.

Obtaining a History

The information gathered when obtaining a history should alert the veterinary team to potential problems and direct the technician's attention to some of the patient's body areas during the examination.

Any given disease tends to be characterized by a certain group of signs. With only one isolated clinical sign, do not jump to conclusions or allow premature assumptions or preconceptions to affect your objectivity when making additional assessments.

The introductory statement

Review the preliminary data (e.g., animal's name and sex) before introducing yourself to the client. If the patient is a new animal to the household or farm or a geriatric patient not seen recently, or if the owner is a new client, confirm this and note it in the medical record. Greet the client by name, make eye contact, shake hands firmly, and smile. Always address the client by an honorific title (e.g., Mrs., Mr.) and his or her last name.

For example, you might say: "Good morning, Mrs. Schwartz. My name is Joe Smith. I'm a veterinary technician and I'll be obtaining a history and performing a preliminary examination on Buffy. Can you please tell me the reason for Buffy's visit today?" You can then validate the preliminary data if needed and go on to obtain the history for the presenting complaint.

Some technicians prefer to address the presenting complaint first, and then validate or confirm the preliminary data. Regardless of which approach you prefer, develop a consistent routine that is comfortable for you and the client and that obtains the necessary data (Box 17-1).

Patient characteristics

The receptionist can obtain certain preliminary data, such as patient characteristics (age, breed, sex, reproductive status). The technician should verify that the patient's age, breed, sex, and reproductive status have been correctly recorded and note any changes since the patient's last visit (e.g., if patient has been spayed or castrated). Pay close attention to the patient's age. Congenital and infectious diseases, parasitism, ingestion of foreign bodies, and intussusceptions are usually predominant in young animals. Degenerative diseases and neoplasia are more common in adult animals. Certain species or breeds are predisposed to particular problems. For example, toy breeds of dogs (e.g., Chihuahuas, Pomeranians) are predisposed to patella luxation and hydrocephalus. Brachycephalic (short-nosed) dogs are predisposed to respiratory problems. Combined immunodeficiency affects Arabian horses. Any predispositions should be considered when formulating a list of differential diagnoses (diagnostic possibilities).

The patient's sex and reproductive status are important, because certain conditions are gender-specific and deter-

---

BOX 17-1

Checklist for Physical Examination

Introduction to the Client

Patient History

- Patient characteristics
- Geographic origin
- Current environment
- Diet
- Previous medical history and vaccination status
- Presenting complaint(s)
- History of chief presenting complaint
- Conclusion

Physical Examination

- General observation
- Recording vital signs

Level of Consciousness

- Respiratory rate and effort
- Heart rate and rhythm
- Indications of perfusion

Systematic Physical Examination (Visual Inspection, Palpation, Percussion, Auscultation)

- Examination of head and neck
- Examination of trunk and forelimbs
- Examination of thorax
- Examination of abdomen
- Examination of skin and lymph nodes
- Examination of hind limbs
- Examination of external genitalia and perineum

---

mine what areas should be given special attention in patient evaluation. For example, in a 10-year-old intact (not spayed) female dog with a history of excessive water consumption and urination, vomiting, and lethargy, pyometra (uterine infection) would be an important differential diagnosis. In a 5-year-old spayed female with the same history, however, diabetes mellitus would be an important differential diagnosis. The incidence of some diseases decreases markedly as a result of ovariohysterectomy (spay) or castration. Dogs spayed at an early age are less likely to develop mammary tumors, and castrated male dogs are at lower risk of developing perianal adenomas.

Geographic origin and prior ownership

Determine where the patient originated (e.g., home, breeder, pet shop, animal shelter, neighboring farm, livestock auction), where it has recently traveled, and if it was recently boarded or shown. This information may indicate if the patient has been exposed to infectious or parasitic diseases.

Current environment

Obtain information about the patient's environment and activities. Is it an indoor or outdoor animal? Is the patient free-roaming or confined to a yard or house? Is it housed in a pasture or in a stable? Free-roaming or pastured animals are at higher risk of exposure to toxins or trauma. Determine if the patient shares the environment with other animals. For example, multiple-cat households and catteries have a higher prevalence of infectious respiratory diseases and feline leukemia virus infection.

Diet

Information about the patient's diet can help rule out nutritional disease. When obtaining dietary information, question the client about the patient's appetite, gain or loss of weight, type of diet (e.g., dry, moist, or table food; total mixed rations; supplements), brand name of food, method of feeding (free choice or individual meals), and amount fed daily.

Past medical history

Past medical history provides information about the patient's health before the current illness. Carefully inquire about and record the dates of previous illnesses and treatment, hospitalization, and surgeries, followed by a brief description of each problem, how it was managed, and how the patient responded to treatment. Ask the client to describe any allergies (environmental, ingestible, or drug-related) and how these were diagnosed. Note any medications the patient is currently receiving. It is important to determine if the client is giving medications as prescribed.

Vaccination status

Question the client about the patient's vaccination status and when any vaccinations were given. Some clients are not familiar with vaccination schedules and may simply report that their animal "has been vaccinated." It is easy to presume that the patient is up-to-date on vaccinations, when in fact the vaccinations were given several years ago. Be aware of recommended intervals for vaccinations and diagnostic tests. For example, inquire when a cat was last assessed for exposure to feline leukemia virus and feline immunodeficiency virus. Ask if a dog has been checked for heartworm infection in the past year, and if and what type of preventive is being used.

The presenting complaint

The *presenting complaint* is the reason the client has sought veterinary care for the animal. For example, the client may say a cow has had diarrhea for three days, is not eating, and is depressed. It is important to remember that *the presenting complaint is what the client perceives the patient's problem to be.* Although the client's fears or anxieties may influence your observations of the animal, pay attention to these concerns. Allow the client to communicate these observations, and then continue with the interview. This tends to relieve a client's anxieties about the animal.

Another important interviewing skill is the ability to assess the source and reliability of the information obtained. A history obtained from second parties presenting the animal for evaluation (friends, neighbors, children) may lack important information that only the client can provide.

It is also important to determine if the client understands the meaning of the medical terms he or she uses to describe the problem. Ask the client to define such terms. For example, "What do you mean when you say the cat regurgitated?" A client may bring in a dog and say that it "just had a stroke." To an experienced veterinary professional, the patient's ataxia, incoordination, head tilt, and horizontal nystagmus may indicate vestibular disease rather than a cerebrovascular accident (stroke). It is important to record the clinical signs observed and not the client's presumptive diagnosis. Be aware that the client's comments, observations, and conclusions are based on his or her experience. We must interpret their comments, observations, and conclusions in light of our professional experience.

Once the presenting complaint is listed, record the information gathered in chronologic order to clarify areas of possible confusion. Separate the client's *observations* from his or her *conclusions*, and amplify certain portions of the complaint that may be important.

History of presenting complaint. The history of the current complaint helps determine when the animal was last normal, if the condition is acute or chronic, what medications and dosages were used previously, how the patient responded to previous therapy, and the duration and progression of clinical signs. The history is best recorded by chronology (i.e., in the order in which events occurred). This provides a better understanding of the sequence and development of the problem. Begin with the first sign of illness observed by the client, and follow its progression to the present time (see Box 17-1).

It is important to determine when the client first noticed the presenting complaint, apart from any other health problems. Some patients might have other ongoing health problems (e.g., flea-bite dermatitis, food allergies) unrelated to the current complaint. Ask for specific information that describes the signs observed (e.g., color, odor, consistency, and volume of vomitus or diarrhea). When the client uses such terms as *somewhat, a little, sometimes,* or *rarely,* ask for clarification. Remember, precise communication is important.

Some clients simply cannot remember when the signs first developed. You may be able to help the client relate the onset of signs to some event. For example, ask, "Was the horse's lameness evident around the Thanksgiving or Christmas holidays?" When obtaining information on the presenting complaint, use open-ended questions that allow the client to describe the problem, rather than simple yes or no questions. The following example illustrates a series of open-ended questions that elucidate the sequences of events and the nature of the problem:

- Why is Buffy being presented? This identifies the presenting complaint.
- When did you first notice the problem? This determines the onset of the problem.
- What was the first sign that you observed, and what did you notice after that initial sign? This helps establish progression of the problem.
- Can you describe in detail the signs you observed? This helps identify clinical signs observed, rather than the client's diagnosis.
- Was there any change in routine or anything new, unusual, or different in Buffy's routine at the time of onset? This helps determine precipitating events.
- Has Buffy been treated for this problem before? How did she respond? This determines the response to previous treatment.

Concluding the history

If any part of the history needs further clarification, it should be done after all of the initial information has been gathered. At this point, you may wish to summarize for the client the most important parts of the history. Encourage the client to correct any misinterpretations, and discuss any additional concerns. Allow the client the final say. At the conclusion of the interview, thank the client and say that you will now perform a physical examination of the patient.

PHYSICAL EXAMINATION

The physical examination assesses the animal's current state of health. The four primary techniques employed during physical examination are inspection, palpation, percussion, and auscultation.

Primary Techniques for Physical Examination

Inspection

Inspection begins with the technician's first contact with the patient and continues throughout the data collection.

Early in the physical examination, the technician visually examines the patient's entire body for structure and function, paying close attention to deviations or abnormalities. Inspection is an active process, not a passive one. The technician must know what to look for and where. It should be done in a systematic manner so that nothing is missed.

Palpation

Palpation involves using the hands and the sense of touch to detect tenderness, altered temperature, texture, vibration, pulsation, masses or swellings, and other changes in body integrity (Fig. 17-2). The sense of touch is most acute using light, intermittent pressure; heavy, prolonged pressure causes loss of sensitivity in the hands of the examiner.

The fingertips are highly sensitive to tactile discrimination. The pads of the fingertips are used to assess turgor (e.g., skin), texture (e.g., hair), position, size, consistency, mobility (e.g., mass or organ), distention (e.g., urinary bladder), pulse rate and quality, tenderness, and pain. Temperature of a skin area is best assessed using the dorsum (back) of a hand or finger. The palm of the hand is more sensitive to vibrations, allowing one to feel such abnormalities as crepitus ("grinding") in a joint.

Palpation can be classified as light or deep. Light palpation of structures such as the abdomen is performed primarily to detect areas of tenderness. Deep palpation is used to assess underlying organs (e.g., liver), while giving careful consideration to the discomfort the procedure may cause the patient.

Terms used to describe structures palpated include doughy (soft, malleable), firm (normal texture of organs), hard (bonelike consistency), fluctuant (soft, elastic, and undulant, as with a cyst or abscess), and emphysematous (air or gas in tissue planes).

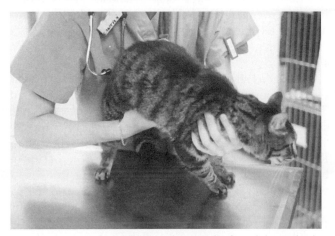

Fig. 17-2 Because of patient size and personal safety, abdominal palpation is used more commonly in small animals than in large animals. In cats and small dogs, one hand can be used to restrain the animal while the other is used for palpation.

Percussion

Percussion is tapping of the body's surface to produce vibration and sound. The sound reflects the density of underlying tissue and size and position of organs. Percussion is most commonly used on the thorax for examining the heart and lungs. It helps determine if a tissue is fluid-filled, air-filled, or solid. Percussion elicits the following five types of sound:

1. *Flatness* (extremely dull sound produced by very dense tissue, such as muscle or bone)
2. *Dullness* (a thudlike sound produced by encapsulated tissue, such as liver or spleen)
3. *Resonance* (a hollow sound, such as that produced by air-filled lungs)
4. *Hyperresonance* (a "booming" sound heard over a gas-filled area, such as an emphysematous lung; this is always abnormal)
5. *Tympany* (a musical or drumlike sound produced by an air-filled organ, such as with gastric dilatation-volvulus)

Thoracic percussion in the standing patient can be used to detect a fluid line, as found in hydrothorax. Percussion ventral to the fluid line produces a dull thud, whereas percussion dorsal to the fluid line produces a resonant or hyperresonant sound.

Abdominal percussion can detect large volumes of air or fluid in the peritoneal cavity. Rhythmic palpation of a fluid-filled abdomen elicits a fluid wave that is transmitted to the opposite side.

Auscultation

Listening to sounds produced by the body is termed auscultation. Auscultation may be direct (with the ear and no instrument) or indirect (using a stethoscope to amplify sounds). The stethoscope allows auscultation of specific areas within a body cavity for assessment of the cardiovascular, respiratory, and gastrointestinal systems (Fig. 17-3).

Abnormal sounds can be recognized only after one has learned to identify the types of sounds normally arising from each body structure and the location in which they are most commonly heard. Proficiency at auscultation requires good hearing, a good-quality stethoscope, and knowledge of how to use a stethoscope correctly. The technician should become familiar with this instrument before attempting to use it with the patient. The stethoscope's chestpiece should have a stiff, flat diaphragm and a bell (Fig. 17-4). The diaphragm is the flat, circular portion of the chestpiece covered by a thin, resilient membrane. It transmits high-pitched sounds, such as those produced by the bowel, lungs, and heart. The bell is not covered by a membrane. It facilitates auscultation of lower-frequency sounds, such as third and fourth sounds of the heart, or what is most commonly termed a "gallop rhythm."

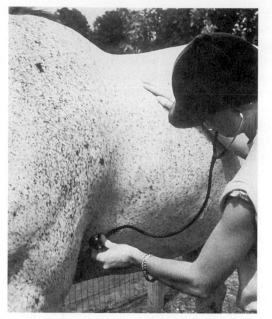

Fig. 17-3 Thoracic auscultation should be performed systematically, evaluating the lungs first and then the heart. The abdomen can also be auscultated to evaluate gastrointestinal sounds.

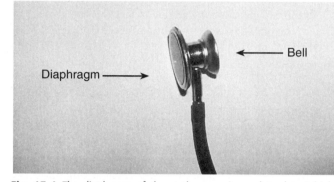

Fig. 17-4 The diaphragm of the stethoscope is used to detect high-pitched sounds, such as heart, bowel, and lung sounds. The bell is used to detect lower-frequency sounds, such as the third and fourth heart sounds.

General Survey

The physical examination begins from the moment the client and the patient enter the examination area. While obtaining the history, the technician should generally observe the patient to note certain characteristics. These are *mentation, general appearance, state of nutrition, symmetry,* and *posture and gait.*

Mentation

The patient's attentiveness or reaction to its environment provides a basis to evaluate the degree of consciousness, depression, excitement, or overreaction to stimuli. The patient's ability to walk or avoid objects can be used to assess vision and balance.

General appearance

Assess the patient's facial expression, size and position of the eyeballs, general body condition (flesh and haircoat), response to commands, and temperament.

State of nutrition

Note if the patient appears in normal body condition, is thin and frail, or is obese. Most patients with chronic disease appear cachexic (wasted). Sunken eyes, temporal muscle atrophy, and excessively loose skin turgor are signs of poor nutrition in chronically ill patients. Long-standing disease, such as renal failure, hyperthyroidism, and cancer, can result in marked wasting.

Symmetry

The body is normally symmetric; note any asymmetry. Observe closely for complementary ("balanced") or noncomplementary conformation of the thorax and abdomen. Note any difference in size or shape of the extremities.

Posture and gait

Walking requires coordination and integrity of the nervous and musculoskeletal systems. Note if the patient can walk, and describe any abnormalities in the gait. Proprioception (sense of body part position), soundness (lack of lameness), and coordination can be quickly assessed.

Vital Signs

Vital signs include the level of consciousness, respiratory rate and effort, heart rate and rhythm, and indications of perfusion. These reflect overall patient status; changes in any vital sign can warn the medical team of impending complications. Vital signs are monitored at regular intervals. The initial findings are used as the baseline, and subsequent findings help establish trends indicating improvement or deterioration. To identify abnormalities, technicians must know the normal ranges for each species, age group, and, sometimes, breed (Table 17-1).

Vital signs should be evaluated in relation to the presenting complaint, history, and current health status. Technicians must know the normal ranges for each vital sign and understand which variations might be considered "normal" with regard to a particular patient's status. Remember that vital signs reflect function of various body systems. For example, when assessing the level of consciousness, pupillary light response, and eye position, to some degree we are assessing the nervous system. All body systems (e.g., neurologic, cardiovascular, and respiratory) contribute to overall function of the individual; failure of one system can lead to compromise of others. For example, in patients with heart disease, a drop in blood pressure can compromise kidney function.

TABLE 17-1

Normal Ranges of Heart Rate, Respiratory Rate, and Rectal Temperature in Adults of Some Domestic Species

	Heart Rate (beats/min)	Respiratory Rate (breaths/min)	Rectal Temperature
Dogs	70-100	0-20	37.5°-39° C
Cats	150-210	8-30	38°-39° C
Hamsters	250-500	35-135	37°-38° C
Guinea pigs	230-280	42-104	37.2°-39.5° C
Rabbits	130-325	30-60	38.5°-40° C
Horses	28-50	8-16	37.5°-38.5° C
Cattle	40-80	12-36	38°-39° C
Sheep	60-120	12-72	39°-40° C
Pigs	58-100	8-18	38°-40° C

Level of consciousness

A declining level of consciousness suggests progressive brain damage and a worsening prognosis. In order of declining consciousness, the levels of consciousness are alert and responsive; depressed; uncontrolled hyperexcitability; stupor; and coma. A depressed patient is conscious but slow to respond to stimuli. A semiconscious patient that can respond to noxious (painful) stimuli is considered stuporous. An unconscious patient that does not respond to any stimuli is in a coma. Of these levels, coma warrants the worst prognosis.

A patient might be conscious yet have abnormal mentation (mental function). These mentation changes can include slow but appropriate responses to stimuli (suggesting severe depression) and inappropriate responses to stimuli (suggesting dementia). Bizarre behavior (e.g., biting at imaginary flies) may also be seen. Patients that are mentally dull exhibit slow responses and are unaware of stimuli.

Changes in level of consciousness or mentation can be caused by metabolic problems (e.g., liver failure, portacaval shunts, hyperglycemia, hypoglycemia, hypernatremia, hyponatremia), hypoxia, hypotension, iatrogenic rapid elevation in serum osmolality (e.g., mannitol overdose, total parenteral nutrition), trauma, toxicity (e.g., ethylene glycol), brain damage (e.g., tumors, infection, inflammation), and drugs (e.g., sedatives, anesthetics). Any pathologic change can lead to brain edema or hemorrhage and result in increased intracranial pressure. When this occurs, the brain is compressed and it malfunctions.

Changes in behavior, the response to stimuli, or posture may be significant. Unconscious patients can be tested by toe pinching to detect their response to this painful stimulus. Any decline in the level of consciousness suggests worsening pathologic changes and warrants immediate neurologic examination and medical or surgical intervention.

Neurologic evaluation can localize and determine the progression of the injury. Pupillary size and response to light are noted. Normal, responsive pupils, or equally constricted (miotic) pupils are associated with damage to the cerebral cortex or subcortical structures. Dilated or midrange fixed pupils are most commonly related to midbrain injury and are a grave sign. Eye position is noted, with ventral or lateral strabismus (crossed eyes) indicating a midbrain lesion. Nystagmus (repeated sweeping movement) is caused by a vestibular problem, either in the inner ear or within the brain stem. In an unconscious patient, changes in posture, with the forelimbs and neck in extensor rigidity (decerebrate rigidity), are a grave neurologic sign, indicating a midbrain lesion.

Respiratory changes imply serious central nervous system damage. A rhythmic waxing and waning of respiration (Cheyne-Stokes respiration) is due to severe, diffuse cortical injury. Apneustic breathing (holding the breath) and uncontrolled hyperventilation indicate a brain stem lesion.

Respiratory rate and effort

The lungs, airways, larynx, pharynx, and nasal passages make up the respiratory tract. The rate, pattern, and effort of breathing are controlled by the brain and respiratory muscles (intercostal muscles and diaphragm).

Respiratory rate and effort can be affected by disease of the respiratory tract, respiratory center of the brain, or respiratory muscles. Thoracic trauma (e.g., diaphragm rupture, pressure on the diaphragm, rib fractures, intercostal muscle damage) can hinder respiration from pain and also by disrupting the mechanics of breathing. Metabolic changes leading to acid-base imbalances and pain can cause abnormal breathing.

The first subtle sign of respiratory distress is increased respiratory rate. This is followed by a change in respiratory pattern, which is determined by the site of the injury or disease. Difficult or labored breathing is called dyspnea. As distress progresses, the patient assumes various postures in attempts to bring relief, followed by open-mouth and labored breathing. With increasing respiratory distress, the patient assumes a posture that aids the respiratory effort. Cats often crouch, with the sternum elevated. Dogs extend their necks, abduct their elbows, and arch their backs. Cyanosis (bluish mucosae) is a late sign of respiratory distress and is often followed quickly by death.

Respiratory patterns can suggest the anatomic site of disease and guide lifesaving intervention. Stridor (loud breathing heard without the aid of a stethoscope) indicates upper airway disease (nasal passages, larynx/pharynx, trachea). Inspiratory stridor should direct investigation to the extrathoracic airways, especially the larynx. Expiratory stridor is usually due to intrathoracic tracheal changes. Rapid, shallow breathing suggests infringement of the pleural space (e.g., by air or fluid). Labored breathing on both inspiration and expiration is most typical of lung parenchymal disease. Distress on expiration, with a short inspiration, directs attention to the small airways.

Auscultation can help distinguish pleural disease from lung disease. Moist lung sounds suggest fluid in lung tissues. Dry, coarse sounds on inspiration and expiration suggest fibrosis of the lung. Absence of lung sounds indicates interruption of sound transmission by air or fluid in the pleural space.

In general, respiratory rates below 8 or above 30 per minute are considered abnormal (see Table 17-1). Low respiratory rates can be caused by trauma to the brain or spinal cord, diseases affecting respiratory drive (e.g., chronic obstructive pulmonary disease, low blood carbon dioxide level), or drugs (e.g., sedatives). Increased respiratory rates can be caused by fever, pain, anxiety, trauma to the brain or chest, metabolic alterations (e.g., alkalosis), pulmonary disease (e.g., pneumonia or edema of the lungs), and drugs (e.g., oxymorphone).

Heart rate

An increase in heart rate and contractility increases the force and volume of blood flow to tissues. Tachycardia can be normal or may be associated with shock, stress, excitement, fever, or hyperthyroidism. However, when the heart rate increases above a critical level, the heart muscle becomes exhausted and coronary perfusion decreases, causing myocardial hypoxia. Cardiac arrhythmias and myocardial failure can result, leading to systemic hypoxia and organ failure.

A decreased heart rate (bradycardia) can decrease cardiac output. Causes of bradycardia include hypothermia, metabolic disorders (e.g., hyperkalemia, hypoglycemia, hypothyroidism), and parasympathetic (vagal) stimulation. Parasympathetic stimulation can occur with brain, pulmonary, and gastrointestinal diseases, or a diseased sinoatrial node. Heart rates below a critical level can lead to tissue hypoxia, organ failure, and death.

Heart rhythm

An arrhythmia is an irregular heartbeat. Arrhythmias can be detected by auscultating the heart. An abnormal conduction system or diseased heart muscle causes an arrhythmia. When ventricular contraction does not forcefully propel blood to the periphery, a pulse deficit is detected.

Not all arrhythmias are pathologic. When the ECG has a P wave associated with most QRS complexes and the QRS complexes are of normal width, the rhythm is termed supraventricular. Sinus arrhythmia is fluctuation of heart rate with respiration, decreasing with expiration and increasing with inspiration; this is normal in dogs. Ventricular rhythm is characterized by QRS complexes that are wide and bizarre and not associated with P waves. Supraventricular and ventricular arrhythmias can be subdivided into bradyarrhythmias or tachyarrhythmias.

Listen to the heart by placing the stethoscope over the left and right side of the patient's thorax at the fourth to sixth intercostal space, while palpating the pulse (Fig. 17-5). Pericardial fluid, pleural air or fluid, severe hypovolemia, or herniated abdominal organs cause muffled heart sounds. Tachycardia, bradycardia, muffled heart sounds, and pulse deficits require immediate attention by the veterinary team.

Indications of perfusion

Mucous membrane color, capillary refill time, pulse strength and quality, and body temperature reflect perfusion of (blood flow to) peripheral tissues. Blood pumped into the aorta during ventricular contraction creates a fluid wave that travels from the heart to the peripheral arteries. This wave is called a pulse. Evaluation of pulse strength is based on the difference between the systolic (heart contracting) and diastolic (heart filling) pressure, called the pulse pressure. With normal pulse pressure, the pulse is easily palpated and strong. When the difference is great, the pulse is bounding. Causes of a bounding pulse include fever, hyperthyroidism, patent ductus arteriosus, and early shock. When the difference is small or the time to maximum systolic pressure is prolonged, the pulse feels weak. Any condition that decreases cardiac output (e.g., late shock, heart failure, arrhythmia) causes a weak pulse.

The pulse is palpated by lightly placing the tips of the index and middle fingers at a site where an artery crosses over bone or firm tissue. The most common pulse points assessed are the femoral and dorsal pedal arteries. In cats, both femoral pulses should be assessed simultaneously to detect caudal aortic obstruction, as seen with a saddle thrombus. In large animals, the pulse can be assessed where the facial artery crosses the ventral border of the mandible.

A bounding pulse may reflect pain, fever, or early shock, and it indicates the need for intervention with analgesics (pain relievers) and fluid replacement. A weak pulse is cause for immediate concern and warrants aggressive measures to

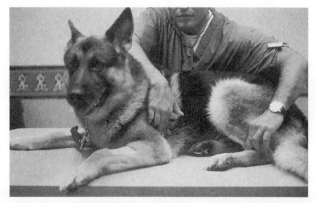

Fig. 17-5 The pulse can be evaluated while the thorax is auscultated. Any difference between heart and pulse is termed a *pulse deficit.*

improve cardiac output (e.g., IV fluids for shock, appropriate cardiac medications for heart failure).

Capillary refill time is the time required for blood to refill capillaries after displacement by finger pressure. Prompt refilling of capillaries depends on cardiac output and vascular tone.

To measure the capillary refill time, apply pressure with the index finger to an unpigmented area of mucous membrane and then release. The time for the color to return to the blanched area is the capillary refill time. Normal values are 1 to 2 seconds. A prolonged capillary refill time (more than 2 seconds) suggests poor peripheral perfusion (e.g., late shock, severe vasodilation or vasoconstriction, pericardial effusion, heart failure). A short capillary refill time (less than 1 second) can be related to anxiety, compensatory shock, fever, and pain.

Although mucous membrane color is most commonly assessed by examining the gums, one can also use the conjunctiva of the eye and the membranes of the vulva and penis. The normal pink color of unpigmented mucous membranes requires adequate blood hemoglobin concentration, tissue oxygen tension, and peripheral capillary blood flow (Table 17-2). Pale gums with prolonged capillary refill time warrant oxygen administration and a rapid search for the underlying cause. Patients with these signs may require aggressive fluid therapy.

Evaluating body temperature

The body maintains its normal temperature by balancing heat production with heat loss through a thermostatic feedback mechanism in the hypothalamus. This mechanism can be altered by disease of the central nervous system or other illness. Chemical substances released in disease can affect the thermoregulatory center and increase the metabolic rate, elevating the body temperature. These chemicals may be pyrogens secreted by bacteria or cytokines associated with inflammation. Brain disease (e.g., cerebral edema, neurosurgery, trauma, tumors) can reset the thermostat to a higher level.

Hyperthermia (increased body temperature) increases tissue oxygen requirements. The body responds by increasing ventilation to release body heat. Cerebral vasoconstriction and brain hypoxia can develop if the blood carbon dioxide levels fall too low from hyperventilation. Cardiac work and oxygen demands increase. Peripheral vessels dilate in an effort to release heat. Damage to vascular cells can lead to disseminated intravascular coagulation, sloughing of the gastrointestinal mucosa, bacterial translocation, and hypovolemia.

Hypothermia (decreased body temperature) reduces the metabolic rate, enzyme functions, oxygen consumption, and the ability of hemoglobin to release oxygen to tissues. Hypothermia can cause peripheral vasoconstriction, decreased heart rate, and hypotension. Gastrointestinal motility is decreased, and ileus (lack of bowel motility) may occur.

Body temperature should be monitored from a single site, usually the rectum (see Table 17-1). Serial readings are more informative than a single reading. Other sites include the axillary and inguinal regions. Readings in these areas generally are 1 to 2 degrees lower than the rectal temperature. Body temperatures can also be measured with an ear probe inserted carefully into the external ear canal. Serial temperatures taken from the same area are more important than single values.

SYSTEMATIC APPROACH TO PHYSICAL EXAMINATION

After the vitals are recorded, proceed to the physical examination, beginning at the tip of the nose and concluding at the tip of the tail. The examination can be divided into several areas: head and neck; trunk and forelimbs; thorax; abdomen; hind limbs, and external genitalia and perineum.

TABLE 17-2

Interpretation of Mucous Membrane Color

Membrane Color	Interpretation	Causes
Pink	Normal	Adequate perfusion and oxygenation or peripheral tissues
Pale	Anemia poor perfusion vasoconstriction	Blood loss, shock vasopressors
Blue	Cyanosis, inadequate oxygenation	Hypoxemia
Brick red	Hyperdynamic perfusion vasodilation	Early shock sepsis, fever systemic inflammatory response syndrome
Icteric	Bilirubin accumulation	Hepatic/biliary disorder, hemolysis
Brown	Methemoglobinemia	Acetaminophen toxicity in cats
Petechiae or ecchymoses	Coagulation disorder	Platelet disorder, disseminated intravascular coagulation, coagulation factor deficiencies

Examination of the Head and Neck

Observing the patient at arm's length allows comparison of the two sides of the face and head for symmetry. Look for unilateral (one-sided) facial paralysis and unilateral or bilateral (two-sided) nasal/ocular discharge, and note any irregularities in head shape or size.

Assess the eyes for size, position, and any discharge. Observe for ectropion (everted eyelids) or entropion (inverted eyelids). Assess pupil size and the response to light. Check the cornea for clarity and contour, looking for scars, ulcers, infiltrates, and pigmentation. Assess the color and condition of the sclera and conjunctiva. Note any signs of jaundice, hemorrhage, or increased vascularization.

Evaluate the nose and nares for symmetry and conformation, as well as evidence of nasal discharge. If there is swelling evident or a history of chronic nasal discharge, determine patency of the nares. If the patient allows it, close the mouth, cover one nostril first and then the other, and assess nasal airflow. Note any areas with increased malleability of facial bones.

Check the lips for areas of inflammation, swelling, masses, or lip-fold pyoderma. Retract the lips and assess the oral mucosa and gingival tissues for color, capillary refill time, inflammation, jaundice, and ulcers. Check for fractured, missing, or loose teeth and periodontal disease. Assess the soft and hard palates for tumors, ulcerations, and foreign bodies.

Evaluate the carriage and position of the ears, thickness and malleability of the pinnae, and cleanliness of the ear canals. Check for odors, fluid, or exudate in the ear canal. Patients exhibiting pain or discomfort during examination of the ear canal should have a more detailed otoscopic examination.

After examining the ears, palpate the cervical and mandibular lymph nodes, salivary glands, larynx, and thyroid gland. Palpate the trachea to determine if it is on the midline. In patients with inspiratory dyspnea, gently palpate the trachea to detect tracheal ring abnormalities. A sustained cough, retching, or gagging after gentle compression of the larynx and trachea is abnormal.

Examination of the Trunk and Forelimbs

Palpate each forelimb, feeling for abnormalities in angulation, deformities, swelling, bleeding, bony protrusions, obvious fractures, or joint luxations. Assess both limbs in weight-bearing and non–weight-bearing positions. Assess for masses or lymph node abnormalities. Palpate for points of tenderness, stiffness, or crepitus at the joints. Note the condition of the feet, nails, or hooves; nail bed or hoof color may give an indication of perfusion. Palpate both brachial pulses for quality and strength. Examine the haircoat for alopecia (hair loss), eruptions, parasites, dryness, or excessive oil. Palpate for any skin masses or lacerations. Assess the elasticity of the skin.

Examination of the Thorax

Observe the patient's respiratory rate, effort, and depth. Look for evidence of dyspnea, such as rapid open-mouth breathing, increased effort, an increased abdominal component, abnormal posture to assist in breathing, and cyanosis.

Observe and palpate the thorax for conformation, symmetry, and movement of the ribs, sternum, or vertebral column. Palpate for masses. Palpate the area between the fourth and sixth intercostal spaces on both sides of the thorax for the point of maximum intensity of the heartbeat and cardiac thrills.

Assess the respiratory tract. Listen for noisy breathing at the mouth and nares without the use of a stethoscope. Use a stethoscope to auscultate the lungs. Divide each side of the thorax (left and right) in four quadrants: *craniodorsal, caudodorsal, cranioventral,* and *caudoventral.* Begin by auscultating the right side at the craniodorsal quadrant, and continue in a clockwise fashion. Then do the same on the left side.

Normal respiratory sounds are described as *vesicular* or *bronchial,* depending on where they are auscultated. Vesicular sounds are heard over normal lung parenchyma and are produced by movement of air through small bronchi, bronchioles, and alveoli. Vesicular sounds are best heard on inspiration. They have been described as resembling the sound made by wind blowing through trees or the sound of rustling leaves. Bronchial sounds are produced by movement of air through the trachea and large bronchi. They are usually heard over the area of the trachea and carina, most noticeably during expiration.

Abnormal lung sounds include crackles (sometimes referred to as rales), wheezes, dull lung sounds, or muffled lung sounds. Crackles are usually caused by air movement through small airways within the lumen reduced by fluid, mucus, or thickened walls. Dry crackles are associated with passage of air through relatively solid material in the bronchi or trachea. Moist crackles are caused by passage of air through fluid material. Crackles are mostly heard in such conditions as pulmonary edema, bronchopneumonia, and pulmonary fibrosis. Wheezes are high-pitched, musical sounds heard mostly on expiration. They are associated with infectious or allergic bronchitis (e.g., asthma in cats). Dull or muffled lung sounds may be due to collapse or consolidation of a lung lobe, tension pneumothorax, pneumomediastinum, hydrothorax, pyothorax, a mass displacing the lung, or diaphragmatic hernia.

Cardiac auscultation can detect murmurs, arrhythmias, and muffled heart sounds. When assessing murmurs, it is important to determine in which quadrant the murmur is the loudest; this helps identify the valvular area involved. Arrhythmias most commonly detected are sinus arrhythmia (normal), atrial fibrillation, heart block, premature ventricular contractions, and gallop rhythm. Muffled heart sounds can be due to obesity, pericardial effusion, pleural effusion, an intrathoracic mass, or diaphragmatic hernia.

Examination of the Abdomen

The abdomen should be inspected for distention, deformity, displacement, symmetry, and bruising. In trauma patients, examine the umbilicus for red discoloration, suggestive of intra-abdominal bleeding. If the abdomen is distended, use percussion to determine if the distention is due to peritoneal effusion, gastric dilatation or volvulus, an intra-abdominal mass, or obesity. Percussion that produces tympanic sounds suggests gastric or small intestinal obstruction and gas entrapment.

Auscultate the abdomen to detect intestinal hypermotility (increased frequency or intensity of intestinal sounds) or hypomotility (decreased frequency or intensity of intestinal sounds). Absence of bowel sounds suggests ileus (lack of intestinal motility) or a fluid-filled abdomen.

The abdomen of most small animals can be readily palpated, but this may not be feasible in patients with tense abdominal muscles. Abdominal palpation in large animals is more in the form of *ballottement*, in which the fist is rhythmically pressed into an area of the abdomen in an attempt to "bump" any large underlying masses or organs.

Palpate the abdomen in an orderly fashion. Divide the abdomen into three areas: cranial, middle, and caudal. Start the procedure at the cranial portion, and conclude at the caudal portion. Palpate the cranial abdomen to assess the stomach, duodenum, biliary structures, liver, and the area of the pancreas (seeking pain on palpation). In the midabdominal area, assess the spleen, kidneys, adrenal glands, mesenteric lymph nodes, and intestines. Organs assessed upon caudal abdominal palpation are the urinary bladder, prostate, uterus (in the intact female if enlarged), and colon. A normal uterus is not ordinarily palpable.

Examination of the Hind Limbs

Palpate each hind limb, feeling for abnormalities in angulation, deformities, swelling, bleeding, bony protrusions, obvious fractures, or joint luxations. Assess both limbs in weight-bearing and non–weight-bearing positions. Assess for masses or lymph node abnormalities. Note the position of the patellas when assessing the stifle. Palpate the popliteal lymph nodes for size and consistency. Palpate for points of tenderness, stiffness, or crepitus at joints. Also evaluate muscle mass and tone.

Palpate the pelvic region for conformation and symmetry. Palpate the vertebral column to assess for deviations and pain.

Examination of External Genitalia and Perineum

In males, inspect the prepuce and penis, noting any discharge. In dogs, expose the penis by retracting the preputial sheath. Look for masses and evidence of trauma, and note any color abnormalities (such as jaundice or bruising). If the patient is intact (not castrated), inspect both testicles for symmetry, size, location (within the scrotum), and conformation. If you detect only one testicle (cryptorchidism), palpate the inguinal area and caudal abdominal region for a retained testicle. A rectal examination to determine texture, size, and conformation of the prostate is done by the veterinarian.

Female genital examination includes inspection and palpation of the mammary glands for tumors or cysts. In the lactating bitch or female dogs in pseudopregnancy, determine if there is evidence of mastitis or milk. In lactating cows, palpate for excessive heat and areas of firmness (induration). A California mastitis test can quickly assess the milk of lactating cows. Inspect the vulva for any discharge (blood, pus), polyps, tumors, or structural defects.

Rectal examination is done with a finger in small animals and with the hand and arm in large animals. Assess the sublumbar lymph nodes in the dorsal aspect of the pelvic canal. Feel for evidence of pelvic fracture and note anal tone and fecal consistency. Check for masses in the pelvic canal and caudal abdomen. In large animals, feel for displaced or distended loops of bowel, and assess the kidneys, if within reach.

Inspect the perianal area for hair mats, hernias, feces, masses, and evidence of discharge. In dogs, palpate for impacted or abscessed anal sacs.

PHYSICAL EXAMINATION IN EMERGENCIES

Triage, Primary Survey, and Secondary Survey

The procedure called *triage* (French for "to sort") is used to classify patients according to the severity of illness or injury to determine their relative priority for treatment. In its original application in combat, triage was used by French military medical personnel to sort wounded soldiers into three categories: those that would survive without immediate treatment; those that would die despite immediate treatment; and those that would survive only if given immediate treatment. Emergency treatment of only the last group (those likely to survive) allowed them to salvage the most lives using limited resources.

In veterinary medicine, triage is used primarily in emergency situations. It can also be used in the critical care setting as a means of prioritization and assessment, and it guides the veterinary care team in efficient delivery of medical and patient care. Using triage, the treatment team focuses initially on life-threatening conditions (e.g., an obstructed airway or massive external hemorrhage) and institutes immediate measures to correct them with the most efficient use of available manpower and skills. A primary survey is used to detect any life-threatening problems.

A secondary survey is used to broaden the evaluation to include all organ systems in a progressive, detailed manner. In triage of multiple patients (e.g., after a barn fire or horse trailer accident, or in a busy emergency clinic), those with a compromised airway, breathing difficulties, and/or circulatory problems (ABCs) should be assessed and treated first.

Vital signs assessed during triage include level of consciousness, respiratory rate and effort, heart rate and rhythm, and indications of perfusion (pulse, mucous membrane color, capillary refill time, temperature). These vital signs can indicate trends of deterioration, warning the team of complications. Vital signs should be assessed at frequent, regular intervals to detect trends, using initial values as the baseline.

In the emergency setting, no disease, injury, or physiologic abnormality should be considered as an isolated entity. The team should consider the current status, physiologic reserve, and potential for deterioration of each organ system or problem, rather than just the primary problem (e.g., fractured femur), and develop a plan of action.

During the primary survey and initial management, life-threatening conditions are addressed in the following order of priority:

1. Airway patency (open airway)
2. Breathing
3. Circulation
4. Neurologic deficit assessment

During the primary survey, neurologic status can be evaluated with the aid of the acronym AVPU: Is the patient Alert and aware of its surroundings? Is it Voice responsive? Is it Pain responsive? Is it Unresponsive?

After the ABC areas have been addressed and resuscitation measures have been initiated, the secondary survey is performed. Vital signs are reassessed, and the patient is rapidly and thoroughly examined from head to tail. The thorax, abdomen, pelvis, and extremities are visually inspected, palpated, and auscultated where appropriate. Neurologic status is repeatedly assessed. Appropriate radiographic and laboratory studies are obtained. Other diagnostic procedures that may be done at this time include, but are not limited to, an ECG, measurement of blood pressure and central venous pressure, and pulse oximetry.

Classification system for triage

When dealing with more than one emergency or critically ill patient, the team can use a classification system based on the nature of the presenting complaint, as well as vital signs assessed during triage.

Class I. Patients in class I must receive treatment immediately and are usually those suffering from acute trauma, respiratory or cardiorespiratory arrest or failure, or airway obstruction, or are unconscious. Class I patients may be dying before your eyes. They are usually in a decompensatory stage of shock. The decompensatory stage of shock is characterized by cyanosis, ashen white mucous membranes, prolonged capillary refill time or no capillary refill, cold skin, a decreased rectal temperature, weak or undetectable femoral pulses, and oliguria (reduced urine production). They may be unconscious, stuporous, or losing consciousness. The bleeding patient may have seizures as a result of low blood pressure if the hemorrhage is substantial.

Class II. Patients in class II are critically ill. These patients are suffering from multiple injuries, shock, or severe bleeding but have adequate respiratory function. They require treatment within minutes to an hour. They may be in a mild state of shock. Mild shock is characterized by pale or ashen mucous membranes, prolonged capillary refill time, cool skin, a decreased rectal temperature, and weak femoral pulses. Class II patients may show tachycardia, oliguria, and altered mentation (e.g., depression, seizures, excitation). Hemorrhage may be profuse or a slow trickle.

Class III. Patients in class III are seriously ill but not critically ill. These patients usually have severe open wounds or fractures, burns, penetrating wounds to the abdomen without active bleeding, or blunt trauma. They are not in shock or exhibiting an altered level of consciousness. They require treatment within a few hours.

Class IV. Patients in class IV are less seriously ill but are still of concern. This classification does not apply to most trauma patients. The mucous membranes may be red or pale pink and capillary refill time under 1 second. The skin and rectal temperatures are normal, and femoral pulses are normal or bounding. These patients often have normal respiration, tachycardia or a normal heart rate, normal urine output, and normal mentation, evidenced by alertness and awareness of their surroundings. Usually these patients are mildly depressed to slightly excited and generally are not actively hemorrhaging. Class IV patients require treatment within 24 hours.

RECOMMENDED READING

Allen DG, Kruth SA, Garvey MS, eds: *Small animal medicine*, Philadelphia, 1991, Lippincott, Williams & Wilkins.

Edwards NE: *Basic principles of electrocardiography: ECG manual for the veterinary technician*, Philadelphia, 1993, Saunders.

Grenvik A, Ayers SM, et al., ed: *Textbook of critical care*, ed 4, Philadelphia, 2000, Saunders.

Hall JB, Schmidt GA, Wood LDH, eds: *Principles of critical care*, New York, 1992, McGraw-Hill.

Harkness JE, Wagner JE, eds: Biology and husbandry. In *The biology and medicine of rabbits and rodents*, ed 4, Philadelphia, 1995, Lippincott, Williams & Wilkins.

Kirby R: Approach to the trauma patient. *Waltham Sympos Treatment Sm Anim Dis: Emerg Crit Care*, 1990.

Lorenz MD, Cornelius LM, eds: *Small animal medical diagnosis*, ed 2, Philadelphia, 1993, Lippincott, Williams & Wilkins.

Low DG: General examination of dogs, *Vet Clin North Am* 1:3-14, 1971.

McQuillan KA, et al., eds: *Trauma nursing, from resuscitation through rehabilitation*, ed 3, Philadelphia, 2001, Saunders.

The Merck veterinary manual: clinical values and procedures, Rahway, N.J., 1998, Merck.

Murtaugh RJ, Kaplan PM, eds: *Veterinary emergency and critical care medicine*, St Louis, 1992, Mosby.

Nelson RW, Couto GC, eds: *Small animal internal medicine*, ed 3, St Louis, 2003, Mosby.

Pratt, PW: *Medical, surgical, and anesthetic nursing*, ed 2, St Louis, 1994, Mosby.

Rivera AM, Rudloff E, Kirby R: Monitoring the ICU patient, *Vet Technician* 17:27-43, 1996.

18

Diagnostic Imaging

Connie M. Han, Cheryl D. Hurd, and Christine Royce-Bretz

Learning Objectives

After reviewing this chapter, the reader should understand the following:

- Anatomy and function of x-ray machines
- Way in which x-rays are produced
- Factors affecting radiographic quality
- Techniques and devices used to optimize radiographic quality
- Dangers of radiation and how to avoid radiation injury
- Procedures used to develop radiographs
- Positioning of animals for radiographs
- Basic physics of ultrasound
- Anatomy and function of ultrasound machines
- Techniques used to produce high-quality sonograms

RADIOGRAPHY
Connie Han and Cheryl Hurd

X-RAY GENERATION

X-rays are a form of electromagnetic radiation. X-rays are similar to visible light, but they have a shorter wavelength. X-rays are generated when fast-moving electrons collide with any form of matter. The x-ray tube of an x-ray machine projects a stream of electrons toward a metal target. The energy of the electrons interacting with the atoms of the target is converted to heat (99%) and x-radiation (1 %). Heat generation in the x-ray tube is a limiting factor in the production of x-rays. This is why high-output x-ray machines have rotating anode x-ray tubes.

X-RAY TUBE ANATOMY

The x-ray tube contains a heated tungsten filament in the *cathode*, where the electrons are generated, and an *anode* containing a tungsten target where x-rays are generated. Both are enclosed in a vacuum-filled glass envelope. A beryllium window in the glass envelope allows x-rays to pass with minimal filtration. An aluminum filter is placed across the window to absorb the low-energy (soft) x-rays, while allowing the more energetic and useful x-rays to form the x-ray beam. The entire tube is surrounded by oil, which acts as an electrical barrier while absorbing heat generated by the tube. The tube and oil are encased in a metal housing to prevent damage to the glass envelope and to absorb stray radiation (Fig. 18-1). The tungsten filament is housed within a focusing cup to focus the beam of electrons on the focal spot of the anode. The focal spot is the tungsten metal plate where the x-rays are generated. The focal spot is oriented at an angle of 11° to 20°.

Anode Heel Effect

Anode heel effect is the unequal distribution of the x-ray beam intensity emitted from the x-ray tube. Tubes with lower target angles (e.g., 11°) have a distribution of x-ray beam intensity that decreases rapidly on the anode side of the tube (Fig. 18-2). This is caused by absorption of the x-ray beam by the target and by anode material. This can be used to advantage when radiographing areas of unequal thickness, such as the thorax or abdomen. By placing the patient's head toward the anode side, the part of the x-ray beam with the higher intensity (cathode side) is directed to the thickest area. This produces a more even film density. The heel effect is most noticeable when large films and short focal-film distances are used.

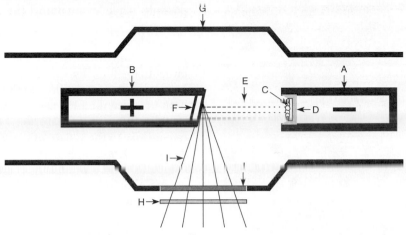

Fig. 18-1 Anatomy of an x-ray tube. **A,** Cathode. **B,** Anode. **C,** Tungsten filament. **D,** Focusing cup. **E,** Accelerating electrons. **F,** Tungsten target. **G,** Glass envelope. **H,** Aluminum filter. **I,** Generated x-rays. **J,** Beryllium window.

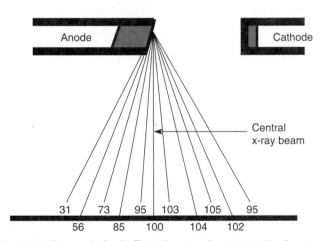

Fig. 18-2 The anode heel effect. The x-ray beam intensity decreases toward the anode side because of absorption by the target and anode material.

RADIOGRAPHIC QUALITY

Radiographic Density

Radiographic density is the degree of blackness on a radiograph. The dark areas are made up of black metallic silver deposits on the finished radiograph. These deposits occur in areas where x-rays have penetrated the patient and exposed the emulsion of the film. Radiographic density can be increased by increasing the mA (milliamperage) or the exposure time. Either one increases the number of x-rays produced by increasing the number of electrons in the electron cloud or the time the electrons are allowed to travel from the cathode to the anode. A higher kilovoltage peak (kVp) yields more radiographic density by increasing the penetrating power of the x-ray beam.

Radiographic Contrast

Radiographic contrast is defined as the differences in radiographic density between adjacent areas on a radiographic image. Radiographs that show a long scale of contrast have a few black and white shades, with many shades of gray. A short scale of contrast has black-and-white shades, with only a few shades of gray in between. For most studies, a long scale of contrast is desirable. Obtaining a long scale of radiographic contrast depends on four factors: subject density, kVp level, film contrast, and film fogging.

Subject density is the ability of the different tissue densities to absorb x-rays. The extent to which x-rays penetrate the various tissues depends on the differences in atomic number and thickness. On radiographs, air is least radiodense, followed in increasing radiodensity by fat, water and muscle, bone and metal, the last being most radiodense (Fig. 18-3). Bone, containing mainly calcium and phosphorus, has a high average atomic number as compared with muscle, which contains mainly hydrogen and nitrogen. Bone absorbs more x-rays than muscle and appears whiter on the finished radiograph. The thickness of the area also affects the number of x-rays absorbed. If you radiograph an area that ranges from 5 to 20 cm in thickness, the 20-cm–thick area absorbs more x-rays than the 5-cm area.

The scale of radiographic contrast can be lengthened or shortened by increasing or decreasing the kVp. As kVp increases, the scale of contrast gets longer (more grays can be visualized). Radiographs made with a high kVp have more exposure latitude, allowing minor errors in technique without affecting the diagnostic quality of the radiograph.

Film contrast also affects radiographic contrast. Some types of film can produce a long scale of contrast or long latitude. Long latitude film allows for more variation in technique while still producing a diagnostic radiograph. The scale of contrast can be shortened by changing the exposure

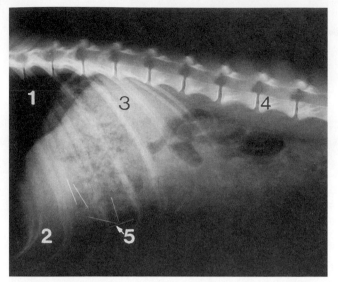

Fig. 18-3 Subject densities: *1,* Air. *2,* Fat. *3,* Water. *4,* Bone. *5,* Metal. Air is least dense, allowing x-rays to penetrate and expose the film. Metal is the most dense, absorbing most of the x-rays and allowing only a few to penetrate, exposing the film.

technique when using long-latitude film. However, the scale of contrast cannot be lengthened when using contrast film (film that produces a short scale of contrast).

Film fogging can greatly decrease radiographic contrast by decreasing the differences in densities between two adjacent shadows. Care must be taken in the storage and handling of x-ray film to prevent fogging. Film can become fogged from low-grade light leaks in the darkroom, scatter radiation, heat, and improper processing.

Radiographic Detail

A diagnostic radiograph is one with good radiographic detail. Radiographic detail is considered to be good when the interfaces between tissues and organs are sharp. Many factors can affect the detail on a radiograph. The most common are patient motion and the penumbra effect.

Patient motion causes loss of detail because of blurred interfaces. A blurred image is generally a result of long exposure time combined with motion of the patient. This can be controlled by using the shortest possible exposure. If the image remains blurred, the patient should be sedated.

A loss of detail is also caused by the penumbra effect. Excessive penumbra causes blurring at the edges of the shadows cast by the x-ray exposure. Three main factors influence the amount of penumbra on a radiograph. Changes in these factors increase or decrease the radiographic detail. The first factor is the size of the focal spot. The larger the focal spot is, the more pronounced the penumbra effect. Decreasing the focal spot size decreases the penumbra; however, this cannot be changed on most equipment. Manufacturers design the focal spot as small as

possible while maintaining the ability to dissipate heat effectively.

Another factor that affects the amount of penumbra is the focal-film distance (FFD). This is the distance from the target to the film. The penumbra effect can be decreased by increasing the focal-film distance (Fig. 18-4). There is a limit to which the FFD can be increased because of what is stated in the inverse square law. The intensity decreases at a rate inverse to the square of the distance. In simpler terms, if the FFD is doubled, the mAs (a product of the milliamperage and exposure time) must increase four times to maintain the same radiographic density. In most cases this is not practical, because the shortest possible exposure times are necessary to counteract patient motion. An FFD of 36 to 40 inches is sufficient to minimize the penumbra effect.

The third factor that affects penumbra is the object-film distance (OFD). This is the distance from the object being imaged to the film. The penumbra is decreased by keeping the OFD as short as possible (Fig. 18-5). Using a combination of these factors, the penumbra can be minimized and good radiographic detail achieved.

Distortion

Foreshortening occurs when the object is not parallel to the recording surface. This distorts size by shortening the length of the object. This occurs mainly when imaging the long bones, such as the humerus or femur. If one end of the bone is farther from the recording surface than the other, the bone appears shorter. The object being radiographed must be parallel to the recording surface and the OFD as short as possible. Increasing the OFD increases the penumbra and greatly magnifies the size of the object. The degree of magnification increases as the distance to the recording surface increases.

It is important to accurately project areas between a series of radiodense and radiolucent objects. The vertebral column is a good example. The vertebrae must be parallel to the recording surface. When radiographing the cervical vertebrae in lateral recumbency, if the patient is allowed to lie naturally, the midcervical vertebrae tend to sag. This produces false narrowing of the intervertebral spaces. A small amount of padding beneath the patient brings the vertebral column parallel to the recording surface. Care must be taken not to use too much padding because this can elevate the spinal column, also producing false narrowing of the intervertebral spaces.

Distortion can also occur when the x-ray beam is not perpendicular to the recording surface. X-rays in the center of the primary beam penetrate perpendicular to the intervertebral spaces. As the distance from the center of the primary beam increases, the x-rays strike the intervertebral spaces at an increasing angle. False narrowing of the intervertebral space occurs because of this increase in distance

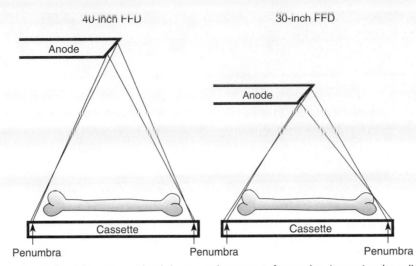

Fig. 18-4 Increasing the focal-film distance (FFD) decreases the amount of penumbra, increasing the radiographic detail.

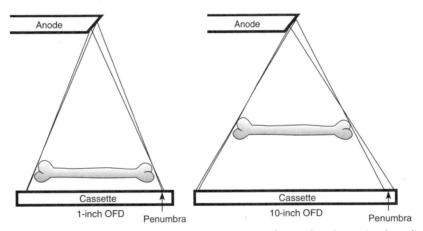

Fig. 18-5 Increasing the object-film distance (OFD) increases the amount of penumbra, decreasing the radiographic detail.

from the center of the primary beam (Fig. 18-6). To combat such distortion, sometimes it is necessary to make multiple images of the vertebral column, centering the primary beam over multiple areas. This type of distortion is also apparent when radiographing complex joints, such as the stifle and elbow. When imaging these areas, be sure the center of the primary beam is directly over the joint.

Scatter Radiation

When an x-ray photon strikes an object, it can do one of three things. It can penetrate the object, be absorbed by the object, or produce scatter radiation. Scatter radiation fogs the film, greatly decreasing the contrast. It also is a safety hazard to patients and personnel. Scatter radiation is projected in all directions. Exposure techniques that use a high kVp produce more scatter radiation. Body parts measuring 10 cm or more produce enough scatter radiation to significantly decrease detail on the radiograph.

Beam-limiting devices are commonly used to decrease scatter radiation by confining the primary beam to the area being examined. Several types of beam-limiting devices are available. *Cones* are lead cylinders placed over the collimator on the x-ray tube head. This restricts the primary beam to the size of cone used. *Diaphragms* are sheets of lead with a rectangular, square, or circular opening that limits the size of the primary beam to the size of diaphragm used. *Collimators* consist of adjustable lead shutters installed in the tube head of the x-ray machine. Finally, *filters* are used to absorb the less penetrating or soft x-rays as they leave the tube head. Filters are made of a thin sheet of aluminum and are placed over the tube window.

Grids

Grids are used to decrease scatter radiation and increase the contrast on the radiograph. As the thickness of the area being imaged increases, the amount of kVp required also

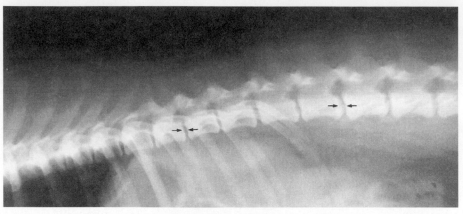

Fig. 18-6 The intervertebral spaces appear narrow toward the edges of the radiograph *(arrows)* as compared with the spaces in the center of the radiograph.

increases. As the kVp increases, more scatter radiation is produced. To minimize scatter radiation, grids are necessary when radiographing areas 10 cm or more in thickness.

A grid is a series of thin, linear strips made of alternating radiodense and radiolucent material. The radiodense strips are made of lead, whereas the radiolucent interspacers are plastic, aluminum, or fiber. The grid is placed between the patient and the cassette. X-rays that penetrate the patient and pass in perfect alignment between the lead strips expose the film. Scatter radiation diverges in all directions and is more likely to be absorbed by one of the lead strips.

The grid also absorbs a portion of the usable x-rays. To compensate for this loss, the number of x-rays generated must be increased by increasing the mAs. Depending on the type of grid used, the increase may be up to 6.6 times the mAs required for the tabletop exposure.

Grids are manufactured with either parallel or focused lead strips arranged in crossed or linear configuration.

Parallel grids have the lead strips placed perpendicular to the grid surface. X-rays and scatter radiation that interact with the lead strips are absorbed, whereas the ones that interact with the interspacers pass through to expose the film. A disadvantage of a parallel grid is that the x-ray beam diverges at increasing angles and is absorbed at the periphery of the grid. This decreases the number of x-rays reaching the film near the grid edges, commonly called grid cutoff.

Focused grids have the lead strips placed at progressively increasing angles to match the divergence of the x-ray beam. By angling the lead strips, cutoff of the primary beam is eliminated and radiographic density is uniform. The grid manufacturer supplies a list of distances, called the grid focal distance. Setting the FFD out of the grid focal distance results in primary beam cutoff on the periphery of the radiograph. Cutoff of the primary beam also occurs if the grid is not perpendicular to or centered with the x-ray tube (Fig. 18-7).

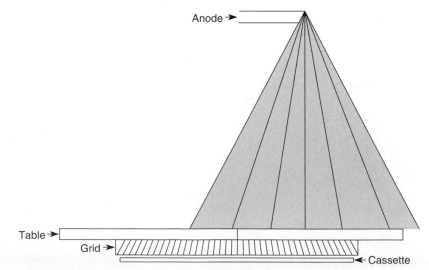
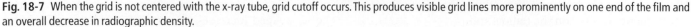

Fig. 18-7 When the grid is not centered with the x-ray tube, grid cutoff occurs. This produces visible grid lines more prominently on one end of the film and an overall decrease in radiographic density.

Linear grids have the lead strips placed parallel to each other and parallel with the length of the table. With linear grids, the primary x-ray beam can be angled along the length of the grid without absorption of x-rays by the lead strips.

Crossed grids have two linear grids placed one on top of the other. The lead strips on the top grid cross those on the bottom grid. This type of grid removes more scatter radiation than the linear grid. However, the tube cannot be tilted without producing cutoff. Because crossed grids contain more lead, more x-rays are absorbed, requiring a higher mAs than used with linear grids.

Grids produce thin white lines on the finished radiograph. Visibility of the grid lines can be decreased in three ways. First, the lead strips can be made as thin as possible while retaining the ability to effectively absorb scatter radiation. The thinner the lead is, the thinner the white line is that it produces on the radiograph.

The second way is to increase the number of grid lines per inch, making the individual lines less visible. To increase the grid lines per inch and keep the thickness of the lead the same, the width of the radiolucent strips must be decreased. This produces a grid with more lead in it, which absorbs more of the primary beam and requires a higher mAs. A grid with 80 to 100 lines per inch is sufficient to make the grid lines less visible.

The third way is by using a Potter-Bucky diaphragm, also called a Bucky. This device sets the grid in motion as the x-rays are generated, blurring the white grid lines on the radiograph. The Bucky is placed in a cabinet beneath the x-ray table, with a tray to hold the cassette. When using a grid in combination with a Bucky, fewer lines per inch are necessary. This allows for use of a lower mAs. One disadvantage of using a Bucky mechanism in veterinary medicine is the noise and vibration it produces. Some animals may object to this and struggle or move during the x-ray exposure.

Air gap technique

Scatter radiation can also be reduced using the air gap technique. This method is most useful in large-animal radiography, where use of a grid cassette may not be possible. With this technique, the FFD is increased to 6 feet and the OFD is increased to 6 inches. By increasing the OFD, the amount of scatter radiation that reaches the cassette is decreased. Increasing the FFD decreases the penumbra and magnification produced by a greater OFD. The air gap acts somewhat like a grid, allowing the scatter radiation to pass by the cassette (Fig. 18-8).

EXPOSURE VARIABLES

Four exposure factors control radiographic density, contrast, and detail. These are mAs, kVp, focal-film distance (FFD), and object-film distance (OFD). Changing one of these factors usually requires adjustments in another factor to maintain the same radiographic density.

mAs

The mAs is a product of the milliamperage and the exposure time. The milliamperage controls the number of electrons in the electron cloud generated at the filament of the

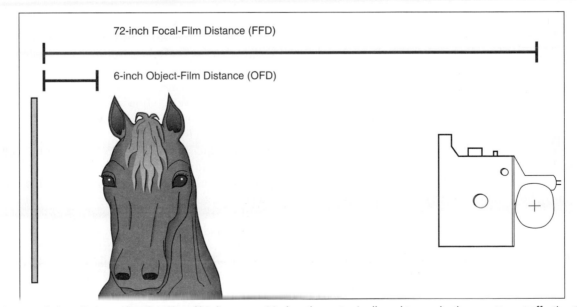

Fig. 18-8 Air gap technique. By increasing the object-film distance to 6 inches, the scatter is allowed to pass by the cassette, not affecting the film. Then, increasing the focal-film distance to 72 inches decreases the magnification and penumbra that occurred from increasing the object-film distance.

cathode. This is done by controlling the temperature of the cathode filament. When the mA is increased, the temperature of the filament is increased, producing more electrons to form the electron cloud. Increasing the mA increases the amount of radiographic density, because more x-rays are generated.

The other factor is the time during which the electrons are allowed to flow from the cathode to the anode. By varying the exposure time, the number of x-rays generated is controlled. Using a longer exposure time allows the electrons more time to cross from the cathode to the anode, generating more x-rays.

Exposure time and mA are inversely related. As mA increases, the exposure time required to maintain the desired number of x-rays generated decreases. Many different combinations of mA and time can be used to produce the same mAs. For example:

$$300 \text{ mA at } \tfrac{1}{60} \text{ sec} = 5 \text{ mAs}$$
$$200 \text{ mA at } \tfrac{1}{40} \text{ sec} = 5 \text{ mAs}$$
$$100 \text{ mA at } \tfrac{1}{20} \text{ sec} = 5 \text{ mAs}$$

When faced with a choice of which mAs to use, always choose the one with the highest mA and the fastest exposure time. The mAs can be used to adjust the radiographic density by following these rules:

- To double the radiographic density, double the mAs.
- To halve the radiographic density, halve the mAs.

Kilovoltage Peak

The kilovoltage peak (kVp) is the voltage applied between the cathode and the anode. It is used to accelerate electrons flowing from the cathode toward the anode side. Increasing the kVp increases the positive charge on the anode. This causes the electrons to move faster, increasing the force of the collision with the target. This produces an x-ray beam with a shorter wavelength and more penetrating power. The correct kVp setting is determined by the thickness of the part being imaged. The thicker the part, the higher the kVp setting, because more penetration is needed. A higher kVp produces a longer scale of contrast and more exposure latitude. A greater exposure latitude allows for more variation in exposure factors, which will still produce a diagnostic radiograph. As with mAs, there are rules when changing the radiographic density with kVp:

- To double the radiographic density, increase the kVp by 20%.
- To halve the radiographic density, decrease the kVp by 16%.

Focal-Film Distance

Focal-film distance (FFD) is the distance from the target to the recording surface (film). For most radiographic procedures, this distance is held constant, around 36 to 40 inches. In some situations, the FFD must be changed. This requires changing one of the other factors to maintain radi-ographic density. The inverse square law states that the intensity of the x-ray beam is inversely proportional to the square of the distance from the source of the x-ray (see p. 360). If the FFD is doubled, the mAs must be increased four times to maintain radiographic density. The same number of x-rays must diverge to cover an area that is four times as large. Changing the FFD does not affect the penetrating power of the beam, so kVp remains constant.

Object-Film Distance

The object-film distance (OFD) is the distance from the object being imaged to the recording surface (film). This distance should be as short as possible to minimize the penumbra effect and the magnification that occurs with a long OFD.

RADIOGRAPHIC FILM AND SCREENS

X-Ray Film

X-ray film consists of three layers: a thin protective layer, an emulsion containing silver halide crystals, and a polyester film base. The first layer is a thin, clear gelatin that acts as a protective coating. This protective material helps protect the sensitive film emulsion. The second layer is the emulsion that contains finely precipitated silver halide crystals in a gelatin base.

The emulsion coats both sides of the film base. This gives the film greater sensitivity, increasing the speed, density, and contrast. By increasing the speed of the film, the exposure required to produce an image can be decreased, thus decreasing exposure of the patient and veterinary personnel. The silver halide emulsion is 90% to 99% silver bromide crystals and 1% to 10% silver iodide crystals. The gelatin that suspends the silver halide crystals is a colloid. It liquefies in high temperatures and remains solid in cool temperatures. When placed in the developing chemicals, the emulsion swells, allowing the chemicals to act on the exposed or sensitized crystals without losing the crystals. Once the emulsion is dry, it hardens again, trapping the black metallic silver. The film base is in the center of the film, giving it support. It does not produce a visible light pattern or absorb the light, although a blue tint has been added to ease eyestrain.

When the silver halide crystals are exposed to electromagnetic radiation, they become more sensitive to chemical change. These sensitized crystals are what make up the *latent image*. When the film is placed into the developer, the latent image is reduced to black metallic silver. The remaining silver halide crystals are removed in the fixer. This produces varying shades of black metallic silver and the clear film base.

Film is sensitive to all types of electromagnetic radiation. These include gamma radiation, particulate radiation (alpha and beta), x-rays, heat, and light. Film is also sensitive to excessive pressure, so care must be taken when handling and storing radiographic film.

The two types of film used in veterinary radiography are *screen-type film* and *direct exposure film*. Screen-type film is more sensitive to the light produced by intensifying screens. Two screen-type films are blue-sensitive film and green-sensitive film. Blue-sensitive film is more sensitive to light emitted from screens containing blue-light–emitting phosphors. Calcium tungstate and some rare-earth phosphors are the most common blue-light–emitting phosphors. They emit light in the ultraviolet, violet, and blue-light range. Green-sensitive film is most sensitive to light from green-light–emitting phosphors. Rare-earth phosphors are the most common green-light–emitting phosphors.

Direct-exposure film is more sensitive to direct x-rays than it is to light. Because it does not use the intensifying effect of the screens, it requires a higher mAs than screen film. General anesthesia or heavy sedation may be necessary to prevent patient motion and blurring on the radiograph because of the higher mAs. Direct-exposure film is mainly used to image the extremities or rostral mandible or maxilla, where good detail is needed. It is packaged in a paper folder enclosed in a stout lightproof envelope. Take care when handling this film, because it is protected only by paper. Pressure artifacts can easily occur. Some direct-exposure film can only be manually processed because of the thickness of the emulsion. However, some types of direct-exposure film can be processed in an automatic developer.

Film speeds are rated as high (regular or fast), average (par), and slow (detail). The faster the film, the more sensitive it is and the lower mAs it requires. High-speed film requires less exposure than slow-speed film to produce a given radiographic density. Film speed is changed by increasing the size of the silver halide crystals. High-speed film has larger silver halide crystals than average-speed or slow-speed film. The drawback to using high-speed film is that, with the larger crystal size, the image has a more granular appearance. This decreases the detail considerably. Average-speed film should be used for most veterinary radiography.

Another important feature in x-ray film is *film latitude*. This is the film's inherent ability to produce shades of gray. Film with long or increased latitude can produce images with a long scale of contrast (many shades of gray). Longer-latitude film is desirable, because it allows for greater exposure errors but still produces a diagnostic radiograph.

Proper storage and handling of the film are important to ensure a good diagnostic radiograph. Unexposed film should be stored in a cool, dry place, away from strong chemical fumes. A base fog can develop if film is stored under adverse conditions over a long period. Film is pressure-sensitive, so it should be stored on end or flat on its side.

Intensifying Screens

Intensifying screens contain fluorescent crystals bound to a cardboard or plastic base. When exposed to x-rays, they emit foci of light. Placing radiographic film in direct contact with the screens accurately records any x-rays that penetrate the patient. Approximately 95% of the film's radiographic density is due to fluorescence of the intensifying screens, and only 5% is due to direct x-ray exposure. For each x-ray photon the screen absorbs, it emits 1000 light photons, amplifying the photographic effect of the x-rays. The film is sandwiched between two screens mounted inside a lightproof cassette. The cassette holds the film in close uniform contact with the screens (Fig. 18-9).

The screens are supported by a plastic or cardboard base. Next to the base is a thin reflecting layer, which reflects the light back toward the film side or front of the screen. The third is the phosphor layer. The two most common phosphors used are calcium tungstate and compounds containing rare-earth elements. Calcium tungstate is a blue-light emitter. Some of the rare-earth phosphors also emit blue light. Lanthanum oxybromide and gadolinium oxysulfide are rare-earth phosphors that emit green light. The rare-earth phosphors differ from calcium tungstate in their increased ability to absorb x-rays and convert them into light energy. Rare earth screens allow shorter exposure time compared with a calcium tungstate screen of the same thickness. Over the phosphor layer is a thin waterproof protective coating that prevents static during cassette loading and unloading, provides physical protection, and provides a surface that can be cleaned.

Intensifying screens are available in three different speeds: high (regular), par (medium), and slow (detail or fine). High-speed screens require less exposure time as

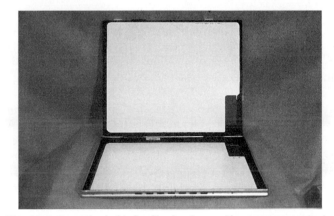

Fig. 18-9 Cassettes hold the film in close uniform contact with the screens.

compared with the par or slow speeds, but detail is decreased. With shorter exposure times, high-speed screens are ideal for imaging soft tissues, such as the thorax and abdomen, which are accompanied by unavoidable movement. Better detail can be achieved with slow-speed screens requiring longer exposure time. When changing from a high-speed screen to a par-speed screen, the mAs must be increased two times. When changing from high speed to slow speed, the mAs must be increased four times to maintain radiographic density.

Proper care of intensifying screens is very important in veterinary radiography. Regular cleaning is necessary to ensure that the screens are free from dirt and foreign material. Such material can block the light emitted from the screens, leaving parts of the film unexposed. The result is a white area on the film in the likeness of the foreign material. Identifying the cassettes on the screens and on the outside of the cassette enables the dirty cassette to be retrieved and cleaned. Processing chemicals can cause permanent damage if the screen surface is not promptly cleaned. The screens should be cleaned with a soft, lint-free cloth and screen-cleaning solution. If a commercial cleaner is not available, warm water is the next best thing. Do not use denatured alcohol or abrasive products, because they can damage the protective coating and phosphor layer. Be sure to allow the screen to completely dry before reloading.

Cassettes are precision instruments and should be handled that way. Do not drop them or set heavy objects on them. This can result in poor film-screen contact and blurring of one area of the image. To check the film-screen contact of your screens, place paper clips over the surface of the cassette. Use enough to completely cover every area. Expose the cassette using 50 to 60 kVp and half the mAs you would use for nongrid extremity. Process the film and view it dry. Any areas with poor film-screen contact are indicated by a blurred image of the paper clips.

X-RAY EQUIPMENT

There are many factors to consider when choosing x-ray equipment. The needs of individual practices vary, depending on species majority, caseload, and degree of technology desired.

There are three basic types of x-ray equipment from which to choose: portable, mobile, and stationary units. A portable unit can be carried to the animal. These machines generally have a fixed mA set by the manufacturer at 15 to 30 mA, a variable kVp ranging from 40 to 90, and exposure times as short as 1/120 second (Fig. 18-10). Portable units are ideal for large-animal extremities but can be used to radiograph some small animals. Because the mA is fixed, the exposure time is changed to increase the radiographic den-

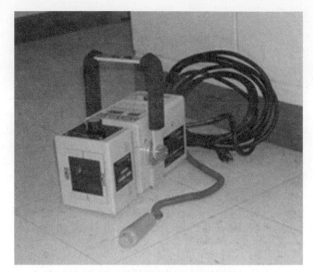

Fig. 18-10 Min X-Ray HF 8015 portable x-ray unit.

sity. For this reason, motion can be a problem for some exposures because of the prolonged exposure times.

The mobile unit can be transported to the patient; however, because of its large size, it is limited to in-hospital use, such as in the treatment room or perhaps in a driveway (Fig. 18-11). These units generally produce a maximum 300 mA, 125 kVp, and 1/120-second exposure. The tube head on a mobile unit can be lowered to the ground for large-animal radiography or suspended above a table for small-animal radiography.

Stationary units are those that are installed in a room with proper shielding for radiography. These units have many different exposure capabilities, depending on the quality desired. A general small-animal practice that does mainly routine radiographic examinations may be well-served by a machine with 300 mA, 125 kVp, and at least 1/60-second output (Fig. 18-12). However, practices that provide specialty services, such as internal medicine or surgery referrals, may require higher-output equipment.

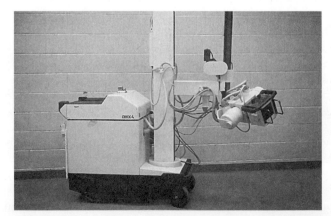

Fig. 18-11 AMX-4 mobile x-ray unit. This unit has been modified to allow the tube head to be lowered to the ground.

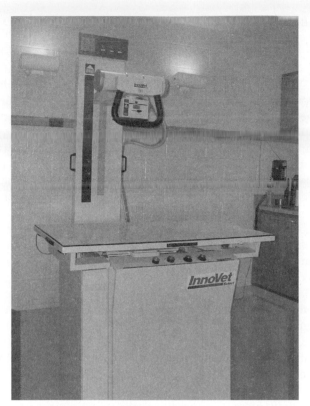

Fig. 18-12 Summit Innovet Select x-ray unit.

Caseload should be taken into account when choosing x-ray equipment. If a practice has an average of 1 to 2 cases requiring radiographs per week, with a majority of large-animal extremities and an occasional small animal film, a portable unit may be considered. If a practice has an average of 3 to 15 radiography cases per week, with a mixture of large and small animals, a mobile unit may be considered. A high-volume practice that radiographs an average of more than 16 cases per week may benefit from a stationary unit.

Accessory equipment used depends on the type of x-ray machine needed. Basic equipment requirements for a stationary x-ray machine include the x-ray–generating system, collimator, grid, table, tube stand, and positioning aids. Because most large-animal extremity radiographs are made with portable or low-output x-ray machines, tube stands and cassette holders should be used. These pieces of accessory equipment allow the individuals to be positioned farther from the primary beam, thus decreasing personal exposure. The cassettes or x-ray tubes should never be handheld.

FLUOROSCOPY

Fluoroscopy uses a device called a fluoroscope to record an x-ray image on a fluorescent screen. Fluoroscopy differs from conventional radiography in several ways. With fluo-roscopy, the x-ray tube is mounted beneath the table and a continual flow of x-rays is directed up toward a fluoroscopic screen. The image is then transferred to a monitor and can be recorded on spot film or videotape. Conventional radiography produces a single exposure from an x-ray tube suspended above the table. The image is captured on radiographic film. Fluoroscopy should never be used in place of radiography. Radiation risks greatly increase with constant x-ray production used in fluoroscopy. One method used to decrease the risk to personnel while using fluoroscopy is to depress the x-ray button intermittently instead of holding it down continuously.

RADIATION SAFETY

Ionizing radiation can be a difficult concept to grasp, because at diagnostic levels it cannot be seen, felt, or heard by the patient or operators. Why is radiation safety important? Radiation ionizes intracellular water. This releases toxic products, which can damage critical components of the cell, such as DNA. When radiation comes in contact with the cells of living tissue, it can:

- Pass through the cells with no effect
- Produce cell damage that is repairable
- Produce cell damage that is not repairable
- Kill the cells

Radiation damages the body in several ways. It may have carcinogenic effects, which means that cancer may develop in body tissues. Effects on the body may be somatic, occurring in future generations. Tissues that are most sensitive to ionizing radiation are those with rapidly growing or reproducing cells. The reproductive organs may suffer from temporary or permanent infertility, decreased hormone production, or mutations. The hematopoietic (blood-forming) cells are relatively sensitive to ionizing radiation. The lymphocytic series of blood cells is most sensitive. Damage to these cells can reduce resistance to infection and cause clotting disorders. The thyroid gland, intestinal epithelium, and lens of the eye are also radiosensitive. There may be an increased incidence of squamous-cell carcinoma with chronic, low-level skin exposure. Radiodermatitis (reddened, dry skin) can result from excessive, chronic, low-level radiation exposure.

The developing fetus is sensitive to the effects of ionizing radiation. The degree of sensitivity depends on the stage of pregnancy and the dose received. The preimplantation period (0 to 9 days) is the most critical time for the embryo regarding intrauterine lethality. The period of organogenesis (10 days to 6 weeks) carries the greatest risk of congenital malformation in the fetus, because this is the critical development period for fetal organs. The fetus may have skeletal or dental malformations. Other abnormalities include microphthalmia (small eyes) and overall growth retardation. A fetal dose greater than 25 rads (0.25 Gray) is recognized as the threshold for significant damage to the fetus (for an explanation of these units of measure, see the Terminology section). The fetal period (6 weeks to term) is the least sensitive time for the fetus; however, growth and mental retardation may still occur. Irradiation after 30 weeks is less likely to cause abnormalities because the sensitivity of the fetus approaches that of the adult.

Terminology

REM stands for Roentgen Equivalent Man. REM is used to express the dose equivalent that results from exposure to ionizing radiation. REM takes into account the quality of radiation, so doses of different kinds of radiation can be compared. Sievert (SV) is the current terminology used to define a REM (1 SV5 100 REM). A millirem (MREM) is equal to 0.001 REM or 1/1000 REM. A *rad* is the Radiation Absorbed Dose. Current terminology is *Gray (GY) (1 GY = 100 rad)*. This chapter concerns x-rays only and not other types of radiation, so rads can be considered equivalent to REMs. Other types of radiation must have a quality factor figured in to determine the dose. MPD is the Maximum Permissible Dose.

The National Council on Radiation Protection and Measurements recommends that the dose for occupationally exposed persons not exceed 5 REM per year. An occupationally exposed individual is one who normally performs his or her work in a restricted access area and has duties that involve exposure to radiation. *ALARA* stands for As Low As Reasonably Attainable. The MPD for nonoccupational persons is 10% of the MPD for occupationally exposed persons, or 0.5 REM per year. This is known as the *ALARA MPD*. Also, a fetus should not receive more than 0.5 REM during the entire gestation period. A pregnant employee who chooses to continue working around radiation-producing devices should wear an additional badge at waist level, underneath the lead gown, to monitor the fetal dose. This badge should not exceed 0.05 REM per month.

There are three important ways to minimize occupational exposure to radiation. The first is *lead shielding*. Lead shielding should be a requirement for all personnel remaining in the room while an exposure is made. Lead gowns, gloves, and thyroid shields should all contain at least 0.5 mm of lead. Lead-based glasses can also be worn to protect the lens of the eye.

Lead apparel is expensive, so it should be handled appropriately. Lead aprons should be draped over a rounded surface, without folds or wrinkles, to prevent cracks in the lead. Lead gloves can be stored with open-ended soup cans inserted to prevent cracks and to provide air circulation to the liners. Lead gloves should be radiographed every 6 months to check for damaged areas. Lead gowns should be checked every 12 months to screen for holes and cracks in the lead. A commonly used technique for this procedure is

5 mAs and 80 kVp. This can be adjusted as needed to attain the proper density in the radiographs.

Another method for decreasing personnel exposure is by *increasing the distance from the primary beam*. Personnel restraining the animal should try to remain as far as possible from the x-ray source during exposure. During exposure, the restrainers should lean back and look away from the beam to protect the lenses of their eyes (Fig. 18-13). Employees should take care to wear lead apparel properly to obtain full protection, unlike the personnel in Fig. 18-14. Placing a glove on top of a hand for protection does not protect the hand from scatter radiation. The scatter can come from any direction, including from under the tabletop.

A third technique for reducing radiation exposure is *reduced exposure time*. Using the fastest film-screen combinations allows reduced exposure time for the patient and personnel. Proper darkroom practices and technique charts allow for consistent production of high-quality films, which reduces the number of repeated radiographs. It is very important to collimate the beam down to the area of interest, because this reduces exposure of personnel to scatter radiation. Cones and diaphragms may also be attached to the tube window to increase detail and reduce scatter radiation. A 2-mm aluminum filter is used at the tube window to filter out soft rays that are too weak to penetrate the patient. If these rays are not filtered out, they scatter about the room, fogging the film and striking personnel.

Each clinic should have a radiation protection supervisor. A veterinary technician can fill this role. Responsibilities include educating personnel on radiation safety, monitoring safety practices, and maintaining a radiologic badge system. The supervisor also maintains x-ray equipment, darkroom facilities, and radiographic records. A good radiation control program consists of safe x-ray equipment, low-exposure techniques, shielding, and monitoring personal radiation exposure (Box 18-1). The x-ray equipment is usually under control of the state government (e.g., State Board of Health). Regulations vary between states, so check with your state government about their policy regarding radiation-producing devices.

DARKROOM TECHNIQUES

Along with a good technique chart, proper darkroom techniques should be followed to ensure consistent production of high-quality radiographs. Properly exposed radiographs can quickly become nondiagnostic with poor film handling and darkroom techniques.

Darkroom Setup

For most veterinary practices, the darkroom does not need to be large or fancy, as long as the layout is designed for efficiency. The room must be just large enough to provide a

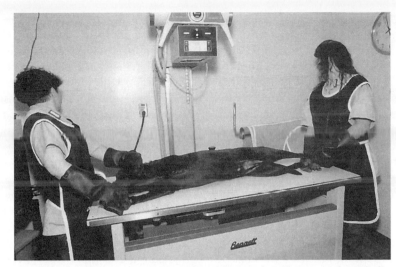

Fig. 18-13 Proper radiation safety practices. The restrainers have increased their distance from the primary beam by leaning back. They are also protecting the lenses of their eyes by looking away.

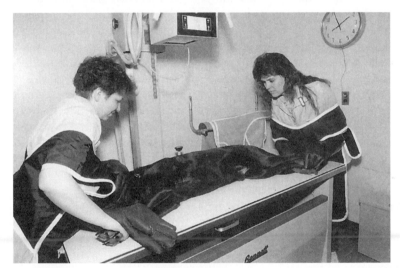

Fig. 18-14 Improper radiation safety practices. The restrainers are leaning in and looking at the patient. Also, one hand is not properly gloved.

BOX 18-1

General Radiation Safety Rules

- Always wear lead gloves and a lead apron when remaining in the room during radiography or fluoroscopy. Lead gowns and lead gloves *must* be worn by all individuals involved in restraint of the animal.
- Always wear a radiation monitoring device on your collar *outside* the apron when working around x-ray equipment. *Note:* Badges should not be exposed to sunlight, dampness, or extreme temperatures. This could cause falsely high readings.
- Never allow any part of your body to be exposed to the primary beam. Lead clothing does not protect against primary beam exposure.

- Always look away from the x-ray beam during an exposure to protect the lens of the eye. Lead-based glasses may be worn for protection.
- Use alternative methods of restraint (drugs, tape, sandbags, etc.) when using high-exposure radiographic techniques.
- Pregnant women and persons under the age of 18 years should not be involved in radiographic procedures.
- Only the people required for restraint should remain in the room when an exposure is made.

"dry bench" area away from the "wet bench" area (Fig. 18-15). The dry bench area is for unloading and loading cassettes and film storage. The wet bench area is for film processing and drying. These areas must be separated to prevent processing chemical splashes from damaging the dry films or sensitive intensifying screens. In a small room, this can be achieved by placing a partition between the two areas. Sufficient electrical outlets should be available to power the safelights, viewboxes, and labeling equipment.

The most important feature of a darkroom is that it must be light tight. White light that leaks around the door, through a blackened window, or around ventilation fans can fog the film. Film is more sensitive after it has been exposed to x-rays, so even low-grade light leaks decrease the quality of the finished radiograph. When checking for light leaks, stand in the darkroom for at least 5 minutes to allow your eyes to adjust to the darkness. Look around the doorframe, ventilation fan, or blackened windows for any signs of white light. When performing this test, vary the intensity of light outside the door. Because work in the darkroom is done with a limited amount of light, painting the walls and ceiling a light color that reflects the available light helps greatly.

The darkroom should have adequate ventilation to prevent volatile chemical fumes from accumulating in the room. These fumes can cause fogging of the film, damage to electrical equipment, and health problems for personnel. A light-tight ventilation fan installed in the ceiling helps remove the fumes and also controls the temperature and humidity in the room. The exhaust from automatic processors and film dryers should also be vented away from the darkroom, because they contain volatile chemical fumes.

Cleanliness is important in the darkroom, because intensifying screens and the film are exposed to this area.

Dirt and hair on countertops can fall into cassettes, causing white artifacts on subsequent radiographs from that cassette. Chemical spills also cause artifacts on the radiographs and damage the intensifying screens. Keeping both wet and dry areas of the darkroom clean prevents these problems. Film hangers for manual processing should also be cleaned regularly. Chemicals that remain on the hanger clips could drip down the next film to be processed, causing an artifact.

Film Identification

Permanent labeling is necessary for all radiographs. Each film must be identified before the film is processed for legal purposes and for certification organizations. The labeling can be done during the exposure or after the exposure, but it must be done before the film is processed. The label should include the clinic name, date, owner's name, address, patient's name, and some patient data, such as age and breed.

There are several methods for film identification. One method is the photo labeler. This uses a cassette containing a leaded window that protects the area during exposure. During identification, the window slides back from the protected area to expose the information on a card. This forms a latent image of the information on the film. Manual printers are similar to photo labelers, except they use a flash of light through an information card to produce a latent image on the film. The manual printer is placed in the darkroom, and the film is taken out of the cassette to be identified. Another method uses lead letters or radiopaque tape. These are placed on the cassette during exposure of the radiograph.

Safelights

Safelight illuminators are important for darkroom processing. A safelight provides sufficient light to work in the room

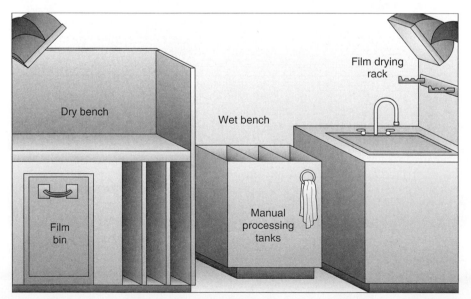

Fig. 18-15 Schematic drawing of a darkroom. Notice the dry bench has been separated from the wet bench by a partition.

but does not cause fogging of the film. Safelights can be mounted to provide light directly or indirectly. With direct lighting, the safelight is mounted at least 48 inches above the workbench and directed toward the workbench. Indirect lighting has the safelight directed toward the ceiling and uses the reflected light to illuminate the room. With indirect lighting, the safelight can be mounted closer to the bench but should be as high as possible (Fig. 18-16).

Many types of safelight filters are available to filter out light in different areas of the light spectrum. The type of film used dictates which filter is necessary. Film that is "blue-light–sensitive" requires a safelight that filters out blue and ultraviolet light. Film that is "green-light–sensitive" requires a safelight to filter both green and blue light. This filter can also be used with blue-light–sensitive film. A red lightbulb should never be used to replace a safelight filter. It does not filter the light; it only colors it. A white frosted 7½- to 10-watt bulb is recommended for most safelight filters.

Periodically check the safelight filter. First, make a moderate exposure on a film using approximately 1 to 2 mAs and 40 to 50 kVp. Film that has been exposed to x-rays is more sensitive to low-grade light, producing an overall fogged appearance. Cover two thirds of the film with black paper or cardboard, and allow the remaining one third to be exposed to the safelight for 30 seconds. This is a little longer than it should take to place the film in an automatic processor or to place the film on a hanger and into the manual tanks. After 30 seconds, uncover another one third of the film and wait 30 more seconds. Repeat the process for the final one third, and develop the film. This test exposes portions of the film to the safelight for 30 seconds, 60 seconds, and 90 seconds. Once the film is dry, look for areas of increased film density. If an increase in density is detected, a close check of the darkroom is necessary. Improper safelight distance, a cracked safelight filter, and light leaking around the filter can all cause film fogging.

Processing Chemistry

Developer

The developer's main function is to convert the sensitized silver halide crystals into black metallic silver. Sensitized silver halide crystals are those that have been exposed to electromagnetic radiation, making them susceptible to chemical change. The developer contains five ingredients: a solvent, reducing agents, restrainer, activator, and a preservative.

Water is used as the *solvent* to keep all the ingredients in solution. It also causes the film emulsion to swell so that the reducing agents can penetrate the sensitized crystals.

Reducing agents change the sensitized silver halide crystals into black metallic silver. The most common reducing agents are a combination of hydroquinone and p-methylaminophenol.

Restrainers are used to protect the unexposed silver halide crystals by preventing the reducing agents from affecting the unsensitized crystals. Potassium bromide and potassium iodide are the most common restrainers. Bromide ions are produced during the exchange between the reducing agents and the sensitized crystals. In a fresh solution, the bromide ions are not available. They are added as a starter solution but are not placed in replenishing solutions. Excessive bromide ions inhibit the reducing agents.

Activators help soften and swell the film's emulsion so that the reducing agents can work effectively. Reducing agents cannot function in an acidic or neutral solution. The

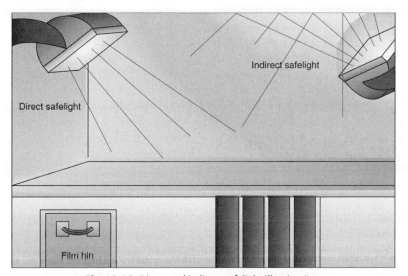

Fig. 18-16 Direct and indirect safelight illumination.

activators, usually a carbonate or hydroxide of sodium or potassium, provide an alkaline pH in the range of 9.8 to 11.4.

Preservatives prevent the solution from rapidly oxidizing. Sodium and potassium sulfite are the most commonly used preservatives.

Developing chemicals are manufactured in two forms: liquid and powder. The liquid form requires dilution with water. The powder form should never be mixed in the darkroom, because the chemical dust contaminates unprotected film, causing artifacts. Always mix the powder in a bucket outside the darkroom, and then finish the dilution in the darkroom.

Fixer

The fixer removes the unchanged silver halide crystals from the film emulsion, leaving the black metallic silver. It also hardens the film emulsion, decreasing the susceptibility to scratches. The fixer contains five ingredients: a solvent, a fixing agent, an acidifier, a hardener, and a preservative.

As with the developer, the *solvent* for the fixer is water. It keeps the ingredients in solution and causes the film emulsion to swell, allowing the fixing agents to reach the unexposed crystals. The *fixing agent* is sodium or ammonium thiosulfate. This clears the remaining silver halide crystals from the film emulsion. The *acidifier* is acetic or sulfuric acid and is used to neutralize any alkaline developer remaining on the film. Ammonium chloride is used as a *hardener.* It hardens and prevents excessive swelling of the film emulsion, shortening the drying time. The final ingredient is the *preservative.* As with the developer, sodium sulfite is used to prevent decomposition of the fixing agents.

Fixer chemicals are manufactured in two forms: liquid and powder. The liquid form requires dilution with water. It is more expensive than the powder form but is more efficient. The powder form requires dissolving and mixing to get it into solution. It should never be mixed in the darkroom, because the chemical dust can contaminate unprotected film, causing artifacts. Always mix the powder in a bucket outside the darkroom and then finish the dilution in the darkroom. Also, the powder requires a longer clearing time than the liquid form.

Manual Processing

Equipment

Manual processing tanks are usually made from stainless steel and are large enough to accept 14-by-17-inch film hangers. Tanks with 5-gallon capacity are sufficient. Plastic or wooden lids are needed to cover the developer and fixer tanks. This reduces the rate of evaporation and oxidation of the chemicals. Separate stirring rods for the developer and fixer are used to mix the chemicals before processing. Also,

an accurate timer and a floating thermometer should be available.

Developing x-ray film is a chemical process that depends on the duration of immersion in the chemicals and the temperature of the chemicals. The recommended time for development is 5 minutes. This allows just enough time for the reducing agents to convert the sensitized silver halide crystals. The temperature of the chemicals is also important. The warmer the temperature, the more the emulsion swells and the faster the chemicals work. Cold temperatures also affect the chemicals by decreasing their ability to penetrate the film emulsion. Manufacturers generally recommend a temperature for the chemicals they produce. Most use 68° F (20° C), with 5 minutes of developing time. For some cases this may not be possible, so the time can be adjusted to compensate for the increase or decrease in temperature. The time can be decreased by 30 seconds for every 2° increase in developer temperature. Also, the time can be increased by 30 seconds for every 2° decrease in developer temperature. This applies only between 65° F (18° C) and 74° F (23° C).

The rinse bath removes developer from the film, preventing carryover into the fixer tank. Agitating the film in the running water bath for 30 seconds adequately removes the developer. The rinse water should be continually exchanged to prevent accumulation of developer. The temperature of the incoming rinse water can often be used to regulate the temperature of the developer and fixer tanks.

The fixing process is also dependent on immersion time and temperature of the chemicals. The standard temperature is 68° F (20° C), and the fixing time is double the developing time. The temperature affects the time the film is left in the fixer. The warmer the chemicals are, the shorter the fixing time is. The film can be removed from the fixer after 30 seconds and viewed with white light. However, it must be placed back into the fixer for the remainder of the time. The clearing time increases as the thickness of the emulsion increases. Direct-exposure film has a thicker emulsion and requires a longer time in the fixer.

The final wash rinses away the processing chemicals. Failure to rinse the film completely results in a film that eventually becomes faded and brown. This is due to oxidation of the chemicals remaining in the film emulsion. The wash tank should have fresh circulating water to decrease the time needed for the final wash. Generally, the wash time is at least 30 minutes. Box 18-2 shows the steps for manual processing.

Maintaining the tanks

There are two methods for maintaining manual processing tanks. The first is the exhausted method. With this method, allow the chemicals to drain back into their respective tanks and not into the wash tank. This permits the exhausted chemicals to remain in the tank, maintaining the chemical levels. The second method is the replenishing method. Do not allow

BOX 18-2

Steps for Manual Processing

- Check chemical temperature (optimal chemical temperature is 68° F (20° C).
- Stir both chemicals.
- Check chemical levels.
- Clean countertops.
- Turn on water to the wash tank.

Processing Individual Films

1. Locate the proper size hanger(s).
2. Set the timer.
3. Turn on the safelight.
4. Turn off the white lights.
5. Unload the cassette and place the film on the hanger.
6. Immerse the film in the developer. The optimal time is 5 minutes at 68° F (20° C).
7. Gently agitate the film to dislodge any air bubbles that may cling the film's surface.
8. Reload the empty cassette.
9. After 5 minutes of developing time, place the film in the wash tank and agitate for 30 seconds.
10. Lift the film out of the wash tank, allowing the excess water to drain back into wash tank.
11. Place the film into the fixer tank and agitate gently to dislodge air bubbles that cling to the surface.
12. Turn on white lights without causing problems after 30 seconds clearing time in the fixer.
13. Place the film in the wash tank for 30 minutes or longer, depending on the amount of water replenishing.
14. After washing the film, let it hang until dry.

Every Three Months

- Completely drain all three tanks.
- Clean the tanks with a 1:32 solution of chlorine bleach and water.
- Rinse the tanks well.
- Refill the tanks with fresh chemicals.

the chemicals to drain back into their respective tanks, but place them in the wash tank. The chemical levels are maintained with replenishing chemicals that are more concentrated than the initial solutions. In this way, the potency and levels of the chemicals can be preserved. With either method, the chemicals should be changed every 3 months.

Automatic Processing

Use of an automatic processor has some advantages over manual processing. Automatic processors can develop film more quickly. They can process and dry a film in 90 to 120 seconds. Also, automatic processors consistently provide high-quality radiographs. This eliminates the need for repeat radiographs because of processing errors.

Automatic processors move the film through the developer, fixer wash bath, and dryers at a uniform rate of speed. Chemicals and film are specially manufactured to withstand the high temperatures involved in automatic processing. The chemicals are kept at temperatures around 95° F (35° C), depending on the type of film and equipment used. The emulsion on film designed for automatic processing is harder than on film designed for manual processing, preventing scratches from the roller. This film can also be manually processed in case of mechanical problems with the automatic processor.

Maintaining the tanks

Small tabletop automatic processors are easily maintained in most veterinary practices. The equipment should be completely cleaned every 3 months. This includes draining and cleaning the tanks. A 1:32 solution of bleach helps to reduce algae and remove chemical buildup. The rollers can be cleaned with a mild detergent and soft sponge. When any cleaning solution is applied to the tanks or rollers, they should be rinsed thoroughly before replacing the chemicals. Also, check the springs and gears for signs of wear and replace if necessary. Wipe the feed tray and top rollers with a clean soft sponge every day. This helps remove dirt, debris, and chemical residue between episodes of routine maintenance.

Silver Recovery

When an exposed film is placed in the developer, the exposed silver halide crystals are converted to black metallic silver. The remaining silver halide crystals are removed from the film in the fixer. Over time, the fixer solution becomes rich with silver that can be reclaimed. Silver recovery systems can be attached to automatic processors to filter and store the silver that would normally be discarded down the drain. The black metallic silver in the radiographs can also be recovered.

The manual processing fixer solution, silver recovery systems, and old radiographs can be sold to companies that reclaim the silver. These companies are usually listed in the *Yellow Pages* under the headings "Gold and Silver Refiners and Dealers."

RADIOGRAPHIC ARTIFACTS

An *artifact* is any unwanted density in the form of blemishes arising from improper handling, exposure, processing, or housekeeping. Artifacts can mimic or mask a disease process or distract from the overall quality of the film.

Before radiographing an animal, check for external changes on the animal. Remove any dirt or mats from the coat. If the coat is wet, dry it as much as possible. Remove any collars, leashes, or halters. Bandage material is visible on radiographs, so remove it if feasible. Boxes 18-3 and 18-4 list common artifact problems.

RADIOGRAPHIC POSITIONING AND TERMINOLOGY

Proper patient positioning is as important as the radiograph itself. Misinterpretations can result from inaccurate positioning. Following is a reference for radiographic procedures conducted in a veterinary hospital.

A basic knowledge of directional terminology is essential when describing radiographic projections. The American College of Veterinary Radiology (ACVR) has standardized the nomenclature for radiographic projections by using currently accepted veterinary anatomic terms. The projections are described by the direction the central ray enters and exits the part being imaged (Fig. 6-1).

- *Ventral (V):* Body area situated toward the underside of quadrupeds.
- *Dorsal (D):* Body area situated toward the back or topline of quadrupeds. Opposite of ventral.
- *Medial (M):* Body area situated toward the median plane or midline.
- *Lateral (L):* Body area situated away from the median plane or midline.
- *Cranial (Cr):* Structures or areas situated toward the head (formerly anterior).
- *Caudal (Cd):* Structures or areas situated toward the tail (formerly posterior).
- *Rostral (R):* Areas on the head situated toward the nose.
- *Palmar (Pa):* Situated on the caudal aspect of the front limb, distal to the antebrachiocarpal joint.
- *Plantar (Pl):* Situated on the caudal aspect of the rear limb, distal to the tarsocrural joint. ·
- *Proximal (Pr):* Situated closer to the point of attachment or origin.
- *Distal (Di):* Situated away from the point of attachment or origin.

Oblique Projections

Oblique projections are used to set off an area that normally would be superimposed over another area. Some rules should be followed when deciding what type of oblique projection is needed and how it is identified.

- *The area of interest should be as close to the cassette as possible.* This decreases magnification and increases detail.
- *Place a marker on the cassette during exposure to indicate the direction of entry and exit of the primary beam.*

Table 18-1 (p. 377) shows the landmarks used to produce radiographs of various body parts.

CONTRAST STUDIES

The purpose of a contrast study is to delineate an organ or area against surrounding soft tissues. They are useful in determining the size, shape, position, location, and function of an organ. The information obtained from a contrast study complements or confirms findings of the survey radiographs. A contrast study should never replace survey radiographs.

With contrast studies, tissues of interest appear either radiopaque or radiolucent on the finished radiograph. Areas that are radiopaque appear white. Positive-contrast agents are radiopaque on a radiograph. Radiolucent areas on the finished radiograph appear black. Negative-contrast agents produce radiolucencies on a radiograph.

Obtaining survey radiographs before doing a contrast study establishes proper exposure technique and proper patient preparation. In addition, a diagnosis may be achieved from survey radiographs, eliminating the need for the contrast study. Because most contrast studies require multiple images, it is very important to label each film with the time and sequence. Always record the amount, type, and administration route of the contrast agent.

Positive-Contrast Media

Positive-contrast media contain elements with a high atomic number. Elements with a high atomic number absorb more x-rays. Thus, fewer x-rays penetrate the patient and expose the film, making a white area on the radiograph. Two common types of positive-contrast agents are barium sulfate and water-soluble organic iodides.

Barium sulfate is commonly used for positive-contrast studies of the gastrointestinal tract. It is insoluble and not affected by gastric secretions. Therefore, it provides good mucosal detail on the radiograph. Barium sulfate preparations are relatively inexpensive and are manufactured in the form of powders, colloid suspensions, or pastes. One disadvantage of using barium sulfate is that it can take 3 or more hours to travel from the stomach to the colon. Also, it can be harmful to the peritoneum, so it should never be used when gastrointestinal perforations are suspected. Barium is insoluble and the body cannot eliminate it, resulting in granulomatous reactions in the abdominal cavity. While administering barium orally, take care to prevent the

BOX 18-3

Causes of Common Radiographic Artifacts that Occur Before Processing

Fogged Film

- Film exposed to excessive scatter radiation. A grid is necessary when radiographing areas measuring 10 cm or more, (overall gray appearance)
- Film exposed to radiation during storage
- Film stored in an area that was too hot or humid
- Film exposed to a safelight filter that was cracked or inappropriate for the type of film used
- Film exposed to a low-grade light leak in a darkroom
- Film expired

Black Crescents or Lines

- Rough handling of film before or after exposure (Fig. 18-17)
- Static electricity caused by low humidity
- Scratched film surface before or after exposure
- Fingerprints from excessive pressure before or after exposure

Black Areas

- Black irregular border on one end of film caused by light exposure while still in the box or film bin
- Black irregular border on multiple sides of the film caused by felt damage in the cassette

White Areas

- Foreign material between the film and screen (Fig. 18-18)

- Chemical spill on the screen, causing permanent damage to the phosphor layer
- Contrast medium on the patient, table, or cassette
- White fingerprints on film from oil or fixer on fingers before processing

Visible Grid Lines

- Grid lines on the entire film from focal-film distance outside the range of the grid's focus
- Grid lines more visible on one end of the film and an overall decrease in radiographic density caused by the grid's not being centered in the primary beam
- Grid lines on the entire film caused by the grid not being perpendicular to the center of the primary beam
- Grid lines more visible in some areas than others from grid damage

Decreased Detail

- Patient motion
- Poor film-screen contact
- Increased object-film distance
- Decreased focal-film distance

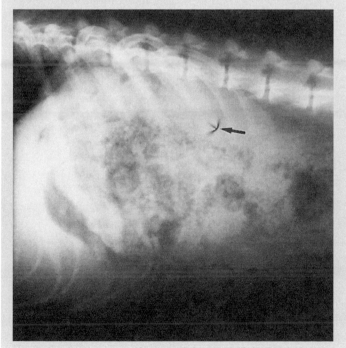

Fig. 18-17 Black crescent from rough handling of the film before or after exposure.

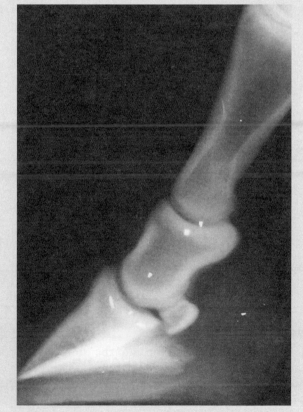

Fig. 18-18 Foreign material between the film and screen blocks light from exposing the film, creating white areas.

BOX 18-4

Causes of Common Radiographic Artifacts that Occur During Manual or Automatic Processing

Increased Radiographic Density with Poor Contrast

- Film overdeveloped (longer than manufacturer recommendation)
- Film developed in hot chemicals. Correct temperature for manual tanks is 68° F (20° C); for automatic processors, it is 95° F (35° C)
- Film overexposed

Decreased Radiographic Density with Poor Contrast

- Film underdeveloped (shorter than manufacturer recommendation)
- Film developed in cold chemicals. Correct temperature for manual tanks is 68° F (20° C), for automatic processors, it is 95° F (35° C)
- Film processed in old or exhausted chemicals
- Film underexposed

Uneven Development

- Lack of stirring allowing chemicals to settle to tank bottom
- Repeated withdrawal of the film from the tank to check on development results
- Uneven chemical levels

Black Areas, Spots, or Streaks

- Identical black areas on two films processed together from films stuck to one another in the fixer and not cleared properly
- Black area on only one film from film sticking to side of tank
- Well-defined spots or streaks from developer splash before processing
- Black lines along the full length of the film and equal distance apart from pressure of rollers in the processor

Defined Areas of Decreased Radiographic Density

- Identical light areas on two films processed together from sticking together in the developer
- Light area on one film from film sticking to the side of the tank during development (Fig. 18-19)
- Air bubbles clinging to the film during development
- Well-defined spots or streaks from fixer splash before processing

Clear Areas or Spots

- Streaks where emulsion scratched away

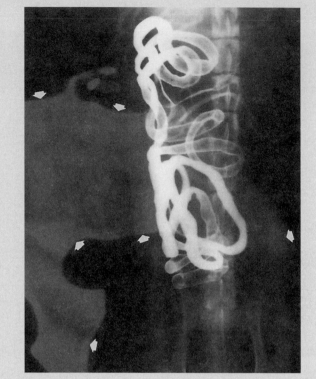

Fig. 18-19 This radiograph stuck to the side of the manual tank while in the developer. The arrows outline the artifact. A light image can still be seen, because the film has emulsion on both sides of the film base. One side developed normally.

- Large clear areas from leaving film in final wash too long and emulsion sliding off film base

Entire Film Clear

- No exposure
- Film placed in fixer before developer

Film Turns Brown

- Improper final wash

---

patient from aspirating barium into the lungs. Aspiration of large amounts can be fatal. Barium sulfate may also aggravate an already obstructed bowel by causing further impactions.

Water-soluble organic iodides in ionic form are also used for positive-contrast procedures. Different forms of the water-soluble organic iodides can be administered intravenously,

orally, or by infusion into a hollow viscus or into the subarachnoid space. Being water-soluble, they are absorbed into the bloodstream and excreted by the kidneys.

A commonly used oral form of ionic water-soluble organic iodide is a solution of meglumine and sodium diatrizoate. It is used when performing contrast studies of the gastrointestinal tract when perforation is suspected. When

TABLE 18-1

Landmarks Used in Producing Radiographs of Various Body Areas

Body Part	Cranial or Proximal Landmark	Caudal or Distal Landmark	Center Landmark	Comments
Thorax	Manubrium sterni	Halfway between xiphoid and last rib	Heart	Expose at peak inspiration
Abdomen	3 rib spaces cranial to xyphoid	Greater trochanter	Last rib	Expose at peak expiration
Shoulder	Midbody scapula	Midshaft humerus	Over joint space	
Humerus	Shoulder joint	Elbow joint	Midshaft	
Elbow	Midshaft humerus	Midshaft radius	Over joint space	
Radius/Ulna	Elbow joint	Carpal joint	Midshaft	
Carpus	Midshaft radius	Midshaft metacarpus	Over joint space	
Metacarpus	Carpal joint	Include digits	Midshaft	
Pelvis	Wings of ilium	Ischium		
Pelvis VD, flexed	Wings of Ilium	Ischium		Pushes stifles cranially
Pelvis VD, extended	Wings of ilium	Stifle joint		Femora parallel to each other and table
Femur	Coxofemoral joint	Stifle joint	Midshaft	
Stifle	Midshaft femur	Midshaft tibia	Over joint space	
Tibia/fibula	Stifle joint	Tarsal joint	Midshaft	
Tarsus	Midshaft tibia	Midshaft metatarsal	Over joint space	
Metatarsus	Tarsal joint	Include digits	Midshaft	
Cervical vertebrae	Base of skull	Spine of scapula		Extend front limbs caudally, collimate width of beam to increase detail
Thoracic vertebrae	Spine of scapula	Halfway between xiphoid and last rib		Collimate width of beam to increase detail
Thoracolumbar vertebrae			Halfway between xiphoid and last rib	Collimate width of beam to increase detail
Lumbar vertebrae	Halfway between xiphoid and last rib	Wings of ilium		Collimate width of beam to increase detail

this agent is administered orally, transit through the gastrointestinal system is rapid, usually within 48 to 60 minutes. However, the hypertonic solution draws fluid into the bowel lumen. Thus, the contrast medium is diluted, decreasing the quality of the study. Fluid loss may further complicate hypovolemia in a dehydrated animal. Water-soluble organic iodides should never be used in place of barium sulfate and should be used only when perforations are suspected.

Ionic water-soluble organic iodides for intravenous use are prepared in various combinations of meglumine and sodium diatrizoate. Diatrizoate can also be infused into hollow organs, such as the urinary bladder, or into fistulous tracts. Sodium diatrizoate is commonly used for excretory urography because it provides better opacification of the kidneys. Nausea, vomiting, or decreased blood pressure can occur when a large bolus of contrast medium is injected intravenously. Ionic water-soluble organic iodides cannot be used for myelography, because they are irritating to the brain and spinal cord.

Nonionic water-soluble organic iodides are used for myelography. Because of their low osmolarity and chemical nature, they cause fewer adverse effects when placed in the subarachnoid space. Three commonly used media are metrizamide, iopamidol, and iohexol. Nonionic water-soluble organic iodides are suitable for myelography and can also be used intravenously. However, they are approximately 10 times more expensive than the ionic media is. Metrizamide is supplied as a powder because it cannot be heat-sterilized and is unstable in solution. Before metrizamide is used, it must be reconstituted and filtered through a 0.22-μ bacteriostatic filter.

Negative-Contrast Media

Negative-contrast agents include air, oxygen, and carbon dioxide. They all have a low atomic number, appearing radiolucent on the finished radiograph. Oxygen and carbon dioxide are more soluble than water. Care must be taken not to overinflate the organs, such as the bladder. Air embolism can occur when air enters ulcerative lesions, causing cardiac arrest.

Double-Contrast Procedures

Double-contrast procedures use both positive- and negative-contrast media to image an organ or area. The most common organs imaged with double-contrast are the urinary bladder, stomach, and colon. In most cases, the negative-contrast medium is added first, then the positive-contrast medium. Mixing negative-contrast medium with positive-contrast medium can cause air bubbles to form, which might be misinterpreted as lesions.

DIAGNOSTIC ULTRASOUND

Diagnostic ultrasound *(ultrasonography)* is a noninvasive method of imaging soft tissues. A transducer sends low-intensity, high-frequency sound waves into the soft tissues, where they interact with tissue interfaces. Some of the sound waves are reflected back to the transducer and some are transmitted into deeper tissues. The sound waves that are reflected back to the transducer *(echoes)* are then analyzed by the computer to produce a gray-scale image. Use of ultrasound in conjunction with radiography gives the veterinarian an excellent diagnostic tool. Radiographs demonstrate the size, shape, and position of the organs. Ultrasound displays the findings found on the radiographs as well as the soft tissue textures and the dynamics of some organs (e.g., motility of the bowel).

Transducers

Ultrasound transducers emit a series of sound pulses and receive the returning echoes. A weak electrical current applied to the piezoelectric crystals incorporated in the transducer causes the crystals to vibrate and produce sound waves. After sending a series of pulses, the crystals are dampened to stop further vibrations. When struck by the returning echoes, the crystals vibrate again, and convert these echoes into electrical energy.

Transducers are available in different configurations, which are mechanical or electronic. The scan plane can either be a *sector scan* (pie-shaped image) or a *linear-array scan* (rectangular image). A mechanically driven sector scan can be produced by a belt and pulley used to wobble a single crystal or rotate multiple crystals across a scan plane. Another method of producing a sector scan is with use of phased-array or annular-array configurations. With *phased-array configuration*, the crystals are pulsed sequentially with a built-in delay to create a "pseudo-sector" scan plane. *Annular array* arranges the crystals in concentric rings. By using electronic phasing of the many crystals, annular-array transducers produce a two-dimensional image by steering the entire array through a sector arc.

Sector scanners are useful when imaging areas limited by ribs, gas-filled bowels, or lungs. The narrow near field and wide far field enable the transducer scan plane to be positioned between or around these structures. Linear-array scanners produce a scan plane by alternately firing groups of crystals in sequence. The pulsing of each group of crystals occurs so rapidly that individual pulses cannot be observed by the human eye. Linear-array scanners are useful in areas with unrestricted window size. The rectangular scan plane is ideal for equine tendons or large or small animal transrectal imaging.

The frequency of the transducer determines the amount of detail or resolution of the image. As frequency increases, the wavelength gets shorter. The shorter the wavelength is, the better the resolution of the image will be.

Transducers are expensive and the most fragile part of ultrasound equipment. Care must be taken when handling them. Avoid hard impacts that can severely damage the sensitive crystals. Prevent exposure to extreme temperature changes. Some transducers are sensitive to certain types of cleaning agents. Always refer to manufacturer's instructions for appropriate cleaning products.

Display Modes

There are three different display modes: A-mode (amplitude mode), B-mode (brightness mode), and M-mode (motion mode).

A-mode

A-mode is the earliest form of ultrasound and is the simplest as far as computer software. With A-mode, the returning echoes are displayed as a series of peaks on a graph. As the intensity of the returning sound increases, the peak at that tissue depth increases. A-mode is not used to show tissue motion or anatomy. The main use in veterinary medicine was to measure the amount of subcutaneous fat in pigs.

B-mode

B-mode uses bright pixels or dots on a screen, whereas A-mode uses peaks on a graph. A dot on the monitor screen corresponds to the depth at which the echo was formed. The degree of brightness is proportional to the intensity of the returning echo. As intensity increases, the brightness of the dot increases. The image that is generated is a two-dimensional anatomic slice that is continually updated. This mode is currently used for diagnostic applications.

M-mode

M-mode is the continuous display of a thin slice of an organ over time. M-mode projects the echoes from a thin beam of sound over a time-oriented baseline. The main use is with echocardiography to assess the size of the heart chambers and the motion of the heart valves and walls.

Terminology Describing Echotexture

The terminology used to describe tissue texture within an ultrasound image is simple. *Echogenic* or *echoic* means that most of the sound is reflected back to the transducer. Echogenic areas appear white on the screen. *Sonolucent* means that most of the sound is transmitted to the deeper tissues, with only a few echoes reflected back to the transducer. Sonolucent areas appear dark on the screen. *Anechoic* is used to describe tissue that transmits all of the sound through to deeper tissues, reflecting none of the sound back to the transducer. Anechoic areas appear black on the screen and are generally fluid-filled structures.

Soft tissues are represented not only as black or white but also as many shades of gray. Additional terminology has been established to describe these areas. *Hyperechoic* is used to describe tissues that reflect more sound back to the transducer than surrounding tissues. Hyperechoic areas appear brighter than surrounding tissues. *Hypoechoic* is used to describe tissues that reflect less sound back to the transducer than surrounding tissues. Hypoechoic areas appear darker than surrounding tissues. *Isoechoic* is used to describe tissue that appears to have the same echotexture on the screen as surrounding tissues (Fig. 18-20).

Terminology has been established to describe areas displayed on the monitor screen. The screen is divided into nine zones, with each zone having its own label. In this way, the sonographer can verbally indicate the area of interest, such as mid field right or near field left.

Patient Preparation

To achieve an optimal acoustic window and produce the best-quality image, the transducer head must be placed in close contact with the skin. The animal's hair must be clipped and in some cases shaved before the study. Occasionally, thin-coated animals can be imaged with minimal preparation. An acoustic coupling gel is used to eliminate the air interface and to improve the acoustic window. Before applying the acoustic coupling gel, wipe the area

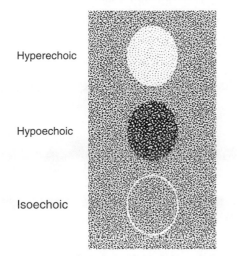

Fig. 18-20 Hyperechoic, hypoechoic, and isoechoic areas.

with alcohol or generous amounts of soapy water to remove any loose hairs, dirt, and skin oils.

Fasting of small animals before abdominal ultrasound examination is recommended. Ingesta and gas in the bowel decrease the amount of the abdomen that can be visualized.

Instrument Controls

Ultrasound equipment has many controls for adjusting the quality of the image. Improper adjustment of any of these can greatly decrease the quality of the image.

Brightness and contrast

The monitor has controls to adjust the brightness and contrast for the image being displayed. If the brightness has been adjusted too high or too low on the monitor, compensating with any other control cannot correct the brightness or darkness. Most machines have a gray bar that displays the gray-scale capability. This capability varies from 16 to 128 shades of gray. The brightness and contrast should be adjusted so that black, white, and all the intermediate shades of gray can be seen.

Depth

The depth control allows for adjustment of the amount of tissue being displayed on the monitor. The depth from the surface of the transducer is measured in centimeters. The area of interest (e.g., kidney, heart) should cover at least two thirds of the screen. Decreasing the amount of depth being displayed causes the area in the near field to become larger.

Gain and power

The gain (overall) and power (output) controls can affect the overall brightness of the image. Gain and power compensate for attenuation of the sound beam as it travels through the tissues. Increasing the gain increases the sensitivity of the transducer to receiving the returning echoes. This can be compared with the volume on a hearing aid. Turning the volume up increases the hearing aid's ability to hear incoming sounds. The power controls the intensity of the sound generated by the transducer. Increasing the power increases the intensity of the sound wave leaving the transducer. The sound is attenuated at the same rate, but a higher-intensity sound wave transmitted into the tissues produces a higher-intensity echo returning to the transducer.

Time gain compensation

The controls that make up the time gain compensation (TGC) are the most important and most often improperly set. The purpose of the TGC is to make like tissues look alike. The intensity of the sound decreases progressively as it returns from deeper tissues. For example, when imaging the liver, three similar reflectors located at 4 cm, 6 cm, and 8 cm of depth should have the same brightness on the monitor. However, because of the attenuation of the echoes returning from the deeper tissues, the brightness gradually decreases. To compensate for the loss of energy, TGC adds increasing amounts of electronic gain to the returning echoes. The three echoes returning from different depths then have the same brightness on the monitor.

The typical controls that make up the TGC are *near field gain* and *far field gain*. The near field gain controls the amount of electronic gain added to the sound returning from the near field. This should be set so that the echoes blend uniformly with those displayed in the mid field. The far field gain controls the amount of electronic gain added to the echoes returning from the far field. With some of the new ultrasound equipment, the TGC is in the form of multiple slide pods. The pods at the top control the near field gain, while the pods closer to the bottom control the mid field and far field.

If proper brightness cannot be achieved, verify the following items. First, check the brightness and contrast controls on the monitor. If the brightness and contrast controls are incorrectly set, changing the TGC cannot compensate for this error. Next, check the power setting to make sure it is not too low. If all controls are set correctly, attempt to improve the acoustic contact with the skin by applying more coupling gel or shaving the clipped area with a razor. If none of these adjustments are productive, change to a lower-frequency transducer. Some resolution is lost, but it is a necessary trade-off when brightness cannot be achieved.

Artifacts

Artifacts can occur during any ultrasound study. Proper identification of these artifacts is important to prevent confusion or misinterpretation. Some artifacts are beneficial in making a diagnosis. Two such artifacts include *acoustic shadowing* and *distance enhancement*. Others, if not readily identified, can be confused as part of the anatomy or a disease process.

Acoustic shadowing occurs when the sound is attenuated or reflected at an acoustic interface (Fig. 18-21). This prevents the sound from being transmitted to the deeper tissues, resulting in no echoes or fewer echoes returning from those areas. Structures that can cause acoustic shadowing include bone, calculi, mineralized tissues, and occasionally fat. For acoustic shadowing to occur, the interface must be in the focal zone of the transducer. If not, the shadowed area may be in with echoes from surrounding tissues as the sound beam diverges. This artifact is more pronounced with higher-frequency transducers.

Distance enhancement occurs when the sound beam traverses a cystic structure (Fig. 18-22). Tissues deep to the cystic structure appear brighter than surrounding tissues. The enhancement occurs because the sound that travels through the fluid-filled areas is less attenuated than

in surrounding tissues. This artifact is useful in establishing that an anechoic or hypoechoic structure is in fact fluid-filled.

Many artifacts have no diagnostic use, though if not identified as artifacts they can lead to confusion. One of these includes the *slice thickness* artifact. This artifact occurs when imaging an anechoic or hypoechoic structure. Echoes are added when the transducer receives echoes with different amplitudes from the same area at the same depth. The

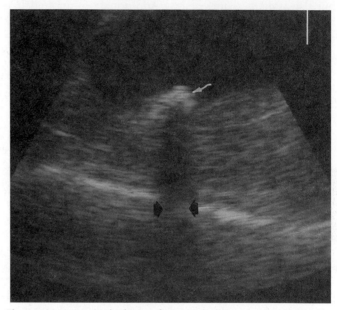

Fig. 18-21 Acoustic shadowing from a calculus in the urinary bladder. The highly reflective surface of the calculus is shown *(white arrow)*. Shadowing caused by the calculus is also shown *(black arrow)*.

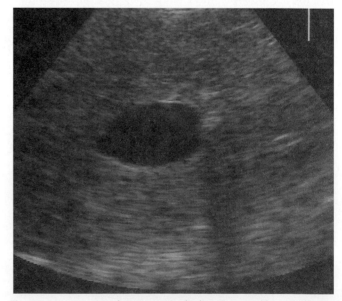

Fig. 18-22 Distance enhancement in the liver is caused by sound waves passing through the fluid-filled gallbladder.

computer then averages these amplitudes and incorporates them in the two-dimensional image. Decreasing the overall gain can minimize this artifact; however, it does not totally eliminate it.

Reverberation occurs when sound is reflected off a highly reflective interface (e.g., soft tissues to air or soft tissues to bone/metal) and then reflected back into the tissues by the surface of the transducer (Fig. 18-23). This bouncing back and forth can continue until the sound energy has completely attenuated. Each time the sound returns to the transducer, it produces an image at a location on the screen that is proportional to the time of travel between the transducer and the reflective interface. This creates a series of lines per equal distance apart on the screen.

The *mirror-image* artifact creates the illusion of liver on the thoracic side of the diaphragm or the appearance of a second heart beyond the lung interface (Fig. 18-24). This artifact can be produced in areas with strongly reflective interfaces. Sound transmitted into the liver is reflected off the diaphragm. Some of those echoes are not reflected directly toward the transducer but back into the liver. In the liver, some of the misdirected echoes are reflected back to the diaphragm and then to the transducer. The computer sees the misdirected echoes as being reflected from the other side of the diaphragm. One way this artifact can be minimized is by decreasing the depth to include only the area of interest.

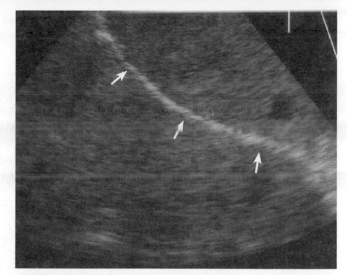

Fig. 18-24 Mirror-image artifact. The arrows indicate the liver/diaphragm to lung interface. The actual liver is in the near field *(top right)*. The far field *(bottom left)* represents the mirror image of the liver.

ENDOSCOPY
Christine Bretz

Veterinary teams are finding that endoscopes are essential tools for diagnosing many conditions and diseases. The opportunity to examine and obtain tissue samples without the invasiveness of surgery makes endoscopy one of the best methods of evaluating the digestive system. Responsibilities of veterinary technicians assisting with endoscopy include selection, care, and maintenance of the endoscopes, and care and positioning of the patient.

TYPES OF ENDOSCOPES

Rigid endoscopes are commonly used for rhinoscopy, cystoscopy, laparoscopy, arthroscopy, vaginoscopy, colonoscopy, and thoroscopy. *Flexible endoscopes* are used for gastrointestinal endoscopy, duodenoscopy, colonoscopy, and bronchoscopy. Flexible endoscopes are also used for percutaneous placement of gastrostomy tubes in small animals.

Rigid Endoscopes

Rigid endoscopes are composed of a metal tube, lenses, and glass rods (Fig. 18-25). They vary in size and characteristics; however, all are composed of a hollow tube containing no fiber bundles. Rigid endoscopes tend to be less expensive than flexible endoscopes, but their uses tend to be limited to that for which they were designed.

Rigid endoscopes should be held by the eyepiece and not by the rod. Even slight bending of the rod section could change the angle of deflection, decreasing the degree of

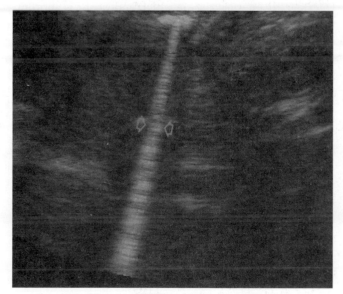

Fig. 18-23 Reverberation artifact caused by gas in the small intestine of a dog. Notice the equally spaced echoic lines *(white arrows)* trailing from the highly reflective interface created by the gas.

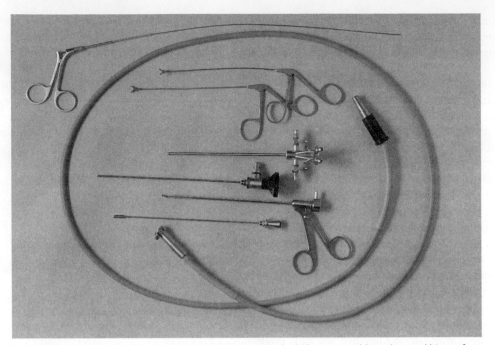

Fig. 18-25 Example of a rigid endoscope used for cystoscopy and rhinoscopy. The light source cable and several biopsy forceps are also shown.

visualization. Rigid endoscopes should never be handled in bunches or piled on top of one another.

Flexible Endoscopes

There are two types of flexible endoscopes: *fiberoptic* and *video*. Fiberoptic endoscopes use glass fiber bundles for transmission of images. These bundles transmit light from the light source to the distal tip of the endoscope. Fiberoptic glass fiber bundles are very fragile and can be damaged easily. Broken fibers show up on the monitor screen as black dots. Too many of these black dots (many broken fiber bundles) can significantly reduce the field of view. For this reason, fiberoptic endoscopes must be handled very carefully and never bent at a sharp angle.

A recent development in veterinary endoscopy is video endoscopes. A microchip located at the distal end of the endoscope records and transmits the image to a computer and then to a monitor screen. The image can be recorded on a VCR, and pictures can be recorded to show the owner and be included in the patient's record. Many operators find the video endoscope more ergonomically pleasing, because the controls are held at the waist and not near the face. Eventually, video endoscopes will replace fiberoptic endoscopes.

PURCHASING AN ENDOSCOPE

Although the cost of an endoscope may be a substantial initial investment, many years of use and its value as a diagnostic tool will make the endoscope more than just a

convenience to the veterinary hospital. The endoscope should pay for itself in the first year. The endoscope's life expectancy is 5 to 10 years.

Commonly associated costs include the intravenous catheter, preprocedure enemas, preanesthetic blood studies and evaluation, the endoscopist's time, anesthesia, and laboratory fees. Skilled technical time involved in the preparation and cleaning of the endoscope must also be considered.

An endoscope of poor quality will rarely be used, so the veterinary team must decide which endoscope is appropriate for the hospital. A good-quality fiberoptic endoscope can be used for many purposes. Reproductive and gastrointestinal endoscopy, colonoscopy, and respiratory procedures can all be performed with one properly functioning endoscope. For most small-animal practice situations, a 110-cm gastroscope/duodenal flexible endoscope should provide sufficient length for dogs and cats.

The diameter of the endoscope is also an important factor. Most human endoscopes are appropriate for endoscopic examination of large dogs; however, a human pediatric endoscope (insertion tube diameter 7.9 to 9 mm) is ideal. Larger endoscopes are difficult to pass into the pyloric canal to the duodenum in small dogs and cats.

Some important characteristics that an endoscope should possess include four-way deflection capability, 180° upward deflection tip, water flush, air insufflation, and suction. Many models can be completely immersed, allowing thorough cleaning and disinfection.

One can easily locate a good-quality, low-cost, used endoscope through a human hospital. These hospitals are constantly updating their equipment and are often willing to sell their relatively new equipment at a reduced price. If you are considering a used endoscope, be sure to check for holes, cracks, or scratches on the insertion tube that might promote leakage of fluids into the endoscope. Look through the eyepiece and check for broken fibers, which appear as small black dots. A few fiber bundles can be expected to break over time, but an excessive number of broken bundles will inhibit visualization. Also check the intensity of the light by attaching the endoscope to the light source. If you purchase a used endoscope from a human hospital, be sure to ask for the operator's manual or other information that accompanies the endoscope. If no information is available, call the manufacturer of the endoscope and request a new operator's manual.

THE ENDOSCOPY ROOM

In an ideal situation, all endoscopic examinations are performed in the same room. This room should preferably be out of the way of hospital traffic. Because the lights are usually dimmed during endoscopic examination to reduce glare on the viewing monitor, a room with curtains or shades is ideal. The room should never be so dark, however, that proper anesthetic monitoring is inhibited.

A sturdy cart with three or four shelves can conveniently store the light source, suction unit, endoscope, and any accessory equipment until ready for use. All necessary equipment should be located near this endoscopy unit so that it can be reached quickly if needed during endoscopy. These items should be meticulously organized. The assisting staff must be able to locate any necessary equipment quickly during a procedure.

To avoid complications and delays, the procedure room should be well stocked before the endoscopic examination begins. All anesthetic equipment must be ready before the procedure begins. Procedure cards or checklists are excellent ways to ensure that each type of endoscopic examination starts with the proper equipment.

ACCESSORY INSTRUMENTS

Accessory instruments can be passed through the working channel of the flexible endoscope and directed to a specific area. The most basic instruments include biopsy forceps, foreign body removal forceps, and a cytology brush (Fig. 18-26).

Endoscopes are fragile and expensive, so personnel must be instructed in their proper care, use, and maintenance before endoscope use. Before each endoscopic examination, be sure each piece of ancillary equipment is functioning properly, and anticipate the need for these pieces of equipment. They should be cleaned as soon as possible after use or the jaws of the forceps may become locked in the closed position. If this occurs, soaking the tip of the biopsy forceps in warm water for 10 to 15 minutes helps to loosen the debris around the jaws.

All personnel involved with endoscopic procedures should wear latex examination gloves. This protects the animal from contamination and also protects the clinician and technician. The endoscope should not be allowed to directly contact the video accessories or any other potentially conductive object; wearing latex gloves offers an added protection against electrical shock.

CLEANING A FLEXIBLE ENDOSCOPE

All endoscopy equipment should be thoroughly cleaned as soon as possible after the procedure. The manufacturer's specific cleaning instructions should be carefully followed. Endoscopes must be handled carefully during cleaning and

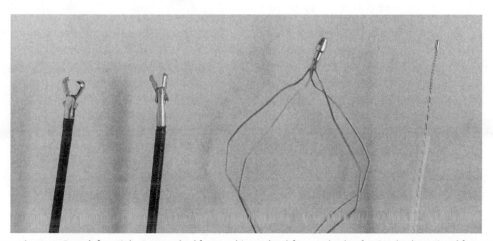

Fig. 18-26 Accessory equipment. *From left to right:* Rat-toothed forceps, biopsy (cup) forceps, basket foreign-body retrieval forceps, and cytology brush.

never placed where they could fall or be bumped. It is also a good idea for the person cleaning the endoscope to wear latex examination gloves. Gather the following supplies:

- Latex examination gloves
- Cleaning solution
- Two large basins for cleaning solution and distilled water
- Distilled water
- Methyl alcohol
- Lint-free gauze pads
- Cotton-tipped applicators
- Channel-cleaning brush

Immediately after the procedure, flush water and then air through the air-water channel of the flexible endoscope. Gently wipe off the insertion tube with a soft gauze or cloth that has been soaked in an approved detergent solution. Do not squeeze the flexible section. Place the distal end of the endoscope in detergent water and suction a small amount through. Alternately suction water and then air a few times. Remove the air-water valve, suction valve, and biopsy cap, and place them in a small amount of cleaning solution to soak. Pass the channel-cleaning brush through the biopsy channel, and suction the channel repeatedly until the brush comes out clean. Clean the brush each time it is passed through the channel.

If the endoscope has a suction cleaning tube, it should then be placed on the biopsy port. Place the end of the suction cleaning tube and the end of the endoscope into a mixture of detergent and water. Cover the suction valve hole with your finger and suction soapy water, then distilled water, and then air to dry the endoscope. Remove the suction cleaning tube, and carefully clean the valve holes with a cotton-tipped swab. Clean and rinse the air-water valve, suction valve, and biopsy cap, and replace them on the endoscope.

It is a good preventive measure to lightly lubricate the air-water and suction valves periodically to prevent cracking. Wipe off the outside of the endoscope with an alcohol-soaked gauze pad. Clean the lenses with an approved lens cleaner by applying some lens cleaner onto a soft gauze pad and rubbing the lens; then rub with a clean gauze pad. Replace any lens caps, light source insertion bar covers, and ETO caps before placing the endoscope back into the cabinet. For proper drying of the biopsy channel, leave the biopsy port in an open position.

Biopsy instruments should be immersed in soapy water, brushed carefully with a cleaning brush, and then rinsed. Check to be sure that the jaws of biopsy instruments are not sticking by carefully opening and then closing them.

STORING AN ENDOSCOPE

The ideal way to store a flexible endoscope is in a hanging position in a well-ventilated cabinet. This allows the endo-

scope to drain completely after cleaning and permits better air movement through the channels. The padded case in which the endoscope was supplied by the manufacturer is another possible storage area; however, little air circulates in these containers and moisture in the channels of the endoscope offers an environment for bacterial growth. Rigid endoscopes are best stored in their original carrying case.

GASTROINTESTINAL ENDOSCOPY

Flexible endoscopes are most commonly used to examine the gastrointestinal tract, including the esophagus. Gastrointestinal endoscopy allows visualization of the upper and lower digestive tract, including its contents.

Patient Preparation

The patient should be fasted for 12 to 24 hours. A longer period of fasting may be required in patients with delayed gastric emptying. An intravenous catheter should be placed and fluid administration started. There are various opinions as to which drugs may impair passage of the endoscope into the duodenum; however, a combination of atropine and morphine is known to make endoscope passage more difficult. Use of these drugs together should be avoided for gastrointestinal endoscopy. Endotracheal intubation and proper endotracheal tube cuff inflation are needed to avoid aspiration of gastric contents in the event of regurgitation.

Place the patient in left lateral recumbency, with a mouth speculum placed to prevent damage to the endoscope from biting. Raise the table to a height that does not require excessive bending of the endoscope near the handpiece (Fig. 18-27). Lubricate the insertion tube with a water-soluble lubricant, such as K-Y Jelly, avoiding the distal end of the endoscope. Use of petroleum-based lubri-

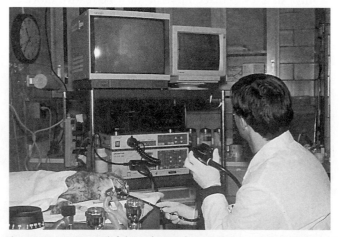

Fig. 18-27 Patient in left lateral recumbency, with a mouth speculum in place. Note that the table is positioned at a height convenient for the endoscopist.

cants, such as Vaseline, is not advised because over time they cause stretching and deterioration of the rubber components of the endoscope. As the endoscope is introduced into the patient's mouth, avoid scraping the endoscope against the teeth in the back of the mouth. Air insufflation is usually needed to facilitate visualization; however, oversufflation may cause overdistention of the stomach or abdomen and can interfere with ventilation.

Obtaining Samples

Tissue samples are obtained by grasping the mucosa with biopsy forceps. The biopsy forceps are passed down the operating channel of the endoscope with the forceps jaws in a closed position. Care must be taken to not open or close the forceps too forcefully, as they can become locked or broken. Also, make sure the jaws of the biopsy forceps are in the closed position before bringing them back out through the biopsy channel of the endoscope; otherwise the accessory equipment and the endoscope may be damaged.

Once a tissue sample is obtained, the specimen is gently teased out of the forceps with a 25-gauge needle or shaken directly from the biopsy forceps into a vial of preservative. If the latter technique is used, the biopsy forceps must be rinsed with water before reinsertion into the endoscope channel.

Upon completion of the gastroscopic examination, the stomach and esophagus are suctioned with the endoscope using gentle external pressure on the abdomen to remove fluids, debris, and excess air.

The endotracheal tube cuff should remain partially inflated when extubating to bring out any remaining material.

COLONOSCOPY

Two types of colonoscopes are available: a rigid colonoscope (Fig. 18-28) and a flexible endoscope. Each requires

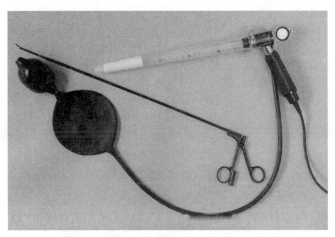

Fig. 18-28 Reusable colonoscope-procto/sigmoidoscope.

different protocols for patient preparation and sedation. *Rigid colonoscopy* allows direct examination of the rectum and descending colon. *Flexible colonoscopy* allows examination of the transverse and ascending colon, cecum, ileocolic valve, and ileum.

Ideally, all feces should be removed from the colon before endoscopic examination; however, this is not always possible. Food should be withheld from the patient for at least 36 hours. Several different colonic cleansing protocols can be used, depending on how cooperative the patient is and the amount of help available. For rigid colonoscopy, a warm-water enema (10 to 20 ml/kg) the evening before the procedure, another enema the following morning, and a final enema 1 hour before the examination usually provide enough cleansing.

To successfully observe the entire colon with a flexible endoscope, the bowel must be completely cleansed before the examination. Colon electrolyte lavage solutions, such as Golytely® (Braintree Laboratories, Braintree, Mass.) or Colyte® (Endlaw Preparations, Farmingdale, N.Y.), are administered orally by stomach tube, usually the day before the procedure. Often a repeat dose is given the morning of the examination. These commercial solutions are superior to traditional soapy water enemas. Rigid colonoscopy can be performed using heavy sedation, but a light plane of anesthesia is usually preferred. The patient is placed in right lateral recumbency, with the table slightly tilted so that any residual material drains away from the endoscopist.

Anesthesia is necessary for flexible colonoscopy. The patient is placed in left lateral recumbency to assist passage of the endoscope into the transverse and ascending colon. Colonic insufflation is used to facilitate passage of the endoscope, and often air escapes through the anal sphincter. If this occurs, manual pressure around the anus by a gloved assistant helps to prevent this escape of air.

AIRWAY ENDOSCOPY

Airway endoscopy allows visualization of the trachea and bronchi. It is most useful when diagnosing collapsed trachea, airway parasitism, and foreign bodies. Tissue samples may also be obtained through the endoscope for histopathologic, cytologic, and microbiologic examinations.

The most common endoscope used for medium-size or large dogs is a small-diameter gastrointestinal endoscope. For smaller dogs and cats, a flexible human pediatric bronchoscope is required. Because bronchoscopes have a smaller working channel, any biopsies obtained are smaller. Before use for lower airway endoscopy, the endoscope must be sterilized according to the manufacturer's guidelines.

General anesthesia is required for lower airway endoscopy. In medium-size to large dogs, the endoscope is passed through a shortened sterile endotracheal tube. Oxygen and/or anesthetic gases can also be delivered to the patient using a bronchoscope tube adapter. The patient must be closely monitored for proper oxygenation and anesthetic depth. A mouth speculum is necessary to prevent damage to the endoscope.

In cats and small dogs, the bronchoscope is passed down the trachea without an endotracheal tube in place. Great care must be taken to evaluate the patient before the procedure, because the patient's airway is occluded by the endoscope. It may become necessary to stop the endoscopy for some time while the patient is oxygenated. Oxygen can also be delivered through the suction channel of the bronchoscope to help prevent hypoxemia.

RECOMMENDED READING

Barr F: *Diagnostic ultrasound in the dog and cat*, London, 1990, Blackwell Scientific.

Brearley MJ et al: *A colour atlas of small animal endoscopy*, St Louis, 1991, Mosby.

Burk RL, Ackerman N: *Small animal radiology and ultrasonography*, ed 2, Philadelphia, 1996, WB Saunders.

Curry TS et al: *Christensen's physics of diagnostic radiology*, ed 4, Philadelphia, 1990, Lea & Febiger.

Han CM, Hurd CD: *Practical diagnostic imaging for the veterinary technician*, St Louis, 2000, Mosby.

Nyland TG, Mattoon JS: *Small animal diagnostic ultrasound*, ed 2, Philadelphia, 2002, WB Saunders.

Tams T: *Small animal endoscopy*, ed 2, St Louis, 1999, Mosby.

Thrall DE: *Textbook of veterinary diagnostic radiology*, ed 4, Philadelphia, 2002, WB Saunders.

Traub-Dargatz JL, Brown CM: *Equine endoscopy*, ed 2, St Louis, 1997, Mosby.

19

Anesthesia and Perioperative Analgesia

C.L. Tyner and Scott W. Rundell

Learning Objectives

After reviewing this chapter, the reader should understand the following:

- The role of veterinary technicians in anesthesia and perioperative pain management
- The significance of and methods for managing perioperative pain
- Goals and fundamentals of anesthesia
- Types of anesthetic agents and their effects, advantages, and disadvantages
- Steps involved in anesthetizing animals
- Equipment used for anesthetizing animals
- Procedures used in medicating and monitoring animals before, during, and after anesthesia

One of the most important areas of veterinary medicine is the management of the pain experienced by our animal patients. Whether due to inflammation from tissue injury (trauma, disease) or the controlled trauma of surgery, pain is debilitating and undesirable.

ROLE OF VETERINARY TECHNICIANS

The involvement of veterinary technicians in managing perioperative pain before, during, and after a procedure is growing profoundly. Technicians are assuming greater responsibilities for the assessment of patients and alleviation of their discomfort, distress, and pain. The concept of pain as a "therapeutic agent" that "keeps the patient from moving around too much" is no longer considered acceptable. In the research setting, the avoidance, recognition, and treatment of discomfort, distress, and pain become a matter of regulatory compliance as well as medical prudence and compassion. In many settings, technicians may assume considerable responsibility for routine anesthesia and monitoring. The alert technician is invaluable in bringing patient distress to the attention of the veterinarian. Given the wide variety of species and situations encountered, this chapter can only provide a foundation on which to build and will focus on surgical anesthesia and perioperative analgesia. It is highly recommended that veterinary technicians involved with these procedures expand their knowledge via the recom-

mended reading and continuing education. The opportunity for specialty certification of technicians in anesthesia exists and may be pursued where appropriate.

INDICATIONS FOR ANESTHESIA, SEDATION, AND ANALGESIA

Anesthesia or sedation is indicated for a wide variety of situations in veterinary medicine. These include restraint of patients, management of acute or chronic pain, and surgical anesthesia. The necessity for chemical restraint of an animal varies tremendously with the species and procedure. Calm, friendly, domestic animals will tolerate more handling than agitated or wild animals. Judgment is required to determine the degree of sedation necessary for patient and personnel comfort and safety. Surgical anesthesia continues to be the central focus of providing intraoperative pain relief. Postoperative analgesia has received increased attention recently and is expected whenever appropriate. Management of chronic pain is an issue of growing concern to owners of geriatric pets. Recent pharmacological innovations have enhanced our ability to provide such relief with increased safety and efficacy.

Coming to Terms With Pain

Pain is defined as an unpleasant sensory or emotional experience associated with actual or potential tissue damage.

Physiologic pain results from the stimulation of nerve endings called *nociceptors*, which are found throughout the tissues. Pain may be classified as *peripheral* (visceral or somatic), *neuropathic* (originating from damaged nerves), *clinical* (ongoing pain), and *idiopathic* (unknown cause).

While we have an understanding of pain from personal experience, we cannot experience it from an animal's perspective. There are difficulties with simply transposing our own feelings onto our patients, especially with nonmammalian species. What is painful to a bird, frog, or fish? Assessment of these conditions has also become a regulatory compliance issue. This is because animal welfare regulations mandate their avoidance in research animals unless specifically allowed by the Institutional Animal Care and Use Committee (IACUC). Even then, there is an expectation for defining a "humane end-point" beyond which animals will not be allowed to experience pain. Hence, the judgment that an animal is in "discomfort, distress, or pain" may determine whether or not one is in violation of federal regulations. There has been quite a debate over the definition of these terms with regard to research animals. In the clinical practice setting, recognizing and alleviating pain is also a growing concern. This has arisen from client demand, recognition of the deleterious effects of pain, and improved methods of pain recognition and relief. However, it is important to know that a universal philosophy of pain management does not exist for all species or situations. Consideration of pain relief for large animal species (especially food animals) is still controversial in some quarters. The old "heavy hand" techniques have not been entirely supplanted by pain-relieving methods. There exists a wide gulf between what is acceptable "on the farm" versus the high degree of concern for pain relief in research animals. Depending on where one is employed, a technician may be required to adapt to various philosophies and concepts of acceptable pain management in animals. However, this is not to suggest that one should simply accept pain as an unavoidable consequence. If one promotes an awareness of its existence and deleterious effects, pain relief will tend to follow.

Effects of Pain

Clinical pain has numerous deleterious effects on the patient. These include the following:

- Immunosuppression
- Increased tissue catabolism
- Reduced healing
- Increased autonomic activity, primarily sympathetic
- Emotional stress/distress

Predicting and Recognizing Pain in Animals

Since we cannot measure pain directly, it is necessary to deduce its existence. Pain recognition is difficult, because responses to pain vary among species and individuals. Some individuals tolerate considerable discomfort without any reaction. Other individuals vocalize loudly when given a minor injection. Anticipation of possible pain enters into the animal's response as well. It is very helpful to know the normal behavior of the individual when assessing them for pain. Changes in behavior may be observed such as shunning or seeking attention, vocalization changes, altered body posture, guarding of painful body parts, altered grooming, inappetence, changes in voiding behavior, or reluctance to move (Box 19-1). Less subjective signs include increased respiration and heart rates, peripheral vasoconstriction, muscle tension, and elevated blood pressure. Obvious inflammation (redness, swelling, and heat) is generally accompanied by pain. Animals recovering from anesthesia are not able to exhibit a normal range of behavioral signs and may be experiencing pain long before it becomes apparent to the observer. Research guidelines indicate that any condition that would cause pain in humans should be assumed to cause pain in animals. Accordingly, we assume that a dog undergoing abdominal surgery would experience as much pain as a person would experience from a comparable procedure, even if the dog does not exhibit "signs of pain." The term *preemptive analgesia* means taking steps to predict and prevent pain before it occurs. It has been demonstrated that pain is more easily managed if analgesics are given before a patient experiences pain.

Pain-Relief Modalities

Pain-relief modalities take advantage of one or more means of preventing or interfering with the development or perception of pain. Refinement of surgical technique to produce less tissue damage will prevent a great deal of postoperative pain. Proponents of performing laser surgery report that postoperative pain is greatly reduced, for example. To the extent that some tissue trauma is inevitable in any surgical procedure, one or more of the following modalities may be utilized before, during, and after the procedure to manage the type and level of pain experienced at that time.

BOX 19-1

Signs of Pain

1. Protection of the affected area (avoids touching; threatens if approached)
2. Vocalization (especially on movement or palpation of affected area)
3. Licking or biting affected area
4. Scratching or shaking affected area
5. Restlessness, pacing
6. Sweating
7. Increased respiratory and/or heart rate

Analgesia

Analgesia is the reduction or absence of pain sensation without loss of other sensations.

In theory, a pure analgesic agent would reduce pain without causing any other effects. In practice, this is not usually the case. Most of the drugs utilized for analgesia cause various other *dose-dependent* effects. A dose-dependent effect varies with the dose of the drug, becoming more intense as the dose increases, or appearing only at higher doses. The opioid analgesic agents produce a dose-dependent sedation (called *narcosis*) that may be quite profound. The nonsteroidal anti-inflammatory drugs (NSAIDs) (especially the older ones) have a tendency to cause GI irritation, ulceration, and bleeding. Newer analgesic agents are designed to have fewer adverse side effects (Table 19-1).

Anesthesia

Anesthesia means "*no feeling*" and may be local, regional, spinal/epidural, or general (supraspinal).

Local anesthesia is induced by infiltrating the immediate area with an agent that interferes with nerve-impulse transmission. It is also called a local block or numbing of the area. The technique of infiltrating an incision site with a local anesthetic agent just before surgery may result in less intraoperative pain from the incision site. Placing a local anesthetic in the open incision just before closing may result in decreased incision site pain during the recovery period.

Regional or *segmental anesthesia* is achieved by blocking the nerve or nerves that supply a region or segment of the body. An injection of a local anesthetic agent is made near the nerve at a point proximal to the region being anesthetized. A paravertebral nerve block is often used to produce regional flank anesthesia in cattle undergoing standing abdominal surgery. Nerve blocks are also commonly used to help diagnose lameness in horses.

Spinal or *epidural anesthesia (or analgesia)* is induced by injecting a local anesthetic or analgesic agent into the subarachnoid or epidural space of the spinal cord. This is typically done at the lumbosacral junction to provide profound analgesia or anesthesia to the pelvis and rear limbs during

fracture repair. *Note:* Animals may perceive numbed body parts with anxiety, and self-mutilation may result. Prevention of these reactions may require tranquilization or sedation.

General anesthesia is the purposeful derangement of a patient's normal physiologic processes to produce a state of unconsciousness, relaxation, analgesia, and/or amnesia. It is induced by administering an anesthetic agent systemically that will be distributed to the brain. The degree to which different agents produce each of these effects varies (Table 19-2). This altered physiologic state may become progressively deranged until it is incompatible with life. Cardiopulmonary depression is the primary derangement to watch for via close monitoring of vital signs. Vigilance at all stages of the anesthetic procedure can warn of an impending crisis, usually with adequate time to take preventive or corrective actions. General anesthetics may be administered by injection (IM or IV) or by inhalation, depending on the agent. When inhalation anesthesia is performed, the animal is usually first induced into general anesthesia with a short-acting injectable agent to facilitate tracheal intubation and induction with the inhalation agent (Table 19-3).

While general anesthesia controls the *perception* of intraoperative pain, one must not equate unconsciousness or unresponsiveness with lack of pain. General anesthetics vary in their analgesic efficacy and may not completely disrupt the nociceptive mechanisms of the nervous system. The astute observer will notice that anesthetized patients may still respond to painful stimuli as evidenced by increased respiratory and heart rates during painful parts of the procedure. Analgesic agents are needed to suppress the physiologic pain mechanisms that remain active during anesthesia. These will also allow a reduction in the dose of general anesthetic needed to maintain anesthesia. In human anesthesiology, there have been recent reports of "awareness" of sound and pain by apparently anesthetized patients. Postoperatively, they are able to repeat conversations overheard during their procedure and describe the experience of searing pain. It is not fully understood if this situation occurs in anesthetized animals or how to recognize it if it does.

TABLE 19-1

Classes of Analgesic Agents

Drug Class	Example
Opioids	Oxymorphone, morphine, fentanyl, butorphanol, buprenorphine
Alpha-2 adrenergic agonists	Xylazine, detomidine, metdetomidine
Nonsteroidal anti-inflammatory drugs (NSAIDs)	Carprofen, aspirin, etodolac, phenylbutazone, flunixin, acetaminophen
Adjunctive agents	Ketamine, acepromazine, diazepam, prednisolone

TABLE 19-2

Injectable General Anesthetics

Drug Class	Example	Comments
Barbiturates	Thiopental Human products: Pentothal Extralabel use: Dogs, cats	Ultrashort-acting thiobarbiturate Concentration: 2% to 5%; store reconstituted product under refrigeration Dosage (if premedicated with tranquilizer/opioid): 5 to 10 mg/kg slowly IV to effect Duration of effects is 5 to 10 minutes but only provides 2- to 3-minute intubation window at minimal doses Used as induction agent for inhalation anesthesia Short action due to redistribution Accumulates in tissue: do not use for anesthetic maintenance Provides minimal analgesia Use small dose, and dilute concentrations in small or debilitated patients with cardiopulmonary, hepatic, or renal compromise May produce arrhythmias and apnea Monitor closely and support ventilation Administer fluids and oxygen to improve outcome Provides smooth transition to unconsciousness Premedication with tranquilizer and opioid reduces dose required Use with caution in sight hounds
Nonbarbiturates	Propofol Veterinary products (canine): Rapinovet, Propofol Human products: Diprivan	Ultrashort-acting alkylphenol, Concentration: 10 mg/ml Used as induction agent for inhalation anesthesia, maintenance for brief procedures Induction dosage: 2 to 6 mg/kg IV over 60 to 90 seconds to effect (if premedicated) Rapid injection causes apnea Duration of effects is 5 to 10 minutes, but only provides 2- to 3-minute intubation window at minimal doses Maintenance dosage: 0.4 to 0.8 mg/kg/min IV infusion in conjunction with benzodiazepine and opioid Highly lipid-soluble Can produce the "five hypos" Short action due to redistribution Tissue accumulation minimal due to rapid metabolism Provides minimal analgesia Not recommended for pregnant or nursing females Provide cardiovascular and pulmonary support Aseptic technique is critical: must be used within 6 hours of opening vial
Dissociative agents	Ketamine Veterinary products (cats, primates): Ketaset, Vetalar, VetaKet	Concentration: 100 mg/ml Dosage: 5 to 30 mg/kg IM or 1 to 6 mg/kg IV (slowly) Duration: 5 to 10 minutes IV 20 to 40 minutes IM

Extralabel uses: Horses, dogs

Causes catatonia, muscle rigidity, possible convulsions if used alone; do not use alone without a tranquilizer

Rapid onset of profound anesthesia with some somatic but poor visceral analgesia

Causes apnea, enhancing hypoxemia and hypercarbemia

Increases heart rate and blood pressure, increasing myocardial oxygen demand

Usually maintains cardiac output and blood pressure better than barbiturates

May increase intracranial and ocular pressure

Avoid in patients with renal, hepatic, or cardiac disease, ocular surgery, and epileptics

Transition to inhalation anesthesia may be rougher than with barbiturates

Apnea reduces uptake of inhalation agent

Animal awakens abruptly when ketamine wears off

Excessive salivation and respiratory secretions may occur.

Dissociative agents are rarely used alone. They are typically combined with other agents that offset the undesirable properties. Examples include:

Ketamine + benzodiazepine:

- Useful combination for canine induction
- Dosage: ketamine at 5 mg/kg and benzodiazepine at 0.25 mg/kg, slowly IV

Others (see recommended reading for details of usage):

- Ketamine + acepromazine + butorphanol
- Ketamine + alpha-2 agonist
- Ketamine + butorphanol

Tiletamine
Telazol (dogs, cats)
Extralabel use: Exotics

The only commercially available dissociative-tranquilizer combination.

Concentration: zolazepam 50 mg/ml and tiletamine 50 mg/ml

Dosage: 2 to 6 mg/kg IV or IM

Rapidly induces surgical plane of anesthesia for 10–20 minutes

Recovery period varies

Tiletamine has longer duration and greater analgesia than ketamine

Large doses can produce apnea, leading to hypoxia and hypercarbia

Excitement may occur during recovery if zolazepam is eliminated from tissues before tiletamine

Administer an additional sedative IV

Recovery may be prolonged with use of large doses if zolazepam is not completely metabolized

Reverse with flumazenil

In cats, tiletamine is often metabolized first; in dogs, zolazepam is usually metabolized first

Very effective in exotic and aggressive patients

In healthy patients, premedication with acepromazine (0.05 to 0.1 mg/kg IM or SC) 15 minutes before Telazol administration may provide 20 to 40 minutes of surgical anesthesia

Recovery varies

TABLE 19-3

Inhalation General Anesthetics

Inhalation Agent	Examples	Characteristics
Methoxyflurane	Veterinary products: Metofane Human products: Penthrane	MAC: 0.23% in dogs and cats Elimination: 50% by metabolism Use has become limited due to popularity of newer agents Slow induction and prolonged recovery Less arrhythmogenic than halothane but more so than isoflurane The most nephrotoxic of the inhalants due to fluoride ion released by metabolism Avoid concurrent use with other nephrotoxic drugs (e.g., aminoglycosides) Do not use on unhealthy animals
Halothane	Veterinary products: Halothane, USP Human products: Fluothane Halothane	MAC: dog, 0.87%; cat, 1.19%; horse, 0.88% Elimination: 20% by metabolism Use declining due to popularity of newer agents Moderately rapid induction and recovery Hepatotoxic and arrhythmogenic Most notable for sensitizing the myocardium to the arrhythmogenic effects of catecholamines Thymol preservative contaminates equipment Decomposes in contact with soda lime.
Isoflurane	Veterinary products: Aerrane, IsoVet, IsoFlo Human products: Isoflurane, Forane	MAC: dog, 1.3%; cat, 1.63%; horse, 1.31% Blood-gas partition coefficient: 1.46 Elimination: 0.17% by metabolism Currently most popular in small-animal practice Provides greatest margin of safety of all currently used gas anesthetics Excellent anesthetic for high-risk patients Indications: liver disease, renal failure, trauma, arrhythmias, cesarean section, old animals, obese animals, hypersensitivity to other anesthetics Stable in contact with soda lime
Sevoflurane	Veterinary products: SevoFlo	MAC: dog, 2.34%; cat, 2.58%; horse, 2.34% Blood-gas partition coefficient: 0.68 Elimination: 3% by metabolism Introduced into veterinary market in 1999 Still very expensive compared with isoflurane Requires a precision vaporizer calibrated for this agent Induction and recovery more rapid than isoflurane due to lower blood solubility Cardiovascular effects similar to isoflurane, with less myocardial sensitization to catecholamines Marked respiratory depression occurs Potential for production of nephrotoxic olefin due to degradation by CO_2 absorbents

Note: All volatile (inhalation) anesthetics decrease cardiac output, and some decrease peripheral vascular resistance in a dose-related fashion. This results in decreased blood pressure.

Sedation and tranquilization

Sedation and tranquilization are terms that are often used interchangeably but actually have different meanings. *Sedation* is a mild to profound degree of CNS depression in which the patient is drowsy but may be aroused by painful stimuli. *Tranquilization* is a state of relaxation and calmness characterized by a lack of anxiety or concern without significant drowsiness. In general, drugs that produce tranquilization at low doses may produce sedation at higher doses. Some sedatives also produce significant analgesia. Hence, it is difficult to refer to a drug strictly as a tranquilizer, sedative, or analgesic agent as any or all of these effects may occur in a dose-dependent fashion. Tranquilizers and sedatives are typically used as preanesthetic medications to calm the patient and reduce the amount of anesthetic needed (Table 19-4).

Alternative pain-relief modalities

Western medicine has depended almost exclusively on pharmacological agents for pain management. However, alternative modalities such as acupuncture, electrical nerve stimulation, magnetic field induction, and neurolysis have gained increasing acceptance. Refer to the recommended reading for information on these pain-relief modalities.

Goals of an Anesthetic-Analgesic Plan

The goals of every anesthetic-analgesic plan are to predict complications, prevent complications, recognize complications when they occur, and correct the complications. Complications can be prevented by using the correct equipment and methods, assuring equipment is in good working order, avoiding drugs that enhance a pre-existing condition, and supporting the specific needs of the patient. Supporting respiration with oxygen enrichment and supporting perfusion with appropriate fluids may be adequate to prevent common arrhythmias or hypotension. Appropriate and timely use of analgesic agents prevents complications associated with pain. Knowledge of pre-existing conditions is essential (see Patient Evaluation section). Promptly recognizing anesthetic complications requires close, continuous monitoring. Specific attention should be paid to the "five hypos" and other predicted complications. (See Anesthetic Monitoring section).

FUNDAMENTALS OF ANESTHESIA

The fundamentals of anesthesia can be summarized as follows:

- Carefully evaluate the medical history, physical examination findings, and laboratory data.
- Prepare for the expected and unexpected. Work with adequately trained personnel.
- Minimize anesthesia time by planning ahead (e.g., prepare the surgical site before anesthesia).
- Carefully select and use the correct dose of anesthetic drugs, based on the patient's health status, species, and breed. Avoid drugs that can enhance pre-existing health problems.
- Avoid administration of induction agents until calming agents have taken effect.
- Re-evaluate and stabilize (if necessary) vital signs before induction.
- Maintain a patent airway and monitor ventilation; support with supplemental oxygen and assisted ventilation.
- Monitor cardiovascular function; support with fluids and oxygen.
- Monitor body temperature; support by preventing heat loss and providing external sources of heat.
- Continually monitor and support all body systems from premedication through recovery.
- Use analgesics to minimize pain and discomfort. Use calming agents to reduce excitement.
- Keep an accurate record of the anesthetic procedure, monitoring efforts, and all major anesthetic events.

STEPS OF ANESTHESIA

Step 1: Patient Evaluation

Patient evaluation means to carefully judge a patient's medical history and physical condition to determine health status and predict potential complications. This is the most important step, because all anesthetic decisions are based on health status. The medical history and physical examination are absolutely critical before anesthesia. All abnormalities discovered should be pursued to determine their potential effect on anesthetic outcome. Patient evaluation includes consideration of patient characteristics, medical history, physical examination, and laboratory data.

Patient characteristics

Patient characteristics such as species, breed, age, and sex may prompt special considerations. Sight hounds (greyhounds, salukis, borzois) are known to be very excitable during induction and have a prolonged recovery period. Brachycephalic breeds (pug, bulldog, Boston terrier) are known to have problems with airway obstruction during recovery. Pediatric patients are prone to hypothermia and hypoglycemia. Geriatric patients may have difficulty metabolizing drugs and typically require more supportive care.

TABLE 19-4

Tranquilizers and Sedatives

Drug Class	Example	Comments
Phenothiazines	Acepromazine Promace (dogs, cats, horses)	Concentration: 10 mg/ml; dilute to 1 mg/ml for small-animal use
		Dosage 0.05 to 0.1 mg/kg IV, IM or SC (3 mg maximum total dose)
		Major tranquilizer, alpha-adrenergic blocker, antiemetic, lowers seizure threshold, no significant analgesia but potentiates or prolongs analgesic effect of analgesic agents, variable sedation
		Potential hypotension/tachycardia due to vasodilation
		Avoid in cardiovascular compromise
		Acepromazine + opioid:
		• Consider anticholinergic: glycopyrrolate IM at 0.01 mg/kg
		Dosage: acepromazine IM at 0.1 mg/kg (3 mg maximum total dose)
		• Wait 10 minutes, then give butorphanol IM at 0.1 to 0.4 mg/kg *or* oxymorphone IM at 0.05 to 0.2 mg/kg (3 mg maximum total dose)
		• Reduce opioid dosage for IV use; administer to effect
		• Used as preanesthetic and for chemical restraint
Alpha-2 agonists	General comments	Sedation, analgesia, anxiolysis, sympatholysis, vasoconstriction
		Arrhythmogenesis
		May induce vomiting during induction (especially if given SC or IM)
		Premedication with anticholinergic prevents bradycardia
		May be used epidurally for analgesia, especially in large animals.
	Xylazine	Alpha-2 to Alpha-1 selectivity: 160:1
	Rompun, Gemini, AnaSed, Sedazine: (different concentrations approved for dogs, cats, horses, deer, elk)	Concentration: Small-animal: 20 mg/mL; Large animal: 100 mg/mL
		Dosage: dogs: 0.25 to 0.5 mg/kg IM; cats: 0.5 to 1 mg/kg IM (max 5 mg dose)
		Onset/duration: 10 to 15 minutes after IM; up to 1 hour of sedation
		Arrhythmogenic effects include bradycardia, AV block, SA block
		Originally used with ketamine
		Rompun-ketamine was a classic combination in dogs and cats for many years; the bradycardia and decreased cardiac output are offset by ketamine's sympathomimetic effects, while the xylazine offset the muscle rigidity of ketamine; newer agents have supplanted this technique somewhat; ruminants are extremely sensitive to alpha-2 agonists, extralabel usage must be cautious
		Xylazine + butorphanol:
		• Dosage: glycopyrrolate IM at 0.01 mg/kg with xylazine IM at 0.2 mg/kg (5 mg maximum total dose)
		• Wait 10 minutes, then give butorphanol IM at 0.1 to 0.4 mg/kg

Detomidine Dormosedan (horses)
Medetomidine Domitor (dogs)

- Reduce dosage for IV use; administer to effect
- Used as preanesthetic and for chemical restraint

Alpha-2 to Alpha-1 selectivity: 260:1
Alpha-2 to Alpha-1 selectivity: 1620:1
Concentration: 1 mg/mL
Dosage for sedation (per label): 750 to 1000 μg/m²BSA
Preanesthetic dosage: 5 to 10 μg/kg IM
>10 g/kg produces sedation and bradycardia
Sedation and analgesia are enhanced by opioids and benzodiazepines

Romifidine

Newest Alpha-2 agonist under investigation

Antagonists

Alpha-2 agonists are antagonized by: yohimbine (Yobine, Antagonil), tolazoline (Tolazine), ?ipamazole (Antisedan)

Benzodiazepines | **General comments**

Minor tranquilizers, muscle relaxation, anticonvulsant, appetite stimulant, little or no sedation, no significant analgesia but potentiates or prolongs effect of analgesic agents, antagonized by flumazenil

Diazepam Schedule IV Valium (human)

Concentration: 5 mg/ml
Dosage 0.2 to 1.0 mg/kg IM
Avoid rapid IV injection; may produce pain and hypotension
Anxiolytic, amnesic, muscle relaxant, anticonvulsant
Useful in central nervous system and cardiac patients
Little sedative effect in healthy animals; may cause profound depression in compromised patients
Do not mix with other agents in same syringe (except ketamine)
Administer cautiously in aggressive patients
Effects may be prolonged effects in hepatic dysfunction
Propylene glycol base may cause arrhythmias
Flumazenil (Romazicon: Roche) is an effective antagonist (0.1 mg/kg IV)

Midazolam Schedule IV Versed (human)

Concentration: 1 mg/ml
Dosage: 0.2–0.4 mg/kg IV
Effects similar to those of diazepam
Water-soluble
More potent, more rapid onset of action, shorter duration of action than diazepam
Excellent choice in critically ill patients
May cause excitement and pain if rapidly administered
Flumazenil is an effective antagonist (0.1 mg/kg IV)

Zolazepam Schedule III

Only available in drug combination Telazol (+tiletamine)
Approved for use in dogs and cats. (See Dissociative agents for information)

Medical history

Patient medical history should include injuries, diseases, past anesthetic complications, and concurrent medication.

Physical examination

The physical examination should include emphasis on the cardiovascular, respiratory, hepatic, renal, and central nervous systems.

Laboratory data

Packed Cell Volume (PCV), total plasma protein level, liver enzymes (especially ALT), bile acids, blood urea nitrogen (BUN), blood glucose, heartworm status, acid-base balance, urinalysis, electrolyte levels, blood gas values, and a blood coagulation profile are all potentially useful in evaluating a patient. Most clinics use a minimum set of laboratory data for most patients and add others when specific concerns arise. Clients are generally given the choice of paying for preanesthetic laboratory tests on the Client Consent Form. It is important to stress the value of preanesthetic screening when counseling a client before a procedure.

Step 2: Patient Preparation

Patient preparation requirements vary, depending on the anticipated procedure. It is also important to prepare for the possibility of unanticipated situations. Standard practice is to withhold food for 8 to 12 hours and water for 2 to 4 hours before anesthetic induction. However, special preparation may be required in complex procedures. Pediatric or smaller patients should have food withheld for only 2 hours before anesthesia. Chronically compromised patients should have their condition stabilized, when possible, before anesthesia. For example, anemic patients (PCV below 20%) should have a transfusion to ensure adequate oxygen-carrying capacity. Dehydrated patients should receive sufficient intravenous fluids to restore hydration status. Patients with low total plasma protein levels (less than 3 g/dl) may benefit from administration of plasma.

Clipping the surgical site and placing an intravenous catheter before induction minimizes anesthesia time. Maintaining patient calmness reduces stress and may lower anesthetic induction requirements. Avoid unnecessary handling and noisy personnel or equipment. Provide an environment free of excitement or anxiety. Oxygenation before and during induction may improve PaO_2 in patients with cardiopulmonary compromise, especially during mask or chamber induction.

Preanesthetic checklists should be completed before all procedures to ensure that appropriate items are readily available, important health issues have been addressed, and all involved persons have communicated. This is especially important in high-volume clinics, when several people are involved in patient evaluation and preparation. Anesthetic induction must not be initiated until the checklist is completed (Box 19-2).

Step 3: Equipment and Supplies

More anesthetic mishaps are attributed to poor planning and preparation than to improper use of drugs. Correct selection, preparation, and use of anesthetic equipment are essential to patient safety. All equipment should be prepared and checked to be in good working order before administration of anesthetic compounds; the need for intubation and oxygenation may occur unexpectedly. The use of a preanesthetic checklist assures that all items are completed before induction (Box 19-3).

Supplies for intravenous fluid administration

Placement of an intravenous catheter is essential for patient safety during anesthesia. Intravenous catheters provide immediate access for intravenous (IV) injection and administration of fluids. Catheters should be placed before induction of anesthesia, when possible, because most anesthetic agents produce hypotension or vasoconstriction and may complicate catheter placement. Appropriately sized catheters, infusion sets, needles, syringes, and other supplies necessary for aseptic catheterization should be arranged for easy access. The correct catheter size is that large enough to deliver large volumes of intravenous fluids (90 ml/kg/hr): 18-gauge for dogs more than 20 lbs; 20-gauge for dogs less than 20 lbs; and 24-gauge for cats. For cats, avoid using the cephalic vein if a front declaw is planned, and the femoral vein if a rear declaw is planned. Large animals (horses, cattle) should have a 16- to 14-gauge catheter placed in the jugular vein.

Infusion sets are available as vented or nonvented sets. *Vented administration sets* are required when using nonvented bottles. *Nonvented administration sets* can be used with plastic fluid bags or vented bottles. Delivery rates of 10 drops/ml, 12 drops/ml, 15 drops/ml, and 60 drops/ml are commonly used in veterinary medicine. Smaller drop sizes improve the accuracy of delivery in smaller patients. Generally, patients weighing less than 10 kg should receive fluids through a "microdrip" (60 drops/ml) infusion set to increase accuracy of fluid delivery. Patients requiring large fluid volumes (e.g., horses) need 10 drops/ml sets. Routine fluid delivery rates during anesthesia should be 5 to 10 ml/kg/hr for larger animals and 10 to 20 ml/kg/hr for smaller animals.

Endotracheal tubes

Endotracheal intubation ensures a patent airway, facilitates patient ventilation, and provides easy delivery of volatile anesthetics. Endotracheal intubation is not necessarily indicated for general anesthesia; however, be prepared for immediate intubation if respiratory complications arise. It is *rarely* a mistake to place an endotracheal tube.

BOX 19-2

Preanesthesia Checklist

Personnel

1. Select personnel and identify roles.
2. Review procedure.
3. Review emergency procedures.

Patient

1. Identify patient properly.
2. Verify patient was fasted (as appropriate).
3. Perform special prep (as needed, e.g., bowel prep).
4. Perform preanesthetic examination (health, sex confirmed).

Drugs

1. Select drugs; confirm they are available.
2. Review routes of drug administration.
3. Check crash cart inventory.

Fluid administration

1. Select IV fluids; maintain at proper temperature.
2. Confirm sufficient fluids available for adverse events.
3. Gather necessary equipment.
   - IV catheters (24 gauge for <5 kg, 20 gauge for 5 to 10 kg, 18 gauge for >10 kg)
   - Injection caps

- Materials for securing IV catheter (tape, adhesive)
- Heparinized saline (2-4 IU/ml), in syringe with needle
- Fluid delivery sets (60 drops/ml for <10 kg, 15 drops/ml for 11-40 kg, 10 drops/ml for >40 kg)

Endotracheal intubation

1. Select and inspect three sizes of endotracheal tube.
2. Gather necessary equipment.
   - Lubricating gel
   - Rolled gauze for securing
   - Laryngoscope and appropriate blades
   - Stylets
   - Lidocaine spray or swab

Equipment

1. Review anesthetic machine checklist (Box 19-3).
2. Select and inspect monitoring equipment.

Miscellaneous supplies

- Ophthalmic ointment
- Circulating warm-water blanket, table insulation, or heated table
- Facemask

BOX 19-3

Checklist for Daily Inspection of Anesthetic Equipment

- Sufficient oxygen available
- Vaporizer filled
- All gas lines correctly connected
- Sufficient CO_2 absorbent time available
- Scavenger system properly connected and operational
- Cuff syringe available
- Attach breathing circuit, tubes, and reservoir bag
- Check for leaks:
  1. Close pop-off valve.
  2. Occlude patient end of breathing circuit (where endotracheal tube attaches).

3. Fill circuit with oxygen to a pressure of 20 cm H_2O.
4. Turn on oxygen flow to 100 ml/min (0.1 L/min).
5. If pressure increases, leaks are within acceptable limits.
6. If pressure drops, increase the flow rate until pressure remains stable.
7. Leaks exceeding 200 ml/min (0.2 L/min) should be corrected via machine maintenance.
8. Open the pop-off valve while occluding Y-piece; pressure should drop to 0 cm H_2O.

Endotracheal tubes should be clean and free of defects or obstructions. If it has an inflatable cuff, it should be checked for leaks. Endotracheal tube diameter and length are important. The diameter should be the largest size that will fit into the trachea with ease. If too large, the larynx and trachea may be traumatized. If too small, the patient will have difficulty breathing through the tube. To illustrate this, try breathing through a soda straw for a couple of minutes. Length is important for two reasons. The inserted tip of the tube should not extend beyond (caudal to) the thoracic inlet, because bronchial intubation may occur. The adapter end of the tube should not extend more than 1 or 2 inches beyond (rostral to) the mouth; limiting the increase of mechanical dead space (Fig. 19-1). Increased

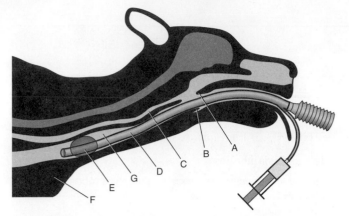

Fig. 19-1 Correct placement of an endotracheal tube. The connector is located near the incisor teeth, minimizing mechanical dead space. The cuffed end is in the cervical trachea, near the thoracic inlet. **A,** Soft palate. **B,** Epiglottis. **C,** Esophagus. **D,** Endotracheal tube. **E,** Inflated cuff. **F,** Thoracic inlet. **G,** Cervical trachea.

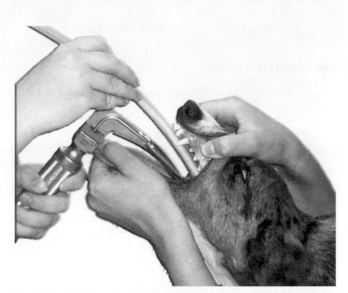

Fig. 19-2 Canine intubation. Proper presentation of a patient and use of a laryngoscope for intubation is shown.

mechanical dead space increases the degree of exhaled gas rebreathing. Stylets may be used to facilitate intubation with small-diameter or very flexible tubes. When using a stylet, the tip should not extend beyond (caudal to) the tip of the endotracheal tube; this prevents damage to or penetration of the trachea. The stylet is removed immediately upon achieving intubation. Secure the endotracheal tube to the maxilla, mandible, or head with gauze or tape to prevent dislodgment or excessive movement during the procedure.

Laryngoscope

The laryngoscope facilitates visualization of the glottis as the endotracheal tube passes through into the trachea. Laryngoscopes consist of a handle and detachable blades in a variety of sizes and shapes. The blade is curved to match the curvature of the tongue and allow even pressure along its length. Avoid the tendency of using only the tip of the blade to depress the tongue, as this puts too much pressure in one place and may cause bruising. Also, the blade should not be used to press down on the epiglottis, as this may damage it and the glottis as well. If the epiglottis is flipped upward or is trapped behind the soft palate, simply lift the soft palate and gently push the epiglottis down with the tip of the endotracheal tube. Pulling the tongue forward also helps to improve visualization of the glottis (Fig. 19-2).

Medical gas supply

Medical gases may be delivered from compressed gas cylinders by central pipeline or by direct attachment to the anesthetic machine. Medical-grade oxygen and nitrous oxide are the commonly used gases in veterinary medicine, although the benefits of nitrous oxide in veterinary practice are limited. The nitrous oxide source must be independent of the oxygen source; nitrous oxide is mixed with oxygen just before passing through the vaporizer.

The most commonly used sizes of compressed medical gas cylinders are the *E cylinder* (4.25 by 26 inches) and the *H cylinder* (9.25 by 51 inches). All medical gas cylinders are color-coded; oxygen cylinders are green, and nitrous oxide cylinders are blue. E cylinders attached directly to the anesthetic machine for backup should be kept in the *off* position until in use to ensure that they remain full until needed.

Pressure regulators attached to the cylinder valve on H cylinders and near the hanger yokes for E cylinders reduce oxygen pressure to the normal working pressure of the anesthetic machine—50 pounds per square inch gauge (PSIG). Pressure reduction is necessary to prevent damage to the anesthetic machine and allows a constant rate of oxygen delivery to the flow meter. Cylinder pressure gauges are associated with the pressure regulator and may be used to estimate the relative volume of gas remaining in a cylinder. Oxygen cylinders contain only compressed oxygen vapors, and the pressure is proportional to the content. The pressure in a fully charged oxygen cylinder, regardless of size, is near 2200 PSIG. A fully charged H cylinder contains 7000 liters of oxygen, and fully charged E cylinders contain 700 liters. A fully charged cylinder of nitrous oxide is 95% liquid; therefore, cylinder contents are not directly proportional to cylinder pressure. Pressure begins to drop only after the liquid is completely vaporized and about 75% of the contents have been used. The remaining gas can be estimated after pressure begins to fall. Fully charged nitrous oxide cylinders have a pressure of 750 PSIG. An H cylinder contains about 16,000 L N_2O, and an E cylinder contains about 1600 L N_2O.

Anesthesia machines

Several companies manufacture anesthesia machines for small and large animal use (Figs. 19-3 and 19-4). Anesthetic

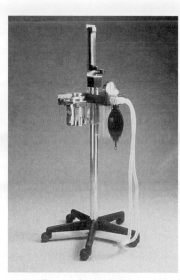

Fig. 19-3 Compact small-animal anesthesia machine. Typical compact small-animal anesthesia machine with pediatric circle breathing circuit. Components include precision vaporizer, flow meter, pressure manometer, oxygen flush valve, CO_2 absorber, common gas outlet, and waste-gas–scavenging device. *(Courtesy Anesco, Inc., Georgetown, Ky.)*

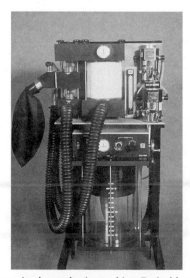

Fig. 19-4 Large-animal anesthesia machine. Typical large-animal anesthesia machine and ventilator, with large-animal breathing circuit, two precision vaporizers, and standard anesthetic machine components. *(Courtesy Anesco, Inc., Georgetown, Ky.)*

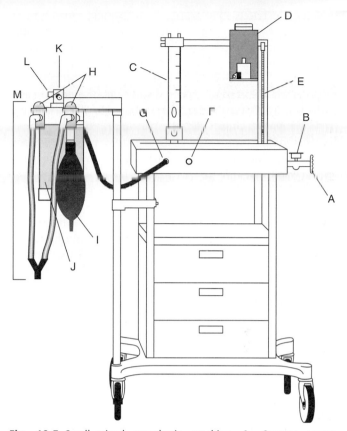

Fig. 19-5 Small-animal anesthesia machine. **A,** Oxygen source. **B,** Oxygen pressure gauge. **C,** Oxygen flow meter. **D,** Precision vaporizer. **E,** Common gas line. **F,** Oxygen flush valve. **G,** Common gas outlet. **H,** Unidirectional dome valves. **I,** Reservoir bag. **J,** Carbon dioxide absorbent canister. **K,** Pressure-relief valve. **L,** Scavenger interface. **M,** Patient rebreathing circuit.

machines deliver a mixture of oxygen and inhalation anesthetic to the breathing circuit. The components of an anesthetic machine are the oxygen source, pressure regulator, oxygen pressure valve, flow meter, vaporizer, and oxygen flush valve (Fig. 19-5).

Flow meters

Flow meters receive medical gases from the pressure regulator. Their purpose is to measure and deliver a constant gas flow to the vaporizer, the common gas outlet, and the breathing circuit. Oxygen enters the flow meter near the bottom and travels upward through a tapered, transparent flow tube. A floating indicator, either a ball or plumb bob, inside the flow tube indicates the amount of gas passing through the control valve. The flow rate is indicated on a scale associated with the flow tube. When the control valve is open, oxygen enters the tube, pushing the floating indicator upward. Where the indicator hovers in equilibrium, the rate of flow is determined by reading the calibrated scale from the center of the ball or the top of the plumb bob.

Flow meters are gas-specific and must not be interchanged; an oxygen flow meter cannot safely be replaced with a nitrous oxide flow meter. Control knobs to regulate flow of medical gases must be distinguishable from each other. Specifically, the oxygen control knob must be green and permanently marked with the word or symbol for oxygen. The valve should be fluted, project beyond other knobs, and be larger in diameter than other knobs.

Flow meters are common sources of leaks and should be checked at regular intervals for cracks in the flow tube. Dirt or static electricity may cause a float to stick, causing flows to be higher or lower than indicated. Excessive tightening easily damages control knobs, leading to expensive repair. Overtightening may prevent the flow meter from closing completely, causing significant leaking in the off position. Leaking may lead to unexpected shortage of medical gases and exhaustion (saturation) of carbon dioxide absorbent from constant flow of gas through the absorbent. Exhausted carbon dioxide absorbent may produce carbon monoxide when exposed to inhalation anesthetics, producing carbon monoxide toxicity manifested as tissue hypoxia.

Vaporizers

Inhalation anesthetic agents are volatile liquids that vaporize at room temperature. The primary function of a vaporizer is controlled enhancement of anesthetic vaporization. Vaporizers in common use are of two general types: precision vaporizers (for use with halothane, isoflurane, sevoflurane) (Fig. 19-6) and nonprecision vaporizers (used for methoxyflurane). Their functional differences apply to the administration of volatile anesthetics (Box 19-4).

Precision vaporizers, designed for a specific anesthetic agent, deliver a constant concentration (%) that is automatically maintained with changing oxygen flow rates and temperature. The percent setting on the control dial approximates delivery to the breathing circuit. Precision vaporizers are designed to function out of the breathing circuit; that is, between the flow meter and the breathing circuit. The inherent safety attributed to precision vaporizers is that the anesthetic concentration delivered to the breathing circuit and patient cannot increase above the vaporizer setting. Precision vaporizers may deliver less than dial settings when flows are very low (250 ml/min or lower) or very

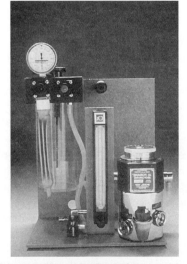

Fig. 19-6 Precision vaporizer. VaporTec Series 5 precision vaporizer, calibrated for volume % delivery of halothane or isoflurane. *(Courtesy Sensor Devices, Inc., Waukesha, Wis.)*

---

high (15 L/min or higher). Examples of precision vaporizers for delivery of halothane and isoflurane include the Fluotec Mark III (Ohmeda) and the Ohio Calibrated Vaporizer (Ohmeda) (Fig. 19-7).

Sevoflurane requires a precision vaporizer calibrated for this agent. One cannot safely use sevoflurane in a vaporizer calibrated for isoflurane. Precision vaporizers are more expensive than nonprecision vaporizers.

Nonprecision vaporizers are rudimentary, allowing some control of vaporization, but delivering an unknown concentration. The dial scale is not a percent concentration, but rather a relative number indicating the amount of fresh gas diverted through the chamber. A lever setting of 0 on the Ohio #8 vaporizer indicates that no gas flows through the chamber, with no anesthetic delivered to the patient. When the lever is set on 10, all of the circuit gases are diverted through the chamber, increasing the anesthetic concentration delivered to the patient. The approximate percent of anesthetic delivered varies with the agent's vapor pressure and temperature, and the patient's minute ventilation. Knowing the precise concentration delivered to the patient is advantageous. However, if one monitors the patient's anesthetic depth and physiological status, simply increasing or decreasing the dial setting in response to observations allows relatively safe delivery of the agent.

Anesthetic concentrations can exceed 12% when administering halothane, isoflurane, or sevoflurane through a nonprecision vaporizer (Ohio or Stephens type) located in the breathing circuit. Concentrations of this magnitude greatly increase the potential for overdosing; this risk outweighs the economy gained by purchase of jar-type vapor-

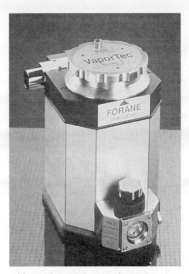

Fig. 19-7 Ohio calibrated vaporizer and circuit manometer. Ohio calibrated vaporizer for vaporization of halothane or isoflurane, with output calibrated in volume % *(left)*. Manometer used to monitor breathing circuit pressure and to check tracheal tube inflation pressure *(center)*. *(Courtesy Sensor Devices, Inc., Waukesha, Wis.)*

izers. There are sufficient concerns with administration of anesthetic agents without the added worry of gross anesthetic overdose.

Nonprecision vaporizers are designed to function in the breathing circuit ("in the circle"). Location of the vaporizer in the circle has disadvantages. The anesthetic concentration may increase over time without change in setting because of positive-pressure ventilation, increased minute ventilation, increased room temperature, and/or low fresh gas flow. High fresh gas flow decreases the anesthetic concentration by dilution of anesthetic in the breathing circuit.

Several hazards are associated with vaporizers. Filling with the incorrect agent can lead to delivery of an excessively high or low concentration of vapor to the patient. Delivering an unknown agent may present varied cardiovascular effects. Tipping the vaporizer may allow liquid agent to enter the fresh gas line, increasing the anesthetic concentration. Overfilling the chamber decreases the volume of vapor available to mix with fresh gas and may allow liquid anesthetic to reach the common gas outlet line. Leaks are also common at the inlet fitting, outlet fitting, filling port, and drain port. Vaporizers incorrectly located in the common gas outlet can deliver excessive anesthetic concentrations when the oxygen flush is activated. The additional flow through the vaporizer (35 to 75 L/min) increases the volume of vapor delivered to the breathing circuit.

Breathing circuits

Medical gases pass from the anesthetic machine to the patient through tubing known as a breathing circuit. Breathing circuits deliver "fresh gases" (oxygen and anesthetic vapor) to the patient and transport exhaled gases from the patient. Carbon dioxide is eliminated from the circuit by *washout* using high gas flow rates and/or soda lime absorption.

Nonrebreathing circuits

Nonrebreathing circuits do not have a carbon dioxide absorber (Fig. 19-8). Removal of carbon dioxide depends on fresh gas flow rates. Properly used, nonrebreathing circuits allow no significant rebreathing of exhaled gases. The point of entry into the circuit, the flow rate, and the expiratory port location determine the amount of carbon dioxide rebreathed. Ultimately, the composition of the inspired gas mixture depends on the fresh gas flow rate. Flow rates near

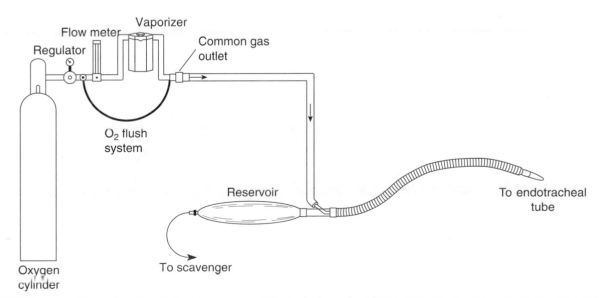

Fig. 19-8 Nonrebreathing system. Anesthetic delivery system with attached nonrebreathing system. *(Courtesy R. Spangler, Morehead State University.)*

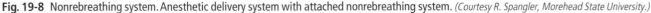

two to three times the patient's minute ventilation are required to prevent rebreathing. Flow rates below two times minute ventilation allow some rebreathing and warrant monitoring for signs of hypoxemia and hypercarbemia.

Nonrebreathing circuits used in veterinary medicine include the *Bain circuit*, *Norman mask elbow*, and *modified Jackson-Reese*. Advantages of nonrebreathing circuits include decreased resistance to breathing, rapid change of inspired anesthetic concentration, light weight, and ease of cleaning and use. Disadvantages are primarily associated with the required high fresh gas flow rates and include increased use of oxygen and anesthetic, enhanced risk of hypothermia, and dehydration (Fig. 19-9).

Rebreathing circuits

The term *rebreathing* means "to breathe again" and refers to exhaled gases (carbon dioxide, oxygen, anesthetic). Rebreathing circuits (circle system) are most commonly used in veterinary practice. The amount of carbon dioxide

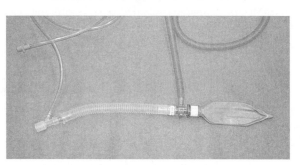

Fig. 19-9 Jackson-Reese Nonrebreathing Circuit.

rebreathed depends on the degree of carbon dioxide absorption and the fresh gas flow rate. The components of the circle system include the absorber, absorbent, fresh gas inlet, unidirectional valves, positive-pressure-relief valve (pop-off valve), manometer, reservoir bag, and a removable set of breathing tubes (Fig. 19-10). Some circuits also have a negative-pressure-relief valve.

Standard breathing tubes are 22 mm in diameter and 1 m long for small-animal patients weighing 7 to 135 kg. Shorter 15-mm–diameter tubes are preferred for patients weighing less than 7 kg. Large-animal tubes are 500 mm in diameter and 1.7 m long. The classic setup uses separate inhalation and exhalation tubes connected via a Y-piece to the endotracheal tube adapter. The Universal F-circuit was developed to place the inhalation tube inside of the exhalation tube. The advantages of this arrangement include warming of inhaled gases by exhaled gases (Fig. 19-11).

Advantages of the rebreathing circuit include conservation of body heat and fluids, reuse of exhaled oxygen and anesthetic gases, and cost-efficient lower flow rates. Disadvantages of the rebreathing circuit include danger of hypercarbia resulting from malfunction of the carbon dioxide absorbent or unidirectional valves, particularly at flow rates low enough to produce a closed system. There also exists a potential for increased work of breathing because of added resistance from faulty unidirectional valves, carbon dioxide absorbent, or faulty pop-off valves. Additionally, there is a slow change in the inspired anesthetic concentration at lower flows.

The *reservoir bag* provides a gas volume sufficient for the patient to inhale maximally without creating negative pressure in the circuit. It is also used for positive-pressure venti-

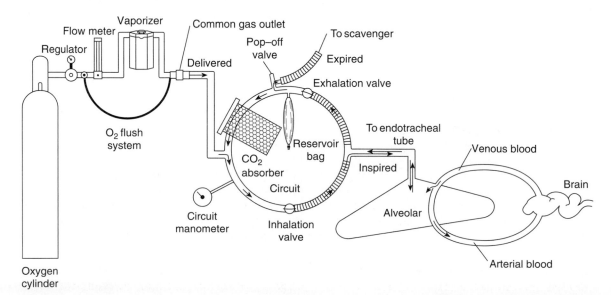

Fig. 19-10 Anesthetic pathway. Anesthetic delivery system showing the pathway traveled by anesthetic, from the vaporizer to the brain. *(Courtesy R. Spangler, Morehead State University.)*

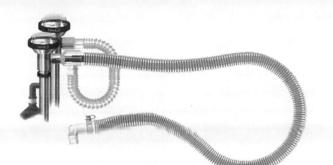

Fig. 19-11 Universal F circuit. This circle breathing system is modified to promote heat exchange between exhaled and inhaled gases and minimize patient heat loss. *(Courtesy of Anesco, Inc., Georgetown, Ky.)*

lation or to inflate the lungs when needed. Reservoir bag sizes of 0.5 to 5 L are used for small animals and 15 to 30 L for large animals. The ideal reservoir bag is five times the patient's normal tidal volume of 10 ml/kg.

The *circuit manometer* is useful to monitor circuit pressure. Excessive circuit pressure (above 4 cm H_2O) may prevent normal respiration and increase intrathoracic pressure, resulting in decreased venous return and a subsequent drop in cardiac output. During positive-pressure ventilation ("bagging"), the manometer allows delivery of the correct circuit pressure. *Barotrauma* (respiratory tract injury from excessive circuit pressure) decreases oxygenation of blood and can rupture lung tissue. Typically, healthy dogs and cats are ventilated to pressures of 15 to 20 cm H_2O to ensure adequate tidal volume. Horses may require positive-pressure ventilation pressures of 30 to 40 cm H_2O to achieve adequate tidal volume. It is vital to note that positive pressure ventilation is not the same as normal physiological inhalation (which is accomplished via negative intrathoracic pressure). When intrathoracic pressure exceeds central venous pressure (approximately 4 cm H_2O), the vena cava collapses and venous return stops. This, in turn, reduces cardiac output. Ventilation rates should not exceed one third of the heart rate to avoid significant cardiac output decrease.

The *positive-pressure-relief (pop-off) valve* prevents excessive pressure in the rebreathing circuit and allows removal of excess waste gases. A common cause of anesthetic mishap is leaving the pop-off valve closed after performing positive-pressure ventilation. The pop-off valve is equipped with a scavenger interface, permitting connection to a waste gas removal system to prevent waste gas discharge into the operating room air.

The *carbon dioxide absorbent* (soda lime or Baralyme) removes carbon dioxide from the breathing circuit by chemical reaction. Inadequate absorbent function may lead to hypercarbia (excessive carbon dioxide in the blood), with resultant increased respiratory rate and initially increased heart rate, followed by cardiovascular depression. The absorbent should be changed after 6 to 8 hours of use, depending on gas flow rates and patient size. Desiccated carbon dioxide absorbents may react with volatile anesthetics, producing carbon monoxide sufficient to cause carbon monoxide toxicity. Precautionary measures to ensure that the absorbent is reasonably fresh include logging of date changed and amount of time used for anesthesia. The absorbent should be changed monthly or every 6 hours of usage, whichever comes first.

The *unidirectional valves* maintain one-way flow of gases within the breathing circuit. This ensures that exhaled gases pass through the carbon dioxide absorbent before reaching the patient again. A recent report of anesthetic complications arising from a malfunctioning exhalation valve and resultant carbon dioxide toxicity is a reminder that any part of the machine can fail unexpectedly. Vigilance and rapid response to complications is always needed.

Anesthetic systems

Taken together, all components of the anesthetic machine and breathing circuit make up an anesthetic system. There are several types of anesthetic systems: *semiclosed*, *closed*, and *open*.

The terms semiclosed and closed refer to operation of rebreathing circuits. A given circuit may be operated as semiclosed or closed. A circuit is semiclosed if oxygen flow is greater than patient oxygen uptake. The circuit is closed if oxygen flow is equal to patient oxygen uptake (4 to 7 ml/kg/min for small animals and 2 to 3 ml/kg/min for large animals). Fig. 19-12 shows small-animal oxygen flow rates. Regardless of the position of the pop-off valve (open or closed), the circuit may be semiclosed or closed. With a closed system, elimination of carbon dioxide is solely dependent on functional carbon dioxide absorbent.

The term open system describes delivery of anesthetic gases via facemask, insufflation, or induction chamber (Fig. 19-13). Open systems are advantageous for very small or aggressive patients. They permit induction by inhalation anesthetics when injectable techniques are contraindicated or impractical. Disadvantages may include prolonged induction time, passage through a stressful excitement phase, inability to monitor the patient, air pollution from waste anesthetics, and increased expense due to high flow. Excitement during inhalation induction, by mask or chamber, increases the anesthetic risk in compromised patients.

Chambers used for induction should be large enough to permit recumbency without compromising respiration. With mask or chamber induction, patients should breathe oxygen-enriched air for several minutes before induction to optimize alveolar oxygen concentration. Chamber induction allows large amounts of waste anesthetic gases to escape into the surgery area. Serious effort to minimize human exposure is prudent. A safety tip is to switch to the facemask

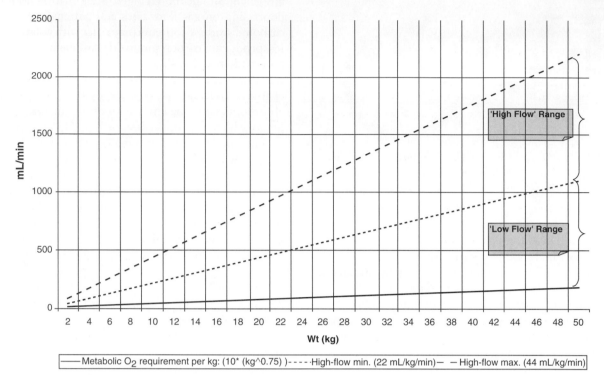

Fig. 19-12 Oxygen flow rates per body weight. Oxygen flow rates for closed, low-flow, and high-flow operation of rebreathing circuits.

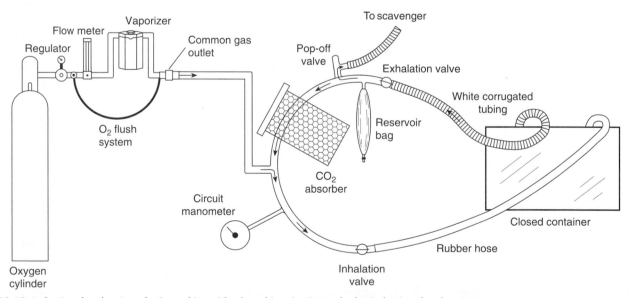

Fig. 19-13 Induction chamber. Anesthetic machine with rebreathing circuit attached to induction chamber. *(Courtesy R. Spangler, Morehead State University.)*

as soon as the patient is manageable. This conserves anesthetic and allows greater control and better monitoring of the patient. Patients should be intubated when sufficiently relaxed; avoiding maintenance by mask except in very short procedures. Maintaining anesthesia via facemask does not permit manual ventilation, may allow aspiration of regurgitated stomach contents, permits leaks around the perimeter causing pollution and inhalation of room air, and increases mechanical dead space. The inhalation agents of choice for open induction are isoflurane or sevoflurane.

Step 4: Preanesthetic Medication

Preanesthetic medication is usually beneficial to the patient and should be considered for all patients. The need is based entirely on patient health status and temperament and drugs selected for induction and maintenance. Selection of preanesthetics is based on the patient's health status, not on the surgical procedure. Various drugs are used for premedication, including calming agents, analgesics, and anticholinergics. Benefits of preanesthetic medication include the following:

- Reduces patient stress and minimizes sympathetic effects, which improves handling during preparation for procedures
- Usually decreases the required dose of induction and maintenance agents
- Facilitates anesthetic induction and maintenance, dampening the sudden changes in anesthetic depth associated with surgical stimulation
- Allows a smoother recovery and reduces pain

Anticholinergics

Anticholinergics block the action of the neurotransmitter acetylcholine at cholinergic receptors in the heart, salivary glands, and smooth muscle fibers throughout the body. Effects may include increased heart rate (with concomitant increase in myocardial oxygen demand), decreased salivation and bronchial secretions, mydriasis (dilated pupils), bronchodilation, decreased gastric and intestinal motility, reduced tear formation, and blocking of vagus-mediated reflexes. Central effects (e.g., sedation or excitement) may occur with anticholinergics that cross the blood-brain barrier.

Atropine and glycopyrrolate (Robinul-V) are the anticholinergics most commonly used in veterinary anesthesia. Anticholinergics are indicated when vagus-mediated reflexes, bradycardia, second-degree AV block, or excessive salivation exist or are anticipated. Because of the expected cardiovascular effects of opioid or alpha-2 agonists (e.g., xylazine) or before reversing the effects of muscle relaxants, an anticholinergic may be indicated. Anticholinergics are used during cardiopulmonary resuscitation (CPR) to alleviate bradyarrhythmias. They are contraindicated in the presence of tachycardia (above 160 beats/min in dogs; above 200 beats/min in cats) or ventricular fibrillation. The introduction of isoflurane and sevoflurane has reduced the incidence of bradyarrhythmias and hence the need to routinely premedicate with anticholinergics. Routine preanesthetic use of anticholinergics was common when halothane was the principle inhalation anesthetic, but it is now considered inappropriate by many anesthesiologists (Table 19-5).

Calming and analgesic agents

Tranquilizers, sedatives, and analgesics (pain relievers) are useful adjuncts to general anesthesia, if given before (preanesthetic), during (maintenance), or after anesthesia (postanesthetic). Patients that are calm, sedated, and free of pain

TABLE 19-5

Anticholinergic Agents

Drug Class	Example	Comments

Anticholinergic	Atropine
	Atropine sulfate injection (dogs, cats, horses, cattle, sheep, swine)
	
	Atropine sulfate injection (human)
	Also available in tablets and
	  ophthalmic ointment
		Concentration: 0.54 mg/ml
		Dosage: 0.02-0.04 mg/kg IV, IM, or SC
		Duration of action: 60 to 90 minutes
		Anticholinergic; use only when indicated
		Prevents vagal effects, bradycardia, heart block, excessive salivation
		Avoid if tachycardia present (dogs, 140/min; cats, 200/min)
		May increase myocardial oxygen consumption
		Indications: before use of narcotics and alpha-2 agonists, muscle relaxant reversal,
		  combat bradycardia or bradyarrhythmias

	Glycopyrrolate Robinul-V (dogs, cats) Robinul (human)	Concentration: 0.2 mg/ml Dosage: 0.01 mg/kg IV, IM, or SC Duration of action: 2 to 4 hours Anticholinergic; use only when indicated Prevents vagal effects, bradycardia, AV block, excessive salivation Does not cross blood-brain barrier; may be less effective in CPR Longer duration of action and fewer side effects than atropine Indications: before use of narcotics and alpha-2 agonists, muscle relaxant reversal, combat bradycardia or bradyarrhythmia

generally require less anesthetic for induction and maintenance. Excited patients or those in pain have higher levels of circulating catecholamines that may increase the likelihood of adverse cardiovascular effects, such as cardiac arrhythmias. Sedation or analgesia may improve recovery from anesthesia. Each of these agents has beneficial as well as adverse effects on physiology.

Drug combinations may have additive, synergistic, complementary, or antagonistic interactions. If the effects are additive or synergistic, less of each drug is needed to produce the desired effect. Complementary effects are useful when a drug lacks a particular effect (e.g., xylazine complements the poor muscle relaxation of ketamine). Drugs commonly used for this purpose fall into several drug categories: phenothiazine derivatives, benzodiazepines, thiazine derivatives, barbiturates, and opioids (Table 19-6).

Step 5: Induction

When gas anesthesia is to be performed, anesthetic induction is the transition from the conscious, preanesthetic state to the level of anesthesia at which the patient may be intubated. The ideal induction agent provides a smooth and calm transition from consciousness to unconsciousness, abolishes oropharyngeal and tracheal reflexes, has a brief duration of effect, produces minimal or no toxicity, and requires minimal metabolism for recovery. Recognize that induction is short-term general anesthesia and that induction agents are frequently used alone to perform short surgical or diagnostic procedures. Balanced anesthesia should be used for procedures lasting longer than the duration of the induction agent or performed in patients with organ dysfunction.

Drugs for anesthetic induction

Several methods are used for induction before inhalation anesthesia, each having advantages and disadvantages. IV administration is preferred in most cases.

IV injection of a thiobarbiturate is a standard induction method before inhalation anesthesia in dogs. Thiopental sodium (Pentothal) is a commonly used thiobarbiturate in veterinary anesthesia. Thiobarbiturates provide rapid, smooth induction of anesthesia, with abolition of oropharyngeal and tracheal reflexes lasting several minutes. Its ultrashort action is due to rapid redistribution from the CNS to the muscle tissue and then the adipose tissue. Repeated injections cause accumulation in the body tissues with saturation eventually occurring; a situation that can result in deadly CNS levels if this drug is used for anesthetic maintenance by repeated injection. The ultrashort barbiturates are Class III controlled substances and must be kept secure.

Propofol is a nonbarbiturate short-acting induction agent. Its action is brief due to redistribution and rapid metabolism by somatic cells. Unlike the thiobarbiturates, it can be used for maintenance via repeated injections and is considered safer for use in sight hounds and patients with compromised liver and kidney function. Its expense and the need to use the entire contents of the vial within 6 hours of opening are limitations in veterinary practice. One advantage is that propofol is not a controlled substance.

Dissociative anesthetics (e.g., ketamine, tiletamine) may be used in combination with acepromazine, alpha-2 agonists, opioids, or a benzodiazepine to induce anesthesia in a wide variety of species. Dissociative agents administered alone may cause extreme excitement or seizures. Telazol (tiletamine + zolazepam) is the only approved dissociative combination on the market. The effects of dissociative combinations last longer than the effects of thiobarbiturates or propofol, affecting the patient well beyond the initial induction period, even into the postoperative recovery period. They are typically used in cats and exotics due to the convenience of intramuscular (IM) administration in these species compared with IV administration. However, they do not completely abolish the oropharyngeal reflexes, may cause excessive respiratory secretions, irregular respirations, rapid heart rate, emergence delirium, and the eyes to remain wide open and prone to drying. Corneal ulceration may occur if ophthalmic ointment is not used to protect the cornea. Dissociative agents have been reclassified as Class III controlled substances in recent years and must be kept secure.

Induction with an inhalant agent (e.g., isoflurane, sevoflurane) via facemask ("masking down") or induction chamber ("tank induction"), with or without preanesthetic medication, is occasionally desirable. Advantages of inhalation induction include avoidance of multiple drugs in the blood and tissues (important for some research protocols), rapid recovery, and ease of induction of very small animals that are difficult to handle (e.g., rats, mice, cats). Disadvantages include slower induction with passage through an excitement phase that may be quite stressful to the patient (and the anesthetist), difficulty restraining and monitoring the patient, high potential for pollution of room air with inhalation anesthetics, and the expense of the high flow rates and anesthetic levels needed. The excitement of inhalation induction increases the risk of anesthetic complications in compromised patients predisposed to cardiac or respiratory insufficiency. In healthy patients, stress-induced catecholamine release may produce cardiopulmonary compromise. If struggling occurs, chamber induction is as stressful as mask induction. The animal may also contort itself into a position that compromises respiration.

Mask or chamber induction requires several minutes of preoxygenation to increase the margin of safety. With chamber induction, large amounts of anesthetic vapor escape into the room air when the chamber is opened. The procedure should ideally be performed under a hood that

TABLE 19-6

Opiates and Opioids

Example	Product	Comments
Opiates, opioids	General comments	Include opioid agonists, opioid agonist-antagonists, and opioid antagonists Opioid portion may be reversed, see Naloxone below Generally sparing to cardiovascular system Depress respiration; assisted ventilation may be necessary May cause excitement and panting Repeated or large doses may produce bradycardia Indicated for relief of postoperative pain; more effective if administered before pain develops
Oxymorphone Schedule II	Numorphan (human)	Concentration: 1.5 mg/ml 10 to 15 times more potent than morphine Dosage: 0.05 to 0.2 mg/kg IV, IM, or SC (3 mg maximum total dose) Reliable pain relief for 2–4 hours
Butorphanol Schedule IV	Torbugesic, Dolorex (10 mg/mL, horses) Torbutrol inj (0.5 mg/mL) and tablets (dogs)	Equine product is typically used extralabel for dogs and cats, diluted appropriately for accurate measurement. 2–5 times more potent than morphine Dosage: 0.2 to 0.5 mg/kg IV, IM, or SC Decreases cough reflex (antitussive) Somewhat reliable for pain relief; combine with a sedative for best results Provides 2–4 hours of analgesia
Buprenorphine	Buprenex (human)	3–5 times more potent than morphine Dosage: 0.005 to 0.01 mg/kg IV or IM Somewhat reliable for relief of pain Provides 4–12 hours of analgesia May cause excitement; combine with a sedative for best results
Morphine Schedule II	Infumorph, Astramorph (human)	Dosage: dogs 0.1 to 0.2 mg/kg IV, IM, or SC; cats 0.05 to 0.1 mg/kg, IM, or SC Duration of action: reliable pain relief for up to 4 hours May cause histamine release or panting; combine with a sedative for best results Epidural administration: 0.1 mg/kg; onset of action within 30 minutes; duration 10–24 hours
Naloxone	P/M Naloxone HCl inj (dogs) Narcan (Human)	Pure narcotic antagonist Dosage: 0.002 to 0.02 mg/kg IM or slowly IV to effect Dilute to 0.4 mg/ml (if needed) with sterile distilled water Observe for return of narcotic effects; redose as needed

removes effluent gases. The tank size should be just large enough to accommodate the animal comfortably. Placing a rat in a cat-sized chamber requires much more anesthetic, oxygen, and time than necessary. One can reduce the dead space in a large chamber with empty plastic bottles. Once anesthesia is induced, the patient should be masked or intubated and maintained on the inhalant anesthetic. When direct inhalant induction is indicated, the agents of choice are isoflurane or sevoflurane. Sevoflurane will induce anesthesia approximately twice as fast as isoflurane.

Step 6: Maintenance

Following induction, the patient must be maintained in the anesthetized state until the procedure is completed. A common misconception is that maintenance involves only keeping the patient from moving during the procedure, regardless of the patient's needs. Maintenance is the management period of the anesthetic procedure. Monitoring and support of organ function are essential during anesthetic maintenance. An anesthetic record provides important documentation of your vigilance, and it notes adverse trends and important events occurring in the perioperative period (Fig. 19-14). A well-organized anesthetic record serves as legal documentation of anesthetic events, drug dosages used, and patient values during anesthesia, and it guides the actions of the anesthetist by tracking trends in cardiopulmonary function.

General considerations

Drugs used for maintenance of anesthesia include inhalant agents and a variety of injectable drugs. Surgical or diagnostic procedures that exceed the duration of the induction agent are best maintained with inhalation anesthesia. Injectable anesthetics are not recommended for long-term maintenance of anesthesia. Repeated injections of the induction agent to maintain anesthesia cause tissue accumulation, with increased risk of adverse events and greater dependence on metabolism for recovery. Steady states of anesthesia and a consistent depth of anesthesia are easier to maintain with inhalants. Once an injection is given it cannot be recovered, while inhalation agents are easily "blown off" via ventilation.

The amount of anesthetic needed to maintain an appropriate level of anesthesia is not a constant. Anesthetic depth is a product of the amount of drug reaching the brain, degree of painful stimulus applied, and patient health status. In a typical abdominal surgical procedure, minimal anesthesia is needed during the surgical preparation, moderate anesthesia during the skin incision, maximal anesthesia during the intra-abdominal phase, and moderate anesthesia during skin suturing. Hypothermia and hypotension reduce anesthetic requirements. If anesthetic administration is not reduced in the presence of hypothermia or hypotension, patients may become too deeply anesthetized, with further compromise of tissue perfusion.

Inhalant anesthetics

Among the inhalant anesthetics commonly used in veterinary medicine are nitrous oxide, methoxyflurane, halothane, isoflurane, and sevoflurane. When mixed with oxygen and inhaled by the patient, they diffuse rapidly into the bloodstream and are then distributed to all body tissues. As the concentration of drug in the brain rises, the CNS becomes progressively depressed. With the loss of consciousness and response to painful stimuli, the patient enters the plane of surgical anesthesia. Further rise of anesthetic concentrations in the brain continues to depress the CNS until vital functions cease and death ensues. The degree of anesthetic depth required by a patient during a particular procedure and the amount of inhalation anesthetic required to achieve and maintain that depth are unpredictable and variable.

Advantages of using inhalant agents include the ease and speed of controlling anesthetic depth, good muscle relaxation, rapid recovery with minimal dependence on metabolism of the agent, and delivery of high levels of oxygen with the agent through an endotracheal tube. Placement of an endotracheal tube provides a patent airway and the ability to support ventilation as needed.

Disadvantages of inhalant agents include the relatively expensive equipment and the knowledge and skill required for their use. Also, halothane sensitizes the myocardium to epinephrine-induced arrhythmias and produces liver damage in some patients. Methoxyflurane produces renal tubular damage. Isoflurane and sevoflurane are the least toxic of these agents, partially because of their small degree of biotransformation in the body.

A drug's *potency* is a measure of how much of the drug is needed to produce a standard effect, as compared with similar agents. For inhalant agents, potency is determined largely by the lipid solubility of the agent and is reflected by the minimum alveolar concentration (MAC). The MAC is defined as the lowest alveolar concentration of anesthetic required to prevent gross, purposeful movement in response to a painful stimulus. The MAC varies with species and individuals. The higher the MAC, the less potent the agent. Ironically, the inhalants with the most rapid induction time (lowest blood-gas solubility) are also the least potent (highest MAC).

Anesthetic delivery, uptake, distribution, and elimination

The relationship between the vaporizer setting and the time required to achieve effective brain levels of anesthetic is fundamental to inhalation anesthesia. Anesthetic delivery, uptake, and distribution are the processes by which the anesthetic reaches its intended site of action, the brain.

The process of getting anesthetic to the pulmonary alveoli is known as anesthetic delivery. Anesthetic uptake is the movement of anesthetic molecules from the pulmonary alveoli into the bloodstream. It is analogous to the

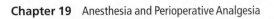

MONITORING	"EARLY WARNING"					RECOVERY PERIOD
Time:	10 20 30 40 50	10 20 30 40 50	10 20 30 40 50	10 20 30 40 50		
AGENTS:	ml/hr	ml/hr	ml/hr	ml/hr		TOTALS
Fluids:						Fluids:
Blood:						Blood:
Plasma:						Plasma:
Meds:						Meds:
Oxygen Flow:						Vaporizer Off:
Vaporizer Setting:						ETT Removed:
End Tidal Conc:						Sternal
Light						Standing

PLANE:		SUPPORT
	Deep	1. None
Anesthesia A	250	2. Heating
	240	3. Fluids
Operation ⊙	230	4. Oxygen
	220	5. ICU
End ⊙⊗	210	6. Other
	200	
End A A	190	COMPLICATIONS
	180	1. None
Systolic P ᴠ	170	2. Arrhythmias
	160	3. Aspiration
Diastolic P ᴧ	150	4. Cardiac Arrest
	140	5. Convulsions
Mean P X	130	6. Cyanosis
	120	7. Death
Heart Rate •	110	8. Excitement
	100	9. Hypothermia
Resp. Rate o	90	10. Injury
	80	11. Laryngospasm
Spont. S	70	12. Panting
	60	13. Regurgitation
Assist. A	50	14. Resp. Arrest
	40	15. Resp. Depression
Ventil. V	30	16. Resp. Obstruction
	20	17. Salivation
	10	18. Other
	0	

| Temperature (°F) |
| E.C.G. |
| pH |
| Pco$_2$ |
| Po$_2$ |
| HCO$_3$ |
| Base Balance |
| Event |

Complications:
1. None
2. Apnea
3. Arrythmias
4. Aspiration
5. Cardiac Arrest
6. Cyanosis
7. Death
8. Hemorrhage
9. Hyperthermia
10. Hypotension
11. Hypothermia
12. Inadequate Relaxation
13. Panting
14. Regurgitation
15. Resp. Arrest
16. Resp. Depression
17. Resp. Obstruct.
18. Salivation
19. Tympany
20. Variable Depth

Assigned to Student Clinician at:_____

Student Anesthetist:

Student Clinician:

Fig. 19-14 Anesthetic monitoring record. Typical anesthetic record for recording information related to an anesthetic procedure.

absorption phase of injectable agents. Anesthetic distribution is the movement of anesthetic molecules throughout the body via the bloodstream and diffusion into the tissues. Movement of gas molecules from the blood into the tissues is also called tissue uptake. Gas molecules must pass sequentially through these phases to reach the brain and produce anesthesia. If any one phase is altered, the chain of events leading to anesthesia is altered.

Anesthetic delivery to the alveoli is determined by the inspired concentration and alveolar minute ventilation. Increased anesthetic concentration in the breathing circuit increases the inspired concentration. The primary means of accomplishing this is by increasing the vaporizer setting. Anesthetic uptake (removal of anesthetic from the alveoli by the blood) is determined by solubility of the agent in blood, cardiac output, and the difference between alveolar and venous partial pressure of anesthetic. Uptake by the blood continually removes anesthetic from the alveoli. The more soluble the agent is in blood, the greater this effect is and the longer it takes to produce anesthesia. This is why less soluble agents like isoflurane and sevoflurane induce anesthesia rapidly.

Vessel-rich tissues include the brain, heart, liver, kidney, lungs, and gastrointestinal tract. These organs make up less than 10% of the body weight but receive 75% of cardiac output. Because of this large volume of blood flow, anesthetic is rapidly distributed to these vessel-rich tissues. Muscle makes up about 50% of body mass and receives nearly 20% of cardiac output. This large tissue group is significant in that, during induction, most of the anesthetic delivered to muscle is removed from the blood. Fat makes up nearly 20% of total body mass but only receives about 4% of cardiac output. Although anesthetics are highly lipid-soluble, low blood flow to this group limits anesthetic uptake, with little effect on induction rate. However, fat continually takes up anesthetic over time, and this must be released upon recovery. Prolonged procedures allow fat to accumulate enough anesthetic to significantly delay recovery. Vessel-poor tissues, such as fascia and ligaments, make up 20% of body mass and receive approximately 1% of the cardiac output. This tissue group has an insignificant effect on anesthetic induction or recovery despite the fact that it is significant in proportion.

In summary, anesthesia does not occur until the brain concentration of anesthetic is sufficient to induce loss of consciousness. The more soluble the anesthetic in the blood, the slower the induction time. Increasing the inspired anesthetic concentration and patient minute ventilation shortens the induction time.

Anesthetic elimination is the reverse of uptake and distribution, wherein anesthetic molecules move from the tissues into the blood, and then into the pulmonary alveoli to be exhaled.

The speed of uptake and elimination is important in inhalation anesthesia, because this determines how rapidly one may alter anesthetic depth. Major factors that determine the speed of uptake are the inhaled concentration of anesthetic, minute ventilation, alveolar diffusion area, the agent's solubility coefficient and molecular weight, pulmonary blood flow, and the anesthetic partial pressure gradient between alveolar gas and plasma.

Specific inhalant agents

Halogenated hydrocarbon anesthetic agents have been used extensively for veterinary anesthesia. These are methoxyflurane (Metofane), halothane (Fluothane), isoflurane (Aerrane), sevoflurane (SevoFlo). Although methoxyflurane and halothane are still in clinical use, isoflurane and sevoflurane now account for the largest proportion of inhalation procedures.

Halothane, isoflurane, and sevoflurane concentrations may rise to lethal levels very easily if they are not strictly controlled. For this reason, they are used in precision vaporizers positioned out of the breathing circuit. With methoxyflurane, maximal vaporization is more difficult to achieve and it may be used in a nonprecision vaporizer in the breathing circuit. Although methoxyflurane has gained a reputation for ease of use and relative safety, its significant disadvantages make isoflurane or sevoflurane the better choices.

Methoxyflurane provides the slowest induction (10 to 15 minutes) and recovery rates (30 minutes to several hours) of these agents because of its high blood-gas solubility coefficient. Sevoflurane, in contrast, has the lowest blood solubility and the fastest induction and recovery rates. Halothane induction requires 3 to 5 minutes, and recovery takes 5 to 20 minutes. Isoflurane induction requires 3 to 5 minutes, and recovery takes less than 5 minutes. Sevoflurane induction and recovery take about half as long as isoflurane.

The degree of metabolism required for elimination of these agents also varies. As much as 50% of methoxyflurane is metabolized by the liver, with 20% of halothane, 0.2% of isoflurane, and 3% of sevoflurane; this partially explains the rapid recovery and low toxicity of isoflurane and sevoflurane. Methoxyflurane has a direct nephrotoxic effect. Halothane has some potential for causing hepatitis. Isoflurane and sevoflurane have no significant toxicity. Methoxyflurane produces the best muscle relaxation of these agents and analgesia. Halothane, isoflurane, and sevoflurane produce adequate muscle relaxation and little analgesia.

Nitrous oxide is occasionally used in veterinary anesthesia as an adjunct to other agents. Its very low blood solubility allows very rapid uptake, distribution, and elimination. Addition of nitrous oxide to an inhalation protocol speeds uptake of the anesthetic gas (a second gas) into the blood, decreasing the time required for induction by inhalant anesthetics. This phenomenon is called the second gas effect. Unfortunately, nitrous oxide is not potent enough to produce general anesthesia alone. It is most commonly used with halothane, permitting a reduction in the amount of halothane required and therefore less occurrence of myocardial depression. There is little to be gained by use of nitrous oxide with isoflurane or sevoflurane.

Use of nitrous oxide requires some caution, because it can diffuse into gas-filled body spaces, causing them to expand. Nitrous oxide is contraindicated in patients with pneumothorax or a diaphragmatic hernia with bowel in the thorax. Diffusion hypoxia may occur during recovery. Rapid movement of nitrous oxide from the blood to alveoli may cause hypoxia by displacing oxygen or by diluting alveolar carbon dioxide, which may decrease respiratory stimulation and ventilation. Adequate ventilation should be maintained and a high flow rate of 100% oxygen used for the first 5 to 10 minutes of recovery after nitrous oxide use.

Step 7: Recovery

Recovery means "to restore to a normal state." This is a reminder that, during anesthesia, patients are in an abnormal state. Vigilance and support of organ function should continue until the patient is satisfactorily recovered from anesthesia. Pain relief and maintenance of a patent airway are important during recovery. The critical period has passed when the body temperature is normal, sternal recumbency is achieved, and oropharyngeal reflexes are restored. However, observation should continue until the patient can stand and is free of all drug effects.

ANESTHETIC MONITORING

Comprehensive monitoring of the anesthetized patient involves observing anesthetic equipment and evaluating the central nervous system, pulmonary function, and cardiovascular function. Early detection of equipment failure and/or depression of vital organ function allows execution of corrective measures, which are more effective than treating complications. Corrective actions to maintain or restore tissue perfusion are determined by integrating information from all body systems. Monitoring anesthesia covers a wide range of parameters and situations. One must "expect the unexpected."

Monitoring of Anesthetic Equipment

Monitoring of anesthetic equipment is the most neglected portion of anesthetic monitoring. The functionality of anesthetic equipment should be carefully tested before and continuously throughout anesthetic procedures. The most common anesthetic complications by far are hypoxemia and inadequate depth. The oxygen source, anesthetic machine, and breathing circuit must be observed for leaks, and carbon dioxide absorbent should be checked to ensure that it is not exhausted.

All anesthetic equipment should be clean, calibrated, and maintained in good working order. During anesthesia, frequently check connections to the patient or anesthetic circuit. Power sources to monitoring equipment and heat sources should be verified throughout the procedure. Be skeptical of sudden changes or erroneous monitoring device readings. Verify monitoring device readings with quick, simple observations, such as mucous membrane color, capillary refill time, pulse rate, and pulse quality. If the blood pressure reads zero but the mucous membranes are pink and well perfused, common sense dictates that the blood pressure reading is probably erroneous.

Monitoring Anesthetic Depth

Monitoring of the CNS includes estimation of anesthetic depth. Anesthetic depth refers to the degree of CNS depression. Typically, as the CNS becomes progressively more depressed, one can observe progressive changes in patient response and condition. For standard anesthetics, these observable signs have been grouped into stages of anesthesia (with some of the stages subdivided into planes). Clinically, it is common to refer to anesthetic depth as *light* if the degree of CNS depression is minimal and *deep* if it is profound (Box 19-5 and Table 19-7.) In reality this assessment is very subjective and requires integration of numerous factors, such as muscle tone, ocular reflexes, heart rate, respiratory rate and depth, and blood pressure. The progressive signs of anesthetic depth vary with the anesthetic drugs used, the species, and the individual patient. One cannot rely on a single sign but must use all available information to evaluate anesthetic depth.

Anesthetic depth is not a steady state, but rather a product of the anesthetic drugs on board, the patient's physiological state, and the degree of surgical stimulation applied to the patient at a particular time. If the anesthetic dose is constant, increased surgical stimulation may quickly result in movement or awakening. Increasing the anesthetic dose to compensate for periods of extreme surgical stimulation

---

BOX 19-5

Progression of Anesthetic Depth

1. Analgesia and amnesia
2. Loss of consciousness and motor coordination
3. Reduced protective reflexes
4. Blockade of afferent stimuli
5. Muscle relaxation
6. Respiratory and cardiovascular depression
7. Depression of cardiovascular and respiratory reflexes
8. Apnea
9. Cardiac arrest

TABLE 19-7

Signs of Anesthetic Depth

	Anesthetic Depth		
	Light	Surgical	Deep
Spontaneous movement	Possible	None	None
Reflex movement	Possible	None	None
Anesthetic	1 MAC	1.1 to 1.5 MAC	1.5 to 2 MAC concentration
Jaw muscle tone	Tense	Moderate	Relaxed
Palpebral reflex	Present	None or slight	None
Globe position	Central	Ventromedial	Central
Corneal moisture	Moist	Moist	Dry
Pupil size	Medium	Reduced	Dilated

may precipitate sudden overdose in the absence of stimulation. In summary, anesthetic depth is dose-dependent; more drug produces more CNS depression. However, the degree to which a given anesthetic dose produces CNS depression (general anesthesia) is quite variable.

Anesthetic depth is sufficient when gross patient movement does not interfere with the procedure being performed. Anesthetic depth is estimated by assessing skeletal muscle tone and selected reflexes. Jaw muscle tone and eye reflexes are useful signs of anesthetic depth and diminish with progression toward deeper planes of anesthesia.

Eye reflexes are frequently used to assess anesthetic depth. Nystagmus and active palpebral reflexes indicate light anesthesia, which is inadequate for most surgical procedures. Absence of the palpebral reflex and presence of the corneal reflex are considered signs of a medium level of anesthesia, at which routine surgical procedures may be performed.

Absence of corneal reflex or drying of the cornea indicates deep anesthesia, in which the patient should be monitored closely for adequate cardiopulmonary function and the anesthetic level lightened if possible. Direct response to surgical stimulation is the most reliable sign of light anesthesia. In many patients, other signs, such as increased rate and depth of respiration, often precede movement.

Monitoring Physiologic Conditions

The patient's physiological conditions are monitored to assure that excessive derangement of vital functions is not developing. This process is focused on the respiratory and cardiovascular systems. The goal is to maintain adequate delivery of oxygenated blood to the tissues.

Perfusion (Latin *perfundere*, meaning "to pour over") refers to the passage of oxygenated blood through body tissues. Poor perfusion may imply poor blood flow and/or poor blood oxygenation. *Shock* is defined as inadequate perfusion. It can be said that death is a late sign of poor perfusion; patients are not normally well-perfused one minute and dead the next. Common complications of poor perfusion, sometimes referred to as the "five hypos," are hypoxemia, hypoventilation/hypercapnia, hypotension, hypovolemia, and hypothermia. This discussion will focus on avoiding the development of these adverse conditions during anesthesia (Box 19-6).

Monitoring respiratory function

Respiratory function is monitored to ensure adequate oxygenation and removal of carbon dioxide from the blood. Respiratory function may be evaluated by respiratory rate, tidal volume, breathing patterns, hemoglobin saturation, end-tidal carbon dioxide, and arterial blood gases. Arterial blood gas analysis, the most reliable method by which to assess respiratory function, is not possible in all clinical settings because it requires an arterial blood sample and special equipment. Equipment useful for monitoring respi-

BOX 19-6

The Five "Hypos"

Hypoxemia	Insufficient oxygenation of the blood (PaO_2 less than 60 mm Hg). A common sign of pulmonary compromise during anesthesia and the reason for oxygen enrichment of inspired air.
Hypoventilation	Reduced rate and depth of ventilation as determined by increased arterial carbon dioxide levels (hypercarbia or hypercapnia) ($PaCO_2$ above 45 mm Hg). Hypercarbia is an early sign of pulmonary compromise.
Hypotension	Inadequate arterial blood pressure. The most common sign of cardiovascular depression. Diastolic/systolic pressures are normally 80/120 mm Hg.
Hypovolemia	Insufficient circulating blood volume. A common cause of hypotension. For this reason, fluid administration is one of the most valuable supportive measures one can provide during anesthesia.
Hypothermia	Abnormally low body temperature (2° to 3° C below normal). A sign of central nervous system and cardiovascular depression.

ratory function includes a blood gas machine, pulse oximeter, end-tidal carbon dioxide analyzer (capnometer), rate monitor, and ventilometer. However, the most essential monitor is a well-prepared, highly skilled individual performing continuous monitoring.

The pulse oximeter measures the percentage of hemoglobin that is saturated with oxygen (oxyhemoglobin). This SpO_2 reading should be 95% to 100% in anesthetized patients breathing an oxygen/anesthetic mixture. A reading of 90% corresponds to an extremely low partial pressure of oxygen in the arterial blood (PaO_2 of 60 mm Hg). Note that an SpO_2 reading of 66% ($\frac{1}{3}$ of hemoglobin not carrying oxygen) is needed before visible cyanosis (blue mucous membranes) occurs in a patient with normal hemoglobin levels (15 gm/dL). The transmissive pulse oximeter probe is usually applied to the tongue, but may be used on any well-perfused, thin, nonpigmented tissue. A reflective probe may be used in the rectum if good mucosal contact is maintained. SpO_2 readings are unreliable in the presence of probe movement or a weak pulse.

The capnometer measures end-tidal carbon dioxide ($ETCO_2$). End tidal means "at the end of expiration," when CO_2 levels of the expired gas are approximately equal to alveolar and arterial CO_2 ($PaCO_2$). The sampling tube is attached to a port on an adapter that fits between the endotracheal tube and the breathing circuit (Fig. 19-15). Levels

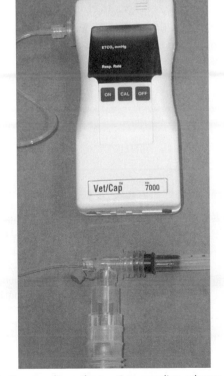

Fig. 19-15 Gas sampling adapter. Gas sampling adapter attached to endotracheal tube with capnometer attached is shown.

for anesthetized patients should be 40 to 45 mm Hg. If higher, hypoventilation exists. Lower levels indicate hyperventilation.

Hearing, vision, and touch can be used to monitor the respiratory system and airway. Good indicators that air is moving in and out of the lungs are auscultation of breathing and lung sounds with a standard or esophageal stethoscope, observation of the chest wall and of the reservoir bag for movement, and feeling the reservoir bag for resistance (Box 19-7). However, air movement does not ensure adequate exchange of oxygen and carbon dioxide between the alveoli and blood. Observation of bright red arterial blood at the surgical site and observing mucous membranes for pinkness are reasonably reliable for determining blood oxygenation. Color changes are not evident until severe hypoxemia exists, however.

Monitoring cardiovascular function

Cardiovascular function is monitored to ensure that cardiac output and forward movement of blood are contributing to tissue perfusion. Cardiovascular function is evaluated by the heart rate, heart sounds, pulse quality and rate, mucous membrane color, and capillary refill time. Electrocardiography is recommended for evaluation of rhythm and conduction disturbances. Comparison of heart rate and pulse rate enables detection of pulse deficits. Blood pressure, urine output, and body temperature are also indicators of cardiovascular function.

All anesthetic drugs used today have dose-dependent cardiovascular depressant effects, such as arrhythmias, decreased contractility, vasodilation, or vasoconstriction. Monitoring the cardiovascular system does not require a grand display of electronic instrumentation. Although mechanical devices are appealing, the senses of touch,

---

BOX 19-7

Informative Auscultatory Sounds

Respiratory sounds

- Partial airway obstruction: increased or decreased sound volume, harshness
- Severe narrowing of airways: stridor, snoring, squeaking, whistling
- Fluid: crepitation
- Excessive fluid: bubbling

Cardiac sounds

- Loudness indicates contractile strength and cardiac output
- Murmurs may mean decreased forward movement of blood
- Simultaneous pulse palpation can reveal arrhythmias

hearing, and vision are extremely useful for evaluation of cardiovascular function. Pulse palpation, capillary refill, blood color, and heart sounds may be determined with simple instrumentation. The stethoscope provides much information useful to estimate cardiovascular status. Monitoring equipment can be used to enhance evaluation of cardiovascular function but can never replace what you observe, feel, or hear (Table 19-8).

Heart rates are easily determined with a simple stethoscope, esophageal stethoscope, or ECG. Counting the rate of the peripheral pulse and the heart rate simultaneously is very useful. Although heart rates vary significantly with patient size and species, the pulse rate and the heart rate should be equal. The presence of a heart sound with an absent or extremely weak pulse indicates a pulse deficit and should be investigated before anesthesia proceeds. Ordinarily, smaller patients have faster heart rates than larger patients of the same species do. Cardiac output (stroke volume × heart rate) is a critical factor in maintaining adequate perfusion. The heart rate alone is of limited value in judging the adequacy of cardiac output. Other factors such as capillary refill time and pulse quality, should be considered as well. Changes in heart rate may indicate adverse anesthetic effects, pain, compensation for decreased blood pressure, or vagal reflex stimulation.

Auscultation. Auscultation of the heart with a standard or esophageal stethoscope can provide valuable information, in addition to the heart rate. The rhythm and loudness of the heartbeat reflect overall cardiovascular function. Heart sounds are easily amplified by inexpensive monitoring devices. These small amplifiers provide the convenience of easily audible heart sounds while freeing the surgeon or technician to move around within the surgical area. Abnormal heart rates, irregular rhythm, and weak or muffled heart sounds may indicate diminished cardiac function. Altered heart rate and irregular rhythm suggest arrhythmias, whereas diminished heart sounds may indicate low cardiac output from myocardial hypoxemia or hypotension. Integrating this information with mucous membrane color, pulse quality, and capillary refill time provides usable information. However, it is a mistake to simply assume that because there is an audible beep or heart sound, everything is fine.

Electrocardiogram. The electrocardiogram (ECG) provides reliable information concerning heart rate and rhythm. The ECG is valuable for diagnosis of specific cardiac arrhythmias. Remember that the ECG is only an indicator of the electrical activity of the heart muscle and alone is a poor indicator of normal contraction or blood flow. Normal contraction requires normal electrical conduction of activating electrical impulses through cardiac muscle tissue. Abnormal or skipped contractions resulting from abnormal electrical activity (ECG) may diminish blood flow, consequently producing pulse deficit. If sufficient skipped beats occur (10 to 12 per minute), perfusion may be significantly affected, requiring organ support. The sequence of adverse events is abnormal ECG, abnormal or skipped beats, decreased blood flow, weak or absent pulse, and finally cardiac arrest.

Pulse. The arterial pulse is the result of a pressure wave generated by cardiac contraction and ejection of blood into the aorta. This pressure wave travels down the arterial blood faster than the blood actually flows. Even though the pulse is not due to blood flow, normal pulse rate and adequate pulse quality are indicators of adequate blood flow. Pulse rate is easily determined by palpation or pulse oxime-

---

TABLE 19-8

Normal Physiologic Values in Dogs, Cats, Horses, and Cattle

	Dogs	Cats	Horses	Cattle
Heart rate	60-160/min	80-200/min	24-50/min	60-120/min
Respiratory rate	20-40/min	20-40/min	8-20/min	20-40/min
Tidal volume	10-20 ml/kg	10-20 ml/kg	10-20 ml/kg	10-20 ml/kg
Minute volume (resp rate × tidal vol)	200-800 ml/kg/min	200-800 ml/kg/min	200-800 ml/kg/min	200-800 ml/kg/min
Blood pH	7.35-7.45	7.35-7.45	7.35-7.45	7.35-7.45
PaO_2	80-110 mm Hg	80-110 mm Hg	80-110 mm Hg	80-110 mm Hg
$PaCO_2$	35-45 mm Hg	35-45 mm Hg	35-45 mm Hg	35-45 mm Hg
HCO_3	22-27 mm Hg	22-27 mm Hg	22-27 mm Hg	22-27 mm Hg
Total CO_2	38-54 mm Hg	38-54 mm Hg	54-72 mm Hg	47-72 mm Hg
Base excess	−4 to +14	−4 to +14 (correct if −5 to −10) −4 to +14	−4 to +14	
Central venous pressure (standing)	3-4 cm H_2O	3-4 cm H_2O	3-4 cm H_2O	3-4 cm H_2O
Central venous pressure (anesthetized, recumbent)	2-7 cm H_2O	15-25 cm H_2O		

ity. The peripheral pulse rate may be less than the heart rate; a situation called *pulse deficit*. Auscultation of the heart while simultaneously palpating the peripheral pulse is an excellent method of recognizing pulse deficits that may be due to cardiac arrhythmias. Significant arrhythmias produce ineffective heartbeats that are audible but do not produce a palpable arterial pulse. Pulse deficits occurring at a rate of 1 per 10 heartbeats (10%) or more may significantly diminish coronary and peripheral perfusion and require immediate attention. Anesthetics produce dose-related decreases in pulse quality. *Pulse quality* describes how the pulse feels when palpated with light digital pressure. Terms that describe pulse quality are: strong, moderate, weak, and thready (means weak). *Pulse pressure* is the difference between systolic and diastolic arterial pressures. The *pulse pressure curve* shows changes in the pulse pressure during the cardiac cycle (Fig. 19-16). Such curves may be obtained from direct arterial pressure monitors. Some pulse oximeters display a pulse curve that looks similar to the pulse pressure curve but is derived from detection of pulsations, not direct pressure. Pulse quality is affected by several factors including vascular tone, vascular fluid volume, systolic/diastolic pressure differences, cardiac stroke volume, cardiac ejection rate, and peripheral location. In general, it is a useful indicator of stroke volume. Frequent causes of decreased pulse quality during anesthesia include hypovolemia, hypotension, and anything that causes decreased cardiac stroke volume. If the pulse weakens, decrease the anesthetic concentration, increase the infusion rate of fluids, determine the underlying cause, and make appropriate corrections.

Mucous membrane color. Mucous membrane color can be used to estimate tissue perfusion and oxygenation. Mucous membranes are normally pink, indicating adequate respiratory and cardiovascular function. Cherry red mucous membranes may be seen with carbon monoxide poisoning.

However, in severe carbon monoxide poisoning, cyanosis may mask the cherry red color. Hemoglobin has 200 times the affinity for carbon monoxide than oxygen, and its presence reduces the oxygen-transporting capability of hemoglobin, resulting in hypoxemia. Carbon monoxide poisoning has occurred during anesthesia of people using halogenated hydrocarbons. There is reason for the same concern in veterinary anesthesia, although it has not yet been reported. Apparently, desiccated soda lime and Baralyme® react with halogenated inhalation anesthetics to produce toxic concentrations of carbon monoxide. The tendency for veterinary clinics to delay changing of carbon dioxide absorbent must be seriously addressed.

Pale mucous membranes indicate vasoconstriction or a decrease in circulating red blood cells. Pale mucous membranes are not always a sign of poor hemodynamic status or shock. Cyanosis is a sign of respiratory insufficiency and an indication of hypoxemia. Absence of blueness does not ensure adequate blood oxygenation. Anemic patients may not have sufficient hemoglobin to produce blueness, even when hypoxia is severe.

Capillary refill time. Capillary refill time (CRT) provides another way to estimate tissue perfusion and oxygenation. It is an indication of cardiovascular tone; it suggests that blood is filling the capillary beds. CRT of less than 2 seconds in small animals and less than 3 seconds in large animals is considered normal. However, in a head-down position or in the presence of vasodilation, patients may have normal or reduced CRT in the presence of severely compromised blood flow. This is especially true in horses, cattle, and other very large patients. Vasoconstriction prolongs the CRT. In summary, the presence of shortened or normal CRT may not be a reliable sign of adequate perfusion, but a prolonged CRT is significant.

Arterial blood pressure. Arterial blood pressure is an indicator of perfusion and cardiac output but not a true measure of blood flow. Anesthetics produce dose-dependent decreases in blood pressure; therefore, monitoring blood pressure during anesthesia is useful for depth determination and evaluation of patient health status. Blood pressure may be determined by direct or indirect methods. Direct or invasive monitoring requires special equipment and placement of an arterial catheter. Indirect or noninvasive methods require special equipment but do not require an invasive arterial catheter to measure blood pressure. Doppler and oscillometric methods are indirect and noninvasive and are frequently used to determine blood pressure in clinical settings. The equipment used to measure blood pressure by noninvasive methods is priced within range of most veterinary facilities.

Low arterial blood pressure may be due to hypovolemia, cardiac depression, or vasodilation. The awake or lightly anesthetized, healthy patient rapidly compensates for hypotension by increasing cardiac output or by increasing

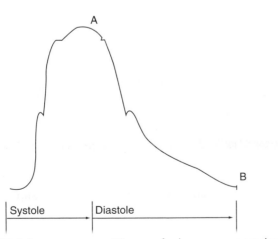

Fig. 19-16 Pulse pressure curve. Diagram of pulse pressure curve shown in relationship to ECG.

vascular tone. However, patients anesthetized to surgical planes of anesthesia may be unable to compensate or maintain acceptable blood pressure because of dose-dependent autonomic nervous system depression produced by anesthetic drugs. In most anesthetized patients, hypotension can be prevented by IV administration of crystalloid fluids at 10 to 20 ml/kg/hr, along with careful monitoring of tissue perfusion and anesthetic depth.

Monitoring body temperature

Monitoring body temperature during anesthesia provides an indication of CNS function and cardiovascular function. Depression of thermoregulatory centers in the brain and decreased blood flow produced by anesthetic agents lead to *hypothermia* (low body temperature). It may be produced in response to various drug combinations, specifically halothane, isoflurane, sevoflurane, succinylcholine, and ketamine. Continuous measurement of core temperature with a rectal or esophageal thermometer warns of significant temperature change.

It is much easier to prevent heat loss than to restore heat. Minimizing potential heat loss requires planning. Minimizing anesthesia time and depth, avoiding cold surfaces and cold scrub solutions, using a circulating-water blanket or hot-water bottles, and warming intravenous fluids help prevent hypothermia. It is also useful to warm and moisturize inspired air, use warm blankets, keep body cavities closed when possible, and use warm irrigation solutions. Fluids, hot-water bottles, or warming blankets should not be warmed to temperatures greater than 40° C or body surfaces may be burned.

Responding to Adverse Events

All adverse events should be brought to the veterinarian's attention immediately. The role of the technician in responding to adverse events is generally that of being prepared to execute the veterinarian's directives quickly and accurately. The administration of drugs to counteract specific conditions should be under the veterinarian's direction. However, some situations simply require a common-sense approach.

Hypothermia

If the body temperature drops below 35° C, decrease the anesthetic concentration, ensure adequate circulation, insulate from cold surfaces, dry the body surface, apply warm blankets and/or hot packs, warm inspired air, and decrease fresh gas flow to minimum requirements.

Tachycardia

When the heart rate exceeds 160 to 180 in dogs (depending on breed) or 200 in cats, tachycardia is occurring. If the patient is not moving (anesthetic depth is adequate), decrease the anesthetic concentration, increase oxygen flow, increase the rate of IV fluid delivery, and support ventilation. If tachycardia persists, prepare for cardiac arrest.

Bradycardia

When the heart rate drops below 60, bradycardia is occurring. Bradycardia caused by alpha agonists may be treated with anticholinergics or a specific alpha antagonist. Opioid-induced bradycardia can be managed with anticholinergics. Bradycardia resulting from excessive anesthetic depth usually responds to a decreased anesthetic concentration and support with oxygen and fluids. Vagus-mediated bradycardia is usually transient and diminishes as vagal stimulation is discontinued. If bradycardia worsens or persists, administration of an anticholinergic may be required, along with fluid administration. Hypothermic patients exhibiting bradycardia must be warmed and may require IV fluid administration to correct bradycardia. Anticholinergics should be avoided in hypothermic patients because of the increased risk of cardiac arrhythmia.

Pain

Pain should be treated with an analgesic that produces less cardiovascular depressant effect than additional general anesthetic.

Hypotension

Hypotension is usually controlled by appropriate fluid administration and lowering the anesthetic concentration.

Hypercarbia

Hypercarbia (hypercapnea) is managed by increasing ventilation ("bagging") to remove carbon dioxide from the patient. In rebreathing circuits, expired soda lime or faulty unidirectional valves may be the cause. In nonrebreathing circuits, the cause may be inadequate flow rate. Excessive mechanical dead space due to an excessively long endotracheal tube or large facemask may contribute to hypercarbia as well.

Hypoxemia

Hypoxemia is initially treated by increasing inspired oxygen concentration and ensuring adequate ventilation. Hypoxemia may be due to a kinked or plugged endotracheal tube or an empty oxygen tank; in such cases, the solution is obvious.

Excessive depth

Excessive anesthetic depth is reversed by decreasing the vaporizer setting, increasing the oxygen flow rate, and ensuring adequate ventilation and circulatory support.

Inadequate depth

Inability to achieve or maintain adequate anesthetic depth is generally due to insufficient delivery of anesthetic to the alveoli. A common cause is breathing around the endotracheal tube or facemask. Other causes include an empty, overfilled, or malfunctioning vaporizer. Inadequate flow rate and vaporizer settings may prolong induction. Inadequate uptake of anesthetic from the alveoli into the bloodstream is also possible.

Endobronchial intubation

This can present with some perplexing signs but is frequently associated with difficulty maintaining adequate ventilation and anesthetic depth. It is easily corrected by withdrawing the endotracheal tube sufficiently to remove it from the bronchus.

Excessive circuit pressure

If the pressure in the breathing circuit exceeds the central venous pressure (approximately 4 cm H_2O), the result is collapse of the thoracic vena cava and reduction of venous return to the heart. Cardiac output cannot exceed venous return, so it decreases as well, leading to hypotension. This is usually caused by a closed or stuck pop-off valve and/or excessive oxygen flow rate. Occlusion of the scavenger system may also be the cause.

INHALATION ANESTHETIC TECHNIQUES

Goals of Proper Technique

A primary goal of proper anesthetic technique is to provide maximum safety for the patient and personnel. Of paramount importance is to minimize or avoid personnel exposure to anesthetic waste gases (Box 19-8). Anesthetic

---

BOX 19-8

Techniques for Minimizing Exposure to Waste Anesthetic Gases

1. Check for and correct leaks in anesthesia machine and breathing circuit.
2. Use a cuffed endotracheal tube of the proper size; inflate cuff if needed.
3. Do not disconnect patient from breathing circuit immediately after anesthesia; if possible, wait several minutes for gases to dissipate.
4. Connect pop-off valve to a scavenger system, preferably one that discharges outdoors.
5. Connect nonrebreathing systems to a scavenger system.
6. Avoid use of chamber or mask-induction techniques.
7. Avoid spilling liquid anesthetic while filling the vaporizer; recap bottle and vaporizer immediately.
8. Maintain adequate ventilation of the area.

---

techniques have evolved to avoid specific problems previously encountered. Although the consequences of error or mishap in any one step of a procedure may seem negligible, the cumulative effects of marginal technique may produce serious consequences. The following selected procedural guidelines should be followed routinely.

Induction Technique

Anesthetic induction may proceed after a vein is catheterized, the equipment is readied, and the surgeon is available. Administration of the induction or maintenance agent should provide a smooth and safe transition to unconsciousness (see Table 19-2). When jaw muscle tone and orolaryngeal reflexes are lost, intubate the patient.

Endotracheal Intubation

Dogs and cats

Dogs and cats are placed in sternal position, with the head and neck extended in a straight line to aid visualization of the larynx. If an assistant is available, have him or her position the head while the anesthetist places the endotracheal tube. A laryngoscope aids intubation. Place the largest tube that will enter the airway without causing trauma or undue stimulation of vagal reflexes, which may induce cardiac arrhythmias. Applying lidocaine to the larynx by spray or with a cotton-tipped swab, especially in cats and swine, facilitates intubation. Cetacaine (benzocaine) spray should not be used because it can cause methemoglobinemia. Lubrication of the cuff with sterile water-soluble lubricant facilitates intubation and protects the tracheal mucosa from drying where the inflated cuff contacts the mucosa. Proper positioning of the endotracheal tube may be confirmed by condensation of respiratory gases on the inside of the tube with expiration, ability to palpate only one tubular structure in the neck (trachea), auscultation of lung sounds when bagging the patient, and the carbon dioxide reading on the capnometer.

Attach the breathing circuit to the endotracheal tube adapter before inflating the cuff (see Endotracheal Cuff Inflation section). Open the oxygen flow meter to deliver 3 L/min, and set the vaporizer to the appropriate delivery concentration (1% to 3%). Secure the tube with gauze or tape to the mandible or maxilla, and begin cardiopulmonary observations. Once the tube is in place and secured, and the system is free of leaks, apply ophthalmic ointment to protect the cornea (if not previously done) and proceed with preparation for the procedure. When moving the patient is required, it is prudent to disconnect the breathing circuit from the endotracheal tube to avoid trauma or dislodgment.

Horses

Horses are intubated similar to small animals, except the horse is placed in lateral recumbency. The oral cavity must be flushed thoroughly with water to remove food and debris before induction and intubation. It is necessary to place an oral speculum between the incisor teeth to prevent biting the tube, causing obstruction of the airway. A tube of the largest diameter that will pass without excessive force is selected. The endotracheal tube is lubricated with copious amounts of water-soluble sterile lubricant and passed through the preinserted speculum, avoiding the sharp edges of the check teeth. Although the glottis cannot be visualized, the tube enters with little difficulty. If difficulty is encountered while blindly intubating, rotating the tube while applying slight pressure usually facilitates tube passage. Box 19-9 presents a summary of techniques used in equine anesthesia.

Endotracheal cuff inflation

The endotracheal tube cuff is inflated to allow positive-pressure ventilation and prevent aspiration in the event of regurgitation. A pressure of 20 to 25 cm H_2O is sufficient for both purposes. *Do not inflate the cuff until the need has been determined.* To determine the need for cuff inflation, perform the following steps:

1. Close the pressure-relief valve and squeeze the reservoir bag while observing the manometer and listening for leakage of gas around the endotracheal tube. Signs of leakage include: a hissing sound as gas escapes around the cuff, inability to hold the pressure at 20 to 25 cm H_2O, the smell of anesthetic agent emanating from the mouth, and/or stertorous breathing from the tube pushing on the side of the larynx.
2. If circuit pressure reaches 25 cm H_2O without leaking around the tube, do not inflate the cuff.
3. If leakage occurs below 25 cm H_2O, inflate the cuff just enough to prevent the leakage. Should the cuff be inflated beyond 25 cm H_2O, the excessive pressure may damage the tracheal mucosa.
4. Changes in the patient's position or a slow leak in the cuff may result in leakage occurring later in the procedure. It is prudent to observe for signs of leakage during routine manual ventilation (bagging).

Tissue damage from traumatic intubation or an overinflated cuff is often manifested as coughing a few days after anesthesia.

Maintenance of Anesthesia

Once the patient is fully anesthetized by the inhalation anesthetic, the induction period is over and the stage of maintenance anesthesia begins. Generally, the anesthetic effects of an ultrashort-acting induction agent will dissipate within a few minutes. By then, the patient needs to be fully anesthetized by the inhalation agent. Ideally, the transition from anesthesia by the induction agent to the inhalation agent will be smooth and uneventful. It must be recognized that the uptake of inhalation anesthetics is dependent on adequate ventilation. If the patient is hypoventilating when first placed on the gas machine, inadequate anesthetic will be taken up to maintain anesthesia once the induction agent dissipates.

Once anesthesia with the inhalant agent is accomplished, the vaporizer setting and oxygen flow should be reduced to maintenance levels. The anesthetist's attention now focuses on monitoring and support of vital organ function. Connect all monitoring instruments, and begin recording all pertinent information on the patient's anesthetic record. Monitoring should be continuous, and data should be recorded every 5 to 10 minutes or when significant changes occur.

The oxygen flow rate used for maintenance depends on the type of breathing circuit used. Nonrebreathing circuits require high flows throughout maintenance, whereas rebreathing circuits may use reduced flows for semiclosed or closed operation.

Flow rates for nonrebreathing systems

Flow rates for nonrebreathing systems must remain high because this is the means by which exhaled CO_2 is flushed away from the patient. Depending on the system used, flow rates of 100 to 300 mL/kg/min or 2 to 3 times the minute ventilation are recommended. Ideally, $ETCO_2$ should be monitored with a capnometer to assure adequate removal of CO_2.

Flow rates for rebreathing systems

As previously mentioned, rebreathing circuits are most commonly used in veterinary practice. The systems are referred to as either *closed* or *open*, depending on the rate of oxygen delivery to the patient.

Closed systems. Maintenance flow rate for a rebreathing circuit operated as a closed system is equal to the patient's calculated oxygen consumption rate:

$$10 \times (kg \times 0.75)/kg$$

At 4 kg, this will be a total flow of 28 ml/min (7 ml/kg/min), while at 38 kg it will be 153 ml/min (4 ml/kg/min). The larger the animal, the lower its per-kilogram oxygen requirement. Oxygen consumption is also affected by body temperature and anesthesia. The advantages of closed-system operation include minimal pollution, economy, and minimal loss of moisture and heat. Disadvantages include slow changes in anesthetic concentration, increased use of the CO_2 absorber, necessity to monitor the system volume closely, inability to use N_2O, dilution due to patient nitrogen output, and necessity of high flow rates during induction.

Semiclosed systems. Maintenance flow rate for a rebreathing circuit operated as a semiclosed system exceeds oxygen requirements. These have traditionally been called *low flow* (up to 22 mL/kg/min), and *high flow* (up to

Quick Reference Guide for Equine Anesthesia

Preparation

1. Withhold food for 24 hours and water for 6 to 12 hours, when possible. Telephone the client to remind about food and water restriction.
2. Obtain the horse's body weight by weighing or chest girth tape measurement for estimation.
3. Avoid or delay elective procedures in horses that are not healthy. Perform a physical examination before administration of any drug. Minimum data should include heart rate, respiratory rate, mucous membrane color, pulse quality, ocular or nasal discharge, lymph nodes, PCV, and total plasma protein assay.
4. Administer fluids to debilitated horses or horses to be anesthetized for long procedures.
5. Use an IV set with a drip chamber. Do not use a simplex.
6. Place an IV catheter.
7. Use a trained technician (rather than a client or barn staff) to assist, monitor vital organ function, and administer drugs.
8. Avoid stress, such as from extreme heat or long trailer rides, before induction of anesthesia.
9. Keep the horse calm before induction of anesthesia.

Sedation and analgesia in standing horses

Xylazine and butorphanol

1. Give xylazine IM or IV at 4 to 7 mg/kg.
2. Wait 10 minutes.
3. Give butorphanol IV at 2 to 5 mg/kg.
4. Monitor sedation and heart rate.
5. Give small IV doses of xylazine and butorphanol as needed.
6. Give xylazine in IV boluses of 50 to 100 mg (maximum of 500 mg/hr).
7. Give butorphanol in IV boluses of 5 to 10 mg (maximum of 50 mg/hr).
8. If patient has difficulty standing, do not administer more drug.

Detomidine and butorphanol

1. Give detomidine IV at 0.02 mg/kg or IM at 0.04 mg/kg.
2. Wait 10 minutes.
3. Give butorphanol IV at 2 to 5 mg/kg.
4. Monitor sedation and heart rate.
5. Give small IV doses of detomidine and butorphanol as needed.
6. Give detomidine in IV boluses of 2 mg (maximum of 20 mg/hr).

7. Give butorphanol in IV boluses of 5 to 10 mg (maximum of 50 mg/hr).
8. If patient has difficulty standing, do not administer more drug.

Anesthetic induction and maintenance

Xylazine and ketamine

1. Give xylazine IV at 1.1 mg/kg. If the horse is not sedated by xylazine, administer 10 to 20 mg (total dose) of diazepam or butorphanol IV, rather than additional xylazine.
2. Give ketamine as an IV bolus at 2.2 mg/kg.
3. Anticipate 8 to 12 minutes of anesthesia.
4. Anesthesia may be prolonged with Triple Drip (see below) or with up to two additional doses of xylazine and ketamine, using half the original dosage. Do not give more than two additional doses.

Diazepam with xylazine and ketamine

1. Give diazepam IM or slowly IV at 0.05 mg/kg.
2. Wait 20 to 40 minutes for maximum effect.
3. Give xylazine IV at 1.1 mg/kg.
4. When the horse is sedated (may occur rapidly), give ketamine as an IV bolus at 2.2 mg/kg.
5. Provides smooth induction, 12 to 20 minutes of anesthesia, and smooth recovery.
6. Anesthesia may be prolonged with Triple Drip.

Butorphanol with xylazine and ketamine

1. Give butorphanol IM or slowly IV at 0.05 mg/kg.
2. Wait 20 minutes.
3. Give xylazine IV at 1.1 mg/kg.
4. When the horse is sedated, give ketamine as an IV bolus at 2.2 mg/kg.
5. Anticipate 12 to 20 minutes of anesthesia and analgesia.
6. Anesthesia may be prolonged with Triple Drip or guaifenesin.

Triple drip

1. Add 1000 to 2000 mg of ketamine (1 to 2 mg/ml) and 500 mg of xylazine (0.05 mg/ml) to 1 liter of 5% guaifenesin (50 mg/ml).
2. Infuse IV at a constant drip rate of approximately 1 to 2 ml/kg/hr.
3. Triple Drip is useful for maintenance following induction with xylazine and dissociative anesthetics.

44 mL/kg/min) rates. Depending on the size of the animal, low flow is up to 3 to 5 times oxygen needs and high flow is up to 6 to 10 times oxygen needs.

The standard practice of using 1 L/min for the maintenance flow rate exceeds the high flow range (22 to 44 ml/kg/min) for animals less than 23 kg and is in the high flow range for animals 23 to 45 kg. Therefore, 1 L/min is excessively expensive financially and physically for the majority of patients less than 45 kg (Fig. 19-12).

The advantages of maintenance flow rates greater than oxygen needs include: less oxygen dilution due to patient nitrogen output, less worry about meeting oxygen needs, less dependence on CO_2 absorber, ability to use N_2O safely, and faster changes in anesthetic concentration. Disadvantages include: greater loss of heat and moisture, and greater expense.

It should be recognized that lower flow rates increase the time it takes to change the anesthetic concentration of the breathing circuit. Any time rapid changes must be made in anesthetic concentration (such as the patient awakening during surgery), a very high flow rate (3 to 4 L/min) must be used in conjunction with an increased vaporizer setting. A good rule to remember is: *The vaporizer setting controls where anesthetic concentration in the circuit is going, and the oxygen flow rate controls how fast it will get there.*

One must also remember that the larger the circuit volume, the more time it takes to alter the anesthetic concentration in the circuit. The use of an excessively large reservoir bag adds unnecessary volume to the circuit that slows changes in anesthetic concentration.

Adjust the vaporizer to provide the desired depth. The correct setting provides just enough anesthetic depth to perform the procedure. Excessive concentrations should be avoided. Begin administration of intravenous fluids as soon as possible (10 to 20 ml/kg/hr).

Throughout maintenance, the patient should be ventilated twice per minute or as needed to maintain a $PaCO_2$ of 40 to 45 mm Hg. This is accomplished by closing the pop-off valve and squeezing the reservoir bag to inflate the lungs to a pressure of 15 to 20 cm H_2O. This artificial "breath" should mimic a normal breath in terms of inspiratory time (do not hold pressure; just inflate and release).

Recovery from Anesthesia

Recovery begins when administration of anesthetic is discontinued. The patient should be maintained on 100% oxygen to ensure oxygenation and allow exhaled anesthetic gases to enter the scavenger system, rather than the room air. As the patient begins to awaken, the endotracheal tube cuff should be deflated and the tie undone. When the patient exhibits swallowing reflexes, the tube should be gently removed. Close observation is essential immediately after extubation, as the patient may regurgitate or have difficulty breathing. Brachycephalic dogs are especially notorious for developing breathing difficulties after extubation.

Fluid administration should continue until recovery is adequate. Premature removal of the IV catheter may result in the inability to quickly administer IV medications in the event of an emergency. Recovery is considered adequate (but not complete) when the body temperature is normal, the patient's vital signs are stable, and sternal recumbency is maintained. Observation should continue until the patient can stand and walk without assistance.

RECOMMENDED READING

Anon: Commentary and recommendations on control of waste anesthetic gases in the workplace, *J Am Vet Med Assoc* 209:75-77, 1996.

Mathews KA: Management of pain, *Vet Clin North Am Small Animal Practice* July 2000. Saunders.

Muir WW et al, *Handbook of veterinary anesthesia*, ed 3, Mosby, 2000.

Riebold TW et al: *Large animal anesthesia: principles and techniques*, ed 2, Ames, Iowa, 1995, Iowa State University Press.

Shaffran N: Defining pain in dogs and cats, *Veterinary Technician*, August 2002.

Short CE: *Principles and practice of veterinary anesthesia*, Baltimore, 1987, Williams & Wilkins.

Thurmon JC, Tranquilli WJ: *Lamb and Jones' veterinary anesthesia*, ed 3, Baltimore, 1996, Williams & Wilkins.

Thurmon et al: *Essentials of small animal anesthesia and analgesia*, Lippincott, 1999.

Tranquilli WJ et al: *Pain management for the small animal practitioner*, Teton NewMedia, 2000. *Note: The CD-ROM version of this book also contains video demonstrations of procedures such as epidural injection.*

20

Principles of Surgical Nursing

Margi Sirois

Learning Objectives

After reviewing this chapter, the reader should understand the following:

- Terminology used in surgery
- Principles of aseptic technique
- Methods used to disinfect and sterilize surgical instruments and supplies
- Procedure for preparing the surgical site and surgical team
- Types of surgical instruments and their uses and maintenance
- Types of suture needles and suture materials

GENERAL SURGICAL PRINCIPLES

The role of the veterinary technician in surgical procedures is quite diverse. During the presurgical period, the veterinary technician is responsible for preparation of the patient, the surgical instruments and equipment, and the surgical environment. During surgery, the veterinary technician is usually responsible for anesthesia of the patient. The veterinary technician often assists the surgeon, either directly by scrubbing in, or indirectly by opening surgical packs, suture materials, and other supplies. It is vital that the veterinary technician know how to function in a sterile surgical environment without causing contamination. In the postsurgical period, the veterinary technician is frequently responsible for postoperative patient care and monitoring, instructing clients on patient care during the recovery period, and removing sutures.

BASIC SURGICAL TERMINOLOGY

Surgical procedures are described using anatomic terms combined with word roots called suffixes (see Chapter 5). The most common suffixes used for describing surgical procedures are in Box 20-1.

Abdominal Incisions

Abdominal surgery is commonly performed in animal species. Entry into the abdomen is usually gained by any of four common abdominal incisions. Named according to its location, each incision offers different advantages and a different exposure of the abdomen (Fig. 20-1).

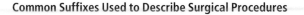

BOX 20-1

Common Suffixes Used to Describe Surgical Procedures

-ectomy = to remove (to excise). For example, a splen*ectomy* is a surgical procedure to remove the spleen.

-otomy = to cut into. For example, a cyst*otomy* (incision into the urinary bladder) is often performed to remove urinary calculi (bladder stones).

-ostomy = surgical creation of an artificial opening. For example, a perineal urethr*ostomy* is a surgical procedure often performed on male cats for relief of urethral obstruction. It involves excision of the penis (pen*ectomy)* and creation of a widened new urethral opening.

-rrhaphy = surgical repair by suturing. For example, abdominal hernio*rrhaphy* is the surgical repair of an abdominal hernia by suturing the defect in the abdominal musculature.

-pexy = surgical fixation. For example, gastro*pexy* (suturing of the stomach to the abdominal wall to fix it in place) is often performed in cases of gastric torsion.

-plasty = surgical alteration of shape or form. For example, pyloro*plasty* enlarges the pyloric orifice of the stomach to facilitate gastric emptying.

A *ventral midline incision* is located on the ventral midline of the animal. It offers excellent exposure of the entire abdominal cavity. Because the abdominal cavity is entered through the linea alba, where the abdominal muscles on each side are joined, the abdominal wall can be closed with a single layer of sutures in the linea alba. Closure of a ventral midline incision must be very secure, because the weight of the abdominal organs exerts tension on the incision when the animal stands. Also, any exertion by the animal can create tension on the suture line.

A *paramedian incision* is located lateral and parallel to the ventral midline of the animal. It is usually used when exposure of only one side of the abdomen is needed, such as for removal of a cryptorchid (retained) testis. The muscles of the abdominal wall are individually incised, so closure of the abdominal wall usually requires multiple layers of sutures.

A *flank incision* is generally performed on either a standing animal or one in lateral recumbency. It is oriented perpendicular to the long axis of the body, caudal to the last rib. A flank incision provides good exposure of the organ(s) immediately deep to (beneath) the incision but does not allow exploration of much of the remainder of the abdomen. It is, therefore, useful for such procedures as rumenotomy and nephrectomy, in which the organ in question lies directly beneath the incision. The muscles of the abdominal wall usually require a multiple-layer closure. In contrast to tension exerted on a ventral midline incision, the weight of the abdominal organs generally tends to keep a flank incision closed rather than pulling it apart.

A *paracostal incision* is oriented parallel to the last rib and offers good exposure of the stomach and spleen in monogastric animals. The muscles of the abdominal wall are usually closed in multiple layers.

Common Surgical Procedures

Soft-tissue procedures

- *Ovariohysterectomy*, commonly referred to as a spay, involves removal of the ovaries and uterus.
- *Cesarean section* is a method of delivering newborn animals in cases of dystocia (difficult labor). It consists of an abdominal incision (flank or ventral midline) and then an incision into the uterus through which the newborn(s) is (are) delivered.
- *Orchiectomy* (castration) is the surgical removal of the testes.
- *Lateral ear resection* is often performed in animals with chronic external ear infection. It involves removal of the lateral wall of the vertical portion of the external ear canal to allow improved ventilation and to establish drainage for exudates.
- *Laparotomy* is an incision into the abdominal cavity, often through the flank. *Celiotomy* is another term for laparotomy.
- *Cystotomy* is an incision into the urinary bladder, frequently for removal of urinary calculi (bladder stones).
- *Gastrotomy* is an incision into a simple stomach, whereas a *rumenotomy* is an incision into a rumen.
- *Gastropexy* involves suturing of the stomach to the abdominal wall to fix it in place. This procedure is frequently done in cases of gastric torsion.
- *Splenectomy* is the removal of the spleen.
- *Thoracotomy* is an incision into the thoracic cavity (chest).
- *Herniorrhaphy* is the surgical repair of a hernia by suturing the abnormal opening(s) closed.
- *Enterotomy* is an incision into the intestine, often for removal of a foreign body.
- *Intestinal resection and anastomosis* involves removal of a portion of the intestine (resection) and suturing the cut ends together to restore the continuity of the intestinal tube (anastomosis).
- *Perineal urethrostomy* involves incision into the urethra and suturing of the splayed urethral edges to the skin to create a larger urethral orifice. This procedure is frequently performed on male cats with recurrent urethral obstruction.
- *Mastectomy* involves removal of part or all of one or more mammary glands.

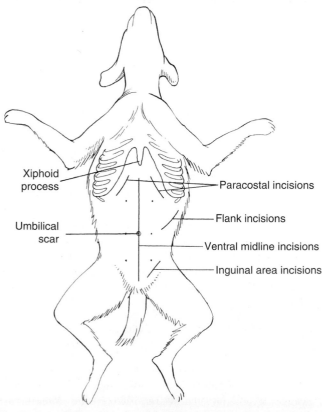

Xiphoid process

Umbilical scar

Paracostal incisions

Flank incisions

Ventral midline incisions

Inguinal area incisions

Fig. 20-1 Surgical incisions for abdominal procedures. *(From Tracy DL:* Small animal surgical nursing, *ed 3, St. Louis, 2000, Mosby.)*

Orthopedic (bone) procedures

- *Onychectomy* is the surgical removal of a claw, commonly called declawing.
- *Intervertebral disk fenestration* is done to remove prolapsed intervertebral disk material causing pressure on the spinal cord.
- *Intramedullary bone pinning* involves insertion of a metal rod (bone pin) into the medullary cavity of a long bone to fix fracture fragments in place.
- *Cranial cruciate ligament repair* is performed when one of the stifle joint ligaments has ruptured. Lack of an intact cranial cruciate ligament creates instability in the stifle, causing abnormal movement. This can damage the joint surfaces of the distal femur and proximal tibia.
- *Femoral head ostectomy* involves amputation of the head of the femur. It is usually performed in animals with severe damage to the femoral head or neck, or with a damaged acetabulum.

PREOPERATIVE AND POSTOPERATIVE CONSIDERATIONS

Preoperative Evaluation

Anesthesia and surgery are very stressful events that put an animal's life at risk. The role of a proper preoperative evaluation is to gather enough pertinent information to minimize that risk. That information can be gathered through a patient history, a physical examination, and appropriate laboratory tests. Chapter 19 contains a more detailed review of preoperative evaluation.

Postoperative Evaluation

The postoperative period should be considered critical for all patients. Because of the possibility of unforeseen complications, it is essential that patients be continually monitored after any type of surgery.

Body temperature

After surgery, every patient should have a rectal temperature measured at least once per day, and preferably two to three times per day. A 1° or 2° increase in rectal temperature for the first few postoperative days is a normal physiologic response to the trauma of major surgery. A higher or more prolonged temperature increase may indicate infection.

Body weight

Daily monitoring of a surgical patient's body weight gives a measure of the animal's nutritional status and general body condition. One of the most frequently neglected aspects of postoperative patient care is provision of adequate nutrition. The healing process after surgery increases an animal's nutritional needs, particularly for protein. Those needs must be met so that healing can proceed without delay.

Attitude

A patient's behavior during the immediate postoperative period can give important information about the amount of pain it is enduring and possible complications that may be developing. If a patient is very depressed, the reasons for that state must be determined and appropriate treatment instituted quickly.

Appetite and thirst

Surgical patients must receive adequate nutrition and fluid intake. Animals should begin eating and drinking as soon as possible after surgery. Lack of interest in food and/or water indicates problems that should be investigated without delay.

Urination and defecation

Elimination patterns give important information about kidney and GI tract function in patients recovering from surgery. Assuming adequate fluid and food intake, urination and defecation should proceed normally.

Appearance of the surgical wound

The surgical incision should be examined at least daily during the immediate postoperative period. It should be evaluated by visual inspection as well as gentle palpation. Such abnormalities as excessive or prolonged bleeding, fluid accumulation, inflammation, and impending *dehiscence* (opening) of the surgical wound can be detected and corrected early if the incision is carefully evaluated.

Postoperative Complications

Hemorrhage

If not quickly corrected, postoperative hemorrhage can lead to serious consequences for an animal, even death from shock. External hemorrhage is usually relatively easy to evaluate and control because it is easily visible. Internal hemorrhage is not readily apparent and, therefore, often more serious. An animal can bleed to death through hemorrhage into the abdominal cavity or thoracic cavity. The status of an animal's cardiovascular system should be frequently monitored during the immediate postoperative period for signs that might indicate hemorrhage. Pulse rate, capillary refill time, temperature of the extremities, and color of the mucous membranes can give valuable information on cardiovascular function.

Seroma and hematoma

Seromas (accumulations of serum) and hematomas (accumulations of blood) beneath the surgical incision are usually caused by "dead space" left in the incision that the body naturally fills with fluid. Small seromas and hematomas are usually of cosmetic importance only, unless the skin sutures tear out. Treatment usually involves drainage of the fluid via needle and syringe and application of a pressure bandage, or resuturing of the incision to eliminate the dead space.

Infection

A persistently or drastically elevated rectal temperature, depressed attitude, poor appetite, or a swollen, inflamed incision are all signs of possible postoperative infection.

Postoperative infections can be superficial, subcutaneous, within a body cavity, or spread throughout the body. Superficial infection often results in a draining wound that does not heal well. Subcutaneous infections frequently progress to abscess formation. Infection in the abdominal cavity (*peritonitis*) or thoracic cavity (*pleuritis*) often results from a penetrating injury or damage to organs in that body cavity. Septicemia is a generalized infection that spreads via the bloodstream. Fortunately, septicemia is not common after surgery.

When the danger of postoperative infection is high, as with long or potentially contaminated procedures, the patient may be given a broad-spectrum antibacterial 24 hours before surgery to achieve an effective blood level. Continue drug use for at least 5 consecutive days after surgery.

Wound dehiscence

Wound dehiscence (disruption of the surgical wound) is one of the most common and serious postoperative complications that can occur. Possible causes of wound dehiscence include the following:

- Suture failure (loosening, untying, breakage)
- Infection
- Tissue weakness (old or debilitated animals, hyperadrenocorticism, prolonged corticosteroid use)
- Mechanical stress (stormy anesthetic recovery, chronic vomiting, chronic cough, excessive activity)
- Poor nutrition

Early signs of surgical wound dehiscence are frequently seen within the first 3 or 4 days after surgery. They may include a serosanguineous discharge from the incision, firm or fluctuant swelling deep to (under) the suture line, and palpation of a hernial ring or loop of bowel beneath the skin.

If only the muscle layer of an abdominal incision breaks down and the skin sutures remain intact, a doughy swelling can be palpated under the skin. This is a serious situation but is not an acute emergency. A bandage should be applied for support, and the suture line should be repaired as soon as possible.

If both the muscle layer and the skin sutures of an abdominal incision break down, the animal can *eviscerate* (abdominal organs protrude through suture line). If evisceration occurs, the involved organs can become bruised and grossly contaminated, and may even be mutilated by the animal itself. This is an acute emergency that must be

attended to immediately. Carefully gather the exteriorized viscera in a towel moistened with physiologic saline and hold them in place near the incision while others are preparing the animal and operating room for the repair.

ASEPTIC TECHNIQUE

Aseptic technique is a term used to describe all of the precautions taken to prevent contamination, and ultimately infection, of a surgical wound. Its purpose is to minimize contamination so that postoperative healing is not delayed.

Contamination and Infection

Contamination of an object or a wound implies the presence of microorganisms within or on it. Contamination of a wound can, but does not necessarily, lead to infection. With infection, microorganisms in the body or a wound multiply and cause harmful effects. Fungal, protozoal, viral, and bacterial organisms can all cause contamination of the surgical area and harmful effects to the patient. Four main factors determine if infection occurs:

- *Number of microorganisms:* There must be sufficient microorganisms to overcome the defenses of the animal
- *Virulence of the microorganisms:* Their ability to cause disease
- *Susceptibility of the animal:* Some individuals have a greater natural resistance to infection than others
- *Route of exposure to the microorganisms:* Some routes of exposure are more likely to result in infection than others

The route of exposure to microorganisms during surgery is determined by the surgical procedure. The factor that can be most significantly influenced is the number of microorganisms that enter the surgical wound, by application of strict aseptic technique before and during surgery. Improper application of methods of sanitation, sterilization, and disinfection can lead to microbial resistance and increase the risk of *nosocomial* (hospital acquired) infection.

Rules of Aseptic Technique

During surgery, aseptic technique protects the exposed tissues of the patient from four main sources of potential contamination: the operative personnel, the surgical instruments and equipment, the patient, and the surgical environment. Proper operating room conduct and adherence to a few general rules will help minimize the possibility of contamination. All personnel must be aware of which items are sterile and which are nonsterile. Sterile items should be grouped together in the operating room and kept separate from nonsterile items. Body movements should be restricted to reduce air currents. Only sterile items should touch patient tissues. When the sterility of an item is in question, always consider it contaminated.

Sterilization and Disinfection

Sterilization refers to the destruction of all microorganisms (bacteria, viruses, spores) on a surface or object. It usually refers to objects that come in contact with sterile tissue or enter the vascular system (e.g., instruments, drapes, catheters, needles). *Disinfection* is the destruction of most pathogenic microorganisms on inanimate (nonliving) objects; *antisepsis* is the destruction of most pathogenic microorganisms on animate (living) objects. Antiseptics are used to kill microorganisms during patient skin preparation and surgical scrubbing; however, the skin cannot be sterilized. Most disinfectants are microbicidal; that is, they kill microbes. Some disinfectants are bacteriostatic; they inhibit the growth of microbes. Common antimicrobial agents are listed in Table 20-1.

Disinfectants can be classified according to their spectrum of activity as:

- Bactericidal (kills bacteria)
- Bacteriostatic (inhibits growth of bacteria)
- Sporicidal (kills bacterial spores)
- Virucidal (kills viruses)
- Fungicidal (kills fungi)

Mode of action

Different physical and chemical methods destroy or inhibit microorganisms in several ways. Some act by damaging microbial cell walls or membranes. Others act by interfering with microbial cell enzyme activity or metabolism or by destroying microbial cell contents by oxidation, hydrolysis, reduction, coagulation, protein denaturation, or the formation of salt. The effectiveness of all microbial control methods depends on the following factors:

- Time: most methods have minimum effective exposure times
- Temperature: most methods are more effective as temperature increases
- Concentration and preparation: chemical methods require appropriate concentrations of agent; disinfectants may be adversely affected by mixing with other chemicals

TABLE 20-1

Common Antimicrobial Chemical Agents

Agents	Major Mode of Action	Applications
Soaps	Disrupt cell membranes and increases permeability	Cleansing, mechanical removal of microorganisms
Detergents	Disrupt cell membranes by combining with lipids and proteins; leak N and P compounds out of cells	Cleansing, bactericidal action
Quarternary ammonium compounds	Cause changes in cell permeability, neutralized phospholipids	
Bisdiguanide compounds (chlorhexidine)	Alter cell-wall permeability, protein precipitation; rapid action broad spectrum	Routine skin preparation
Povidone-iodophor compounds	Damage cell wall, forms reactive ions and protein complexes; rapid action	Routine skin preparation
Phenols		
Phenol, cresols, lysol, hexylresorcinol	Bactericidal; denaturation and precipitation of proteins	Disinfection of laboratory equipment, instruments, bench tops, garbage pails, toilets
Bis-phenols (hexachlorophene)	Bacteriostatic	Deodorants in soaps, inhibition of gram-positive bacteria; require repeated use
Oxidizing agents		
Cl_2 and sodium hypochlorite (bleach)	Bactericidal, oxidation of SH and NH_2 groups	Purification of water, kennel sanitation
Iodine	Bactericidal, oxidation of indole nucleus of enzymes or coenzymes	Skin disinfection, especially as tincture
H_2O_2 (hydrogen peroxide)	Bacteriostatic; mildly bactericidal	Antisepsis of cuts, minor wounds
Heavy metals		
$HgCl_2$ (zinc)	Highly bacteriostatic; precipitation of proteins	Antisepsis of cuts, minor wounds
$AgNO_3$, silver nitrate	Stops minor bleeding	

Modified from Hunter P: *General microbiology: the student's textbook*, St Louis, 1977, Mosby, p 191.

- Organisms: type, number, and stage of growth of target organisms
- Surface: physical and chemical properties of the surface to be treated may interfere with the method's activity; some surfaces are damaged by certain methods
- Organic debris or other soils: if present, will dilute, render ineffective, or interfere with many control methods
- Method of application: items may be sprayed, swabbed, or immersed in disinfectants; cotton and some synthetic materials used to apply or store chemicals may reduce their activity

Methods used for control of microorganisms consist of chemical and physical methods. Physical methods include dry heat, moist heat, radiation, filtration, and ultrasonic vibration. Of these methods, only moist heat, in the form of steam under pressure, is routinely used for sterilization in the veterinary clinic. Chemical control methods include application of soaps, detergents, disinfectants, and gases.

QUALITY CONTROL FOR STERILIZATION AND DISINFECTION

The effectiveness of any method of microbial control must be monitored regularly. Verification of the effectiveness of microbial control should be performed at least monthly. Simply placing an item in a sterilizer and initiating the sterilization process does not ensure sterility. Improper cleaning may cause the failure to achieve sterility (if an item cannot be disassembled and all surfaces cleaned, it cannot be sterilized). Mechanical failure of the sterilizing system, improper use of sterilizing equipment, improper wrapping, poor loading technique, and/or failure to understand the underlying concepts of sterilization processes may also cause the failure to achieve sterility.

Sterilization indicators allow monitoring of the effectiveness of sterilization. Indicators undergo either a chemical or biologic change in response to some combination of time and temperature. Some autoclaves contain recording thermometers. These display the temperature of the autoclave chamber. The operator can then verify that the correct temperature has been achieved during the cycle. Some autoclaves are equipped with printed tape of chamber temperatures and pressures. Steam, dry heat, and chemical sterilization chambers may contain temperature sensors that are placed in the part of a test pack that is most inaccessible to steam penetration.

Chemical Indicators

Chemical indicators are generally paper strips or tape impregnated with a material that changes color when a certain temperature is reached (Fig. 20-2). The chemical responds when a certain heat, pressure, or humidity has been attained. Most also indicate that a specific duration of exposure has been achieved, which is critical to the sterilization process. Therefore, it is important to remember that *chemical indicators do not indicate sterility. Their response indicates only that certain conditions for sterility have been met.* Chemical indicators can be used with autoclaves and ethylene oxide systems and must be placed deep inside packs before sterilization. Autoclave tape (Fig. 20-3) is used to secure surgical packs. The tape incorporates an indicator that changes color when sterilization temperatures have been reached. The color change in autoclave tape does not allow for evaluation of duration of exposure to sterilization conditions.

Biological Testing

Since the purpose of the sterilization procedures is to eliminate the hardiest microorganisms, the presence or absence of bacterial spores can help verify proper sterilization conditions. To perform a biological test of sterility conditions, commercially available bacterial spores are exposed to autoclave or ethylene oxide and then cultured. Bacterial spores should be killed by sterilization, so no bacterial colonies should be present after culturing. This is the recommended method for verification of proper autoclave operation in veterinary clinics.

Another test used to verify sterility is the surface sampling technique. The procedure involves swabbing the test surface (i.e., surgical equipment) with a sterile swab. The swab is then transferred to a suitable media plate for growth. This method is recommended for ensuring proper disinfection of surgical suites in veterinary clinics.

Steam Sterilization

Several types of autoclaves are available. Gravity displacement autoclaves involve water that is heated in a chamber. The continued application of heat by an electric element creates pressure within the chamber; the pressure raises the boiling point of the water, and thus the ultimate temperature of the steam. These are the most common type of autoclave in veterinary clinics and are known as gravity displacement autoclaves because the steam gradually displaces the air contained within the chamber—the air is forced out through a vent (Fig. 20-4). A prevacuum autoclave is a much larger and more costly machine that is equipped with a boiler to generate steam and a vacuum system. Air is forced out of the loaded chamber by means of the vacuum pump. Steam at 121° C (250° F) or more is introduced into the chamber; the steam immediately fills the chamber to eliminate the vacuum.

Pressurized steam is the most efficient and common method of sterilization used in veterinary clinics. Steam destroys microbes via cellular protein denaturation. To destroy all living microorganisms, the correct relationship among temperature, pressure, and exposure time is critical. If steam is contained in a closed compartment under

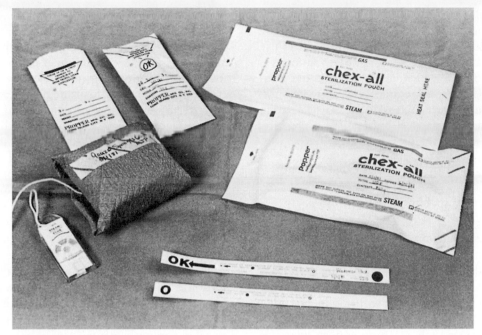

Fig. 20-2 Sterilization indicators. Compare pairs of envelopes, bags, and strips to note color changes that occur during steam sterilization. *(From Tracy DL: Small animal surgical nursing, ed 3, St. Louis, 2000, Mosby.)*

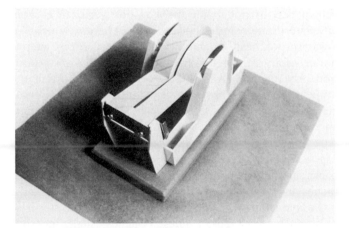

Fig. 20-3 Steam sterilization indicator tape. The roll of tape *(left)* is impregnated with dye that will turn black when exposed to high temperature during sterilization. *(Courtesy Ohio State University.)*

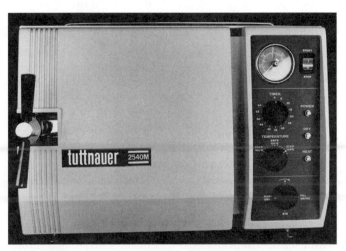

Fig. 20-4 Steam autoclave, countertop model. Chamber will hold one surgical gown pack or one surgical instrument pack each cycle. *(From Tracy DL: Small animal surgical nursing, ed 3, St Louis, 2000, Mosby.)*

increased pressure, the temperature increases as long as the volume of the compartment remains the same. If items are exposed long enough to steam at a specified temperature and pressure, they become sterile. The unit used to create this environment of high-temperature, pressurized steam is called an autoclave.

Autoclaves consistently achieve complete sterility, and are inexpensive and easy to operate. They are safe for most surgical instruments and equipment, drapes and gowns,

suture materials, sponges, and some plastics and rubbers. Achieving complete sterility depends on saturated steam of the appropriate temperature having contact with all objects within the autoclave for a sufficient length of time. Heat is the killing agent in the autoclave, and steam is the vector that supplies the heat and promotes penetration of the heat. Pressure is the means to create adequately heated steam. Complete sterilization of most items is achieved after 9 to 15 minutes of exposure to 121° C (250° F). The temperature of steam at sea level is 100° C (212° F); an increase in pressure results in an increase in the temperature of the steam. The minimum effective pressure of the autoclave is 15 psi, which provides steam at 121° C (250° F). Many autoclaves attain pressures of 35 psi, which creates a steam temperature of 135° C (275° F). Exposure times must allow penetration and exposure of all surfaces to 121° C (250° F) steam. Exposure time can be decreased by increasing pressure, which increases steam temperature.

CARE AND MAINTENANCE OF SURGICAL INSTRUMENTS AND SUPPLIES

Good surgical instruments are a valuable investment and must be used and maintained properly to prevent corrosion, pitting, and/or discoloration. Instruments should be rinsed in cool water as soon after the surgical procedure as possible to avoid drying of blood, tissue, saline, or other foreign matter on them. Many manufacturers recommend that instruments are rinsed, cleaned, and sterilized in distilled or deionized water, because tap water contains minerals that may cause discoloration and staining. If tap water is used for rinsing, instruments should be dried thoroughly to avoid staining. Instruments with multiple components should be disassembled before cleaning. Delicate instruments should be cleaned and sterilized separately. All surgical supplies and equipment that come in to contact with the patient or other surgical equipment, such as Mayo instrument stands, must be cleaned and disinfected before use.

Instrument Cleaning

Ultrasonic and enzymatic methods of cleaning are effective and efficient. Before putting soiled instruments in an ultrasonic cleaner, they should be washed in cleaning solution to remove all visible debris. Dissimilar metals (e.g., chrome and stainless steel) should not be mixed in the same cycle. All instruments should be placed in the ultrasonic cleaner with their ratchets and boxlocks open. Instruments should not be piled on top of each other to avoid damaging delicate instruments. They should be removed from the cleaner, rinsed, and dried at the completion of the cycle.

If an ultrasonic cleaner is not available, instruments should be manually cleaned as thoroughly as possible, paying particular attention to boxlocks, serrations, and hinges. Nylon brushes and cool cleaning solution may be used for most instruments. Rasps and serrated parts of instruments may require a wire brush. A cleaning solution with a neutral pH should be used to avoid staining. Cleaning solutions should be prepared as instructed by the manufacturer and changed frequently. Enzymatic solutions may be used to remove proteinaceous materials from general surgical instruments and endoscopic equipment.

Instrument Lubricating and Autoclaving

Autoclaving is not a substitute for proper instrument cleaning. Before they are autoclaved, instruments with boxlocks and hinges and power equipment should be lubricated with instrument milk or surgical lubricants. Do not use industrial oils to lubricate instruments because they interfere with steam sterilization. All instruments should be allowed to thoroughly air-dry before packing them into a surgical pack. The procedure for wrapping items is based on enhancing the ease of sterilization and preserving sterility of the item, not for convenience or personal preference. Before they are packed, instruments are separated and placed in order of their intended use. If steam or gas sterilization is used, the selected wrap should be penetrable by steam/gas, impermeable to microbes, durable, and flexible.

Specific guidelines should be followed when preparing packs for steam and gas sterilization to allow maximal penetration. Small items may be wrapped, sterilized, and stored in heat-sealable paper/plastic peel pouches. Items to be gas-sterilized are wrapped in heat-sealable plastic peel pouches or tubing or muslin wrap.

Packed instruments can be placed in a tray or wrapped individually. The pack is wrapped using at least two layers of material. A presterilization wrap for steam sterilization consists of two thicknesses of two-layer muslin or nonwoven (paper) barrier materials. The poststerilization wrap (after sterilization and proper cooldown period) consists of a waterproof, heat-sealable plastic dust cover; this wrap is not necessary if the item is used within 24 hours of sterilization. Always take care to wrap packs tightly so that the drape material does not contact the inner wall of the autoclave. The instrument pack is sealed with autoclave tape and labeled with date, contents, and operator. Autoclave tape provides verification that the *outside* of the pack was exposed to appropriate sterilization temperatures. Surgical packs should not exceed 30 by 30 by 50 cm (12 by 12 by 20 inches) in size and 5.5 kg (12 lb) in weight.

Individual instruments can also be placed into sterilization pouches (Fig. 20-5). These pouches usually incorporate a chemical sterilization indicator. Many sterilization pouches are transparent, allowing easy visualization of contents. The pouches are often self-sealing, or you may use autoclave tape to close the pouch. Always mark items with the date that the item was autoclaved.

For steam and gas sterilization, instruments should be organized on a lint-free towel placed on the bottom of a perforated metal instrument tray. A chemical sterilization indicator is included in every pack. This provides verification that the inside of the pack was exposed to appropriate sterilization temperatures for the correct amount of time.

Instruments with boxlocks should be placed in the autoclave closed but not locked. A 3- to 5-mm space between instruments is recommended for proper steam/gas circulation. Complex instruments should be disassembled when

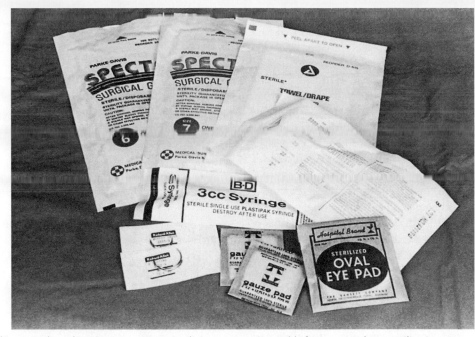

Fig. 20-5 Presterilized items packaged in paper. For average in-clinic use, paper is suitable for steam and gas sterilization. *(From Tracy DL: Small animal surgical nursing, ed 3, St Louis, 2000, Mosby.)*

possible, and power equipment should be lubricated before sterilization. Items with a lumen should have a small amount of water flushed through them immediately before steam sterilization, because water vaporizes and forces air out of the lumen. Conversely, moisture left in tubing placed in a gas sterilizer may decrease the sterilization efficacy below the lethal point. Containers (e.g., saline bowl) should be placed with the open end facing up or horizontally; containers with lids should have the lid slightly ajar. Multiple basins should be stacked with a towel between each. A standard count of radiopaque surgical sponges should be included in each pack. A sterilization indicator is placed in the center of each pack before wrapping. Solutions should be steam-sterilized separately from instruments using the slow-exhaust phase. Linens may be steam-sterilized.

Wrapping Instrument Packs

To properly wrap instrument packs, place a large unfolded wrap diagonally in front of you. Place the instrument tray in the center of the wrap so that an imaginary line drawn from one corner of the wrap to the opposite corner is perpendicular to the two sides of the instrument tray. Fold the corner of the wrap that is closest to you over the instrument tray and to its far edge. Fold the right corner over the pack as illustrated in Fig. 20-6. Then, fold the left corner similarly. Turn the pack around, and fold the final corner of the

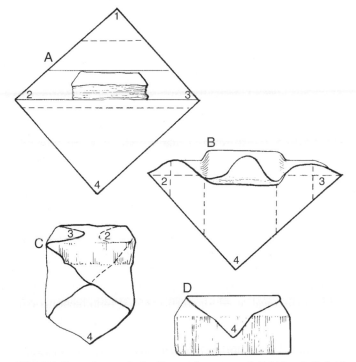

Fig 20-6 General wrap. **A,** Position pack contents. **B,** Fold flap 1. **C,** Fold flaps 2 and 3. **D,** Fold flap 4 as shown, or fold under on the dotted line. Pack is then ready to be sealed and labeled. *(From Tracy DL: Small animal surgical nursing, ed 3, St Louis, 2000, Mosby.)*

wrap over the tray, tucking it tightly under the previous two folds. Fold the tip of the final fold so that it is exposed for easy unwrapping. Wrap the pack in a second layer of cloth or paper in a similar manner. Secure the last corner of the outer wrap with autoclave tape; fold one end of the tape on itself so that it can be easily grasped and removed. Label the tape with the current date, date of expiration (optional), contents, and whether it is to be gas- or steam-sterilized.

Packs may not be completely sterilized if they are wrapped too tightly or improperly loaded in the autoclave or gas sterilizer container. Instrument packs should be positioned vertically (on edge) and longitudinally in an autoclave. Heavy packs should be placed at the periphery, where steam enters the chamber. Allow a small amount of air space between each pack to facilitate steam flow (1 to 2 inches between each pack and surrounding walls). Load linen packs so that the fabric layers are oriented vertically (on edge). Do not stack linen packs on top of one another, because the increased thickness decreases steam penetration. Careful attention to exact standards for preparing, packaging, and loading of supplies is necessary for effective steam and gas sterilization.

Gas Sterilization

Ethylene oxide is a flammable, explosive liquid that becomes an effective sterilizing agent when mixed with carbon dioxide or freon. Equipment that cannot withstand the extreme temperature and pressures of steam sterilization (e.g., endoscopes, cameras, plastics, power cables) can be safely sterilized with ethylene oxide. Environmental and safety hazards associated with ethylene oxide are numerous and severe. It is critical to the safety of the patient and hospital personnel that all materials sterilized with ethylene oxide are aerated in a well-ventilated area for a minimum of 7 days or 12 to 18 hours in an aerator.

Items should be clean and dry before ethylene oxide sterilization; moisture and organic material bond with ethylene oxide and leave a toxic residue. If an item cannot be disassembled and all surfaces cleaned, it cannot be sterilized. Items are packed and loaded loosely to allow gas circulation. Complex items (e.g., power equipment) are disassembled before processing. Items that cannot be sterilized with ethylene oxide include acrylics, some pharmaceutical items, and solutions.

Cold Chemical Sterilization

Liquid chemicals used for sterilization should be noncorrosive to the items being sterilized. These items are usually placed in a special tray kept in the surgery area (Fig. 20-7). Glutaraldehyde solution is noncorrosive and provides a safe means of sterilizing delicate, lensed instruments (endoscopes, cystoscopes, bronchoscopes). Most equipment that can be safely immersed in water can be safely immersed in 3% glutaraldehyde. Table 20-2 lists some commonly used

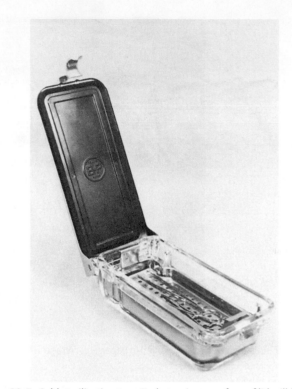

Fig. 20-7   Cold sterilization tray. Gasket on inner surface of lid will form a seal when lid is closed, preventing air-carried microbes from contaminating contents and preventing evaporation of chemical disinfectant solution. *(From Tracy DL:* Small animal surgical nursing, *ed 3, St Louis, 2000, Mosby.)*

cold sterilization agents. Items for sterilization should be clean and dry; the presence of organic matter (e.g., blood, pus, saliva) may prevent penetration of instrument crevices or joints. Residual water causes chemical dilution. Complex instruments should be disassembled before immersion. Immersion times suggested by the manufacturer should be followed (e.g., for sterilization in 3% glutaraldehyde for 10 hours at 20° to 25° C (68° to 77° F); for disinfection for 10 minutes at 20° to 25° C (68° to 77° F)). After the appropriate immersion time, instruments should be rinsed thoroughly with sterile water and dried with sterile towels to avoid damaging the patients' tissues.

Folding and Wrapping Gowns

Surgical gowns should be folded so that they can be easily donned without breaking sterile technique (Fig. 20-8). Place the gown on a clean, flat surface with the front of the gown facing up. Fold the sleeves neatly toward the center of the gown with the cuffs of the sleeves facing the bottom hem. Fold the sides to the center so that the side seams are aligned with the sleeve seams. Then, fold the gown in half longitudinally (sleeves inside the gown) (Fig. 20-8, *B*). Ties should be placed so that they can be touched without contaminating the gown. Starting with the bottom hem of the gown, fanfold it toward the neck. Fanfolding allows compact storage and simple unfolding. Fold a hand towel in half

TABLE 20-2

Antimicrobial Activity of Commonly Used Cold "Sterilants"

Agent	Bacteria	Tubercle bacilli	Spores	Fungi	Viruses
		Destructive Action Against			
Alcohol-ethyl (70% to 90%)	+	+	0	+	+
Alcohol-Isopropyl (70% to 90%)	++	+	0	+	±
Alcohol-iodine (2%)	++	+	±	+	+
Formalin (37%)	+	+	+	+	+
Glutaraldehyde (buffered, 2%) (Cidex)	++	+	++	+	+
Iodine (2% to 5% aqueous)	++	+	±	+	+
Iodophors (1%) (povidone-iodine complex)	+	+	±	±	+
Mercurials (Merthiolate)	±	0	0	+	±
Phenolic derivatives (0.5% to 3%)	+	+	0	+	±
Quats (benzalkonium chloride, 1:750 to 1:1000)	++	0	0	+	0

++, Very good; +, good; ±, fair (greater concentration or more time needed); 0, no activity.

horizontally and fanfold it into about four folds. Place it on top of the folded gown, leaving one corner turned back to allow it to be easily grasped. Wrap the gown and towel in two layers of paper or cloth wrap as previously described.

Folding and Wrapping Drapes

Drapes should be folded so that the fenestration can be properly positioned over the surgical site without contaminating the drape (Fig. 20-9). Lay the drape out flat with the ends of the fenestration perpendicular and the sides of the fenestration parallel to you. Grasp the end of the drape closest to you and fanfold one half of the drape toward the center. Be sure the edge of the drape is on top to allow it to be easily grasped during unfolding. Then, turn the drape around and fanfold the other half toward the center, similarly). Next, fanfold one end of the drape to the center; repeat with the other end. Note that when the drape is properly folded, the fenestration is on the ventral outermost aspect of the drape. Fold the drape in half and wrap it in two layers of paper or cloth wrap as described above.

Storing Sterilized Items

Packs are allowed to cool and dry individually on racks when removed from the autoclave; placing instrument packs on top of each other during cooling may promote condensation of moisture, resulting in contamination via strike-through (wick action). After sterile packs are completely dry, they should be stored in waterproof dust covers in closed cabinets (rather than uncovered on open shelves) to protect them from moisture or exposure to particulate matter, such as dust-borne bacteria. Sterile packs are labeled with the date on which the item was sterilized and a control lot number to trace a nonsterile item. Heat-sealed waterproof dust covers are placed on items not routinely used. The shelf life of a sterilized pack varies with the type of outer wrap (Table 20-3).

PREPARATION OF THE OPERATIVE SITE

Surgery puts a patient at risk for nosocomial (hospital-acquired) infections. Because most surgical infections develop from bacteria that enter the incision during surgery, proper preparation of the surgical site is crucial to reduce the likelihood of infection. Resident skin flora (particularly *Staphylococcus aureus* and *Streptococcus* spp.) are the most common source of surgical wound contaminants. Although it is impossible to sterilize skin without impairing its natural protective function and interfering with wound healing, proper preoperative preparation reduces the likelihood of infection.

Before preparing the patient for surgery, verify the patient's identity, surgical procedure being performed, and surgical site. It is useful to bathe the animal the day before the surgical procedure to remove loose hair, debris, and external parasites. Preparing patients for surgery includes clipping hair and scrubbing the skin at the surgical site. These procedures should be performed outside of the surgical suite. Always clip hair in the direction of the hair growth and keep the clipper blade parallel to the skin. This will minimize the likelihood of irritation to the patient's skin (commonly referred to as "clipper burn"). Once hair is removed, a small

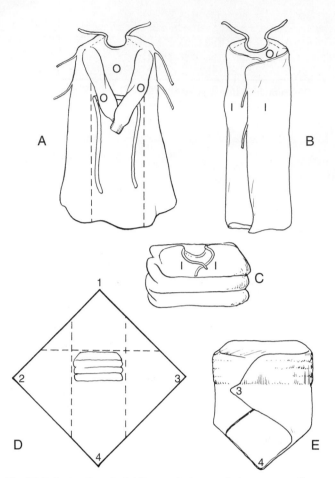

Fig. 20-8 Instructions for folding surgical gown. **A,** Lay gown on flat surface. Avoid large wrinkles because they may affect donning gown. **B,** Fold gown lengthwise. **C,** Make an accordion pleat. **D,** Position gown in the center of wrap. **E,** Wrap by folding flaps in sequence: *O,* outer (sterile) surface of gown when worn; *I,* inner (nonsterile) surface of gown when worn. *(From Tracy DL:* Small animal surgical nursing, *ed 3, St Louis, 2000, Mosby.)*

handheld vacuum can be utilized to remove the clipped hair from the area.

The extent and location of hair removal is based on the type of surgical procedure to be performed (Fig. 20-10). Hair should be liberally clipped around the proposed incision site so that the incision can be extended within a sterile field. A general guideline is to clip 20 cm on each side of the incision. The hair can be removed most effectively with an Oster-type clipper and a #40 clipper blade. Patients with a dense haircoat may be clipped first with a coarse blade (#10). The higher the blade number is, the shorter the remaining hair. Clippers should be held using a "pencil grip," and initial clipping should be done with the grain of the hair-growth pattern. Subsequent clipping should be against the pattern of hair growth to obtain a closer clip. Depilatory creams are less traumatic than other hair-removal methods, but they induce a mild dermal lymphocytic reaction. They are most useful in irregular areas where adequate hair clipping is difficult. Razors are occasionally used for hair removal (e.g., around the eye), but they cause microlacerations in skin that may increase irritation and promote infection. After hair has been clipped from the site, loose hair is removed with a vacuum. To enhance manipulation of limbs during surgery, a "hanging-leg" preparation may be done. This requires that the limb be circumferentially clipped; the limb is hung from an intravenous pole during preparation to allow the sides of the limb to be scrubbed (Fig. 20-11).

Before transporting the animal to the surgical site, the incision is given a general cleansing scrub and ophthalmic antibiotic ointment or lubricant is placed on the cornea and conjunctiva. In male dogs undergoing abdominal procedures, the prepuce should be flushed with an antiseptic solution. The skin is scrubbed with germicidal soap to

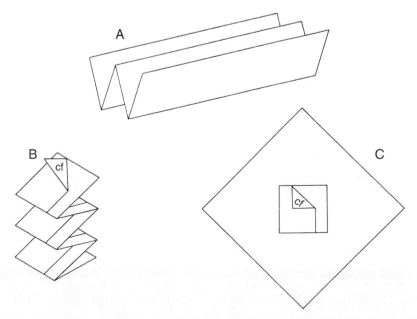

Fig. 20-9 Accordion pleat technique for folding soft goods before wrapping for sterilization. **A,** Fold item lengthwise as shown. **B,** Fold item as shown. **C,** Position item to wrap as shown. Corner fold *(cf)* will facilitate lifting drape when pack is opened and minimize chances of contamination. *(From Tracy DL:* Small animal surgical nursing, *ed 3, St Louis, 2000, Mosby.)*

Recommended Storage Times for Sterilized Packs*

Wrapper	Shelf life
Double-wrapped, two-layer muslin	4 weeks
Double-wrapped, two-layer muslin, heat-sealed in dust covers after sterilization	6 months
Double-wrapped, two-layer muslin, tape-sealed in dust covers after sterilization	2 months
Double-wrapped nonwoven barrier materials (paper)	6 months
Paper/plastic-peel pouches, heat-sealed	1 year
Plastic peel pouches, heat-sealed	1 year

*Note that sterilized items from hospitals adopting event-related sterility assurance have an indefinite shelf life.

remove debris and reduce bacterial populations in preparation for surgery. The area is lathered well until all dirt and oils are removed. This is a generous scrub that often encompasses the hair surrounding the operation site to remove unattached hair and dander that may be disturbed during draping.

Commonly used scrubbing solutions include iodophors, chlorhexidine, alcohols, hexachlorophene, and quaternary ammonium salts. Alcohol is not effective against spores, but it rapidly kills bacteria and acts as a defatting agent. Using alcohol alone is not recommended, but it is commonly used in conjunction with povidone-iodine. Hexachlorophene and quaternary ammonium salts are less effective than other available agents.

Positioning

Before sterile application of the epidermal germicide, the animal is moved to the operating room and positioned so that the operative site is accessible to the surgeon and secured with ropes, sandbags, troughs, or tape. The animal is generally placed on a water-circulating heating pad (Fig. 20-12); if electrocautery is being used, a ground plate should be positioned under the patient.

Sterile Skin Preparation

Sterile preparation of the surgical site begins after transporting and positioning the animal on the operating table. Scrubbing the skin for surgery is a multistep process. Once the hair is clipped, the patient's skin should be washed with mild soap and water to remove gross dirt. A surgical scrub can then be performed. An appropriate antiseptic solution

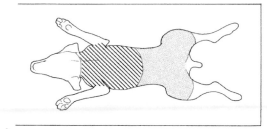

A

☒ Thoracic procedures
☐ Abdominal procedures

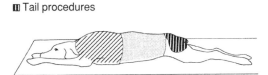

B

☒ Thoracic or cervical spine procedures
☐ Postmesenteric or lumbar spine procedures
▥ Tail procedures

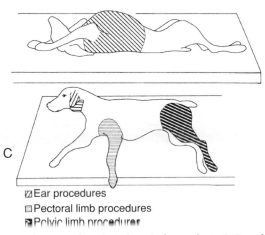

C

☒ Ear procedures
☐ Pectoral limb procedures
▥ Pelvic limb procedures

Fig. 20-10 Hair-removal patterns for selected surgical procedures. **A,** Dorsal recumbency. **B,** Sternal recumbency. **C,** Lateral recumbency. *(From Tracy DL: Small animal surgical nursing, ed 3, St Louis, 2000, Mosby.)*

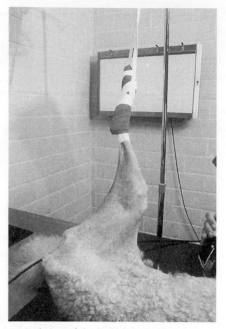

Fig. 20-11 Manipulation of the limb during orthopedic procedures may be facilitated with a "hanging-leg" preparation. The limb is clipped circumferentially and carefully suspended from an intravenous pole with tape. *(From Fossum TW: Small animal surgery, ed 2, St Louis, 2002, Mosby.)*

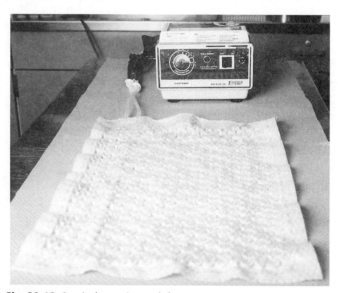

Fig. 20-12 Surgical warming pad that uses water at a preset temperature. *(Courtesy Angell Memorial Hospital.)*

should be applied using sterile gauze. Gauze sponges for use in the surgical site preparation are sterilized in a pack, along with bowls into which the germicides can be poured. Sponges are handled with sterile sponge forceps or the gloved hand, using aseptic technique. The dominant hand should be used to perform the sterile preparation, while the less dominant hand is used to retrieve sponges from the prep bowl. Transferring the sterile sponges to the dominant hand before scrubbing the site helps ensure that the hand picking up the sponges remains sterile during the procedure. The scrub should begin at the intended incision and continue out in concentric circles to an area at least two inches larger than the expected size of the sterile field needed (Fig. 20-13). The scrub should be completed three times and may incorporate a rinse with alcohol or sterile water between each scrub. Sponges are discarded after reaching the periphery. This will minimize the possible transfer of bacteria to the incision site. Frequently, when using povidone-iodine and alcohol, the site is scrubbed alternatively with each solution three times to allow for 5 minutes of contact time. However, using alcohol between the povidone-iodine scrubs decreases contact time of povidone-iodine with skin and may decrease its efficacy. Excess solution on the table or accumulated in body "pockets" should be blotted with a sterile towel or sponges. When the final povidone-iodine scrub is completed, a 10% povidone-iodine solution should be sprayed or painted on the site. If chlorhexidine is the preparation solution, it remains in contact with the skin at the end of the preparation procedure or may be rinsed with saline. Because chlorhexidine binds to keratin, contact time is less critical than with povidone-iodine. Two 30-second applications are considered adequate for antimicrobial activity. The patient can be moved into the surgical suite by covering the scrubbed site with sterile gauze.

PREPARATION OF THE SURGICAL TEAM

Surgical Attire

All persons entering the operating room suite, regardless of whether a surgery is in progress or not, should be appropriately clothed. To minimize microbial contamination from operating room personnel, wear scrub clothes rather than street clothes in the operating suite. With two-piece pantsuits, tuck loose-fitting tops into the trousers. Tunic

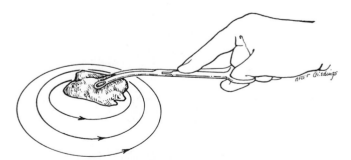

Fig. 20-13 Direction for applying preparations used in skin scrub of patient. Sponge is directed in a circular motion beginning over site of incision and radiating outward.

tops that fit close to the body may be worn outside the trousers. The sleeves of the top should be short enough to allow the hands and arms to be scrubbed. Pants should have an elastic waist or drawstring closure. Nonscrubbed personnel should wear long-sleeved jackets over their scrub clothes. Jackets should be buttoned or snapped closed during use to minimize the risk of the edges inadvertently contaminating sterile surfaces. Scrub clothes should be laundered between wearings and changed if they are visibly soiled or wet to prevent transfer of microorganisms to the environment. Wearing scrub clothes outside the surgical environment increases microbial contamination. If a scrub suit must be worn outside the surgery room, a laboratory coat or single-use gown should be used to cover it.

Other surgical attire includes hair coverings, masks, shoe covers, gowns, and gloves. Hair is a significant carrier of bacteria; when left uncovered, it collects bacteria. Because bacterial shedding from hair increases surgical wound infection rates, complete hair coverage is necessary. Even when surgery is not in progress, caps and masks should be worn in the surgical suite. Caps should completely cover all scalp and facial hair, and masks should cover the mouth and nostrils (Fig. 20-14). Sideburns and/or beards necessitate a hood for complete coverage. Skullcaps that fail to cover the side hair above the ears and hair at the nape of the neck should not be worn.

Any footwear that is comfortable can be worn in the surgery area. Shoe covers should be donned when first entering the surgical area and should be worn when leaving it to keep shoes clean. New shoe covers are donned when returning to the surgical area. Shoe covers are generally made of reusable or disposable materials that are water-repellent and resist tearing.

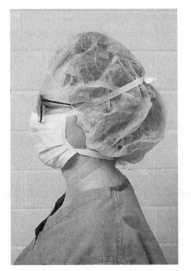

Fig. 20-14 Hair should be covered by a bouffant-style surgical cap. This is the correct way to tie a surgical mask. (*From Fossum TW:* Small animal surgery, *ed 2, St Louis, 2002, Mosby.*)

Masks, constructed from lint-free material containing a hydrophilic filter web sandwiched between two outer layers, should be worn whenever entering a sterile area. Their major function is to filter and contain droplets of microorganisms expelled from the mouth and nasopharynx during talking, sneezing, and coughing. Masks must be fitted over the mouth and nose and secured in a manner that prevents venting. The dorsal aspect of the mask is secured by shaping the reinforcing top edge tightly around the nose.

Surgical gowns may be reusable and made of woven materials (usually cotton), or disposable. Disposable (single-use) gowns are nonwoven and made directly from fibers rather than yarn. Loosely woven cotton is commonly used for reusable gowns. This fabric is instantly permeable to bacteria when it becomes wet. Fewer microorganisms contaminate the surgical environment when disposable (single-use) nonwoven materials are used.

The Surgical Scrub

Surgical scrubbing cleans the hands and forearms to reduce the numbers of bacteria that come in contact with the wound from scrubbed personnel during surgery. All sterile surgical team members must perform a hand and arm scrub before entering the surgical suite. Objectives of a surgical scrub include mechanical removal of dirt and oil, reduction of the transient bacterial population (bacteria deposited from the environment), and reduction of the skin's resident bacterial population. Relying on latex gloves alone (without a surgical scrub) to prevent microbial contamination is not recommended; up to 50% of surgical gloves contain holes at the completion of surgery. This proportion may increase with long or difficult surgeries.

Antimicrobial soaps or detergents used for scrubbing should be rapid-acting, broad-spectrum, and nonirritating, and they should inhibit rapid rebound microbial growth. They should not depend on accumulation for activity. The most commonly used surgical scrub solutions are chlorhexidine gluconate, povidone-iodine, and hexachlorophene.

Surgical scrubs physically separate microbes from skin and inactivate them via contact with the antimicrobial solution. Two accepted methods of performing a surgical scrub are the *anatomic timed scrub* (5-minute scrub) and the *counted brush stroke method* (strokes per surface area of skin) (Box 20-2). Recommendations vary regarding the number of times one should lather and rinse during the scrub, number of strokes per surface area, and time spent on each surface. A sequential approach will help ensure that all skin surfaces are properly scrubbed (Fig. 20-15). However, both methods ensure sufficient exposure of all skin surfaces to friction and antimicrobial solutions.

If the hands and arms are grossly soiled, lengthen scrub time or increase brush counts. However, avoid skin irritation or abrasion; this causes bacteria residing in deeper

BOX 20-2

Surgical Scrub Procedure

- Locate scrub brushes, antibacterial soap, nail cleaners.
- Remove watches, bracelets, and rings.
- Wet hands and forearms thoroughly.
- Apply 2-3 pumps of antimicrobial soap to hands, and wash hands and forearms.
- Clean nails and beneath nails with a nail cleaner under running water.
- Rinse arms and forearms.
- Apply 2-3 pumps of antimicrobial soap to hand and forearms.
- Apply 2-3 pumps of antimicrobial soap to sterile scrub brush.

Anatomic timed method

- Start timing; scrub each side of each finger, between fingers, and back and front to the hand for 2 minutes.

- Proceed to scrub the arms, keeping the hand higher than the arm.

- Scrub each side of the arm to 3 inches above the elbow for 1 minute.
- Total scrub time is 2 to 3 minutes per hand and arm.

Counted brush stroke method

- Apply 30 strokes (one stroke consists of up and down or back and forth motion) to the very tips of your fingers and thumb.
- Divide each finger and thumb into 4 parts and apply 20 strokes to each of the 4 surfaces, including the finger webs.
- Scrub from the tip of the finger to the wrist when scrubbing the thumb, index, and small fingers.
- Divide your forearm into 4 planes and apply 20 strokes to each surface.

- Rinse the scrub brush well under running water and transfer the brush to your scrubbed hand. Do not rinse the scrubbed hand and arm at this time.
- Repeat the process on your other hand and arm.
- When both hands and arms have been scrubbed, drop the scrub brush in the sink.
- Starting with the fingertips of one hand, rinse under running water by moving your fingertips up and out of the water stream and allowing the rest of your arm to be rinsed off on the way out of the stream.
- Allow the water to run from fingertips to elbows
- Never allow fingertips to fall below the level of your elbow.
- Never shake your hands to shed excess water, allow the water to drip from your elbows.
- Rinse off your other hand similarly.
- Hold your hands upright and in front of you so that they can be seen, and proceed to the gowning and gloving area.

tissues (e.g., around base of hair follicles) to become more superficial, increasing the number of potentially infective organisms on the skin surface. Contact time between the antimicrobial soap or detergent should be based on documentation of product efficacy in the scientific literature. An initial 5- to 7-minute scrub for the first case of the day, followed by a 2- to 3-minute scrub between additional surgical operations, is generally adequate.

Before scrubbing, remove all jewelry (including watches) from your hands and forearms, because they are reservoirs for bacteria. Fingernails should be free of polish and trimmed short, and cuticles should be in good condition. Artificial nails (bondings, tips, wrappings, tapes) should never be worn. More gram-negative bacteria have been cultured from the fingertips of personnel wearing artificial nails than from personnel with natural nails, both before and after handwashing. Fungi residing between an artificial

nail and the natural nail can contaminate the surgical wound. Hands and forearms should be free of open lesions and breaks in skin integrity, because such skin infections may contaminate surgical wounds.

Once the scrub has been started, nonsterile items cannot be handled without breaking sterility. If your hands or arms inadvertently touch a nonsterile object (including surgical personnel), repeat the scrub. During and after scrubbing, keep the hands higher than the elbows. This allows water and soap to flow from the cleanest area (hands) to a less clean area (elbow). A single scrub brush can generally be used for the entire procedure. No difference has been documented in the effectiveness of a sterilized reusable brush and disposable polyurethane brush/sponge combination.

When the scrub has been completed, dry the hands and arms with a sterile towel. When picking up the sterile towel from the table, take care not to drip water on the gown

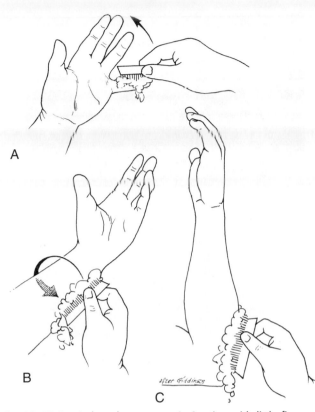

Fig. 20-15 Surgical scrub sequence. **A,** Starting with little finger and working across to thumb, scrub all surfaces of each digit. **B,** Scrub forearm, again scrubbing entire circumference. **C,** Scrub elbow area to 2 inches above elbow, including all surfaces. *(From Tracy DL: Small animal surgical nursing, ed 3, St Louis, 2000, Mosby.)*

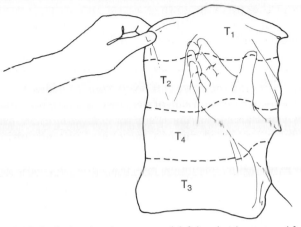

Fig. 20-16 To dry hands using one towel, left hand picks up towel from sterile field and drapes towel over right hand. Use T_1 to dry left hand, T_2 to dry left forearm and elbow. Dried left hand picks up towel at corner of T_4 and dries right hand using T_4, then forearm and elbow using T_3. *(From Tracy DL: Small animal surgical nursing, ed 3, St Louis, 2000, Mosby.)*

beneath it, and then step back from the table. Hold the towel lengthwise and dry one hand and arm, working from hand to elbow with one end of the towel; use a blotting motion (Fig. 20-16). Bend over at the waist when drying the arms so that the end of the towel will not brush against your scrub suit. After one hand and arm are dry, move the dry hand to the opposite end of the towel. Dry the other hand and arm in a similar manner. Drop the towel into the proper receptacle or on the floor if a receptacle is not provided. Do not lower your hands below waist level.

Gowning

Gowns are another barrier between the skin of the surgical team and the patient. They should be constructed of a material that prevents passage of microorganisms between sterile and nonsterile areas. Gowns should be resistant to fluid, lint accumulation, stretching, and tearing (especially at the forearm, elbow, and abdominal areas) and should be comfortable, economical, and fire-resistant. Reusable or single-use disposable gowns are available.

Gowning and gloving should occur away from the surgical table and the patient to avoid dripping water onto the sterile field and contaminating it. Gowns are folded so that the inside of the gown faces outward (see Fig. 20-8). Grasp the gown firmly, and gently lift it away from the table. Step back from the sterile table to allow room for gowning. Hold the gown at the shoulders, and allow it to gently unfold. Do not shake the gown, because this increases the risk of contamination. Once the gown is opened, locate the armholes and guide each arm through the sleeves. Keep your hands within the cuffs of the gown. Have another person pull the gown up over your shoulders, and secure it by closing the neck fasteners and tying the inside waist tie. If a sterile-back gown is used, do not secure the front tie until you have donned sterile gloves.

Gloving

Latex rubber gloves are another barrier between the surgical team and the patient; however, they are not a substitute for proper scrubbing methods. If the glove of a properly scrubbed hand is perforated during a surgical procedure, bacteria are rarely cultured from the punctured glove. Lubricating agents for latex gloves, such as magnesium silicate (talcum) or cornstarch, allow gloves to slide more easily onto the hand. Unfortunately, these agents cause considerable irritation to various tissues, even if gloves are vigorously rinsed in sterile saline before surgery. Therefore, the surgeon should use gloves in which the inner surfaces are lubricated with an adherent coating of hydrogel.

Closed Gloving

This method ensures that the hand never comes in contact with the outside of the gown or glove. Working through the gown sleeve (your bare hand must not be allowed to touch the cuff of the gown or outside surface of the glove), pick up one glove from the wrapper. Lay the glove palm down over the cuff of the gown, with the thumb and fingers of the glove facing your elbow (Fig. 20-17, *A*). Working

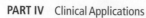

though the cuff of the gown, grasp the cuff of the glove with your index finger and thumb. With your other hand still inside the cuff of the gown, take hold of the opposite side of the edge of the glove between your index finger and thumb. Lift the cuff of the glove up and over the gown cuff and hand, bringing the glove cuff below your knuckles. Release and come to the palm side of the glove and take hold of the gown and glove, pulling them toward your elbow while pushing your hand through the gown cuff and into the glove (Fig. 20-17, *B*). Proceed with the opposite hand, using the same technique. Do not allow the bare hand being gloved to contact the gown cuff edge or sterile glove on the opposite hand.

Open gloving

The open method of gloving is used when only the hands must be covered (e.g., as for urinary catheterization, bone marrow biopsy, sterile patient preparation) or during sur-

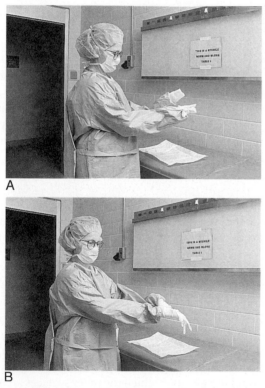

Fig. 20-17 Closed gloving. Working through the gown sleeve, pick up one glove from the wrapper. **A,** Lay the glove palm-down over the cuff of the gown, with the thumb and fingers of the glove facing your elbows. Grasp the cuff of the glove with your index finger and thumb. With the index finger and thumb of the other hand (within the cuff), grasp the opposite side of the edge of the glove. Lift the cuff of the glove up and over the gown cuff and hand. **B,** Release, move to the palm side of the glove, and grasp the gown and glove, pulling them toward the elbow while pushing the hand through the cuff and into the glove. Proceed with the opposite hand using the same technique. *(From Fossum TW:* Small animal surgery, *ed 2, St Louis, 2002, Mosby.)*

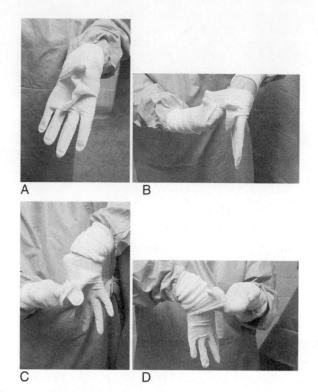

Fig. 20-18 Open gloving when one hand is sterile. Open the glove wrapper and pick up the correct glove at the folded edge with your sterile hand. Gently insert your hand into the glove until your fingers are in the fingers of the glove. **A,** Place your thumb inside the thumb of the glove and hook the cuff of the glove over your thumb. Release the glove. **B,** Place the fingers of your sterile hand under the cuff at the palm of the glove, and **C,** bend the wrist of the hand being gloved 90°. **D,** Gently walk your fingers to the front of the cuff while pulling the cuff up and over your gown. *(From Fossum TW:* Small animal surgery, *ed 2, St Louis, 2002, Mosby.)*

gery when one glove becomes contaminated and must be changed. It should not be used routinely for gowning and gloving. If one hand is contaminated during surgery, have the glove removed as described below. Open the glove wrapper and pick up the correct glove at the folded edge with your sterile hand. Gently insert your hand into the glove until your fingers are in the fingers of the glove. Do not allow the glove to roll up over the back of your hand. Place your thumb inside the thumb of the glove and hook the cuff of the glove over your thumb (Fig. 20-18, *A*). Release the glove. Place the fingers of your sterile hand under the cuff at the palm of the glove (Fig. 20-18, *B*), and bend the wrist of the hand being gloved 90°, pointing the fingers down (Fig. 20-18, *C*). Gently walk your fingers around to the front of the cuff (Fig. 20-18, *C*) while pulling the cuff up and over your gown (Fig. 20-18, *D*).

If both gloves are being donned, pick up one glove by its inner cuff with the opposite hand (Fig. 20-19, *A*). Do not touch the glove wrapper with your bare hand. Slide the glove onto the opposite hand; leave the cuff down. Using

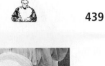

the partially gloved hand, slide your fingers into the outer side of the opposite glove cuff (Fig. 20-19, *B*). Slide your hand into the glove and unfold the cuff; do not touch the bare arm as the cuff is unfolded. With your gloved hand, slide the fingers under the outside edge of the opposite cuff and unfold it.

Assisted Gloving

When gloving another person, the person assisting with the gloving should have on a sterile gown and/or gloves. The assistant's hands should not touch the nonsterile surface of the person being gloved. If both gloves are being replaced, have the assistant pick up one glove and place his or her fingers and thumb under the cuff of the glove (Fig. 20-20, *A*). With the thumb of the glove facing you, have the assistant hold the glove open for you to slip your hand into (Fig. 20-20, *B*). The assistant then brings the cuff of the glove up and over the cuff of your gown and gently lets it go. The assistant picks up the other glove. Assist him or her by holding the cuff of the glove open with the fingers of your sterile hand, while putting your ungloved hand into the open glove (Fig. 20-20, *C*). The assistant keeps his or her thumbs under the cuff while you thrust your hand into it. Ensure

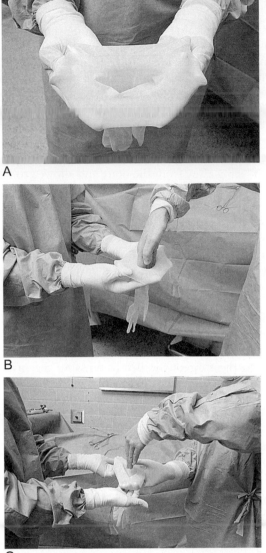

Fig. 20-20 Assisted gloving. **A,** Have an assistant pick up one glove and place his or her fingers and thumb under the cuff of the glove. **B,** With the thumb of the glove facing you, slip your hand into the glove. Have the assistant bring the cuff of the glove up and over the cuff of your gown, and gently let it go. Have the assistant pick up the other glove. **C,** Assist him or her by holding the cuff of the glove open with the fingers of your sterile hand, while inserting your ungloved hand into the open glove. The assistant keeps his or her thumbs under the cuff while you thrust your hand into it. *(From Fossum TW: Small animal surgery, ed 2, St Louis, 2002, Mosby.)*

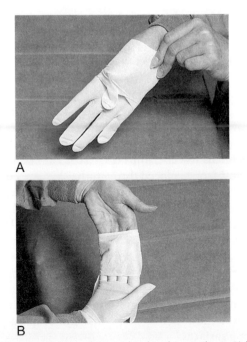

Fig. 20-19 Open gloving when neither hand is sterile. **A,** Pick up one glove by its inner cuff with the opposite hand. Slide the glove onto the opposite hand; leave the cuff down. **B,** Using the partially gloved hand, slide your fingers into the outer side of the opposite glove cuff. Slide your hand into the glove and unfold the cuff; do not touch your bare arm as the cuff is unfolded. With the gloved hand, slide your fingers under the outside edge of the opposite cuff and unfold it. *(From Fossum TW: Small animal surgery, ed 2, St Louis, 2002, Mosby.)*

that the glove cuff is above your gown cuff before the assistant gently releases it (he or she should not let the cuff snap sharply). If only one glove is being replaced, the assistant picks up the glove with the palm facing away from you. Assist the gloving process as described above for the second hand by placing your sterile hand under the cuff.

SURGICAL ASSISTING

The sterile surgical assistant must don a sterile gown and gloves before entering the surgical suite. Closed or open gloving can be used. Care must be taken not to contaminate the gown by brushing against tables or other individuals when entering the surgical suite.

A circulating assistant (nonsterile) should be available to place needed supplies and equipment onto the Mayo stand. All personnel should have cap and mask on before placing sterile items onto the Mayo stand. Materials should be opened facing away from the body and allowed to fall onto the stand so that the assistant's arms are not directly over the top of the Mayo stand. The surgical assistant should arrange the instruments and supplies on the Mayo stand before the start of surgery. The assistant may also be responsible for operating the surgical suction and passing and holding instruments for the surgeon. A circulating (nonsterile) assistant should be present to provide any additional items that may be needed by the surgeon.

The technician must be familiar with the procedure to be performed and be able to anticipate the instruments and supplies that the surgeon may need. Instruments should be passed to the surgeon by firmly pressing the instrument into the surgeon's hand. Instruments are usually passed so that they will be placed in the surgeon's hand in a ready-to-use position. Curved instruments are passed with their concave side up.

The veterinary technician is also responsible for assuring that the surgical lighting is focused on the surgical site and that the site remains dry. Blotting the site gently with gauze sponges or removing excess blood and tissue fluid can be used to accomplish this task. When a body cavity is opened, sponges should be counted at the beginning of the procedure (before the first incision) and before closure to ensure that none have been inadvertently left in the body cavity. Contaminated instruments or soiled sponges should not be placed back on the instrument table. Surgical assistants may also be required to hold clamps on tissues or vessels. Always handle tissues gently and keep tissues moistened with sterile saline when they are removed from body cavities.

Draping and Organizing the Instrument Table

Instrument tables should be height-adjustable to allow them to be positioned within reach of surgical personnel. The instrument table should not be opened until the animal has been positioned on the surgical table and draped. Large, water-impermeable table drapes should be used to cover the entire instrument table. To open these drapes, the drape and outer wrap are positioned on the instrument table, the exposed undersurface of the drape is gently grasped, and the ends and then the sides are unfolded. Once the drape has been opened, nonsterile personnel should not reach over it. *Mayo stands* are often used in procedures that require additional instruments (e.g., bone plating); specially designed Mayo stand covers are available to cover these tables. When the instrument pack has been opened, instruments should be positioned so that they can be readily retrieved. The instrument layout is generally determined by the surgeon's preference, but grouping similar instruments (e.g., scissors, retractors) facilitates their use.

Draping

Once the animal has been positioned and the skin prepared, the animal is ready to be draped. The drapes maintain a sterile field around the operative site. If electrocautery is being used, sufficient time should elapse between skin preparation and application of drapes to permit complete evaporation of flammable substances (e.g., alcohol) from the skin. If an abdominal incision extends to the pubis in males, the prepuce should be clamped to one side with a sterile towel clamp.

Draping is performed by a gowned and gloved surgical team member and begins with placement of field drapes (quarter drapes) to isolate the unprepared portion of the animal. These towels should be placed one at a time at the periphery of the prepared area. Field (quarter) drapes may be lint-free towels or disposable, nonabsorbent towels. Drapes should not be flipped, fanned, or shaken, because rapid movement of drapes creates air currents on which dust, lint, and droplet nuclei can migrate. Drapes, supplies, and equipment extending over or dropping below table level should be considered nonsterile because they are not within the surgeon's visual field and their sterility cannot be verified.

Once the towels are placed, they should not be readjusted toward the incision site, because this carries bacteria onto the prepared skin. Towels are secured at the corners with Bachhaus towel clamps (Fig. 20-21). The tips of the towel clamps, once placed through the skin, are considered nonsterile and should be handled appropriately. Generally, field towels do not cover the edges of the table; do not brush a sterile gown against this nonsterile field. When the animal and incision site are protected by field drapes, final draping can be performed (Figs. 20-22 and 20-23). A large drape is placed over the animal and entire surgical table to provide a continuous sterile field. Cloth drapes should have an appropriately sized and positioned opening that can be placed over the incision site, while the drape covers the remaining surfaces.

To drape a limb, place field drapes and secure them as described above to isolate the surgical site or the proximal aspect of the limb, if the leg is hung (Fig. 20-24). A nonsterile member of the surgical team holds the unprepared area of the limb, and the tape holding the elevated limb is cut. The limb is presented to the sterile surgical member so that it may be taken with a hand in a sterile stockinette or towel.

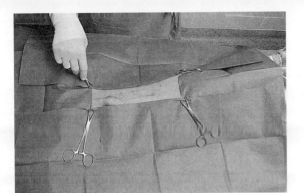

Fig. 20-21 Secure field drapes at the corners with sterile Bachhaus towel clamps. The tips of the towel clamps, once placed through the skin, are considered nonsterile and should be handled appropriately. *(From Fossum TW: Small animal surgery, ed 2, St Louis, 2002, Mosby.)*

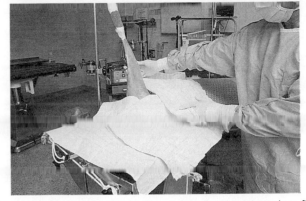

Fig. 20-24 When performing a "hanging-leg" preparation, place field drapes around the limb as illustrated and secure them with towel clamps. *(From Fossum TW: Small animal surgery, ed 2, St Louis, 2002, Mosby.)*

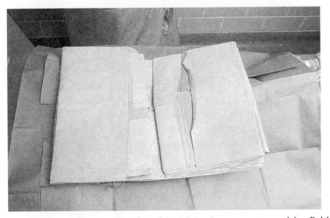

Fig. 20-22 When the animal and incision site are protected by field drapes, final draping can be performed. Place the large drape with the center (or fenestration) over the surgical site and unfold it. To avoid contaminating the drape, do not hold it in the air while unfolding it. *(From Fossum TW: Small animal surgery, ed 2, St Louis, 2002, Mosby.)*

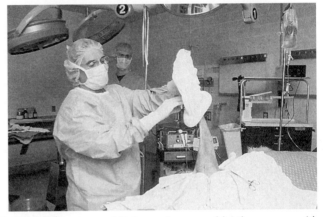

Fig. 20-25 The prepared limb may be grasped by the surgeon with a hand covered by a sterile stockinette. The stockinette is carefully unrolled down the limb and secured with towel clamps. *(From Fossum TW: Small animal surgery, ed 2, St Louis, 2002, Mosby.)*

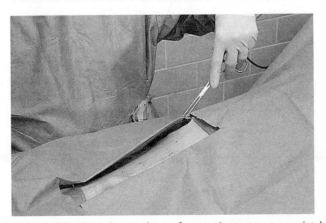

Fig. 20-23 If the drape does not have a fenestration, cut an appropriately sized hole. The edges of the drape can be secured to the field drapes with Allis tissue forceps (not towel clamps). Do not cut holes through the outer drape. *(From Fossum TW: Small animal surgery, ed 2, St Louis, 2002, Mosby.)*

The limb should not be turned loose until it is securely held by the sterile surgical team member. If a stockinette is used, it should be carefully unrolled down the limb and secured with towel clamps (Fig. 20-25). If a sterile towel is used, the limb should be carefully wrapped with the towel before securing it to skin with a towel clamp. Water-impermeable (disposable) towels (plus the towel clamp) should then be covered with sterile Kling. If a cloth towel is used, it (and the towel clamp) should be covered with sterile Vetrap. The limb is now ready to be placed through a fenestration of a lap or fanfold drape, and the drape secured (Fig. 20-26). The end of the stockinette is wrapped with sterile Vetrap.

Unwrapping or Opening Sterile Items

Unwrapping sterile linen or paper packs

If you are right-handed, hold the pack in your left hand (and vice versa). Using the right hand, unfold one corner of

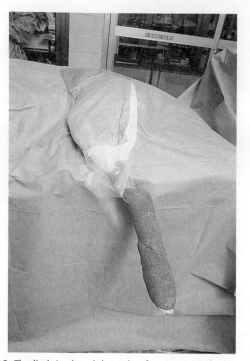

Fig. 20-26 The limb is placed through a fenestration of a lap or fanfold drape, and the drape is secured. A plastic adhesive drape has been applied to the skin and surrounding drapes. *(From Fossum TW:* Small animal surgery, *ed 2, St Louis, 2002, Mosby.)*

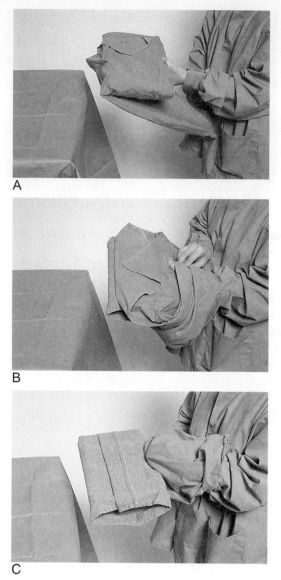

Fig. 20-27 To unwrap a sterile linen or paper pack that can be held during distribution, hold the pack in your right hand if you are left-handed (and vice versa). **A,** Using your right hand, unfold one corner of the wrap at a time. **B,** Secure each corner in the palm of your left hand to keep the corners from recoiling and contaminating the contents. **C,** Hold the final corner with your right hand; your hand should be completely covered by the wrap. When the pack is fully exposed and all corners of the wrap are secured, gently drop it onto the sterile field, being careful not to allow your hand and arm to reach across or over the sterile field. *(From Fossum TW:* Small animal surgery, *ed 2, St Louis, 2002, Mosby.)*

the outside wrap at a time (Fig. 20-27, *A*), being careful to secure each corner in the palm of the left hand to keep them from recoiling and contaminating the contents (Fig. 20-27, *B*). Hold the final corner with your right hand. When the pack is fully exposed and all corners of the wrap secured (Fig. 20-27, *C*), gently drop the pack onto the sterile field, being careful to not allow your hand and arm to reach across or over the sterile field. Or, have a sterile team member grasp the item and place it on the instrument table.

Unwrapping Sterile Items in Paper or Plastic or Plastic Peel-Back Pouches

Identify the edges of the peel-back wrapper, and carefully separate them. Peel the edges of the wrapper back slowly and symmetrically to ensure the sterile item does not contact the torn edge of the wrapper, which is nonsterile (Fig. 20-28, *A*). If the item is small, place it on the sterile area as previously described, being careful not to lean across the sterile table (Fig. 20-28, *B*). If the item is long or cumbersome, have a sterile team member grasp it and gently pull it from the peel-back wrapper, taking care not to brush the item against the peeled edge of the wrapper. Packages containing scalpel blades and suture material are opened similarly.

SURGICAL INSTRUMENTS

Scalpels and Blades

Scalpels are the primary cutting instrument used to incise tissue (Fig. 20-29). Reusable scalpel handles (Nos. 3 and 4) with detachable blades are most commonly used in veteri-

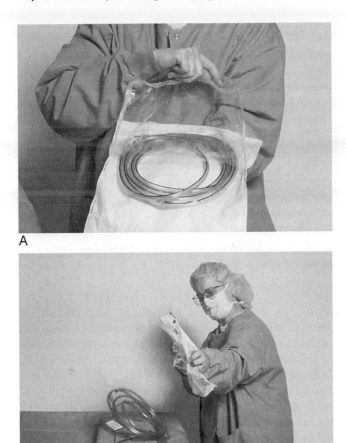

A

B

Fig. 20-28 A, To unwrap a sterile item in a plastic peel-back pouch, identify the edges of the peel-back wrapper and carefully separate them. Peel the edges of the wrapper back slowly and symmetrically to ensure the sterile item does not contact the torn edge of the wrapper, which is nonsterile. **B,** Do not lean over the table when placing the item on the sterile table. *(From Fossum TW: Small animal surgery, ed 2, St Louis, 2002, Mosby.)*

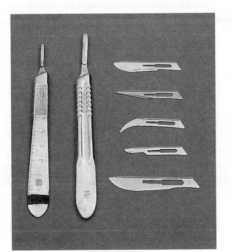

Fig. 20-29 Scalpel handles (No. 3, *left*; No. 4, *right*) and blades *(top to bottom):* No. 10, 11, 12, 15, and 20. *(From Fossum TW: Small animal surgery, ed 2, St Louis, 2002, Mosby.)*

nary medicine, disposable handles and blades are also available. Blades are available in various sizes and shapes, depending on the task for which they are used. Scalpels are usually used in a "slide cutting" fashion, with pressure applied to the knife blade at a right angle to the direction of scalpel pressure.

Laser scalpel

Laser is an acronym for Light Amplification by the Stimulated Emission of Radiation. Laser technology has been used to treat patients for nearly two decades safely and effectively. The most commonly used surgical laser is a carbon dioxide laser that produces an invisible beam of light that vaporizes the water normally found in the skin and other soft tissue. Lasers have the unique ability to both coagulate and cut tissue. The technician's role in laser surgery may include practice management duties, client communication, and laser safety duties. Although there are a variety of lasers, the most common types used in veterinary practice are carbon dioxide (CO_2) and diode. Diode laser energy is delivered through a quartz fiber instead of being reflected through an articulated arm or waveguide. Quartz fibers are generally more flexible and resilient than waveguides and can be inserted through an endoscope for minimally invasive procedures. Laser-tissue interaction is the other significant difference. The CO_2 laser is completely absorbed by water, which limits the effect to visible tissue. The diode wavelength is minimally absorbed by water and may affect tissue as deep as 10 mm below the surface in the free-beam mode.

Because a laser seals nerve endings and small blood vessels as it cuts, there is less bleeding and pain. Since laser scalpels do not crush, tear, or bruise tissue as traditional scalpels do, swelling is minimized. The laser is ideal for a wide variety of surgical procedures for dogs, cats, birds, reptiles, exotics, horses, and other pets. Laser surgery is commonly used in soft-tissue surgical procedures, such as cat declaws, spays, neuters, amputations, oral/dental procedures, dermatology, and avian and exotic procedures.

Electroscalpel

The electroscalpel functions by passing an electrical current through the unit to the patient's tissues. This causes microcoagulation of tissue proteins as the unit cuts the tissue.

Scissors

Scissors are available in a variety of shapes, sizes, and weights, and are generally classified according to the type of points (blunt-blunt, sharp-sharp, sharp-blunt), blade shape (straight, curved), or cutting edge (plain, serrated) (Fig. 20-30). Curved scissors offer greater maneuverability and visibility, whereas straight scissors provide the greatest mechanical advantage

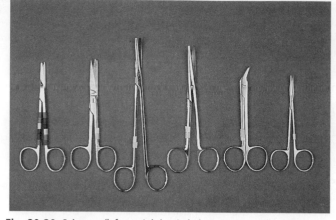

Fig. 20-30 Scissors *(left to right):* stitch (suture removal), sharp/blunt, Metzenbaum, Mayo, wire, tenotomy. *(From Fossum TW: Small animal surgery, ed 2, St Louis, 2002, Mosby.)*

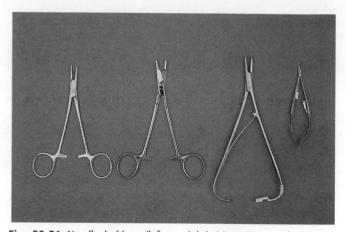

Fig. 20-31 Needle holders *(left to right):* Mayo-Hegar, Olsen-Hegar, Mathieu, Castroviejo. *(From Fossum TW: Small animal surgery, ed 2, St Louis, 2002, Mosby.)*

for cutting tough or thick tissue. *Metzenbaum* or *Mayo scissors* are most commonly used in surgery. Metzenbaum scissors are more delicate and should be reserved for fine, thin tissues. Mayo scissors are used for cutting heavy tissues, such as fascia. Tissue scissors should not be used to cut suture material; suture scissors should be used. *Suture scissors* used in the operating room are different from *suture removal scissors.* The latter have a concavity at the top of one blade that prevents the suture from being lifted excessively during removal. Delicate scissors, such as *tenotomy scissors* or *iris scissors,* are often used in ophthalmic procedures and other surgeries, where fine, precise cuts are necessary. *Bandage scissors* have a blunt tip that, when introduced under the bandage edge, reduces the risk of cutting the underlying skin.

Needle Holders

Needle holders are used to grasp and manipulate curved needles (Fig. 20-31). *Mayo-Hegar* and *Olsen-Hegar needle holders* have a ratchet lock just distal to the thumb. *Castroviejo needle holders* have a spring-and-latch mechanism for locking. *Mathieu needle holders* have a ratchet lock at the proximal end of the handles of the holder, permitting locking and unlocking simply by a progressive squeezing together of the needle holder handles.

Tissue Forceps

Tissue forceps are used to clamp and hold tissue and blood vessels. Thumb forceps are tweezerlike, nonlocking tissue forceps used to grasp tissue (Fig. 20-32). The proximal ends are joined to allow the grasping ends to spring open or to be squeezed together. They are available in a variety of shapes and sizes; tips (grasping ends) may be pointed, flattened, rounded, smooth, or serrated, or have small or large teeth. Tissue forceps with large teeth should not be used to handle tissue that is easily traumatized; smooth tips are recommended with delicate tissue (e.g., blood vessels). The most

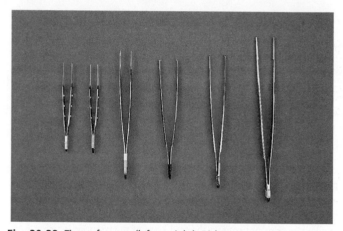

Fig. 20-32 Tissue forceps *(left to right):* Bishop-Harmon (smooth tip), Bishop-Harmon (toothed), Brown-Adson, tissue, serrated, DeBakey. *(From Fossum TW: Small animal surgery, ed 2, St Louis, 2002, Mosby.)*

commonly used tissue forceps, *Brown-Adson,* have small serrations on the tips that cause minimal trauma but hold tissue securely. *Allis* tissue forceps (Fig. 20-33) and *Babcock* forceps (Fig. 20-34) are also for tissue grasping and retraction.

Hemostatic Forceps

Hemostatic forceps, commonly called *hemostats,* are crushing instruments used to clamp blood vessels (Fig. 20-35). They are available with straight or curved tips and vary in size from smaller (3-inch) *mosquito hemostats* with transverse jaw serrations, to larger (9-inch) *angiotribes.* Serrations on the jaws of larger hemostatic forceps may be transverse, longitudinal, or diagonal, or a combination of these. Longitudinal serrations are generally gentler on tissue than cross serrations. Serrations usually extend from the tips of the jaws to the boxlocks, but on *Kelly forceps,* transverse (horizontal) serrations extend over only the distal portion of the jaws. Similarly sized *Crile forceps* have transverse

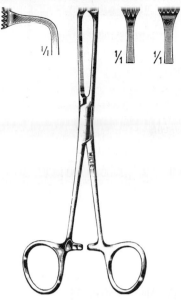

Fig. 20-33   Allis tissue forceps. *(Courtesy Miltex.)*

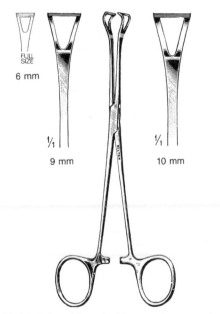

Fig. 20-34   Babcock intestinal forceps. *(Courtesy Miltex.)*

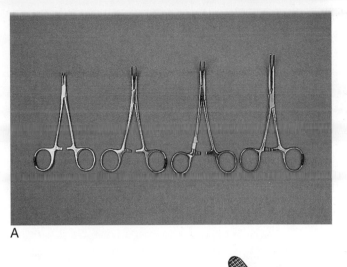

A

B

Fig. 20-35   A, Hemostatic forceps *(left to right):* mosquito hemostats, Kelly, Crile, Carmalt. **B**, Tip detail. *(From Fossum TW:* Small animal surgery, *ed 2, St Louis, 2002, Mosby.)*

serrations that extend the entire jaw length. Kelly and Crile forceps are used on larger vessels. *Rochester-Carmalt forceps* are larger crushing forceps, often used to control large tissue bundles (e.g., during ovariohysterectomy). They have longitudinal grooves with cross grooves at the tip ends to prevent tissue slippage.

Curved hemostats should be placed on tissue with the curve facing up. The smallest hemostatic forceps that will accomplish the job should be used to grasp as little tissue as possible to minimize trauma. To avoid having fingers momentarily trapped within the rings of hemostats, place fingertips on the forceps finger rings or insert fingers into the rings only as far as the first joint.

Retractors

Retractors are used to retract tissue and improve exposure. The ends of handheld retractors may be hooked, curved, spatula-shaped, or toothed. Some handheld retractors may be bent (i.e., malleable) to conform to the structure being retracted or area of the body in which retraction is being performed. *Senn (rake) retractors* are double-ended retractors (Fig. 20-36). One end has three fingerlike, curved prongs; the other end is a flat, curved blade. Self-retaining retractors maintain tension on tissues and are held open with a boxlock (e.g., *Gelpi, Weitlaner*) or other device (e.g., set-screw). Examples of the latter are *Balfour retractors* and *Finochietto retractors*. Balfour retractors are generally used

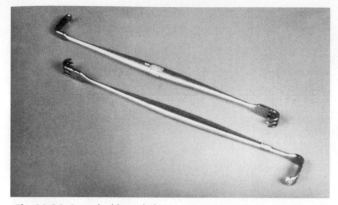

Fig. 20-36 Senn double-ended retractor. *(Courtesy Ohio State University.)*

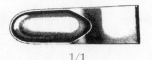

Fig. 20-37 Adson rongeur. *(Courtesy Richards Manufacturing.)*

to retract the abdominal wall, whereas Finochietto retractors are commonly used during thoracotomies.

Miscellaneous Instruments

Instruments are available to suction fluid; clamp drapes or tissues; cut and remove bone pieces *(rongeurs—*Fig. 20-37); hold bones during fracture repair; scrape surfaces of dense tissue *(curettes);* remove periosteum *(periosteal elevators—*Fig. 20-38); cut or shape bone and cartilage *(osteotomes* and *chisels);* and bore holes in bone *(trephines).*

Instruments for Large-Animal Surgery

Dehorning instruments

Various instruments, including gouges and saws, are used to remove horns from cattle (Fig. 20-39). The smaller instruments are used on calves. Saws are generally used to remove the horns of adult cattle.

Castrating instruments

An *emasculator* is used in open castrations to crush and sever the spermatic cord (Fig. 20-40). An *emasculatome* is used to accomplish the same thing through the intact skin during closed castrations, particularly when fly infestation is likely to be a problem.

WOUND CLOSURE AND HEMOSTASIS

The word *suture* refers to any strand of material that is used to approximate tissues or ligate blood vessels. The ideal suture material is easy to handle; reacts minimally in tissue; inhibits bacterial growth; holds securely when knotted; resists shrinking in tissues; is noncapillary, nonallergenic, noncarcinogenic, and nonferromagnetic; and is absorbed with minimal reaction after the tissue has healed. Such an ideal suture material does not exist; therefore, surgeons must choose one that most closely approximates the ideal for a given procedure and/or tissue to be sutured.

Monofilament sutures are made of a single strand of material. They create less tissue drag than multifilament suture material and do not have interstitial spaces that may harbor bacteria. Care should be used in handling monofilament

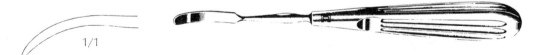

Fig. 20-38 Joseph periosteal elevator. *(Courtesy Richards Manufacturing.)*

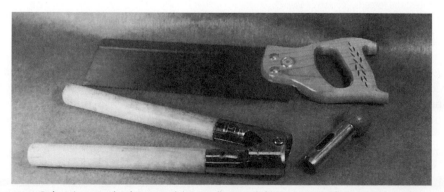

Fig. 20-39 Dehorning instruments: Dehorning saw *(top);* Barnes dehorner *(bottom left),* horn gouge *(bottom right). (From Pratt PW:* Medical surgical and anesthetic nursing for veterinary technicians, *St Louis, 1994, Mosby.)*

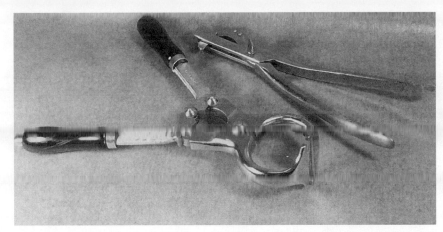

Fig. 20-40 Castration instruments: emasculatome *(bottom left)* and emasculator *(top right)*. *(From Pratt PW: Medical surgical and anesthetic nursing for veterinary technicians, St Louis, 1994, Mosby.)*

sutures because nicking or damaging them with forceps or needle holders weakens them and predisposes to breakage. *Multifilament sutures* consist of several strands that are twisted or braided together. Multifilament sutures are generally more pliable and flexible than monofilament sutures. They may be coated to decrease tissue drag and enhance handling characteristics.

The most commonly used standard for suture size is the U.S.P. (United States Pharmacopeia), which denotes suture diameters from fine to coarse according to a numeric scale. Size 10-0 material has the smallest diameter (finest), and size 7 has the largest diameter (coarsest). U.S.P. uses different size notations for various suture materials (Table 20-4). As the suture diameter decreases, its tensile strength decreases. Stainless-steel wire is usually sized according to the metric or U.S.P. scale, or by the Brown and Sharpe wire gauge.

Absorbable Suture Materials

Absorbable suture materials lose most of their tensile strength within 60 days after placement in tissue and eventually are absorbed from the site and replaced by

---

TABLE 20-4

Systems Used to Indicate Suture Sizes

Diameter (mm)	Metric Gauge	Synthetic Suture Materials (U.S.P.)	Surgical Gut (U.S.P.)	Wire Gauge (Brown and Sharpe)
0.02	0.2	10-0		
0.03	0.3	9-0		
0.04	0.4	8-0		
0.05	0.5	7-0	8-0	41
0.07	0.7	6-0	7-0	38-40
0.1	1	5-0	6-0	35
0.15	1.5	4-0	5-0	32-34
0.2	2	3-0	4-0	30
0.3	3	2-0	3-0	28
0.35	3.5	0	2-0	26
0.4	4	1	0	25
0.5	5	2	1	24
0.6	6	3, 4	2	22
0.7	7	5	3	20
0.8	8	6	4	19
0.9	9	7		18

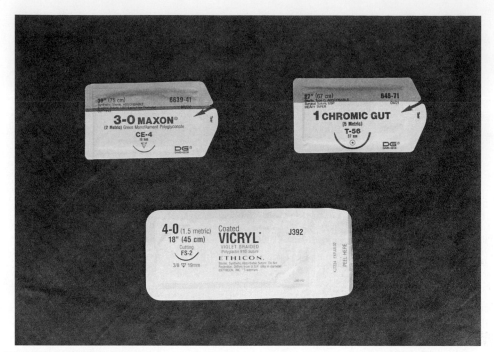

Fig. 20-41 Examples of absorbable suture materials. *(From Tracy DL:* Small animal surgical nursing, *ed 3, St Louis, 2000, Mosby.)*

healthy tissue during the healing process. Absorbable sutures are used when sutures must be buried within body cavities (Fig. 20-41).

Surgical gut

Surgical gut is commonly called *catgut*. Surgical gut is made from the submucosa of sheep intestine or the serosa of bovine intestine. It comprises approximately 90% collagen. *Plain surgical gut* is broken down by phagocytosis and elicits a marked inflammatory reaction, as compared with other materials. "Tanning," by exposure to chrome or aldehyde, slows absorption. Surgical gut so treated is called *chromic surgical gut*. Surgical gut is rapidly absorbed from infected sites or where it is exposed to digestive enzymes. Knots in surgical gut may loosen when wet.

Synthetic absorbable materials

Synthetic absorbable materials (e.g., polyglycolic acid, polyglactin 910, polydioxanone, polyglyconate) are generally broken down by hydrolysis. There is minimal tissue reaction to synthetic absorbable suture materials. The rate of tensile strength loss and rate of absorption are fairly constant in different tissues. Infection or exposure to digestive enzymes does not significantly influence their rates of absorption.

Nonabsorbable Suture Materials

There are four basic groups of nonabsorbable suture materials: organic sutures, braided synthetic sutures, monofilament synthetic sutures, and metallic sutures (Fig. 20-42).

Organic nonabsorbable materials

Silk is the most common organic nonabsorbable suture material, used as a braided multifilament suture that is coated or not coated. Silk has excellent handling characteristics and is often used in cardiovascular procedures; however, it does not maintain significant tensile strength after 6 months in tissues and is therefore contraindicated for use with vascular grafts. It should also be avoided in contaminated sites, because it increases the likelihood of wound infection. *Cotton* suture has less tissue reaction than silk but supports bacterial growth and is not generally used for skin closure.

Synthetic nonabsorbable materials

Synthetic nonabsorbable suture materials are available as braided multifilament (e.g., polyester, coated caprolactam) or monofilament (e.g., polypropylene, polyamide, poly-olefins, polybutester) threads. They are typically strong and induce minimal tissue reaction. Nonabsorbable suture materials consisting of an inner core and an outer sheath (e.g., Supramid) should not be buried in tissues, because the outer sheath tends to degenerate, allowing bacteria to migrate to the inner core. This predisposes to infection and fistula formation.

Metallic sutures

Stainless steel is the most commonly used metallic suture. It is available as monofilament wire or twisted multifilament wire. The tissue reaction to stainless steel is generally minimal; however, the knot ends evoke an inflammatory reaction. Wire tends to cut tissue and may fragment. It is stable

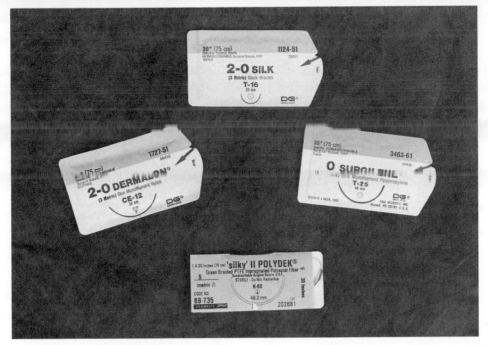

Fig. 20-42 Examples of nonabsorbable suture materials. *(From Tracy DL:* Small animal surgical nursing, *ed 3, St Louis, 2000, Mosby.)*

in contaminated wounds and is the standard for judging knot security and tissue reaction to suture materials.

Suture Needles

Suture needles are available in a wide variety of shapes and sizes. The type of suture needle used depends on the characteristics of the tissue to be sutured (penetrability, density, elasticity, thickness), wound topography (deep, narrow), and characteristics of the needle (type of eye, length, diameter). Most surgical needles are made from stainless steel because it is strong and corrosion free and does not harbor bacteria.

The three basic components of a suture needle are the attachment end (swaged or eyed), body, and point (Fig. 20-43, *A*). Suture material must be threaded onto *eyed needles.* Because a double-strand of suture is pulled through the tissue, a larger hole is created than when a swaged needle is used. Eyed needles may be closed (round, oblong, or square) or French (with a slit from the inside of the eye to the end of the needle for ease of threading) (Fig. 20-43, *B*). Eyed needles are threaded from the inside curvature. With *swaged needles*, the needle and suture are joined in a continuous unit, minimizing tissue trauma and increasing ease of use.

The needle body comes in a variety of shapes (Fig. 20-43, *C*). Tissue type, and depth and size of the wound determine the appropriate needle shape. *Straight (Keith) needles* are generally used in accessible places where the needle can be manipulated directly with the fingers (e.g., placement of pursestring sutures in the rectum). *Curved needles* are manipulated with needle holders. The depth and diameter of the wound are important when selecting the

most appropriate curved needle. One-fourth circle needles are primarily used in ophthalmic procedures. Three-eighths and one-half circle needles are the most commonly used surgical needles in veterinary medicine (e.g., abdominal closure). Three-eighths circle needles are more easily manipulated than one-half circle needles because they require less manipulation of the wrist. However, because of the larger arc of manipulation required, they are awkward to use in deep or inaccessible locations. A one-half circle or five-eighths circle needle, despite requiring more wrist manipulation, is easier to use in confined locations.

The needle point (cutting, taper, reverse-cutting; Fig. 20-43, *D*) determines the sharpness of a needle and type of tissue in which the needle is used. *Cutting needles* generally have two or three opposing cutting edges. They are used in tissues that are difficult to penetrate (e.g., skin). With conventional cutting needles, the third cutting edge is on the inside (concave) curvature of the needle. The location of the inside cutting edge may promote "cut-out" of tissue because it cuts toward the edges of the wound or incision. Reverse-cutting needles have a third cutting edge located on the outer (convex) curvature of the needle. This makes them stronger than similarly sized conventional cutting needles, and reduces the risk of tissue cut-out. Side-cutting needles (spatula needles) are flat on the top and bottom. They are generally used in ophthalmic procedures.

Tapered needles (round needles) have a sharp tip that pierces and spreads tissues without cutting them. They are generally used in easily penetrated tissues (e.g., intestine, subcutaneous tissues, fascia). Tapercut (Ethicon) needles

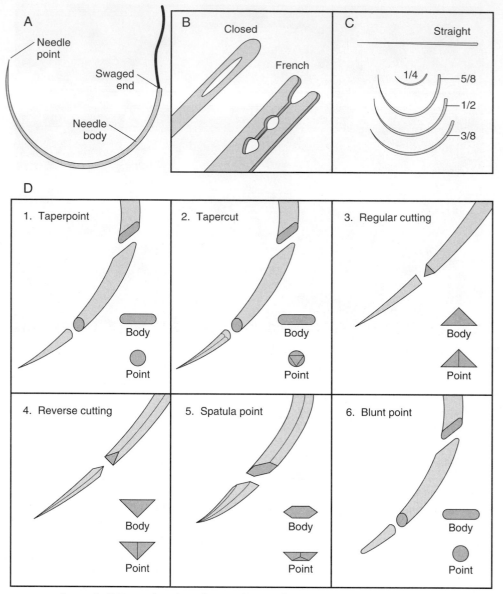

Fig. 20-43 **A,** Basic components of a needle. **B,** Types of eyed needles. **C** and **D,** Needle body shapes and sizes. *(From Fossum TW: Small animal surgery, ed 2, St Louis, 2002, Mosby.)*

have a reverse-cutting edge tip and a taper-point body. They are generally used for suturing dense, tough fibrous tissue (e.g., tendon) and for some cardiovascular procedures (e.g., vascular grafts). *Blunt-point needles* have a rounded, blunt point that can dissect through friable tissue without cutting. They are occasionally used for suturing soft, parenchymal organs (e.g., liver, kidney).

OTHER MATERIALS USED IN WOUND CLOSURE

Tissue Adhesives

Cyanoacrylates ("super glues") are commonly used for tissue adhesion during some procedures (e.g., declawing, tail docking, ear cropping). Products advocated for use in veterinary patients include Tissueglue (GRX Medical), Vetbond (3M), and Nexabond (Tri-Point Medical). These adhesives rapidly polymerize in the presence of moisture and produce a strong flexible bond. Adhesion of tissue edges generally takes less than 15 seconds but may be delayed by excessive hemorrhage. Persistence of the glue in the dermis may result in granuloma formation or wound dehiscence, and placement in an infected site may cause fistulation.

Ligating Clips and Staples

Metal *clips* (Hemoclips, Ligaclips) may be used for vessel ligation (Fig. 20-44). They are particularly useful when the vessel is difficult to reach or when multiple vessels must be ligated. Use of ligating clips on vessels more than 11 mm in

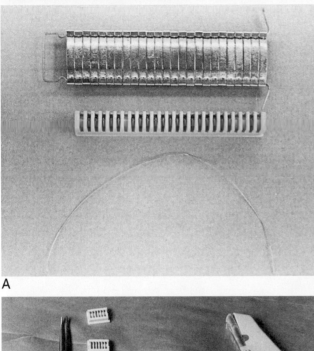

A

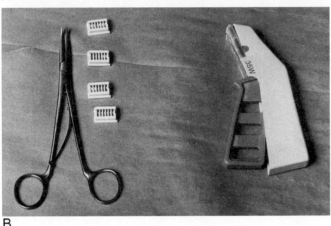

B

Fig. 20-44 Large **(A)** and small **(B)** hemostatic clips. *(From Tracy DL: Small animal surgical nursing, ed 3, St Louis, 2000, Mosby.)*

diameter is not recommended. The vessel should be dissected free of surrounding tissue before the clip is applied, and 2 to 3 mm of vessel should extend beyond the clip to prevent slippage. The vessel should be one-third to two-thirds the size of the clip.

Metal *staples* (e.g., Michel clips) are used to appose wound edges or attach drapes to the skin. Care must be used to ensure that the staple is appropriately bent so that, when staples are used for skin closure, the animal cannot easily remove them. A special staple remover facilitates clip removal after healing.

Surgical Mesh

Surgical mesh may be used to repair hernias (e.g., perineal hernias) or reinforce traumatized or devitalized tissues (abdominal hernias). Occasionally it is used to replace excised traumatized or neoplastic tissues. Surgical mesh is available in nonabsorbable (Mersilene, Prolene) or absorbable (Vicryl, Dexon) forms.

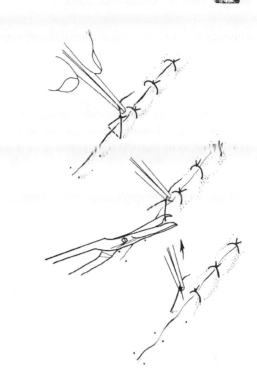

Fig. 20-45 One of free suture ends is gently elevated, and the "hook" of suture scissors is placed inside the loop to cut the suture. After the loop has been cut, suture is removed by continuing to elevate the free end away from the skin. *(From Tracy DL: Small animal surgical nursing, ed 3, St Louis, 2000, Mosby.)*

Hemostatic Techniques and Materials

Hemostasis, or the arrest of bleeding, allows visualization of the surgical site and prevents life-threatening hemorrhage. Low-pressure hemorrhage from small vessels can be controlled by applying pressure to the bleeding points with a gauze sponge. Once a thrombus has formed, the sponge should be gently removed to avoid disrupting clots. Large vessels must be ligated (tied off). Hemostatic agents used to control hemorrhage during surgery include bone wax and hemostatic materials made of gelatin or cellulose (e.g., Surgicel, Gelfoam).

Electrocoagulation can be used to achieve hemostasis in vessels less than 2 mm in diameter; larger vessels should be ligated. The term electrocautery is often erroneously used in place of electrocoagulation. With electrocautery, the needle tip or scalpel is heated before it is applied to the tissue; with electrocoagulation, heat is generated in the tissue as a high-frequency current is passed through it. Excessive use of electrocautery or electrocoagulation retards healing.

SUTURE REMOVAL

Skin incisions are usually closed with nonabsorbable suture material. Because they are not absorbed, nonabsorbable sutures are removed once healing is sufficient to prevent wound dehiscence, usually after 10 to 14 days. However, delayed healing, as in very debilitated animals, may require that sutures be left in place for longer periods. Additionally, if fibrosis is desired (e.g., aural hematoma), delayed suture removal may be considered.

Skin suture removal is begun by grasping one or both of the suture ends, which were deliberately left long for that purpose, and pulling the knot away from the skin (Fig. 20-45). Using suture-removal scissors, cut one of the two strands of suture beneath the knot at the skin surface, and pull the suture out. It is important that only one of the strands is cut to avoid leaving some of the suture material buried beneath the skin, where it could act as an irritant.

RECOMMENDED READING

Pratt PW: *Medical, surgical, and anesthetic nursing for veterinary technicians*, St Louis, 1994, Mosby.
Tracy DL: *Small animal surgical nursing*, ed 3, St Louis, 2000, Mosby.

21

Emergency and Critical Care

Harold Davis, Jr.

Learning Objectives

After reviewing this chapter, the reader should understand the following:

- The role of the veterinary technician on the emergency health care team
- Considerations for rendering first aid to injured or critically ill animals
- Steps in evaluating injured or critically ill animals

- Procedures used to perform vital functions in injured or critically ill patients
- Methods used to monitor the condition of critically ill patients
- Placement and care of catheters, chest tubes, and tracheostomy tubes.
- Procedures used in maintaining recumbent patients
- Procedures used in rendering emergency care in specific medical situations

---

Emergency and critical care is an emerging specialty in veterinary medicine. While emergencies have always existed in veterinary medicine, the American Veterinary Medical Association recognized emergency and critical care as a distinct specialty in the late 1980s. In January 1996, The North American Veterinary Technicians Association (now the National Association of Veterinary Technicians of America) recognized the Academy of Veterinary Emergency and Critical Care Technicians (AVECCT) as the first specialty for veterinary technicians. There are many similarities between emergency and critical care, but there are also differences. As defined by the Veterinary Emergency and Critical Care Society (VECCS), *emergency care* is an action directed toward the assessment, treatment, and stabilization of a patient with an urgent medical problem. *Critical care* is the ongoing treatment of a patient with a life-threatening or potentially life-threatening illness or injury whose condition is likely to change on a moment-to-moment or hour-to-hour basis. Such patients require intense and often constant monitoring, reassessment, and treatment.

The veterinary technician is a front-line member of the health care team. A team approach is mandatory for optimal care of a critically ill patient. For the veterinary technician to excel in emergency and critical care, he or she should have an understanding of the pathophysiology of the disease process in order to understand the patient's current condition and to anticipate developing problems in the

patient or the needs of the veterinarian. The technician should be adept at placing a variety of catheters: peripheral and central venous, arterial, and urinary. He or she should also be cognizant of problems involved with the maintenance of asepsis and the patency of such catheters. The technician should be observant and recognize any untoward changes in the patient's condition in order to alert the clinician of the changes, document them, and be prepared to take action. He or she should be familiar with a variety of lifesaving procedures regardless of whether they are performed exclusively by the veterinarian. The technician should be capable of taking diagnostic radiographs and performing basic laboratory tests. He or she must be compassionate and supportive in order to interact with owners under stressful conditions. The technician is primarily responsible for organizing and controlling chaos.

EMERGENCY READINESS AND PREPARATION

Facility

Clinic facilities should be set up and organized to handle any emergency. This may be an area in the clinic designated for emergency management of patients or a mobile "crash cart" system (Fig. 21-1). When selecting an area, consider the space available; is there enough room for the emergency team (three or more people) and equipment? An

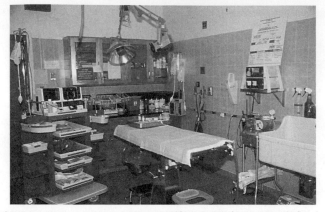

Fig. 21-1 Emergency receiving room. The room is large enough for the emergency team. It has good lighting, emergency equipment (ECG, defibrillator, crash cart, suction, and oxygen), and is in proximity to the patient.

oxygen source should be readily available. Good lighting is a must; it facilitates examination of the patient, endotracheal intubation and visualization of veins, and minor surgical procedures. The area designated for the management of the emergency patient should be centralized and stocked with key emergency supplies and equipment (e.g., ECG, defibrillator, suction). Supplies should be organized for easy accessibility. A crash cart/kit may be as simple as a fishing tackle box or as elaborate as a mobile tool chest. Crash carts/kits make the resuscitation endeavor more efficient. The emergency area should be checked at the beginning of each shift and restocked immediately after each use. VECCS has developed suggested guidelines for equipping and stocking veterinary emergency facilities.

Staff

The emergency team should be composed of at least three people, including veterinarian(s), veterinary technician(s), and other clinic support staff. The team should be prepared to work together. To this end, it is helpful to hold emergency drill sessions so that people can become familiar with specific tasks and procedures. This is also the time to review and update treatment protocols. Treatment protocols or guidelines help maximize efficiency. Protocols should be developed for common problems, but with flexibility to allow modification for specific clinical situations.

Client

Pet owners should be made aware of primary and backup emergency services available in their area. They should know the location, hours of operation, and telephone numbers. As a service to the client, the veterinary staff can hold basic first aid courses. The client should be instructed in recognition of illness/injury; basic care of wounds; foreign bodies; toxins; trauma; and the safe transport of an injured patient. The client should be taught how to put together and use a pet first aid kit. Prehospital care can often influence the final outcome of an emergency.

HOSPITAL CARE

Triage

Triage is the prioritization of treatment based on medical need. On initial presentation to the hospital, the veterinary technician may be the first to receive the patient. It is his or her responsibility to triage the patient(s). While approaching the patient, visually assess ventilation effort, pattern, and any audible airway sounds; the presence of blood, vomitus, or other foreign material about the patient; and the patient's posture and level of consciousness (LOC).

Initial Evaluation

The initial management of the emergency patient requires immediate assessment and therapy. Therapy often begins before "obtaining" or "making" a diagnosis. Following the initial assessment and resuscitation (primary survey), the secondary survey and plans for definitive management are accomplished.

Primary Survey and Resuscitation

The primary survey is an initial brief assessment of the patient (the *ABCDE*s): *A* for airway, *B* for breathing, *C* for circulation, *D* for dysfunction or disability of the central nervous system, and *E* for whole-body examination. When a life-threatening problem is identified during the primary survey, resuscitative action should be instituted immediately.

Airway/Breathing

First, airway and adequacy of ventilation should be assessed by *visualization*, *palpation*, and *auscultation*. Life-threatening airway/breathing problems may be due to apnea, airway obstruction, open chest wounds, severe pneumothorax, or hemothorax. Clinical signs associated with inadequate ventilation vary depending on severity of respiratory compromise. They include stridor, intercostal retraction, decreased breath sounds, restlessness and/or anxiety, minimal or absent chest wall motion, cyanosis (late sign), absence of air exchange from the nose or mouth, and labored use of accessory muscles of respiration.

Normally the patient should have a free, easy, and regular ventilatory pattern. The patient should not be exerting an extraordinary amount of effort. Tidal volume should be adequate. The mucous membrane color should be pink; cyanotic or blue mucous membranes indicate hypoxemia, which is a decrease in blood oxygen content. Cyanosis is an unreliable indicator of hypoxia; it is always a late sign and does not occur in severe anemia. The chest wall should be palpated for integrity and wounds. Normal lungs should sound clear over a large area of the lung fields. Suspect large airway obstruction (foreign body, laryngeal paralysis) in patients with loud sonorous or squeaking sounds on inspiration or expiration or if the chest wall retracts during inspiration. Suspect a lower airway obstruction (asthma) if you hear wheezes or if the patient exhibits a prolonged expiration. Pleural filling defects (pneumothorax, pleural effusion, diaphragmatic hernia) should be considered if the breath and heart sounds are diminished or absent. Crackles suggest fluid-filled airways (pulmonary edema, pneumonia, tracheobronchial fluid).

If an upper airway obstruction is suspected, the mouth and pharynx should be examined for easily removable foreign bodies. If the patient will not permit the examination, or the foreign body cannot be removed, preoxygenation and rapid safe anesthetic induction may be indicated. If the obstruction cannot be removed, the patient should be intubated (oral or tracheostomy) in an attempt to bypass the obstruction. If the patient is apneic, mechanical or manual ventilation will be required. Initial ventilatory requirements are as follows:

- Rate: 10 to 15 breaths per minute
- Inspiratory time: approximately 1 second
- Proximal airway pressure: 15 to 20 cm H_2O, or a tidal volume of 10 to 20 ml/kg

If the patient has an open chest wound, it can be temporarily closed manually, or by placing a generous globule of ointment and a sterile dressing over the wound. Thoracentesis or thoracostomy tube placement should be performed to relieve respiratory distress resulting from pleural filling defects.

Circulation

Circulation is assessed by visualization, palpation, and auscultation. The signs of inadequate perfusion (shock) include increased heart rate (an effort to increase cardiac output); poor pulse quality (indicates poor pulse pressure or stroke volume); and pale mucous membranes, prolonged capillary refill time, and decreased appendage temperature (indicators of poor peripheral perfusion). Inadequate perfusion may be due to hypovolemia as a result of external or concealed blood loss (loss into body cavity or limb). It may also be due to pump failure (intrinsic heart failure, arrhythmias, cardiac tamponade).

Dysfunction/Disability

Dysfunction/disability of the nervous system is assessed via visualization and palpation. The patient's LOC, pupillary light reflex, posture, and response to pain (superficial and/or deep) are particularly important.

The terms normal, obtunded, stupor, and comatose, are used to characterize the LOC but are not specific for a particular type of neural lesion. Pupils are normally equal in size and respond quickly to light. Pupillary constriction, dilation, or anisocoria with a diminished pupillary light reflex, in the absence of ocular trauma, is indicative of neurological involvement. Abnormal postures such as decerebrate, decerebellate rigidity, and Schiff-Sherrington should be noted. Decerebrate and decerebellate rigidity are characterized by extensor rigidity in the front limbs and opisthotonos. The rear limbs are in extensor rigidity in the decerebrate posture and flexed or extended in decerebellate. The decerebrate patient is unconscious, while the decerebellate patient exhibits varying levels of obtundation. Decerebellate rigidity progressing to decerebrate rigidity suggests an extension of the damage to the brain stem. The Schiff-Sherrington posture is extensor rigidity of the forelimbs with flaccid hind limbs. This posture indicates a lesion at T2-L4. It is also a poor prognostic sign when a patient does not perceive pain. Pricking or pinching the skin will test superficial pain. Applying a strong noxious stimulus to the toes or a joint will test deep pain. The patient should show some visible response indicating conscious recognition of the stimulus, such as vocalizing, turning and looking, or turning and biting. This is important because the withdrawal of the appendage alone is a spinal reflex and does not warrant against a more proximal spinal cord lesion.

Nonambulatory traumatized patients should be treated as spinal trauma patients until proven otherwise (e.g., avoid spinal flexion or twisting; use a board for patient transfer; use tape; use drugs; get a lateral spinal radiograph).

Examination

During this final phase of the primary survey, a rapid whole-body examination is performed. Major lacerations may be uncovered and areas of bruising noted. Areas of bruising that appear to be worsening may be indicative of active bleeding. Abdominal girth should also be measured if intra-abdominal bleeding is suspected.

Secondary Survey

The secondary survey is the timely, systematic, and directed evaluation of each body system for injury or other signs of illness, after initial stabilization. The *ABCDEs* are quickly reviewed to ensure that no new problems have developed. A thorough head-to-tail physical examination and history are completed. Finally, a comprehensive plan of diagnostics and monitoring is developed.

Definitive Management

A review is made of the initial ancillary diagnostics that were performed (e.g., radiographs, ECG, lab data), and a management plan is developed. The plan may result in emergency surgery or temporary stabilization of fractures and continued monitoring.

EMERGENCIES

Cardiovascular Emergencies

Hypovolemic shock

Hypovolemic shock can be a sequela to a variety of problems such as protracted vomiting/diarrhea, trauma, sepsis, or gastric dilatation volvulus due to a decreased intravascular volume. As a result of the decreased intravascular volume, venous return to the heart is decreased, which results in decreased ventricular filling (preload). This causes a decreased stroke volume (amount of blood ejected by the ventricle with each contraction) and cardiac output (product of stroke volume and heart rate; the volume of blood ejected by the heart per unit of time). The end result is inadequate tissue perfusion and oxygenation. Peripheral vasoconstriction, in an attempt to maintain arterial blood pressure, further compromises peripheral tissue perfusion.

Fluid therapy must be initiated to improve tissue perfusion and return cardiovascular parameters to normal. Intravenous (IV) catheter(s) are placed. The placement of a jugular catheter allows measurement of central venous pressure, which may be beneficial in guiding fluid resuscitation. If difficulty is encountered in placing the catheter percutaneously, consider performing a cut-down or placing an intraosseous catheter. Absorption of fluids via the bone marrow is rapid. In addition to fluids, some drugs may also be administered via this route.

Fluid resuscitation is the cornerstone of shock therapy. Fluid options for fluid resuscitation include isotonic, polyionic crystalloids, (solutions with electrolyte concentrations similar to plasma [Lactated Ringers, Normasol R, Plasmalyte 148, Normal Saline]), and colloids (Plasma, Dextran 70 [6% Gentran: Baxter], Hetastarch [6% Hetastarch: Abbott], and whole blood). Initially, crystalloids are used in the treatment of shock. The shock dose of crystalloids is 80 to 90 ml/kg and 50 to 55 ml/kg in the dog and cat, respectively (equivalent to one blood volume). It may be necessary to administer 0.5 to 1.5 times the blood volume to resuscitate the patient. In about 30 minutes, 75% to 80% of the crystalloids shift from the intravascular space into the interstitial space. Colloids are better blood volume expanders; 50% to 80% of the infused volume remains in the intravascular space for a longer period of time. Colloids should be administered when crystalloids are not improving or maintaining blood volume. Blood and/or plasma are given in sufficient quantities to maintain the packed cell volume above 25% and a total protein above 4.0 mg/dl. Colloids are dosed at 10 to 40 ml/kg and 5 to 20 ml/kg in the dog and cat, respectively.

Hypertonic saline (7.0% Sodium Chloride Injection USP: Sanofi Animal Health) has been recommended for use in shock therapy for cases in which it is difficult to administer large volumes of fluids rapidly enough to resuscitate the patient. Hypertonic saline causes fluid shifts from the intracellular space to the extracellular (including intravascular) space resulting in improved venous return and cardiac output. Hypertonic saline may have other beneficial cardiovascular effects as well. The recommended dose range is 4 to 6 ml/kg over 5 minutes. Crystalloids should be administered at 50% of the "shock" dose when synthetic colloids or hypertonic saline is used to avoid fluid overloading of the patient.

Sympathomimetics, such as dopamine (Dopamine HCL Injection: Abbott) and dobutamine (Dobutrex: Eli Lilly), are indicated when the patient is unresponsive to vigorous fluid therapy and when blood pressure, vasomotor tone, and tissue perfusion have not returned to acceptable levels. These drugs support myocardial contractility and blood pressure with minimal vasoconstriction. Blood pressure monitoring is important for the knowledgeable administration of these drugs. The effects of dopamine are dose-dependent: 1 to 5 µg/kg/min for the dopaminergic effect (dilate renal, mesenteric, and coronary vascular beds). Cats, as opposed to people and dogs, do not appear to have renal dopaminergic receptors. Beta 1 activity (positive inotropic) is seen at a dose range of 5 to 10 µg/kg/min, and dosages greater than 10 µg/kg/min cause alpha-receptor stimulation (vasoconstriction). Dobutamine has primarily beta activity. It has minimal effect on heart rate and peripheral vascular resistance except at higher dosages. The dose range is 5 to 15 µg/kg/min. Sympathomimetics should not be used as a substitute for adequate volume restoration.

Congestive heart failure

Heart failure is the inability of the heart to supply adequate blood flow to meet the body's metabolic needs. "Congestive" heart failure occurs when increased pulmonary (left side) or systemic venous (right side) and capillary pressures increase, causing fluids to leak from the capillary beds resulting in edema (peripheral and pulmonary) or effusions (ascites, pleural, and pericardial).

Left-sided congestive heart failure (LCHF) manifests dyspnea, tachypnea, orthopnea, cough (cats rarely), the appearance of a pink frothy serosanguinous fluid at the nostrils, cyanosis, and weakness. Tachycardia and arrhythmias resulting from myocardial pathology may be noted. The clinical manifestations of right-sided congestive heart failure (RCHF) include jugular distention, pleural effusion, hepatomegaly, hepatojugular reflux (sustained pressure is applied to the abdomen with one or both hands, causing the jugular veins to be distended), ascites, and peripheral edema.

Radiographs, echocardiography, and electrocardiography are useful aids in diagnosing heart failure. Radiographically, chamber enlargement, evidence of pulmonary edema, and pericardial and pleural effusions support the diagnosis of heart failure. Echocardiography is useful in diagnosing valvular disease, chamber size, atrial and ventricular function, and the recognition of pulmonary vascular distention. Fluid in the pericardial sac is an excellent contrast medium for assessing cardiac structures during ultrasound. Electrocardiography changes in wave-form amplitude, axis deviation, rhythm, and electrical alternans can further support the diagnosis of heart failure, but their absence does not rule out heart failure.

Minimizing stress should be part of the therapeutic plan when treating heart failure patients, especially patients that are hemodynamically unstable. In some instances of patient excitement, sedation may be beneficial. Oxygen therapy improves oxygenation and decreases the work of breathing. Oxygen may be administered via mask, nasal catheter, or oxygen cage. The patient should not be stressed or excited by the oxygen administration technique. In the case of LCHF, the goal is to reduce preload (the end-diastolic ventricular volume) and/or afterload (the arterial blood pressure resistance against which the heart has to pump). Administration of vasodilators such as nitroglycerine (venodilator), and nitroprusside (venous and arteriolar dilator) reduce preload. Hydralazine (arteriolar dilator) is used to decrease afterload. ACE inhibitors (arterial and venous dilator) do not act quickly enough to be useful in the emergency treatment of heart failure patients. In addition to its ability to clear pulmonary edema, furosemide also reduces venous pressure or preload. Drugs such as dopamine, dobutamine, and amrinone (also known as inamrinone) be used to increase contractility of the heart. Therapy in RCHF may be directed at removing pleural fluid (commonly in cats) and/or pericardial fluid and ascites (rare in cats). A thoracentesis has both diagnostic and therapeutic value and is indicated when there is a significant thoracic fluid accumulation. Abdominocentesis is indicated when fluid accumulation impairs ventilation or venous return, or causes patient discomfort. Pericardiocentesis should be performed when pericardial effusion impairs cardiac output. If cardiac output is severely compromised in the face of pericardial effusion, shock doses of fluids should be administered. The fluids increase cardiac filling pressure. Repeated physical examinations determine the effectiveness of therapy. Patients with respiratory distress secondary to heart failure often appear anxious and are often unwilling to sit or lie down. They will also be tachypneic and may have cyanotic mucous membranes. If therapy is effective, resolution of the respiratory distress will be evident as a decrease in respiratory rate and an improvement in attitude and mucous membrane color. The use of vasoactive drugs necessitates the monitoring of systemic blood pressure. The ECG is useful in monitoring heart rate and rhythm. The use of furosemide should result in increased urine production. Urine output should be documented and/or serial body weights obtained. Furosemide

can alter acid base and electrolytes; therefore, they should also be monitored. Excessive furosemide-induced dehydration can lead to prerenal azotemia. Packed cell volume/total solids, urine specific gravity, and blood urea nitrogen (BUN) or creatinine should be monitored.

Aortic thromboembolism

Aortic thromboembolism occurs when an aggregation of platelets and fibrin with entrapped cells migrates and lodges at a distant site in the circulatory system. In feline aortic thromboembolism, the thrombus usually resides within the lumen of the left atrium or is attached to the endocardial surface of the left atrium. The embolus breaks loose and occludes one or more branches of the aorta at the aortic trifurcation. This condition is usually referred to as a *saddle thrombus*.

Clinical signs associated with aortic thromboembolism vary with the location of the embolus. In the case of a saddle thrombus, pain, pallor, paresis, poikilothermy, and pulselessness of one or both of the hind limbs may be observed. The muscles of the rear limb may be affected and are commonly swollen and turgid, particularly the gastrocnemius. Cats with aortic thromboembolism commonly have myocardial disease. Blockage of the aorta can cause hypertension and an increase in afterload to the left ventricle, resulting in increased left heart filling pressure and pulmonary edema. Consequently cats may present with dyspnea.

Diagnostic tests should be directed at determining the underlying cause that led to the thromboembolic event. This may include the standard minimum database (CBC, chemistry, and UA); cardiac workup (ECG, echocardiography, chest radiographs); and coagulation profile. Tests that might be considered specific and sensitive for thromboembolism include: doppler flow studies, ultrasound to visualize the thrombus, and angiography (selective and nonselective). Compare the toenail bed color of the rear paws with the front paws. The rear paws may be cyanotic. In some cases, cutting the toenail of the affected limb to the "quick" may be helpful in diagnosing the problem (there is no bleeding). Cats with severely compromised blood flow will ooze black-colored blood from the cut nail.

Emergency therapy is directed at treating the underlying cause. In some instances, the patient will present with heart failure, which will certainly need to be addressed. If fluid therapy is given, care should be exercised not to aggravate or produce heart failure. If pain is present, analgesia will be required. Analgesic options include butorphanol and oxymorphone. Thrombolytic and anticoagulant therapy may be considered to lyse the thrombus and prevent further thrombi formation, respectively.

Acute Abdomen Emergencies

The "acute abdomen" is not a specific entity, but refers to any disease or disorder that causes the rapid onset of abdominal distress. The primary sign is abdominal pain. One may also see lethargy or collapse, anorexia, fever, dehydration, vomiting, diarrhea, abdominal distension, dysuria, or unusual posturing. Causes of an "acute abdomen" include: intestinal obstruction/overdistention (gastric dilatation/volvulus, foreign body, and intussusception); organ displacement (diaphragmatic/abdominal hernias, uterine/splenic torsion); infection/inflammation (parvo virus, pancreatitis, peritonitis, and pyometra), and trauma (visceral perforation, bladder rupture). In addition to initial evaluation and stabilization, additional diagnostics may be required such as repeated physical examinations, radiographic procedures (plain and contrast), laboratory (CBC, chemistry, blood gases, and electrolytes), and diagnostic peritoneal lavage. Therapy is directed at the cause of the acute abdomen.

Poisonings and Intoxications

Diagnosis is based primarily on history and clinical signs. Once the veterinarian is reasonably confident that a toxin is involved, efforts are made to identify the type of toxin, prevent further exposure and absorption, treat the symptoms, and give the specific antidote. Clinical signs of a poisoning or intoxication are diverse and overlapping due to the variety of such agents to which an animal may be exposed. General, nonspecific signs may include such findings as obtundation and weakness, anorexia, and gastrointestinal signs such as vomiting and diarrhea. CNS excitation (nervousness, apprehension, hypersensitivity, and seizures) may be seen with common poisons such as strychnine, metaldehyde, moldy food products, ivermectin in Collie breeds, chocolate, cocaine, marijuana, amphetamine, toxic mushrooms, and vitamin D-analog rodenticides. Hemorrhage may be seen with vitamin K antagonist rodenticides. Miosis and muscle tremors may be seen with organophosphate, carbamate, pyrethrins, or nicotine intoxication. Salivation may be seen with CNS excitants or with irritating or corrosive ingestions such as household cleaning products or muriatic acid.

If the animal has the toxin on its skin, it will need to be bathed to diminish further exposure. If the toxin was recently ingested, it should be removed from the stomach, as follows:

1. Induce vomiting if it has been two hours or less since the ingestion. Do not induce vomiting if the patient has CNS depression or seizure activity, or has ingested petroleum distillates.
2. Perform gastric lavage, following induction of anesthesia and endotracheal intubation. A stomach tube is passed, and several cycles of warm water are injected and aspirated until the return fluid is clear. Following emesis or lavage, the patient is given activated charcoal to absorb the remaining toxin in the stomach and intestines. If the toxin is identified, then a specific

antidote may be given. The technician will play a vital role in the supportive care of the patient. It will be necessary to maintain respiratory and cardiovascular function, body temperature, acid base balance, and control of the CNS. Some toxins may result in hyperactivity or seizures, requiring the need for sedation or anesthesia.

Urogenital Emergencies

Azotemia

Azotemia is an increase in waste products in the blood (BUN and creatine). Azotemia is categorized as prerenal (inadequate renal blood flow), renal (renal disease), and postrenal (urinary tract obstruction or perforation). Patients with prerenal azotemia show an increase in BUN and creatinine but maintain the ability to concentrate urine to a specific gravity greater than 1.035. Conditions that may predispose the patient to prerenal azotemia include dehydration, hypotension (low blood pressure), hypovolemia, and congestive heart failure. Acute renal failure (ARF) is a clinical syndrome, which results in a rapid decline in renal function. In renal failure, the kidneys are unable to adequately excrete metabolic waste and regulate fluid, electrolyte, and acid base balance. Causes of renal azotemia include toxins (aminoglycoside, ethylene glycol), renal hypoperfusion, and infectious agents (*Leptospira* spp). Postrenal azotemia occurs when the urinary pathway is obstructed preventing adequate urine flow, or from rupture of the urinary tract causing spillage of urine into the abdomen. Causes of postrenal azotemia include urethral plugs (common emergency in the male cat) and urolithiasis (urinary stones).

Acute renal failure

Clinical signs of ARF include lethargy, anorexia, dehydration, vomiting, diarrhea, dysuria (difficult urination), oliguria (decreased urine production), and anuria (lack of urine production). Additional diagnostics may be required such as repeated physical examinations, laboratory (CBC, chemistry, urinalysis, blood gases and electrolytes), radiographic procedures (plain and contrast), and ultrasonography. The objectives of treatment of ARF are to minimize further renal injury, promote diuresis if oliguria exists, and combat metabolic consequences of uremia. Hemodialysis has been used successfully to treat ARF resulting from toxic and infectious agents. Hemodialysis uses an artificial kidney to reduce azotemia, and correct fluid, electrolyte, and acid-base imbalances. There are approximately four hemodialysis units in the United States (two in California, one each in New York and Massachusetts). Peritoneal dialysis is an alternative that can be accomplished in most practice settings. Like hemodialysis, it is technically demanding and labor-intensive. The peritoneum is used as a semipermeable membrane. A peritoneal dialysis catheter is placed in the abdomen. A fluid (dialysate) is infused into the abdomen and allowed to dwell for 30 to 60 minutes. The dialysate is drained, and along with it comes solutes such as urea. The technician should be familiar with urinary and IV catheter placement and management. Measurement of central venous pressure may help guide the delivery of the fluid therapy plan. Nursing care includes monitoring "ins and outs." It is helpful to weigh the patient several times per day. Acute changes in body weight are usually related to fluid gains or losses.

Feline lower urinary tract disease (FLUTD) with obstruction

Dysuria, anuria, hematuria, inappropriate voiding, incessant grooming of the perineum, vocalizing, vomiting, bladder distention, and abdominal pain are signs consistent with FLUTD with obstruction. The narrow urethra of the male cat becomes obstructed with a mucoproteinaceous plug and/or urethroliths. In addition to postrenal azotemia, urinary obstruction leads to impaired excretion of potassium and hydrogen ions, resulting in hyperkalemia and metabolic acidosis. Vomiting and anorexia may cause volume depletion.

The immediate therapeutic goal is to relieve the obstruction and correct the metabolic abnormalities. The patient's condition will dictate treatment priorities. Relieving the obstruction is required for resolution of azotemia and hyperkalemia. In cases in which hyperkalemia and hypovolemia are life-threatening, cardioprotective treatments and fluid resuscitation become top priority. Therapeutic options to protect the heart from toxic effects of hyperkalemia include administration of calcium and/or insulin and 50% dextrose. The administration of calcium antagonizes the effects of potassium on the heart. Regular insulin and dextrose administration causes potassium to shift from the extracellular fluid (ECF) to the intracellular fluid. The insulin dextrose combination has a slightly slower onset of action when compared to calcium administration, but a longer duration of action. In addition to volume restoration, fluid therapy with crystalloids will dilute potassium in the ECF.

Very sick cats with urethral obstruction probably will not require sedation to relieve the obstruction. The obstruction may be relieved by gently massaging the penis or by passing an open-ended tomcat catheter and flushing (retropulsing) the urethra with saline. Once the obstruction is relieved, a soft urinary catheter is placed until it is determined that it can be removed. The catheter should be attached to a closed urinary collection system to prevent infection and to monitor urine production. Cats commonly exhibit a postobstructive diuresis; a high fluid administration rate will be required to meet urine losses. Fluids are given to correct dehydration and to meet normal maintenance requirements as well as to match urine output. Potassium supplementation is neces-

sary because of the potential development of hypokalemia secondary to the post-obstruction diuresis. Eventually, fluids will be tapered off.

Dystocia

Dystocia is rare in the queen but not uncommon in the bitch. The two primary causes of dystocia are either maternal (poor straining effort [uterine inertia], anatomic abnormalities), or fetal (fetal oversize, malposition). Dystocia can be characterized as any of the following:

- Active straining for more than 30 to 60 minutes without delivery of a fetus
- Resting, without straining for more than four hours between deliveries with known retained fetuses
- Intermittent weak contractions for more than two hours

Diagnosis and the mode of therapy are based on thorough history and physical examination. Radiography and, if available, ultrasonography, may aid in the decision-making process. Three options are available for the management of the dystocia patient; they include medical intervention (use of oxytocin, calcium, and glucose), manual manipulation, and surgery.

Pyometra

A pyometra is an infection in the uterus. It is caused by hormonally-induced changes in progesterone or exogenous estrogens. Patients may be depressed and septic or clinically normal. Clinical signs include lethargy, anorexia, dehydration, vomiting, diarrhea, polyuria, polydipsia, and vaginal discharge (with open pyometra). Laboratory tests (CBC, chemistry, urinalysis, cytology and culture, blood gases, and electrolytes) and imaging (radiographs and ultrasonography) aid in the diagnosis of the disease. Pyometras may be surgically or medically managed. Surgery is the treatment of choice. Treatment choice is based on the condition, age, and breeding value of the animal. The patient will need to be supported with intensive fluid therapy and good basic nursing care.

Endocrine System Emergencies

Diabetic ketoacidosis

Diabetic ketoacidosis (DKA) is one of the more common endocrine emergencies. A patient presenting with DKA is glucosuric, hyperglycemic, ketonuric, ketonemic, hypovolemic, and acidotic. DKA is the result of altered carbohydrate, protein, and fat metabolism due to insulin deficiency. Clinical signs include, polyuria (PU), polydipsia (PD), polyphagia (excessive ingestion of food), weight loss, depression, weakness, tachypnea, vomiting, and sweet acetone odor to the breath. The goals of initial therapy are to correct ketonemia and acidosis, blood glucose, hyperosmolality, dehydration, and electrolyte abnormalities (through insulin and fluid therapy).

Hypoadrenocorticism (Addisonian crisis)

Hypoadrenocorticism is a deficiency in the production of mineralocorticoid and/or glucocorticoid steroid hormones. Hypoadrenocorticism occurs in the dog and is rare in the cat. Owner's complaints are rather nonspecific and may include: anorexia, lethargy, vomiting, weakness, weight loss, and diarrhea, with waxing and waning signs. Physical findings may include mental depression, weakness, collapse, decreased body temperature, and bradycardia. Many of the signs may be attributed to decreased tissue perfusion and electrolyte abnormalities. Diagnosis is confirmed by performing an ACTH stimulation test. Other laboratory findings may include hyperkalemia, hyponatremia, sodium/potassium ratio less than 27:1, and usually less than 20:1, azotemia, metabolic acidosis, and normocytic normochromic anemia. The Addisonian crisis is a medical emergency; supportive therapy is often begun before a definitive diagnosis is made. Therapy includes fluid resuscitation, usually with normal saline. If the patient is hypoglycemic, hyperkalemic, or has metabolic acidosis, the appropriate therapy is undertaken. Monitoring entails repeated physical examinations, ECG monitoring, blood pressure and central venous pressure measurements, and acid-base and electrolyte measurements.

EMERGENCY PROCEDURES

Technicians should be familiar with the variety of lifesaving emergency procedures available. The technician should be prepared to render the procedures they are allowed to perform, or be prepared to assist the veterinarian. The technician should know the indications for each procedure; what equipment will be necessary; how the procedure is performed; potential complications; and nursing implications of the procedure whether it goes well or not.

Endotracheal Intubation

Endotracheal intubation is a basic but important technique that can easily be mastered with practice (Chapter 19).

Tracheostomy Tube Placement

Usually an endotracheal tube is placed first. Then preparation is made to place the tracheostomy tube under controlled, aseptic conditions (Box 21-1). The veterinary technician should set up for the procedure, prepare the patient, assist in the placement, and provide pre- and post-tracheostomy wound and tube care.

Thoracentesis

Thoracentesis is useful for collection of pleural fluid to obtain samples for diagnostic laboratory evaluation or for alleviation of respiratory distress. This procedure may be used for patients with respiratory distress and decreased to absent lung sounds. In an emergency situation, a technician can perform the procedure (Box 21-2).

Chest Tube Placement

Chest tubes are placed to relieve progressive pneumothorax and to relieve progressive pleural effusion (Box 21-3).

OXYGEN THERAPY

Overview

Hypoxemia is defined as deficient oxygenation of the blood. Hypoxemia is a result of impaired gas exchange due to small airway and alveolar collapse, an excessive ventilation/perfusion mismatch, or both. Oxygen therapy may be beneficial. The goal of oxygen therapy is to provide adequate blood oxygenation, using the lowest possible inspired oxygen concentrations. The best method for assessing oxygenation is analysis of arterial blood gases. Pulse oximetry (SPO_2) can also be used to assess oxygenation. Clinical signs of hypoxia include cyanosis, dyspnea, tachypnea, tachycardia, and anxiety.

Indications

- Hypoxemia; $PaO_2 < 60$ mm Hg
- Dyspnea

Methods of Oxygen Administration

There are a variety of methods of oxygen delivery. The method selected depends on expected duration of therapy, demeanor of the patient, and equipment availability. Available methods include face mask, oxygen hood, oxygen cage, and nasal insufflation.

Face mask

Face masks are readily available and easy to use. Masks are only good for short-term use. High-inspired oxygen concentrations can be obtained if a properly fitted face mask is used. Unfortunately, patients often fight the face mask (unless obtunded) thereby increasing oxygen consumption and diminishing the effects of the oxygen therapy. The patient's face and nose should fill the mask as much as possible to reduce the amount of dead space in the mask. Increased dead space will increase the work of breathing. Sometimes it is helpful to remove the rubber diaphragm from the face mask to achieve a better fit and achieve better patient cooperation.

Oxygen hood

An alternative to the face mask is a clear plastic bag placed over the head of a patient with an oxygen hose placed near the animal's nose. The bag remains open along the animal's neck to allow the gas to escape. A flow rate of 5 to 8 liters per minute is used. It has been reported that animals toler-

BOX 21-1

procedure

Tracheostomy Tube Placement

Indications

- Airway obstruction
- To facilitate long-term access to the airway and positive pressure ventilation

Materials

- Several tracheostomy tubes (one size smaller and larger than the estimated size)
- Surgical kit
- Sterile drapes
- Bandage material
- Sandbags (to aid in patient positioning)

There are many types of tracheostomy tubes available. We use the Shiley adult (Fig. 21-2) and pediatric tracheostomy tubes. The adult tube consists of an outer tube with fixation flanges and an inner cannula. The tube is soft and pliable, and is nonirritating to the tissues. It has a high volume low-pressure cuff. The inner cannula is removed for cleaning. An obturator is included to assist in the smooth placement of the tracheostomy tube. The pediatric tube is cuffless and does not have an inner cannula. An endotracheal tube can be substituted for a tracheostomy tube and is often cut to decrease dead space and resistance.

Procedure

1. Sedate the patient if necessary. Place the patient in dorsal recumbency, and position as straight as possible. Place a sandbag or roll of towels underneath the neck to cause dorsoflexion of the cervical region. Make a wide clip over the region of the incision site, and prepare the skin antiseptically.
2. The clinician will make a midline skin incision from approximately the first to the fourth tracheal ring. Blunt dissection is continued until the trachea is clearly exposed. Three types of tracheal incisions have been used: transverse, tracheal flap, and vertical. It may be helpful to place sutures around a tracheal ring, above and below the opening (in the transverse incision). The suture is left in place for the duration of the tracheostomy. Sutures help to manipulate tracheal rings during intubation and re-intubation if the tube becomes dislodged.
3. Clean the trachea of blood and mucus before intubation.
4. Insert the tracheostomy tube and inflate the cuff.
5. Close the skin incision (not tightly around the tube), and tie the tube securely around the patient's neck with umbilical tape or other material.

6. Drape a sterile 4-by-4 inch gauze around the tube to absorb serum and secretions from the ostomy site.

Complications

- Tube obstruction with mucus (Fig. 21-3).
- Tube dislodgement from the trachea
- Infection of the incision site
- Tracheal stenosis as a result of an oversized tracheostomy tube, torqued tube positioning, excessive tracheal tube movement, or excessive cuff inflation.

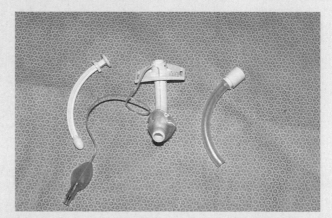

Fig. 21-2 Shiley tracheostomy tube *(center)* with obturator *(left)* and inner canula *(right)*. The inner canula fits into the tracheostomy tube.

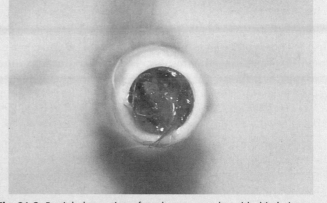

Fig. 21-3 Partial obstruction of tracheostomy tube with dried airway secretions and mucous.

ate this bag/hood method when they resist the oxygen mask.

Oxygen cage

A good oxygen cage should have the following features: it must have a system for eliminating carbon dioxide; deliver a known amount of oxygen in a concentration beneficial to the patient (40% to 50%); and a mechanism for controlling temperature (21° C [70° F]) and humidity (50%). The disadvantages of oxygen cages are: expense to purchase and operate; minimal access to the patient by caregivers; and difficulty accommodating large patients.

BOX 21-2

procedure

Thoracentesis

Indications

- Pneumothorax
- Pleural effusion

Materials

- Butterfly catheter, hypodermic needle, or over-the-needle catheter
- Three-way stopcock
- 3 ml syringe (if procedure is done to obtain diagnostic sample)
- 35 or 60 ml syringe (if procedure is done to remove a substantial amount of fluids)
- IV extension set
- Surgical prep solution and scrub

Procedure

1. Clip and prep area where thoracentesis is to be performed (dorsally for the collection of air or ventrally for fluid).
2. After putting on sterile gloves, assemble catheter, needle or butterfly, stopcock, and syringe (Fig. 21-4). Palpate anterior edge of rib.
3. Insert the needle into the pleural space so that it comes to lie on the pleural surface of the palpated rib; the bevel is directed away from the rib.
4. Aspirate using gentle pressure.

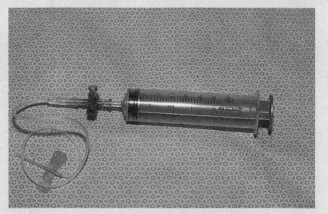

Fig. 21-4 Thoracentesis equipment. A syringe is attached to a stopcock and butterfly catheter, as shown. If the butterfly catheter is too small, IV extension tubing attached to a needle or an over-the-needle IV catheter may be used.

Complications

- Iatrogenic lung trauma and pneumothorax
- Iatrogenic hemothorax

Nasal oxygen

Nasal oxygen is an excellent way to provide oxygen therapy. It does not require an expensive O_2 cage. Also, you can use supplies found in your clinic, you have direct access to your patients at all times, and it is well tolerated by most patients (Box 21-4).

Intraosseous fluid or drug administration

In the event vascular access cannot be obtained, the establishment of an intraosseous line is a reasonable alternative. Intraosseous fluid or drug administration is the administration of fluids or drugs via the bone marrow and into the circulatory system (Box 21-5).

Jugular Catheterization

Jugular catheterization is a technique that all veterinary technicians should feel comfortable performing (Box 21-6). There are times when using a central vein offers more advantages than a peripheral vein. Large central veins also allow the administration of hypertonic solutions. The jugular catheter is well tolerated by veterinary patients. It allows for uninterrupted flow of the IV infusion.

Diagnostic Peritoneal Lavage

Diagnostic peritoneal lavage is useful in diagnosing some abdominal disorders when other diagnostic tests are equivocal. It is not indicated when there is historical, physical, or radiographic evidence of the need for an exploratory laparotomy. Fluid is infused into the abdomen via a peritoneal lavage catheter. The fluid is recovered and analyzed. This procedure is helpful in diagnosing abdominal hemorrhage, ruptured bowel, peritonitis, and bladder rupture (Box 21-7).

CRITICAL CARE

Once the patient has made the transition from the crisis or emergency care phase, critical care nursing may be required. Critical care patients require moment-to-moment monitoring and nursing care. The technician should be able to monitor, reassess, and respond to the patient's needs in an appropriate manner as the condition changes. In addition, the veterinary technician should be knowledgeable in fluid therapy (Chapter 23) and critical care nursing protocols.

BOX 21-3

procedure

Chest Tube Placement

Indications

- To relieve progressive pneumothorax
- To relieve progressive pleural effusion

Materials

- Chest tube
- 2% lidocaine
- Surgical kit
- Suture material
- Sterile gloves
- Sterile drapes
- Bandaging material

Commercial chest tubes come in a variety of sizes with and without trocars. You can use 14- to 16-French tubes for cats and very small dogs; 18- to 22-F tubes for small dogs; 22- to 28-F tubes for medium to large dogs; and 28- to 36-F tubes for very large dogs. If necessary, red rubber or Foley catheters may be used. It may be beneficial to add a few more holes to the chest tube.

Procedure

1. Clip and prepare caudal dorsal quadrant of the chest wall for surgery.
2. Have an assistant grasp skin along the entire lateral chest wall just caudal to the elbow and pull it forward and downward.
3. Locate an intercostal space about 8 or 9 high on the chest wall (about junction of upper ⅓ and lower ⅔ of the chest wall).
4. Inject lidocaine along path of the skin and intercostal muscle incision.
5. Make a skin incision 1½ times the length of the tube diameter.
6. Make an intercostal relief incision, but do not penetrate the pleura.
7. Penetrate the pleura with a blunt object so as not to lacerate the lung.
8. Insert the chest tube through the chest wall and into the pleural space (Fig. 21-5). Guide the tube in a cranial ventral

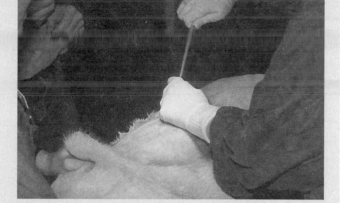

Fig. 21-5 Insertion of a chest tube. Note the skin being pulled forward by the assistant to facilitate the creation of a subcutaneous tunnel.

direction at about a 45 degree angle. If a trocar is used, pull it back from the tip of the chest tube as soon as pleura is penetrated. When the tube is in the desired location, remove the trocar and clamp the tube.

9. Have an assistant release the skin creating a tunnel that prevents air from entering the pleural space.
10. Verify the position of the chest tube with the trocar on the outside of the chest.
11. Secure the chest tube to the chest wall, and apply a triple antibiotic dressing.
12. A chest radiograph may be taken to verify the position of the tube. This is not necessary if the tube is draining properly, but must be done if the tube is not draining properly.

Complications

- Infection
- Laceration of intercostal artery
- Lung trauma/pneumothorax
- Trauma to heart and great vessels/hemorrhage
- Subcutaneous emphysema

Patient Assessment/Monitoring

A great deal of the veterinary technician's responsibility lies with patient monitoring during the definitive management phase.

Cardiovascular system

Assessment of the cardiovascular system may begin with the heart rate. A normal heart rate for a dog is 100 to 140 beats per minute. For a cat, it is 110 to 140 beats per minute. There are several reasons for tachycardia (hypovolemia, fever, excitement, exercise, and pain) and bradycardia (high vagal tone, severe electrolyte disturbances, and atrioventricular conduction blocks). If arrhythmias are auscultated, then an ECG is indicated. The ECG measures electrical activity; it does not measure mechanical activity. Indicators of peripheral perfusion include: mucous membrane color, capillary refill time (normal CRT 1 to 2 seconds), urine output, and appendage temperature. A full strong pulse indicates a good pulse pressure and stroke volume.

BOX 21-4

procedure

Nasal Catheter Placement

Indications

Therapy for patients with hypoxemia

Materials

- Red rubber urinary catheter or 5-F infant feeding tube (for cats and small dogs) or 8-F tube (for medium to large dogs)
- 2% lidocaine
- Lubricating jelly
- Suture material
- ½-inch tape
- Unheated bubble humidifier
- Extension tubing
- Oxygen source

Procedure

1. Place a few drops of 2% lidocaine in the nostril. Wait 30 to 60 seconds, and repeat.
2. Select a catheter of appropriate size. Measure the distance from the tip of the nose to the medial canthus of the eye. Mark the catheter at the tip of the nostril.
3. Lubricate the catheter with sterile lubricating jelly. Insert and direct the catheter ventromedially into the nostril until you reach the mark on the catheter.
4. The catheter can then be brought out around the alar notch and sutured to the skin at that point. Position the catheter back over the head, and suture it to the top of the head.

Oxygen Administration

1. Fill a bubble through humidifier with sterile water, and attach it to an oxygen source.
2. Attach this to the nasal catheter. (Flow rates of 50 to 200 ml/kg per minute are usually effective in increasing inspired oxygen concentration to 40% or greater. The goal is to see improved mucous membrane color, decreased anxiety, decreased breathing and/or heart rate, decreased magnitude of respiratory distress, and improved PaO_2 or SPO_2 to an acceptable level.)

Complications

- Gastric distension
- Epistaxis
- Serous or mucoid nasal discharge
- Decreased mucus clearance without humidification
- Patient discomfort

BOX 21-5

procedure

Intraosseous Tube Placement

Indications

- Circulatory collapse
- Thrombosed veins
- Edematous states/obesity
- Severe burns
- Very small patients

Materials

- 2% lidocaine
- Scalpel blade
- 18- to 22-gauge spinal needle (for small or young animals with soft bones) or bone marrow needle (for most adult dogs and cats)
- 12 ml syringe

Procedure

The most common access sites include the trochanteric fossa of the femur, the greater tubercle of the humerus, the wing of the ilium, and the medial surface of the tibial crest.

1. Clip and aseptically prepare insertion site.
2. Inject lidocaine into the skin and periosteum.
3. Make a small stab incision into the skin. Advance the spinal or bone marrow needle by rotation and steady pressure into the selected site.
4. Verify that the needle is securely lodged in the bone and that the tip is in the medullary cavity of the bone. Attach the syringe to the needle, and apply gentle suction. A small amount of bone marrow/blood should be aspirated into the barrel of the syringe.
5. Flush the needle with heparinized saline, and observe the site for subcutaneous infiltration.
6. Once the placement of the needle is confirmed, attach the IV set and begin the fluid infusion.
7. Cover the insertion site with betadine or triple antibiotic ointment.
8. Administer fluids with gravity flow or under pressure.

Complications

- Osteomyelitis (rare) related to the use of hypertonic solutions, faulty technique, or prolonged infusion.

BOX 21-6

procedure

Jugular Catheter Placement

Indications

- To facilitate the administration of fluids and medications
- To measure central venous pressure
- To facilitate blood sample collection

Materials

- Through-the-needle catheter and T-Port (over-the-needle catheter systems may be used, but they are easy to contaminate; be sure to use a sterile drape)
- Heparinized saline and 6 ml syringe
- Sterile gloves, drapes, suture material, and surgical set
- Bandaging material

Procedure

1. Clip a wide area of hair over the catheterization site. (The area should be wide enough to prevent contamination during catheterization procedure.) Prepare the catheterization site just as you would a surgical site. Wear sterile gloves if necessary to prevent contamination to either the catheter or catheter site. Use sterile drapes to widen the sterile field.
2. Placement of the jugular catheter is best performed with the patient in lateral recumbency with a sandbag or roll of towels under the shoulder/neck area. The patient's head is extended, and the forelimbs are pulled caudally by an assistant. It is important that the patient is positioned properly and the vein immobilized. If the vein is not immobilized properly, it may roll laterally or wrinkle longitudinally.
3. Have an assistant hold off the vein by pressing into the thoracic inlet with one or two fingers; this should cause the vein to engorge and "stand up." Introduce the needle into the subcutaneous space. Position the needle tip over the vein, and align it as close as possible to the longitudinal axis of the vein. Insert the needle tip into the vein. (You may need to apply a little angle to the needle in order to pick up the vein wall.) A flashback of blood into the catheter system should be noted when the needle has entered the lumen of the vein. This may not occur if the venous pressure is low. Once you determine that the entire needle tip is in the vein, advance the catheter through the needle into the vein. Once the catheter is placed, apply pressure over the catheter site and back the needle out. Once the bleeding has stopped, secure a needle guard around the needle. Aspirate the catheter to confirm proper placement and to clear the catheter of air; then flush it with heparinized saline. If blood cannot be aspirated, withdraw the catheter slowly until it can.
4. Cap the catheter with an injection cap or T-port and again flush with heparinized saline. Staple or suture the catheter close to the insertion site. Cover the insertion site with a sterile 2-by-2 inch gauze pad or adhesive bandage. Finally, secure the catheter with an occlusive bandage.

Complications

- Sepsis (cellulitis, septicemia)
- Phlebitis
- Thrombosis (vein, catheter lumen)
- Bleeding
- Catheter backs out

BOX 21-7

procedure

Diagnostic Peritoneal Lavage

Indications

Diagnosis of abdominal hemorrhage, ruptured bowel, peritonitis, and bladder rupture

Materials

- Peritoneal lavage catheter or over-the-needle catheter
- Lactated ringer's or normal saline
- IV administration and/or extension sets
- Surgical kit
- Sterile gloves
- Lab collection tubes

Procedure

1. After the bladder is emptied, clip and prepare the skin caudal to the umbilicus.
2. Infiltrate the skin and abdominal wall with lidocaine.
3. Make a small incision through the skin, subcutaneous tissue, and superficial abdominal fascia.
4. Insert the catheter through the incision, and direct it caudally and dorsally.
5. Infuse 20 ml/kg of warmed lactated ringer's or normal saline into the abdomen. Gently rock the patient from side to side for a few minutes.
6. Collect the fluid aseptically as it flows freely from the catheter; fluid removal may require gentle aspiration.
7. Remove the catheter if the fluid is clear; Otherwise, suture it in place and use as needed.
8. If necessary, perform gross, cytological, and biochemical analysis on the sample.

Complications

- Infection
- Iatrogenic hemorrhage or viscous perforation

Arterial blood pressure is the product of cardiac output, systemic vascular resistance, and blood volume. Normal systolic, mean, and diastolic blood pressure are approximately 100 to 160 mm Hg, 80 to 120 mm Hg, and 60 to 100 mm Hg, respectively. Noninvasive methods of measuring blood pressure include ultrasonic Doppler and oscillometric devices. The doppler detects flow of blood through an artery and converts this to an audible signal. When an occlusive cuff is applied to a limb and inflated, flow is occluded. The cuff pressure is slowly decreased while looking at a sphygmomanometer. With the first sound of flow, the pressure reading from the sphygmomanometer is noted; this approximates systolic pressure. Dinamap blood pressure units utilize the oscillometric technique. A cuff is applied to a limb and automatically inflated; the cuff detects oscillations in the underlying artery. As the cuff is gradually deflated, oscillations are detected. The first detected pulsation is the systolic pressure; the point at which the maximum pulsation is detected is the mean blood pressure; and the point at which oscillations diminish or disappear is the diastolic pressure. The invasive technique requires the placement of an arterial catheter and attachment to a monitoring device.

Central venous pressure (CVP) measures the ability of the heart to pump the quantity of blood returned to it. CVP is also an estimate of the relationship between blood volume and blood volume capacity. Normal CVP ranges between 0 and 10 cm H_2O. A CVP less than 0 suggests that the patient is vasodilated or hypovolemic. A CVP greater than 10 cm H_2O may be due to fluid overload, right heart failure, venoconstriction, cardiac tamponade, or positive pressure ventilation. CVP measurements require the placement of a jugular catheter, such that its tip lies in the anterior vena cava; the catheter is attached to a water manometer or transducer. To measure the CVP, the water manometer is filled three quarters of the way full. The fluids are then allowed to flow from the manometer into the patient. Small fluctuations in the fluid meniscus synchronous with heart beat and ventilation should be evident. The zero reference point is established by drawing an imaginary horizontal line from the thoracic inlet to the manometer. Once the fluid level stabilizes, the difference between the actual fluid level in the manometer and the zero reference point is the CVP measurement. For example, if the fluid level in the manometer is 12 and the zero reference point is 5, the CVP is 7 cm H_2O.

Respiratory system

Assessment of the respiratory system includes answering questions such as the following:
- Is the rate and tidal volume adequate?
- Is the breathing effort smooth and easy, or labored?
- Is the breathing pattern regular?
- Are you able to auscultate normal breath sounds? (Abnormal breath sounds may be described as *crackles, wheezes, squeaks, muffled,* or *quiet.*)

- Is the patient able to meet its ventilation and oxygenation requirements?

Arterial blood gases (ABG) are an excellent way to assess ventilation and oxygenation. $PaCO_2$ (normal: 35 to 45 mm Hg) tells how well the patient is ventilating. PaO_2 (normal: 80 to 100 mm Hg breathing room air) tells how well the patient is oxygenating. Sometimes arrangements can be made to run ABGs through a local human hospital. Recently, new inexpensive portable blood analyzers have been developed. The I-Stat (Heska, Fort Collins, Colo.) and IRMA (Diametrics, St Paul, Minn.) blood analyzers have the capability to run blood gases and electrolytes as well as other tests. It is financially and technically feasible for use in private practice. Pulse oximetry is a noninvasive technique that continuously measures arterial oxygen saturation in the blood (normal SpO_2 is greater than 95%). Corrective measures should be undertaken when the SaO_2 is 90% or less. An SaO_2 of 90% equates to a PaO_2 of 60 mm Hg that indicates severe hypoxemia. There are a variety of pulse oximeters that work well in the veterinary patient.

Central nervous system

Assessment of mental status includes observing whether the patient is conscious, unconscious, or somewhere in between. Patients that are conscious on presentation should be monitored to assure that their level of consciousness does not change for the worse. Pupils should be equal in size and reactive to light. Pupils are considered abnormal if they show any combination of unresponsiveness, dilation, constriction, or asymmetry in the absence of ocular trauma. Irregular breathing patterns indicate brain stem disease. The patient should be observed for abnormal postures such as opisthotonus.

Fluids in and fluids out

Urinary output is a reflection of tissue perfusion. If the kidneys are producing urine, then other organs are probably also being perfused. The normal urinary output is 1 to 2 ml/kg per hour. Ideally, it is important to quantitate the urine output. There are several techniques for urinary collection. Some examples include the following:
- Placing a urinary catheter and using a closed collection system
- Walking the patient and collecting the urine in a bowl
- Weighing a disposable diaper and placing it underneath the penis or vulva in a recumbent patient so that the patient urinates onto the diaper. The difference between the wet and dry weight is the urine (1 gram of urine equates to 1 milliliter of urine)
- Weighing the litter pan pre- and posturination and again obtaining the difference for urine output

In addition to quantitation of urine, it is also helpful to quantitate defecation and emesis; this can provide you with a better picture of your total fluid balance. Weight gains and losses should be monitored on a daily basis. Acute changes in weight are usually a result of fluid changes as opposed to muscle mass.

The fluid losses should be compared to fluid intake; they should just about balance out. Any large discrepancy in the "ins and outs" may be significant.

Temperature

A deep rectal or esophageal thermometer monitors core temperature. Early recognition of hypothermia or hyperthermia and establishing trends in the patient's status is also important. The normal temperature for a dog or cat is 38.3° C to 39.2° C. In the neonate, the normal body temperature is 35.6° C to 36.1° C during the first week of life. By the second week, they can maintain their temperature from 36.7° C to 37.8° C. By the fourth week, their thermal regulation is mature.

Hypothermia is a temperature below 38.3° C. Causes of hypothermia include prolonged exposure to a cold environment and central thermoregulation impairment. Hyperthermia is a temperature above 39.2° C . The causes for hyperthermia include a hot environment with poor ventilation, a response to infection or inflammation, and thermoregulatory dysfunction.

Charting

It is important to monitor trends. Use a charting system to help you keep track of the trends. It need not be elaborate, but it should allow you to see all parameters measured.

Critical Care Nursing Protocols

Veterinarians and technicians should hold rounds at the beginning of each day or shift. Rounds give you the opportunity to talk about the patients.

The technician should perform a basic physical examination on each patient as soon as possible at the start of the day or shift. This will give you a baseline for comparison regarding the patient's progresses throughout the day. In addition to temperature, pulse, and respiration, the lungs should be auscultated, the bladder should be palpated, and mentation should be noted. Also check the operation of all IV and urinary catheters, other monitoring apparatus, and the cleanliness of the patient and bedding.

Check emergency supplies and equipment to be sure that all emergency drugs are present and have not expired, and that the equipment is functional. Pay special attention to endotracheal tubes and cuffs, and oxygen supply.

IV catheter care

IV catheter care should be performed every 48 hours or on an as-needed basis. The catheter dressing should be removed and the site inspected. Signs of phlebitis (inflammation of a vein) may include erythema; a thickened, sensitive vein; and an apparent increase in skin temperature over the vein. Signs of thrombosis include a vein that stands up without being held off and a thick cordlike feeling to the vein. When signs of phlebitis or thrombosis are apparent, the catheter should be removed and a new one placed at a different site. While flushing the catheter with heparinized saline, the insertion site should be observed for leaking of fluid at the insertion site and pain upon injection. If either is observed, the catheter should be removed and replaced with a new one at another insertion site. If any portion of the catheter is exposed, it should be noted in the record. If no apparent problems are noted, the catheter site should be cleaned with a Betadine solution or chlorhexidine solution. When the catheter site is dry, cover the insertion site with a sterile 2 by 2 gauze pad. Then rebandage the catheter in your routine fashion. Traditionally, IV catheters are changed at 72 hours. However, if catheter care is performed on a regular basis and there are no apparent problems, then the catheter may remain in place beyond 72 hours. It has been shown that the likelihood of phlebitis increases the longer catheters are left in place.

IV catheters should be observed several times per day. If the catheter bandage is found to be wet, then the reason should be identified and the bandage should be changed. Swelling distal to the catheter is usually indicative of a tight bandage. Swelling proximal to the catheter may be due to infiltration.

Sterility of IV administration sets must be maintained. Disconnection of the administration set is made only when essential. Administration sets and fluids should not hang any longer than 48 hours. If suspected contamination occurs, the fluid system should be changed immediately.

Urinary catheter care

Urinary catheter care is performed every 8 hours. It entails cleaning the prepuce or vulva and its surrounding area with a mild soap and water rinse. The sheath or vestibule is then flushed with either weak tea-colored betadine solution or 0.05% chlorhexidine solution. Apply betadine ointment with a cotton swab to the sheath or vulvar opening. The urinary catheter should be kept clean, especially in the female patient where the catheter is in proximity to the rectum.

The urinary catheter should be attached to a closed collection system to decrease the chance of a urinary tract infection (UTI). Do not disconnect the urinary catheter from the collection system. The system is drained every 2 to 4 hours. Urinary collection bags may be obtained commercially, or you can use an empty, sterile fluid bag. The addition of 3% hydrogen peroxide to the urinary collection system has been shown to decrease the incidence of UTI. Add 5 to 10 ml of hydrogen peroxide to the urinary collection system to minimize bacterial growth in the collection bag. Hydrogen peroxide is contraindicated when the patient has gross hematuria (blood in the urine). The hydrogen peroxide reacts with the red blood cells causing a gas to form and preventing urine flow.

Chest drain/gastrostomy tube care

The procedure for chest drain and gastrostomy tube care is much like IV catheter care. The bandage is removed and the insertion site is inspected every 24 to 48 hours. The site is cleaned and rebandaged.

Tracheostomy tube management

Patients with indwelling tracheostomy tubes require observation 24 hours per day. It is important to minimize tracheal trauma by the tube or cuff and to provide airway humidity, clear airway secretions, and prevent infection.

Minimizing tracheal trauma. When the tracheostomy tube is placed, it should be secured firmly and double-tied around the patient's neck. This helps prevent movement and torque from being applied to the tracheostomy tube, causing irritation and trauma to the trachea. The tracheostomy tube cuff should be a high-volume, low-pressure cuff. To prevent tracheal mucosal damage, the cuff should not be overinflated.

Airway humidification. Because the artificial airway bypasses the patient's natural ability to warm and humidify the inspired air, it is important to provide humidity. Humidification may be accomplished by nebulization or, in the absence of nebulization, instilling saline down the tracheostomy tube. In addition to airway humidification, be sure the patient is systemically hydrated. This is important in the mobilization of airway secretions.

Nebulization is the production of particulate water droplets. In general, the smaller the particle, the deeper into the airway will be the deposition. However, very small particles (0.25 to 1.0 micron) tend not to deposit. Particles larger than 10 microns are deposited primarily in the upper airway, while smaller particles (2 to 10 microns) are deposited in the lower airway. Small particles (1 to 3 microns) are deposited to a large extent in the alveolar sacs. Nebulization therapy is used to promote bronchial drainage with minimal irritation by depositing large quantities of bland substances such as saline. Nebulization promotes bronchial drainage by liquefying thick respiratory secretions.

Ultrasonic nebulizers increase the water content of inspired gas. Ultrasonic nebulizers are electrically driven units that convert electric energy into high-frequency vibrations that are, in turn, transmitted to the nebulizer reservoir. A fine, dense, cool fog with a particle size less than 5 microns in diameter is produced.

Jet nebulizers pass a high-velocity gas stream across the top of a capillary tube that is immersed in saline. The saline is drawn up the tube and broken into particles. Baffling of the particles causes the larger ones to drop out of the gas stream. Smaller droplets remain in the gas stream and are delivered to the patient. Particle size ranges between 0.5 and 30 microns.

Coupage is a technique that may be used in conjunction with nebulization to promote removal of respiratory secretions. The patient is allowed to stand, sit sternal, or lie in lateral recumbency. The hands should be slightly cupped with the fingers and thumbs together. In this position, the hands are placed on the chest wall, clapping the chest wall over the involved lung. Coupage is delivered primarily by flexion and extension of the wrist and elbows. Coupage should be maintained for 3 to 5 minutes in a steady even fashion.

Tracheal suctioning. In addition to nebulization and coupage, the tracheostomy tube or tracheal tube should be suctioned at regular intervals. The purpose of suctioning is to clear the secretions from the trachea down to the primary bronchi. Due to the artificial airway, the patient is unable to clear secretions because of the interruption of the mucociliary escalator and the inability to cough.

The suctioning procedure should be atraumatic and sterile. The airway should be nebulized before suctioning to liquefy secretions. The patient is preoxygenated before suctioning to prevent hypoxemia. The suction catheter is passed down the trachea (without suction) until resistance is met. Then the catheter is withdrawn a few millimeters, and suction is applied. As the catheter is withdrawn, a rotating or winding motion is used. Suction is applied no longer than 10 to 15 seconds to minimize hypoxemia and small airway collapse. The patient is then hyperinflated (sighed) with 100% oxygen. The character of the secretions is observed. If the secretions are minimal or thick, then approximately 0.2 ml/kg of saline is injected into the trachea, the lungs are again hyperinflated several times with oxygen, and the suctioning is repeated. If the secretions are coming back readily, there will be no need to inject saline. The entire suction procedure is repeated several times, especially if it is very productive. It is important to oxygenate and hyperinflate the patient immediately before and immediately after each suctioning attempt. The suctioning procedure should be stopped immediately if the patient displays excessive discomfort, restlessness, or changes in cardiac or respiratory rhythm.

Infection control. The site around the tracheostomy tube should be inspected for signs of infection every 8 hours. In addition, the site should be cleaned with hydrogen peroxide and covered with a gauze pad.

Blood transfusion

Transfusions with whole blood or its components are indicated in acute blood loss, chronic anemia, thrombocytopenia, hypoproteinemia, and coagulopathies. Transfusions are not an innocuous procedure; there are several complications that can occur. The patient may be subject to either an immune-mediated, or nonimmune-mediated reaction. This discussion will focus on the administration of whole blood and its components and not the collection and storage. The following is a protocol, which is currently used in the Small Animal Intensive Care Unit at the University of California at Davis.

Pretransfusion. If the IV catheter is already in place, then it should be checked for patency. If the catheter is leaking or if there is any doubt about catheter patency, then a new catheter should be placed.

If possible, the stored blood or plasma should be warmed; the administration of refrigerated blood will lower the animal's body temperature. Blood or plasma may be warmed in a water bath or a dry incubator; the temperature should not exceed 37° C (99° F). Temperatures in excess of 42° C (107° F) will cause fibrinogen precipitation and or autoagglutination.

A baseline TPR should be taken, and the blood transfusion started.

During the transfusion. Whole blood or its components is usually administered at a rate of about 5 to 10 ml/kg/hr but may be administered much faster in severely hypovolemic patients. The first hour of the transfusion should be given at half of the desired rate. This will allow for observation of incompatibility reactions. If no problems occur during this test period, the rate of the transfusion may be increased to the desired rate. The drip rate should be checked frequently. Refrigerated blood has a high viscosity and will infuse slower. Therefore, when the blood is warmed you may have to adjust the flow rate.

The patient should be observed continuously for a transfusion reaction; the TPR should be performed hourly.

The clinical signs for immune-mediated reactions include the following:
- Restlessness
- Nausea/salivation
- Vomiting
- Fever
- Tachycardia
- Urticaria
- Muscle tremors
- Tachypnea

The clinical signs for nonimmune-mediated reactions include the following:
- Sepsis
- Vascular overload
- Coagulopathies
- Microembolism
- Citrate intoxication (hypocalcemia)
- Hypothermia

The earlier a reaction occurs in the transfusion, the more severe the reaction. In the event of a mild reaction (vomiting, fever, restlessness), the transfusion should be slowed down. Antihistamines, steroids, and supportive care may be indicated. With severe reactions, the blood transfusion should be stopped.

Care of the recumbent patient

Patients suffering neurological, orthopedic, or traumatic problems can be recumbent for prolonged periods of time. The recumbent patient should be turned every 2 to 4 hours.

Turning the patient prevents the formation of decubital ulcers and atelectasis of the lungs. Decubital ulcers develop over bony prominences as a result of continuous pressure and ischemic damage to the skin. Atelectasis is small airway and alveolar collapse.

Bedding is an important factor in the prevention of decubital ulcers. Fleece pads or blankets work well. The use of elevated grates helps separate the patient from urine on the cage floor. Disposable diapers help to reduce the number of fleece pads used. Diapers are excellent for absorbing urine and keeping the patient dry, and they also allow quantitation of urine production (weigh the diapers before and after urination). Air and water mattresses have also been advocated for use in the prevention of decubital ulcers.

If an animal becomes urine-soaked, it should be bathed immediately. This will prevent urine scalding. Once the skin has been dried, apply Desitin ointment or powder to help protect the skin.

Passive range of movement (PROM) and muscle massage should be instituted unless contraindicated. PROM involves moving the limbs back and forth and flexing the joints. It may help improve muscle tone. If peripheral edema is present, massage may be helpful in reducing the edema.

Nosocomial infection

Nosocomial infections are hospital-acquired infections. Factors that predispose a patient to a hospital-acquired infection include age (geriatric or neonate), immunosuppression, diagnostic and therapeutic invasive procedures, antimicrobial therapy, and long-term hospitalization. Examples of nosocomial infections include *Escherichia coli*, *Klebsiella*, *Salmonella*, canine parvovirus, and feline panleukopenia.

Ways to help reduce the chance of hospital-acquired infection include the following:
- Diligent handwashing by staff before handling medications, fluids, and IV lines, and between patients
- Swabbing injection ports with alcohol before administering IV medication
- Use of disposable thermometer sheaths
- Disinfection of patient care equipment (clipper blades, ECG leads and clips, endotracheal tubes, and breathing circuits)
- Disinfection of environmental surfaces
- Aseptic technique in catheter/tube placements (IV, urinary, and chest)
- Treating patients with known infections last when doing treatment rounds

Patient's mental well being

Take the time to make friends with the patient before treatment (poking, sticking, and prodding). This may set the tone for further encounters. It is helpful to talk and pet the patient when treatments are not due. Then the patient will not assume that every time you open the cage door it means poking and prodding.

Taking a patient out on a walk can do a lot to lift its spirits. Since many dogs do not like to urinate in their cage, this will give them the opportunity to do so. With cats, try and position their cage near a window so they can get some sun.

It is important for patients to have time to rest. In a 24-hour ICU, a patient may have treatments every hour. If at all possible, treatments should be grouped so that the patient has some time to rest.

If a patient will not eat, it may be helpful to find out what the patient likes to eat normally. Also, it may be helpful to find out what time the patient eats when at home.

SUMMARY

Veterinary technicians will find that the responsibilities in emergency and critical care nursing are challenging and diverse. The technician must have a thorough understanding of emergency conditions to better meet the needs of the patient. The technician is the vital link between the veterinarian and the patient. Competent nursing care will increase the odds for patient recovery.

RECOMMENDED READING

Battaglia AM, ed: *Small animal emergency and critical care*. WB Saunders, Philadelphia, 2001.

Murtaugh RJ, ed: *Quick look series in veterinary medicine: critical care*. Teton NewMedia, Jackson Hole, Wyo., 2002.

Winfield WE, Raffe MR, eds: *The veterinary ICU book*. Teton NewMedia, Jackson Hole, Wyo., 2002.

22

Management of Wounds, Fractures, and Other Injuries

Katie Samuelsen

Learning Objectives

After reviewing this chapter, the reader should understand the following:

- Phases of wound healing
- Categories of wounds

- Principles of first-aid treatment of wounds
- Principles of wound closure
- Types and application of bandages
- Types and application of splints and casts
- Ways in which specific types of wounds are managed

A wound is a disruption of cellular and anatomic functional continuity. Wound healing is the restoration of this continuity. Acute wounds are those induced by surgery or trauma that heal normally, with healing time determined by the depth and size of the lesion. Examples of acute wounds include surgical incisions, blunt trauma, bite wounds, burns, gunshots, and avulsion injuries. Chronic wounds have various causes and, as determined by their underlying pathology, may take months or years to heal completely. Decubital ulcers (pressure sores), diabetic ulcers, and vascular ulcers are examples of chronic wounds.

WOUND HEALING

Phases of Wound Healing

Most healing of soft tissue occurs as a result of epithelial regeneration and fibroplasia, both of which occur simultaneously. The epidermis serves as a barrier from the environment and is necessary for optimal appearance, function, and protection. A bed of granulation tissue is required for migration of epithelium across the defect. The four phases of soft tissue wound healing are the *inflammatory phase*, the

The authors acknowledge and appreciate the original contribution of Samuel M. Fassig, whose work has been incorporated into this chapter.

debridement phase, the *repair phase*, and the *maturation phase*. The phases of wound healing are overlapping events; a wound may have more than one phase occurring at the same time. Table 22-1 summarizes the phases of wound healing. Details on tissue response to injury are presented in Chapter 8.

Types of Wound Healing

Relatively clean, minor wounds, such as small lacerations, heal by *primary* or *first-intention healing*. The tissues can be pulled together with sutures, and healing progresses without complication. Wounds that are larger, more complicated, or infected may need to heal by *second intention*. In this case, the wound is left open and allowed to heal from the inner areas to the outer surface. Although sometimes necessary, second-intention healing is a less desirable method of healing.

Some large or grossly contaminated wounds are allowed to heal initially by second intention and then are closed with sutures. After a healthy granulation bed is formed and infection is no longer present, the granulation bed is closed with sutures. This is described as *third-intention healing*. Very large wounds treated with third-intention methods may heal more rapidly than if allowed to heal by second intention.

First-intention healing of fractures is primary bone healing, with rigid internal fixation (e.g., pins, plates). Second-intention ("normal") healing of fractures is by callus formation, using no internal fixation.

TABLE 22-1

Events in the Three Phases of Wound Healing

Exudative-Inflammatory-Debridement Phase	Proliferation-Collagen Phase	Remodeling-Maturation Phase
Inflammation starts immediately and predominates for up to 6 hours	Starts at 12 to 36 hours after injury	Starts after about 2 weeks
This phase can last for several weeks	Fibroblasts and endothelial cells proliferate	Lasts 2 to 3 weeks in rapidly healing tissues (viscera)
Acute vasoconstriction followed by vasodilation	Neutrophils decrease while macrophages increase	Can last for years in slowly healing tissues (bone, tendon, ligament)
Plasma proteins leak from vessels into interstitial space	Collagen synthesis starts after 4 to 6 days	Slow increase in tensile strength
Leukocytes (neutrophils, monocytes, macrophages) exit blood vessels	Components of granulation tissue become engaged in healing; endothelial buds grow into damaged or intact blood vessels; mesenchymal cells follow the budding endothelium, secreting ground substance	Equilibrium of collagen synthesis and breakdown
Fibroblasts differentiate		Collagen cross-linking slowly increases tissue strength
Endothelial cells begin to proliferate		

Wound healing is impaired by numerous factors, including infection, debris and necrotic tissue, old age, malnutrition, poor perfusion, drugs (e.g., corticosteroids), and hypothermia.

Wound Contamination and Infection

Wound contamination is not the same as wound infection. Microorganisms in the environment contaminate all wounds, even those created during surgery using strict aseptic technique. Initially, these organisms are loosely attached to tissues and do not invade adjacent tissue; there is no host immune response to these organisms. With time, the microorganisms multiply. Infection is the process by which organisms bind to tissue, multiply, and then invade viable tissue, eliciting an immune response. Tissue infection depends on the number and pathogenicity (or virulence) of the microorganisms. In general, a wound is infected when the number of microorganisms reaches 100,000 per gram of tissue or milliliter of fluid. At these numbers, the microorganisms have exceeded the host's defense mechanisms to control them. If the patient is presented for treatment more than 12 hours after injury, any wounds should be considered infected. Infection is characterized by: erythema, edema, pus, fever, elevated neutrophil count, pain, change in color of exudate, or uncharacteristic odor. Contaminated wounds may become infected under the following circumstances:

- Foreign bodies are present (e.g., organic material, bone fragments, suture material, glove powder, bone plates, and screws).
- Excessive necrotic tissue is left in the wound.
- Excessive bleeding results in higher levels of ferric ion necessary for bacterial replication.

- Local tissue defenses are impeded (e.g., excessive hemoglobin in burn patients or patients receiving immunosuppressive drugs).
- The vascular supply is altered.
- Dirt and debris are present.

Appropriate treatment soon after injury is important to avoid infection.

Wound Categories

Open traumatic wounds can be categorized according to the degree of contamination present (Table 22-2). Management of these wounds varies according to the severity of the injury and the patient's condition. In general, wounds that are grossly contaminated and/or dirty may not be good candidates for primary closure. Until contamination and infection can be eliminated, open wound management is necessary. Dead and dying tissues must be excised (debrided) to minimize the potential for bacterial infection and create a viable wound bed.

Use of Antibacterials

The decision to use antibacterials systemically or topically in a surgical wound depends on several preoperative factors, including the patient's condition and immune status, the nature of the surgery (emergency versus elective), location of the wound (orthopedic versus abdominal), predicted duration of the surgical procedure, the surgeon's experience, and the environment in which the procedure is performed.

It is generally thought that antibacterials are not needed for patients in good health with an adequate immune status undergoing a relatively short (less than 90 minutes) elective orthopedic or soft tissue surgical procedure (not abdominal), performed by an experienced surgeon using aseptic technique in a clean surgical facility.

TABLE 22-2

Categories of Wounds

Type of Wound	Description
Clean	• Surgical wounds • Elective incisions • Highly vascular tissues not predisposed to infection
Clean-contaminated	• Minor contamination evident • Surgical wounds with minor break in aseptic technique • Elective surgery in tissues with normal resident bacterial flora (e.g., gastrointestinal tract, respiratory tract, or genitourinary tract) • No spillage of organ contents
Contaminated	• Moderate contamination evident • Fresh traumatic injuries, open fractures, penetrating wounds • Surgery with gross spillage of organ contents • Presence of bile or infected urine • Surgical wounds with major break in aseptic technique
Dirty	• Grossly contaminated or infected • Contaminated traumatic wounds more than 4 hours old • Perforated viscera, abscess, necrotic tissue, foreign material

In clean surgical wounds, preoperative antibacterials should be considered in cases of shock, severe systemic trauma, long procedures, traumatic procedures, poor blood supply, foreign bodies, dead space (seromas, hematomas), malnutrition, obesity, or other factors altering host defense mechanisms. When systemic (injected) antibacterials are used, they are most effective if administered just before surgery or shortly after surgery is begun.

Traumatic wounds, as opposed to "clean" surgical wounds, may contain devitalized tissue and/or foreign material and are contaminated by microorganisms. Traumatized tissue provides a suitable environment for bacterial multiplication and provides a route of entry for penetration of pathogens into adjacent viable tissue. Chronic (long-standing) wounds offer an ideal environment for bacterial proliferation, with copious wound fluid, necrotic tissue, and deep cracks and crevices on the wound surface. In such cases, antibacterials with a broad spectrum of antimicrobial activity are given systemically.

It is likely that we often do more harm than good by applying topical medications to wounds. The adverse effect of these products on wound healing is independent of their antimicrobial action. Generally, water-soluble antibacterial products tend to impede wound healing more than do ointments or creams. Solutions tend to evaporate, contributing to drying of the wound surface. Ointments and creams remain in contact with the wound longer than solutions, preventing drying of the wound surface. A clean wound in a healthy patient can heal optimally without application of ointments, salves, etc. Certain topical products may be beneficial at times; however, a focus on aseptic technique and appropriate "clean" management of wounds is more appropriate.

WOUND MANAGEMENT

First Aid

In the field and/or before transport to a treatment facility, the wound should be protected with a bandage. An occlusive bandage is preferred. This type of bandage controls hemorrhage, prevents additional contamination, and provides immobilization of the extremity. Open fractures should be splinted. In open or compound fractures, exposed bone should not be forced into position below the skin. This avoids additional soft tissue trauma and reduces chances of deep tissue contamination. The wound should be evaluated for antimicrobial therapy at the treatment facility. The wound should be protected during preparation of the surrounding area (e.g., clipping and scrubbing).

Wound Assessment

Wound assessment includes evaluation of the wound's location, size, and depth; exudate (drainage); tissue in the wound bed; and any signs of infection. Wound management revolves around three considerations: cleansing, closing, and covering. Control of hemorrhage is usually the first step in wound management. After initial hemostasis, it is important to evaluate the wound for bacterial contamination and the potential for bacterial growth. To avoid introduction of microorganisms, the wound should be cleaned under aseptic or at least sanitary conditions.

Clipping

In initial wound treatment, the wound must be protected while areas around the wound are clipped and cleaned. Before the area around the wound is clipped and cleaned, cover the wound with a water-soluble sterile ointment (e.g., K-Y Lubricating Jelly, Johnson & Johnson, New Brunswick, N.J.) or moistened sterile gauze sponges. This helps to prevent loose hair from further contaminating the wound. The wound can also be temporarily closed with towel clamps or a continuous suture. This may require analgesia. Before clipping and shaving areas around head or face wounds, an ophthalmic ointment should be instilled in the conjunctival sac to protect the cornea and conjunctiva.

If the patient is covered with dirt and debris (and is not in critical condition), it should be bathed before clipping. This reduces further contamination. (Clipper blades also stay sharper longer when cutting clean hair.) Clipping removes sources of contamination (e.g., hair, dirt, and debris) and allows better visualization of the wound. Two pairs of clipper blades are advantageous; the second set of blades is disinfected for use in areas of elective surgical sites. Hair at wound edges may be trimmed with scissors or a handheld No. 10 scalpel blade dipped in mineral oil, K-Y Jelly, or water so that the hair sticks to the blade and does not enter the wound.

Scrubbing

After the area around the wound has been clipped, replace the gauze sponges or gel over the wound. Gently scrub the surrounding intact skin, not the wound itself. The most commonly used surgical scrubs for skin preparation contain an antimicrobial agent plus a detergent/surfactant, such as chlorhexidine (Nolvasan, Fort Dodge) or povidine-iodine (Betadine, Purdue Frederick). Rinsing with saline or 70% isopropyl alcohol does not seem to influence the antimicrobial effect.

Wound Lavage

Cleansing and debridement of a wound begins after the surrounding area has been cleaned. Obvious foreign bodies and gross contamination must be removed. Usually, a non-caustic solution is used to clean the wound without creating further irritation. Lavaging with a sterile solution and gentle scrubbing are the primary methods used for cleaning the wound. Take care not to use forceful lavage or scrub too vigorously; this may force bacteria into the wound and spread contamination. Often more than one session of lavage and additional debridement may be necessary to remove debris and necrotic tissue. Bandaging with wet wound dressing can facilitate this process. As a general rule, wound lavage should be discontinued before the tissues take on a "water-logged" appearance.

Lavage solutions are most effective when delivered with a fluid jet impacting the wound with a pressure of at least 7 pounds per square inch (psi). This can be achieved by forcefully expelling solution from a 35- to 60-ml syringe through an 18-gauge needle. Lavage solutions can also be delivered using a spray bottle or Water Pik. The Water Pik should be used with care, as it can deliver fluids at up to 70 psi. Adequate fluid pressure cannot be achieved with gravity flow, a bulb syringe, or a turkey baster.

Isotonic ("normal") saline, lactated Ringer's solution, or plain Ringer's solution may be used for lavage. These physiologic (isotonic, isosmotic, and sterile) solutions do not damage tissue but have no antibacterial properties.

Povidone-iodine solution is commonly used to lavage wounds because of its broad antimicrobial spectrum. Dilutions of povidone-iodine in the range of 1% to 2% are more potent and more rapidly bactericidal than commercial 10% povidone-iodine solution, because dilution makes more "free iodine" available. A 1% solution can be prepared by diluting 1 part commercial 10% povidone-iodine with 9 parts sterile water or electrolyte solution. The bactericidal effect of povidone-iodine lasts only 4 to 6 hours. It is inactivated by blood, exudate, and organic soil, reducing the period of residual action. The detergent form of povidone-iodine (scrub) is deleterious to wound tissues, causing irritation and potentiation of wound infection.

Chlorhexidine diacetate solution has a broad antimicrobial spectrum and is commonly used on small animals. In dogs, it is more effective against *Staphylococcus aureus* than is povidone-iodine. When chlorhexidine is applied to intact skin, the antimicrobial effect is immediate, with a lasting residual effect. Prolonged tissue contact with solutions of 0.5% or more concentrated solutions may be harmful. Currently, 0.05% chlorhexidine solutions are recommended for use in wound lavage. A 0.05% solution can be prepared by diluting 1 part 2% stock solution with 40 parts water. Chlorhexidine has sustained residual activity. Systemic absorption, toxicosis, and inactivation by organic material do not seem to be problematic.

Hydrogen peroxide is commonly used as a foaming wound irrigant. It has little antimicrobial effect, except on some anaerobes. It is more effective as a sporicide. In concentrations of 3% and more, hydrogen peroxide is damaging to tissues. It also causes thrombosis in the microvasculature adjacent to the wound margins, impairing proliferation of blood vessels. Hydrogen peroxide should be reserved for one-time initial irrigation of dirty wounds. It should not be delivered to wounds under pressure, because its foaming action forces debris between tissue planes, enlarging the wound and allowing accumulation of air in tissues.

Anesthesia and Analgesia

After preparation of the surrounding area, the wound is prepared for analgesia and debridement. Local, regional, or general anesthesia may be used for wound management.

General anesthesia is preferred if the patient can tolerate it. Tranquilizers or sedatives (e.g., xylaxine, acepromazine, diazepam) are often used in conjunction with local and regional anesthesia.

Local anesthetics, such as lidocaine and bupivacaine, are used for pain control if the patient is not a candidate for general anesthesia. It may be beneficial to lavage a wound initially with 2% lidocaine for 1 or 2 minutes before irrigating to make removal of foreign bodies less painful. Local anesthetics do not usually offer analgesia sufficient for surgical debridement.

Epinephrine is included in some local anesthetic products. It causes vasoconstriction and helps reduce hemorrhage and prolong the anesthetic effect. Epinephrine may cause tissue necrosis along the wound edge, adversely affect tissue defenses, and potentiate infection. In general, local anesthetics containing epinephrine should not be used in wound care.

Debridement

Debridement is the removal of devitalized or necrotic tissue. Necrotic tissue must be removed, as epithelium will not migrate over nonviable tissue, a wound will not contract without debridement, and necrotic tissue may act as a growth medium for bacteria. Debridement also removes sources of contamination, infection, and mechanical obstructions to healing.

Debridement is complete when the wound bed consists of only healthy tissue, commonly referred to as a "clean wound." However, this does not mean the wound is free of bacteria. Acute traumatic wounds are usually debrided to facilitate surgical closure, whereas chronic wounds are usually debrided to reduce the risk of infection and facilitate second-intention healing.

Wounds are usually debrided by mechanical means, such as with surgical instruments, irrigation, and dry-to-dry or wet-to-dry dressings. Nonmechanical debridement techniques include application of enzymatic agents or chemicals. In many cases, a combination of techniques is used.

Debridement should be performed as an aseptic procedure. To protect the wound from further contamination, sterile surgical gloves and mask should be worn and the area draped. Ideally, several sets of sterile instruments should be used to prevent reintroducing contaminated instruments into the wound.

After a wound is cleansed and free of devitalized tissue, the surgeon explores the wound using sterile techniques. Other diagnostic procedures, such as radiographic studies using contrast materials, collection and assessment of fluid samples, and cytologic examination, may be performed to assist in the overall evaluation. Once this process is completed, a decision is made regarding how the wound will be managed, including if drainage is required. If primary closure is elected, decisions are made concerning anesthesia, antibacterials, nonsteroidal anti-inflammatory drugs, tetanus status (if the injured animal is a horse), and bandaging (if required). The wound is then prepared for suturing.

Drainage

Drains implanted in a wound provide an escape path for unwanted air and/or wound fluids, thus preventing or reducing seroma or hematoma formation in tissue pockets or dead space. Accumulation of exudate in a wound favors infection. Excessive fluid prevents phagocytic cells from reaching bacteria within a wound and provides a medium for bacterial growth. Drains are needed when wounds produce fluids and exudates for several days after initial treatment. They are indicated as follows:

- For treatment of an abscess cavity
- When foreign material and nonviable tissue are present and cannot be excised
- When contamination is inevitable (e.g., wounds near anal area)
- To obliterate dead space
- As a prophylaxis against anticipated fluid or air collection after a surgical procedure

Penrose drains are made of soft latex rubber. Their sizes range from ¼ to 1 inch in diameter and 12 to 18 inches long. They provide a simple conduit for gravity flow. If a bandage covers the drain, there may be some capillary action. Fluid flows through the drain's lumen and around the tube and is related to the surface area of the tubing. The fenestrations (holes) in the drain decrease the surface area and reduce its effectiveness. Cutting the Penrose drain in half lengthwise increases the surface area by 100%. Penrose drains should not be left in place for more than 3 to 5 days, because most gravitational drainage has subsided by that time.

Closed-suction drains provide drainage with a vacuum applied to the drain lumen with no air vent. Closed-suction drains allow wounds and dressings to stay dry, prevent bacterial movement through and around the drain, afford continuous drainage, and eliminate the need for irrigation.

These drains help hold the skin grafts in contact with the granulating wound bed to enhance revascularization. Excessively high negative pressure in the drain system can injure tissue. The vacuum for these drain systems can be generated by glass vacuum bottles, a compressible plastic canister (Hemovac), a compressible plastic canister with two one-way valves (Drevac), or a simple syringe (usually a modified 60-ml syringe) (Fig. 22-1).

Gauze or umbilical tape "setons" may be passed into a wound opening to keep the wound from closing before all exudates have drained. They are unsatisfactory for drainage purposes because they do not promote drainage once the gauze is saturated. They act as wicks, retaining bacterial contaminants, and can be mechanically irritating.

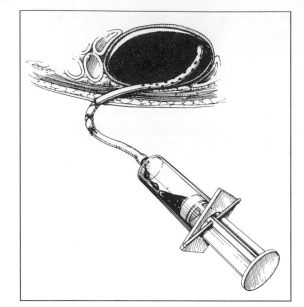

Fig. 22-1 Fluids can be drained by periodic aspiration with a syringe attached to the drain.

Box 22-1 presents guidelines for and complications of drain use.

WOUND CLOSURE

The patient's ability to tolerate anesthesia influences initial wound management. It is usually best to close fresh wounds as quickly as possible, when the risk of infection and complications is very low. Wounds with minor contamination may be cleaned, debrided, and closed. Sometimes a drain is installed to facilitate removal of tissue fluids associated with significant soft tissue trauma. Wounds that require optimal wound drainage because of gross contamination, tissue necrosis, and/or infection are managed as open wounds until they can be closed at a later time. Table 22-3 summarizes the types of closure used with different types of wounds.

A wound should be closed only when the veterinarian is certain that all devitalized and contaminated tissue has been removed and there is adequate skin to appose the wound edges. Veterinarians should consider covering the wound and allowing it to heal by second intention or delayed closure. Unfortunately, wounds are sometimes closed prematurely, resulting in *dehiscence* (opening) and infection a few days later. If there is any doubt about the advisability of a surgical closure, the clinician should cover the wound with a proper dressing and manage the wound with frequent dressing changes (at least daily), lavage, debridement, and reassessment as required.

BOX 22-1   *procedure*

Guidelines for Drain Use

Procedure

- Provide adequate drainage, using the fewest possible drains with the least number of drain holes.
- Clip a generous area of skin around the drain to prevent contamination of the drain end by hair.
- Do not tunnel the drain too far subcutaneously before entering the wound pocket; this may collapse the drain and prevent proper drainage.
- To minimize the chance of misplaced drains, record the number and size of drains used in the patient, and count them again when the drains are removed.
- Make the stab incision for the drain exit large enough to allow adequate drainage.
- Make the drain exit through a separate stab incision; drains that exit the primary wound/incision may cause dehiscence.
- Place the drain dorsoventrally to allow drainage through the dependent opening.
- Bandage the drain, if possible, to increase drainage by capillary action and prevent ascending infection, self-mutilation, and premature drain removal.
- Use radiopaque drains (evident on radiographs).
- Suture the drain to the skin at the point of exit.

Complications

- Infection from bacteria ascending the drain
- Drain obstruction
- Retention of the drain if the exposed portion of the drain retracts under the skin, requiring surgical removal
- Foreign-body reaction
- Damage to surrounding tissues
- Pain
- Premature loss and/or removal by the patient
- Delayed healing, with increased possibility of wound dehiscence or formation of a fistulous tract

---

Closure With Sutures

When wound closures requires suturing, certain fundamental considerations apply:
- Potential tissue reaction to the suture material must be acceptable.
- The suture material need not be stronger than the tissue in which it is placed.
- The sutures should retain their strength until healing keeps the wound edges together.
- Suture patterns should not impair blood supply to the wound.
- Knots should be tied securely with sufficient but not excessive "throws."

TABLE 22-3

Types of Wound Closures

Type of Closure	Type of Wound Healing	Conditions of Use
Primary closure	First-intention healing	• Wound closed with sutures or staples • Full-thickness apposition of wound edges • Tissues in direct apposition • Minimal edema • No local infection • No serious discharge • Minimal scar formation • Rapid healing
Nonclosure	Second-intention healing	• Wound left open because of infection, extensive trauma, tissue loss, or incorrect apposition of tissues • Healing by contraction and epithelialization, from inner layers to outer surface • Contraction starts after around 72 hours and stops when wound edges meet or tension exceeds strength of contraction • Epithelialization starts within 24 hours after injury and requires a moist, oxygen-rich environment • Delayed by healing
Delayed primary closure	Form of third-intention healing	• Closure 3 to 5 days after cleaning and debridement, but before granulation tissue forms • Wound strength and rate of healing not affected by delaying primary closure
Secondary closure	Form of third-intention healing	• Closure after more than 3 to 5 days after granulation tissue has formed in the wound bed
	Third-intention healing	• Safe method for repair of dirty, contaminated, or infected wounds with extensive tissue damage • Allows for management of infection or necrosis before closure • Surgeon debrides damaged tissue and wound is closed, with accurate apposition of tissues
Adnexal re-epithelialization	Second-intention healing	• Partial-thickness skin loss with epithelialization primarily from compound hair follicles ("road burns")

In selecting suture material, considerations include suture construction (monofilament, braided), suture material (absorbable, nonabsorbable), suture size (diameter), suture pattern, knot type, and needle type. Chapter 20 presents detailed information on suture materials.

Nonclosure

In second-intention healing (nonclosure), the wound is not sutured but heals by contraction and epithelialization. Second-intention healing is selected for wounds involving significant tissue loss. In horses, it is especially useful for wounds of the neck, body, and proximal limbs. Although these wounds are prepared with the same care as for primary closure and delayed primary closure, wounds of the extremities in horses are often left uncovered or managed with a pressure bandage or a cast. If left open to heal by second intention, the wound should be cleaned daily at first to remove accumulated exudate. Skin distal to the wound is also cleaned and protected with petroleum jelly or a similar product to prevent skin maceration ("serum burns").

Second-intention healing in horses

Wounds of the distal limbs of horses (carpus and distally) with large tissue deficits present a special problem, mainly the formation of excessive granulation tissue (Fig. 22-2). With newly formed moist granulation tissue protruding slightly above the skin edges, application of a corticosteroid-antibacterial combination ointment with an overlying pressure bandage can control granulation tissue growth. The topical corticosteroids seem to have little effect on wound healing and epithelialization at this early stage. If the granulation tissue is mature and protrudes well above the skin surface to form a fibrogranuloma, sharp excision is preferred. If excessive granulation tissue must be

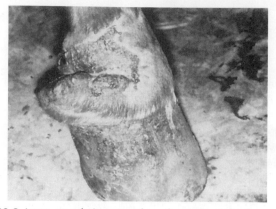

Fig. 22-2 Large granulating wound on the pastern of a horse. *(From Colahan PT et al:* Equine medicine and surgery, *ed 4, St Louis, 1991, Mosby.)*

excised with a scalpel, a pressure bandage is applied immediately after excision to control the considerable hemorrhage. Several hours after surgery, this bandage must be changed.

Topical application of caustics (e.g., silver nitrate or triple dye) and astringents can remove and prevent formation of granulation tissue by chemically destroying it. This destructive chemical action is indiscriminate, however, and also harms migrating epithelial cells. Often this prolongs healing and produces more scarring than sharp resection, bandaging, and casting. Large wounds of the distal extremities with skin deficits tend to heal very slowly due to reduced blood supply, increased movement, and excessive contamination. They heal by formation of scar tissue covered with a thin layer of easily damaged epithelial cells. Skin grafting is often recommended in these cases.

COVERING WOUNDS

Nature provides "natural bandages" as a part of normal healing. A partial-thickness wound that forms a blister rarely becomes infected and heals more rapidly if the blister is not broken. The scab of a full-thickness wound and the *eschar* (necrotic layer that sloughs off) of a burn also serve as natural bandages. The scab protects from external contamination, maintains internal homeostasis, and provides a surface beneath which cell migration and movement of skin edges occur. The eschar of large burn wounds serves as a biologic dressing that is protective and is considered by many surgeons superior to artificial bandaging materials.

Principles of Bandage Application

In veterinary application, bandages have the following functions:

- Protect wounds
- Hold clean or sterile dressings in place
- Absorb exudate and debride a wound
- Serve as a vehicle for therapeutic agents
- Serve as an indicator of wound secretions
- Pack the wound
- Provide support for bony anatomic structures
- Support and stabilize soft tissue
- Secure splints
- Prevent weight bearing
- Provide compression to control hemorrhage, dead space, and tissue edema
- Discourage self-grooming
- Restrict motion to eliminate stress of the wound edges
- Provide patient comfort
- Provide an aesthetic appearance

The basic principles of bandage application are as follows:

1. *Properly prepare the area before application of a bandage.* This may require clipping of the hair, wound debridement, and/or cleaning of surrounding skin.
2. *Use porous materials where possible.* This allows circulation of air and escape of excessive moisture.
3. *Use absorbent materials where exudates may be a problem.* Change absorbent dressings when they become saturated and before saturation is evident externally.
4. *Use appropriate materials of adequate width* to avoid producing a tourniquet effect.
5. *Apply bandage materials as smoothly as possible.* Ridges and lumps lead to skin irritation and necrosis.
6. *Secure protective wound pads to the skin* so that they do not shift from the site.
7. *Check bandages frequently* to determine if there is persistent swelling, skin discoloration, or coolness. A bandage applied too tightly can impair circulation, resulting in serious damage to soft tissues.
8. *Instruct clients on basic care of bandages and signs of bandage failure.* This includes the physical appearance of the bandage, as well as behavior of the patient.

Ideally, materials used for bandaging should have the following properties:

- Permeable to oxygen and other gases
- Conform to body contours
- Acceptable appearance
- Inert
- Long storage life
- Inexpensive
- Easily sterilized
- Unaffected by disinfecting and cleaning solutions
- Nonflammable
- Will not shred (so particles do not contaminate the wound)
- Compatible with topical therapeutic agents
- Will not adhere to the wound but can remove exudate and debris from the wound
- Maintains a moist wound surface that is free from exudate

Bandage Components

In most situations, bandages are generally composed of three layers, each with its own properties and function. The *primary layer* rests on the wound and may or may not be adherent. The *secondary layer* provides absorbency and padding. The *tertiary layer* is the outer layer that holds the underlying layers in place. This is usually the only layer the client sees. Clients often judge the quality of treatment solely on the appearance of this outer bandage layer.

Primary layer

The primary layer is in contact with the wound itself. When debridement is the goal, an adherent layer is used for the primary bandage. Once the wound is in the proliferation phase and granulation tissue has formed, use a nonadherent dressing to avoid disruption of the new tissue. The primary layer should be sterile and comfortable, allow fluids to pass to the secondary layer, protect the wound from exogenous contamination, and be nontoxic and nonirritating to tissue.

Adherent bandaging material, such as sterile gauze sponges with wide mesh openings and noncotton filler, can be used to provide debridement during the early stage of wound healing. This layer removes devitalized tissue and wound exudate when it is taken off during a bandage change. Adherent dressings may be wet or dry, depending on the nature of the wound. Some bandages are applied wet and then allowed to dry. Use of an adherent primary layer should be discontinued after the wound has been cleared of necrotic debris and heavy exudate.

If loose necrotic tissue or foreign material is present on the surface of the wound, a *dry-to-dry* dressing may be the best type to use. Dry gauze with a large mesh is placed directly on the wound. An absorbent layer is placed over this primary layer, and fluid is absorbed from the wound and allowed to dry. Necrotic material adheres to the gauze and is removed with the bandage. Although this type of bandage removes tissue debris, bandage removal is very painful and may also remove viable tissue. For this reason, dry-to-dry dressings should be used only when necessary.

If the exudate is especially viscous or if dried foreign matter must be removed, a *wet-to-dry* dressing may be appropriate. The bandage is applied wet, which dilutes the exudate for absorption. As the bandage dries, the foreign material adheres to the bandage and is later removed with the bandage. Solutions used to wet the primary layer include physiologic (0.9%) saline or a water-soluble bacteriostatic or bactericidal compound, such as 0.05% chlorhexidine diacetate solution (Nolvasan, Fort Dodge, Wilmington, Ohio).

For wounds with copious exudate or transudate, a *wet-to-dry* dressing may be best. Wet dressings absorb fluid more rapidly than dry dressings. They may be used to transport heat to a wound and/or enhance capillary action to promote wound drainage. A water-soluble bacteriostatic or bactericidal solution can be used to wet the dressing to help control microorganisms. The primary layer is applied wet and kept wet after the secondary and tertiary layers have been applied. This bandage is also removed wet. Wet-to-wet dressings cause less pain than dry dressings when removed; by using a warm solution, patient comfort is increased. A disadvantage is that these bandages tend to cause tissue maceration and have little debriding capacity.

A nonadherent primary layer is indicated during the reparative stage of wound healing, with formation of granulation tissue and production of a more serosanguineous exudate. In the early repair stage, petrolatum-impregnated products can be used in the presence of exudate and when little or no epithelialization has taken place. Later, when there is little fluid and during epithelialization, nonadherent dressings are indicated. Nonadherent dressings are used to cover lacerations, skin graft donor sites, minor burns, abrasions, and surgical incisions. The main goal is to minimize tissue injury upon removal. They do not absorb much fluid; draining wounds usually require a secondary dressing. Examples of nonadherent dressing materials include Adaptic (Johnson & Johnson), Release (Johnson & Johnson), and Telfa adhesive pads (Kendall/Curity). These semiocclusive, nonadherent materials leave the granulation bed undisturbed yet still move fluid away from the wound.

Secondary layer

The secondary (intermediate) layer provides support and moves exudate or transudate away from the wound. Materials used in this layer include gauze bandaging material (e.g., Sof-Band, Kling, Sof-Kling, Johnson & Johnson), cast padding, and bandaging cotton.

The secondary layer should be thick enough to absorb moisture, pad the wound from trauma, and inhibit wound movement. If the bandage allows evaporation of fluid from absorbed exudate, this partially dry environment retards bacterial growth. With wounds producing copious fluids, evaporation does not keep the bandage dry. If such a moist bandage is not changed frequently, the wound fluids serve as a growth medium for bacteria.

Tertiary layer

The tertiary (outer) layer holds the underlying bandage layers in place. Materials used in this layer include adhesive tapes (e.g., Zonas,® Johnson & Johnson), elastic bandages (Elastikon,® Johnson & Johnson, New Brunswick, N.J.; Vetrap,® 3M; Conform,® Kendall; Medi-Rip,® CoNco Medical), and conforming stretch gauze. This layer should be applied carefully to provide support without constricting.

Porous adhesive tape allows evaporation of fluid from the bandage. It can also allow movement of fluid (e.g., saliva, rainwater) into the wound, which may be undesirable. Waterproof adhesive tape repels water but also prevents evaporation. If the wound is producing considerable exudate, the tissues may become macerated from retained fluids. The resultant damp environment favors bacterial growth.

Elastic adhesive tape is compliant and applies continuous, dynamic pressure to the wound as the patient moves. Elastic tape products should be wrapped over the underlying bandage materials carefully to apply even but not excessive pressure. Elastic adhesive tapes tend to adhere to themselves, so minimal external taping is needed. Self-adherent products (e.g., Vetrap, MediRip) have no adhesive undercoat. Although these products tend to adhere to themselves, in veterinary practice, some external tape is usually required at the ends to keep the bandage from coming apart during movement.

ORTHOPEDIC BANDAGES AND SPLINTS

Robert Jones Compression Bandage

The Robert Jones compression bandage is illustrated in Fig. 22-3.

Indications

The Robert Jones bandage is generally used in large and small animals to temporarily immobilize fractures distal to the elbow or tarsus, support injured soft and bony tissues, and prevent excessive swelling. It may be modified to incorporate the thorax or pelvis to provide additional stabilization of more proximal limb fractures. It absorbs exudates, decreases or prevents edema and swelling through compression, and reduces (but does not totally inhibit) movement of fracture fragments. It is an excellent emergency treatment for distal limb injuries, reduces or prevents limb swelling postoperatively, and absorbs drainage before or after surgery. In horses, the Robert Jones bandage is used as an emergency method for treating fractures and tendon and ligament disruptions until repair can be made. It is used to immobilize a limb to protect from further damage through weight bearing or motion.

Materials

- 1-inch adhesive tape
- Dressing for primary layer if needed
- Cotton rolls (1 lb cotton/10 kg body weight in small animals)
- 4- to 8-inch Kling or roll gauze
- 4- to 8-inch elastic or Ace-type bandage

Technique

In small animals, suspend the limb vertically, if possible; this allows gravity to work. Dress any wounds; Telfa type of material is preferred. Apply porous tape stirrups, extending

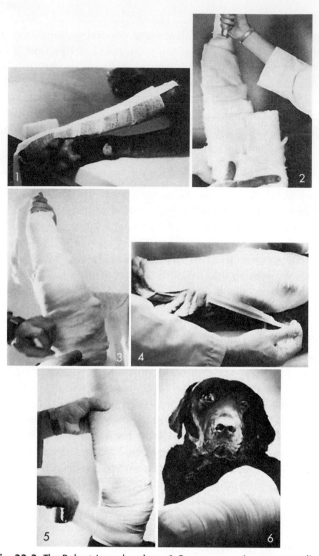

Fig. 22-3 The Robert Jones bandage. *1,* Porous tape stirrups are applied to the dorsal and palmar aspects of the leg, extending from the elbow or knee to well beyond the toes. A layer of stretch Sof-Kling® is applied over the stirrups. *2,* With the limb suspended, roll cotton is applied, beginning at the foot and moving proximally up the limb to the axilla or groin, overlapping each pass. *3,* Wide Sof-Kling® is stretched as tightly as possible over the cotton, overlapping each pass. *4,* Each stirrup is reflected proximally. *5,* Elastikon® tape is applied, starting at the foot and working proximally, stretching the tape as tightly as possible. *6,* The completed bandage should be firm. *(Courtesy Mallinckrodt Veterinary.)*

to the elbow or knee and considerably past the toes. Apply a snug layer of Sof-Kling to prevent slippage. Unroll cotton to remove the separation paper, then reroll before application. Apply cotton to the limb, starting at the foot and extending to the groin or axilla, overlapping one quarter to one half the width of the roll. An assistant should hold the limb in extreme abduction to facilitate this process. Wrap the cotton as tightly as possible, with no wrinkles or twists. The object is to make the limb into a straight cylinder.

Wrap the cotton with Kling or Sof-Kling gauze as tightly as possible, again overlapping half the width of the roll. Separate the tape stirrups to the sides of the bulky bandage. This provides a small opening to assess blood flow to the toes. Apply self-adherent elastic adhesive tape, an Ace-type bandage, or vet-wrap type material, starting at the toes and working proximally, overlapping by about half the width. The completed bandage should be very firm and should produce a sound similar to a ripe watermelon when thumped.

Stirrups are not used in horses. Apply rolls of cotton to the limb, from the distal limb proximally, in gradual spirals to the proximal forearm. The proximal edge of the bandage should extend as far proximally as possible. It is most important to start the bandage on the inside of the leg. If started on the back, it may damage the tendon. Apply five to eight consecutive rolls of cotton with firm pressure. When the final layer has been applied, the bandage should be of even thickness throughout its length. Secure the bandage in place with one or two layers of 6-inch gauze. The tertiary layer consists of an elastic bandage covered with a 4-inch elastic adhesive tape and or vet-wrap material as the final wrap. Apply the elastic adhesive tape, overlapping by about half, in several layers, depending on the strength and durability of the bandage desired. Then apply the adhesive bandage layer. This bandage requires six to eight rolls of Ace elastic bandage, six or seven rolls of Elastikon, four to six rolls of Sof-Kling, Kling or other conforming bandage, and a roll of porous tape to secure the ends of each roll of Ace elastic bandage used.

Precautions

The Robert Jones bandage may act as a heavy pendulum if used for injuries proximal to the elbow or stifle unless modified. It should never be used as a definitive fracture treatment for any type of fracture.

Soft Padded and Coaptation Bandages

Indications

These bandages include the Schanz soft padded bandage, the Mesa-Meta Splint, the coaptation bandage made with a thermoplastic splint (Orthoplast, Johnson & Johnson), fiberglass strips (C-Splint, Johnson & Johnson), or other casting materials. The Schanz soft padded bandage is the most commonly used limb bandage. It is designed to cover abrasions and lacerations, and to provide light support following long bone or joint surgery.

Materials

- Wound dressing for the primary layer
- 2-inch porous adhesive tape
- Kling
- Splint of appropriate size (width, curvature, length)

- Cast padding or soft bandage (e.g., Sof-Band bulky bandage)
- Elastic self-adherent tertiary layer (e.g., Elastikon, Vetrap)

Technique

Apply a primary dressing to the wound area. Form stirrups of porous tape to prevent bandage slippage. Apply the stirrups on the medial and lateral surfaces of the limb, leaving a tab on the distal end, if possible, to be pulled apart later. Apply cast padding snugly to the limb, starting at the foot and moving proximally, overlapping one-quarter to one-half the roll width, to a point proximal to the elbow joint. Apply a layer of Sof-Kling or other conforming bandage in the same manner. Separate the tape stirrups and attach them to their respective sides. Apply adherent elastic bandage tape, being careful not to pull the tape too tightly. Pulling the tape to its elastic limits can compromise the circulation of the limb. Leave the toes exposed to allow assessment of circulation.

The soft padded bandage may be modified to provide additional support of a limb by incorporating splint materials. The resultant bandages can support the limb distally to the elbow or hock. They are generally used to provide additional support for fractures or other orthopedic injuries after surgical intervention. For some types of fractures, they may be used as the primary means of stabilization.

Precautions

Bandages in this category should not be used for fractures near the elbow or tibiotarsal joint, severely comminuted or collapsing fractures, or as definitive treatment for ligament or tendon ruptures.

Spica Splint

The spica splint is a semirigid splint bandage. It is usually brought over the trunk to immobilize the elbow or shoulder. It is made from casting material or a thermoplastic splint fitted to the lateral portion of the limb, incorporated into a padded bandage, and fixed to the limb with conforming gauze and surgical porous or elastic adherent tape.

Schroeder-Thomas Splint

The Schroeder-Thomas splint is an external weight-bearing device. It is best used for closed fractures of the radius/ulna or tibia/fibula in young dogs. These fractures heal rapidly with moderate stabilization. It is also of value in elbow dislocations, because the elbow can be held in position following reduction. Fractures proximal to the elbow or stifle are better repaired by internal fixation than with the Schroeder-Thomas splint. After surgical bone or joint repair, this device can provide additional stabilization and restrict movement of the limb. It is best if the aluminum splint rod is custom made for each individual patient.

Ehmer Sling

The Ehmer Sling is illustrated in Fig. 22-4.

Indications

An Ehmer sling is applied after reduction of hip luxation. It maintains the hip joint in flexion, abduction, and internal rotation; the sling provides limited abduction. The Ehmer sling helps keep the femoral head deeply seated within the acetabulum by internally rotating and abducting the hip.

Materials

- 4-inch Elastikon
- 2-inch nonporous adhesive tape

Technique

The traditional Ehmer sling is based on a modified figure-8 bandage. First wrap cast padding around the metatarsal area. Then cover it with elastic adherent tape (Elastikon). Manually flex the stifle, trying to keep the femur rotated slightly inwards. Continue the Elastikon from the metatarsal region passing it medial to the stifle. Pass the tape over the stifle and medially, to the hock, creating a figure-8 pattern. Repeat several times. Cover the limb completely with several more wraps of tape. Abduct the limb by then passing the Elastikon dorsally over the back and fully around the body, incorporating the knee into the wrap. A towel may be used just above the leg on the abdomen to decrease the chances of swelling and rubbing of the bandage. Then cover the whole bandage with white tape. Monitor for swelling resulting from impaired circulation.

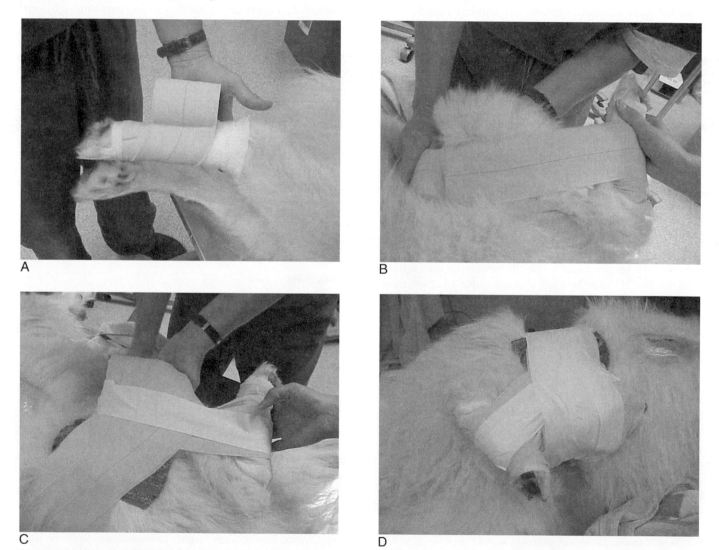

Fig. 22-4 Application of Ehmer Sling. **A,** Cast padding is first wrapped around the metatarsal region and then covered with Elastikon® tape. **B,** The leg is flexed, and the Elastikon® is then continued around the whole leg in a figure-8 pattern. **C,** The wrap is extended around the abdomen (with a towel inserted in this picture) and then covered with white (nonelastic) tape. **D,** The finished product is shown.

Modified Ehmer Sling

Indications

The modified version maintains hip flexion and abduction but no internal rotation. The modified Ehmer sling can be adjusted to ensure abduction and relieve swelling by simply cutting the tape, repositioning it, and retaping. These adjustments cannot be made easily with the traditional Ehmer sling.

Materials

- 4-inch Elastikon
- 2-inch nonporous adhesive tape

Technique

Place the elastic wrap around the metatarsals, from medial to lateral, without encircling the limb, and adhere the tape to itself. Carry the tape dorsally and cranially to encircle the trunk at the level of the caudal thorax, and anchor it to the body around the caudal ribs. This location avoids compression of the abdomen and avoids the prepuce in male dogs. Applying tension to the wrap before encircling the trunk provides both hip joint flexion and abduction. Before encircling the trunk, pull the skin from the dorsal back toward the affected limb to prevent the limb from dropping into an abducted position. Once the elastic wrap is secured, apply 2-inch waterproof tape, covering the elastic wrap and eliminating any stretch of the elastic material. Apply the waterproof tape, fanning outward from the metatarsal area to the trunk. This ensures that the stifle joint remains covered and medial to the bandage.

Velpeau Sling

Indications

The Velpeau sling prevents weight bearing on the forelimb by cradling the forelimb against the shoulder and chest wall. It is indicated for scapular fractures not requiring open reduction and internal fixation, postoperative splintage of scapular fractures and shoulder dislocations, and ligament and joint capsule injuries of the shoulder joint.

Materials

- 6-inch Kling gauze, Elastikon, Ace bandage, or Vetrap

Technique

Slightly flex the carpus and metacarpus to a comfortable position and wrap them. Comfortably flex the antebrachium across the cranial chest wall (with paw pointing toward the opposite scapulohumeral joint). Apply additional wraps around the chest and flexed limb. This bandage is well tolerated for prolonged periods.

Precautions

The Velpeau sling should not be used in patients with internal or external thoracic trauma or disease; respiratory compromise; limbs with swelling, edema, or cellulitis; lateral luxation of the scapulohumeral joint; scapular neck fractures; or fractures involving the scapulohumeral joint.

CASTS

Indications

Casts are simple and very effective devices for providing support for some fractures in companion animals. Indications include external fixation of noncollapsing fractures of the radius, ulna, tibia, metacarpals, and digits; as an adjunct to internal fixation, including arthrodesis; immobilization of a limb after tendon repair or surgery; protection from self-mutilation; and restriction of motion after plastic or reconstructive surgery.

Bending forces, primarily transmitted perpendicularly to the long axis of a bone, are well neutralized by a cast. Rotational, compressive, shearing, and tensile forces transmitted parallel to the long axis of a bone are poorly neutralized by a cast. Incomplete or minimally displaced, transverse, or short oblique diaphyseal fractures of the radius/ulna and tibia/fibula, especially in younger animals, are ideally suited for cast fixation.

Materials

For many years, plaster was the only cast material available. Disadvantages of plaster casts included heavy weight, permeability to water, and susceptibility to breakage and mutilation.

Fiberglass casting material is now widely used because of its light weight, rigidity, ventilation, and waterproof characteristics. In small animals, fiberglass casts are highly effective for external fracture fixation and as an adjunct to internal fixation techniques (e.g., pinning, plating). Equine practitioners use fiberglass casts to protect heel bulb and flexor tendon lacerations, protect granulation tissue beds in wounds, and treat laminitis. Casts are also used after surgical fracture repair and in management of midbody sesamoid fractures following a bone graft, by keeping the leg in a flexed position. In neonatal calves, fiberglass casts have proven to be of value for external fixation of forelimb fractures caused by assisted deliveries in dystocia.

Technique

Proper application of a fiberglass cast requires practice and experience (Fig. 22-5). Patient movement during application can create pressure points. General anesthesia is required for cast application. The skin of the affected area should be clean and dry before casting. If a hoof is to be

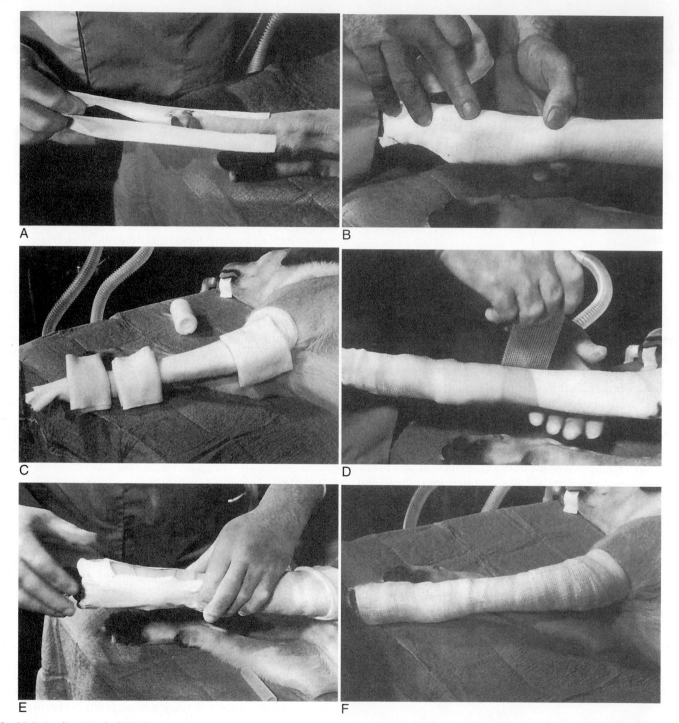

Fig. 22-5 Application of a fiberglass cast. **A,** Stirrups of porous taper applied to the dorsal and palmar aspects of the limb, extending well beyond the toes. **B,** A stockinette is applied over the limb, with excess material at the proximal and distal ends. **C,** Padding material is applied to cover bony protuberances. **D,** After the rolled fiberglass casting material has been soaked in warm water and excess water squeezed out, the material is rolled onto the limb, beginning at the toes and working proximally, overlapping each pass. **E,** The stockinette ends and the tape stirrups are reflected onto the limb and are incorporated into the cast by two or three more overlying layers of fiberglass. **F,** The completed cast can be molded by hand during the last few minutes before setting. *(Courtesy Mallinckrodt Veterinary.)*

covered with fiberglass casting material, it should be cleaned and disinfected to prevent foot rot and thrush. Surgical incisions, lacerations, or wounds should be debrided and, if indicated, sutured and covered with a sterile nonadherent primary dressing. Cast padding should be kept to a minimum and applied only at pressure points. Cast padding is used infrequently in equine and bovine patients.

The cast should be of sufficient length to immobilize the joints proximal and distal to the lesion. Assistants should be advised to use the flat portion of the hand to support the limb during cast application to prevent indentations that may cause pressure sores. Any sharp edges at proximal and distal ends of the cast should be well padded. For horses and cattle, tape should be placed around the proximal rim of the cast to prevent foreign material from entering between cast and skin. If horses or cattle are to be kept outside after casting, the hoof should be covered with a rubber boot to prevent excessive moisture from entering the cast. Clients must be instructed about observing the cast, cast care, adverse clinical signs, and limiting the patient's activity.

Maintaining Bandages, Splints, and Casts

A trained staff member should examine every bandage, splint, cast, or orthopedic appliance every 6 to 8 hours during the first day after application. The device should be removed immediately if evidence of constriction is detected.

Home Care of Bandages

It is important to involve clients in wound management, especially for outpatients. Clients play a significant role in detection of adverse conditions affecting the bandage. Many problems can be avoided by taking the time to instruct clients on care of the bandage, splint, or cast placed on their animal. An information sheet with home care instructions is often helpful (e.g., Erlewein and Kuhns: *Instructions for veterinary clients*, St Louis, 1996, Mosby). However, an instruction sheet cannot replace face-to-face communication between the client and veterinary staff. Before leaving the clinic, the client must be shown how to check the bandage or orthopedic appliance. It is often a good idea to telephone the client the next day to inquire about any problems.

Bandage, Cast, and Splint Removal

To remove the bandages, it is often easiest and safest to carefully cut the outer layer with scissors or a scalpel blade and then tear the cotton material from distal to proximal along the lateral aspect of the extremity, rather than trying to cut the cotton with bandage scissors. Casts are typically removed with an oscillating saw (e.g., Stryker). Splints can be removed with bandage scissors. With bandages or casts around any body part, be sure to determine the exact location of underlying structures before cutting the bandage. It is very easy to cut off the tip of an ear, toe, foot pad, or the tail if the area is not identified before cutting.

MANAGEMENT OF SPECIFIC WOUND TYPES

Penetrating Wounds

Gunshot wounds

High-velocity rifles and the more powerful handguns generate tremendous explosive kinetic energy that can shatter bone, cause massive tissue destruction, and propel fragments of metal and bone into surrounding soft tissue. High-velocity projectiles also destroy tissue by shock waves or cavitation. Large exit wounds are common. Treatment of high-velocity missile wounds generally requires extensive debridement that creates a considerable tissue defect. This prolongs the healing time and usually requires more elaborate reconstructive procedures than low-velocity wounds.

Bullets from most handguns are considered low-velocity projectiles; however, they can inflict serious injuries at close range. Handgun bullets produce an entry wound, with or without an exit wound. As these missiles travel through tissues, they create a tract via crushing and laceration, damaging only tissues contacted by the projectile. When these wounds are confined to soft tissues, they may require little or no exploration or debridement, unless vital or important structures are involved. The tract is considered contaminated by bacteria. Clipping of hair around the wound, local wound cleaning, lavage, and application of topical dressings may suffice. Easily accessible projectiles may be removed. Retention of projectiles in the hypodermis, fascia, or muscle poses little health threat to the patient. If perforation or penetration involves the abdomen, surgical exploration is required. Missile fragments in joints should be removed.

Shotguns fire multiple small pellets or a single large slug. At close range, shotguns are among the most lethal and traumatic of weapons, causing massive tissue destruction. At extremely close range, the wadding of the explosive charge may be driven into the tissues.

Arrow wounds

Broad-head arrows, used for hunting, have razor-sharp blades to lacerate vessels and vascular visceral tissues. Field-point arrows, usually used for target practice, have a rounded point about the size of the arrow shaft. They can penetrate deeply but do not lacerate tissues like broad-head hunting arrows.

Deeply embedded arrows, especially broad-heads, are best removed surgically by the veterinarian, not the client. Clients may cut short arrow shafts with a bolt cutter to transport the patient to the veterinary facility. The client should be discouraged from pulling the arrow out before transport to the clinic. The shaft end of some arrows is threaded for changing heads. If the arrow's head is accessible to the clinician, it can be grasped with a forceps and unthreaded from the shaft to facilitate removal.

Thorough examination is essential to identification and management of injuries caused by projectiles. This includes radiographs of the involved body region. Abdominal cavity wounds require surgical exploration to prevent bacterial peritonitis resulting from perforation of the bowel. Penetrating thoracic wounds generally do not require exploration unless there is significant hemorrhage, pneumothorax, or esophageal involvement.

Snakebites

Treatment of snakebites is directed toward preventing and controlling shock, neutralizing venom, minimizing necrosis, and preventing secondary infection. Fatal snakebites are more common in dogs than in any other domestic animal. Dogs are typically bitten in the head region. Because of their size, horses and cattle rarely die from snakebites; however, swelling on the muzzle, head, or neck can produce dyspnea and then death. Domestic animals vary in their sensitivity to the venom of pit vipers.

In North America, venomous snakes of the Crotalidae group, sometimes listed as a subfamily of Viperidae, are most commonly encountered in bite cases. These include the copperhead, cottonmouth, and rattlesnake. Clients should be instructed to bring the *dead* snake along with the bitten animal when possible, without mutilating the snake's head, because it may be needed for identification.

Systemic effects of envenomation include hypotension, shock, lethargy, salivation, lymph node pain, weakness, muscle fasciculations, and possible respiratory depression. Venomous snakebites often produce tissue necrosis and require reconstructive surgery. Tissue damage varies with the depth of bite and amount of venom injected. Local signs include fang puncture wounds (one or two), bleeding, swelling, tissue discoloration, and pain. The severity of envenomation cannot be judged by local signs alone.

Diphenhydramine hydrochloride (Benadryl, Parke-Davis) is often given as a pretreatment (10 mg for small dogs and cats, 25 mg for large dogs). After an intravenous catheter has been placed and fluid administration (lactated Ringer's solution, physiologic saline, colloids) has commenced, give half the dose subcutaneously and the remainder intravenously.

Antivenin (polyvalent for Crotalidae, Fort Dodge Laboratories) should be given, as soon as possible, according to package insert recommendations. Antivenin can prevent systemic reactions and limit tissue necrosis. Although antivenin is expensive, it helps prevent large necrotic sloughs and may reduce costs associated with reconstructive surgery.

Necrotic snakebite wounds should be managed as an open infected wound during sloughing. Broad-spectrum antibacterial therapy is warranted to help prevent wound infection; tetanus antitoxin should be given. When sloughing is complete and healthy granulation tissue has formed, the wound should be assessed for possible reconstruction, grafting, or management as an open wound.

Burns

Thermal burns

Thermal burns caused by exposure to excessive heat are classified according to their depth. First-degree burns are superficial and involve only the epidermis. Except in pigs, first-degree burns in animals do not form vesicles or blisters, as commonly seen in humans. Third-degree burns destroy the full thickness of the skin. They form a dark brown, insensitive, leathery covering called an *eschar*. Second-degree burns fall between these two classifications.

Burn patients may be sedated to relieve pain and provide restraint if cardiovascular function is stable. Fluid therapy with a balanced electrolyte solution or lactated Ringer's solution should be used to treat shock associated with burns.

If started soon after injury, application of ice/cold water compresses or submersion in ice water may relieve pain and arrest progression of the burn. Hair should be clipped or removed from the burned surface and the area washed gently with a detergent antiseptic. The antiprostaglandin effects of topical aloe vera products may reduce the severity of burns.

Burns should be carefully debrided. In first-degree and second-degree burns, cleaning the burn may constitute debridement. A third-degree eschar may retain infection under it and prevent wound contraction. As the eschar separates from underlying tissue during healing, it should be removed with scissors. This is painful, and the patient's pain tolerance should be considered. After the eschar has been removed from second-degree and third-degree burns, topical antibacterial medication (e.g., silver sulfadiazine or bacitracin cream) and light bandages are applied. Bandages are changed at least twice daily. Occlusive dressings and ointments are usually contraindicated. The prognosis depends on the total area of the burn, depth of penetration, location, and age and condition of the patient.

Electrical burns

Electrical burns occur most often when animals chew on electrical cords. The most common signs are tissue damage with necrosis, cardiac dysrhythmias, and acute pulmonary edema. Often, there is charring of tissue at the point of contact (e.g., lips or mouth). Because the electrical current may flow along blood vessels to tissues, ischemic demarcation and sloughing often occur two or three weeks later. Managing lip and mouth injuries associated with electrical burns requires debridement and possibly reconstructive surgery.

Chemical burns

Chemical burns cause denaturation and coagulation of tissue protein. They often produce hard and soft eschars, with underlying ulcers. They may also be deeper and more extensive than they initially appear. Chemical burns are managed in much the same manner as thermal burns, with reconstruction or open wound healing.

Bite wounds

Bite wounds usually appear as punctures, lacerations, or avulsions of skin flaps. Massive subcutaneous and muscle contamination, maceration, dead space, serum accumulation, and infection leading to abscess formation (especially in cats) may develop in underlying tissues. Bite wounds in cats commonly form abscesses and draining sinuses. These should be surgically explored, lavaged, and initially managed as a dirty wound. Systemic antibacterials should be used in bite wound patients.

Decubital Ulcers

Decubital ulcers ("pressure sores") are open wounds that develop over bony prominences as a result of pressure in patients recumbent for long periods. Pressure sores can also develop over bony prominences covered by a cast or bandage as a result of insufficient or loose padding or overly tight application of the cast or bandage.

Decubital ulcers should be cleaned thoroughly with a surgical scrub and debrided when necessary.

Following cleaning, the area should be completely dried. Astringents (e.g., Burrow's solution) can be used to help dry the lesion. The decubital ulcer should be padded to prevent further pressure injury by use of a soft padded bandage held in the shape of a donut, with the ulcer in the center. These protective bandages leave the ulcer open to the air and relieve pressure. Use of antibacterial agents may be considered; however, decubital ulcers heal best if kept clean and dry.

In recumbent patients, decubital ulcers can be prevented using the following measures:

- Provide sufficient soft padding or bedding material. This can include water pads, air mattresses, artificial fleece, rubber grids, straw, and towels. The material should be disposable or washable.
- Change the patient's position frequently. Turn the patient from side to side. Intermittent use of slings or carts may be considered.
- Periodically check the skin over bony prominences for signs of ulcer formation. These include hyperemia, moisture, and easily epilated hair.
- Keep the skin clean and dry. Bathe the patient frequently.
- Provide a well-balanced, high-protein diet.
- Apply casts and bandages correctly. Safeguard bony prominences with adequate padding.

RECOMMENDED READING

Bojrab MJ: *A handbook on veterinary wound management*, Ashland, Ohio, 1994, KenVet.

Fossum TW: *Small animal surgery*, ed 2, St Louis, 2002, Mosby.

Gfeller RW, Crowe DT: Emergency care of traumatic wounds, *Vet Clin North Am Small Anim Prac* 24:1249-1274, 1994.

Pavletic MM: The clinician's guide to basic wound management, *Proc North Am Vet Conf* 1996, pp 512-513.

Stashak TS: *Equine wound management*, Philadelphia, 1991, Lea & Febiger.

Swaim SF, Henderson RA: *Small animal wound management*, ed 2, Philadelphia, 1997, Lippincott, Williams and Wilkins.

23

Fluid Therapy and Blood Transfusions

Donna A. Oakley

Learning Objectives

After reviewing this chapter, the reader should understand the following:

- Fluid distribution in the body
- Methods of assessing hydration status
- Indications for fluid therapy
- Types of fluids used in fluid therapy
- Methods of assessing bleeding patients
- Types of blood products used in transfusion medicine
- Blood groups of dogs and cats
- Techniques used in blood collection, crossmatching, and transfusion
- Signs of adverse reactions to blood transfusion

FLUID THERAPY

Fluid therapy is one of the most commonly used supportive measures in veterinary medicine and is an important aspect of virtually every critical care case. It is primarily used to correct fluid deficits, electrolyte disturbances, and acid-base imbalances. In order to understand the need and value of fluid support, and to recognize and manage patients with fluid and electrolyte disorders, one must have a basic understanding of the physiology of fluid balance.

Fluid Distribution

Approximately 60% of the body is composed of fluid, often referred to as *total body water (TBW)*. Three major fluid compartments make up TBW: intracellular fluid within the cells; interstitial fluid between the cells; and intravascular fluid, or plasma, within the blood vessels. About two thirds of TBW is intracellular fluid *(ICF)*. The remaining third, called extracellular fluid *(ECF)*, is composed of interstitial fluid (75%) and plasma (25%) (Fig. 23-1). Some extracellular fluids can collect in various parts of the body secondary to infection, injury, or compromised circulation. These fluids, referred to as third-space fluids, have no functional use (e.g., pleural effusions [fluid between lung pleura], pericardial effusions [fluid within the pericardial sac], ascites [fluid within peritoneal cavity], and generalized edema).

The ECF is in constant motion throughout the body. It allows the nutrients, oxygen, and electrolytes necessary for the maintenance of cellular life to reach cells, and removes waste products as well. These regulatory functions performed by the body contribute to the maintenance of a consistent internal environment, referred to as *homeostasis*.

The chemical composition of the ECF and the ICF is very different, and these differences are extremely important to the life and function of each cell, as well as the regulation of all body systems. Water and electrolytes continually move in and out of cells working in concert to maintain water balance. The process of the movement of water across a cell membrane is called *osmosis*. When the concentration of solutes is greater on one side of the membrane than the other, water moves through the membrane toward the side with a greater concentration. How much and how quickly this movement occurs is dependent on the composition of the solutes in solution and the permeability characteristics of the membrane between the two compartments. A certain amount of pressure is required to stop this process completely and is referred to as the *osmotic pressure*. The concentration of these osmotically active particles (e.g., sodium, potassium) in solution is called *osmolality*. The normal serum osmolality in the dog and the cat is approximately 300 mOsm/kg.

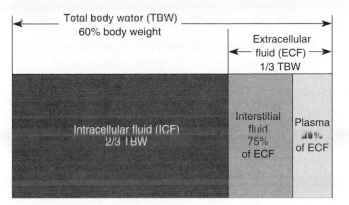

Fig. 23-1 Fluid compartments of the body. (Adapted from Vander: *Human physiology: the mechanisms of body function*, ed 4, New York, 1985, McGraw-Hill.)

Electrolytes

Electrolytes are active chemicals or elements within all body fluids, each playing a role in the maintenance of normal body functions. Many organs are involved in the homeostatic mechanisms that maintain electrolyte balance. In the clinical setting, electrolyte balance refers to the maintenance of normal serum concentrations. Measuring the concentration of electrolytes in the ICF is difficult; therefore, measuring serum concentrations (i.e., ECF) is used to assess and manage patients with imbalances.

The major extracellular electrolytes are sodium, chloride, and bicarbonate. Sodium is the most abundant and important of the extracellular ions in that the distribution of body water is influenced by sodium more than by any other electrolyte. Because sodium attracts water, it is the primary factor responsible for determining extracellular fluid volume and osmotic pressure. Maintaining a balance of sodium intake and excretion (via the kidney) is critical in controlling ECF volume.

Low extracellular sodium concentration creates a low osmolality and will therefore cause an influx of water into cells. Clinical signs associated with low sodium levels, or *hyponatremia*, are usually neurologic in origin and include generalized muscular weakness, lethargy or mental depression, nausea, inappetence, and hypotension. *Hypernatremia*, or sodium excess, can be seen as a result of water loss (dehydration). This is associated with an osmotic movement of water out of cells. The clinical signs are also primarily neurologic and include excessive thirst, muscle weakness, disorientation, seizures, and possible coma. Hypernatremia is a less frequently encountered condition.

The major intracellular electrolytes are potassium, magnesium, and phosphorous. ICF also contains sodium but in much smaller amounts than outside the cell. Potassium is the dominant intracellular ion and is responsible for osmotic pressure within the ICF. It plays an important role in normal cell metabolism and is necessary for the maintenance of several body functions, most importantly the generation of

electrical potentials in muscles and nerves. Relatively small changes in serum potassium concentration can alter nervous and cardiac functions; therefore, serum potassium levels must be maintained within very close limits.

Abnormal serum potassium concentrations occur frequently in animals with fluid disturbances. *Hypokalemia*, or low serum potassium, is the most frequently encountered potassium abnormality and usually requires supplementation in hospitalized patients. Causes include decreased intake (e.g., anorexia or restricted diet), excessive loss (e.g., gastrointestinal, urinary, or third space loss), and movement from extracellular fluid to intracellular fluid (e.g., with alkalosis). The distribution of potassium between ECF and ICF can be affected by serum pH. Animals experiencing an increase in pH (alkalosis) may become hypokalemic due to potassium being driven into the cells.

When serum levels begin to drop, potassium will leave the cells to increase the serum concentration. Serum potassium will therefore decrease only after a considerable loss of total body potassium. Since we can only measure serum potassium, it is difficult to accurately assess total body deficits. Many animals with hypokalemia have no clinical signs unless depletion is severe. Muscle weakness, polyuria, and polydipsia can be seen in some patients. Also, potassium depletion can impair insulin release, ultimately affecting glucose levels.

Hyperkalemia, or high serum potassium concentration, is less commonly encountered than hypokalemia, but can be life-threatening. Potassium is normally excreted by the kidney; therefore, hyperkalemia is often encountered in animals where renal excretion is impaired. Hyperkalemia is most commonly seen with urethral obstruction in cats, but also with anuric or oliguric renal failure, Addison's disease, or excess potassium delivery during IV fluid therapy. Given that serum potassium levels are inversely related to serum pH, animals experiencing a decrease in pH (acidosis) may become hyperkalemic due to potassium being driven out of cells. Clinical signs of hyperkalemia include classic ECG changes representing a weakness in myocardial contractility and bradycardia.

Acid-Base Balance

Acid-base balance is the regulation of hydrogen ion concentration in body fluid. The slightest change in the concentration of this ion can cause marked alterations in chemical reactions in the cells. Because of this, regulation of hydrogen is one of the most important aspects of homeostasis.

Hydrogen ion concentration is expressed as pH. A low pH corresponds with a high hydrogen ion concentration and is referred to as *acidosis*. A high pH corresponds with a low hydrogen ion concentration and is referred to as *alkalosis*. The normal pH of arterial blood is 7.4; the pH of venous blood and interstitial fluid is approximately 7.35. The body must maintain the slightly alkaline pH of blood within this range as major complications in life support can occur if the pH falls below 7.2 or rises above 7.6 for more than a few hours.

The three primary systems that help control acid-base balance are blood buffers, lungs, and kidneys. These systems will be utilized based on the severity of the impending acidosis or alkalosis. Within seconds of any change in hydrogen ion concentration, buffer systems within all body fluids will bind with any acid or alkali. Secondly, if the hydrogen ion concentration increases, the respiratory center is stimulated to increase the respiratory rate. With an increase in respiration, there comes an increase in the amount of carbon dioxide removed from the body. This process will ultimately help to return the hydrogen ion concentration to normal. This system requires more time (approximately 10 minutes) than the buffer system in readjusting these levels. The most powerful regulatory system, the kidneys, requires up to several days to readjust the concentration of hydrogen. The kidneys achieve regulation by readjusting the pH of the urine, and thereby readjusting the pH of body fluid.

CLINICAL ASPECTS OF FLUID THERAPY

Determining the Need for Fluid Therapy

Determining the need for fluid administration requires assessment of the patient's state of hydration (Table 23-1)

TABLE 23-1

Clinical Estimation of Degree of Dehydration

Degree of Dehydration	Clinical Signs
< 5%	Not clinically detectable
5% to 6%	Subtle loss of skin elasticity
6% to 8%	Obvious delay in return of tented skin to normal position
	Slightly prolonged capillary refill time
	Eyes possibly sunken in orbits
	Possibly dry mucous membranes
10% to 12%	Skin remains tented
	Very prolonged capillary refill time
	Eyes sunken in orbits
	Dry mucous membranes
	Possibly signs of shock (tachycardia, cool extremities, rapid, weak pulse)
12% to 15%	Obvious signs of shock
	Death imminent

From Muir WW, DiBartola SP: *Fluid therapy.* In Kirk RW: *Current veterinary therapy VIII,* Philadelphia, 1983, WB Saunders.

and estimation of fluid deficits through subjective patient evaluation. Formulation of a fluid therapy regimen is based on information gathered from an accurate history, a thorough physical examination, and laboratory tests.

History

A complete history helps to establish the presence of fluid deficits (dehydration and/or hypovolemia). The history should include information on the patient's food and water intake (i.e., polydipsia, anorexia), routinely and currently. Any information regarding urination (i.e., polyuria), defecation (including diarrhea), and vomiting is useful. Ensure that there is no history of trauma or evidence of hemorrhage. To help assess the degree of dehydration, consider exposure to extreme environmental heat, excessive exercise, fever, panting, and the period over which losses have occurred, including the amount and frequency of fluid losses. Information pertaining to medication the animal has been or is currently taking can be useful. Some medications can have potentially harmful or complicating side effects.

Physical examination

A complete physical examination can help define the avenue of fluid loss. Dehydration and hypoperfusion are the most frequently encountered conditions; however, not all dehydrated patients are hypovolemic, and not all hypovolemic patients are dehydrated. Animals should be assessed for signs that will help determine which of these processes or combination thereof is in progress.

Certain physical signs can help estimate hydration status, including dry, tacky mucous membranes, skin turgor, position of the eye in the orbit, body temperature, evidence of decreased peripheral circulation (e.g., poor pulse quality), and changes in body weight (see Table 23-1).

The cardiovascular and respiratory system should be carefully evaluated. Assessment of perfusion is based on mucous membrane color, capillary refill time, heart rate, and pulse rate, pulse strength, and pulse character. Most of these assessments are subjective. For this reason, monitoring is more accurate when serial examinations are performed consistently by an experienced member of the health care team and results are monitored in relation to one another.

Normal mucous membranes are pink and moist to the touch but can range in color from pale to cyanotic to muddy or injected. Dry oral mucous membranes may result from panting and should be evaluated in addition to other values or mucous membranes. The degree of dehydration in patients that are vomiting and salivating can be underestimated if one relies solely on mucous membrane assessment.

Capillary refill time (CRT) provides an indication of peripheral perfusion. Pressure is applied to the pink mucosa of the gum or the inner lip and then released. The time required for the blanched area to return to pink should he 1 to 2 seconds. Prolonged refill time is suggestive of compromised tissue perfusion and shock. Rapid refill time of less than 1 second is usually associated with tachycardia as a result of the heart's attempt to increase cardiac output in compensating for hypovolemia.

Pulse rate and intensity provide information regarding heart rate and perfusion pressure. Technicians should become proficient at assessment, accurate interpretation, and monitoring of pulse intensity. Most easily accessible and palpable are the femoral, dorsal metatarsal, and ulnar arteries. A skilled technician can learn to use pulse pressure in estimating blood pressure when more advanced equipment is not available.

The heart and lungs should be auscultated before the onset of fluid therapy and frequently throughout treatment. Cardiac auscultation allows detection of heart murmurs and arrhythmias. Palpation of a peripheral pulse while auscultating the heart helps detect pulse deficits. If a compromise in cardiac function is suspected, the approach to fluid therapy may require adjustment. On pulmonary auscultation, crackling sounds indicate fluid accumulation in the alveoli or bronchioles, suggesting edema or overhydration. Wheezing sounds are usually a result of some degree of airway obstruction. When wheezing sounds are detected during auscultation, the stethoscope should always be placed over the trachea to determine whether the same sounds can be heard in this area as those heard over the lung fields. If present, the sounds most likely can be classified as referred upper respiratory noise. Conversely, absence of lung sounds is abnormal and may suggest consolidation of lung tissue, as in pneumonia. The depth of respiration, along with the rate and effort, should also be noted.

Skin turgor is not the most accurate way to detect or estimate dehydration. In addition to tissue hydration, it is affected by the amount of subcutaneous fat and elastic tissue present. The most commonly tested area is over the trunk; avoiding the loose skin of the neck region and the top of the head. The skin is lifted a short distance (tented) and then released, monitoring its return to the initial position. Normal skin returns to its position immediately. The skin of dehydrated animals may show varying degrees of slow return to the initial position. The skin turgor of obese animals may appear normal despite dehydration due to excessive stores of subcutaneous fat. Likewise, the skin of emaciated animals lacks subcutaneous fat and elastic tissue and, therefore, may lead to an overestimation of dehydration.

Obtaining the patient's body weight is an important aspect of the physical exam. An acute decrease in body weight is expected in animals that experience some type of water loss. Dehydration can be more accurately assessed if the patient's current body weight can be compared with a weight obtained before the presenting episode. A change in body weight of 1 kg represents a gain or loss of 1 L of fluid. Frequent, serial body weight measurement is a good moni-

toring tool for continued fluid loss during treatment. Keep in mind that third-space fluid loss can occur from the ECF into the gastrointestinal tract and thoracic or peritoneal cavities without creating a change in body weight. Auscultation and abdominal palpation may help determine the presence of third-space losses.

The normal urine output in an animal is 1 to 2 ml/kg/hr. Urine output is a reflection of cardiac function, circulating blood volume, perfusion, and function of the kidneys and lower urinary tract. Urine production should be monitored in patients when abnormalities of these factors are suspected or confirmed. It is very important to monitor the amount of urine being produced as it relates to the amount of fluid being administered. Fluid intake and output records may provide an estimate of the balance between fluid loss and fluid replacement, keeping in mind they are sometimes inaccurate. Evaluation of hydration status is necessary before proper assessment of urine production. Dehydrated patients require fluid replacement before oliguria (urine production of less than 1 ml/kg/hr) is confirmed. Once patients are adequately hydrated and blood pressure is returned to normal, the presence of oliguria may suggest renal failure.

Hypothermic and hyperthermic patients have complications that require adjustments in fluid therapy and close monitoring during temperature alterations. When a change in body temperature occurs in a previously stable animal, potential causes must be investigated.

Spontaneous hypothermia can result from heat loss (e.g., extreme environmental cold, surgery), impaired heat production (e.g., underlying disease), or toxicosis (e.g., ethylene glycol ingestion, drug therapy). In response to decreased cardiac output, hypothermic animals will attempt to conserve heat by shunting blood from the peripheral vasculature and the gastrointestinal tract. Cardiovascular and respiratory support and monitoring must be instituted before initiating warming procedures. A rapid increase in body temperature may lead to peripheral vasodilation and hypotension, further complicating the situation at hand.

Spontaneous hyperthermia can be due to poor environmental ventilation (animals confined in automobiles), heat prostration, inflammatory response, or abnormalities of the thermoregulatory center. Dehydration (as a result of excessive panting) and hypovolemia (secondary to decreased cardiac output) may occur in any of these situations; therefore, fluid therapy is a crucial part of the therapeutic plan.

Laboratory tests

Laboratory tests may be vital in establishing the nature and extent of fluid imbalances and in monitoring treatment. Serial determinations of the hematocrit (packed cell volume) and total plasma protein level are important for establishing a trend and adjusting therapy. A decreasing hematocrit and total plasma protein level can suggest acute or chronic bleeding or hemodilution. Patients with a low serum protein level (hypoproteinemia) are in danger of losing fluid from the intravascular space into the interstitium because of low intravascular oncotic pressure. Once the protein level falls below 3.5 g/dl or the albumin level below 2.0 g/dl, colloid administration should be considered. An increasing hematocrit and total plasma protein level can indicate fluid loss from the intravascular space, ultimately resulting in dehydration. These two values should routinely be evaluated together to avoid misleading information that could be obtained from evaluation of either value alone.

Serum chemistry profiles can be performed to determine the functional status of certain organs (e.g., liver, kidneys, pancreas). The results will assist with patient evaluation, determining the need for electrolyte replacement therapy, detecting complications, and ruling out other diseases.

Urine specific gravity is a measurement of solids in solution and indicates the kidney's ability to concentrate urine. In a normal animal, the specific gravity depends on fluid intake and urine output. An increased urine specific gravity is most likely to occur in animals with decreased water intake. Upon rehydration, the urine specific gravity should decrease. Urine specific gravity should be measured before, during, and after fluid therapy to help evaluate kidney function.

Fluid Choices

The goal of fluid therapy is to restore body fluid losses, reestablish normal blood volume, improve tissue perfusion, and facilitate administration of certain drugs and therapeutics. Many considerations are integrated into a fluid choice (e.g., tonicity, amount of glucose, electrolyte balance, acidity, osmotic pressure, oxygen-carrying capability). The choice is based on the composition of fluid lost from the body, abnormalities requiring correction, and the severity and type of fluid depletion that has occurred. There are three main groups of fluids to choose from (i.e., crystalloids, artificial colloids, and blood products), and they can be used individually or in a variety of combinations. The choice, composition, and volume of fluid being administered typically require adjustment throughout the course of treatment.

Crystalloids

Crystalloid solutions (e.g., lactated Ringer's solution, 0.9% NaCl, Normosol-R) contain small molecules that, when in solution, can pass through a semipermeable membrane and enter all body compartments. Crystalloid solutions contain sodium as their major osmotically active particle and are categorized as *balanced* if similar in composition to plasma (e.g., lactated Ringer's solution, Normosol-R), or *unbalanced* if the electrolyte composition differs from that of plasma (e.g., 5% dextrose in water, 0.9% NaCl). For example, lactated Ringer's solution and Normosol-R contain sodium, chloride, potassium, calcium, and lactate in similar concentrations as found in plasma. Although these solutions are comparable with plasma in regard to their electrolyte composition, they do not contain phosphorus, proteins, or other oncotic substances.

A fluid into which normal body cells can be placed without causing either shrinkage or swelling of the cells (i.e., similar concentration) is said to be *isotonic* (e.g., 0.9% sodium chloride); a solution that causes cells to swell is said to be *hypotonic* (e.g., 0.45% sodium chloride with 2.5% dextrose); a solution that causes cells to shrink is said to be *hypertonic* (e.g., 7% sodium chloride). The tonicity of a solution will determine its distribution following IV infusion. Crystalloid solutions can be isotonic, hypotonic, or hypertonic.

When using isotonic crystalloid fluid solutions, one must remember that they pass readily through the blood vessel wall. Approximately 25% of the fluid will remain in the vasculature 30 minutes postinfusion, and 75% is redistributed to the interstitium. Although volume restoration can be achieved with crystalloid solutions, effectiveness may be short-term. In some cases, it is difficult, if not impossible, to administer adequate volumes of crystalloid fluids to reverse the hypovolemic state. If volume depletion does not resolve or recurs, administration of colloid solutions may need to be incorporated into the treatment plan. As a direct result, hemodilution is a common concern when utilizing crystalloid therapy only. The addition of a colloid solution has been shown to decrease the volume of additional fluid administration.

Crystalloid solutions can also be classified as to whether they meet replacement or maintenance needs. *Replacement* solutions have a composition similar to that of plasma, with high sodium and low potassium (e.g., lactated Ringer's solution, Normosol-R). *Maintenance* solutions differ from plasma in that they contain less sodium and more potassium (e.g., Normosol-M). The most commonly used crystalloid solutions are balanced replacement solutions. When replacement solutions are used for maintenance therapy or in animals with conditions causing loss of potassium, supplementation of potassium may be necessary.

Hypertonic saline solutions can be used in cases where rapid re-expansion of the vascular volume is needed (e.g., hypotensive shock). These solutions (e.g., 7% to 7.5% strengths) provide intravascular volume expansion by recruiting interstitial and intracellular fluid. The effects are short-lived and can begin to dissipate in as little as 30 minutes. Hypertonic saline is often combined with a colloid solution (e.g., dextran, hydroxyethyl starch) to help prolong its effects. Because the interstitial space and intracellular fluid volumes are utilized by hypertonic saline, this fluid solution should not be used in severely dehydrated animals.

Artificial colloids

There are three main types of artificial colloid solutions: hydroxyethyl starches, dextrans, and gelatins. These solutions contain large molecules that do not readily pass through a semipermeable membrane. When colloid solutions are administered IV, their distribution is primarily limited to the intravascular compartment, making them more effective than crystalloids at expanding blood volume. Ultimately, these solutions increase osmotic pressure and, therefore, are used in conditions in which the vascular space cannot retain an adequate fluid volume (e.g., hypoproteinemia). Albumin, the molecule responsible for providing oncotic pressure in the natural state, has a molecular weight of 69 kD. Hydroxyethyl starches (e.g., Hetastarch, Pentastarch) are the most commonly used artificial colloid and have a much wider range of molecular weights, with an average of 450 kD. The dextrans (e.g., Dextran 40, Dextran 70) have a molecular weight of 40 to 70 kD. The gelatins (e.g., Gelofusin, Haemaccel, Vetaplasm), used least frequently in veterinary medicine, have a molecular weight of approximately 30 kD.

Many factors influence the duration of action of artificial colloids, including species of animal, dosage, specific colloid formulation, preinfusion intravascular volume status, and microvascular permeability. Although artificial colloids are more expensive, they are more cost-effective in that they promote better tissue perfusion and maintain colloid oncotic pressure at a lower infusion volume. As a rule of thumb, colloids should be used in combination with crystalloid solutions to support the fluid shift from the extravascular to the intravascular compartment. Also, crystalloids are held in the vascular space more effectively by the osmotic pressure of the colloids. One limitation with artificial colloid solutions is their potential to cause or aggravate coagulopathies. Patients receiving these solutions should be monitored accordingly.

Note: Blood products are covered in the Whole Blood and Blood Components section.

Indications for Fluid Therapy

Fluid therapy is an important aspect in the treatment of many hospitalized patients. Dehydration and hypovolemia are the two most common indications for fluid therapy. It is important to understand the differences in these pathologies as well as in their treatments. Dehydration is the loss of total body water with preservation of the vascular volume. Hypovolemia occurs when the vascular volume is not large enough to preserve cardiac output. Animals can be dehydrated and have normal intravascular volume, or they can have normal hydration but be hypovolemic. A good example of this is a dog that has been hit by a car and presents with a weak, rapid pulse as a result of intraabdominal hemorrhage. This patient is not dehydrated but has hypovolemia. Although dehydration can, and must, be corrected slowly so as not to overexpand the vascular space, hypovolemia requires rapid re-expansion of the vascular space.

Hemorrhage

A significant loss of blood over minutes to hours results in hypovolemia and potential cardiovascular collapse. The therapeutic goal in the treatment of acute hemorrhagic hypovolemia is to stop hemorrhage and support the cardiovascular system. Aggressive, rapid restoration of vascular volume must be instituted while preventing further blood loss if possible.

When choosing resuscitation fluid for vascular space replacement, volume and composition are critical in determining the effectiveness of volume expansion and duration of its effect. Following blood loss, the intravascular space is depleted, and only later does interstitial fluid shift from the extravascular into the intravascular space, providing much-needed volume. Early in the hemorrhagic situation, focus should be placed on replenishing intravascular space losses. This can be accomplished easily using crystalloid fluid solutions. Crystalloid solutions also enter the extravascular space and, therefore, it is necessary to administer two to three times the amount of crystalloid as the volume lost. Risk of fluid overload is of concern when a large volume of crystalloids are administered, especially in geriatric patients or patients with some degree of cardiovascular compromise. Colloid solutions should be considered when there is a need to maintain intravascular oncotic pressure without administering large volumes of fluid. Most often, crystalloid solutions are recommended initially in the treatment of acute blood loss. If blood loss continues and a substantial portion of the blood volume is depleted, colloid solutions can be added.

The symptoms that occur following hemorrhage are a result of blood volume depletion, not a decrease in red blood cell mass. Unfortunately, volume expansion will further dilute any hemoglobin remaining within the circulation. Although intravascular volume expansion will improve tissue perfusion, patient assessment will help determine whether enough hemoglobin is present to provide oxygenation to vital organs. The need for transfusion should be based on clinical assessment of the signs of anemia, as there is no magic laboratory number at which a patient must be transfused. Red cell replacement is not necessary during initial therapy of acute blood loss. The aggressiveness of therapy will depend on the volume of blood lost, the rapidity at which it was lost, and the patient's condition.

Shock

Shock is a condition in which systemic blood pressure is inadequate to deliver oxygen and nutrients to vital tissues and organs. Although the causes of shock vary, the end result of poor perfusion and impaired cellular metabolism are life-threatening. Treatment of the patient in shock is directed at identifying the cause, with focus on restoring blood volume and improving tissue perfusion. Fluid therapy is the foundation of a treatment plan. However, this syndrome affects multiple body systems, and individual patients will respond differently. Thorough patient assessment and continual monitoring is essential for proper adjustment to fluid choice, volume, and rate.

Dehydration

Dehydration is the loss of body water, often accompanied by electrolyte imbalances. Excessive loss of body fluid or lack of water intake may occur in any one or combination of the following conditions:

- Diarrhea
- Prolonged vomiting
- Prolonged fever
- Sequestration of gastrointestinal fluid
- Sweating
- Exudating burns or open wounds
- Chronic blood loss
- Uncontrolled polyuria (if there is inadequate water intake to compensate for the loss)
- Lack of access to water
- Inability to drink
- Nervous system disturbances
- Systemic illness
- Anorexia

The degree of dehydration can be roughly estimated by clinical assessment (see Table 23-1).

Maintenance fluids

In healthy animals at rest, the daily intake of water, nutrients, and minerals matches the daily loss of these substances. *Sensible water loss* refers to that lost through the urine and feces. *Insensible water loss* includes water lost through the respiratory tract (e.g., panting). Normal fluid losses are approximately 40 to 60 ml/kg/day, with urinary losses accounting for approximately 20 ml/kg/day, fecal losses for 5 ml/kg/day, and respiratory and transcutaneous losses for 15 ml/kg/day.

These losses are balanced daily through drinking water, water in food, and metabolic breakdown of fat, carbohydrate, and protein. To maintain body fluid volume, an animal's daily intake of fluid must equal the sum of sensible and insensible losses. This is defined as the daily maintenance fluid requirement. Maintenance fluid requirements may be calculated from charts that relate body weight to basal metabolic rate (Fig. 23-2).

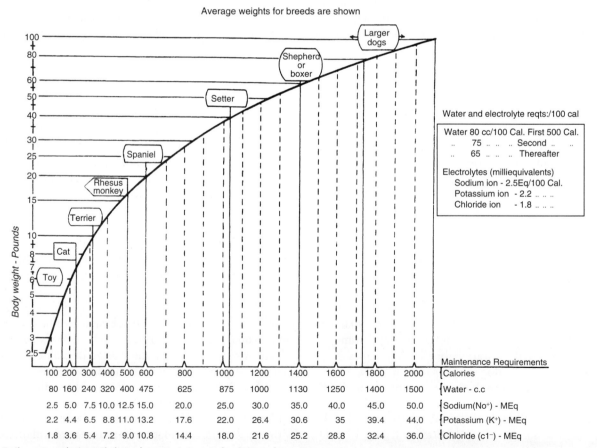

Fig. 23-2 Daily water, calorie, and electrolyte requirements for dogs and cats. (From Harrison JB et al: Fluid and electrolyte therapy in small animals, *J Am Vet Med Assoc* 137:638, 1960.)

Maintenance requirements should be provided with a solution intended for maintenance therapy (e.g., Normosol-M or 0.45% NaCl with KCl). This is especially important for patients receiving maintenance therapy only, given their potassium needs will not be met with a replacement solution. Once patients are returned to a normal state of hydration, maintenance fluids can be administered per os, subcutaneously, intraosseously, or intravenously (PO, SQ, IO, or IV, respectively).

Correcting electrolyte imbalances

Dehydration and known disease processes can cause predictable electrolyte changes in the body. These imbalances are most often corrected through fluid therapy. The fluid choice, additive solutions, and administration route and rate are dependent on the disease, patient status, and laboratory values. If additives of any type are incorporated into the main fluid source, the fluid bag should be labeled to note the additive and its concentration and amount, and the person adding the solution should initial the date and time of addition.

Hypokalemia frequently occurs in animals with fluid disturbances, and supplementation is often required. The dosage and route of potassium supplementation will depend on the cause and severity of the deficiency. IV administration can be used to correct severe potassium deficiencies. The rate of potassium-augmented fluid infusion depends on the amount of potassium added to the fluid. The maximum rate of potassium supplementation in fluids is 0.5 mEq/kg/hr (Table 23-2). Potassium should never be administered in an undiluted form directly into the circulation because of the potential risk of cardiac arrest. Fluid with potassium in concentrations up to 30 to 35 mEq/L can be administered subcutaneously without discomfort or irritation.

Diuresis

Certain diseases (e.g., kidney disease) and treatments (e.g., chemotherapy) require diuresis (increased fluid loss through the kidneys) as part of the therapeutic plan. Diuresis is achieved through placement of IV catheters and institution of aggressive fluid therapy. Patients undergoing diuresis should be monitored closely for signs of overhydration. If there is some question as to adequate renal function, an indwelling urinary catheter should be placed and maintained so urine output can be measured and fluid therapy adjusted accordingly.

Drug therapy

In medicine today, many drugs are available in IV solution. If medication is administered directly to the circulation, rapid uptake of the drug can have an overall positive or negative effect. Drugs administered IV will potentially have a much quicker effect with greater impact; therefore, IV doses are often lower than those administered by other routes. Most drugs can be vascularly irritating, so dilution to an appropriate and acceptable concentration is important (e.g., antibiotics, chemotherapeutic agents).

Routes of Fluid Administration

There are many routes through which fluid solutions can be administered. An appropriate route is chosen after careful evaluation of the following several factors

- Fluid loss
- Volume of fluid loss
- Rate of fluid loss (acute vs. chronic)
- Fluid solution selected for administration
- Volume and rate of administration
- Patient status

These factors will be influenced by the cause and severity of the condition. In small-animal medicine, medical, practical, and economic considerations may affect the fluid solution chosen and administration route used.

Oral

Oral fluid therapy can be used if the gastrointestinal tract is working properly (no vomiting, diarrhea, or gastrointestinal obstruction). Unfortunately, this route cannot be used to correct severe fluid deficits in critically ill patients in need of rapid fluid and electrolyte delivery. If the patient is only mildly dehydrated and will eat and drink, and there is no evidence of vomiting, the oral route is an ideal choice for fluid delivery. It should also be the route of choice for animals with maintenance needs only and not requiring replacement fluids or sustaining ongoing losses.

Animals sometimes voluntarily drink any of several commercially available human electrolyte products. If the patient does not drink the fluid, it can be administered via syringe into the mouth, nasogastric tube, pharyngostomy tube, percutaneous gastrostomy tube, or jejunostomy tube.

TABLE 23-2

Guidelines for Intravenous Potassium (K) Supplementation[*]

Serum Potassium Level	KCl Safely Added to 250 ml of Fluid	Maximal Rate of Infusion
<2.0 mEq/L	20 mEq	6 ml/kg/hr
2.1 to 2.5 mEq/L	15 mEq	8 ml/kg/hr
2.6 to 3.0 mEq/L	10 mEq	12 ml/kg/hr
3.1 to 3.5 mEq/L	7 mEq	16 ml/kg/hr

[*]The infusion rate should not exceed 0.5 mEq/kg/hr. (From Muir WW, DiBartola SP: *Fluid therapy*. In Kirk RW: *Current veterinary therapy VIII*, Philadelphia, 1983, WB Saunders.)

Consideration must be given to the amount of stress imposed on the patient when incorporating this into the treatment plan.

Subcutaneous

Subcutaneous fluid administration is frequently employed. Advantages of this method include ease of administration, reduced cost, and avoidance of problems potentially encountered with IV administration. The subcutaneous route is the delivery method of choice when small volumes are needed, such as maintenance requirements in small animals. When animals are being weaned from IV fluid therapy and would recuperate much more quickly at home, owners can be instructed on how to administer subcutaneous fluids.

Subcutaneous fluid administration cannot be used in animals that require large replacement volumes, or in animals that are severely dehydrated or hypothermic. These conditions cause peripheral vasoconstriction, ultimately reducing the fluid absorption rate. Absorption may also be prolonged in animals that are hypotensive. The most effective approach to rehydrate the patient is by initially using the IV route to improve circulation to the subcutaneous tissues.

Fluids are usually administered in subcutaneous space over the dorsal neck and cranial trunk, where loose connective tissue is abundant. The areas where the limbs join the trunk should be avoided, because fluid can gravitate into the limbs and cause discomfort. Warming the fluids before infusion encourages absorption and benefits hypothermic animals. There are limitations as to the volume that can be mechanically infused under the skin. The volume that can be administered via injection or gravity flow varies from animal to animal. Usually 50 to 150 ml can be infused at each SQ site, depending on the elasticity of the skin. If larger volumes are required, multiple sites may be used and treatment repeated every few hours.

To avoid skin sloughing, administer only nonirritating, isotonic fluids subcutaneously. A solution of 5% dextrose in water (D5W) should not be given SQ. This fluid is devoid of electrolytes; when the fluid is not immediately absorbed, electrolytes from the body can equilibrate into the pooled fluid and potentially initiate or aggravate electrolyte imbalances.

Intravenous

The IV route of fluid administration is preferable when treating animals that are critically ill, severely dehydrated, or hypovolemic, or are experiencing some electrolyte or metabolic disorder. Vascular access supplies the most direct route to plasma volume and, therefore, fluid administered IV has the most rapid effect on blood volume. If fluid loss is acute, it is important to replace deficits rapidly. If fluid losses have occurred over an extended period, the body has had time to adjust, and slow fluid replacement is generally all that is required. IV delivery allows titration of fluids to meet requirements of the patient. Because of direct access to the venous system, complications are more numerous than with other routes (e.g., infection, phlebitis, hematoma formation, thrombosis).

In a healthy patient, there are many superficial veins that can be easily cannulated. The catheter site selection is determined after careful consideration of many factors: patient status, vascular accessibility, operator experience, therapeutic goals, and risk of infection. The cephalic, medial femoral, and saphenous veins are easy to prepare, catheterize, and bandage for fluid administration. Peripheral venous catheters are sufficient in many patients, but often in critical patients other routes are required. During hypovolemia, peripheral vessels may vasoconstrict or simply not have the volume required to distend sufficiently for cannulation and; therefore, a central venous catheter is the best recourse. Central venous catheters may be placed in the jugular vein and the caudal vena cava (via the femoral vein). Isotonic and hypotonic solutions can be easily administered through any vein, but hypertonic solutions must be delivered through a central vessel. These vessels have higher blood flow and, therefore, any hemolytic effects of the fluid can be minimized by dilution with the blood. Central venous catheters allow for the administration of hypertonic solutions or irritating drugs, direct monitoring of venous pressure, and a port for blood sampling.

The size of the catheter is also an important consideration. Rate of flow through a catheter is controlled by three factors: patient's blood pressure, resistance in administration system (e.g., catheter size and placement), and the pressure or height of the fluid source. The resistance to flow of the catheter is dependent on its length and diameter. For rapid fluid administration, the largest, shortest catheter practical is the best. The maximal fluid flow rate increases as the radius of the catheter lumen is increased. For routine maintenance treatment, the smallest gauge catheter that provides adequate flow should be used.

Intraosseous

Intraosseous catheters provide excellent access to the peripheral circulation, with absorption equivalent to that of IV infusion. Fluids can be administered via a needle or catheter introduced into the intramedullary space. The bones of choice for placement include the femur, humerus, and wing of the ilium. This is an excellent method for fluid delivery in young animals or in animals where vascular access is a problem. Fluids administered through the intramedullary space are almost immediately available to the general circulation, and all solutions can be given, regardless of their composition. One limitation is the rate at which fluids can be delivered. Also, a major complication associated with this route is the potential for introduction of infection, resulting in osteomyelitis. Secure placement of the intraosseous catheter can be a challenge but is of utmost importance to maintain vascular access and decrease infection risk.

Volume and Rate of Fluid Administration

Once vascular access has been achieved, the decision of fluid volume and rate must be made. Fluids are in many ways drugs, and as such have dosages. The difference between drugs and fluids, however, is that the body requires various amounts of fluid in various metabolic states. In patients with ongoing losses, fluid dosages may need to change. Because of this, fluid therapy requires frequent evaluation and adjustments to achieve the proper balance of fluids. There are some basic guidelines to assist in calculating requirements: blood pressure must be maintained, dehydration and ongoing losses must be replaced, acid/base and electrolyte balance must be maintained, and maintenance fluids must be supplied.

Many factors influence the rate of fluid administration (e.g., disease process, rate of fluid loss, severity of clinical signs, fluid composition and delivery route, cardiac and renal function). Patients with poor perfusion because of severe dehydration or hypovolemia must be given immediate and rapid IV fluid replacements. The goal is to restore intravascular fluid volume and improve tissue perfusion as quickly as possible, as long as the cardiopulmonary and renal systems can handle the fluid load. Animals with marginal cardiovascular function cannot tolerate rapid fluid infusion, so their deficits must be restored with greater care. Acute fluid therapy is used in emergency situations to rapidly replace plasma volume in animals with hypovolemia. Chronic fluid therapy is used to replace fluid deficits (dehydration without hypovolemia), provide maintenance requirements, and compensate for ongoing losses.

Patients with brittle cardiovascular systems or compromised renal function are excellent candidates for CVP monitoring. Central venous pressure (CVP) reflects the heart's ability to accommodate fluid administration. It is regulated by a balance between the ability of the right heart to pump blood to the lungs and the tendency for blood to flow from peripheral vessels back into the right atrium. Valuable information regarding the relationship among intravascular volume, venous return, and right heart function can indirectly be provided with these measurements. CVP monitoring can be useful as a clinical guide for determining rate of fluid administration, but not as an indication of fluid volume to be replaced.

Acute fluid therapy

Patients experiencing mild to moderate hypoperfusion usually require crystalloid infusion rates of 20 to 60 ml/kg/hr. Patients who are critically ill, in shock, severely dehydrated, or poorly perfused may require crystalloid infusion rates of 60 to 90 ml/kg/hr. Flow rates even higher than this may be required in some instances. *The key to determining fluid rates is to reassess the patient and then reassess the fluid rate.* In some cases, hourly adjustments must be made to the fluid rate to support the patient. Fluid rates and volumes are usually reduced by one half to one third for cats requiring acute IV fluid support.

The maximum rate of fluid administration is usually limited by mechanical ability to administer fluids. In a life-threatening situation, two or more catheters may be used simultaneously to administer large volumes of fluid. In addition, a commercially available pressure infusion cuff allows rapid delivery of fluid, but pressure should not exceed 300 mm Hg. Care should be taken to not introduce air into the system and risk infection or air emboli.

In hypoproteinemic animals, caution should be exercised with the rate of administration, even when the patient is severely dehydrated or poorly perfused. Diminished colloid in the vascular space results in less retention of fluid in the circulation, ultimately risking development of edema and respiratory compromise.

Chronic fluid therapy

Most fluid deficits can be replaced with fluid administration over 12 to 24 hours, depending on the underlying disease process and the severity and duration of the dehydration. In general, it is better to overestimate rather than underestimate the replacement volume, unless the patient has some underlying restrictive condition (e.g., cardiac or renal disease). A fluid plan should address the amount of fluid lost before presentation (i.e., replacement), daily maintenance requirements, and ongoing fluid losses. Pre-existing fluid deficits are usually replaced with IV fluid formulated for replacement (e.g., Normosol-R or lactated Ringer's).

daily fluid requirement = replacement + maintenance + ongoing losses

A simple formula utilizing the % dehydration scale and body weight can help define the replacement volume:

fluid deficit (ml) = % dehydration × body weight (kg) × 10

Maintenance requirements are estimated by body weight and are 40 to 60 ml/kg/day, or approximately 2 ml/kg/hr. Maintenance requirements should be provided with a solution intended for maintenance therapy (e.g., Normosol-M or 0.45% NaCl with KCl). This is especially important for patients receiving maintenance therapy only, given their potassium needs will not be met with a replacement solution.

Ongoing fluid losses should be estimated from the daily volume of urine, diarrhea, vomiting, tube drainage, etc. The calculated amount should be divided over 24 hours and added to the maintenance fluid dose. Replacement solutions are given to compensate for ongoing losses. Box 23-1 shows calculations of fluid requirements for a hypothetical case.

BOX 23-1

procedure

Calculating Daily Fluid Requirements in a Hypothetical Case

Patient

5-month-old, 20-kg Rottweiler

History

- 3 days of anorexia, lethargy
- 2 days of vomiting and diarrhea, 5 to 6 times/day, becoming bloody
- No vaccinations

Physical examination findings

- Depression
- Heart rate: 140 beats/minute
- Pulse: weak to moderate
- Capillary refill time: 1 to 2 seconds
- Tented skin slowly returns to normal position

Replacement requirements

% dehydration × body weight × 10 = fluid deficit

$8 \times 20 \times 10 = 1600$ ml

Maintenance requirements

Maintenance requirement = 40 to 60 ml/kg/day

$50 \times 20 = 1000$ ml/day

Ongoing losses

Ongoing losses = losses in diarrhea and vomitus

Estimated diarrhea volume/episode = 100 ml

5 episodes/day = 500 ml

Estimated vomitus volume/episode = 50 ml

5 episodes/day = 250 ml

Ongoing losses 500 + 250 = 750 ml/day

Daily fluid requirement

Daily fluid requirement = fluid deficit + maintenance + ongoing losses

= 1600 + 1000 + 750

= 3350 ml/day

= 3350 ml over 24 hr/day

Infusion rate = 140 ml/hr

Patients receiving fluid support should be closely monitored for signs of overhydration. These include restlessness, shivering, tachycardia, serous nasal or ocular discharge, respiratory distress, pulmonary crackles or rales, coughing as a result of pulmonary edema, vomiting, and diarrhea. Fluid administration must then be slowed or stopped, depending on the severity of clinical signs.

TOTAL PARENTERAL NUTRITION

Fluid therapy should be considered as the first supportive measure in re-establishing nutritional balance. Only after the primary goals of rehydration, replacement of electrolytes, and normalization of acid-base balance should parenteral feeding be introduced. As a rule of thumb, animals that have been off food for 3 to 5 days should be considered candidates for total parenteral nutrition (TPN).

Parenteral nutrition is indicated for patients that are severely malnourished and cannot meet nutritional needs adequately using the oral or enteral route. Ideally, nutrition should be maintained via the gastrointestinal tract. If any part of the alimentary tract is nonfunctional, nutrients can be infused IV for some time. Total parenteral nutrition is not an innocuous treatment. Complicating factors associated with TPN include: placement and use of a central catheter dedicated solely to administration of TPN solution; potential septic and mechanical problems if the catheter is not placed and maintained properly; possible metabolic disturbances as a result of TPN solution composition, concentration, and administration; and expense. The three main ingredients of a TPN solution are dextrose, amino acids, and lipids. Dextrose supplies the calories; amino acids supply protein, nitrogen, and electrolytes; and lipid emulsions serve as a concentrated energy source. Because TPN solutions are hypertonic, they must be infused into a central vein (e.g., jugular, medial, femoral) to allow for rapid dilution of the fluid. Because of the high level of nutrients in TPN solutions, they should be infused slowly to prevent possible rebound hypoglycemia.

TRANSFUSION MEDICINE

Proficiency in transfusion therapy and blood banking techniques is an invaluable skill for veterinary technicians as blood products are used in treatment of many patients with hematologic disorders. Education is clearly the link to ensuring the overall quality of all aspects of blood banking and transfusion services as a safe and adequate supply of blood components for transfusion is indispensable.

Clinical Evaluation of Bleeding

When a patient presents with abnormal bleeding, it is important to determine the cause. Although it is the responsibility of the veterinarian to diagnose and choose an appropriate therapy for these patients, the veterinary technician should be knowledgeable and anticipate the needs of the veterinarian and, most importantly, the patient. This requires a basic understanding of the physiology of hemostasis.

Hemostasis

Hemostasis, the body's balancing mechanism of arresting hemorrhage while simultaneously maintaining blood flow within the vascular compartment, occurs through a complex series of events involving the vessels, platelets, plasma coagulation factors, and the fibrinolytic system. The role that each component plays in hemostasis is dependent on the size of the vessel and the amount of damage that has occurred. Bleeding in smaller vessels (e.g., normal wear and tear on capillaries) may be controlled by a simple response involving the vessels and platelets, referred to as *primary hemostasis*, during which platelets adhere to the injured area and form a complete but unstable plug.

With greater damage and/or damage to larger vessels, *secondary hemostasis*, involving plasma coagulation factors, becomes necessary to arrest bleeding. Plasma coagulation factors are produced in the liver and circulate in the blood in the inactive form. They become activated only when exposed to certain substances (tissues or platelet phospholipids). The end result of activation of the clotting cascade (i.e., intrinsic, extrinsic, and common pathways) is the creation of *fibrin*, a threadlike protein. The fibrin threads form an insoluble meshwork over the site of the platelet plug, consolidating and stabilizing the clot.

The final step in the hemostatic process is fibrinolysis. Once the vessel is healed, fibrinolytic enzymes digest the clot that has been formed, restoring normal blood flow. Clot lysis produces small pieces of fibrin, referred to as fibrin split products (FSPs) or fibrin degradation products (FDPs), which are cleared from circulation by the liver. Small levels of FSPs always appear in the circulation as a result of bleeding and clotting secondary to normal wear-and-tear on vessels. FSP levels increase during episodes of excessive bleeding with diffuse coagulation (disseminated intravascular coagulation or DIC) and in patients with compromised liver function. Following clot digestion, vessel wall endothelium is re-established and returned to its original state.

An accurate history, thorough physical examination, and certain laboratory tests must be performed to accurately evaluate bleeding patients, determine a diagnosis, and define a therapeutic plan.

History

A complete history is critical in beginning a workup for a hemostatic defect. In veterinary medicine, all pertinent information regarding patient history must be gathered from the owners. Obtaining and assessing a complete and detailed history will help define the nature, severity, and duration of clinical signs and aid in making a correct diagnosis. Attention to detail allows the clinician to establish probability for each possible differential early in the diagnostic process.

Questions should be clear and thought-provoking. Devising a list of questions for owners to review may incite them to think of important, most likely not obvious facts. Does the patient have any previously diagnosed diseases? For example, animals with liver failure may have compromised clotting because the liver produces clotting factors. Is the patient currently on any medication? A list of prescription or over-the-counter medications should be included, as many drugs have potentially harmful or complicating side effects, resulting in a toxic effect on red blood cells, white blood cells, and platelets. Complete vaccination history should not be overlooked, because a relationship between recent vaccination and onset of immune-mediated hemolytic anemia (IMHA) has been demonstrated. The patient's environmental history may suggest potential exposure to toxic substances such as anticoagulant rodenticide poisons or lead. Also, many organic and other substances (e.g., onions, zinc) can cause hemolytic conditions. Tick exposure should also be investigated.

It is vital to evaluate the current bleeding episode. Determine whether the bleeding is localized to one site or is multifocal. Is this the patient's first bleeding episode, or is there a history of bleeding tendency? These facts can help characterize if the bleeding is a result of an acquired or hereditary disorder. The breed may suggest specific coagulopathies. Any information the owner may have regarding breed history can provide helpful clues. Many breeders are becoming educated in regard to bleeding disorders that affect their breed and, specifically, their family line.

Physical examination

A complete physical examination and multiple monitoring procedures are required to properly assess the patient in a bleeding crisis. Optimal assessment cannot be based on the result of a single parameter, but is based on the results of several physical exam findings and monitored parameters, which should always be evaluated in relation to one another.

During physical exam, certain clinical signs may help determine the origin of the bleeding episode. Small surface bleeds (e.g., petechiation, ecchymosis, epistaxis, hematuria) are usually suggestive of platelet or vascular abnormalities. Larger bleeds or bleeding into body cavities (e.g., hematoma formation, hemarthroses, deep-muscle hemorrhage) are suggestive of clotting factor deficiencies. A combination of these clinical signs is not uncommon.

In anemic patients, the development and progression of clinical signs depends on the rapidity of onset, degree, and cause of anemia, as well as the patient's physical activity. Common physical findings are those associated with a decrease in red cell mass: lethargy, weakness, pale mucous membranes, tachycardia, tachypnea, and bounding pulses. The cardiovascular and respiratory system should be carefully evaluated. Assessment of perfusion is based on mucous membrane color; capillary refill time (CRT); heart rate; and pulse rate, strength, and character. Normal mucous membranes are pink and moist to the touch, but can range in color (e.g., pale, injected, cyanotic) dependent on patient status. CRT is determined by applying pressure to a non-pigmented area of the gum or lip, and then released. The time required for the blanched area to return to pink should be 1 to 2 seconds. A rapid CRT (less than 1 second) is a result of vasodilation (e.g., compensatory stage of shock, fever, anxiety); prolonged CRT (greater than 2 seconds) is a result of vasoconstriction and suggests poor tissue perfusion (e.g., decompensatory stage of shock, hypovolemia, heart failure). CRT may be difficult to assess in an anemic patient due to the paleness of the gums. Arterial pulses should be monitored routinely for rate, rhythm volume, and synchronicity with the heart rate. Weak and rapid pulses suggest poor perfusion (e.g., hypovolemic shock) and severe dehydration; bounding pulses suggest anemia. Assessment of respiratory rate and effort, as well as careful auscultation, may help differentiate between decreased oxygen-carrying capability and possible compromised lung function. In a severe anemic state, a low-grade systolic flow murmur may occur secondary to decreased blood viscosity. Monitoring these parameters in unison with one another will lend information regarding severity of the bleed and the presence of potentially life-threatening complications.

Laboratory tests

Although information obtained from the history and specific clinical signs may suggest a diagnosis, certain laboratory tests are necessary for definitive diagnosis. Laboratory tests should be performed ASAP and therapy instituted promptly after test samples are obtained.

Anemia is suggested when one or more of the red cell parameters are below normal for the age, sex, and breed of the species concerned. Of these red cell parameters, packed cell volume (PCV) provides a simple, quick, and accurate means of detecting anemia. The degree of anemia varies with the nature, extent, and duration of the disease process.

Serial PCV determinations may help demonstrate progression or stabilization of bleeding, taking into account that the body takes a certain amount of time to equilibrate following an acute bleeding episode. Note that dehydration and splenic contraction can mask anemia, whereas hemodilution from IV fluid therapy may cause a temporary reduction in PCV. Evaluating both PCV and total plasma protein (TPP) levels may help in differentiating these variables (Table 23-3).

Normal platelet count is 150,000 to 400,000/μl. Abnormal bleeding may occur with platelet counts below 40,000/μl; however, each patient varies and some patients with a platelet count of 2,000/μl may not exhibit clinical signs associated with bleeding. The thrombocytopenic patient requires special care (e.g., extra cage padding, avoidance of central vessels for blood collection, extended application of pressure to venipuncture sites). In a patient exhibiting signs of surface bleeding with a normal platelet count, consideration should be given to the function of platelets, and similar precautions may be required.

Certain tests are available to monitor coagulation in patients with suspected coagulopathies. Prothrombin time (PT) measures extrinsic and common clotting pathway activity, whereas activated partial thromboplastin time (APTT) measures intrinsic and common pathway activity. Prolongation of PT/APTT will be seen when clotting factors are depleted below 30% of normal. PT and APTT samples should be collected and processed carefully to avoid potential sample errors. Atraumatic venipuncture and smooth blood flow into collection tubes are necessary to avoid extraneous clotting mechanism activation. Samples should be processed immediately after collection and frozen before being sent to an outside laboratory.

Elevation in FSPs occurs with excessive bleeding and fibrinolysis, and in animals with severe liver dysfunction. Interpreted in conjunction with the PT, aPTT, and platelet count, elevated FSP levels are useful as a diagnostic indicator of **disseminated intravascular coagulation (DIC)**.

TABLE 23-3

Differentiating Causes of Hypovolemia

	PCV	TPP
Dehydration	Increase	Increase
Acute blood loss, hemodilution	Decrease	Decrease
Splenic contraction	Increase	Normal
Hemolytic anemias	Decrease	Normal
Anemia caused by decreased production or hemolysis	Decrease	Normal
Blood loss anemia*	Decrease	Decrease

*Both decreases caused by loss of erythrocytes *and* plasma proteins, as well as the compensatory shift of fluid from the interstitial space to the intravascular compartment.

Practical hemostatic tests

The following are simple, in-house tests requiring no specialized equipment. They are quick, inexpensive, practical tests that allow recognition and characterization of hemostatic defects. These tests are often referred to as "cage-side," in that they provide results almost immediately.

Platelet estimation. An estimate of platelet number from a stained blood smear is much quicker than an actual platelet count. With some practice, platelet estimation can be reasonably accurate. After routine preparation and staining, the blood smear is first scanned to ensure that platelets are evenly distributed on the smear and there is no platelet clumping. The average number of platelets in 5 to 10 oil-immersion fields is determined to estimate platelet numbers; approximately 8 to 12 platelets should be seen per field. This should be adequate to categorize platelet numbers as very low, low, normal, or high. One platelet per oil-immersion field represents approximately 20,000 platelets. An estimated platelet count can quickly detect thrombocytopenia in an emergency situation, but a true platelet count is necessary to classify the severity of the depletion.

Bleeding time. Bleeding time is the time it takes for bleeding to stop after severing a vessel. The bleeding time test most often used in veterinary medicine is the buccal mucosal bleeding time (BMBT) (Box 23-2).

The BMBT assesses platelet and vascular contribution to hemostasis, thereby evaluating primary hemostasis. A disposable template with two spring-loaded blades is used to produce standardized incisions in the buccal mucosal surface of the upper lip. The blades create 5-mm-long by 1-mm-deep incisions. The duration of bleeding from these incisions is monitored. Normal bleeding time in the dog and cat is less than 4 minutes and 2 minutes, respectively.

The BMBT is a screening test. As with any screening test, it is not 100% sensitive and, therefore, not all primary hemostatic defects will be discovered. This test also will not differentiate between vascular defects or platelet function defects. The BMBT is prolonged in cases of thrombocytopenia/thrombopathia, von Willebrand disease, uremia, and aspirin therapy. BMBT should not be performed on any patient that is known to be thrombocytopenic. Although it does have limitations, there are several advantages to this test. Commercial bleeding time devices are readily available and inexpensive. The templates are standardized and therefore, results are reproducible. It is a simple and quick test to perform, and the results are almost immediately available. Patients seem to tolerate the procedure well, eliminating need for chemical restraint. The incisions produced are well above the concentrated pain fibers in the lip. Sometimes the animal will reflex upon hearing the noise the scalpels make when released from the device, but the procedure itself is not painful.

Activated clotting time. Activated clotting time (ACT) is a simple, inexpensive screening test for severe

---

BOX 23-2 *procedure*

Determining Buccal Mucosal Bleeding Time

Materials
- Bleeding time device
- Gauze strip
- Filter paper or gauze sponges
- Timing device

Procedure

1. Place animal in lateral recumbency.
2. Expose mucosal surface of upper lip. Position a gauze strip around the maxilla to fold up the upper lip. Tie the strip gently, just tight enough to partially block venous return.
3. The incision site should be void of surface vessels and slightly inclined so that shed blood from the incision can flow freely toward the mouth. Place bleeding time device flush against mucosal surface, applying as little pressure as possible, and press tab to release scalpels.
4. Let stab incisions bleed freely, *undisturbed*, and time until bleeding stops. Excessive blood should be blotted as often as necessary to avoid blood flow into the patient's mouth. Place either filter paper or gauze sponge approximately 3 to 4 mm below the incision, taking care not to disturb the incision site and any clot that may be forming.
5. The end point is recorded when the edge of the filter paper/sponge does not soak up free-flowing blood. The bleeding time is the mean bleeding time for the two incisions.

---

abnormalities in the intrinsic and common pathways of the clotting cascade (Box 23-3). It evaluates the same pathways as the APTT, but is less sensitive in detecting factor deficiencies. Normal ACT is 60 to 110 seconds in dogs and 50 to 75 seconds in cats.

The ACT is prolonged with severe factor deficiency in the intrinsic and/or common clotting pathway (e.g., hemophilia), in the presence of inhibitors (e.g., heparin, warfarin), or in cases of severe thrombocytopenia resulting from lack of platelet phospholipid (mild prolongation of 10 to 20 seconds). The ACT is inexpensive, easily learned, quick to perform, reproducible, and provides immediate results. It is a very useful measurement of coagulation in emergency situations. In most situations, the ACT should be followed up with an APTT.

WHOLE BLOOD AND BLOOD COMPONENTS

Blood comprises two portions: the cellular portion (red blood cells, white blood cells, platelets) and plasma, which acts as a carrier medium for the cells, proteins, gases, nutrients, and waste products. Each component of blood has a

BOX 23-3 *procedure*

Determining Activated Clotting Time

Materials

- Vacutainer sleeve
- Vacutainer single-collection needle
- ACT tube containing diatomaceous earth
- 37° C electric heat block (can substitute hot water bath)

Procedure

1. Warm ACT tube in heat block to 37° C for approximately 3 minutes.
2. Perform clean venipuncture on an unthrombosed vessel. Discard the first few drops of blood to eliminate tissue thromboplastin, the tissue factor responsible for activation of the extrinsic pathway.
3. Puncture the ACT tube with the distal needle, and collect approximately 2 ml of blood. Begin timing as soon as blood enters the tube.
4. After collection, invert the tube several times to mix with diatomaceous earth and place in heating block.
5. After 30 seconds from start of timing, gently tilt the tube and examine for clot formation. Return tube to heat block and repeat procedure every 10 seconds.
6. The ACT time is the time from collection of blood in the tube to *initial* clot formation. In the dog, the normal is 60 to 110 seconds. In the cat, the normal is 50 to 75 seconds.

specific function. Certain diseases necessitate replacement of one or any combination of these components (Table 23-4).

With the availability of variable speed, temperature-controlled centrifuges and the advent of plastic storage bags with integral tubing for collection, processing, and administration, specific blood component therapy is possible. The goal in veterinary transfusion medicine is to limit whole-blood transfusion and to use component therapy whenever possible. Whole blood can be stored or processed into one or more of the following components: red blood cells, platelets, plasma, and cryoprecipitate. Blood components permit specific replacement therapy for specific disorders, reduce the number of transfusion reactions as a result of diminished exposure to foreign material, and decrease the amount of time needed to transfuse. Most importantly, appropriate therapeutic use of blood components increases the number of patients who benefit from this limited resource.

Fresh Whole Blood

Initial collection yields fresh whole blood (FWB) and is considered *fresh* for up to 8 hours after collection. Fresh whole blood provides red blood cells (RBCs), white blood cells (WBCs), platelets, plasma proteins, and coagulation factors. Certain components in blood are more fragile than others, and these become less effective over time and with changes in ambient temperature. Platelet and coagulation factor efficacy becomes compromised once whole blood is refrigerated; therefore, to achieve the full benefit of all components, administer fresh blood immediately after collection.

Fresh whole blood is transfused into actively bleeding, anemic animals with thrombocytopenia/thrombopathia, anemia with coagulopathies, (DIC), and massive hemorrhage. Massive hemorrhage is defined as a loss approaching or exceeding 1 total blood volume within a 24-hour period. In cases of severe hemorrhage, administration of all components may be necessary to support the patient.

Stored Whole Blood

Following collection, whole blood must be processed into components or at least refrigerated at 4° C within 8 hours. After 24-hour storage of whole blood, platelet function is lost and the concentration of labile coagulation factors decreases. The product is then defined as stored whole blood (SWB) and provides RBCs and plasma proteins (albumin and globulins). The length of time a unit of whole blood can be stored under refrigeration is dependent on the anticoagulant-preservative solution used in collection. With the well-documented advantages in the use of blood components in human and veterinary medicine and the improved availability of these products as a result of commercial blood banks, the use of whole blood is no longer considered the treatment of choice. The use of whole blood, fresh or stored, is not recommended in severe chronic anemia. Chronically anemic patients may have a reduced red blood cell mass but have compensated over time by increasing their plasma volume to meet their total blood volume. Administration of whole blood may expose these patients to the risk of volume overload, especially in patients with pre-existing cardiac disease or renal compromise. If available, however, stored whole blood can be used in patients that require intravascular volume expansion as well as improved oxygen-carrying capability.

Packed Red Blood Cells

Packed red blood cells (pRBC) is the component of choice for increasing red cell mass in patients who require oxygen-carrying support. Decreased red cell mass may be caused by decreased bone marrow production, increased destruction, or surgical or traumatic bleeding. Although it seems logical that blood loss should be replaced with whole blood, replacing blood volume with pRBC and crystalloid or colloid solutions adequately treats most blood loss. This is often adequate therapy for the majority of acutely bleeding patients. Transfusion of pRBC is not recommended in

TABLE 23-4

Components of Transfusion Therapy

Contents	Indication	Shelf Life	Preparation	Comments
Fresh Whole Blood (FWB)				
RBC, plasma proteins, all coagulation factors, WBC, platelets (~ Hct 40% to 50%)	Acute active hemorrhage; hypovolemic shock; thrombocytopenia with active bleeding	Less than 8 hours following initial collection	Use immediately following collection (refrigeration compromises platelet function)	Restores blood volume and oxygen-carrying capacity; may help control microvascular bleeding in patients with thrombocytopenia/thrombopathia
Stored Whole Blood (SWB)				
RBC, plasma proteins (~ Hct 40% to 50%)	Anemia with hypoproteinemia; hypovolemic shock	Greater than 8 hours old and up to 35 days (dependent on anticoagulant-preservative solution used); refrigerate at 1° C to 6° C	Allow to come to room temperature (temperatures exceeding 37° C will result in hemolysis and bacterial proliferation)	Restores blood volume and oxygen-carrying capacity; WBC and platelets not functional; F V and VIII diminished; not recommended for chronic anemia
Packed Red Blood Cells (PRBC)				
RBC, reduced plasma (~ Hct 80%)	Increased red cell mass in symptomatic anemia	Dependent on anticoagulant-preservative solution used; refrigerate at 1° C to 6° C	Allow to come to room temperature (temperatures exceeding 37° C will result in hemolysis and bacterial proliferation); may reconstitute with 0.9% NaCl before administration	Same oxygen-carrying capacity as whole blood, but less volume
Packed Red Blood Cells (PRBC), Adenine-Saline Added				
RBC, reduced plasma, 100 ml additive solution (~ Hct 60%)	Increased red cell mass in symptomatic anemia	30 to 35 days; refrigerate at 1° C to 6° C	Allow to come to room temperature (temperatures exceeding 37° C will result in hemolysis and bacterial proliferation)	Additive solution extends shelf life of PRBC by improving storage environment; reduces viscosity for infusion
Platelet-Rich Plasma/Platelet Concentrate				
Platelets, few RBCs and WBCs, some plasma	Life-threatening bleeding due to thrombocytopenia/thrombopathia	5 days at 22° C; intermittent agitation required	Administer immediately following collection and preparation	Do not refrigerate; usually requires multiple units for measurable increase
Fresh Frozen Plasma (FFP)				
Plasma, albumin, all coagulation factors	Treatment of coagulation disorders/factor deficiencies; liver disease, DIC, anticoagulant rodenticide toxicity	1 year frozen at −20° C or below	Thaw in 37° C warm water bath (temperatures exceeding 37° C will result in protein denaturation and bacterial proliferation)	Frozen within 8 hours following collection; no platelets; can be relabeled as FP after 1 year for additional 4 years; must be administered within 4 hours

Continued

TABLE 23-4

Components of Transfusion Therapy—Cont'd

Contents	Indication	Shelf Life	Preparation	Comments
				following thawing; do not refreeze once room temperature is reached
FROZEN PLASMA (FP)				
Plasma, albumin, stable coagulation factors	Treatment of stable coagulation factor deficiencies	5 years frozen at −20° C or below	Thaw in 37° C warm water bath (temperatures exceeding 37° C will result in protein denaturation and bacterial proliferation)	Frozen after more than 8 hours following collection or relabeled FFP after 1 year; no platelets; can be used to treat some cases of acute hypoproteinemia; must be administered within 4 hours following thawing; do not refreeze once room temperature is reached
CRYOPRECIPITATE (CRYO)				
Factor VIII, vWF, fibrinogen, fibronectin	Hemophilia A; von Willebrand disease; hypofibrinogenemia	1 year frozen at −20° C or below	Thaw in 37° C warm water bath (temperatures exceeding 37° C will result in protein denaturation and bacterial proliferation)	Must be administered within 4 hours following thawing; do not refreeze once room temperature is reached

patients who are well-compensated for their anemia (e.g., chronic renal failure). The decision to perform red blood cell transfusion should never be based solely on hematocrit or hemoglobin levels. Patients should be properly evaluated, and pRBC administration should be based primarily on clinical status (e.g., tachycardia, poor pulse quality, respiratory distress, lethargy).

Packed RBCs can be harvested from whole blood (fresh or stored) by the use of a refrigerated centrifuge (5000 G for 5 minutes at 4° C [39° F]). If a refrigerated centrifuge is not available, RBCs can be harvested by allowing whole blood to separate by sedimentation over one to two days. After sedimentation, the plasma is removed and placed in a sterile transfer pack. Ideally, packed RBCs should be reconstituted with a nutrient solution before storage to maintain the cells in a healthier environment. This extends storage time; also, reconstitution of the RBCs reduces viscosity during administration. Packed RBCs can be refrigerated at 4° C, with storage time determined by the anticoagulant-preservative or additive solution used in collection and processing. If a nutrient solution is not used at the time of processing, packed RBCs can be reconstituted with 100 ml of 0.9% NaCl before administration to reduce viscosity.

Reconstitution with nonisotonic fluids may cause RBC damage.

Platelet-Rich Plasma

Platelet-rich plasma (PRP) is harvested from a unit of FWB that is less than 8 hours old and has not been cooled below 20° to 24° C (68° to 75° F) ("light spin," 1000 G for 4 minutes at room temperature). Refrigerated platelets do not maintain function or viability as well as platelets stored at room temperature. The PRP may be administered following centrifugation, or the platelets can be concentrated by further centrifugation and removal of most of the supernatant plasma. Under optimal conditions, platelets prepared from a single unit of FWB administered to a 30-kg dog should result in an increase in the patient's platelet count of 10,000/µl.

The major indication for platelet transfusion is to stop bleeding in patients with low platelet numbers and/or impaired function. These patients experience bleeding when inadequate numbers (or diminished function) of platelets are available to form a platelet plug. A significant volume is needed to measurably increase platelet numbers in larger patients. In some patients, however, bleeding stops after platelet transfusion without a measurable increase in platelet number. Because of the impracticality associated with production of this component, in veterinary medicine we routinely treat thrombocytopenia/thrombopathia accompanied by active bleeding with fresh whole blood, through which the patient receives both platelets and RBCs. In conditions causing platelet destruction, such as idiopathic thrombocytopenic purpura, transfused platelets survive only minutes rather than days. If the patient is acutely bleeding into a vital structure (e.g., brain, myocardium, pleural cavity), platelet transfusion may be warranted. In most instances, however, medical management is most often the treatment of choice.

Fresh-Frozen Plasma/Frozen Plasma

In addition to water and electrolytes, plasma contains albumin, globulins, coagulation factors, and other proteins. Plasma is primarily used for its coagulation factor value; it does not contain functional platelets. Most coagulation proteins are stable at 1° C to 6° C (33° to 43° F), with the exception of factors V and VIII. In order to maintain adequate levels of all factors, plasma must be harvested from a unit of whole blood and frozen at −20° C (−4° F) or below within 8 hours from the time of initial collection. We refer to this as fresh-frozen plasma (FFP). FFP will retain its coagulation factor efficacy for a period of 12 months provided it is maintained at the appropriate temperature. FFP can be used to treat most coagulation factor deficiencies (e.g., DIC, liver disease, anticoagulant rodenticide toxicity) and other conditions (e.g., pancreatitis). FFP is not recommended for use as a blood volume expander or for protein replacement in animals with chronic hypoproteinemia.

If FFP is not used within 12 months, it can be relabeled as frozen plasma (FP) and stored for an additional 4 years. Also, plasma may be separated from a unit of whole blood at anytime during storage. When stored at −20° C (−4° F) or below, this component is called FP and may be kept for up to 5 years. If not frozen, it is called liquid plasma (LP) and has a shelf life not exceeding 5 days following the expiration date of the WB from which it was harvested. Plasma prepared from outdated WB may have higher levels of ammonia than FFP as a result of longer contact with red blood cells before its preparation.

FP and LP may have varying levels of the more stable coagulation factors, as well as albumin, but they do not contain functional platelets or the labile coagulation factors V and VIII. FP and LP can be used to treat stable clotting factor deficiencies and certain cases of acute hypoproteinemia (e.g., parvoviral enteritis). If animals are severely or chronically protein-deficient, plasma must be administered in large volumes in order to have a measurable impact in managing the acute effects of hypoproteinemia (i.e., pulmonary edema, pleural effusion). In this case, synthetic colloid solutions should be considered because they are readily available and more effective in increasing oncotic pressure. As with FFP, FP and LP are not recommended for use as a blood volume expander.

Cryoprecipitate

Cryoprecipitate is harvested from fresh-frozen plasma within 12 months of collection by thawing the plasma at 4° C (39° F) until it is of slushy consistency (approximately 12 to 18 hours). The slurried plasma is then centrifuged (5000 G for 6 minutes at 4° C [39° F]). The liquid plasma is expressed into a satellite bag using a plasma extractor, leaving behind a white, foamy precipitate (mostly adhered to the bag) and approximately 50 ml of liquid plasma. This precipitate provides von Willebrand factor, factor VIII:C, fibrinogen, and fibronectin. Cryoprecipitate can be frozen at −20° C (−4° F) or below and has a shelf life of 1 year from the date of collection. Cryoprecipitate can be used in patients diagnosed with von Willebrand disease and hemophilia A.

Oxyglobin Solution

Oxyglobin® is a sterile solution of purified, polymerized bovine hemoglobin (13 g/dL) in a modified Lactated Ringer's solution. Oxyglobin increases oxygen delivery to tissues as a result of an increased oxygen content in the blood. Traditionally, RBC hemoglobin carries 98% of the circulating oxygen and plasma carries only 2%. The administration of oxyglobin increases the plasma hemoglobin concentration, shifting the majority of the oxygen content of the blood to the plasma. Oxygen uptake and unloading occurs more readily with oxyglobin than RBCs, facilitating delivery of oxygen to tissues. Additionally, Oxyglobin has a low viscosity, which enhances perfusion to the tissues. There is no need for blood typing or crossmatching with Oxyglobin.

Oxyglobin is indicated for the treatment of anemia in dogs. In addition to providing oxygen-carrying support, this hemoglobin solution has been proven to exert a colloidal effect; therefore, administration of Oxyglobin is not recommended in dogs with cardiac or renal disease because of the potential for volume overload. A transient discoloration (yellow to red) of mucous membranes, sclera, urine, and skin may be noted. Monitoring of patients receiving. Oxyglobin requires measurement of hemoglobin rather than PCV to determine its effect on oxygen-carrying support.

BLOOD TYPES

Canine Blood Types

Thirteen specific antigens, or blood types, have been identified on the surface of canine RBCs identified as dog erythrocyte antigen (DEA) 1.1, 1.2, and 3 to 13.

The canine *universal donor* blood type is DEA 1.1-negative, and, ideally, should also be DEA 1.2- and DEA 7-negative. The most severe antigen-antibody reaction can be seen after transfusion with these antigens, most specifically DEA 1.1. Significant naturally occurring alloantibodies are not seen in dogs; therefore, antigen-antibody reactions are not likely to occur after an initial transfusion. However, dogs that are DEA 1.1-, 1.2-, and 7-negative can develop alloantibodies to DEA 1.1, 1.2, and 7 from a mismatched transfusion. This can occur within 4 to 14 days after an initial transfusion. These antibodies can potentially destroy the donor's RBCs (i.e., delayed hemolytic transfusion reaction), ultimately minimizing the benefits of the transfusion.

Ideally, all transfusion recipients should be blood-typed and crossmatched before transfusion. Blood that is DEA 1.1-positive should be administered only to dogs that are DEA 1.1-positive. Veterinary practices can easily and economically test for this antigen using a commercial card blood-typing kit (Fig. 23-3). If typing is unavailable or in an emergency situation, recipients should be crossmatched with universal donors before transfusion to avoid sensitization to the DEA 1.1 antigen. Because of the absence of clinically significant naturally occurring alloantibodies in dogs, the initial crossmatch performed on a dog that has not previously been transfused should yield a compatible result. However, crossmatching is important with subsequent transfusions.

Feline Blood Types

One blood group system, the AB system, has been recognized in cats. It contains three blood types: A, B, and the extremely rare AB. These blood types represent antigens on the RBC surface. Nearly all domestic shorthair and domestic longhair cats have type A blood, the most common. Many purebred cats (and some domestic shorthairs) have type B blood. The proportion of A and B types varies among cat breeds and also nationally and internationally.

Cats differ from dogs in that they have significant, naturally occurring alloantibodies against the other blood type. Cats with type B blood appear to have very strong naturally occurring anti-A alloantibodies, whereas type A cats have relatively weak anti-B alloantibodies. These alloantibodies can cause the following serious problems:

- Cats with relatively rare type B blood can experience potentially fatal transfusion reactions if they are transfused with the common type A blood.
- If a queen with type B blood is bred to a type A tom and the mating produces kittens with type A blood, the antibodies in the colostrum of the queen destroy the RBCs in the kittens (a condition called *neonatal isoerythrolysis*).

Following administration of type B blood to a type A cat, there may not be any obvious clinical reaction, but the transfused red cells have a half-life of only approximately 2 days. Ultimately, this is of no benefit to the patient. With transfusion of type A blood to a type B cat, the type A RBCs survive only minutes to hours and clinical signs are severe and sometimes fatal. Administration of a small amount of blood to test for incompatibility is no longer an acceptable procedure. Life-threatening acute hemolytic transfusion reactions can be observed with administration of as little as 1 ml of AB-incompatible blood. These reactions can be avoided by typing and crossmatching the blood of donors and patients. A simple test using whole blood and blood-typing reagents is available (Fig. 23-4). Blood-typing cards similar to those used in dogs are also commercially available, yielding accurate results in minutes. Because of the presence of naturally occurring alloantibodies, there is no universal donor type in cats. All feline blood donors and recipients must be blood-typed, and only typed, matched blood should be administered. The extremely rare blood type AB cat can be safely transfused with type A blood.

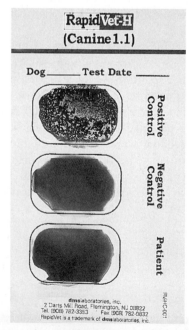

Fig. 23-3 Commercial canine blood typing card using DEA 1.1. *(Available from dms Laboratories, Flemington, N.J.)*

SOURCES OF DONOR BLOOD

Historically, veterinarians have relied on donors living within the hospital facility as a source of blood for transfusion purposes. The cost of an in-house donor is often overlooked, and the charges for a unit of blood are severely underestimated. In the past few years, several commercial blood banks have been established to help meet blood transfusion needs in primarily small-animal medicine. Purchasing products from these banks and maintaining an inventory within the facility are much more efficient and

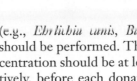

| blood type | red blood cell agglutination with | |
	anti-A serum	anti-B reagent
type A	strong	none
type B	none	strong
type AB	strong	strong

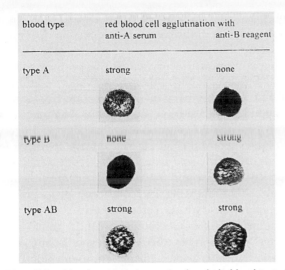

Fig. 23-4 Feline blood typing using a simple whole blood test. Anti-A serum is collected from any type B cat. The anti-B reagent is lectin triticum vulgaris. *(Available from Dr. Urs Giger, Veterinary Hospital of the University of Pennsylvania, Philadelphia, Penn.)*

cost-effective than maintaining a donor colony within the hospital. Using employee-owned personal pets and healthy client-owned animals as blood donors is a good alternative to maintaining in-house donors. For reasons to be discussed, this type of program is more practical for dogs than cats.

Canine Blood Donors

Blood donors can be recruited through employee personal pets, client-owned animals, breeders, and organized dog clubs. Many owners are happy to volunteer their animal for periodic blood donation (e.g., three to four times yearly) once they understand the need for blood products in veterinary medicine. Nevertheless, potential donors may carry illnesses that could possibly affect the safety of the donation process and/or the safety and quality of the blood products, thereby further compromising the patient. For this reason, it is important to verify donor health status through a brief history, physical exam, and appropriate laboratory testing, all of which are performed on the day of the donation.

There are specific requirements canine donors must meet as well before being accepted as a volunteer donor. Donors must be a minimum of 1 year of age and weigh at least 25 kg to allow for the collection of a full unit (i.e., 450 ml +/− 10%). They should be healthy; have a current vaccination status for distemper, hepatitis, parainfluenza, parvovirus, and rabies; and not be on medication at the time of donation (excluding heartworm and flea preventative). As canine donors are not sedated for blood collection, good temperament is required for successful donation. On an annual basis, a complete blood count, chemistry profile, and testing for geographically specific infectious agents

(e.g., *Ehrlichia canis*, *Babesia canis*, *Dirofilariasis immitis*) should be performed. The hematocrit or hemoglobin concentration should be at least >40% or >13.5 gm/dl, respectively, before each donation. Donors can be screened for von Willebrand factor antigen levels to identify the population of the donor pool that has the highest plasma concentration of this platelet adhesion protein for use in patients with von Willebrand disease. Blood donor dogs should be typed for DEA 1.1, and possibly others (DEA 1.2 and 7).

Feline Blood Donors

At present, there are few commercial feline blood banks. In addition, volunteer programs for cats hold many risks. Although blood can be collected from dogs with minimum restraint, most donor cats must be sedated for blood collection. There are legal ramifications associated with sedating personal pets for blood donation. Another concern is that cats can harbor infectious agents more readily than dogs. Because of this, only 100% indoor cats should be used.

Feline blood donors should be large, good-natured, lean, young adults weighing at least 5 kg. Good health can be verified through history, physical exam, and routine laboratory testing. Donors should have current vaccination status for rhinotracheitis, calicivirus, panleukopenia, and rabies. Annual laboratory screening should include a complete blood count, serum chemistry profile, and screening for feline leukemia virus, feline immunodeficiency virus, feline infectious peritonitis virus, and *Hemobartonella felis*. Before each donation, the hematocrit (>35%) or hemoglobin (>11 g/dl) should be checked.

BLOOD COLLECTION

The recommended collection site is the jugular vein. Because of this vein's size and increased blood flow, RBC trauma is minimized during collection. Blood should be collected via a single venipuncture to avoid cell damage and excessive activation of coagulation factors. Strict aseptic technique and use of sterile equipment minimize the possibility of bacterial contamination.

Anticoagulant-Preservative Solutions

There are several anticoagulants, anticoagulant-preservatives, and additive solutions available for blood collection for transfusion purposes. The primary goal of preservative solutions is to maintain red cell viability during storage and to lengthen the survival of red cells post-transfusion. According to American Association of Blood Banking standards, 75% of transfused red blood cells must survive for 24 hours following infusion in order for the transfusion to be considered acceptable and successful. The longer cells are stored, the more viability decreases. Predetermined storage times are based on studies that have investigated adverse biochemical changes that take place during red cell storage. These changes, referred to as the storage lesion, ultimately lead to a loss of red cell function and decreased viability. Storage time will vary with the anticoagulant-preservative solution used:

Citrate-phosphate-dextrose-adenine (CPDA-1)

- RBC 2,3 DPG and ATP better maintained
- Best anticoagulant preservative solution. Canine and feline whole blood may be stored for 35 days; canine pRBCs may be stored for 21 days
- Used at ratio of 1 ml CPDA-1 to 7 to 9 ml blood

Citrate-phosphate-dextrose (CPD)

- Whole blood and pRBCs may be stored for 21 to 28 days
- Used at ratio of 1 ml CPD to 7 to 9 ml blood

Acid-citrate-dextrose (ACD)

- Whole blood and pRBCs may be stored for 21 to 28 days
- Used at ratio of 1 ml ACD to 7 to 9 ml blood

Heparin

- Not recommended for transfusion purposes

Additive solutions*

- Protein-free solution added to red cells after plasma removal from unit of whole blood
- Canine pRBCs may be stored for approximately 35 days Such as *Adsol*,® Fenwal Laboratories, Baxter Healthcare Corporation, Deerfield, Ill; *Nutricel*,® Miles, Inc., Pharmaceutical Division, West Haven, Conn.; *Optisol*,® Terumo Medical Corporation, Somerset, N.J.)

Blood Collection Systems

Whole blood is most often collected into commercially available plastic bags (Baxter Healthcare Corporation, Fenwal Division; Miles, Inc., Cutter Biological Division, Elkhart, Ind.; Terumo Medical Corporation, Somerset, N.J.). These sterile bags are considered "closed" collection systems in that they allow for collection, preparation, and storage of blood and blood components without exposure to the environment, diminishing the risk of bacterial contamination to the product. These systems are available in a variety of configurations that will determine blood component preparation and storage. All of these systems meet human blood banking standards and have been tested successfully in veterinary medicine. Vacuum chambers that allow for more rapid collection into blood collection bags are available.

A single bag is used for collection of blood to be administered as whole blood. It consists of a main collection bag containing anticoagulant-preservative solution and integral tubing with an attached 16-gauge needle. This system is not recommended for component preparation in that the bag must be entered to harvest components, risking bacterial contamination. If the bag is entered, the product must be used within 24 hours.

Other collection systems consist of a primary collection bag containing an anticoagulant-preservative solution, usually CPD, and one, two, or three satellite bags intended for component preparation. One satellite bag may contain 100 ml of an additive solution used for RBC reconstitution after plasma removal (Fig. 23-5). Additive solutions (e.g., saline, dextrose, adenine) extend storage time by enhancing packed RBC survival and function. All bags are attached via integral tubing, allowing for collection, processing, and storage of products within a closed system.

Vacuum glass bottles containing ACD anticoagulant-preservative solution have been the most popular collection system used in veterinary medicine. Although blood collection is easier with this system, there are many limitations and disadvantages: this is considered an "open" collection system; the glass activates platelets and certain clotting factors, the foam created during collection will disrupt the red cell surface and cause hemolysis, and component preparation is not possible. For these reasons, vacuum glass bottles are not recommended.

In the dog, blood may be collected using commercially made blood-collection bags (Box 23-4); however, the size of these systems prohibit their use in cats. Currently, smaller closed collection systems are not available. In addition, blood component preparation would be difficult due to the small volume collected from feline donors. Recommendations have been made to utilize the 450-ml CPDA-1 whole-blood collection system used in dogs. The majority of anticoagulant is expressed from the main collection pack into a satellite container via integral tubing. The remainder

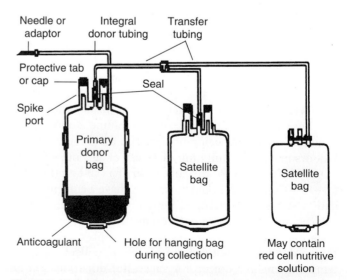

Fig. 23-5 Triple blood collection bag for use in preparing blood components. *(From Hohenhaus AE: Transfusion medicine, Prob Vet Med 4, 1992).*

BOX 23-4

procedure

Canine and Equine Blood Collection Using Commercial Bags

Materials:

- Commercial blood collection bag (450 ml) with 16-gauge needle
- Tube stripper
- Heat sealer, sealer clips/crimper

Procedure:

1. Clip the hair over the jugular groove and surgically prepare the area.
2. Restrain the donor securely but comfortably (dogs in right lateral recumbency, horses standing).
3. Apply pressure at the thoracic inlet to facilitate visualization and palpation of the jugular vein.
4. Perform venipuncture using the 16-gauge needle attached to the main collection bag. The bag should be positioned lower than the animal to aid gravitational flow.
5. Periodically invert the bag gently to mix the blood with anticoagulant solution. The collection bag should be weighed intermittently to ensure that an appropriate volume of blood is collected (1 ml of blood weighs approximately 1 g). One unit of blood should contain 450 ml of blood ± 10%

(i.e., weighs 405 to 495 g). If lesser amounts are collected (300 to 405 ml), only the RBCs can be used after plasma removal because of concern for excessive citrate in plasma and possible resultant hypocalcemia in certain patients (e.g., liver disease, severe hypothermia).

6. When the bag is full, remove the needle from the jugular vein and apply pressure over the venipuncture site to prevent hematoma formation. The donor should remain recumbent (dogs) or quietly restrained (horses) until clotting has occurred.
7. Strip remaining blood from the tubing into the bag and mix it with anticoagulant solution (Fig. 23-6, *A*).
8. Allow the tubing to refill with anticoagulated blood and clamp the distal end with a heat sealer clip (Fig. 23-6, *B* and *C*).
9. Section the entire length of the collection tubing into 3- or 4-inch segments to be used for subsequent crossmatches (Fig. 23-6, *D*).
10. Label the bag with donor identification, date of collection, date of expiration, blood type, unit volume, and anticoagulant used.

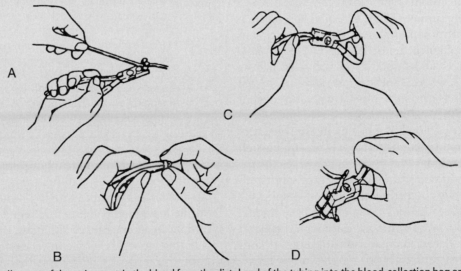

Fig. 23-6 A, Using the roller part of the stripper, strip the blood from the distal end of the tubing into the blood-collection bag and allow it to mix with the anticoagulated blood. **B,** To seal the donor bag and tubing, fold the tubing and place a sealer clip over the folded tubing. **C,** Crimp the sealing clip. Repeat this for as many tubing segments as needed. **D,** Cut the tubing between each sealed segment to obtain samples for crossmatching. *(From Hohenhaus AE: Transfusion medicine,* Prob Vet Med 4, *1992.)*

---

of anticoagulant-preservative solution in the collection tubing will be appropriate for one unit of blood, defined as approximately 40 to 50 milliliters of whole blood. This maintains the system as a "closed" system. Because of the size of the collection bag and its attached 16-gauge needle, this approach is less than optimal.

Alternatively, blood can be collected utilizing separate, single syringes. A 19/21-gauge butterfly catheter attached to a three-way stopcock and sterile 10- to 30-milliliter syringes containing anticoagulant may be used. During collection, the syringes should be gently inverted to allow for mixing of blood and anticoagulant, preventing clot formation. Blood collection utilizing this technique is effective, but considered an "open" system. Following collection, blood can be transferred from the syringes into an empty sterile bag, or transfer pack, making delivery more efficient. Products collected via syringe are not intended for storage.

Cats in need of transfusion support have most often received FWB. This is because of the lack of commercially-prepared closed blood-collection systems for cats, the difficulty in preparing blood components from small whole-blood units, and limited storage time allowed for blood collected with an "open system."

BLOOD ADMINISTRATION

Blood Typing and Crossmatching

Ideally, patients should be blood-typed and crossmatched before any blood transfusion. If blood typing reagents or cards are not available, at the very least a blood crossmatch test should be done. Blood typing determines the blood group antigen on the surface of RBCs. A blood crossmatch test is used to identify antibodies in donor or recipient plasma against recipient or donor RBCs. The *major blood crossmatch test* detects alloantibodies in recipient plasma against donor RBCs, whereas the *minor blood crossmatch test* detects alloantibodies in donor plasma against recipient RBCs (Box 23-5). If there is evidence of macroscopic agglutination of the patient's blood (rarely seen in cats) or severe hemolysis of the patient's blood sample, a blood crossmatch test cannot be performed.

Dogs being transfused for the first time (not sensitized) can have a serologically compatible crossmatch, despite differing blood types, because they often do not have significant, naturally occurring alloantibody. Although the blood crossmatch test can detect many incompatibilities, it does not guarantee against future sensitization. A blood crossmatch test should always be performed in dogs that were previously transfused. If neither crossmatching nor typing is available, or it is an emergency situation with no time for crossmatching, universal donor blood should be given to the dog. All feline patients with unknown blood type should be crossmatched.

Preparing Blood for Transfusion

Refrigerated blood may be gently warmed by allowing it to sit at room temperature for approximately 30 minutes. Properly administered cold blood will not increase the

---

BOX 23-5   *procedure*

Blood Crossmatching

Materials:

anticoagulated blood from donor and recipient
centrifuge
test tubes
0.9% sodium chloride
microscope slides

Procedure

1. Collect 2 ml of EDTA-anticoagulated blood each from the donor and recipient.
2. Centrifuge the blood samples for 1 minute at 3000 G. Remove the plasma to prelabeled tubes.
3. Make a 2% RBC suspension by mixing 0.1 ml of the RBCs and 5 ml of 0.9% saline solution. Mix the suspension.
4. Centrifuge the suspension for 1 minute and discard the supernatant. Resuspend the RBCs in another 5 ml of 0.9% saline and centrifuge. Repeat this washing procedure three times.
5. Place two drops of the recipients plasma and two drops of the donor's RBC suspension in a 3-ml test tube: this is the *major* part of the crossmatching. Then place two drops each of the recipient RBC suspension and the donor's plasma in another 3-ml test tube; this is the *minor* part of the crossmatch. Mix well and incubate the tubes for 30 minutes at room temperature.
6. For controls, use the donor's and recipient's own cells and plasma following the same procedures as above. Centrifuge for 1 minute at 3000 G. You now have a total of four tubes.
7. *Reading the crossmatch:* Grossly check for agglutination and hemolysis, and then place a drop on a slide and examine microscopically at 40× agglutination.

---

chance of a transfusion reaction, but large amounts of cold blood infused rapidly can induce hypothermia and cardiac arrhythmias. Warming of RBC products is recommended for neonates and patients that require large-volume transfusion. In an emergency situation, the tubing of the blood administration set can be immersed in a warm-water bath (not to exceed 37° C [99° F]) so that the blood is warmed as it passes through the tubing. The entire unit should not be warmed at one time. Frozen products should be thawed in a 37° C [99° F] warm-water bath. Blood products should not be exposed to temperatures exceeding 42° C (108° F); this results in damage to RBCs and denaturation of blood proteins. Warming RBC products or thawing plasma products in a microwave oven is not recommended.

Transfusion Volume

The aim of transfusion in anemic patients is to correct the clinical signs rather than return the PCV to normal.

The volume of blood administered is dependent on the onset and degree of anemia, clinical status of the patient, and body weight. There is no magic laboratory number at which a patient must be transfused. For practical purposes, feline patients initially receive one unit of whole blood (35 to 50 ml) or one unit of pRBC (20 to 25 ml), based on product availability. Clinical evaluation of the patient post transfusion will determine if further blood product support is necessary. The following are guidelines to use when calculating the volume of whole blood or plasma needed:

- PCV rise (%) × patient body weight in pounds = ml whole blood needed
- 10 to 20 ml/kg = ml whole blood needed
- 6 to 10 ml/kg = ml pRBCs needed
- 6 to 10 ml/kg = ml FFP needed

Administration Routes

Blood and blood components are best administered IV, making the infused RBCs or plasma products immediately available to the general circulation. Intraosseous infusion is used in puppies or kittens when vascular access is difficult or unsuccessful. When delivering blood products intraosseously, infused cells and proteins are available to the general circulation within minutes. The most common sites for intraosseous catheter placement are the trochanteric fossa of the femur, the wing of the ilium, and the shaft of the humerus. Care should be taken in placement of these catheters because of the risk of osteomyelitis.

Administration Rates

Administration rates vary. For example, a patient with massive hemorrhage may require a more rapid transfusion than a normovolemic patient with chronic anemia. Blood should not be administered at a rate exceeding 22 ml/kg/hr. However, the infusion rate is less critical in a hypovolemic animal than in a normovolemic animal, where circulatory overload is a potential problem. Animals with cardiovascular compromise cannot tolerate infusion rates above 4 ml/kg/hr.

Initially in all patients, blood should be delivered slowly (1 ml/kg during the first 15 minutes) while monitoring for signs of an acute transfusion reaction. The blood product should then be infused as quickly as will be tolerated; infusion of a single unit of blood or blood component should not take longer than 4 hours. Before infusion, baseline values of attitude, rectal temperature, pulse rate and quality, respiratory rate and character, mucous membrane color, capillary refill time, hematocrit, total plasma protein, and plasma and urine color should be recorded. Patients should be monitored closely during transfusion, and parameters should be checked every 30 minutes. Blood values should be checked after transfusion to ensure that the desired effect has been achieved.

Transfusion Reactions

Patients should be carefully monitored for any adverse reactions during and for several weeks following transfusion. Transfusion reactions can be immune-mediated or nonimmune-mediated in origin.

Immune-mediated reactions can be hemolytic, with either acute or delayed presentation. Hemolytic transfusion reactions are the most serious but are rare. In acute situations, intravascular hemolysis is due to pre-existing alloantibodies, as seen in the mismatched transfusion of feline type-A blood to a cat with type-B blood, or in previously sensitized DEA 1.1-negative dogs receiving DEA 1.1-positive blood. Clinical signs include fever, tachycardia, weakness, tremors, vomiting, collapse, hemoglobinemia, and hemoglobinuria. The most common hemolytic transfusion reaction is delayed in presentation and can be exhibited 2 to 21 days post-transfusion.

Nonhemolytic transfusion reactions are a result of antibodies to white blood cells, platelets, or plasma proteins. These reactions are most often transient in nature and do not cause life-threatening situations. Clinical signs include anaphylaxis, urticaria, pruritus, fever, and neurologic signs. Vomiting can be noted with any type of transfusion reaction. Patients receiving blood products should be fasted before administration to avoid this potential complication.

There are a variety of factors associated with nonimmune-mediated transfusion reactions. Any type of trauma to the RBCs can cause hemolysis (e.g., overheating, freezing, warming and then rechilling, mixing RBC products with nonisotonic solutions, and collecting or infusing blood through small needles or catheters). Bacterial pyrogens and sepsis can be a complication of improperly collected and stored blood. Dark brown to black supernatant plasma in stored blood indicates digested hemoglobin from bacterial growth. Any blood with discolored supernatant should be immediately discarded. Citrate intoxication may occur when the citrate/blood volume ratio is disproportionate or in massively transfused patients, particularly in patients with liver dysfunction. Common signs include tremors, cardiac arrhythmias, and decreased cardiac output. This compromised state can be confirmed by obtaining an ionized serum calcium level. If citrate toxicity if suspected, blood administration should be discontinued and calcium gluconate administered IV.

It is imperative to administer the appropriate volume of blood to each patient. One should only use the blood component necessary to treat the specific disorder, and cardiovascular status should be assessed before determining required volume and administration rate. Because blood is a colloid solution, vascular overload is a potential complication of transfusion. Clinical signs include coughing (as a result of pulmonary edema), dyspnea, cyanosis, tachycardia, and vomiting. If volume overload is of concern, blood administration should be temporarily discontinued and supportive care instituted.

All blood products should be filtered in order to help prevent thromboembolic complications. Standard blood infusion sets have in-line filters with a pore size of approximately 170 to 260 microns. A filter of this size will trap cells, cellular debris, and coagulated protein. Trapped debris combined with room temperature conditions may promote proliferation of any bacteria that may be present. Infusion sets may be used for several units of blood products, or for a maximum time of 4 hours.

RECOMMENDED READING

Bell FW, Osborne CA: Maintenance fluid therapy. In Kirk RW, ed: *Current veterinary therapy X, small animal practice*, Philadelphia, 1989, WB Saunders.

Cotter SM, ed: *Comparative transfusion medicine. Advances in veterinary science and comparative medicine*, Volume 36, San Diego, 1991, Academic Press.

DiBartola SP: *Fluid therapy in small animal practice*, ed 2, Philadelphia, 2000, WB Saunders.

Guyton AC: *Human physiology of mechanisms of disease*, ed 6, Philadelphia, 1997, WB Saunders.

Hohenhaus AE, ed: *Transfusion medicine, problems in veterinary medicine*, Philadelphia, 1992, JB Lippincott.

Hughes D: Fluid therapy. In King L, Hammond R, eds: *Manual of canine and feline emergency and critical care*, United Kingdon, 1999, British Small Animal Veterinary Association.

Kirby R, Rudioff E: Fluid therapy, electrolytes, and acid-base control. In Ettinger SJ, Feldman EC, eds: *Textbook of veterinary internal medicine*, ed 5, Philadelphia, 2000, WB Saunders.

Kristensen AT, Feldman BF, eds: *The Veterinary Clinics of North America, Small animal practice: canine and feline transfusion medicine*, Philadelphia, 1995, WB Saunders.

Oakley DA: Establishing and monitoring central venous pressure in the critical patient, *Vet Tech* 1:40-46, 1987.

Oakley DA: Small animal transfusion medicine. In Battaglia AM, ed: *Small animal emergency and critical care*, St Louis, 2001, WB Saunders.

Oakley DA: Hematologic emergencies. In Battaglia AM, ed: *Small animal emergency and critical care*, Philadelphia, 2001, WB Saunders.

Walker RH, ed: *Technical manual of the American Association of Blood Banks*, ed 14, Arlington, 1996, American Association of Blood Banks.

24

Dentistry

Kathy A. Sylvester

Learning Objectives

After reviewing this chapter, the reader should understand the following:

- Anatomy of teeth
- Terms used to describe teeth and their surfaces
- Dental formulas of companion animals

- Instruments used in dentistry
- Procedures used in dental prophylaxis
- Treatments for common dental problems
- Safety in the dental operatory
- Marketing veterinary dentistry by utilizing technicians

As much as in any field in veterinary medicine, the role a technician can play in dentistry can be extremely important. In many practices, the technician provides the majority of hands-on care, particularly in performing dental prophylaxis or teeth cleaning. The technician may also take history, perform the initial examination, and inform the clinician of any pertinent facts. The patient's health depends on the technician's ability to assess the situation, call attention to specific problems, and provide quality care. The technician may also discuss dental hygiene and home care with the client. Depending on the "dental IQ" and skills of the technician, the service provided can be of great benefit or detriment to the patient.

Although the oral cavity may not seem to be an important part of the body, its role in the overall health of the patient can be quite significant. Oral and dental disease not only affects local structures but also contributes to many systemic problems (Fig. 24-1), particularly when bacteremia originating from the mouth has profound effects on other organs. A patient with oral problems may not eat well or groom its body, and halitosis may make the patient an unwelcome guest. There is a high proportion of veterinary patients with dental problems. Up to 85% of dogs and 70% of cats over 3 years of age show some indication of active periodontal inflammation. If only 50% of clients sought professional help, it would have a tremendous effect on practice income.

The importance of veterinary dentistry and its role in patient health should never be minimized. Veterinary commitment is to provide the best health care for patients, and this goal certainly includes care of the oral cavity.

ORAL ANATOMY

As with every other body system, it is essential to know the normal anatomic structures of the oral cavity, and how they are to function. Knowing this, one can determine whether a certain condition is abnormal and if further assessment is necessary.

Teeth

Teeth are the primary functional structures of the oral cavity. A mature tooth can be divided into the exposed crown and the "submerged" root portions that join at the neck of the tooth (cementoenamel junction, or CEJ) (Fig. 24-2). The enamel covering of the crown is the hardest substance in the body (96% inorganic) and is made of hydroxyapatite crystals. A layer of cementum covers the root. Cementum is closer in composition (45% to 50% inorganic) to bone than enamel. Because cementoblasts also participate in the initial formation of cementum, cementum also regenerates, unlike enamel. Underlying the enamel and cementum for the entire length of the tooth is a layer of dentin (70% inorganic, 30% organic collagen fibers and water). Although the dentin layer is very thin in immature teeth, odontoblasts from pulpal tissue continue to manufacture dentin in

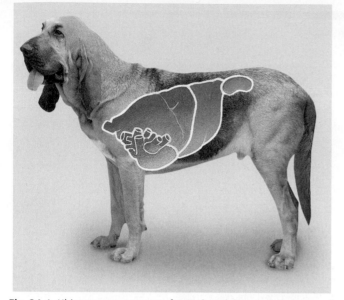

Fig. 24-1 Ultimate consequences of periodontal disease. Left untreated, periodontal disease has serious implications for canine health. Besides breath odor and unpleasant appearance of teeth, periodontal disease inevitably leads to tooth loss. There can be a loss of appetite leading to weight loss. The problems of periodontal disease can affect the liver, kidneys, and heart. Less commonly, the lungs can be affected by the persistent invasion of toxins and bacteria into the bloodstream. *(From "How to prevent tooth loss"; courtesy Pharmacia Animal Health.)*

a tubular pattern throughout the life of the tooth. This makes the dentinal walls progressively thicker and the canal space of the tooth narrower as the tooth matures.

The internal canal space surrounded and protected by the dentin is called the *pulp cavity* for the entire tooth; the *pulp chamber*, including pulpal horns, for the crown; and the *root canal* for the root. This internal space, or pulp cavity, houses the blood vessels, nerves, and connective tissue that serve the tooth. These pulpal structures enter the tooth in small animals at the apical, or root tip end, often through the *delta foramina*, a formation with many small openings. These pulpal tissues provide oxygen and nutrients through the blood vessels, contain cells instrumental in laying down and removing dentin (odontoblasts and odontoclasts), and have nerves to conduct impulses in response to various stimuli.

Although teeth can "sense" a variety of stimuli from cold to heat (depending on the health or sensitivity of the teeth) and pressure, the animal only feels the sense of pain. This is a good defense mechanism, because if a tooth is compromised to the extent that it is sensitive to cold or heat, the resulting pain may alert a client to the denture problem.

Both *deciduous* (primary) and *permanent* (adult) teeth arise from a ridge of dental laminar epithelium. In a young animal with deciduous teeth, the permanent tooth buds are located adjacent to them underneath the *gingiva* (gum). Any stimu-

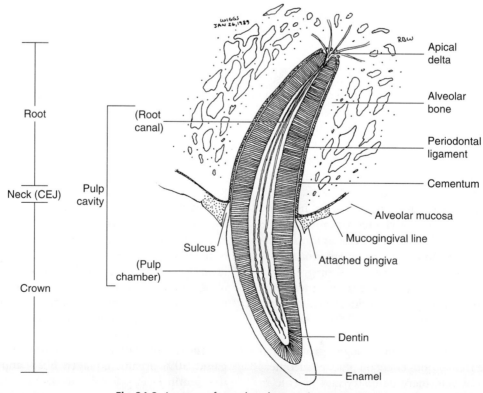

Fig. 24-2 Anatomy of a tooth and supporting structures.

lus, from generalized infection (distemper) or fever to a local infection from an abscessed deciduous tooth, can affect development of the permanent tooth, much like a developing fetus in the uterus. Deciduous teeth are often shed in sequence as the permanent teeth erupt. This sequence can be influenced by many factors, including genetics, nutrition, and trauma. If a deciduous tooth is still present when a permanent tooth is erupting, the deciduous tooth should be carefully extracted to avoid deflection of the adult tooth into an abnormal position (see Orthodontics section).

Skull types and related problems

There are three recognized skull types in dogs and cats. By recognizing these types, you can identify the problems that are inherent with their dentition and ideally pretreat them.

Mesaticephalic. This is the most common skull type. Poodles, Labradors, and shorthair cats best illustrate this skull type. One problem seen in the toy breeds is loose incisors. This is due to the fact that there is less bone in the rostral jaw due to the small size of the mouth. Thus, gingival recession, tooth mobility, and the potential for fractured jaws occur more quickly in these breeds.

Brachycephalic. Boxers, Pugs, and Persian cats best illustrate this skull type. They have short, wide heads that cause increased tooth crowding, causing the teeth to rotate or overlap. This in turn causes a higher incidence of periodontal disease.

Dolichocephalic. The long, narrow skulls of the collie and greyhound best illustrate this skull type. The genetic abnormality called *Posterior crossbite* can be found in these breeds. Performing a routine cleaning on their teeth often seems endless because of the length of the jaw.

Dental formulas

A dental formula (Box 24-1) is a way of expressing the normal number and arrangement of deciduous and permanent teeth in a species. By knowing the dental formula for a species, you can determine when there are an inappropriate number of teeth or a variation in tooth eruption times.

Although some breeds have specific tooth numbers and placement (see Orthodontics and Dental Records sections), in most animals the important thing to note is the presence of healthy, functional dentition. A few missing teeth may not pose a problem, as long as they are not embedded. A few extra teeth can sometimes fit in nicely, as long as overcrowding does not predispose the area to food accumulation and periodontal disease. Tooth form and structure may also vary at times, from reduced crown size to extra roots. As long as the root canal (pulp cavity) system is intact and viable, however, the tooth should remain functional.

Directional terms

It is important to be able to describe where on a tooth or in the oral cavity a lesion exists. Directional terms may be

---

BOX 24-1

Dental Formulas for Cats and Dogs

Cats

Deciduous: 23 (Id $\frac{3}{3}$; Cd $\frac{1}{1}$; Pd $\frac{3}{2}$) 5 26

Permanent: 23 (I $\frac{3}{3}$, C $\frac{1}{1}$, P $\frac{3}{2}$, M $\frac{1}{1}$) 5 30

Time of Eruption

	Deciduous	Permanent
Incisors	2 to 3 weeks	3 to 4 months
Canines	3 to 4 weeks	4 to 5 months
Premolars	3 to 6 weeks	4 to 6 months
Molars	4 to 6 months	

Dogs

Deciduous: 23 (Id $\frac{3}{3}$; Cd $\frac{1}{1}$; Pd $\frac{3}{3}$) 28

Permanent: 23 (I $\frac{3}{3}$; C $\frac{1}{1}$; P $\frac{4}{4}$; M $\frac{2}{3}$) 42

Time of Eruption

	Deciduous	Permanent
Incisors	3 to 5 weeks	3 to 5 months
Canines	3 to 6 weeks	3.5 to 6 months
Premolars	4 to 10 weeks	3.5 to 6 months
Molars	3.5 to 7 months	

---

helpful in noting lesions in the patient's record. In addition, certain dental abnormalities may also be defined (Box 24-2). Fig. 24-3 shows directional terms pertaining to teeth.

Periodontium

The supporting structure around the teeth, or *periodontium*, maintains the stability of the teeth in the oral cavity. The periodontium includes the gingiva, the cementum of the root, the periodontal ligament (goes from the cementum to the alveolar socket), and the alveolar bone or socket (see Fig. 24-2). The mandible and maxilla have a series of depressions, or sockets, in the alveolar ridge to house the root structures. The periodontal ligament stabilizes the tooth within the socket and absorbs some of the shock of the occlusal forces generated during chewing. The cementum must remain healthy to maintain attachment of the periodontal ligament to the tooth. Covering all of these structures is the gingival mucosa.

The specialized tissue of the attached gingiva immediately adjacent to the tooth structure provides the first line of defense against bacteria for the rest of the periodontium. The attached gingiva is histologically different from the looser alveolar mucosa. Interdigitations of connective tissue (*rete pegs*) provide firm attachment to the underlying periosteum of the alveolar bone. Without this specialized

BOX 24-2

Dental Terminology

Dental Directional Terms	**Dental Abnormalities**
Mesial: surface of tooth toward the rostral midline	Macrodontia: oversized crown
Distal: surface of tooth away from the rostral midline	Microdontia: reduced crown
Palatal: surface of tooth toward the palate (maxillary arcade)	Dilacerated: distorted (twisted) crown or root
Lingual: surface of tooth toward the tongue (mandibular arcade)	Dens-in-dente: enamel layer "folds" into itself/tooth
Labial: surface of tooth toward the lips	Enamel pearls: beads of enamel at CEJ, furcation
Buccal: surface of tooth toward the cheeks	Fusion tooth: fusion of two tooth buds during formation
Facial: labial and/or buccal surface	Gemination: complete tooth duplication but incomplete split
Occlusal: surface of tooth facing a tooth in opposite jaw	Twinning: complete tooth duplication and split
Interproximal: surface between two teeth	Enamel hypocalcification ("hypoplasia"): enamel pitting/discoloration
Apical: toward the apex (root)	Hypodontia: some teeth missing
Coronal: toward the crown	Oligodontia: most teeth missing
Supragingival: above the gum line	Anodontia: all teeth missing
Subgingival: below the gum line	Supernumerary: extra tooth/teeth
Mucogingival line (MGL): junction of the attached gingival and mucosa	
Cemento-enamel junction (CEJ): area where the enamel and the cementum meet	

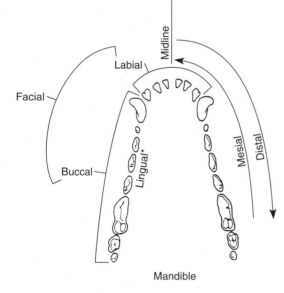

*Or palatal in the maxilla

Fig. 24-3 Directional terms used in dentistry.

keratinized epithelium, bacteria can readily attack the underlying periodontal ligament and bone. A minimum of 1 to 2 mm of attached gingiva is necessary to provide this protection and can be measured from the mucogingival line that delineates its connection to the alveolar mucosa. This mucogingival line is most readily apparent on the facial or buccal surfaces of the teeth.

The free edge, or *gingival margin*, of this epithelial collar is often not directly attached to the tooth, although it can be very close to the teeth in a cat's mouth. The space between the tooth and the free gingiva is termed the *gingival sulcus*. At the depth of the sulcus, the junctional epithelium attaches to the tooth. A sulcus depth of up to about 2 to 3 mm is considered normal in dogs (depending on patient size); sulcus depth should not be more than 0.5 to 1.0 mm in cats without a concurrent disease process. Any variation in sulcus pocket depth should alert the technician to potential problems (see Periodontal Disease section).

PERIODONTAL DISEASE

Periodontal disease is the most common oral disease in pets and is probably the most common infectious process in the body. Bacteria are normally found in the oral cavity as a component of plaque. Plaque is a soft mixture of bacteria and mucopolysaccharides (carbohydrates) that adheres to the tooth. These carbohydrate molecules are very sticky and act as a matrix. The bacteria and associated endotoxins in the plaque initiate the inflammatory process in the gingival tissue (gingivitis). The inflammation may start as a mild gingivitis with edema and redness of the free gingival margin. If the inflammation is limited to this region and there is no attachment loss, it can be reversible with appropriate therapy (stage I periodontal disease: gingivitis). A slight increase in sulcus depth is typically attributable to swollen gingival margins and usually resolves when the edema subsides.

More extensive involvement of the periodontal ligament without intervention leads to periodontitis and subsequent attachment loss, as evidenced by an increased pocket depth and bone loss (stage II periodontal disease: periodontitis). Stage II periodontal disease consists of pockets up to 5 mm deep in dogs (1 mm in cats) or up to approximately 25% attachment loss. Pockets up to 9 mm deep (1.5 mm in cats) and 50% attachment loss is characteristic of stage III periodontal disease. Stage IV periodontal disease shows greater than 9-mm pocket depth and over 50% attachment loss. Often there are different stages of periodontal disease in different areas of a patient's mouth.

The bacteria associated with reversible gingivitis are generally located above the gum line (supragingivally) and tend to be aerobic, gram-positive, nonmotile cocci. As the disease progresses, the periodontal pockets enlarge, and bacteria work their way into the deeper structures. The bacterial flora in these deeper tissues tends to be more anaerobic, gram-negative, motile bacilli. The damage from bacteria and associated toxins can be significant, but the body's response with influx of many neutrophils, lymphocytes, and plasma cells can cause as much or more tissue destruction than the bacteria. Therefore, the primary goals of treating periodontal disease are controlling bacterial populations, minimizing pocket depth, and maintaining healthy attached gingiva.

Dental Instruments

Although antibiotics and anti-inflammatories have their place in treating periodontal disease, mechanical removal of plaque, calculus, bacteria, and abnormal tissue with dental instruments is the focus of treatment. A wide variety of equipment is available to help manage periodontal disease.

Power scaling units

The most commonly used scaling unit in veterinary dentistry is the ultrasonic scaler. The magnetostrictive scaler works through vibrations of the metal stacks that cause the tip to rotate at around 45,000 Hz, with continuous emission of an aerosolizing water spray. This vibration helps to remove the tartar or calculus from the teeth. Piezoelectric ultrasonic scalers use the vibrations generated from electrical current running through a quartz crystal. Newer ceramic models show promise with potentially less damage, but these are fairly expensive. Ultrasonic scalers produce heat, and a constant water flow is essential to keep the instrument cool. Fig. 24-4 shows a tabletop scaling and polishing unit.

Sonic scalers vibrate at 16,000 to 20,000 Hz generated from the pressurized air of a high-speed handpiece.

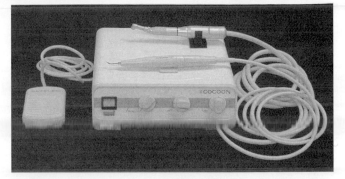

Fig. 24-4 Tabletop scaling and polishing unit. *(Courtesy C-Med Surgical.)*

Although sonic scalers do not produce excessive heat, the water spray is helpful to flush debris from the tooth surface. A soft steel rotary bur with six cutting flutes rotates at 300,000 rpm on a high-speed handpiece. This produces a frequency similar to that of an ultrasonic unit, but it is potentially very damaging to the tooth. Although power scaling units can quickly remove tartar, if improperly used they can generate excessive heat, even with adequate water flow, and can damage the tooth structure inadvertently.

Hand-scaling instruments

Although power equipment is certainly faster, at times hand-scaling instruments may be a better choice. Hand instruments used for scaling include scalers and curettes. Although hand-scaling instruments are available in various types, the most typical form is a *sickle scaler*. These instruments, with their sharp tip and triangular cross-section (Fig. 24-5), can be used to scale calculus off the crown of the tooth. Sickle scalers should never be used subgingivally because of the potential for gum damage.

The instrument of choice for removing subgingival deposits is the curette, with rounded toe and back (see Fig. 24-5). With small to moderate subgingival pockets less than 5 mm deep, the curette can be gently introduced into the pocket and used to scale the root surface and debride the lining of the soft tissue.

The working end of scalers and curettes must be sharpened at least after every use; dull instruments only burnish the calculus instead of removing it. Although the face of the instrument can be sharpened with a conical sharpening stone, it is usually best to use an oiled flat stone, drawing the working edge across at a 110-degree angle to approximate the angle of the head.

Other hand instruments that are essential in evaluation of periodontal disease are periodontal explorers and probes. A *periodontal explorer* has a sharp, thin tip, often curved into a "shepherd's crook." This tactile instrument is used in human dentistry to detect softened areas of enamel that are starting to decay. Carious lesions are not as common in dogs and cats due to less occlusal surfaces in the

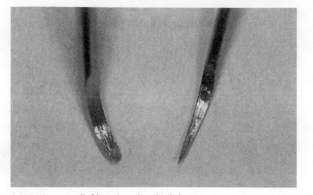

Fig. 24-5 Curette *(left)* and scaler *(right)*. *(From Harvey CE, Emily PP: Small animal dentistry, St Louis, 1993, Mosby.)*

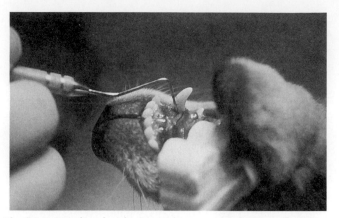

Fig. 24-7 Periodontal probe inserted into a palatal pocket of an upper canine tooth.

mouth. The instrument is used to detect roughened areas or residual calculus on the tooth surface; resorptive areas (feline or canine odontoclastic resorptive lesions called CORLS or FORLS); and open canals in broken teeth.

The *periodontal probe* is an even more important tool in assessment of periodontal disease. Probes are marked in varying millimeter increments, with either notches or color changes on the working end, which can be round or flat (Fig. 24-6). A probe can be gently introduced into the gingival sulcus to determine the depth of any pocket (Fig. 24-7). Measurements at up to six sites around a tooth's circumference give an indication of any increased pocket depth, which can then be noted on the record. Careful attention should be made to place this tool gently into the sulcus as the operator can create a "pocket" if too much pressure is applied.

Polishing Equipment

Polishing equipment is another essential tool in treatment of periodontal disease (see Fig. 24-4). Scaling roughens the enamel surface of a tooth; this must be polished to produce a smooth surface that slows accumulation of plaque. Battery-operated polishing instruments can be used, but these typically do not last long. Rotary hand tools (Dremel-type) can be used to power the polishing handpiece, but

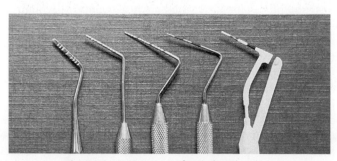

Fig. 24-6 Various types of periodontal probes.

rotational speed must be controllable and maintained at less than 3000 rpm. Micromotor units often have the option of using a prophy angle, or the slow-speed handpiece of an air-driven unit can be used.

ORAL RADIOGRAPHY

Radiographic equipment is essential for a quality dental practice. Although one may purchase expensive dental radiographic equipment, it is possible to do oral radiography using standard equipment with intraoral films and rapid developer/fixer solutions.

Extraoral films and oblique projections can be used for survey films, but these generally produce some degree of superimposition of other oral structures over the area to be viewed. Small, flexible intraoral films can be used with the standard radiographic unit with few variations. Intraoral films provide excellent detail, and superimposition of other oral structures is rarely a problem, unless positioning was incorrect. The unit can be used with the radiographic head positioned at a 36- to 40-inch focal distance for $\frac{2}{5}$ to $\frac{3}{5}$ of a second at 100 mA. It is preferable if the radiographic head is mobile, however, to decrease the focal distance to 12 inches and the exposure time to $\frac{1}{10}$ to $\frac{1}{15}$ of a second to minimize distortion and exposure. Depending on the equipment, the kVp may vary from 65 for a small dog or cat up to 85 for a large breed (Fig. 24-8).

The intraoral films come in a variety of small sizes (0, 1, 2, 3, 4); No. 2 film *(periapical)* is most commonly used (Fig. 24-9). No. 4 film *(occlusal)* measures 2 by 3 inches and can be used to view a larger area of the incisors and canines or the nasal cavity (also for small rodents, birds, and cat feet). These nonscreened, double-emulsion films are encased in a black paper sleeve with a lead foil back sheet that helps prevent back scatter produced by x-rays bouncing back off the table. A paper or plastic covering protects

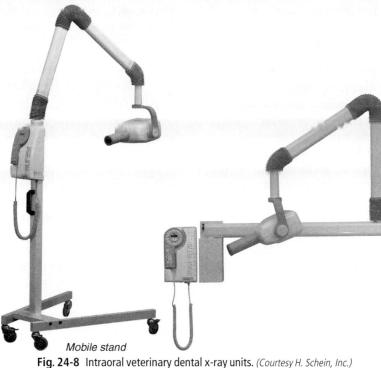

Mobile stand

Fig. 24-8 Intraoral veterinary dental x-ray units. *(Courtesy H. Schein, Inc.)*

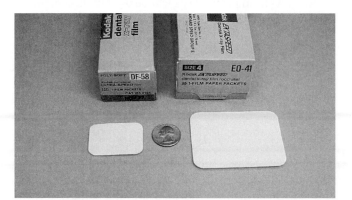

Fig. 24-9 Intraoral films: size 2 *(left)* and size 4 *(right).*

30 seconds, using fresh developing solutions. After a water rinse, fixing time is in the same range, so a film can be developed in less than 1 minute. This makes use of dental films very convenient. Rapid development time is particularly important when multiple films must be made.

The difficulty of oral radiography lies in positioning the film and the patient to obtain an image with the least distortion. A *parallel technique* is used only with the mandibular premolars/molars, when the film can be placed parallel to the teeth, with a corner pressing down into the intermandibular space. With the film so positioned, the x-ray head can then be aimed perpendicular to the parallel items.

the films until after exposure, when they are removed before developing.

Dental films can be developed in standard tanks or automatic processors (taped to the lead end of a larger film). They take the same amount of time and volume of developing solutions as for a larger film. These smaller films can sometimes be lost in standard developing tanks. As an option, rapid dental developer and fixer solutions can be used in individual containers, either in the existing darkroom or in a chairside developer at the dental station (Fig. 24-10). After rehydrating the emulsification of the film in water for 3 to 5 seconds, developing time ranges from 15 to

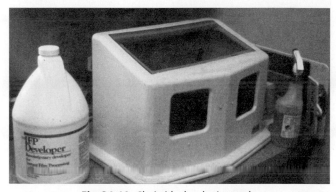

Fig. 24-10 Chairside developing tank.

Elsewhere in the oral cavity, the film cannot be positioned directly against the object to be viewed, particularly in the maxilla, due to the shape of the palate. To accommodate for this obstacle, the *bisecting angle technique* can be used to minimize distortion that is inherent when the film cannot be placed parallel to the tooth.

If the x-ray beam is aimed perpendicular to the film, the tooth image will be shortened; if it is aimed perpendicular to the long axis of the tooth, the image will be elongated. Therefore, if the beam is aimed midway between the two positions, the image should approximate the size of the tooth itself. One way to visualize this is to imagine an angle formed by the line of the film and the line of the long axis of the tooth or its root. Once this angle is assessed, a line that would bisect this angle is determined. By aiming the beam perpendicular to this bisecting line, the image will closely approximate the tooth size. To better visualize the angle when working on the buccal teeth, one should stand facing the nose of the animal. To determine the angle of the rostral teeth, stand at the patient's side (Fig. 24-11). Sometimes better visualization is achieved by working with models or using 3 cotton-tipped applicator sticks to elongate the 3 axis until you are more familiar with the technique. Certain corrections must be made when taking x-rays of the maxillary premolars and molars in the cat. Due to its prominent zygomatic arch, if one followed the standard bisecting angle rule there would be superimposition of the arch over these teeth. In order to avoid this, the operator must come in at a steeper angle, thus creating elongated teeth but no interference from the cat's zygomatic arch.

A dental radiographic unit with a mobile head is optimal to attain these positions, but a standard radiographic unit can sometimes be adjusted accordingly. If the unit is not mobile, the patient's head can be positioned so that the determined bisecting line is parallel to the table, thus becoming perpendicular to the beam. Once exposed and

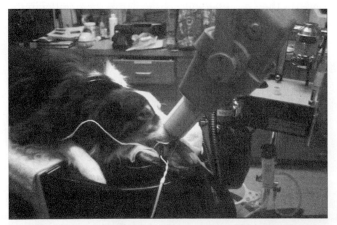

Fig. 24-11 Intraoral x-ray of a dog's rostral jaw utilizing bisecting angle technique.

developed, these films reveal many problems that otherwise might not have been grossly visible, particularly during routine prophylaxis.

PROPHYLAXIS AND PERIODONTAL THERAPY

Because periodontal disease is the most common oral problem in dogs and cats, it is safe to say that periodontal treatment is the most frequent oral/dental procedure performed in a practice. The primary goals of periodontal therapy include removing any accumulations of plaque, calculus, and diseased tissue, and trying to minimize gingival pocket depth while maintaining at least 1 to 2 mm of attached gingiva.

The term *prophylaxis* is often used to describe the process of cleaning the teeth by removing plaque and calculus. The true meaning of the word is "prevention." However, there are relatively few patients to which this term applies. When there is merely accumulation of plaque and calculus with reversible gingivitis, a thorough cleaning helps to prevent further periodontal disease at that time. If there is any indication of extended periodontitis, particularly with any attachment loss, the more appropriate terminology is *periodontal therapy*. Not only is this term more correct, it also helps impress upon clients the level of care necessary for the patient. The term prophylaxis will be used in this chapter to avoid confusion.

Procedure

The steps of a complete prophylaxis should be followed in a systematic manner to avoid missing any particular step. The first step is removal of any grossly visible plaque and calculus on the crowns of the teeth. After this process, the patient's mouth may look greatly improved, but it is only the beginning of adequate treatment. One must remember that most of the periodontal disease process is occurring below the gingiva, in the sulcus or pocket. A concentrated effort should be made to thoroughly evaluate the oral cavity for any periodontal pockets, no matter how slight, and to adequately clean each area.

The legal definition of oral surgery and how much a technician is legally able to perform subgingivally varies among states. In some areas, any work that is to be done under the gum line is considered oral surgery, and legally must be performed by the veterinarian. In other locales, a technician may gently clean areas of slightly increased sulcus depth using curettes to remove any subgingival debris. The American Veterinary Dental College has published a position statement that defines the areas of the mouth on which a technician can work and the procedures a technician can perform.

Smaller curettes can be used in pockets up to 5 mm in depth in a process known as *closed root planing*. In this technique, the curette is gently introduced into the sulcus down to the depth of the junctional epithelial attachment. The cutting edge of the curette is then adjusted to engage the surface of the root, and the curette is withdrawn from the pocket in a pulling action. Repeating the process in varying directions in a cross-hatched pattern (horizontal, vertical, oblique) on the tooth surface ensures thorough cleaning of the root surface. The goal is to remove all calculus, debris, and diseased tissue without removing excessive amounts of normal cementum. The term *periodontal debridement* is sometimes used, instead of root planing, to denote a more controlled therapy. The curette can also be used in the pocket by changing the position of the working head to gently debride the inner lining of the soft tissue with slight digital pressure from the outside. This subgingival curettage removes infected or necrotic pieces of gingiva lining the sulcus, and any associated debris.

Once the pocket area has been adequately cleaned, it should be gently irrigated with sterile saline or dilute chlorhexidine or fluoride to remove any remnants of calculus or tissue that may cause a periodontal abscess if left in the pocket. It is best to use a blunt, side-slot needle for irrigation to minimize damage to the soft tissue and avoid forceful extrusion of fluids into the junctional epithelium. A gentle air blast or flow can open the pocket slightly to allow better visualization of the root surface. At that time, remaining areas of calculus deposition show up as a chalky white residue. Further insurance toward healing of the area can be achieved by the placement of an antibiotic/polymer gel product into the pocket. Veterinarians have had success with regained periodontal ligament attachment and decreased pocket depth when using this product under prescribed conditions. Results vary from patient to patient, but benefits can be seen by decreased anaerobic bacteria colonization even if a patient does not regain significant attachment. This is due to the presence of doxycycline (Fig. 24-12).

POLISHING

All scaled tooth surfaces should be polished to minimize any roughening of the enamel that would predispose the area to accelerated plaque accumulation. Generally, a medium to fine prophy paste can be used, applying enough pressure to gently splay the foot of the prophy cup against the tooth. Lack of sufficient paste and use of excessive pressure or time spent on the tooth should be avoided, because this can cause overheating and enamel damage. The speed of the prophy angle should be at approximately 1500 rpm, not to exceed 3000 rpm. After polishing, a final irrigation should be performed to flush out any remaining debris or prophy paste.

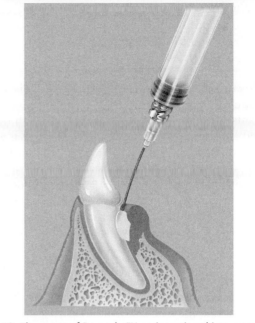

Fig. 24-12 Placement of Doxyrobe™ perioceutic gel into a periodontal pocket. *(From "How to prevent tooth loss"; courtesy Pharmacia Animal Health.)*

FLUORIDE APPLICATION

Although there is some difference of opinion on use of fluoride in the oral cavity, its antibacterial properties and use on sensitive teeth because of enamel wear or after root planing are some considerations. It is best to limit any possibility of fluoride ingestion; in an anesthetized patient, more control is possible. After the final irrigation, the tooth surfaces should be dried, particularly when using sodium fluoride. The fluoride should be placed on the tooth with a small brush (if a gel) to avoid excessive application. It may be more difficult to control the exact amount when using a form, but an attempt should be made not to leave excessive material in the oral cavity. After the appropriate time, the fluoride should be blown off the teeth with air or wiped off—never rinsed away, because this would inactivate the effects of the fluoride. If there is an indication for home use of fluoride, the client should be instructed to apply it carefully and therefore limit the amount of fluoride that could be ingested by the patient. There has been some discussion of placing fluoride on the teeth of juvenile patients, especially when they have come in to have persistent or retained deciduous teeth removed. The thought is that this initial application can help toughen the enamel. Again, careful consideration should be made to prevent overingestion of fluoride, especially in a young patient.

Sealants

Sealants are used almost universally in human dentistry, and are gaining more acceptance in animal dentistry. A sealant is a plastic product that is applied to the chewing surfaces of teeth. The purpose is to act as a barrier and prevent decay and the adherence of plaque (the precursor to calculus). As animals are not usually bothered with or decay or traditional cavities, the benefits are seen more from slowing the progression of periodontal disease (see Periodontal Disease section).

Sealants are relatively easy to apply. The teeth that will be sealed are cleaned. Next an acid etch solution is applied to the tooth surface. This will roughen the surface and allow the sealant to adhere. The sealant is then applied to the tooth with a brush. It will then harden with or without the aid of a curing light to form a barrier on the tooth.

In humans, these sealants remain intact for many years when exposed to normal chewing. It has not been determined whether these sealants will hold up to the forces of an animal's daily chewing in the long term. A Canadian company has recently introduced a take-home sealant kit for clients to reapply on a weekly basis. This may be a more successful option for follow-up home care if it proves effective, especially for clients who do not like to brush.

DENTAL RECORDS

Throughout the process of the prophylaxis, the mouth is continuously evaluated for any abnormalities. Although notations can be made at any time during the procedure, it is often best to review the entire oral cavity after prophylaxis and ensure that all items are noted on the record. Recording observations in the dental chart should follow a systematic order to avoid missing any details. Many forms of dental records are available, including complete record sheets, stickers to affix to the records, and even ink stamps. Any variations in tooth appearance, pocket depth, or other abnormalities should be recorded, along with the appropriate treatment. Individual teeth can be described using several techniques, but be sure to use a consistent style. In longhand terms, the tooth should be described as deciduous or permanent, which quadrant (right or left, mandibular or maxillary), and number and type (first, second, etc.; incisor, canine, premolar, or molar).

A shorthand method uses the abbreviation for the tooth (I, C, P, M) and its numbered position around the tooth, depending on quadrant. For example, the upper-left second incisor is noted as ^{2}I. Canine teeth can be designated with the number 1, and deciduous teeth can be designated with a lowercase letter (which can be hard to distinguish from an uppercase letter) or by using the letter *d* (e.g., Id, Cd, Pd, Md).

The triadan system can also be used, particularly when using a computer system, as it relies on a three-digit code. The first digit (hundreds) signifies the quadrant (upper-right 100; upper-left 200; lower-left 300; lower-right 400).

The last two digits indicate the tooth number, starting with 01 to 03 for incisors, 04 for canines, 05 to 08 for premolars, and 09 to 11 for molars. Dogs and cats do not have 11 teeth in each quadrant (although pigs do), so some variation will be seen in the numbering systems for various species. Deciduous teeth can be identified with the triadan system using 500 for the upper-right quadrant, 600 for the upper-left, 700 for the lower-left, and 800 for the lower-right. When charting, an orientation trick to keep in mind is the "rule of 4s and 9s." All number 4 teeth indicate a canine tooth (e.g., 104, 204). All number 9 teeth indicate a first molar (e.g., 109, 209). This also makes charting easier when a tooth is missing or a supernumerary tooth is present. Further delineations of tooth number are less obvious. Current anatomic guidelines state that there are no "deciduous molars," so all deciduous teeth caudal to the canines are considered premolars. Examples of triadan numbering are as follows:

- 104–C^1: right maxillary canine
- 307–$_3$P: left mandibular third premolar
- 802–Id$_2$: deciduous right mandibular second incisor

On a dental chart, many symbols can be used to designate specific problems observed. Any system can be used, as long as it is consistent and the information can be readily interpreted. Some commonly used abbreviations and symbols are listed in Box 24-3.

The depth of periodontal sulci or pockets should be measured at six sites around the tooth, taking particular care to evaluate the palatal aspect of the maxillary canines. Often pockets can exist with no external sign of a problem, so the examination should be thorough.

RADIOGRAPHS

Radiographs should always be made in animals with periodontal disease to evaluate bone loss, with "neck lesions" to evaluate root integrity, with crown fracture or discoloration to look for apical problems, and any time a problem is suspected. Extensive lesions not apparent grossly can be hidden subgingivally, so radiographs can be very useful (Box 24-4). Some practices find it very useful to offer "survey" or complete mouth x-rays. These films help the veterinarian to visualize problems not apparent to the naked eye.

HOME DENTAL CARE

Routine home care is an important part of maintaining oral health. The technician is often responsible for instructing the client on the type and frequency of recommended home dental care. *Brushing* is the best way to remove plaque from the tooth surface before it calcifies into calculus.

BOX 24-3

Common Dental Abbreviations and Symbols for Charting the Mouth

X: extracted
O: missing
FE: furcation exposure, or *F1, F2, F3,* graded *1:* furcation detected; *2:* probe passes into furcation; *3:* probe passes through furcation
RE: root exposure
\: tooth fracture; also *fxo* for open fracture, pulp exposed; *fxc* for closed fracture, no pulp evident
GH: gingival hyperplasia, charted as *H* followed by number to designate mm (e.g., *H1, H2*)
C: calculus, charted as *C/H-heavy, C/M-moderate, C/S-slight*—an objective decision
CLL, CNL, FRL: cervical line lesion; cervical neck lesion; feline resorptive lesion (*stage 1 to 4*)
EH: enamel hypocalcification (hypoplasia)
S: supernumerary tooth
GR: gingival recession, charted as *GR* followed by a number to designate mm (e.g., *GR1, GR2*)
M: mobility, graded *1:* slight; *2:* moderate; *3:* severe with loss of attachment; *4:* no longer functional and extraction candidate (e.g., *M1, M2, M3*)
Gingival scores: O: healthy; *I:* mild gingivitis with slight bleeding upon probing; *II:* moderate gingivitis with edema and erythema and some bleeding; *III:* severe gingivitis with swelling, pustular discharge, pocket formation, bleeding, erythema

BOX 24-4

Reasons for Using Dental X-rays

- Gingival pockets greater than 1 mm in a cat
- Gingival pockets greater than 3 mm in a dog
- Areas of facial swelling/especially below the eye
- Periodontal disease, grade 2, 3, or 4
- Chronic discharge from one or both nares
- Evaluation of tooth undergoing root canal or pulp capping procedure
- Evaluating fractured tooth or jaw
- Oral bony or soft-tissue growths
- Malocclusion/supernumerary or deciduous teeth
- Malformed teeth

A soft-bristle, disposable toothbrush is ideal for most patients. Many fine brushes for pets are on the market, particularly some of the smaller brushes for cats, but even children's toothbrushes are useful for some patients. It may take some training to accustom a patient and client to routine brushing, so a gradual, gentle beginning is recommended. Teaching a young animal to tolerate brushing is much easier for both client and pet. Encourage new puppy and kitten owners to make toothbrushing part of their pet's daily routine, so the animal becomes used to the task and the client succeeds. Working with older pets requires more diligence, but it can also have a successful outcome.

The client can begin by touching the pet more around the mouth and head, gently keeping the mouth closed with one hand and lifting the lips with the other. A soft washcloth or gauze can be used to carefully wipe the outer surface of the teeth. In dogs, garlic powder or canned meat can be used on the cloth to make the experience more pleasant; the liquid from water-packed canned tuna can be used with cats. Once the patient accepts the initial attempts, a soft toothbrush can be introduced to the regimen.

Depending on the individual, the patient may immediately accept flavored toothpaste, or it may have to become accustomed to toothpaste. Human toothpastes should not be used because of their fluoride and detergent content. Most patients do not spit out the excess but swallow it instead. Baking soda products should be avoided in older or cardiac patients because of the potential for sodium overload. Daily brushing is ideal for good oral hygiene, but even two to three times per week can make a big difference.

Other oral products include solutions and gels, such as chlorhexidine and fluorides, to reduce bacterial populations in the mouth. Chlorhexidine products work best when retained in the mouth for a minute or more, so the more viscous gels or gingival patches are more efficient. Though fluoride helps control oral bacteria and helps prevent carious lesions, it should not be overused, because excessive ingestion can cause toxicity. Zinc ascorbate liquids and gels can aid healing of soft tissue after oral surgery and can be useful for patients that will not tolerate toothbrushing.

FOOD AND CHEW TOYS

Different food products vary in efficacy in controlling plaque and tartar. There seems to be some benefit of hard foods over soft, though the result of studies may conflict. Newer products have a specialized fiber composition to help clean the teeth as the food is eaten, or contain substances that discourage mineralization of plaque.

Chew toys can also help reduce accumulation of plaque and calculus, especially the more fibrous, "chewy" objects. Extremely hard objects, such as cattle hooves and bones, ice, and even tennis balls, can cause severe wear of teeth and even fractures. It is sometimes difficult to find the correct balance for an animal that is a heavy chewer; a product may not break the teeth, but it often does not last long. Finding the right chew toy can sometimes be a challenge for the client. For dogs that continue to chew harder objects, the carnassial teeth (upper fourth premolar, lower first molar) should be regularly inspected for fractures.

TREATMENT OF COMMON ORAL PROBLEMS

As discussed previously, the periodontal examination should be quite thorough. At the time of pocket evaluation, the amount of exposed root should be noted, because the combined degree of root exposure and pocket depth gives the most accurate assessment of total attachment loss. In other words, if the gingival margin starts 2 mm below the neck of the tooth and there is an additional 4 mm in pocket depth, the attachment is a total of 6 mm below the normal placement. These measurements should consider the size of the patient to determine the percentage of attachment loss in comparison with the normal degree of attachment for that size of animal.

PERIODONTAL SURGERY

In cases of gingival hyperplasia, there can be increased pocket depth without attachment loss because of falsely "elevated" gingival margins. Typically, resection of the excessive tissue using periodontal probes to determine the normal extent of the sulcus can restore a more normal amount of attached gingiva without excessive pocket depth that could predispose to periodontal disease.

If pockets more than 5 mm deep are associated with attachment loss and extensive periodontal disease (Fig. 24-13), closed-root planing is typically not helpful, as the curettes cannot effectively reach the depths. The veterinarian should perform periodontal surgery, including releasing gingival flaps to expose the area and to provide access for proper therapy. Specialized procedures can be performed to graft or move (pedicle flap) healthy attached gingiva to replace areas with less than 2 mm of tissue. In areas with sufficient gingiva and moderately deep pockets, some gingiva can be excised to reduce pocket depths, as seen with gingival hyperplasia. If the amount of attached gingiva is barely sufficient but a significant pocket is present, releasing and then suturing the gingiva back at a lower position on the tooth after cleaning the roots and bone (apically repositioned flap) can preserve the remaining gingiva while reducing pocket depth.

Procedures can be done to stimulate formation of bone or periodontal ligament. With deep pockets, a gingival flap can be performed to expose the site for cleaning. Barrier material or a membrane is placed to keep soft tissue from growing into the site. The palatal area of the upper canine teeth (see Fig. 24-7) is especially important, because exten-

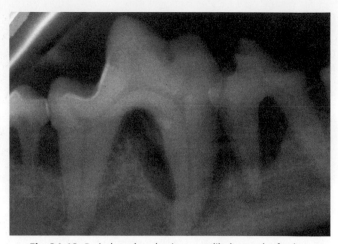

Fig. 24-13 Periodontal pocket in a mandibular tooth of a dog.

sive bone loss on the palatal surface can expose the nasal cavity, causing an oronasal fistula. If a fistula is suspected in a deep pocket there, a gentle stream of water can be flushed into the region to see if there is communication with the nasal passages. If bone loss is extensive enough for fistulation, periodontal ligament regeneration is not possible and the tooth must be extracted.

Simple closure of the area is not adequate because of the tension placed on the sutures every time the animal breathes. A mucoperiosteal flap from the remaining gingiva and alveolar mucosa may be elevated from the underlying attachment to prevent tension and the defect sutured. With chronic or large openings, a flap can be harvested from the palate for additional repair.

TOOTH EXTRACTION

If attachment loss or accompanying infection is too advanced to warrant additional therapy, the tooth can be extracted. The decision to extract a tooth should consider several factors, particularly in borderline cases. If the client is committed to perform home care, some periodontal procedures can be performed to save a tooth that would otherwise be sacrificed. Furcation exposure is not always a criterion for extraction if the client can regularly clean the area and keep it free of debris. On the other hand, specialized procedures, particularly flaps and regenerative ones, should not be performed if the commitment to home care is lacking. Selection of the teeth to be extracted may also depend on the function of the tooth. Some teeth are considered more "strategic" than others, such as the canines and carnassial teeth (upper fourth premolars and lower first molars in dogs and cats) (Fig. 24-14). These teeth tend to be more vital in function or structure than small teeth and may warrant additional effort in their preservation. In addition, early periodontal disease of smaller teeth that may

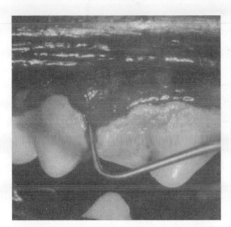

Fig. 24-14 Periodontal pocket in a maxillary premolar of a dog. A probe can be inserted subgingivally into the pocket formed by the loss of attachment to the gum tissue. *(From "How to prevent tooth loss"; courtesy Pharmacia Animal Health.)*

affect adjacent strategic teeth may lead a practitioner to decide on extraction of the nonstrategic teeth.

Retained deciduous teeth should be extracted (Fig. 24-15). There should *never* be two teeth (deciduous or permanent) growing in the same place at the same time. Clients should be instructed to monitor the progress of eruption of permanent teeth. If a deciduous tooth has not been exfoliated (shed), it should be extracted. If it remains in the mouth during eruption of that permanent tooth, the permanent tooth will be deflected to an abnormal position. Most permanent teeth erupt in a more lingual position when a deciduous tooth is retained, including the incisors and the lower canines. These displaced permanent teeth can be malpositioned enough to impinge on the palate

(base narrow). The permanent upper canines, however, erupt more mesial (rostral) to their normal position, sometimes even pointing straight forward and often impinging on the space that the lower canine would normally occupy, thereby displacing that tooth.

Another indication for deciduous tooth removal is when a deciduous malocclusion would impede normal growth of the jaws. Examples include base-narrow mandibular deciduous canines hitting the palate, or upper incisors located lingual to the corresponding lower incisors. If these situations can be discovered in young animals (8 to 12 weeks of age), careful extraction of the teeth can often resolve the malocclusion and allow the jaws to grow to their proper length. If there is a genetic predisposition for the jaw to be abnormal, however, this procedure will not change the eventual outcome.

Deciduous teeth should also be extracted if they are broken or discolored and abscessed. The close proximity of the permanent tooth bud under the gingival surface makes it very susceptible to infection from the deciduous tooth. The position of the permanent tooth bud close to the deciduous tooth necessitates careful extraction of deciduous teeth. Even with careful elevation of the deciduous tooth during extraction, the permanent tooth structure and position can be altered.

Permanent teeth should also be extracted with care. Extractions can be challenging and even frustrating, so the veterinarian should handle most cases, depending on state laws. Certainly, a loose single-rooted tooth poses no problem; however, solidly anchored multirooted teeth often require gingival flaps, sectioning the tooth into single-root fragments, and good elevation technique to adequately remove the tooth without damaging surrounding tissue.

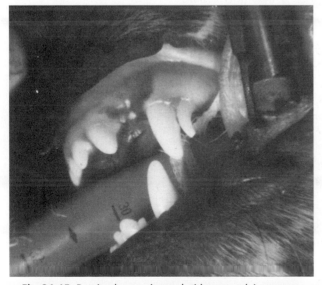

Fig. 24-15 Retained or persistent deciduous tooth in a puppy.

ROOT CANAL THERAPY

Any permanent tooth with nonvital or compromised pulp (fracture with open canal) that will not receive endodontic (root canal) therapy should be extracted. Except for a tooth that has been recently fractured, especially in a young animal that can have vital pulpotomy/pulp capping performed to preserve the rest of the pulp, any tooth with an open canal or gray to purple discoloration should be considered nonvital. In order to illustrate this point in an exam room, or to forewarn a client about the possibility of a "dead" tooth, a penlight can be pointed at the tooth in question. If the tooth is vital, the light will transluminate the tooth. A nonvital tooth will appear opaque. Nonvital pulp provides substrate for bacterial growth, which can allow bacteria to enter the bloodstream. If a root canal is not performed to remove the infected pulp and seal the canal, the tooth must be extracted. Such a tooth should never be ignored because it does not seem to bother the patient. Animal patients may tolerate pain and discomfort better than humans do, but it does not excuse ignoring a potentially dangerous situation. Once such teeth are treated, the animal often shows improvement (eating or feeling better), even though the client noticed no abnormal signs previously. A root canal procedure can preserve the structure of the tooth by removing the potential for ongoing infection. Also, metal or metal and porcelain crowns can be placed on the tooth to provide additional strength.

Excessive tooth wear can expose the pulp canal, necessitating some form of treatment. If the wear is gradual, odontoblasts in the pulp tissue manufacture additional dentin to protect the pulp as it retreats. A dark spot on a worn tooth that is smooth, hard, and solid is most likely reparative dentin and the pulp is probably still protected. Radiographs should be made in these cases and in cases with minor fractures without pulpal exposure, because even if the pulp cavity is not open, the pulp tissue still may be compromised and eventually die, necessitating treatment. Radiographic signs of a nonvital pulp with extension of infection into the bone around the root include a periapical lucency or halo around the apex (Fig. 24-16).

CARIES

The teeth can also be compromised by carious lesions or cavities, though caries are not as common in dogs and cats as in humans. Occasionally a carious lesion is seen on the occlusal surface of the upper first molar (see Hand Scaling Instruments section). The sharp tip of the explorer tends to penetrate this region of dark, soft enamel. Very shallow lesions that do not extend into the pulp cavity can be debrided and restored with amalgam or composites. By the time most carious lesions are detected, however, there is extensive damage to the tooth and extraction may be the only option.

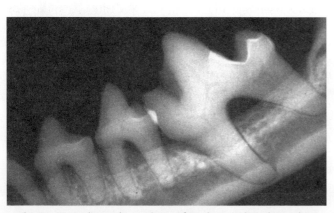

Fig. 24-16 Radiographic evidence of an abscessed tooth in a dog.

RESORPTIVE LESIONS IN ANIMALS

The teeth of certain animals (wild and domestic cats, dogs, rats, mice, marmosets, and pigs) can develop resorptive lesions, known as *cervical line lesions*, or odontoclastic resorptive lesions. For the purpose of this discussion, we will describe feline and canine resorptive lesions (FORLS or CORLS) (Table 24-1). Although these lesions can be found in various areas of the teeth, the most typical presentation is a loss of tooth structure at or near the neck or cervical region of the tooth, frequently on the buccal surface (Fig. 24-17), but sometimes on the lingual or palatal surface. These may be grossly apparent or may be hidden by overlying calculus or an area of hyperplastic, reddened gingiva that grows into the space created. They often become apparent during prophylaxis, as the patient "twitches" or "chatters" when the area is touched by the scaler, even under general anesthesia. The cause of these painful lesions is unknown, but they tend to be progressive, even with attempts at treatment. Restoration of an affected tooth, generally with a glass ionomer, should be performed only with very early lesions that affect just the enamel and some of the dentin. Even lesions that appear shallow often exhibit radiographic signs of root resorption, which is an indication for extraction of the tooth. Affected teeth are often *ankylosed* (joined) to the underlying bone and are difficult to remove intact. Difficult to extract or fragile teeth that do not exhibit clinical signs of infection can be atomized (or have the crown amputated) just apical to the level of the alveolar bone. This is sometimes a less lengthy procedure

TABLE 24-1		

Classes of Resorptive Lesions

Stage	Description	Treatment
Stage 1	Areas of erosion in the enamel	Use cavity varnish to seal dentinal tubules and harden enamel
Stage 2	Lesions have penetrated the enamel and dentin	Restore with composite or glass ionomer cavity varnish; may only last 2 years
Stage 3	Tooth has eroded into the endodontic system	Root canal with restoration; more likely tooth extraction
Stage 4	Severe erosion apparent in crown and root structures	Extract tooth
Stage 5	Crown is totally resorbed	No treatment unless area is inflamed, then extract root

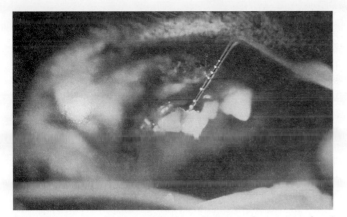

Fig. 24-17 Erosive lesion on the buccal aspect of an upper fourth premolar.

for both patient and veterinarian. Careful attention should be made to smooth out all protruding bone spicules as these will cut into the gingiva and cause the animal pain. In cats with an inflamed mouth (stomatitis or faucitis), every effort should be made to remove the entire tooth structure.

Even without resorptive lesions, sometimes tooth extraction is the only effective treatment for cats with severe stomatitis (Fig. 24-18). In less severe cases, regular prophylaxis and home care, combined with use of antibiotics and anti-inflammatories as indicated, can often help control the inflammation. In cats that eventually become nonresponsive to such conservative treatment, removal of all teeth (and therefore the surfaces that plaque can adhere to) may substantially decrease the amount of inflammation.

Extraction of the caudal teeth (molars and premolars) is sometimes sufficient, particularly when the cat will no longer be chewing on the inflamed tissue. Some affected cats, however, require extraction of all teeth. Certain breeds, such as Abyssinians, Maine coon cats, and some of the Oriental breeds, are predisposed to stomatitis, but it can occur in any cat. Cats with stomatitis should be checked for infection with feline leukemia virus, Bartonella, or feline immunodeficiency virus before any treatment is given, particularly with anti-inflammatories.

CONGENITAL PROBLEMS

Animals may be born with oral defects, because of either a genetic influence or stimuli during fetal development. Some of these lesions may be quite obvious, as with a puppy that cannot nurse or has milk coming out of its nose after nursing due to a cleft palate. The genetic defect, called *microglossia* or "bird tongue," may not be readily apparent (Fig. 24-19). Affected patients have a small tongue and cannot adequately nurse; they often weaken quickly. Unless microglossia is diagnosed, failure of these puppies to thrive may be attributed to the "fading puppy" syndrome.

Another congenital dental problem seen in dogs is *wry mouth*. This is a condition in which one side of the skull grows faster than the other, causing the mouth to have an uneven appearance. Other congenital abnormalities include a variation in tooth number (Fig. 24-20), certain developmental tumors, pitting in the enamel (enamel hypoplasia), malocclusions such as posterior crossbite, and other inherited defects of the oral cavity such as gray Collie syndrome.

ORAL TRAUMA

Trauma to the head can cause significant damage to the oral cavity. With any trauma, the patient's condition must be

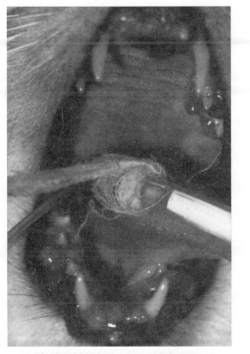

Fig. 24-18 Severe stomatitis in a cat.

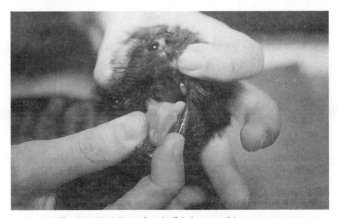

Fig. 24-19 Microglossia (bird tongue) in a puppy.

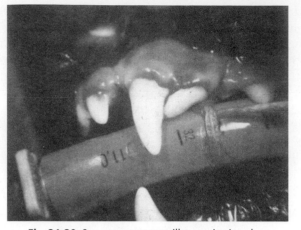

Fig. 24-20 Supernumerary maxillary canine in a dog.

stabilized before any corrective oral work can be attempted. Fractured teeth are one of the most common results of trauma. Teeth can be fractured by external sources of trauma, but more commonly they are fractured by chewing on hard objects, such as bones, cattle hooves, or even ice. External trauma frequently damages other tissues in the mouth, so the soft tissue and bones of the head and mouth should be carefully examined.

A tooth can also be avulsed (lost or ejected) from the socket. If handled correctly and in a timely fashion, an avulsed tooth can be reimplanted into the socket to preserve it. An avulsed tooth should immediately be placed in sterile saline, and the reimplantation procedure should be performed as quickly as possible. If saline is not available, the client can place the tooth in cold milk until reaching the clinic. After reimplantation, the tooth will also need endodontic treatment. If the previous presence of the tooth must be documented for legal or breed registry reasons (i.e., some working breeds, Schutzen dogs), a preoperative radiograph can demonstrate the empty alveolus or a retained root if the crown has broken off.

Mandibular or maxillary fractures often occur with severe head trauma. Many basic techniques of fracture reduction have been attempted in the oral cavity, but certain long bone fracture repair techniques do not adapt well to this region. The mandibular canal is not suitable for intramedullary pinning. External fixators, screws, plates, and pins often damage root structures when placed improperly. In addition, fracture reduction and stabilization are not the only considerations. Restoring normal occlusion must also be addressed when repairing these fractures. Interdental or transosseous wiring, with or without use of acrylics, is often employed for stabilization. Additional injuries, such as palate separation or temporomandibular joint (TMJ) luxation, must be addressed accordingly.

Soft tissue trauma should be thoroughly evaluated and addressed in conjunction with any bony or dental injuries. Depending on the degree of damage, the region should be flushed and cleaned of debris and nonvital tissue, and tissues sutured in their proper position if possible, without interfering with occlusion or mastication. All attempts should be made to preserve as much attached gingiva as possible when it is involved.

A degloving type of injury to the rostral portion of the mandibular (lower) lip can occur as it is nearly scraped off the mandible. Often the soft tissue must be sutured by securing it around the mandibular canine teeth. Soft-tissue injury in the sublingual area can go undetected. By gently pressing a finger up into the intermandibular area while opening the patient's mouth, the tongue can be elevated and the area beneath can be better visualized. Lacerations, ulcerations, foreign bodies, and even tumors can be better assessed using this method.

The oral cavity can be a common location for foreign bodies, particularly in young animals that indiscriminately chew on objects. Foreign bodies can lodge anywhere in the mouth, such as rib bones lodged against the palate; round bones stuck behind the canines or around the mandible; fish hooks, needles, or tacks penetrating the lips or palate; or string or fishing line caught around the base of the tongue. With smaller foreign bodies, such as burrs or plant awns, the object may not be visible because it is embedded in granulomatous tissue, sometimes coalescing into a large lesion if multiple burrs are embedded, such as in the tongue. Radiographs are always indicated if a foreign body is suspected.

Chewing on electrical cords can cause significant damage and burns in the oral cavity, not to mention serious damage to internal organs and severe pulmonary edema. Conservative debridement of necrotic tissue can help to preserve as much normal oral tissue as possible. Burns and ulcerations from ingestion of caustic chemicals can be moderate to severe, depending on the compound and degree of exposure. As with any other oral injuries, supportive care must be provided until the animal can comfortably eat and drink.

ORAL TUMORS

As both veterinary staff and clients continue to improve their dental "IQ" and as pets are living longer lives, oral tumors are more likely to be detected. Unless the client is doing regular home care or examining the pet often, oral tumors often have grown to a large size before they are detected. Considering the aggressive biologic nature of malignant oral tumors, by the time the tumor is diagnosed, it may have already metastasized (spread to other body areas).

The most common oral malignancy of dogs is *melanosarcoma* (Fig. 24-21). Melanosarcoma is more prevalent in older (more than 10 years of age), male dogs with dark pigmentation of the skin and mucosae, and in certain breeds (e.g., Cocker Spaniels). These tumors grow rapidly and can be found on the gingiva, palate, tongue, or lips. By the time of detection, they have most likely metastasized throughout the lymphatics or to the lungs, so thoracic radiographs should be made. Although aggressive resection combined with chemotherapy and/or radiation therapy can increase the anticipated survival rates, melanosarcoma still warrants a guarded prognosis.

Another common oral tumor in dogs is the *fibrosarcoma*, which can be seen in larger dogs, often on the palate. These are typically firm, and sometimes flat and ulcerated. Fibrosarcomas are locally invasive but slow to metastasize, and they tend to recur after resection. *Squamous-cell carcinoma* in dogs shows variable biologic characteristics, depending on its site in the oral cavity. Tonsillar forms are extremely invasive, often metastasize, and warrant a grave prognosis. Nontonsillar squamous-cell carcinomas are often found on the buccal mucosa or tongue. If found in the rostral oral cavity, these tumors tend to be less aggressive than tumors found in the caudal portion of the mouth. Squamous-cell carcinoma is the most common oral tumor seen in cats (Fig. 24-22). They have a variable presentation in cats, depending on the site. Cats can also have fibrosarcomas, but melanosarcomas are rare in cats.

Of the benign tumors found, the *epulis* is probably the most frequently seen. The fibromatous epulis and the ossifying epulis can often be treated adequately with excision and extraction of the associated teeth (they arise from the periodontal ligament). These tumors are usually found above the free gingival margin. The acanthomatous epulis or ameloblastoma tends to be a more locally invasive tumor, requiring more radical surgery to address the problem. These tumors tend to invade the bone adjacent to the

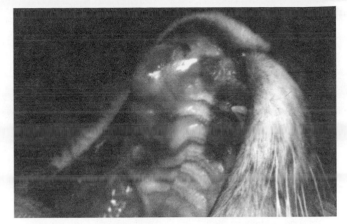

Fig. 24-22 Squamous-cell carcinoma in a cat.

tumor and may cause pain and destruction of the bone if left untreated. These tumors are generally found on the anterior part of the mandible. Treatment of choice for epulis is complete removal of the oral mass with wide (more than 1 centimeter) margins and further evaluation by a pathologist. *Viral papillomatosis* and some developmental tumors (e.g., odontoma, dentigerous cyst) are also seen in dogs.

ORTHODONTICS

Orthodontics is the branch of dentistry concerned with prevention or correction of *malocclusion* (improper bite). In veterinary dentistry, orthodontics involves assessment of a patient's occlusion to determine whether orthodontic measures can help alleviate pain and discomfort and provide a more normal bite (Table 24-2).

The relationship between the upper and lower incisors is usually evaluated. Looking at the premolars can better assess the relationship between the upper and lower arcades. Ideally, the upper and lower incisors should meet in a *scissors* fashion, with the upper incisors slightly rostral to the lower incisors. The American Kennel Club permits many breeds to have a *level bite*, with the incisal edges of the incisors contacting; this can be an uncomfortable situation. Brachycephalic (pug-nosed) breeds have a reverse scissors bite, with the lower incisors rostral to the upper incisors. This is considered normal within certain limits for these breeds.

When the relationship of the maxilla and mandible is correct, the lower canine tooth is positioned directly between the upper canine and upper corner incisor, with equal spacing on either side (mesial and distal aspects) of the lower canine. The premolars should also be positioned in an "interdigitation" with the cusp tip of the rostral mandibular premolars, like a pair of pinking shears.

Animals with properly aligned upper and lower arcades (premolar interdigitation, canine placement) may have

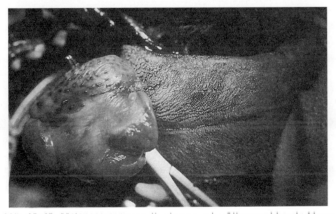

Fig. 24-21 Melanosarcoma on the tongue of a 10-year-old male Chow Chow.

TABLE 24-2

Common Dental Malocclusions and Treatment

Malocclusion	Recommended Treatment
Wry mouth	None—see Congenital Problems section
Anterior crossbite—reverse scissor bite involving incisors	Movement with elastic bands and arch wire
Posterior crossbite—mandibular premolars buccally occluded with maxillary teeth	None—see Congenital Problems section
Base narrow canines—mandibular canines displaced palatally, penetrate palate	Use an inclined plane to deflect buccally or shorten crowns of canines
Lance canines—"tusk teeth" canines deflected rostrally	Extraction or movement with brackets, buttons, or elastics
Overbite (parrot mouth or overshot jaw)—maxillary teeth extend beyond mandibular teeth	Crown reduction with vital pulpotomy of mandibular canines or orthodontic movement
Underbite (undershot jaw or prognathism)—mandibular teeth in front of maxillary teeth	Crown reduction with vital pulpotomy of maxillary canines if ulceration noted
Level bite—incisors in maxilla and mandible meet end-to-end; considered normal in some breeds; causes wear and stress on TMJ	Treat as underbite, if necessary
Open bite—mouth unable to close due to other malocclusions	Check size and location of teeth, TMJ, or potential congenital problems

misplaced individual incisor teeth, as from retained deciduous teeth, that cause a maxillary incisor to erupt palatal to its normal position. Such *anterior crossbites* can sometimes be uncomfortable and result in abnormal wear to the teeth, even causing them to be sensitive.

Retention of deciduous teeth can also influence another malocclusion, when the mandibular canines are deflected lingually, often to the extent that they contact the palate. If the soft tissue contact is at the edge of the palate, excision of the gingival "groove" that is formed may be sufficient to relieve the problem. When teeth contact the palate with full force, some form of correction is necessary to relieve pain. The offending teeth can be extracted, the coronal height can be reduced (with vital pulpotomy and pulp capping), or orthodontic movement with incline planes can be considered. Any extensive work requires specialized training, as well as client commitment to home care while the orthodontic appliance is in place.

Rostral or mesial deviation of an upper canine tooth can occur as a result of retention of its deciduous counterpart. The prevalence tends to be higher in certain breeds, such as Shelties and Italian Greyhounds (lance tooth), indicating possible genetic involvement. Rostral positioning of this tooth can also result in lateral or buccal displacement of the lower canine. Orthodontic movement can help resolve these problems.

With any malocclusion or orthodontic case, the genetic implications should always be thoroughly discussed with the client. It must be stressed that correction is done only to relieve any pain or discomfort the patient may be experiencing. If the abnormality appears to be inherited, the client should be counseled against breeding the animal. In addition to the forms of malocclusion previously discussed, many other inherited problems warrant serious consideration of the patient's breeding potential. For example, consider a patient with what appears to be a normal scissors bite, with the lower canine positioned tightly against the upper corner incisor. This indicates a mandible that is relatively longer than the maxilla, but held in place by the canines' position. Such an individual may produce offspring with a distinct malocclusion. Orthodontic correction should never be done to conceal or camouflage an abnormality.

SYSTEMIC PROBLEMS AFFECTING THE ORAL CAVITY

The mouth is sometimes the first, or the most noticeable, place where certain systemic diseases or conditions become apparent. The gingival mucosa, with its high vascularity, shows distinct changes when anemia (pale), lack of oxygen (cyanotic), toxicity (chocolate brown), or bleeding abnormalities (petechia) are present.

Gingival ulcerations may be present with renal disease (e.g., uremia), during certain infections (e.g., calicivirus), or as a sequel to immunodeficiency (e.g., feline immunodeficiency virus). Hyperparathyroidism, either primary or secondary to severe renal disease, causes "rubber jaw" when the calcium in the bones is depleted. The bones of affected animals are less radiodense, and the teeth appear to be "floating" without jaw contact. There may be swelling and softening of the maxilla and mandible. Autoimmune diseases (e.g., pemphigus vulgaris, bullous pemphigoid) often have oral signs. Recognizing abnormalities in the oral cavity alerts the veterinary staff to potential problems else-where in the body.

DENTISTRY IN OTHER SPECIES

Rabbits and Rodents

Animals other than dogs and cats are occasionally presented for specific oral problems. Rodents and rabbits have specific oral and dental needs related to the structure and function of the teeth and mouth. Rodents and rabbits have four prominent incisor teeth for gnawing. Rabbits also have two additional small maxillary incisors called peg teeth, caudal to the large ones. These incisor teeth have very long "root" structures, and grow continuously for the life of the animal. They are termed *aradicular hypsodont teeth*, because the apex never closes into a distinct root structure. As the animal chews on rough or abrasive objects, the teeth wear down but continue to erupt. In rabbits and some rodents (e.g., chinchillas, guinea pigs), the cheek teeth (premolars and molars) also grow continuously.

Continuous growth of the incisors poses no problems when the patient has a normal occlusion; however, problems arise when there is a malocclusion and the upper and lower teeth do not meet correctly. If this is the case, particularly with the incisors, the teeth do not wear down in the proper manner, and they overgrow, often causing a worse malocclusion. These teeth must be trimmed every 6 to 8 weeks to prevent additional problems of cheek teeth overgrowth.

These teeth are best cut with a bur on a high-speed handpiece; such instruments as nail trimmers can break or split a tooth, exposing the pulp cavity. Another alternative to frequent trimmings is the extraction of all four incisors, which can be challenging with their long, curved roots. The use of small instruments and even blunted hypodermic needles (25- to 18-gauge) with gentle elevation around the tooth can often successfully remove these teeth. Special rabbit/rodent extraction forceps and molar cutters are now available to make these procedures less traumatic (Fig. 24-23).

Other oral problems, such as periodontal disease, can occur in these small pets. This can be quite challenging, particularly if the problem is in the caudal portion of the

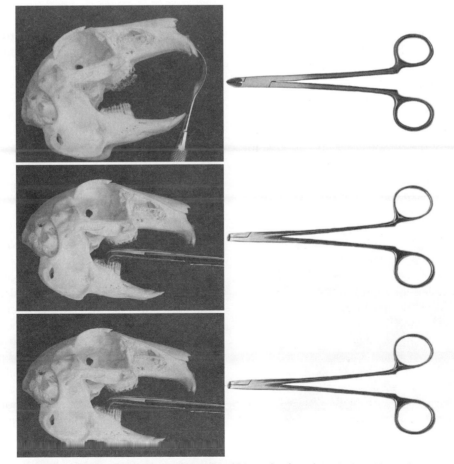

Fig. 24-23 Extraction forceps for use in rabbits and rodents. *(Courtesy H. Schein, Inc.)*

oral cavity, because the mouth opening is quite restrictive in rabbits and rodents. By using rodent mouth gags, cheek dilators, and tongue depressors, the operator can better visualize the oral cavity and treat the problem accordingly (Fig. 24-24).

Horses

It should be noted that the continually growing teeth of rabbits and rodents are different from the teeth found in horses and some other herbivores. In horses, the teeth are considered to be continually erupting but not continually growing. These teeth continue to erupt, but without further growth at the root (Table 24-3). Tooth length diminishes as the animal ages and the erupted tooth is worn away. These can be described as *radicular hypsodont teeth* (long-crowned, with a root), in comparison with the teeth of rodents and lagomorphs (aradicular hypsodont) or dogs and cats (brachyodont, short-crowned).

Horses can also experience overgrowth of incisors and cheek teeth, particularly when the teeth wear unevenly. This uneven wear forms sharp hooks or ridges that must be periodically filed down (*floated*). It should also be pointed out that horses have additional teeth known as *wolf teeth*. These small teeth are located in front of the second premolar and usually are only present in the maxilla. The amount of wolf teeth may vary from one horse to another. Although they may not routinely cause problems, veterinarians usually remove them to avoid problems. Table 24-4 lists dental procedures performed on horses at various ages.

SAFETY IN THE WORKPLACE

In addition to the safety precautions that you observe for patients, it is also necessary to protect yourself against potential dangers. Wearing goggles or other protective eyewear will prevent shards of teeth or aerosolized bacteria from entering your eye. A HEPA mask will keep the same

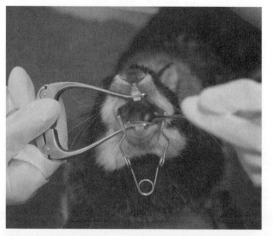

Fig. 24-24 Rodent mouth gags and cheek dilator. *(Courtesy H. Schein, Inc.)*

TABLE 24-3

Tooth Eruption Times in Horses

Deciduous Teeth	Eruption Time
1st incisors (centrals)	Birth to first week
2nd incisors (intermediates)	4 to 6 weeks
3rd incisors (corners)	6 to 9 months
1st, 2nd, and 3rd premolars (cheek teeth)	Birth to first 2 weeks for all premolars
Permanent Teeth	**Eruption Time**
1st incisors (centrals)	2 ½ years
2nd incisors (intermediates)	3 ½ years
3rd incisors (corners)	4 ½ years
Canines (bridle)	4 to 5 years
Wolf teeth (1st premolars)	5 to 6 months
2nd premolars (1st cheek teeth)	2 ½ years
3rd premolars (2nd cheek teeth)	3 years
4th premolars (3rd cheek teeth)	4 years
1st molars (4th cheek teeth)	9 to 12 months
2nd molars (5th cheek teeth)	2 years
3rd molars (6th cheek teeth)	3 ½ to 4 years

From *"Dental Care,"* American Association of Equine Practitioners, Bayer Corporation, 1995.

bacteria from entering your respiratory system and causing bronchial infection. We also recommend latex gloves to protect your hands from bacteria and other contaminants. Many advocate full sterile dress. This allows the technician to remove contaminated clothes without bringing home germs or passing them to another patient. Prerinsing the patient's mouth with a dilute chlorhexidine acetate solution will cut down on some bacteria. Even pretreating the patient 24 to 48 hours before the procedure with an antibiotic, such as clindamycin, can cut down on the number of aerosolized bacteria. Antibiotics that are administered prior to or during dental procedures can help reduce the risk of systemic infection by oral flora.

Special solutions are also available to use in your scaling and polishing units. This prevents the buildup of biofilm in the dental lines, which ultimately can prevent a hazard for the operator. Research has indicated the seriousness of having stagnant water run through dental lines. There is an increased risk of nosocomial infections in patients and personnel from poorly maintained dental equipment. In an article presented in 1997 at the Worldwide Companion Animal Dental Forum, Jeffrey Williams, BVS, MRCVS, PhD, cited numerous examples of how biofilm and "suckback" of bacteria from a patient's mouth contributes to the extensive bacterial population in dental lines. He made several suggestions for correcting the problem or diminishing the bacteria count. Suggestions included using filters and disinfected tubing, and driving hot air through the tubes.

TABLE 24-4

Dental Procedures Performed on Horses at Various Ages

Age	Examine for Necessary Dentistry	Dental Procedure
2 to 3 years	1. 1st premolar vestige (wolf teeth) 2. 1st deciduous premolar (upper and lower) 3. Hard swelling on ventral surface of mandible beneath 1st premolar 4. Cuts or abrasions on inside of cheek in region of 2nd premolars and molars 5. Sharp protuberances on all premolars and molars	1. Remove wolf teeth if present 2. Remove deciduous teeth if ready. If not, file off corners and points of premolars 3. Make radiographs. Extract retained temporary premolar if present 4. Lightly float or dress all molars and premolars if necessary 5. Rasp protuberances down to level of other teeth in the arcade
3 to 4 years	1. 1, 2, 3, and 5 above 2. 2nd deciduous premolar (upper and lower)	1. 1, 2, 4, and 5 above 2. Remove if present and ready
4 to 5 years	1. 1, 4, and 5 above 2. 3rd deciduous premolar	1. 1, 4, and 5 above 2. Remove if present and ready
5 years and older	1. 1, 4, and 5 above 2. Uneven growth and "wavy" arcade 3. Unusually long molars and premolars	1. 1, 4, and 5 above 2. 1, 4, and 5 above 3. Unusually long molars and premolars may have to be cut if they cannot be filed down

From Baker GJ: *Diseases of the teeth*. In Colahan PT, et al: *Equine medicine and surgery*, ed 4, St Louis, 1991, Mosby.

MARKETING IN VETERINARY DENTISTRY

With veterinary dentistry gaining popularity across the nation, veterinarians are facing a different type of problem—"selling" the dental procedure. As they become more proficient in these specialized dental procedures, veterinarians are concluding that they want to be fairly compensated for their time. This is where a trained and certified dental technician becomes an invaluable asset to a practice. Dental procedures can be time-consuming, and it may not be necessary for a veterinarian to be present during the whole procedure. A dental technician can successfully navigate the mouth by scaling and polishing, observing abnormalities (soft tissue or tooth-related), and taking radiographs of suspicious areas. This can be timesaving for the veterinarian. For the client, it can be the difference between an expensive and an affordable procedure. Most veterinarians who charge average prices for dental procedures are confronted with resistance from clients due to cost. The veterinarian and technician should be schooled in the benefits of regular dental care and why the client's commitment to home care is important. A patient may be able to keep a tooth that may have been considered for extraction if a client is willing to cooperate. This may involve serious brushing using chlorhexidine gel and monthly "pulsing" (using a low-dose antibiotic such as clindamycin hydrochloride for 5 days per month to maintain a healthier mouth).

Using a dental technician in exam rooms for pre-exams can also start a dialogue about dental care. Again, while doing a pre-exam, a dental technician may notice a problem in a patient's mouth. The technician may suggest dental care and how dental cleanings are done. A toothbrushing session may follow. By the time the veterinarian comes into

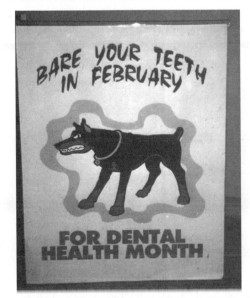

Fig. 24-25 Poster used in marketing dentistry during Dental Health Month. *(Courtesy Rutherford Animal Hospital, N.J.)*

the room, the client will be ready and enthusiastic to focus on dental care.

Dental technicians can also be involved in "marketing" dental procedures. The technician can draw attention to special events, such as Dental Health Month. Posters and giveaways can also complement these events (Fig. 24-25).

Utilizing a technician efficiently in the dental operatory, as well as on the "front lines" can be the difference between a static practice and a growing practice with a profitable and recognized dental department.

RECOMMENDED READING

Bellows J: *The practice of veterinary dentistry*, Ames, Iowa, 1999, Iowa State University Press.

Crossley CA, Penman S: *BSAVA manual of small animal dentistry*, ed 2, Ames, Iowa, 1996, Iowa State University Press.

Eisner, C: *Dentistry: creating a profit center*, Lakewood, Colo., 1999, AAHA Press.

Harvey CE, Emily PP: *Small animal dentistry*, St Louis, 1993, Mosby.

Holmstrom SE, Front P, Gammon RL: *Veterinary dental techniques*, ed 2, Philadelphia, 1998, WB Saunders.

Kesel ML: *Veterinary dentistry for the small animal technician*, Ames, Iowa, 2000, Iowa State University Press.

Mulligan TW, Aller MS, Williams CA: *Atlas of canine and feline dental radiography*, Trenton, 1998, Veterinary Learning Systems.

Wiggs RB, Lobprise HB: *Oral disease (33): Dental disease (52)*. In Norsworthy GD: *Feline practice*, Philadelphia, 1993, JB Lippincott.

Wiggs RB, Lobprise HB: *Veterinary dentistry: principles and practice*, Philadelphia, 1997, JB Lippincott.

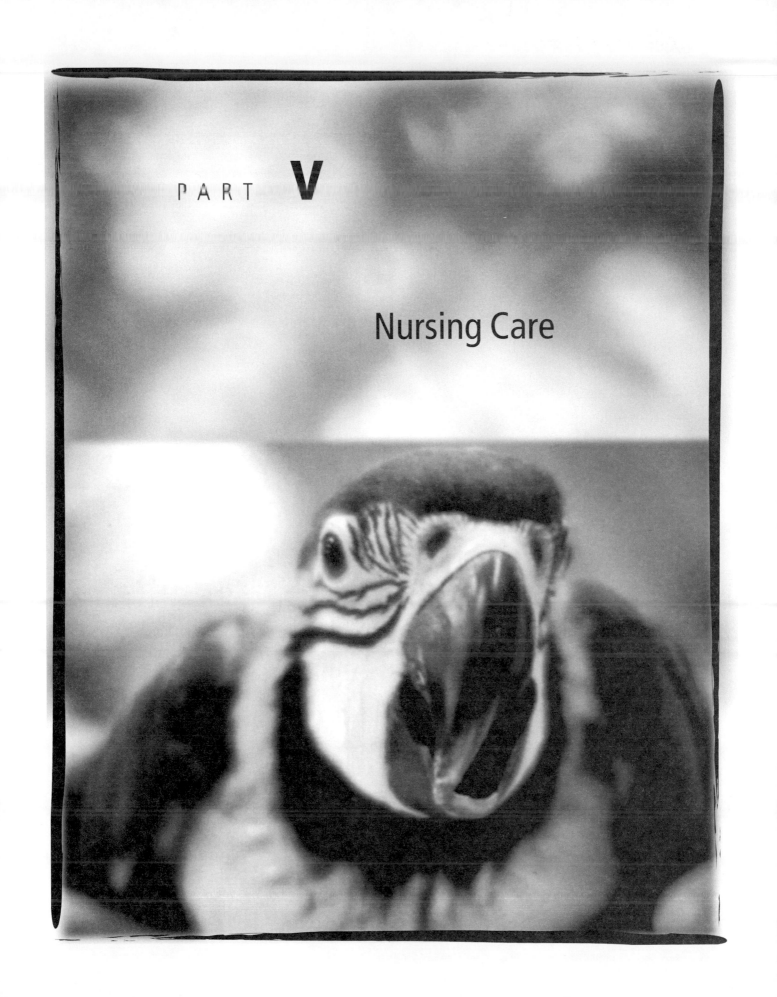

PART **V**

Nursing Care

25

Nursing Care of Dogs and Cats

Vivian Tiffany

Learning Objectives

After reviewing this chapter, the reader should understand the following:

- Techniques used in general nursing care of dogs and cats
- Procedures used in grooming and in skin, nail, and ear care
- Routes of administration of medication
- Methods of parenteral administration
- Methods of intravenous catheterization

- Methods of urethral catheterization
- Methods of orogastric and nasogastric intubation
- Methods of respiratory support
- Procedures used in rehabilitative therapy
- Procedures used in the care of recumbent patients
- Procedures used in the care of critical patients
- Procedures used in the care of neonatal puppies and kittens
- Procedures used in the care of geriatric dogs and cats

GENERAL CARE OF DOGS AND CATS

Attending to Physical Needs

Companion animals should be kept in clean, dry, comfortable, and secure housing. Every effort should be made to eliminate environmental stress. Each animal should be adequately identified with cage cards and paper ID neckbands. Soiled cages should be cleaned promptly with approved disinfectants and the bedding replaced. Exercise should be scheduled and carried out when permitted. Clean water and food should be supplied if medically permitted. The veterinary nurse is instrumental in providing physical comfort and safety to hospitalized patients.

Attending to Psychological Needs

Develop a friendship with the patient by always talking gently and quietly. When interacting, place yourself on the patient's level by sitting on the cage edge or squatting to pet and stroke the chest or chin. Repeat this at every opportunity. Establish a rapport with the patient. At treatment times, double the amount of positive interaction, especially when the procedure or treatment involves pain or discomfort. Patients respond positively to gentle reassurance and

The authors acknowledge and appreciate the original contribution of Cathy Winters, Elizabeth A. Gorecki, Autumn P. Davidson, and Barbara J. Deeb—whose work has been incorporated into this chapter.

support. If the patient's condition permits, provide special snacks or food. Each patient has individual needs, and it requires observation and often client input to help make hospitalization as positive as possible.

Monitoring Vital Signs and Elimination

Assessing attitude or mentation

Assessment of a patient's attitude can provide important information on care and treatment. Is the patient alert, depressed, sedated (recovering from anesthesia), agitated, quiet, or comatose? Pain may be assessed depending on the patient's attitude. Signs of pain may include anorexia and depression. Other signs include whimpering or crying, sharp yipping when moved or touched, growling when approached, anxiety, avoidance behavior, restlessness, frequent repositioning in the cage, reluctance to lie down, arching of the spine, limping or non–weight-bearing on a limb, and chewing at a specific area.

Monitoring weight

Weigh each patient daily, at the same time and on the same scale, to help monitor hydration and nutrition status (Fig. 25-1).

Monitoring body temperature

Get a baseline temperature on every patient. Body temperature can be monitored rectally with a standard mercury

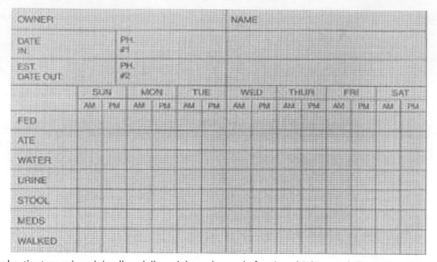

OWNER				NAME										
DATE IN.		PH. #1												
EST. DATE OUT		PH. #2												
	SUN		MON		TUE		WED		THUR		FRI		SAT	
	AM	PM	AM	PM	AM	PM	AM	PM	AM	PM	AM	PM	AM	PM
FED														
ATE														
WATER														
URINE														
STOOL														
MEDS														
WALKED														

Fig. 25-1 Stable, hospitalized patients require minimally a daily weight and record of eating, drinking and elimination. This example of a cage card is conveniently graphed for recording this information. It is also a sticker, and can be applied to the permanent medical record after use.

thermometer, a battery-operated digital thermometer, or an electronic probe for continuous monitoring rectally or in the ear canal. Leave the thermometer in the rectum for 2 or 3 minutes (count the pulse and respiratory rates while waiting), and record the temperature. Temperature change can be an early sign of metabolic status. It can decrease in renal failure and increase in bacterial infection. Monitoring temperature can be an important indicator and early sign of an improving or deteriorating condition.

Maintenance of normal body temperature (normothermia) involves regulating the external environment as well as the internal environment of the patient. Hypothermia (subnormal body temperature) can occur with shock, after anesthesia or surgery, and with low environmental temperatures. Hypothermia can be combated with a circulating warm-water blanket (not an electric heating pad), a warm-water bottle, a warmed towel or blanket, a warm bath, a blow dryer, a heat lamp, or an incubator. Fluids may be warmed to 37° C (98.6° F) and slowly infused intravenously (IV).

Monitor the rectal temperature at least hourly. Discontinue warming when the rectal temperature approaches the normal range. Do not overheat the patient. Most water blankets can be adjusted (lowered) to normal body temperature to maintain normothermia and not overheat patients. Always have a towel or pad between the water blanket and the patient. Electric heating pads are not recommended because of the possibility of electric shock, overheating, and burns. If a heat lamp is used, the patient must be able to move away from the heat source. When using an incubator, extreme care must be taken to avoid overheating the patient.

Hyperthermia (abnormally high body temperature) may occur with infection, inflammation, brain lesions (loss of thermoregulation), heat stroke, seizures, stress, and excita-tion. Patients with extreme and persistent hyperthermia require constant monitoring. Hyperthermia can be controlled with ice wrapped in towels, a fan, alcohol application, a cool-water enema, and cool drinking water. Discontinue cooling when the rectal temperature reaches 39.5° C (103° F). Do not overcool the patient.

Monitoring pulse

Assessment of pulse quality and rate can help determine the patient's medical status and guide the course of treatment. Auscultate the heart while palpating the pulse. A pulse deficit (more heartbeats than pulse beats) indicates an arrhythmia. Pulses can be described as *absent, weak,* and *thready, normal, bounding,* or *irregular.*

If there is any question about heart rate or pulse quality, monitor the patient with an electrocardiogram (ECG). Place the patient in right lateral recumbency and attach alligator clips to the skin caudal to the elbows and on the stifles. Alcohol on the contact points will help with transmission. If the clips are color-coded, the right front is white, the left front is black, the right rear is green, and the left rear is red. Assess the ECG to determine if continuous monitoring is advisable.

Monitoring respiration

Auscultate the patient's lungs, starting at the cranial thorax and working toward the caudal thorax. Normal respiration is quiet. Nervousness, heat, pain, hypoxia, lung disease, or heart problems can increase the respiratory rate. Metabolic alkalosis may cause a decreased rate. Increased respiratory sounds or short, shallow, rapid breathing can indicate pulmonary or bronchial disease. Patient posture is noted as a part of respiratory evaluation. Dyspnea (labored breathing) may be manifested as extension of the neck, refusal to lie down, and open-mouthed breathing. Note the quality of the patient's breathing. Is the patient having difficulty on inspiration or expiration? Is the breathing abdominal?

Monitoring urine production

Urination frequency is recorded on stable patients and possibly measured on critical ones. Walk dogs regularly and record any urination. Note frequency of urination for cats by cleaning the litter box. Patients on IV fluids may have an increased amount of urine production with brief periods of diuresis.

The veterinary nurse is important in reporting frequency, type of stream, and gross analysis of the urine. Further laboratory analysis and methods of collection are explained in detail in Chapter 13. The urinalysis can aid, diagnosis, and monitor response to treatment. Urine production and composition reflect perfusion, renal function, hydration status, bladder function, and endocrine function.

Measuring urine production. Normal urine output is 1 to 2 ml/kg/hr. Dogs can be taken outside to urinate if no urinary catheter is in place to collect and measure urine. Walk ambulatory canine patients outside every 4 hours during the day to eliminate. A bedpan works well for catching the urine. Pour the urine into a graduated container to measure. Disposable pads or diapers can be used in recumbent patients to facilitate cleaning and measure urine output by weight. Weigh the dry diaper. After a patient urinates, remove the diaper and weigh it. Subtract the initial weight of the diaper from the total weight; the remainder is the weight of the urine. Convert the weight to milliliters to determine approximate urine output.

Urinary catheterization permits accurate measurement of urine output, facilitates collection of urine for analysis, promotes cleanliness of recumbent patients, and reduces exposure of other patients or personnel to contaminated urine (e.g., leptospirosis, chemotherapy). For patients with bladder dysfunction, a urinary catheter and collection system also keeps the bladder empty. In cats with lower urinary tract disease, urinary catheters prevent reobstruction. Cats without urinary catheters can have their urine output quantitated by using an empty litter pan, paper litter, or diapers. The paper litter and the litter pan should be weighed before placing it in the cage.

Manual expression of the bladder may be necessary for patients that cannot completely empty the bladder. This will keep the bladder empty, improve bladder tone, and decrease the chance of urinary tract infection. Carefully take nonambulatory patients outside on a gurney, assist the patient to stand, and, if necessary, have the bladder expressed to stimulate urination. Bladder expression keeps the patient clean and reduces the chance of urine scalding.

Gastrointestinal Monitoring

Monitor all excretions (urine, feces, vomit, saliva) from the patient and record a description (including estimated quantity) on the patient's chart. The color and content of feces (e.g., yellow, green, coffee-ground, black, red with frank blood, mucoid, partially digested food, undigested food, watery, voluminous, projectile, foul-smelling) can aid diagnosis. Regurgitation must be differentiated from vomiting. For patients that do not or cannot drink water, calculated fluid losses may be replaced with IV fluids.

The patient's body must be kept clean and free of body waste and excretions. Cleaning and flushing the oral cavity with saline can help prevent or heal oral ulcers. Flushing any vomitus out of the mouth also helps the patient feel better. Moisten the patient's mouth with a gauze sponge and water if the patient cannot take food or water per os. The skin around the mouth should be kept clean of vomitus and saliva to prevent scalding and secondary bacterial infections.

Patients with diarrhea must be kept as clean and dry as possible. Clean the cage or run thoroughly and replace any soiled bedding. If a recumbent patient must be turned every few hours, be sure to place the patient down on the correct side. Face the recumbent patient with its head toward the cage door. The patient should be able to see activity and not be forced to face a wall. Also, the nurse must be able to see the patient's head to monitor attitude, mucous membrane color, and respiration. Frequent walks outside to eliminate can help the patient feel better and reduce cage cleanup.

Patients that have not had a bowel movement in the past 2 days but are still eating should be closely monitored and encouraged to eliminate. Take the patient outside on a long leash or to an outdoor run, or provide a larger litter box or different litter. Diet changes may be necessary (e.g., canned food, addition of fiber). Enemas may be indicated if constipation is diagnosed. Any tenesmus (straining to defecate) should be reported to the veterinarian.

Nutritional Support

Proper nutritional support is an important aspect of therapy for hospitalized patients. Sick or injured patients need good nutritional support to counteract the immunosuppressive effects of sepsis, neoplasia, chemotherapy, anesthesia, and surgery. This support enhances wound healing and minimizes the length of hospitalization without significant weight loss and muscle atrophy. Initiation of nutritional support early in the course of hospitalization is crucial for a successful outcome. Refer to Chapter 7 for detailed information on nutritional support for hospitalized patients.

Grooming and Skin Care

Some hospitalized patients develop skin problems (e.g., decubital ulcers, pyoderma, urine scald, dry scaly skin) because of recumbency, urinary or fecal incontinence, or general lack of appropriate care. Others are healthy until they are admitted for trauma. Regardless of the reason for admittance to the hospital, all patients require routine grooming and skin care. Patients also feel better when kept clean and dry.

When a patient is admitted and its condition has been stabilized, any vomit, diarrhea, urine, or blood should be removed from the skin to prevent secondary infections. Skin care of the hospitalized patient involves bathing to remove body fluids, skin oil, or exudates; brushing to prevent mat formation; padding to prevent decubital ulcer formation; and medicating affected areas of skin. Before the patient is discharged from the hospital, such routine procedures as toenail trimming, anal sac expression, and ear cleaning should be performed before a final bath.

Skin care

Many critically ill patients are too weak or unable to get up to relieve themselves. Urine and fecal scalding develops if these patients are not cleaned after each occurrence. However, use good judgment before partially or completely bathing a critically ill patient. For example, if a dyspneic patient in an oxygen cage urinates on itself, remove the soiled bedding and spot-clean the patient. Do not jeopardize the patient's overall health to completely bathe the patient; also, do not let the patient continue to lie in body waste without attempting to clean it.

Long hair should be trimmed to prevent moisture from being trapped and causing a secondary infection. Carefully shave the hair around the perianal and inguinal areas for ease of cleaning. Avoid nicking or cutting the patient with the clippers. Apply a light tail wrap on longhaired patients with diarrhea to help keep the tail clean and prevent scalding. Wrap the tail loosely, and incorporate some of the hair to keep the wrap in place. Change the wrap after each episode of diarrhea.

Patients with minor soiling can be spot-cleaned with mild solutions (e.g., Peri-Wash, Sween). Continuous diarrhea can cause perineal irritation and ulceration and ascending urinary tract infections. A complete bath is recommended when large areas are soiled. Clean contaminated incision areas gently with water and a washcloth. Soak off any dried organic material. Pat the incision dry. Remove as much organic material from the patient as possible before placing in a bathtub and bathing. Apply a light layer of triple antibiotic ointment to the incision to prevent contact with water and shampoo.

Recumbent patients can be kept cleaner and drier if a urinary catheter is placed to prevent urine scald. If the patient is large, transfer the patient on a gurney to a tub with a grate placed over it, or slide the patient out of the cage onto a rack elevated above a floor drain. Have shampoo, several buckets of warm water, and towels ready before starting. If the patient does not have a urinary catheter, encourage urination before bathing. Express the bladder if the patient is incontinent. If the patient has not defecated in days, enemas or digital removal of feces may be necessary. Use this opportunity to make the patient more comfortable before bathing. Cover any clean and dry bandages with plastic to reduce the need for bandaging after the bath. Change any contaminated bandages.

Wet the patient on the exposed side, apply shampoo, and scrub gently with the hands. Rinse thoroughly and turn the patient to the other side. Repeat the shampooing. Remove all wet and soiled bandages at this time. Clean and completely dry the areas under the bandages before replacing. Squeeze excess water from the fur and towel dry. Use a blow dryer to dry the exposed side; then turn the patient over and repeat on the other side. Completely dry the patient with a handheld dryer or cage dryer.

Using a comb or brush while drying the patient decreases drying time. Use care when brushing thin-skinned patients with a slicker brush. The wire bristles can scratch the skin easily. Remove mats with scissors or electric clippers while the hair is dry, preferably before bathing. Before replacing the patient back in the cage, make sure the patient is completely dry and all irritated areas on the skin are examined, shaved if necessary, cleaned, and treated appropriately. Ointments, creams, lotions, drying solutions, or powders can be reapplied at this time. For recumbent patients, place clean towels or padding between the patient's legs to aerate the skin, make the patient more comfortable, and prevent scrotal edema. Roll stockinette into a donut-shape to pad any decubital ulcers.

Patients who are vomiting should have the hair on their face and front legs kept clean or trimmed, and their mouth rinsed of vomit.

Bathing

Baths are given to clean the entire patient. Coat conditioners are applied after shampooing and towel drying. Trim the toenails, express the anal sacs (dogs), and clean the ears (dogs) before bathing. Wear a gown or apron for bathing. Have all supplies ready and within reach before placing the patient in a tub: shampoo, bucket, washcloth, towels, conditioning spray, clippers or scissors if necessary, brush and comb, blow dryer, and cologne. Dilute the cleansing shampoo with water for easier application and lathering.

Dogs and cats can be placed directly into a tub. Some cats will not tolerate a sprayer hose and do better if placed in a tub already partially filled with water. Use a cup to pour water over the body, starting at the neck (not over the head). Allow the patient to move around in the tub unless it becomes too frantic. Holding the cat gently by the scruff is usually all of the restraint necessary. A second person may be needed for restraint if the patient becomes agitated or fractious. Never leave a patient unattended in the tub.

Starting at the base of the head, soak the patient with warm water before applying shampoo. In cats, some medicated shampoos can cause toxicity. Always read the directions before applying shampoo. Any cleaning needed for the head can be done with a wet cloth after the body is bathed. If shampoo inadvertently gets into the eyes, rinse with sterile saline. Rub in the shampoo gently down to the skin and work into lather. Rinse thoroughly and remove excess water from the patient before towel drying. Medicated dips can be applied at this time. Place the patient on a table at waist level to blow-dry and brush out. If using a cage dryer, place the setting on low or warm. Patients can become overheated quickly if left unattended with a dryer on high setting. Monitor patients frequently during drying. Medicated shampoos may be antiseptic, moisturizing, degreasing (keratolytic and keratoplastic), antipruritic, antifungal, or insecticidal. Patients with bacterial dermatitis may need to be carefully shaved before shampooing. Avoid clipper burns and irritating the skin when shaving with a number 40 blade. The goal for bathing patients with seborrhea is to remove the scales and crusts while decreasing oiliness. Massaging the shampoo into the coat disperses the medication while loosening scales and crusts. Contact time for therapeutic shampoos is important, so be sure to read the directions for recommendations.

Insecticidal spot-ons, sprays, powders, or mousses may be applied after drying. It is contraindicated to use dryers after some therapeutic dips. Read the directions on the dip for these recommendations. Numerous spot-on treatments are available. However, their efficacy can be affected by improper application. Read and follow all directions, and be able to educate the client with their proper use as well.

Some insecticidal dips are still in use. Pay strict attention to the package insert. Insecticides may cause toxicities in cats and certain dog breeds, such as Collies, Shelties, and Old English Sheepdogs. Signs of toxicity include vomiting, diarrhea, excessive salivation, bradycardia, miosis, ataxia, and seizures; these need immediate medical attention. Mildly affected patients can be rebathed with a nonmedicated shampoo to remove any remaining insecticide on the fur. Rinse and dry thoroughly.

Nail care

The claws or nails of cats and dogs are regularly trimmed to prevent ingrown nails, injury from traumatic nail fractures, and impaired walking from overlong nails that impinge on the footpads. Trimming also minimizes damage to the environment (e.g., bedding and padding) and injury to handlers and other patients. The nail should not extend beyond the level of the footpad and should be trimmed accordingly. However, patients that do not have their nails trimmed routinely can have an overlong *quick* or ungual blood vessel that bleeds with trimming; this vessel will gradually regress with frequent nail trimming. To avoid injury of veterinary staff, cats should have their claws trimmed before starting any procedure.

Purposely quicking the nails (cutting the nail short, causing bleeding) is unnecessarily cruel and painful. Quicking is viewed unfavorably by clients and causes the patient to resist subsequent nail trimming. Unless the patient has a history of painful nail trims, most animals do not dislike nail trimming (Fig. 25-2).

The patient should be in lateral or sternal recumbency or sitting. It may be necessary to have an assistant help restrain the patient. Hold the toe between thumb and forefinger, with the foot grasped firmly in that hand. Push the toe distally to extend the nail, and allow the guillotine trimmer to slide over the tip of the nail (Fig 25-3)

The nail should be cut cleanly, with no frayed edges; smooth off any rough edges with nail file or dremel (Fig. 25-4). After trimming, examine each nail for bleeding before going on to the next nail. Examine each foot to ensure that all nails, including the dewclaws, have been trimmed cleanly and are not frayed.

If the quick is accidentally cut, apply a cauterizing agent, such as silver nitrate applicators or Quick Stop powder (Figs. 25-5 and 25-6). Place the tip of the applicator directly on the quick and apply pressure. If no cauterizing agent is available, apply pressure with a cotton ball or gauze sponge directly on the quick to gradually stop the bleeding. Silver nitrate application may cause discomfort, so be prepared for the patient to attempt to withdraw the foot.

Anal sac care

The anal sacs are paired sacs located beneath the skin on either side of the anus at the 4 o'clock and 8 o'clock positions. Each sac has a duct opening directly into the terminal rectum. The anal sacs normally empty their malodorous secretions during defecation. Occasionally, patients (rarely cats) may not be able to empty the anal sacs naturally and develop painful distention or impaction of the anal sacs. Signs include "scooting" on the hindquarters and licking of the anal area. The anal sacs of dogs can be expressed

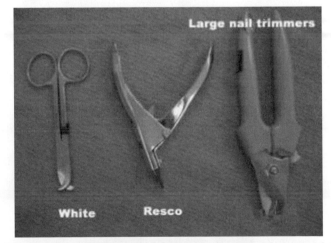

Fig. 25-2 Nail trimmers are available in a variety of styles and sizes. Guillotine-type trimmers (Resco) are available in regular and large sizes. The blade can be replaced when it becomes dull. Scissors-type trimmers (White) work well for ingrown nails, for nails of puppies and kittens, and for cat claws. Always ensure that trimmers are clean and sharp.

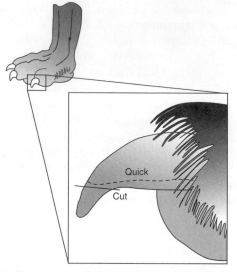

Fig. 25-3 Position all types of trimmer blades within 2 mm from the end of the quick. With a swift, smooth motion, cut the nail just distal to the quick. In patients with white nails, the quick is visible and easy to avoid. In those with dark nails, pare the end of the nail down a bit at a time until a clearer or lighter color appears in the cross-section of the nail. This is the tip of the quick. Compare the remaining untrimmed dark nails with the trimmed nail for proper length of trim.

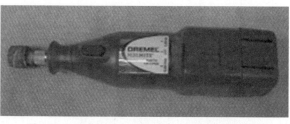

Fig. 25-4 A dremel is used to remove jagged edges.

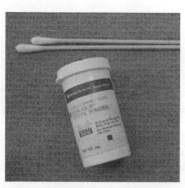

Fig. 25-5 Quick stop.

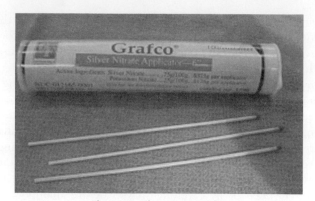

Fig. 25-6 Silver nitrate sticks.

(emptied manually) as a routine part of grooming, as part of the physical examination, and before bathing. The anal sacs are emptied with the dog restrained in the standing position. Anal sac expression may cause discomfort, and a muzzle may be necessary.

For internal anal sac expression, wear exam gloves that are well lubricated with a water-soluble lubricant or 2% lidocaine jelly. With the handler holding the tail dorsally or laterally, insert the first joint of the index finger into the rectum and gently palpate the anal sac between thumb (externally) and forefinger. Gently massage with light to moderate pressure, milking the secretions medially into the anal opening; repeat on the other side. Notify the veterinarian of any unusual secretions. Clean the perineum with a deodorizer or spot cleaner if not bathing immediately after expression.

For external anal sac expression, place a gauze sponge or paper towel over the anus while applying gentle, firm pressure craniomedially against the perineum. Examine the secretions, and repeat on the opposite side. External expression does not completely empty the anal sacs but may cause less discomfort than internal expression.

Anal sac abscesses may need to be treated with hot packs to the perineum, instilling medication into the anal sacs, drains, or surgical intervention. Patients with recent rectal surgery should not have the anal sacs expressed.

Ear care

Before cleaning ears, visually examine the external ear canal and tympanic membrane for any irregularity. Cleaning the ears and instilling medication without examination may cause further damage to the tympanic membrane and result in loss of hearing, loss of vestibular function, or facial nerve paralysis. The tympanic membrane must be intact before any products other than saline or water are instilled into the ear. Note any redness, discharge, ulceration, excessive tissue formation, narrowing (stenosis) of the canal, abnormal odor, or debris in the outer ear and on the pinna. These could indicate a bacterial or yeast infection, ear mite infestation, or tumor. Thickening of the pinna could indicate an aural hematoma. Signs of ear disease include excessive shaking of the head, scratching at the ears, head tilt, and ataxia.

If the patient has an ear problem, examine the less affected ear first. Most patients tolerate ear examination with minimal restraint while sitting or in sternal recumbency. Patients with painful ears or chronic ear disease require general anesthesia for ear examination and cleaning. It is important to use a separate clean otoscope cone for each ear to avoid contaminating a normal ear with organisms from an infected ear.

Grasp the pinna and carefully insert the otoscope cone into the ear canal. Straighten the ear canal by gently pulling the pinna laterally, while advancing the otoscope cone into the canal to visualize the tympanic membrane. Occasionally, the ear canal is occluded with debris and must be cleaned and flushed with saline to visualize the tympanic membrane. If cultures or cytologic samples are required, obtain the samples *before* cleaning the ears.

Some dog breeds, such as Poodles, have hair growth in the ear canal. This hair traps moisture and debris and increases the likelihood of infection. Hair in the ear canal should be plucked out with hemostats or the fingertips, a few strands at a time. This procedure may be painful, so appropriate restraint of the head is necessary. Sedation or tranquilization may be necessary. Grasp a few hairs at a time with the hemostats and quickly pluck the hair out. Grasping too much hair in the hemostats is painful and may cause more inflammation.

Ensure the tympanic membrane is intact before any cleaning. Most cleaning solutions are ototoxic if the tympanic membrane is not intact. If the membrane is not intact, use a saline solution to clean the ears. Antimicrobial agents may be used if the membrane is intact. Various ceruminolytics are available for breaking up debris and cleansing. Cleansing products with a drying agent are good for cleaning the ears of dogs with long, droopy ears, such as Poodles and Cocker Spaniels (Box 25-1).

It is good public relations to have the patient look and feel better upon discharge than when it was admitted. Examine every patient before discharge to ensure that all extraneous bandages are removed; it is bathed, groomed, de-matted, and smelling good; and the nails are trimmed, ears cleaned, and anal sacs expressed. Brush one last time, and spray with a lightly scented spray. Educating clients on proper skin care and grooming can prevent many problems and keep patients in better health.

ADMINISTERING MEDICATIONS

Topical Administration

Medication applied to the skin provides a local effect and is also absorbed through the skin. Shaving and cleaning the

---

BOX 25-1 *procedure*

Cleaning a Dog's Ears

Materials

- Basin
- Bulb syringe
- Cotton balls or cotton swabs
- Hemostats
- Ceruminolytic agents, saline solution, cleansing solution, or dilute vinegar

Procedure

1. Tip the head and ear slightly ventrally, grasp the pinna, and place the solution into the ear canal, with the bulb syringe directed ventromedially into the canal. Have the basin ready below the ear to catch the excess.
2. Massage the base of the ear to distribute the cleansing solution and loosen any debris. Flush the ear again. Use cotton balls on a hemostat to clean the debris in the ear canal. Never insert cotton-tipped swabs into the canal of an inadequately restrained patient. Use cotton swabs for the external ear canal and interior of the pinna only. Allow the patient to shake its head occasionally to loosen more debris. Flush and clean the ears until debris is no longer visible. Dry the ear canal with cotton balls.
3. Examine the ears with an otoscope, and apply any medications necessary. Massage the ear canal to distribute the medication evenly and thoroughly.

---

area or parting the hair before application facilitates absorption of the medication. Wear exam gloves and/or plastic aprons when giving a medicated bath or applying topical medication. Topical medications include the following:

- Medicated shampoos for skin disease
- Fentanyl transdermal patches for analgesia
- Spot-on flea and tick control
- Topical anesthetics
- Nitroglycerin ointment
- Other antibiotic and cortisone creams or ointments

Oral Administration

Oral administration is the route most commonly used to administer medications. Medications given orally are metabolized slowly; another route of administration is necessary if more rapid absorption is required. The patient must be able to swallow and have normal digestive function if medication is given per os (PO, by mouth).

Oral medications are available in tablet, capsule, and liquid form. If necessary, tablets can be crushed or capsule contents dissolved in water and given with a syringe or feeding tube. Compounding pharmacies are now available to make medicine solutions with tasty flavorings. If the patient has a good appetite, the medication may be placed in a meatball of canned food (this does not work well with sick cats). If the oral cavity is damaged, bypass it by crushing the medication and mixing with water, or administering the medication directly into the gastrointestinal tract via naso-gastric or gastrostomy tube.

A pilling device can be used to avoid being bitten. This is a plastic rod with a rubber-tipped plunger to hold the med-ication. Hemostats should not be used to administer med-ication, because they can damage the teeth or soft palate. Instruct clients how to correctly administer oral medication and how to check the patient's mouth to ensure that all medications have been swallowed.

Place small patients at waist level and large dogs on the floor. Prepare cats by grasping the upper jaw over the top of the head and tipping the head back. The lower jaw will drop open, or use the middle finger of the dominant hand to pry it open slightly. Holding the pill between the thumb and fore-finger, place it in the center groove of the tongue, at the back of the throat. Do not scratch the soft palate with your fingers. With aggressive cats, a towel or cat bag may be necessary.

For dogs, grasp the muzzle using the fingers and thumb to press the skin against the teeth (Fig. 25-7). Slip the thumb of the left hand into the mouth and press up on the hard palate, keeping the lips against the teeth. Place the pill on the base of the tongue at the back of the throat. Keep the head slightly elevated, close the mouth, and hold it shut, while rubbing the throat until the patient swallows. Facilitate swal-lowing by blowing into the patient's nose. After administer-ing medication, always examine the patient's mouth to ensure complete swallowing of the medication.

To administer liquid medication in a syringe, tilt the head back slightly and pull the lips outward slightly to form a pocket (Fig. 25-8). Place the syringe between the lips and

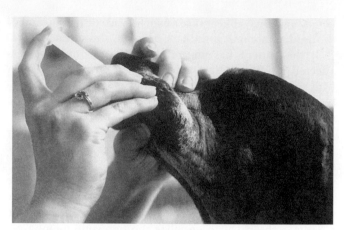

Fig. 25-8 Oral administration of a liquid. *(From Pratt:* Medical, surgical and anesthetic nursing for veterinary technicians, *ed 2, St Louis, 1994, Mosby.)*

back teeth so that the liquid flows between the molars to the throat. Administer the liquid slowly in small boluses to allow the patient to swallow and not aspirate.

Rectal Administration

An enema introduces fluids into the rectum and colon to stimulate bowel activity, evacuate the large intestine for diagnostic procedures, and irrigate the colon (Box 25-2). Enemas soften feces and stimulate colonic motility. Tap water or saline adds bulk, whereas petrolatum oils soften, lubricate, and promote evacuation of hardened feces. Glycerin and water, mild soap and water, or commercial enema preparations can also be used for enema solutions. However, phosphate enemas (e.g., Fleet) should not be administered to cats or small dogs. Large volumes of warm water are administered with a bucket elevated above the patient and attached to soft red rubber tubing. Smaller

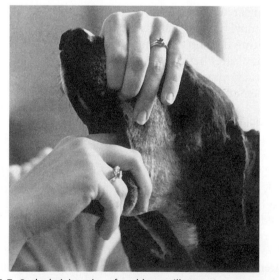

Fig. 25-7 Oral administration of a tablet or pill. *(From Pratt:* Medical, surgical and anesthetic nursing for veterinary technicians, *ed 2, St Louis, 1994, Mosby.)*

| BOX 25-2 | *procedure* |

Giving an Enema

Procedure

1. For an evacuation enema, place the patient in a tub, run, or large cage. Lubricate the tubing with water-soluble lubricating jelly.
2. Wearing gloves and with the patient restrained in a stand-ing position, insert the lubricated tube into the rectum, at least 5 cm cranial to the anal sphincter, and administer the solution slowly. Water enemas to evacuate the bowel are safely given at 10 to 20 ml/kg of body weight. Rapid administration may cause the patient to vomit.
3. Remove the tubing from the rectum, and allow the patient to evacuate in a large area. This may take minutes to hours.

volumes can be administered with a 60-ml syringe attached to the tubing. The solution should be at room temperature or tepid.

Enemas are contraindicated if the bowel is perforated or recent colon surgery has been performed. Complications of enema administration include perforating the colon and leakage of fluid into the peritoneal cavity, vomiting if fluid is administered too quickly, and hemorrhage if the colon is irritated.

Nasal Administration

Some medications may be administered into the nasal cavity to be absorbed through the nasal mucosa. Occasionally, a nasal canula is inserted through the nares to administer oxygen and humidified air to the lungs; nasoesophageal and nasogastric tubes are inserted to provide nutrition. Respiratory vaccines and local anesthetics also may be placed into the nasal passages. Nasal administration via syringe or dropper is usually not stressful, and most dogs and cats tolerate it very well.

Have all medications and materials ready and within reach before starting. With the patient in sternal recumbency or sitting, tip the patient's head back so that the nose is slightly elevated, and instill the medication into the nares (Fig. 25-9). It may be helpful to cover the eyes during the procedure with the hand that is holding the head back. Once the medication is administered, keep the nose elevated until the medication is absorbed through the mucosa.

Ophthalmic Application

Medication can be applied topically onto the eye to treat the cornea, conjunctiva, and anterior chamber. Ophthalmic medications are available in liquid and ointment forms. Most eye conditions are very painful and may require restraint for application. Before applying the medication, the eye must be cleaned of any exudates. Use an ophthalmic irrigating solution and cotton balls to clean the surrounding area. A clean comb can be invaluable when removing exudate from hair surrounding the eye. Have all materials and medications ready and within reach before restraining the patient.

Restrain the patient in a sternal position or sitting, with the head tipped back and the nose pointed toward the ceiling. Grasp the muzzle to prevent the patient from moving its head. Gently clean the eye area with wet cotton balls. Flush the cornea and conjunctival sac by everting the eyelids and applying a gentle stream of irrigating solution from medial to lateral. If excessive ocular discharge has caused irritation of surrounding skin, apply a thin layer of petrolatum-based ointment onto the skin.

Ophthalmic solutions are easier to administer but may need to be administered more frequently than ointments. Most solutions are applied every few hours to maintain their effect. With the dropper or bottle held 1 or 2 inches above the eye and the upper eyelid pulled up, apply the solution directly onto the sclera; then release the eyelid (Fig. 25-10). To avoid contaminating the dropper bottle or tube, do not touch the eye or eyelid with it. If more than one solution is to be applied, wait a few minutes between applications. If both a solution and an ointment are to be used, apply the solution several minutes before the ointment.

Ointment is slightly more difficult to apply. Ointments are usually applied every 4 to 6 hours; they do not wash out but may soil the skin around the eye. The ointment tube must be held close to, but *not in contact with*, the eye. Evert the eyelid, and place a ⅛ - or ¼-inch strip of ointment medial to lateral onto the cornea or lower border of the eyelid, ensuring not to touch the tube to the eye or eyelid (Fig. 25-11).

Otic Application

Liquids can be instilled into the ear canal to medicate or clean the ear. The ear should be cleaned before instilling medication to ensure that the medication is absorbed and fully dispersed. Otoscopic examination is necessary to ensure that the tympanic membrane is intact before cleaning the ear or applying medication. Obtain culture or cytologic samples, if necessary, before the ears are cleaned.

Most patients tolerate medication of the ear with minimal restraint. Start with the less affected ear first, to avoid contaminating the other ear. To straighten the ear canal, apply lateral tension on the pinna (earflap). Instill the medication into the external ear canal, and massage the base of the ear to disperse it.

Parenteral Administration

Fluids and medications administered parenterally are injected via sterile syringe and needle or through a catheter.

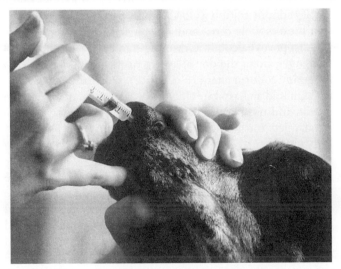

Fig. 25-9 Intranasal administration of medication or vaccines. Note that the head is elevated to allow flow of the medication into the nasal passages. *(From Pratt P:* Medical, surgical and anesthetic nursing for veterinary technicians, *ed 2, St Louis, 1994, Mosby.)*

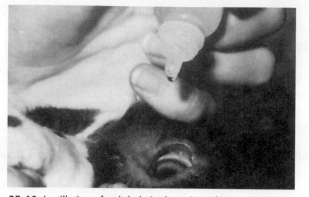

Fig. 25-10 Instillation of ophthalmic drops into the eye. Note that the container does not touch the eye. *(From Pratt P:* Medical, surgical and anesthetic nursing for veterinary technicians, *ed 2, St Louis, 1994, Mosby.)*

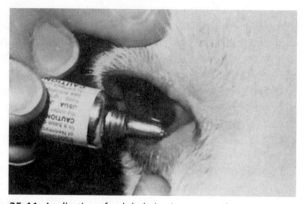

Fig. 25-11 Application of ophthalmic ointment to the eye. *(From Pratt P: Medical, surgical and anesthetic nursing for veterinary technicians, ed 2, St Louis, 1994, Mosby.)*

Parenteral routes include *intradermal* (ID), *subcutaneous* (SQ), *intramuscular* (IM), *intravenous* (IV), *intraosseous* (IO), *epidural*, and *intraperitoneal* (IP). Local inflammation, infection, nerve damage, anaphylactic or allergic reactions, and necrosis at the injection site are possible complications of parenteral administration.

Before aspirating medications into a syringe, swab the rubber stopper of the medication vial with alcohol. Select the appropriate syringe and needle size for the dose and route chosen (22- to 27-gauge for ID, 18- to 22-gauge for SQ, 22-gauge for IM, 20- to 25-gauge for IV, and 20- to 22-gauge for IP). Aspirate the medication into the syringe, hold the syringe vertically, and tap it to expel any air bubbles. Keep the needle covered while preparing the site for injection.

Intradermal administration

ID injections are used primarily for skin testing and local anesthesia. Skin testing may require sedating the patient before placing in lateral recumbency; local anesthesia may or may not require sedation.

Prepare the skin for testing by shaving a large area over the lateral thorax or abdomen, being careful to prevent "clipper burn." Do not use antiseptics to clean the area. For local anesthesia of wounds, skin biopsy, and excision of small lesions, shave and prepare the area as for surgery.

Hold the skin taut between the thumb and forefinger of the left hand, and insert the needle (bevel up) into the skin at an angle of approximately 10 degrees. The bevel of the needle should be within the dermis and not visible. Inject a small amount of allergen or local anesthetic intradermally to form a bleb at the site. If no bleb forms, the injection may have been SQ and not ID.

Subcutaneous administration

SQ injections are used for sustained absorption of fluids and medications and administration of some vaccines. Medication and fluids are absorbed slowly over 20 or 30 minutes, or longer for larger volumes of fluids (6 to 8 hours). Clients can easily be taught to give SQ injections of medication (e.g., insulin) and fluids to patients at home.

Fluids are not readily absorbed when injected SQ in severely dehydrated, "shocky," or debilitated patients. The IV route should be used in such cases. Hypertonic, caustic, or irritating solutions administered SQ can cause damage and sloughing of the skin and should not be administered by this route. Read the package insert before administering medications subcutaneously.

Large volumes of room-temperature fluids may be administered by gravity flow via fluid bag and administration set with a needle attached. This allows for patient comfort during the long process of administering larger volumes of fluid. Change the needle with each injection site change to prevent abscess. Restrain the patient in a comfortable sitting, standing, or sternal position. Most cats and dogs tolerate SQ administration well. Carefully part the hair, clean the skin if excessively dirty, and apply a skin antiseptic, such as 70% isopropyl alcohol. Grasp the skin between thumb and forefinger along the dorsal aspect of the neck or back, and lift gently to form a tent (Fig. 25-12). Insert the needle into the skin fold and aspirate. If blood is aspirated, withdraw the needle and use another injection site. If no blood is aspirated, inject the medication or fluids slowly.

Multiple injection sites can be used along the dorsum and lateral to the spine. Between 50 and 100 ml of fluid may be safely injected at each site without discomfort. Remove the needle, gently pinch the injection site, and massage the area. This prevents leakage and facilitates dispersal and absorption of fluid or medication. Large volumes of fluid may gradually migrate ventrally before being absorbed completely.

Intramuscular administration

Muscles are more vascular than subcutaneous tissue, and medication is more readily absorbed after IM administra-

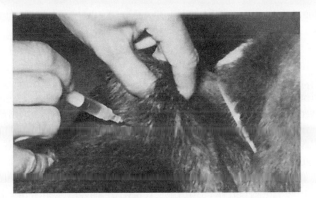

Fig. 25-12 Subcutaneous injections can be given at the back of the neck, with the skin grasped to form a tent. *(From Pratt P: Medical, surgical and anesthetic nursing for veterinary technicians, ed 2, St Louis, 1994, Mosby.)*

tion than if given SQ. However, muscle tissue cannot accommodate more than 2 to 5 ml of medication at any one site, and IM injections can be painful. Slow to moderate rates of administration with small-gauge (22- to 25-gauge) needles may be less painful than rapid injections. Intramuscular administration is never used for fluid therapy. Some medications that are poorly soluble and mildly irritating can be administered IM but not SQ or IV. Large muscle groups are used for IM injections, such as the epaxial muscles lateral to the dorsal spinous process of lumbar vertebrae 3 to 5, quadriceps muscles of the cranial thigh, and triceps muscles caudal to the humerus (Fig. 25-13). The epaxial muscles are the best site for IM injections in small patients. The semimembranosus/semitendinosus muscles on the caudal thigh should be avoided because of possible sciatic nerve damage from incorrect IM injection. If that muscle group must be used, insert the needle at a 45-degree angle directed caudad to avoid the sciatic nerve. Repeated IM injections should be alternated between muscle groups and given on different sides of the body.

Proper patient restraint is necessary to avoid painful injections. Restrain the patient's head and body during IM administration. After locating the muscle group by palpation, swab the injection site with a disinfectant. With the needle attached to the syringe, quickly insert the needle 1 to 2 cm at a 45-degree to 90-degree angle. Aspirate the syringe to ensure that the needle is not placed in a blood vessel. If blood is aspirated, withdraw the needle and insert into a different site. This step is crucial when injecting potent medications, oil-based drugs, or microcrystalline suspensions. If no blood is aspirated, inject the medication at a slow to moderate rate. Remove the needle and massage the muscle to disperse the medication.

Intravenous administration

Medications and fluids administered IV are rapidly absorbed and reach a higher blood level faster than by other routes. Large volumes of solutions may be given in a short time. Caustic, irritating, or hypertonic medications can be given IV with fewer problems than with other routes. IV injections typically do not produce a lasting effect unless a continual infusion is given. A general rule is that if the solution is opaque, it cannot be safely given IV, except for parenteral nutrient solutions and propofol. Vaccines are never administered IV.

Drugs can be given IV with a syringe and needle, winged infusion set, or catheter (Box 25-3). The most commonly used veins for IV administration using a syringe and needle are the cephalic vein and the saphenous vein. Restrain the patient sitting or in sternal recumbency if the cephalic vessel is being used, and in lateral recumbency if the saphenous vessel is used.

Patient restraint is very important if using a syringe and needle for administration of medication. The limb being used must remain immobile during administration. Any movement of the patient may lacerate the vessel with the needle and/or result in extravascular administration of

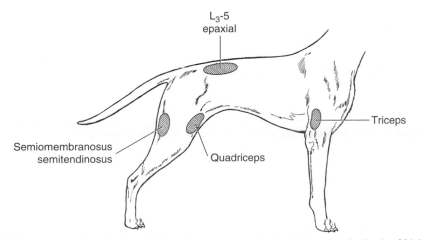

Fig. 25-13 Sites for intramuscular injection. The preferred site is the epaxial muscles lateral to the third to fifth lumbar vertebrae.

BOX 25-3

procedure

Intravenous Injection

Procedure

1. Have an assistant restrain the patient, immobilize the limb, and occlude the vessel proximal to the administration site to distend the vein. Shave the venipuncture site to easily visualize the vessel, if necessary. Prepare the site using 70% alcohol swabs to moisten the hair, clean the skin, and aid visualization of the vein. Surgical preparation of the site is not necessary for IV administration with a syringe and needle, unlike catheter placement.
2. Grasp the metacarpal/metatarsal area, and straighten the leg.
3. Using a 20- to 22-gauge needle attached to a syringe full of medication, direct the bevel of the needle up and insert the needle at a 30° angle through the skin and into the vessel lumen. Aspirate blood into the syringe to ensure venipuncture. Redirect the needle into the vessel, if necessary.
4. Once the needle is in the vessel, have the assistant release pressure on the vein while still holding the limb immobile.
5. Inject the medication slowly or rapidly, depending on the drug (e.g., thiopental is injected fairly rapidly; chemotherapeutic agents are given slowly).
6. After the medication is administered, withdraw the needle and apply pressure at the venipuncture site. A light compression bandage can minimize hematoma formation.

medication. When injecting a caustic or irritating solution, an IV catheter should be placed to prevent extravascular injection.

Always attempt venipuncture at a distal point on the limb. If the needle lacerates the vessel, moving more proximally or using another vein may be indicated. Light pressure should be applied at all venipuncture sites to prevent hematoma formation. To place a needle into small, rolling vessels or vessels surrounded by fat (i.e., in obese patients), insert the needle into the skin lateral to the vessel and then puncture the vessel.

Intraosseous administration

IO administration is used to inject medication and fluids in small patients in which an IV cannot be placed. It is performed with a needle or catheter inserted into the trochanteric fossa of the femur, the tibial tuberosity, or the greater tubercle of the humerus. It is helpful to use a stylet so as to avoid clogging the needle with bone. Intraosseous catheters can be painful and should be replaced every 72 hours.

Intraperitoneal administration

IP administration provides faster but sustained absorption of fluids and medications than with SQ administration. Medication or fluids may be administered into the peritoneal space in neonates with vessels too small for IV catheterization, or in patients needing peritoneal lavage (e.g., with pancreatitis). Irritating medications cannot be given intraperitoneally but blood transfusions may be given IP if an IV catheter cannot be placed. Debilitated or hypovolemic patients do not absorb IP fluids or medication readily.

Peritoneal lavage is performed with a peritoneal catheter set; IP fluids can be administered with a syringe and needle or standard IV catheter placed into the peritoneal space. To avoid hypothermia in neonates and critically ill patients, fluids should always be slightly warmer than room temperature. Cool fluids may be given IP to combat hyperthermia in adult patients. Complications of IP injection include peritonitis and perforation of the intestines, bladder, or other abdominal organs. A flexible catheter is less likely to cause damage than a needle. Aseptic technique must be used to avoid contamination of the abdomen.

Have all materials ready before placing the patient in lateral or dorsal recumbency. Shave and prepare the ventral abdominal midline caudal to the umbilicus, using triple applications of surgical soap and alcohol. Using a 22- to 25-gauge needle attached to a syringe, or a 22-gauge IV catheter, insert the needle or catheter into the abdominal cavity in a caudal direction. Aspirate; if fluid or bowel contents are aspirated, withdraw and use a new needle and syringe. If nothing is aspirated, inject the fluid slowly and then withdraw the needle or catheter.

Epidural Administration

Epidural administration is used for injection of analgesics and anesthetics. Injection of local anesthetics or analgesics into the lumbosacral junction (L7-S1) provides complete analgesia and muscle relaxation caudal to the block.

Intravenous Catheterization

Intravenous catheters provide access to circulating blood for administration of medication, fluids, nutrients, and blood products, as well as monitoring blood pressure and collecting blood samples. Catheters are available in a wide variety of lengths and diameters (Fig. 25-14). Types of catheters include winged infusion needles (butterfly catheters), over-the-needle catheters, and through-the-needle catheters. Common insertion sites are the cephalic vein, the saphenous vein, and the jugular vein. The medial or lateral auricular (ear) vein may be used in some patients (Fig. 25-15).

The longer the catheter, the more stable it is in the vessel and the less likely it is to cause mechanical irritation with resulting phlebitis. A short, peripheral over-the-needle catheter may be inserted distal to an area of flexion, such as

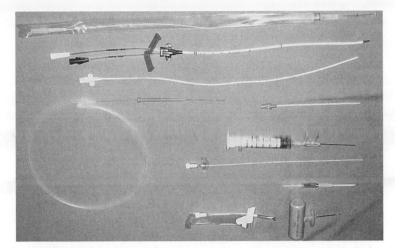

Fig. 25-14 Variety of catheters for administration of fluids and liquid medication. *Top to bottom:* Through-the-needle catheter (Intracath, Becton Dickinson); over-the-guidewire double-lumen catheter (Double-Lumen Arrow, Arrow International); over-the-guidewire single-lumen catheter (Single-Lumen Arrow, Arrow International) with vessel dilator directly below and guidewire to the left; breakaway needle introducer with syringe attached for the L-Cath (Luther Medical Products); through-the-needle catheter with a breakaway needle (L-Cath, Luther Medical Products); over-the-needle catheter (Insyte, Becton Dickinson); pediatric through-the-needle catheter with breakaway needle (Pediatric L-Cath, Luther Medical Products) *(lower left);* and intraosseous catheter.

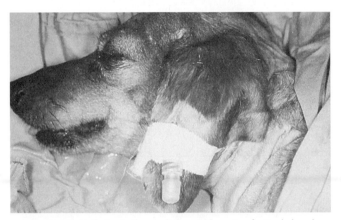

Fig. 25-15 Catheter in the medial auricular vein of a Dachshund.

in a cephalic vein distal to the elbow. A central catheter placed in a large vessel, such as the jugular vein, is less likely to cause mechanical or chemical irritation.

The diameter (gauge) of the catheter depends on the diameter of the vessel. Large-diameter catheters placed in small vessels can compromise venous return and cause phlebitis. Small-diameter catheters decrease the flow rate of fluid delivery but do not compromise venous return. A fluid pump can facilitate delivery of fluids through a small catheter. Small-diameter catheters are easily occluded with fibrin clots, and blood sample collection is not recommended. Winged infusion (butterfly) catheters are indicated for patients that need numerous IV infusions of medications (e.g., chemotherapeutic agents) but not long-

term fluid therapy. Several medications can be given if the catheter is flushed with 0.9% saline between infusions of each medication. These catheters are simple to insert and cause fewest local infections; however, they can cause irritation and may perforate the vessel. Winged infusion catheters require constant monitoring while in place; stabilization of the catheter can be difficult. Once the blood starts flowing into the catheter tubing, attach the heparinized saline-filled syringe, aspirate the air out of the tubing, and flush to ensure catheter patency before administering medications. Administer the medication while holding the leg and the catheter steady. Occasionally aspirate to check catheter patency while administering medications. Once the medication has been administered, flush the tubing and the catheter with heparinized saline before removing the catheter. If multiple drugs are to be administered, flush between medications with heparinized saline. If any type of catheter is used for fluid administration, cap the catheter end with an injection cap and flush it with heparinized saline solution four times daily to prevent clot formation. Over-the-needle peripheral catheters are quick and relatively atraumatic to place, inexpensive, and easily stabilized with a light bandage (Box 25-4). They are used for infusion of fluids, medication, anesthetics, and blood products. They can be left in place for 72 hours before changing to another vessel. Unless care is taken during placement, the catheter can easily be contaminated (Fig 25-16). These catheters usually cannot be used for blood sampling. Complications that can occur with short over-the-needle catheters are easy removal by the patients and SQ infusion of fluids.

BOX 25-4

procedure

Peripheral Intravenous Catheter Insertion

Materials

- Catheter of appropriate type, length, and diameter
- Clippers with a #40 blade
- Cotton balls or gauze sponges soaked in povidone-iodine or chlorhexidine gluconate.
- Cotton balls or gauze sponges soaked in 70% isopropyl alcohol
- Dry, sterile gauze sponges
- Two pieces of ½-inch-wide porous adhesive tape that are long enough to go around the patient's limb two times (or ½-inch-wide roll of tape that has been unrolled and then loosely rerolled)
- Two pieces of 1-inch-wide porous adhesive tape that are long enough to go around the patient's limb two times (or 1-inch-wide roll of tape that has been unrolled and then loosely rerolled)
- Povidone-iodine ointment
- 2- or 3-inch roll of Kling (Johnson & Johnson)
- 2- or 4-inch roll of Vetwrap (3M)
- Extension set primed with heparinized saline (2 I.U. of heparin/1 ml of 0.9% saline) or the fluids to be administered
- Injection cap

Procedure

1. Shave approximately 1 clipper blade width on each side of the vessel, with the shaved length (proximal to distal) approximately twice that of the width. This allows a second attempt at catheterization more proximal than the first.

2. Prepare the insertion site using a surgical soap and antiseptic.

3. While the handler occludes the vessel, grasp the limb with the left hand while the right hand holds the catheter with the bevel directed up.

4. With an over-the-needle catheter, perform direct venipuncture by holding the catheter at a 15-degree to 30-degree angle over the vein, puncturing the skin, and advancing the catheter needle into the vessel in a single, quick, smooth motion. Hold the catheter needle at a 45-degree angle slightly distal and to one side of the desired site of catheter entry into the vessel to perform indirect venipuncture. Once the catheter needle is inserted into the skin, decrease the angle of the needle, advance the catheter needle into the vein, and slide the catheter into the vessel. If the catheter does not advance into the vessel, replace the catheter and attempt catheterization more proximal than the first attempt. With a winged infusion catheter, grasp the wings between thumb and forefinger and advance directly into the vessel, keeping the vessel steady until the catheter is stabilized. Tape the catheter in place using ½-inch tape attached to the wings and wrapped around the limb.

5. Once the catheter is advanced to the hub, remove the catheter needle and hold the catheter in place while attaching the injection cap or primed extension set. Flush a small amount of fluid or heparinized saline into the vessel to ensure catheter patency. For very small, pediatric patients, monitor the amount of fluid used to flush the catheter.

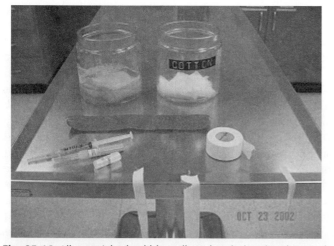

Fig. 25-16 All materials should be collected and placed within reach before skin preparation and catheter placement is begun.

Proper skin preparation before catheter placement is essential to prevent phlebitis and infection. Strict aseptic technique must be followed during catheterization to avoid sepsis. Ensure proper handwashing after clipping and before catheter placement. Sterile surgical gloves may be indicated by the patient's condition. All catheters must be secured with tape or sutures and covered with a light bandage to protect the insertion site. Winged infusion catheters require only taping. Occlude the selected vessel to raise the pressure in the vessel and allow for easier visualization and palpation. For the cephalic vein, the handler supports the patient's elbow with the fingers, while placing the thumb over the vessel on the medial side and rotating it laterally. Occlude the lateral saphenous vein by placing one hand on top of and around the stifle, medial to lateral; occlude the medial saphenous by applying pressure on the vessel in the inguinal area and stabilizing the stifle.

To reduce movement of the catheter and decrease the likelihood of phlebitis, secure it in the vessel (Figs. 25-17 and 25-18). Anchor a piece of ½-inch tape around the catheter hub, and loosely wrap it around the limb. Place a second piece of tape, sticky-side-down, underneath the catheter hub and wrap it around the limb. If the tape is wrapped too tightly, the foot will swell and become painful, and the patient will chew at the catheter. If the tape is not placed immediately distal to the catheter insertion point and stuck to the hair, the catheter may back out of the vessel.

For an over-the-needle jugular catheter in a pediatric patient, wrap the rerolled ½-inch tape around the catheter hub and secure it loosely around the neck.

Conscientious nursing care of the catheter is necessary to maintain a catheter and prevent complications from catheterization. Catheter management can prevent sepsis, the most serious complication associated with catheters. Chemical or mechanical irritation, or contamination of the catheter during placement can cause phlebitis, or local venous inflammation. Signs of phlebitis include swelling at the catheter site, redness, pain, thickening, or irritation of the vessel. Indwelling catheters can cause septicemia, thrombosis, or bacterial endocarditis. Signs of septicemia and bacterial endocarditis include cardiac arrhythmias, injected mucous membranes, fever, and leukocytosis.

It is important to keep the catheter bandage clean and dry. Ensure that the catheter and extension set is clear of blood clots. Establish a closed administration system to prevent contamination. Measure the patient's body tem-

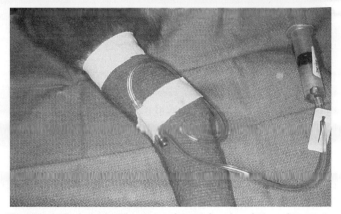

Fig. 25-18 The lateral saphenous catheter is bandaged. Note the security loop in the extension set.

perature at least once daily. Monitor the site proximal to the catheter for signs of phlebitis or subcutaneous fluid accumulation, and check the toes for swelling. Remove the catheter at the first sign of phlebitis, sepsis, or catheter malfunction. Routine changing of the catheter depends on hospital policy for the type of catheter placed. Catheters not in constant use should be flushed with heparinized saline several times per day. When the catheter bandage becomes wet or soiled with organic material, it must be changed and the catheter evaluated for problems. The catheter may need to be covered with plastic to keep clean in incontinent patients. Swabbing the injection port with alcohol or a disinfectant before flushing or injecting medications can help decrease the chance of sepsis. Kinked or malfunctioning catheters and extension tubing with blood clots occluding the ports must be replaced.

The amount of time a catheter can be safely left in place is controversial. Depending on the established hospital policy, a short peripheral catheter is usually moved to another vessel (and a new catheter inserted) every 72 hours. Leaving it in place longer can contribute to phlebitis. Continuous rotation of the veins used allows indefinite IV catheterization for therapy. Central catheters may be left in place for an extended period, with routine catheter bandage changes, provided the catheter is still functional.

Patients receiving hyperalimentation require a central catheter for nutritional support and an additional peripheral catheter for medication and fluid therapy. Another central catheter is also necessary if central venous pressure (CVP) monitoring or blood sampling is required. Placement of one multilumen central catheter for CVP monitoring, blood sampling, nutritional support, fluid therapy, and medication administration reduces the need for a second catheter and can be maintained for long periods.

Central catheters are long catheters made of an inert material that causes little tissue reaction and can be left in for extended periods. Placement in the cranial or caudal

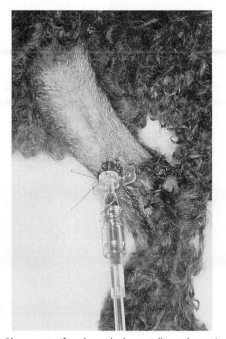

Fig. 25-17 Placement of a through-the-needle catheter in the lateral saphenous vessel. The catheter has been secured with sutures, and an extension set has been attached.

vena cava does not compromise venous return and decreases the possibility of phlebitis from mechanical irritation. Two types of central catheters are the *over-the-guidewire* catheter and the *through-the-needle* catheter. Placement in large vessels allows greater dilution of hypertonic fluids, rapid infusion rates, administration of blood products, blood sampling, and central venous pressure monitoring. However, the cost of these catheters may be prohibitive for short-term (less than 3 days) fluid therapy. The length of central catheters needed to reach the cranial or caudal vena cava depends on the size of the patient. For jugular catheterization, the handler immobilizes the patient's head while placing one finger in the thoracic inlet and applying pressure on the vessel. For jugular insertion, measure from the insertion point to the third intercostal space; for a saphenous insertion, measure from the insertion point to the seventh lumbar vertebra.

The catheter should be inserted in a long, straight vessel with no nearby infection, scars, lesions, wounds, or fractures, and little chance of the patient's contaminating the catheter insertion site. The catheter should be placed in the distal part of the vessel, away from any area of flexion and inserted toward the heart. Once placement is achieved, the catheter is sutured or bandaged in.

Urinary Tract Catheterization

Urinary catheters provide access to the urinary bladder via the urethra to do the following:

- Administer radiographic contrast material directly into the bladder
- Collect urine for urinalysis
- Relieve urethral obstruction
- Maintain urine flow
- Provide a closed urinary collection system for precise monitoring of urine output, collection of contaminated urine, and patient cleanliness

Urinary catheters are available in a variety of materials, diameters, and lengths (Figs. 25-19 and 25-20).

Metal urethral catheters can be used to temporarily catheterize a female dog but can cause hematuria and injury to the urethra and bladder. Olive-tipped metal catheters can be used to relieve an obstruction at the tip of a male cat's penis.

Careful placement of the most flexible, smallest-diameter catheter minimizes trauma to the urethra and bladder. However, an overly small catheter diameter may allow leakage of urine around the catheter. Before placement, always examine the catheter for defects, and test the bulb of Foley catheters by gently inflating with sterile water or saline.

Measure the distance from the tip of the penis or vulva to the neck of the bladder before placing the catheter. Catheters that are too rigid or long can traumatize the wall of the bladder (Fig. 25-21). Flexible catheters that are too long or advanced too far into the bladder can become

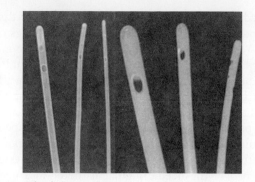

Fig. 25-19 Polyethylene catheters are semirigid, made as small as a 3½ French, and used to bypass strictures or backflush urethral calculi. This catheter is recommended for temporary use because it can be irritating to the urethra and bladder. Flexible rubber or silicone catheters for temporary or long-term use can prevent urethral trauma. Placement is slightly more difficult with flexible catheters but can be managed by first freezing the catheter to stiffen it, or by using a metal or plastic stylet or guidewire.

kinked, knotted, or folded within the bladder and may require surgical removal. Foley catheters that are too short or inflated in the urethra and not in the bladder can damage the urethra.

In patients with a possible ruptured bladder, urethral stricture, or urolithiasis (bladder stones), air or radiographic contrast material may be administered through a urethral catheter to evaluate the bladder and urethra. When percutaneous cystocentesis is difficult or impossible, a urinary catheter may be passed aseptically to collect urine. Once the catheter is placed, a syringe is attached to the catheter, the sample is aspirated, and the urinary catheter is removed. Patients with lower urinary tract disease, urolithiasis, or urethral stricture require a more rigid urinary catheter placed initially to pass the problem area in the urethra, then a softer, more flexible urinary catheter placed for continuous urine collection. Patients with bladder atony need a urinary catheter to keep the bladder small and to prevent urine retention. Large, nonambulatory patients with leg, pelvic, or spinal fractures or recent spinal surgery

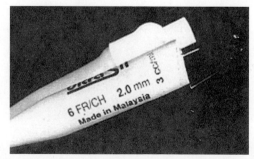

Fig. 25-20 Foley catheters are flexible catheters with an inflatable bulb at the tip to prevent the catheter from slipping out of the bladder. These catheters come in sizes as small as 5 French.

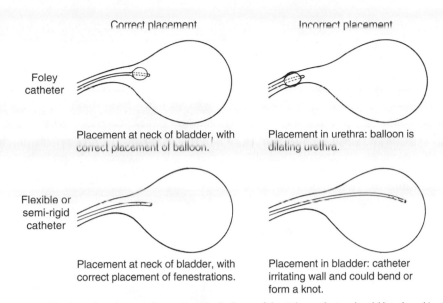

Correct placement | Incorrect placement

Foley catheter

Placement at neck of bladder, with correct placement of balloon.

Placement in urethra: balloon is dilating urethra.

Flexible or semi-rigid catheter

Placement at neck of bladder, with correct placement of fenestrations.

Placement in bladder: catheter irritating wall and could bend or form a knot.

Fig. 25-21 Correct and incorrect positioning of a urinary catheter. *Top:* The balloon of the Foley catheter should be placed in the neck of the bladder *(left)*, rather than in the urethra *(right)*. *Bottom:* The tip of a flexible or semirigid catheter should be placed in the neck of the bladder *(left)*, rather than against the bladder wall *(right)*, where it can bend or cause irritation.

require a urinary catheter collection system to avoid moving the patient excessively for nursing care (Fig. 25-22).

Complications of urethral catheterization include iatrogenic ascending urinary tract infections, catheter breakage, and trauma to the urethra or bladder. Urinary catheters must be placed aseptically. Indwelling urinary catheters that are left open and exposed can lead to infection. A closed urinary system can decrease infection rates. Changing the collection system every 72 hours (only if it is easy to replace the urinary catheter) also helps prevent infection. Daily nursing duties include inspecting the system for kinks and blood clots, cleansing the vulva or pre-

puce with an antiseptic, and emptying the urine bag at scheduled times.

Most healthy cats require sedation or general anesthesia to place a urinary catheter, but very sick cats may not require chemical restraint. Most dogs do not require chemical restraint and can be physically restrained. All patients should be placed in lateral recumbency for urinary catheterization. However, female dogs may also remain standing or be placed in sternal recumbency, with the vulva and pelvic limbs over the edge of the table for ease of placement. Male cats may also be placed in dorsal or lateral recumbency.

In female dogs, urinary catheters can be placed by visualization of the urethral orifice or by palpation. Palpation is usually tolerated better in canine patients and allows the catheter to be placed as quickly and easily as the visual method. The vagina of a cat or small dog may be too small for palpation, but a small, sterile, slit otoscope can be used with a light source to visualize the papilla for placement of a flexible urinary catheter with or without a stylet. A semirigid urinary catheter may be placed with the "blind" technique but can cause trauma to the tissues. Usually a Foley catheter is placed in females. The smallest Foley (5 French) can be placed in female cats. Before placing a urinary catheter, gather all materials needed (Box 25-5). Clip long hair around the prepuce or vulva, and clean the immediate area. Wear sterile gloves when handling the catheter, and use sterile water-soluble lubricant to prevent contamination of the catheter. Use of sterile 2% lidocaine jelly on the gloves, speculum, and urinary catheter minimizes patient discomfort.

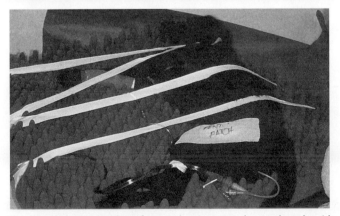

Fig. 25-22 Patient with a fractured spine, taped to a board, with a urinary catheter in place for cleanliness and maintenance of bladder function. Note that the board is padded with rubber egg crates.

BOX 25-5

procedure

Urinary Catheterization

Materials

- Clippers with a #40 blade
- Sterile gauze sponges
- Cleaning solution (Nolvasan, Fort Dodge; Phisohex, Winthrop)
- Sterile water-soluble lubricating jelly (K-Y, or lidocaine jelly)
- Sterile gloves
- Urinary catheter of appropriate type and size
- 20- or 22-gauge wire, flexible wire stylet, or plastic stylet for very flexible catheters
- Light source and sterile speculum for female patients
- Urinary collection system and connecting tubes
- Material to stabilize the urinary catheter in place (1-inch tape, suture material, gauze sponges, Kling, 3-inch elastic tape)

Procedure

Catheter Placement in Male Dogs

1. Shave the hair around the prepuce and apply thumb pressure caudad where the prepuce attaches to the abdomen. Retract the prepuce to expose the distal glans penis (Fig. 25-23). Clean away exudates with the gauze sponges and cleaning solution. Have an assistant continue to hold the penis in this manner during catheterization.
2. With gloves on, place lubricating jelly onto the tip of the urinary catheter and insert the catheter into the distal urethral orifice. Advance the catheter into the bladder until urine flows out continuously, then advance 1 to 2 cm farther to place all catheter fenestrations in the bladder.
3. For Foley catheters, advance the catheter 4 or 5 cm farther to ensure the balloon is in the bladder. Inflate the balloon slowly with saline so that it does not burst (Fig. 25-24). To minimize the length of catheter in the bladder, gently withdraw the Foley catheter until the balloon halts withdrawal.

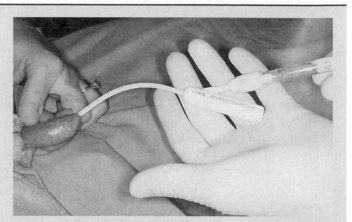

Fig. 25-24 Placement of a Foley catheter in a male dog. The balloon is filled with sterile saline. Sterile gloves are worn during placement.

4. To place urinary catheters aseptically, without gloves, keep the catheter in its sterile package while advancing the tip into the urethra. A paper tab can be made with the package and used to advance the catheter without directly touching the catheter. Avoid touching the penis with the paper tab. Advance the catheter as directed in steps 2 and 3.
5. Once the catheter is placed and urine is flowing freely, release the os penis and allow the prepuce to retract over the glans penis. Secure the catheter as described in the text.

Catheter Placement in Male Cats

1. Clean the perineal area without saturating the fur. Have an assistant extrude the penis from the prepuce by placing the thumb and index finger on each side of the prepuce and applying gentle pressure toward the ischium.
2. With gloves on, place lubricating jelly on the catheter tip and insert it into the penis. The catheter will not be able to advance beyond 1 or 2 cm because of the curve of the penile urethra. To straighten the penile urethra, allow the penis to retract into the prepuce, then gently pull the prepuce distally while advancing the catheter through the urethra into the bladder. Continue to advance the catheter until urine flows freely.
3. Allow the prepuce to cover the penis with the catheter in place. Attach elastic tape to the catheter if no suture wings are available on the catheter. Suture the urinary catheter to the prepuce, then attach the collection system. Always have a security loop attached to the patient to avoid excessive pressure on the catheter. Apply an Elizabethan collar before the patient awakens.

Catheter Placement in Female Dogs (by Visualization)

1. Shave the excess hair away from the vulva and clean the perineal area.

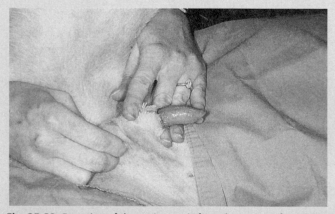

Fig. 25-23 Extrusion of the canine penis from the prepuce for urinary catheterization.

BOX 25-5   *procedure*

Urinary Catheterization—cont'd

2. For placement of the urinary catheter by visualization, lubricate a sterile speculum, catheter tip, and stylet tip. Insert the stylet into the catheter. A slight bend in the stylet approximately 1 cm from the tip may help direct the catheter ventrally into the urethral orifice.

3. Gently place the speculum into the vagina, and direct it dorsally and then cranially until the angle becomes more horizontal. Do not insert the speculum very far in female cats. Look through the speculum while slowly backing out of the vagina. The urethral orifice is on the ventral aspect of the vagina, cranial to the vulva.

4. Holding the speculum and light source steady, guide the urinary catheter and stylet gently through the speculum into the urethral orifice (see Fig. 25-25). Gently advance the catheter through the urethral orifice into the bladder. Once the catheter is placed and urine is flowing freely, advance the catheter 1 or 2 cm farther to ensure that the fenestrations or the entire balloon is in the bladder and inflate the balloon if using a Foley catheter.

5. Remove the speculum from the vagina, and back the Foley catheter out until the balloon stops at the neck of the bladder. If using the sterile slit otoscope cone, remove the cone from the catheter by sliding the catheter through the slit. If using a red rubber or non-Foley catheter in a cat, attach butterfly wings to the catheter before suturing to the perineal area. Attach the extension of the collection system to the leg of the patient Place an Elizabethan collar if necessary.

Catheter Placement in Female Dogs (by Palpation)

1. For placement of a urinary catheter in a female by palpation, apply sterile lubricating jelly to the gloved fingertip, catheter tip, and, if using a stylet, the stylet tip. If the patient is small, using the smallest digit to palpate is least painful for the patient. Once the stylet tip is inserted into the catheter, bending it may facilitate placement of the catheter. However,

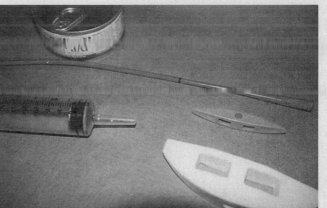

Fig. 25-25 A speculum is used to keep the mouth slightly open and allow for passage of the tube. In addition to the speculum, a roll of tape or syringe casing may be used.

this is not necessary, because the catheter is directed into the orifice with the fingertip. A stylet may or may not be used, depending on the preference of the person placing the catheter.

2. Identify the urethral papilla; it is a firm, round mass on the ventral aspect of the vagina 3 to 5 cm cranial to the vulva in dogs. Bend the tip of the finger just cranial to the papilla to guide the catheter into the urethral orifice. Insert the catheter into the vagina and ventrally into the urethra and on into the bladder.

3. Once the catheter is advanced into the bladder, remove the finger and inflate the balloon of the Foley catheter. Back the urinary catheter out gently until the balloon stops at the neck of the bladder. Attach the urinary system to the catheter and tape it to the patient.

For urinary catheters without suture wings or balloons, make a butterfly wing with elastic tape around the catheter approximately 0.5 cm from the tip of the prepuce. Suture the tape wings on each side of the prepuce. Attach the urinary catheter collection system aseptically. Depending on the patient and the type of catheter placed, a light abdominal wrap may be necessary. For male dogs, place an abdominal bandage (not necessary for Foley catheters) to keep the urinary catheter straight and clean. Place gauze sponges between the prepuce and abdomen for padding. Secure 1-inch tape around the catheter, and wrap the tape loosely around the abdomen. Cover the prepuce and urinary catheter connections with Kling wrapped around the abdomen. Create a security loop by looping the catheter extension tubing and taping it to the patient's abdomen. The extension is then attached to one of the rear legs. For male dogs with Foley catheters, attach 1-inch porous tape around the distal end of the catheter, and loosely wrap it around the abdomen with a security loop in the catheter extension.

Female dogs have the extension attached to the rear leg, with enough slack to prevent tension on the catheter during movement. Cats have the extension tubing looped and attached to the tail or rear leg. Place the collection bag below the level of the patient to prevent backflow of urine into the bladder.

Orogastric Intubation

Orogastric tubes are inserted through the mouth to the stomach and used for administering liquid medication or barium, short-term feeding of gruel-type diets, and flushing of the stomach (gastric lavage). The patient should have a swallowing reflex to prevent aspiration upon regurgitation. Another cause of aspiration is passing the orogastric tube into the trachea, instead of the esophagus, and administering the medication.

A soft, flexible feeding tube is used, of appropriate diameter and length and with a slightly rounded tip. Premeasure the distance from the tip of the nose to just caudal to the last rib. Mark the tube with a piece of tape or permanent marker. Lubricate the tube with water-soluble lubricating jelly.

Place the patient in sternal recumbency or sitting, with the speculum in place (see Fig. 25-25). Two people may need to restrain the patient if chemical restraint is not used. Elevate the head slightly and extend the neck, while passing the tube slowly and gently into the esophagus. Palpate the neck to ensure esophageal placement. Inadvertent passage of the tube and subsequent administration of medication into the trachea may result in severe lung damage and possibly death. Once the tube reaches the line marked, inject air through the tube and auscultate for air bubbling in the stomach or inject a small amount of sterile saline and listen for a cough. Gas may be smelled as it exits the tube. If the tube cannot be passed to the line marked on the tube, withdraw it and try again. Administer the fluid with a syringe, and flush the tube with a small amount of water or air to empty the tube of medication. Occlude or kink the end of the tubing to prevent spilling of liquid into mouth or trachea while the tube is being removed.

Nasoesophageal Intubation

Restrain the patient in sternal recumbency or sitting, with the head held level or slightly elevated. Anesthetize the nostril with 1 to 2 drops of topical ophthalmic anesthetic. While waiting for the topical anesthetic to take effect, lubricate the tip of the feeding tube with a water-soluble lubricant or 5% lidocaine jelly.

Premeasure the tube from the tip of the nose to midthorax, and mark with a permanent marker. Place the tip of the tube in the nares, and direct the tube medially and ventrally. After the tip has been inserted 1 or 2 cm into the nostril, direct the tube caudoventrally into the esophagus. When the tube is inserted to the premeasured line, infuse a small amount of sterile saline into the tube. If coughing occurs, the tube is probably in the trachea. Remove and reinsert the tube. If no coughing occurs, aspirate the syringe. If air is removed from the tube, the tube may be in the trachea. If negative pressure is evident, the tube is in the esophagus. If fluid is aspirated, the tube is in the stomach. If there is any question of tube location, make a lateral radiograph to determine placement.

Move the proximal end of the tube laterally alongside the nares, place a small strip of elastic tape around the tube, and either suture or glue it alongside the nares. The tube

may be sutured without tape using a series of handties around the tube. Move the tube caudad between the eyes, and suture or glue it in place. Cap the end of the tube to prevent air from entering. Apply an Elizabethan collar to prevent the patient from removing the feeding tube (Fig. 25-26). Evaluate the sutures, or glue at each feeding to ensure that the tube is stable and not malpositioned.

To remove the tube, flush it with air to clear fluid out of the tube. Remove the sutures, or gently pull the glued tube away from the skin, and pull the tube out of the nose.

Endotracheal Administration

Oxygen, inhalant anesthetics, medication, and small volumes of fluid can be administered through the trachea for direct absorption through the mucosa or for diagnostic evaluation of tracheal/bronchial secretions (tracheal wash). Placement of an endotracheal tube allows direct administration of oxygen or anesthetics. Humidification and nebulization for respiratory therapy can be administered through an oxygen mask, nasal insufflation tube, tracheostomy tube, or endotracheal tube. Medications may be placed into the humidifier/nebulizer for direct administration, by aerosolization, to the bronchioles. For diagnostic evaluations of bronchial secretions, a sterile polypropylene catheter can be inserted through the skin and tracheal rings (transtracheal wash). To avoid respiratory distress, fluid volumes injected depend on the patient's size.

NURSING CARE OF RECUMBENT PATIENTS

A number of conditions can cause recumbency in patients, including pelvic fractures, head trauma, and herniated intervertebral discs. A major concern in recumbent patients is formation of decubital ulcers (e.g., bed sores, pressure sores). The best treatment is prevention. Patients should

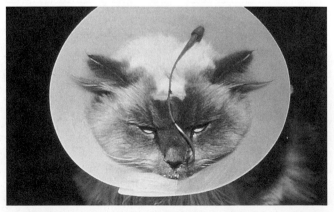

Fig. 25-26 Cat with a nasoesophageal tube sutured in place. An Elizabethan collar has been applied to prevent dislodgment of the tube. *(Courtesy Dr. Nancy Poy, Michigan State University.)*

be kept clean. Urine and feces should not be allowed to remain on the skin and haircoat. Poor sanitation promotes skin breakdown and formation of decubital ulcers. Frequent baths should be given, and the patient should be dried completely. Shaving the hair around the perineal region on patients with incontinence or diarrhea will save time in baths and drying. Sponge baths can be done instead.

Decubital ulcers develop rapidly (within 2 or 3 days) but heal slowly. Once the underlying muscle and/or bone are exposed, it can become infected. Small, superficial ulcers can be managed conservatively with doughnut bandages and topical astringents and antibiotics. Ointments with a petroleum base are not recommended, because these can harbor bacteria. Deep, extensive ulcers require surgical treatment. This may include wound debridement, placement of drains, and secondary closure. If bone is exposed, take proper care to prevent the periosteum from drying. Prevention and treatment of infection are essential. Areas affected most are the sternum, shoulders, sides of the fifth digits, stifles, and hips.

Preventative Care

Turning

Turning patients every 2 to 4 hours helps prevent formation of ulcers and dependent pulmonary atelectasis. Check pressure points after turning. Redness should be temporary; if redness persists 30 minutes or longer, decrease the time on that side. After a position change, stimulate areas over pressure points by massaging to increase circulation to the areas.

Padding

Padding the recumbent patient is essential in preventing the formation (and treatment) of decubital ulcers. Paralyzed patients frequently thrash about; padding helps prevent them from harming themselves. Place padding in the cages for patients with paralysis or paresis, seizures, vestibular problems, encephalopathy resulting from neoplasia of the brain, orthopedic disease, or metabolic disease. Place padding in the doors and walls of cages for patients with vestibular disease, neoplasia of the brain, or frequent seizures.

Types of padding include fleece pads, sponge rubber egg crates, diapers, and waterbeds. Household items, such as blankets, sheets, and foam rubber placed in plastic bags, can be used as padding. Fleece pads are synthetic sheepskins. They are washable, absorbent, very soft, and airy. These can be combined with other forms of padding. If used alone, they are best for patients under 25 pounds. Foam rubber egg crates are especially good for larger patients (see Fig. 25-22). A disadvantage, however, is that they act like a sponge, absorbing urine and water. Place them in plastic bags to keep them clean and dry. Clients can purchase these

crates at medical supply stores or in the bedding department of retail stores.

Waterbeds are especially good in preventing decubital ulcers. Animal waterbeds are made in various sizes, so most standard veterinary cages will accommodate them. The bed should be placed in a cage of nearly the same area so that the patient will not fall off and become stuck between the bed and the cage wall. Animal waterbeds are thermostatically heated and provide warmth and comfort to patients. If they become unplugged, they require about 12 hours to heat up before they can be used. Temperature can be adjusted easily to prevent the patient from becoming overheated or cold. Heat eases muscle soreness, stimulates circulation, and helps the patient relax. Waterbeds should never be used without turning on the heat. A cold waterbed draws heat from the patient and produces hypothermia.

Place disposable diapers or bed pads on top of all padding to help keep the padding clean. Use of diapers saves valuable nursing time. Soiled diapers are simply thrown away, leaving the underlying padding reasonably clean and dry. In pet stores, they are called puppy-training pads.

Bladder maintenance

Every effort should be made to promote voluntary urination to minimize expressing the bladder and catheterization. Taking the patient outside may stimulate or promote voluntary urination. Before expressing, allow the patient to urinate. Attention should be given to bladder size, the act of urination, and the amount, color, and odor of the urine. When leg muscle function starts to return, some bladder function usually returns, also. Time should be allowed for the patient to totally evacuate its bladder.

Palpate the bladder with even, steady pressure. Sudden movement may cause the patient to tense the abdominal muscles. In toy breeds and cats, it is easier to use one hand. Use both hands for larger breeds. Placing patients on their side is easier than trying to hold them up while expressing the bladder, especially if the patient starts to struggle. Once the bladder is palpated, apply pressure. Several seconds may be required to override the sphincter tone, especially in patients with neurologic injury.

A urinary catheter and collection set may be used for a paralyzed patient for better nursing care. The urinary catheter should be left in place only 3 to 4 days because of the risk of infection. If hematuria or some other change in urine color develops, consider removing the catheter. The risk of infection can be decreased if the patient is catheterized only when necessary. The major disadvantage is the time required to catheterize the patient.

Bowel maintenance

Keep a record of the patient's bowel movements (Fig. 25-27). An enema may be required if the patient becomes

Client:	Date:
Patient:	
Breed:	
Sex:	Problem list:
Age/DOB:	
Weight:	

Food:

H2O:

	Food	H20	1	2	3	4	5	6	7	8	9	comments
7am												
8am												
9am												
10am												
11am												
12n												
1pm												
2pm												
3pm												
4pm												
5pm												
6pm												
7pm												
8pm												
9pm												
10pm												
11pm												
12pm												

Veterinarian:

Telephone/beeper:

A

Fig. 25-27 Successful implementation of nursing care can be improved with the use of flowcharts or critical care daily sheets. **A,** Blank form.

Client: Smith	Problem list. HBC, facial trauma, has
Patient: Reggie	Esophageal feeding tube.
Breed: DSH	
Sex: M/N	
Age/DOB: approx 6-8 yr	
Weight: 9.0 #	

Food. NPO

H2O: NPO

1) A/D gruel :60 ml
4 X day via tube

2) Water flush:
20 ml 4 X day via
tube

3) Clavamos drops
1 ml BID via tube

4) Hycodan 5 mg
¼ t BID via tube

5) Pred 5mg SID
via tube

6) BNP ou TID

7) Atropine ophth
ou SID

8) Pred Acetate
ophth OS TID

	Food	H20	1	2	3	4	5	6	7	8	9	comments
7am												
8am												
9am												
10am												
11am												
12n												
1pm												
2pm												
3pm												
4pm												
5pm												
6pm												
7pm												
8pm												
9pm												
10pm												
11pm												
12pm												

B

Fig. 25-27 Cont'd B, Form filled out with daily orders. The nurse checks off medications as given and includes any comments on the patient.

constipated. This is not generally the case, however. If the patient has a flaccid anal sphincter, nursing care and adequate sanitation can be especially difficult. The hindquarters of longhaired dogs and cats should be clipped closely to ensure that feces do not smear or entangle in the haircoat. Clipping also facilitates bathing and drying if the patient becomes soiled.

NURSING CARE OF CRITICAL PATIENTS

Head Trauma and Seizure Patients

Continuous monitoring of semicomatose or comatose patients is necessary. Monitoring includes heart rate, respiration, temperature, mucous membrane color, and neurologic function. Re-evaluation is done every 15 to 60 minutes, depending on deterioration or improvement. Patients with *status epilepticus* (continuous seizures) or head trauma usually have increased intracranial pressure. Cerebral edema peaks at 24 to 48 hours after trauma and can last up to 96 hours. Extending and elevating the head and neck help cerebral venous outflow. Care should be taken not to occlude the jugular veins.

Excessive fluid therapy and hypoxia contribute to cerebral edema. Fluid therapy should be administered only to maintain hydration and normal blood pressure (after shock treatment). To combat potential hypoxia, oxygen should be given by mask, nasal catheter, or oxygen cage. If intubation is required, it should be done as quickly and smoothly as possible. Struggling and coughing increase intracranial pressure.

Caloric needs for these patients can increase as much as 2½ times. A high-calorie diet is recommended. Patients in stuporous or comatose states can receive nutrition by nasogastric tube, percutaneous enterogastric tube, or IV.

Spinal Trauma

Clients calling with concerns that their pets may have sustained spinal trauma should be told to place them on some form of board. They can use duct tape to help stabilize the patient. If the patient is not brought to the clinic on a board, the patient should be placed on one immediately. Assessments, treatments, and diagnostics should be done with the patient on the board until the patient is stabilized. Only lateral views and across-table radiographs should be made.

Blood Pressure Monitoring

Blood pressure monitoring is also used in assessment of critically ill patients. Blood pressure is the pressure exerted by the blood on the wall of the vessel. The systolic pressure is the maximum force caused by contraction of the left ventricle of the heart. Diastolic pressure is the minimum force during the relaxation phase, when the aortic and pulmonic valves are closed. Direct blood pressure monitoring requires an arterial catheter connected via IV extension tubing to an external monitor. For intermittent indirect blood pressure monitoring by Doppler, the ultrasound probe is placed over a peripheral artery and the pressure cuff is placed proximal to the probe. Manually inflate the cuff until the sound of the blood flow stops, then deflate the cuff until the first sound is heard. The systolic pressure is read from the manometer when the first sound is heard. The diastolic pressure is read when the sound changes. It can be difficult to detect this change; therefore, the diastolic pressure reading may not be possible with this method.

Central Venous Pressure

CVP is the pressure within the cranial vena cava. It reflects the condition of the cardiovascular system and is influenced by many factors, including blood volume and cardiac function. The CVP is monitored in patients receiving large volumes of IV fluids, with poor cardiac or renal function, or with encephalopathies. It is monitored by catheterization of the cranial vena cava via the jugular vein. The catheter is connected to a fluid-filled column (manometer) and a source of fluid (syringe or bag). Normal central venous pressure is less than 5 cm water; however, the trend of CVP changes is more important than a single reading.

Pain Control

Analgesia (pain relief) can speed recovery and improve the patient's mental status. Pain can cause cardiovascular and respiratory irregularities, aggression, and hysteria. The ability to recognize a patient in pain and provide pain relief can prevent the patient from harming itself or the handler, improve patient health, and shorten the length of hospitalization.

Individual patients react differently to pain. If the patient is resting quietly in a cage, signs of pain may not be detected unless a physical examination is performed. Signs may include anorexia, depression, mydriasis (dilated pupils), partially closed eyes, third eyelid protrusion, tachypnea (increased respiratory rate), tachycardia (increased heart rate), pale mucous membranes, and ptyalism (excessive salivation). Other signs include whimpering or crying, sharp yipping when moved or touched, growling when approached, anxiety, avoidance behavior, restlessness, frequent repositioning in the cage, reluctance to lie down, arching of the spine, limping or non–weight-bearing on a limb, and chewing at a specific area.

Attempt to determine the location and severity of the pain, and, if possible, eliminate the cause or factors contributing to the pain. Application of heat or cold to the affected area, additional padding or bedding, massage, quietly speaking to the patient while stroking, and hand feeding highly palatable food may be of comfort to the patient. Monitor the patient at regular intervals for change in the degree of pain.

When using medication to control pain, consult the package insert for the onset of analgesic effect. The route used may alter the onset and duration of action. For example, pain may be relieved immediately with IV analgesia, but the duration of action is short.

The common practice of waiting until a specified time has elapsed between doses of analgesic medication is not humane. Pre-emptive application of pain management is more effective than giving the drug after the pain is present. At the conclusion of surgery, administer systemic, regional, epidural, or local analgesia before the patient is removed from inhalation anesthesia. A fentanyl citrate skin patch can be applied for pain relief. Other analgesics can be administered systemically or locally.

Respiratory Support

Respiration supplies body cells with oxygen and eliminates carbon dioxide from the body. Dyspnea is difficult or labored breathing resulting from airway obstruction (e.g., infection, neoplasia, laryngeal paralysis, asthma), changes in the lungs or thorax (i.e., metastasis, pneumothorax, diaphragmatic hernia, pneumonia, pleural effusion), or cardiovascular or hematologic abnormalities (e.g., anemia, heart failure, heartworm disease).

Respiratory therapy can improve or maintain pulmonary function and tissue oxygenation. The therapeutic objective is to maintain alveolar ventilation (with oxygen, ventilator therapy, or chest tube placement), control secretions (by decreasing production and increasing clearance), and normalize pulmonary reflexes.

Respiratory support may involve placement of an oxygen mask, nasal insufflation tube, tracheostomy tube, or endotracheal tube, or placing the patient in an oxygen cage or on a ventilator to provide oxygen to the lungs and prevent hypoxia. It may also involve placement of a chest tube to remove fluid or air surrounding the lungs and allow expansion of the lungs.

Oxygen mask

An oxygen mask placed over the mouth and nose provides the patient with 100% oxygen. This is for temporary use only. Some patients may not tolerate the mask but may tolerate a hood made from an Elizabethan collar covered with clear plastic. Oxygen can be delivered through a hole in the collar. A clear plastic bag may also be placed loosely over the patient's head with oxygen tubing entering the hood near the patient's nose or mouth. Use caution with this method. Ensure that oxygen is always flowing into the hood.

Oxygen cage

Patients in acute respiratory distress can be placed in an incubator or oxygen cage. The cage provides an environment with stable temperature, humidity, and oxygen. The temperature should be adjusted to make the patient comfortable and the humidity kept at 10% to 60%, while oxygen is delivered to provide 40% oxygen in the environment (normal room air contains 20.9% oxygen). A major drawback to using the oxygen cage is limited access to the patient. If the cage is opened, the percentage of oxygen in the air immediately drops and the patient may become dyspneic. Use pillows to prop the patient in sternal recumbency in the oxygen cage.

Nasal insufflation is an easy way to provide oxygen without causing undue stress to the patient (Fig. 25-28). An oxygen flow rate of 100 ml/kg/min provides approximately 40% oxygen to the patient. Nasal insufflation allows full access to the patient without decreasing or stopping the flow of oxygen during treatment procedures. Some patients may not tolerate a nasal insufflation tube and require an Elizabethan collar to prevent removal of the tube. Oxygen administered through a tube placed in the nasal cavity must be humidified to prevent drying of the respiratory mucosa. A humidification unit can be attached to the flow meter.

Chest tube

Chest tubes are placed through the chest wall into the pleural space to remove fluid or air from around the lungs, allowing the lungs to expand maximally. The chest tube must be securely attached (sutured) to the patient to prevent inadvertent leakage of air into the chest by accidental removal of the chest tube. More than one clamp (e.g.,

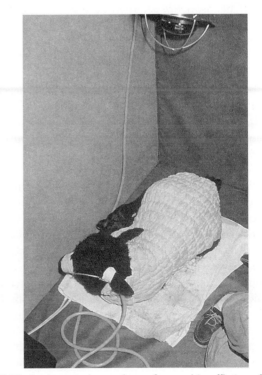

Fig. 25-28 Cat in sternal recumbency for nasal insufflation of oxygen. Note that the head is elevated to aid ventilation. The tubing is connected to a humidification unit attached to a flow meter.

hemostats with padded jaws) and a three-way stopcock should be placed on the chest tube to prevent leakage of air into the pleural cavity between aspirations. Aseptic removal of fluid or air from the chest prevents secondary infections.

The bandage securing the chest tube in place should be tight enough (or attached to the patient with tape) to prevent slippage, but loose enough to allow the patient to breathe. Always cover the jaws of the hemostat and the three-way stopcock with an easily removed layer of tape. This will prevent the hemostats or the stopcock from catching on anything and becoming dislodged. If the patient is left unattended with a chest tube in place, an Elizabethan collar should be placed to prevent tube removal by the patient. Always check the bandage and the chest tube for security when aspirating.

Control of respiratory secretions

Nasal and pulmonary secretions may be decreased with systemic or topical administration of antibiotics, antifungals, or corticosteroids. Patients with pulmonary edema are treated during nebulization with antifoaming agents. Dried secretions may be rehydrated and loosened by aerosolization/nebulization with saline and cleared by coupage or physical therapy.

Ultrasonic nebulization. Ultrasonic nebulization provides humidification of inspired gases and promotes mobilization of the mucous layer to aid removal of secretions. In conjunction with percussion and vibration, postural drainage (using gravity) moves secretions from small airways into the bronchi, where they can be coughed up. Exercise and stimulation of the cough reflex (e.g., by tracheal manipulation) also improves clearance of secretions.

Ultrasonic nebulizers produce a dense mist of microdroplets. They are used to administer medication (e.g., bronchodilators, antibiotics, detergents, mucolytics) directly to the lungs, humidify air inhaled by the patient, hydrate and loosen dried bronchial secretions, restore the epithelium in the lungs, and promote coughing. Effective nebulization must also be accompanied by other physical therapy techniques (e.g., coupage, postural drainage, exercise, cough stimulation) to be effective in clearing the lungs. Nebulization for 15 to 30 minutes every 4 to 6 hours, with additional respiratory therapy, is more effective than continuous ultrasonic aerosolization. Nebulizer equipment should be cleaned and all removable parts sterilized before use on each patient. Each patient should have a separate sterile fluid reservoir and hose leading from the nebulizer. Sterile fluids should be used whenever possible. Complications can also occur if the dried secretions are not suctioned immediately after nebulization therapy. The patient can become more dyspneic from swelling of the rehydrated secretions. The patient should never be left unattended once ultrasonic nebulization therapy has begun. Fluid overload may occur in pediatric patients on continuous therapy; therefore, always use intermittent nebulization therapy.

The nebulizer hose may be attached to an oxygen mask for direct administration to the patient. Patients that do not tolerate a facemask may allow an Elizabethan collar to be placed and covered with plastic to form a tent over the head. The nebulizer hose can be attached to the tent to permit aerosolization of the patient. Another method of administration is by covering the cage door with plastic and nebulizing the cage. A cage specifically for nebulization may be used, but this can cause cross-contamination between patients if the unit is not thoroughly cleaned between uses.

Respiratory physiotherapy

Immediately after nebulization, the rehydrated, loosened secretions must be mobilized and cleared out of the lungs using physiotherapy. *Coupage* (percussion and vibration) and tracheal manipulation to stimulate the cough reflex, postural drainage, and mild exercise (to improve tidal ventilation) are methods of physiotherapy.

Percussion is the creation of waves of air to loosen secretions in the lungs. *Vibration* is high-frequency compression of the chest wall. For manual percussion, the cupped hands are clapped against each side of the chest, trapping air between the hands and the chest wall, starting with the caudal lung lobes and working cranially to move the secretions out of the tract. Care must be taken to strike the chest wall without causing discomfort or bruising. Percussion may be contraindicated in patients with a bleeding disorder, fractured ribs, or fragile bones. Rhythmic percussion loosens and mobilizes secretions; postural drainage, exercise, and coughing help expel the secretions.

Recumbent patients may be turned to the other side or placed sternally, with the head lower than the chest to augment gravitational drainage of secretions. After nebulization and coupage, dogs may be walked outside to help increase drainage of secretions. Cats may be placed in a large cage to encourage physical activity, which increases clearance of secretions.

REHABILITATION AND PHYSICAL THERAPY

Rehabilitation is an extremely important part of medical management. Patients that receive some form of rehabilitative treatment recover faster than those that do not. The type of therapy used depends upon the severity of the problem and condition of the patient. Rehabilitation therapy can prevent decubital ulcers, enhance blood and lymphatic circulation, prevent muscle contracture, maintain muscle tone and joint flexibility, produce relaxation, and reduce pain. Although some types of rehabilitation can be expensive, most are not. Many are easy to perform, so clients can do them at home. This helps keep costs down, or, if done in the clinic, does not require significant overhead. Types of rehabilitation therapy include thermal therapy, passive exercise, and active exercise.

Local Hypothermia/Cold Therapy

Hypothermia is most effective during the first 24 to 48 hours after surgical procedures and after acute soft-tissue contusions, muscle/tendon strains, and ligament sprains or lacerations. The cold decreases the tissue temperature, which decreases pain perception and reduces nerve conduction and muscle spasms. Local vasoconstriction also helps decrease edema.

Local hypothermia can be as easy as applying an ice pack to the affected area. These can be the cold packs used for shipping by drug companies, ice cubes wrapped in a towel, or continuous surface cooling blankets. Cold packs should be covered with a towel; ice should be placed in a plastic leakproof bag wrapped in a towel. Applications should be for 5 to 10 minutes, two to four times per day. Treatment should not exceed 30 minutes. Edema may become more severe if treatments exceed 30 minutes. Open wounds must be protected with a sterile, water-impermeable dressing to avoid contamination; use light pressure and avoid excessive cold. If the condition worsens at any point, discontinue treatment.

Local Hyperthermia/Heat Therapy

Hyperthermia is applied 48 to 72 hours after injury. Caution should be used when applying heat. Patients with sensory nerve involvement and those recovering from anesthesia may sustain thermal injuries. Before applying hot packs or a hot towel, place a form of insulation, such as a towel, on the skin. The hot pack should be 40° to 45° C (104° to 113° F) and applied for 10 minutes, two to four times per day. Check the skin every 1 to 2 minutes to see if it is overly hot. If so, another towel should be placed over the treatment area.

The therapeutic benefits of hyperthermia include muscle relaxation, pain relief, localized vasodilation, and localized increase in metabolic rate. This form of treatment is contraindicated for acute injuries, because it increases edema. Some of the different forms of heat treatments are radiant heat (applied with infrared lamps), ultrasound, and some forms of warm-water hydrotherapy.

Combination Therapy

Combination therapy is used in the latter stages of healing and can be used with other forms of physical therapy. Heat applied before massage or exercise can improve muscle relaxation and circulation. Cold applied to the injured area after exercise helps decrease swelling and pain. If the patient has just had surgery, it is best to wait 2 to 3 days before beginning physical therapy.

Passive Exercise

The patient in passive exercise requires no voluntary muscle activity. Two forms of passive exercise include massage and range of motion (ROM).

Massage

Massage is used to rehabilitate patients with diseases of the bone, muscle, joints, nerves, and skin, as well as patients with decubital ulcers. Massage can be administered a couple of days after surgery. The patient that is treated medically can also receive massage, but care should be taken to prevent aggravating an existing lesion. Massage can also be done after a session of active therapy (combination therapy).

The primary objective of massage is to increase flow of blood and nutrients to the tissue, which in turn will provide quicker elimination of wastes. Deeper forms of massage can decrease the chances of fibrosis. Massage contraindications include acute inflammation of soft tissue, bones, and joints, recent fractures, sprains, foreign bodies under the skin, hemorrhage or lymphangitis, advanced skin diseases, fever or heat stroke, round incision sites, and torn muscles.

Consider the following factors when administering massage:

- Direction of the massage (should always be toward venous return)
- Amount of pressure used (start with superficial pressure and gradually work to deeper muscles)
- Duration of massage
- Rate and rhythm of massage (depends on the type used)
- Frequency of massage

In *effleurage*, strokes are given with the palm and fingers, slowly and lightly, just like petting. Gradually increase the pressure of the strokes. This produces a calming effect, which allows the patient to relax. This also allows the patient to become accustomed to the therapist. With light strokes, apply fifteen per minute; with heavy strokes, apply five per minute. Give 5- to 10-minute sessions of effleurage. This type of massage enhances draining of veins and lymph channels.

With *fingertip massage*, use two or three fingers and keep them close together. Do not lose contact with the skin. Massage slowly and gently in a circular motion, increasing the pressure as the patient relaxes. This massages underlying muscles. Massage for 5 to 10 minutes.

Petrissage, or deep massage, is used on the back, flank, and chest. The skin is lifted, pulled, and rolled between the fingers and thumb, like rolling dough. For the shoulder, thigh, and limbs, the deeper muscles and tendons can be kneaded between the thumb and fingers of the right hand, while the left hand holds the limb and occasionally flexes and extends it. The kneading movements should be slow and rhythmic. Muscle is compressed from side to side and always in the direction of venous return. Deep massage enhances circulation, stretches muscles and tendons, and prevents adhesions and contracture.

Friction massage is fast, invigorating, circular massage given with the first two or three fingers. Massage at a rate of one circular motion every second, gradually increasing to twice that rate. This massage helps loosen superficial scar tissue and adhesions, as well as remove loose hair from the coat.

Stretch pressure massage combines pressure on a muscle with a stretching motion. This type of massage provides mechanical deformation of the skin and elongation of underlying muscle fibers and spindles. It helps maintain skin compliance and benefits muscle.

Range-of-motion therapy

Range-of-motion therapy helps maintain the proper range of motion of a limb by minimizing muscle and joint contraction from disuse. Take the affected limb and slowly move it through its normal range, ensuring not to hyperextend the limb. Treatment should be for 5 or 10 minutes, two to four times per day. Range of motion can be combined with other forms of rehabilitation.

For patients with orthopedic injuries/conditions and muscle contractions, a slow controlled movement should be applied. Caution should be used not to overstress the limb, because this may loosen fixation devices or cause muscle/tendon/ligament damage.

Active Exercise

The intent of active exercise is to stimulate as much voluntary activity as possible. Voluntary muscle contraction is the most beneficial form of therapy. Most patients must be supported with a towel/stockinette used as a sling or supporting them at the base of the tail (Figs. 25-29 and 25-30). Exercise carts and hoists can also be used to help them walk (Fig. 25-31). These exercises should be done on textured surfaces, because most patients slip or slide on tile floors. Treatment time depends on the patient. Once you notice the patient becoming tired, treatment should end. This

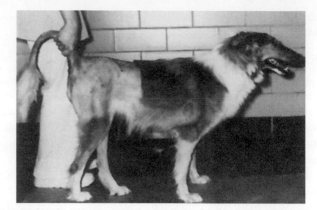

Fig. 25-30 The tail is used to support the hindquarters during active exercise therapy of dogs with caudal paresis. Note that the tail is grasped at its base so as to avoid tail injury.

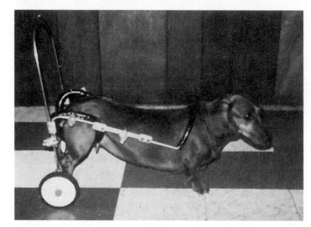

Fig. 25-31 A commercially available cart used for dogs with caudal paralysis.

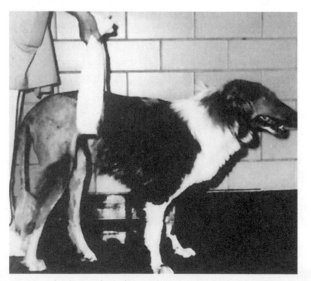

Fig. 25-29 A bath towel can be used to support the hindquarters during active exercise of patients with caudal paresis.

may be as short as 1 to 2 minutes. Within the first few weeks, treatment should not exceed 20 minutes.

Standing exercises are done when the patient starts supporting weight. Allow the patient to do so for as long as possible. It may be only 1 or 2 seconds in the beginning. After the patient sinks back down, pick it up and repeat for as long as possible. As the patient becomes stronger and can support its total weight, gently apply downward pressure over the hips or shoulders. This helps strengthen the muscles as the patient attempts to resist.

Walking exercises are performed when the patient starts to regain voluntary muscle movements or with a paraplegic patient. Although a patient may only have function of the forelimbs, exercising should begin again as soon as possible. A leash should always be used to restrict the patient's activity.

Hydrotherapy

Hydrotherapy provides passive and active therapy. Passive hydrotherapy is provided with a whirlpool, whereas active hydrotherapy is swimming (underwater exercise). Patients may be fearful of the water; allow time to acclimate the patient to the water.

Contraindications of hydrotherapy include peripheral vascular disease, acute injury, acute inflammation, fever, recent surgery, hemorrhage, cardiac disorders, and respiratory disorders. Hydrotherapy should not begin until at least 5 days following surgery. Wait 10 to 30 days for patients treated medically. Before placing the patient in a tub, check the water temperature to be sure it is appropriate. Never leave a patient alone in a tub!

A patient with an elevated temperature should not be treated with warm-water therapy until its temperature has been normal for 72 hours. Patients with respiratory or cardiac insufficiency should not be treated.

Whirlpool therapy provides a vigorous hydromassage. This massaging effect helps in removing dirt, necrotic tissue, and purulent exudates, and can also help fight infection if povidone-iodine is added. It speeds wound healing, reduces hyperesthesia of the skin, and may facilitate urination and defecation.

Before putting the patient in the whirlpool, remove all bandage material. During treatment, the water surface should be skimmed to remove hair and other debris. The water temperature should be 39° to 41° C (102° to 105° F). Caution should be taken not to scald the patient. For the first treatment, have the patient sit in the tub for 5 minutes to become accustomed to immersion. Increase each treatment in duration, ending with a 20-minute treatment after several days.

Swimming is an excellent form of physical therapy. Buoyancy and hydrostatic pressure in a pool provide support and allow voluntary exercise with a minimum of effort. Patients with paresis must be helped through the motions of walking or swimming. Weights can be added to the patient's legs to build strength and endurance. Water also creates resistance to movement, which helps strengthen weakened muscles as exercise sessions continue. Because a patient produces heat while exercising, the water temperature should be 27° to 32° C (80° to 90° F).

NURSING CARE OF NEONATAL PATIENTS

Examination

Signs of distress or disease in neonates are usually nonspecific, most commonly including continuous vocalization, ineffective nursing, and restlessness. Careful examination of the neonate and its environment can yield specific clues. The normal neonate is warm to the touch and is vigorous and vocal in its objection to handling. Body temperature ranges from 35.5° to 36.5° C. Mucous membranes are pink to red, and moist. Capillary refill time is less than 2 seconds.

Respiration is regular (15 to 35 breaths per minute), and no fluid is auscultated over the lung fields. Minimal clear nasal discharge may be evident. The heart rate is rapid, usually 180 to 250 beats per minute. Normal hydration is evidenced by normal skin turgor. Urination and defecation are easily elicited by gentle stimulation of the anogenital area with a moistened cotton ball. The umbilical area is normally not inflamed, and the anus and genitalia are clean. The limbs and paws, including nails (claws), should be well-developed and properly oriented. The haircoat is full, shiny, and free of parasites or fecal contamination. The bedding of the nest box should not show evidence of diarrhea.

Resuscitation

Resuscitation of the neonate is necessary when the bitch or queen fails or is unable to perform this (such as after cesarean section or with maternal behavioral problems), or when a puppy or kitten does not respond to typical maternal manipulation (licking and nuzzling by the bitch or queen). An airway free of amniotic fluid, placental membranes, and meconium (first neonatal feces) should be established within 3 to 5 minutes after birth. Remove the placental membranes first, if present, by tearing from the neonate's face. Clear the oral cavity and trachea by swabbing with cotton-tipped applicators or gentle suction with a bulb syringe. To assist removal of airway fluids by centrifugal force, carefully swing the neonate headfirst in a downward arc while supporting the head and trunk in a towel. Perform the swinging action with the hands only and not by whole-arm movement. Clearing the airway prevents aspiration of potentially damaging meconium-containing fluids.

Stimulate respiration by thoracic and facial massage with a dry, warm towel. If cyanosis persists, supply oxygen with a small facemask. The size of most canine and feline neonates precludes nasal oxygen insufflation and intubation, but positive-pressure ventilation can be achieved with a properly fitted facemask. Care should be taken not to overinflate the neonatal lungs. External cardiac massage is performed if the heart rate is very low (less than 80 to 100 beats per minute) or not detectable. The umbilical cord should be clamped and ligated if bleeding and coated with tincture of iodine (Fig. 25-32). Tincture of iodine is preferable to povidone-iodine because it is more astringent (drying) because of its alcohol content. Gut suture material (2-0 or 3-0) is ideal for ligation of the umbilical cord.

The neonate should be completely dried and warmed. Immediate suckling is encouraged, because it provides colostrum (first milk), calories, and glucose, sparing the neonate's limited glycogen stores. If nursing is not immediately available, glucose should be provided via oral administration of one or two drops of Karo (corn) syrup. SQ administration of 5% dextrose (2 to 4 ml/kg) is possible, but this runs the risk of abscess.

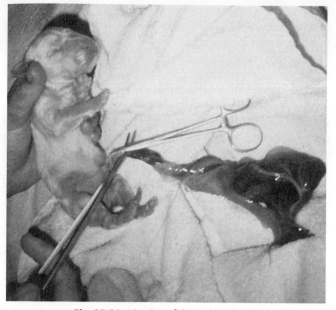

Fig. 25-32 Ligation of the umbilical cord

The SQ route is convenient for delivery of balanced, preservative-free electrolyte solutions to mildly dehydrated puppies and kittens, but it is not adequate for dehydrated individuals. Intravenous catheterization of the jugular vein in kittens and small-breed puppies, or the cephalic vein in larger neonatal puppies is possible. The IO route of fluid administration is optimal in very small neonates; it permits rapid administration of large volumes of fluids to the venous system via the bone marrow sinusoids and medullary venous channels. The trochanteric fossa of the femur and the greater tubercle of the humerus are preferred sites. An 18- to 20-gauge spinal needle is advanced into the marrow cavity and secured to the skin. Oral administration of fluids is useful for neonates without gastric disorders (not vomiting), but it is also not adequate for dehydrated individuals. Fluids administered by any route should be first warmed to body temperature.

Poorly responsive neonates can benefit from drug therapy. For the purposes of drug dosing, normal puppies weigh 100 to 700 g (0.1 to 0.7 kg) at birth, whereas normal kittens weigh approximately 100 g (0.1 kg). Reversal of the effects of any narcotic or barbiturate anesthetic agent used during anesthesia of the dam can improve the status of neonates born by cesarean section. Naloxone, a narcotic antagonist, and doxapram, a respiratory stimulant, can be administered (0.1 to 0.2 ml) into the tongue (or other muscle) or umbilical vein of the neonate.

Apnea (lack of breathing) that lasts longer than 5 minutes can warrant therapeutic intervention to correct acidemia and provide substrate for myocardial metabolism. Sodium bicarbonate, diluted 1:1 with 5% dextrose (0.5 mEq/ml), can be administered at 0.5 to 1 mEq/kg via the umbilical vein, over 2 to 4 minutes. Prolonged bradycardia or cardiac standstill can be treated with epinephrine (1:10,000 solution given IV at 0.1 ml/kg) and atropine (0.03 mg/kg IM or IV).

The ambient temperature of neonates during the first few weeks of life (30° to 32° C [86° to 89.6° F]) can be maintained with an infrared lamp, positioned 6 feet above the draft-free nest box, illuminating half of the area available to the dam and neonates. Heating pads can cause thermal burns, so their use is discouraged. The temperature within the nest box should be monitored with a thermometer. Hypothermia of neonates predisposes to hypoglycemia, hypoxemia, and poor digestive function. Nest box surfaces should be lined with smooth, nonporous materials to facilitate cleaning and avoid abrading the neonates.

Disinfectants used on nest box surfaces must not leave caustic or toxic residues. Bedding material should not impair respiration or obscure neonates from the dam's view, but it should provide good footing and absorb wastes. Shredded, unprinted newspaper and washable terrycloth toweling are superior.

Acquired disorders of the postpartum period include immunodeficiencies, malnutrition, and infectious disease. Orphaned neonates are at increased risk. Neonatal congenital immunodeficiencies associated with thymus dysfunction have been proposed. Acquired immunodeficiency results from failure of passive transfer of maternally derived antibodies, acquired primarily by ingestion of colostrum during the first 24 hours of life. Acquired immunodeficiencies also occur secondary to distemper and parvoviral infections and dietary zinc deficiencies.

Neonatal malnutrition can result from poor milk production or quality, crowding, and ineffectual nursing. Malnutrition is evidenced by failure to gain weight steadily. The birth weight should double by 12 days of age. Rotating neonates in the whelping box gives smaller, weaker individuals first access to the teats. Supplemental feeding with commercially available artificial bitch and queen milk is often indicated. Approximately 22 to 26 kcal per 100 g of body weight should be fed daily. Commercial milk replacers generally provide 1 to 1.24 kcal/ml of formula. The neonate should receive 13 to 22 ml of formula per 100 g of body weight, divided into four meals daily, over the first 4 weeks of life.

Neonates rarely nurse effectively from artificial nipples and bottles because of problems with equipment size and shape, as well as milk flow and variable suckling reflexes. Gastric intubation is preferred. Large-bore, soft, red rubber catheters, cut to proper length (from mouth to stomach), minimize inadvertent tracheal intubation (Fig. 25-33). Frequent small-volume feedings reduce the risk of regurgitation and aspiration. Commercial milk substitutes are closer to bitch or queen milk than most homemade recipes. Milk should be warmed to body temperature just

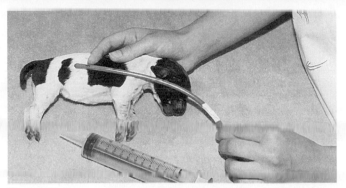

Fig. 25-33 Proper measurement of feeding tube length for an orphan puppy.

before administration. Hand-fed neonates should be weighed daily.

NURSING CARE OF GERIATRIC PATIENTS

The Effects of Aging

Old age brings about numerous gradual degenerative changes. Body weight increases, skin loses elasticity and becomes dry and scaly, and the haircoat becomes dull and sparse. Footpads become hyperkeratinized, and nails become brittle. In carnivores, dental calculus increases; in older rabbits or rodents, dental malocclusion becomes more common. Digestion is less efficient, and reduced colonic motility leads to constipation.

Cardiac output decreases with age, usually as a result of mitral valve insufficiency. The lungs lose elasticity, and increased susceptibility to respiratory infection can lead to chronic obstructive pulmonary disease, chronic bronchitis, bronchiectasis, and emphysema. Diminished kidney function leads to polydipsia, polyuria, urinary incontinence, anemia, and wasting. In addition, muscle and bone atrophy may also occur. Degenerative joint disease and vertebral spondylosis are common in older patients. Changes in the nervous system lead to loss of short-term memory, changes in sleep patterns, and incontinence. Hearing, vision, and taste decrease; the sense of smell is preserved to some extent in most aged companion animals. Altered immune function leads to reduced antibody response to antigens, autoimmune diseases, and a higher incidence of neoplasia.

Geriatric pets are less able to adjust to stressful conditions, and some react with stereotypic, destructive, or aggressive behaviors or depression and anorexia. Separation anxiety or excessive vocalization is certainly a consideration whenever the geriatric patient is hospitalized. A patient with failing vision or hearing is more apt to be startled and overreact aggressively. Housesoiling is another common geriatric problem. Musculoskeletal disease may make movement to the appropriate place for elimination difficult or painful. Inappropriate elimination caused by medical problems must be differentiated from that related to behavior.

Geriatric Criteria

When the changes described above have taken a toll on the patient's well being, that patient can be considered *geriatric*. The age at which this occurs depends on the expected life span of the species, as well as various individual factors. In general, species that grow to large size live longer than smaller mammals. If there is wide variation in size within a species, such as with the many dog breeds, smaller breeds tend to live longer than larger breeds.

Handling

When providing nursing care for a geriatric companion animal, assume that the effects of aging are affecting the health and behavior of the patient. Old pets brought to the veterinary hospital may be overly anxious and have problems, such as impaired vision and hearing; painful joints; thin bones; weak muscles; poor kidney function; congestive heart failure; chronic bronchitis; decreased liver, pancreatic, and gastrointestinal function; periodontal disease; malodorous breath; flaky skin; and a sparse haircoat.

Schedule office visits for geriatric patients during less busy times of the day and week. Never rush examinations or sample collection. Take time for discussion with the client. Handle the geriatric patient gently and deliberately. Avoid sudden movements. Let the patient know where you are at all times; this is especially important with old horses, because they may be more prone to kick or bolt. Keep your hands on the patient and gently stroke it. Be careful while moving or manipulating the limbs. If the patient is to be left at the hospital, expect separation anxiety. Placing the patient's blanket or food dish or a piece of the clients' clothing in the cage or run may help reduce stress. Polydipsia and polyuria necessitate attention to the water supply and may require more frequent cleaning of the enclosure. If possible, do not leave a geriatric patient unattended overnight in the hospital.

Drug Therapy

Age-related organ and metabolic changes affect drug absorption, disposition, and excretion. These alterations should be considered to ensure efficacy and avoid toxicity during drug therapy. Absorption of orally administered drugs is affected by an increase in gastric pH, loss of intestinal absorptive surface area, prolonged intestinal transit time, and decreased blood flow to the liver and gastrointestinal tract. Absorption of parenterally administered drugs is affected by increased fat deposits and decreased vascularity.

While body fat increases, muscle and body fluid decrease in many older patients. Lipophilic drugs, such as some anesthetics, will be distributed more to body fat and less to the plasma, altering their effects and rate of elimination. Hydrophilic drugs, such as aminoglycosides, accumulate less in fat-containing tissues and more in plasma. Renal excretion of drugs may be reduced; reducing dosing frequency or reducing the drug dose can reduce the likelihood of nephrotoxicity.

Anesthesia

A geriatric patient requiring anesthesia should be thoroughly examined and have a panel of laboratory tests performed (e.g., CBC, blood chemistry panel) to obtain baseline blood values. The doses of preanesthetics and anesthetics may need to be altered and usually reduced. Drugs with profound effects on the cardiovascular system should be avoided. Of the inhalant anesthetics, isoflurane is preferred. It has minimal effects on cardiac, renal, and hepatic function, and it provides rapid induction and recovery. Chapter 19 contains detailed information on anesthetic agents available for geriatric patients. Special care must be taken when handling anesthetized geriatric patients. The patient's airway should never be compromised. The patient should be supported and handled with extreme care especially when unconscious.

Client Education

Aging affects all patients, but the effects of aging on each individual vary. You can prevent serious problems by knowing the history of the geriatric patient and scheduling regular physical examinations with appropriate laboratory tests. Veterinary technicians should educate the client on the effects of aging and the special requirements of geriatric patients. Technicians should discuss diet, body condition, grooming, dental problems, vaccinations, internal parasites, and the value of regular examinations. Solicit questions from the client during office visits or field calls, and periodically contact the client to inquire about the patient's well-being. A health care program for the geriatric patient is more apt to be implemented by clients if they are convinced of the benefits.

Euthanasia Methods

The term *euthanasia* is derived from the Greek *eu-*, meaning "good," and *thanatos-*, meaning "death." The goal is to provide the patient with a quick and painless death, while minimizing stress and anxiety. Considerations that help determine the method of euthanasia include the following:

- Safety of the individual performing the task
- Safety of the patient
- Ability of the agent to produce rapid loss of consciousness and death without pain, distress, or anxiety
- Reliability and availability of the agent
- Age and species limitations

Depending on the technique used, death is produced by hypoxia, depression of neurons vital for life's function, or disruption of brain activity.

Patients can be euthanized by inhalation or injection methods. An enclosed chamber or induction mask is used to deliver inhalant anesthetics such as isoflurane. Inhalant anesthetics can also be used to render a patient unconscious while a second method is used to cause death. Intravenous injection of an anesthetic (barbiturates) is the most rapid and reliable, and a very desirable method for performing euthanasia. Sedate anxious, wild, or aggressive patients before intravenous administration of any euthanasia agent. Once the patient is sufficiently sedated, an IV or butterfly catheter will provide a controlled means for administration of the barbiturate. In small patients (less than 7 kg), intraperitoneal injection is acceptable, provided the euthanasia agent is nonirritating. Intracardiac injection is acceptable for a patient that is heavily sedated, anesthetized, or comatose.

When it becomes necessary to euthanize a patient, induce death as quickly and painlessly as possible. Only trained and qualified individuals should perform the euthanasia. When a necropsy is to be performed immediately after euthanasia, use a method of euthanasia that causes the least amount of artifactual changes in the tissues and leaves the patient as intact as possible.

26

Nursing Care of Horses

Terry N. Teeple

Learning Objectives

After reviewing this chapter, the reader should understand the following:

- Principles of feeding, watering, exercising, and bedding of horses
- Procedures used in grooming and foot care

- Techniques used in general nursing care of horses
- Procedures used in caring for recumbent horses
- Methods of sample collection for laboratory analysis
- Routes of administration of medication
- Procedures used in intravenous catheterization of horses

GENERAL CARE OF HORSES

Feeding and Watering

Proper feeding and watering of horses is a critical component of good nursing care. In addition to providing the usual maintenance requirements, the food and water given to sick or injured patients should meet their added nutritional requirements for healing.

Hospitalized horses often have special dietary needs. Their diseases can often create a catabolic state. Horses may require extra calories to maintain their weight. Horses that can chew and swallow normally should be fed their usual diet if their disease permits. Good-quality alfalfa or grass hay, such as timothy hay, can be fed. Good-quality oat hay is also a suitable feed. Horses with gastrointestinal disturbances, such as colic or diarrhea, need special consideration. Horses recovering from impactions may need more laxative feeds, such as alfalfa hay, grass pasture, and even bran mashes. Horses with diarrhea or ones that have had an operation because of colic may benefit from a diet that is not quite so rich, such as timothy or oat hay. Hay pellets or cubes that contain alfalfa or a mixture of alfalfa and Bermuda or oat hay can also be used. If added carbohydrate is needed, a pelleted feed that also contains grains may be fed.

Pelleted feed produces less dust and may be better for horses with heaves or for those suffering from respiratory allergies or pneumonia. Horses recovering from gastrointestinal ulceration may also need to be fed a pelleted ration, because the increased fiber and stem in hay may irritate and exacerbate certain kinds of ulcers. Pellets soaked to make gruel can be fed to horses with oral lesions, facial fractures, dental problems, or recurrent episodes of choke. Feed softened in this manner is easier for the horse to chew and swallow. Horses with neuromuscular disorders, such as botulism, may be unable to chew and swallow normally. For these patients, a pelleted ration that has been soaked in water may be the only type of feed they can eat.

Fresh, clean water should be available at all times. Many horses will require 10 to 15 gallons of water daily. Therefore, providing a continuous supply of water becomes critical in meeting this requirement. Some horses can learn to use an automatic watering cup that refills as it drinks, however, water buckets or tubs are usually used. When supplying water to buckets or tubs, the water level should be checked at least twice per day to ensure a continuous supply is available.

Bedding

Horses can be bedded on a variety of materials. It is important that the bedding be clean, as dust-free as possible, and relatively deep. Another important consideration when choosing bedding is its usefulness as a fertilizer after composting. Pine shavings are adequate for most patients, but they tend to be very dusty. This may not be acceptable for horses with open wounds or respiratory disorders. Pine shavings with minimal dust or shredded paper bedding is preferable for horses with severe respiratory problems. It is best to obtain wood shavings from a known source to prevent accidental exposure to black walnut shavings, which can cause laminitis when the horse stands in the shavings. Black walnut wood is darker than pine but can be difficult to recognize if the bedding is soiled or if multiple types of wood chips have been mixed. Straw bedding is often used for mares with newborn foals. Bedding should always be deep unless the horse has a problem that necessitates a firmer surface for standing. Regardless of the type of bedding used, it should be kept very clean by removing soiled bedding at least once daily. The use of rubber stall mats reduces the amount of bedding that has to be used.

Recumbent adult horses must have very deep bedding to help prevent formation of decubital ulcers (pressure sores). Alternatively, large mattresses or specially designed waterbeds may be used. Critically ill foals can be kept on mattresses with waterproof covers and fleece pads to keep them clean and dry. It may be necessary to clean the stall or change the bedding each time the horse or foal urinates or defecates if the patient is recumbent. Strategically placed diapers or absorbent mats may help reduce the number of bedding changes needed with a recumbent foal.

Fly Control

The best method of fly control is to maintain a clean barn with frequent manure removal. Various topical fly sprays are available. Those containing permethrins, pyrethrins, or citronella are safest for sick horses. Fly repellents containing organophosphates should not be applied to debilitated horses or foals. Overhead fly systems that release fly repellents at regular intervals can also minimize the fly population. A soft cloth can be used to apply fly repellent to the horse's face, taking care to apply the repellent around the eyes without getting any into the eyes. Fly masks are available for the face and the ears of sensitive patients. A fly sheet can also be used to cover most of the body, except the distal parts of the legs.

Exercise

Adult horses and foals should have some form of exercise daily unless their medical problem requires stall rest. Walking on soft dirt or grass surfaces is preferable to walking on concrete or asphalt. Foals may be allowed to run freely alongside the mare if they do not have a condition that warrants more restricted activity, and if the area is properly fenced with no hazards, such as drains or moving vehicles. If the foal's activity must be controlled, the foal can be walked using a halter and a rope around its hindquarters in the area of the semimembranosus and semitendinosus muscles. Good judgment and caution are needed to prevent the foal from rearing and flipping over

backward. To walk a neonate whose exercise should be limited, place one arm in front of its chest and one arm behind the foal to cradle it while walking. Alternatively, an adult horse halter can be used over the foal's body like a harness, with the nose piece around the foal's neck, the buckle strapped around the ventral thorax, and the rope clip located on the caudodorsal portion of the foal's back. The hind end of the foal may still need to be supported.

Grooming

Equine patients should be groomed daily, unless the horse has a condition whereby vigorous grooming would be painful or damaging (e.g., severe skin infections, cutaneous burns). A rubber currycomb should be used in a circular motion to remove dried sweat or mud. Next, use a stiff-bristled brush to remove dirt and loose hair. If stiff brushes and rubber currycombs are used on the horse's face and distal limbs, use them gently; overly vigorous grooming may be uncomfortable for the horse. Metal currycombs should not be used on the horse's head or distal limbs. Use a soft brush to finish removing loose hair and dirt. If needed, use a damp or dry cloth to remove the remaining dust from the horse's coat. Use a stiff brush, hairbrush, or metal mane comb on the tail and mane.

Hoof Picking

A horse's hooves should be picked clean daily. Most adult horses raise the foot when a hand is run down the caudal aspect of the distal limb and gentle pressure is exerted over the caudal aspect of the limb at the level of the distal splint bones. The hoof is then cleaned with a hoof pick by removing debris from the lateral and central sulci, starting at the heel and working toward the toe, and then from the rest of the hoof (Fig. 26-1). A degenerative condition called *thrush* is common in feet that are infrequently cleaned, or if the horse stands for long periods in damp bedding or muddy soil. Thrush may occur secondary to a bacterial infection and appears as black, malodorous material in the region of the frog. A 10% Na hypochlorite (bleach) solution or 2% iodine solution can be applied to the lateral and central sulci to dry the foot and kill the bacteria. Commercial formulations containing formaldehyde or copper sulfate can also be used. Take care to avoid spilling caustic solutions on the coronary band or other parts of the horse's leg. The technician should wear gloves to protect herself/himself from the solutions. Some patients with severe thrush require foot trimming to remove diseased hoof tissue and wraps to help keep the foot clean and dry during the length of the treatment program.

MONITORING PATIENTS

Hospitalized patients must be monitored regularly for changes in their condition. Horses that are slightly ill can

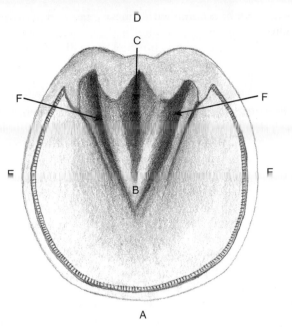

Fig. 26-1 Ventral view of the equine hoof. **A,** Toe. **B,** Frog. **C,** Central sulcus or cleft of the frog. **D,** Heel. **E,** The quarters. **F,** Lateral sulci.

develop more severe and even life-threatening illness while receiving treatment. For instance, a horse receiving antibiotic therapy for a mild respiratory infection can develop life-threatening diarrhea from changes in bowel microflora. A horse receiving nonsteroidal antiinflammatory drugs for an orthopedic problem can develop gastrointestinal ulceration or renal dysfunction secondary to the antiinflammatory medication, particularly if the patient is not eating and drinking normally.

The heart rate, respiratory rate, rectal temperature, mucous membrane color, capillary refill time, attitude, digital pulses, urine and fecal output, gastrointestinal motility, and appetite should all be monitored at least once or twice daily. Critically ill neonates require more frequent monitoring, sometimes as often as every 2 hours, as their condition can deteriorate rapidly. Adult horses should be weighed at admission with a walk-on scale, if available, or a weight tape can be used to estimate the horse's weight. Neonates should be weighed at admission and then daily. Most newborn foals can be weighed by picking them up and weighing the handler and foal together on a conventional scale and then subtracting the handler's weight. This may not be feasible with larger foals.

CARE OF RECUMBENT HORSES

Nursing care for recumbent patients must be meticulous. Caring for a horse that is unable to rise is tedious and often unrewarding. Horses that remain recumbent for prolonged periods eventually develop various complications, regardless of the primary disease. Because of the weight of the horse, several people are needed to frequently turn it from one side to the other. This is usually done with long ropes *looped,* not tied, around the pasterns so that the handlers can stand farther from the limbs of the horse, or by using a winch and harness, when available. If the size of the horse permits, flex the horse's legs up next to its body than to roll its torso over the flexed legs. It is preferable to rolling the horse over on its back, which this may cause a twisted intestine. When a horse is turned from one side to another, it often kicks, which can be very dangerous for anyone standing in the vicinity. No one should stand within striking range of the limbs of a recumbent horse. The patient must be turned as frequently as possible to prevent development of decubital ulcers on the skin and edema and congestion in the dependent portion of the lung. Helmets can be applied to horses that tend to flail about and hit their heads against the wall or ground. The technician should also pay particular attention to the eyes of a recumbent patient since the corneas can become ulcerated if the patient rubs its eyes on the ground.

The primary disease should be resolved as quickly as possible so that the patient may once again stand. If the horse can stand only with assistance, the hind limbs can be supported by suspending a rope attached to the tail from a ceiling beam. The head may also need to be supported. Commercial slings are available that provide support for horses that have some ability to support themselves but require additional help. A sling cannot be used for horses with flaccid paralysis or other conditions that make them unable to support themselves at all, because they can only slump down in the sling. Slings must be well-padded to prevent development of pressure sores.

Regardless of how meticulous the nursing care, decubital ulcers may develop over bony prominences, such as the tuber coxae, carpus, hock, shoulder joint, or elbow. These must be cleaned with a mild antibacterial soap. Topical antibacterial powders or sprays can also be used. A spray that creates a "breathable" bandage may provide the best protection. Any bony protuberance that can be protected by wraps should be wrapped. It is important to keep the patient clean and dry. Frequent cleaning can help to prevent urine scalding and reduce the severity of decubital ulcers. Additional bedding may also help minimize the formation of decubital sores.

The recumbent patient may not eat or drink well. Soft, highly palatable feeds should be offered. If mashes are offered but not eaten, they must be replaced frequently to ensure palatability. Fresh, clean water should be offered to the recumbent patient every 2 hours, if possible. It may be necessary to give a recumbent patient food and water by nasogastric tube to prevent aspiration of feed or water into the lungs. If possible, it is preferable to feed the horse while it is in a more sternal position. Infusion of IV fluids may be required in more debilitated or dehydrated patients.

Bandaging

Materials needed to bandage the distal limbs include cotton quilts or sheet cottons (three), and track wraps, brown roll gauze, or a type of conforming bandage material. Leg wraps can be used to protect a wound, to give additional support, or to cover a medicated area. The wrap should be applied with even pressure so that the tendons running along the caudal aspect of the leg (superficial and deep digital flexor tendons) are protected and pressure is evenly applied over the entire length of the tendons.

To start, wrap a quilt or some other thick padding around the leg. Sheet cotton can be used; at least three sheets are needed for sufficient padding. Start the wrap at the front portion of the leg. Then bring the quilt across the outside of the leg, around the back, and then inside the leg, maintaining even tension at all times (Fig. 26-2, *A* and *B*). Once the quilt is in place, use a track wrap brown gauze roll or other type of outer wrap. The same principle is followed, with the wrap being placed from lateral toward medial across the back of the leg. It is best to start this part of the wrap near the bottom of the leg (distally) and work up (proximally) (Fig. 26-2, *C*, *D*, and *E*).

Secure the outer wrap with Velcro attachments, ties, or adhesive tape. If adhesive tape is used, the ends should not overlap, because the tape is relatively inelastic and may produce uneven pressure across the tendons. If roll gauze is used, it can be secured with adhesive tape; alternatively, an additional layer can be applied using a conforming bandage wrap. When the wrap is finished, a small strip of padding should be visible in the innermost layer of the wrap both proximally and distally. Care must be taken to ensure that the wrap is snug but not too tight. Two fingers should be able to fit snugly between the leg and the wrap, but the wrap should feel firm and should not slip down the leg. If the wrap is applied to protect a wound, antibacterial ointment and a nonstick dressing must first be applied to the area and held in place with a layer of stretch gauze.

If the full length of the leg must be wrapped, an additional wrap can be applied so that it overlaps the lower limb wrap to some extent. This additional wrap is applied in a similar manner. The proximal wrap should overlap the distal wrap and extend to the mid-radius area. Often, a piece of the wrap is cut out over the accessory carpal bone to prevent development of pressure sores over this bone. This is more difficult to do on the hind leg, because special consideration must be given to the highly movable hock joint. Often the conforming bandage material is applied in a figure-8 fashion around the hock so that only the sheet cotton contacts the point of the hock.

Foot Wraps

There are many ways to wrap feet. First, pick the foot clean. Then wash and dry, if necessary. If medication is required, apply it and cover the foot with a gauze sponge secured with a layer of rolled gauze (Fig. 26-3, *A*, *B*, and *C*). If padding is

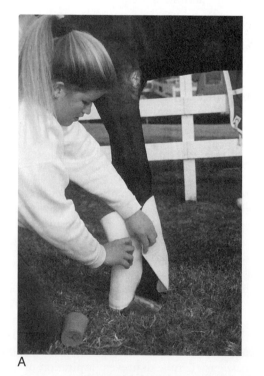

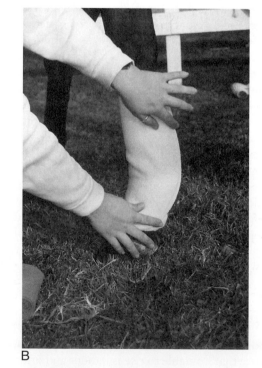

A   B

Fig. 26-2 A through **E,** Application of a wrap to the distal limb of a standing horse.

needed for protection, wrap roll cotton or two to three sheets of cotton around the foot (Fig. 26-3, *D* and *E*). Next, secure the sheet cotton with rolled brown gauze or stretch gauze. Apply it in figure-8 fashion to make the sheet cottons lie flat across the bottom of the foot (Fig. 26-3, *F, G,* and *H*). Finally, apply elastic tape or duct tape to provide

additional support and protection, and to secure the bandage in place (Fig. 26-3, *I* and *J*). It is very important to have the ground surface of the foot wrap flat, rather than convex and bulging, so that even pressure is applied to the bottom of the foot. If no padding is needed and the foot wrap is being used to apply medication to an area of the foot, the

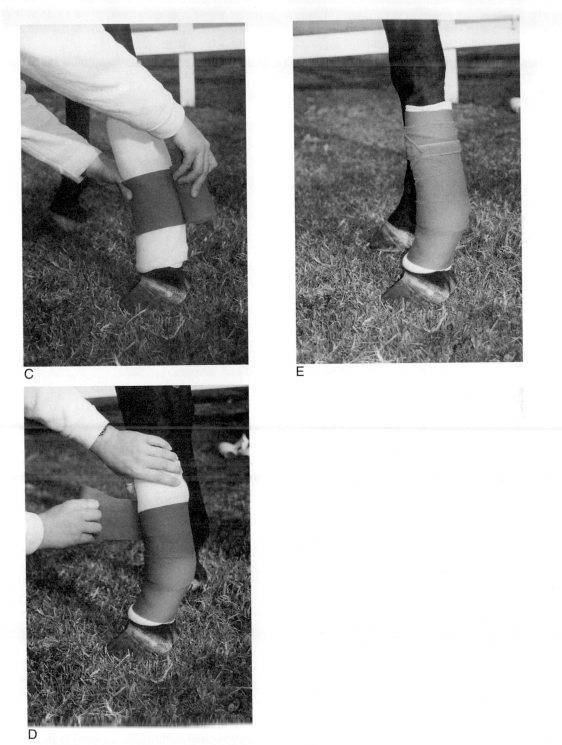

C

E

D

Fig. 26-2 Cont'd

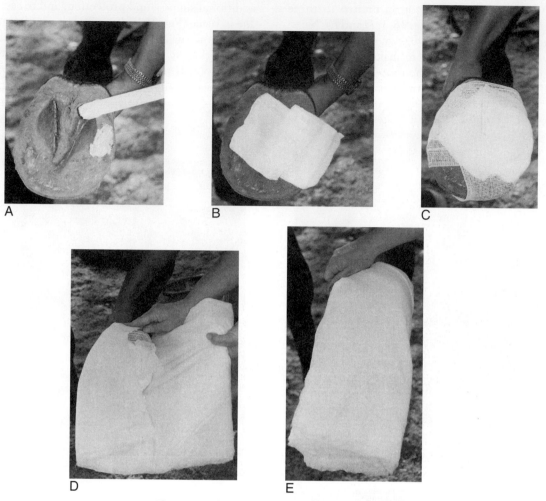

Fig. 26-3 A through **J,** Application of a foot wrap.

duct tape or a conforming bandage material can be applied directly to the foot after a nonstick dressing or gauze sponge is placed over the medication.

Be careful not to wrap up over the coronary band if no protective padding is in place, because excessive pressure directly on the coronary band can reduce circulation to hoof tissues and cause damage or sloughing of the hoof. If there is any question about the amount of pressure on the coronary band, one or more vertical slits can be cut in the bandage where it covers the coronary band to relieve pressure.

Tail Bandages

Tail wraps can consist of stall bandages, rolled brown gauze, or even commercial tail bags. If the tail wrap is to be left on the horse for many days, it is important to ensure that the wrap does not extend proximally to include the tail bones (coccygeal vertebrae). This is because the tail has little muscular padding, and a tight wrap can occlude blood circulation to the tail and create a tissue slough or loss of the entire tail. If it is necessary to wrap more proximally on the tail, loosely apply a nonconstricting wrap and change it daily.

At times, it is necessary to wrap the tail of a horse with severe diarrhea to keep the tail clean. This can be done using a plastic rectal sleeve. Holes can be cut in the sleeve to help keep the tail from "sweating." First braid the tail hair. Then tie the sleeve at the most proximal part of the braid, or anchor the sleeve to the most proximal part of the tail with a strip of adhesive tape or duct tape placed lengthwise from the sleeve cranially along the midline of the back.

The tail may also need to be wrapped when a mare is about to foal or for a reproductive examination. Apply rolled brown gauze, starting at the tail head (proximal area) and working distally, being sure to incorporate all of the tail hairs within the wrap. When the wrap reaches just distal to the last tail bone, the remaining tail hairs can be folded and incorporated within this section of the wrap. The brown gauze is then tied to itself to end and secure the wrap.

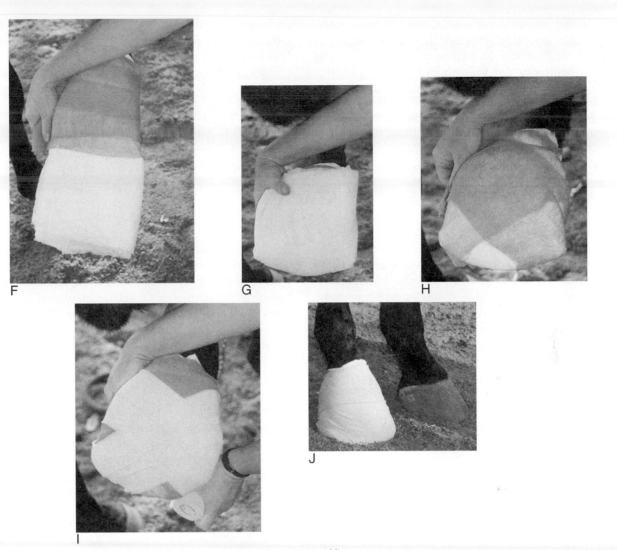

Fig. 26-3 Cont'd

Abdominal Bandages

It may be necessary to wrap a horse's abdomen to protect a wound or an abdominal incision following colic surgery. Place a sterile nonstick pad over the wound. Next, place a dressing made from large folded sheet cotton against the sterile dressing. Wrap a conforming bandage material around the abdomen and over the back to hold the bandage in place. It may be necessary to use four to six rolls of this material when applying a full abdominal bandage.

Padding in the form of leg rolls or quilts should be used across the horse's back to protect the skin if the backbone is prominent. Because pressure is applied with the wrap, skin necrosis can occur in this area if there is little muscle or fat across the back. The same application principles are used as for leg wraps. The material is applied evenly, starting at the cranial part of the abdomen and working caudad. It is applied snugly to provide support, but not too tight. Each layer of the material should overlap the last pass until the wrap is completed. This type of wrap is very expensive and usually does not need changing unless there is excessive drainage, or if the wound or incision must be evaluated. Thoracic wraps can be applied in a similar manner to cover a thoracic wound or protect a thoracic drain. Chapter 22 contains detailed information on wound management and bandaging.

COLLECTING BLOOD SAMPLES

To obtain a blood sample from a horse, properly restrain the patient. The jugular vein is most commonly used to obtain blood samples and lies directly under the skin in the jugular furrow. The vein should be entered at the most cranial one third of the neck, where the vein is more superficial and somewhat better separated from the carotid artery. The jugular vein and carotid artery exit the thoracic inlet closely together but become more separated as the vessels course cranially toward the head.

The vein is distended by occluding it with a thumb placed proximal (ventral) to the venipuncture site. Once the vein fills, a 20-gauge or larger needle, attached to a syringe, is quickly and smoothly inserted. The entire length of the needle's shaft should be well-seated in the vein. The syringe is then aspirated to withdraw the sample (Fig. 26-4). Alternatively, use a double-ended blood-collection needle. Insert the unsheathed longer portion into the vein, and attach the collection vials to the shorter, sheathed end. The vacuum within the collection vials allows the blood to flow freely into the vial. For either method, the needle is removed after pressure on the vein has been released. Releasing the pressure prior to removing the needle reduces the chance of developing a hematoma.

In a seriously ill horse, the jugular veins may need to be preserved to allow continued venous access for delivery of medications and fluids. In this case, another site should be used for routine blood collection. A venous sinus ventral to the facial crest can be used for obtaining blood samples. It should be entered just caudal to its midpoint between the medial canthus of the eye and the rostral end of the facial crest, just ventral to the facial crest. Only experienced technicians or veterinarians should attempt this because of the proximity to the horse's eye. Care must be taken to avoid inadvertently puncturing the eyeball if the horse turns its head suddenly.

ADMINISTRATION OF MEDICATION

Oral Administration

Medications that are in liquid form and required in only small doses may be administered with a dose syringe or a

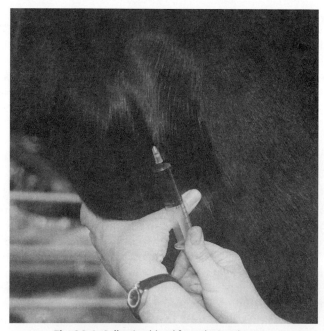

Fig. 26-4 Collecting blood from the jugular vein.

syringe with the locking tip removed. Place the syringe through the side of the mouth in the area of the diastema, or interdental space (space between the incisors and premolars). Deposit the medication on the caudal portion of the tongue, if possible. Medications in pill form can be crushed with a mortar and pestle and then mixed with something sweet, such as molasses, and given in a similar manner. It is best not to mix medication with the feed, because horses often eat around the medication and do not consume the full dose. Medication that must be given in large volumes requires use of a nasogastric tube for delivery into the stomach.

Nasogastric Intubation

A horse that cannot chew or swallow normally, but with a functional gastrointestinal tract, can be fed and hydrated through a *nasogastric tube*. Nasogastric intubation should be done in the presence of a veterinarian until the technician has become proficient in the technique. Feeding through a nasogastric tube requires a larger-bore stomach tube than does water administration. Before the procedure, determine the length of tube necessary to reach the stomach. First, lubricate the tube with a water-soluble lubricating jelly (K-Y Jelly) or even plain water. Then, insert the tube into the nostril with one hand. Use the other hand to guide the tube through the most ventral portion of the nasal passage, the ventral meatus. Care must be taken to ensure that the tube is directed caudoventrally, because it will not easily pass into the pharynx if it is inserted into the middle or dorsal meatus. Never force the tube if it will not pass easily. If the tube strikes the ethmoturbinates as it is being passed through the ventral meatus to the pharynx, the nasal membranes may bleed profusely. This may happen if the horse moves at the wrong moment, or if the technician or veterinarian is not careful.

After you insert the tube to the level of the pharynx, lower the horse's head and flex the neck slightly to facilitate entrance of the tube into the esophagus and not the trachea. Pass the tube into the esophagus as the horse swallows. If the horse will not swallow, gently move the tube back and forth to stimulate swallowing. If the tube passes into the trachea by mistake, the horse may cough and resist. However, sedated or severely debilitated horses may not resist or cough if the tube is erroneously placed into the trachea. If the trachea is grasped in one hand and moved back and forth, the tube can be felt rattling within the cartilaginous structure. The tube will not rattle if it is in the esophagus, because this is a collapsible structure composed of striated and smooth muscle. If the tube is in the esophagus, it can often be seen on the left side of the neck near the jugular furrow as it is being passed. If the tube cannot be seen, it can be palpated as it passes through the esophagus. The tube may be difficult to pass if the horse has an esophageal obstruction. Care should be used, because the esophagus may be ruptured by overaggressive nasogastric intubation. The tube should be passed caudad, all the way into the stomach, but never forced.

Once the tube enters the stomach, the typical sweet and slightly fetid odor of the stomach contents may be discernible through the tube. No material should be pumped through the stomach tube unless you are absolutely certain that the tube is in the stomach and not in the trachea. Horses cannot vomit, so always check for excessive gastric contents (gastric reflux) before administering fluid, feed, or medication. Create a siphon effect to check for gastric reflux by injecting a small amount of water into the tube with a stomach pump or dose syringes and disconnecting the pump or syringe to see if fluid or ingesta flows freely back out of the tube. If excessive fluid or ingesta is present, it may be necessary to medicate the horse at a later time, when no reflux is present. Overfilling the stomach can result in gastric rupture and death. The adult horse's stomach can hold 8 to 15 liters, but this varies between horses.

Administer medication or fluid by gravity flow through a funnel, when possible, to prevent overfilling of the stomach. If a stomach pump must be used to administer water or mineral oil, disconnect it periodically to check for increased pressure and backflow of fluid out of the stomach tube. Before the nasogastric tube is withdrawn, remove all of the fluid from the tube. This can be done by pumping or blowing a small amount of air through the tube while it is still in the stomach and then kinking the end of the tube or placing a finger over the end while it is being removed. This prevents the horse from aspirating fluid into the lungs as the tube is being removed.

Administer water through the nasogastric tube to rehydrate a horse. If IV administration of fluids is not possible or practical, the stomach tube can be taped where it exits the nostril and then taped to the horse's halter. Then wrap the tube around and tape it in one additional site on the halter to minimize movement. A syringe or cork can be placed in the end of the tube to prevent air from filling the stomach. Water can be given every 2 hours or as needed in this manner. Horses must not be allowed to eat or drink with a large-bore stomach tube in place, because they cannot adequately protect their airway when they swallow.

Parenteral Injections

Drugs and other liquids can be injected into a muscle (IM) or vein (IV), under the skin (SQ), or into a layer of the skin (ID). Some medications can be given by multiple routes, either IV or IM. It is very important to know which routes of administration are acceptable for each drug administered, because injection by an inappropriate route can have harmful or even lethal effects on a horse. For example, procaine penicillin should be given only IM. If this medication is given IV, the procaine component may cause excitation, seizures, and death. Some medications, such as phenylbuta-

zone, should be administered intravenously only. These medications can be very caustic and cause tissue sloughing if administered outside the vein (perivascular) or in the muscle.

Intradermal injections

Rarely an injection must be given into the upper layers of the skin. Some forms of allergy testing use intradermal injections of allergens. A very small amount of test material, usually 0.1 to 1 ml, is injected using a 25-gauge, ⅝-inch needle. Clean the skin with alcohol if necessary, and insert the needle into the skin (not underneath it). Withdraw the plunger slightly to ensure that a blood vessel has not been entered. If no blood is aspirated, the medication is injected. Because the medication is being injected into the skin, a small bleb, called a *wheal*, becomes visible in the skin.

Subcutaneous injections

Occasionally medications are injected SQ. These medications are usually given in smaller doses, such as for allergy desensitization. A 20- or 21-gauge, 1-inch needle should be used. Any area where the skin can easily be lifted from the underlying muscle and fascia may be used; the lateral aspect of the neck where IM injections are also given is a suitable site. First clean the skin with alcohol if necessary, and then pull it laterally to form a "tent." Then insert the needle under the skin. Always aspirate to ensure that no blood enters the syringe; then inject.

Intramuscular injections

Various sites can be used for IM injections. The safest muscle for technicians to use is in the neck area. The neck muscles of the horse can be used only for administering small volumes of medication. The area to be used is a triangular portion on the side of the neck formed by the ligamentum nuchae dorsally, the spine ventrally, and the scapula caudad (Fig. 26-5). Another common area for IM injection is in the semitendinosus and semimembranosus muscles of the hind leg. (This is the preferred site for IM injections in neonates.) However, this is a very vulnerable position for the technician; horses that are known to kick should not be injected at this site. If this site becomes infected and an abscess forms, this is the easiest area to establish adequate drainage to allow for healing. An alternative site is in the gluteal (hip) muscles. This allows the person giving the injection to stand in a somewhat safer position, but if the horse develops an abscess subsequent to a gluteal injection, it can be very difficult to establish adequate drainage. There should always be a handler available to restrain the horse's head when administering IM injections.

A 16- or 18-gauge, 1.5-inch needle should be used for IM injections in adults. A 20-gauge, 1-inch needle should be used for small equines and neonates. The site is cleaned with alcohol if necessary, and the needle, without an

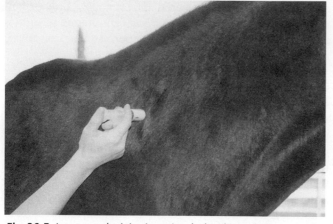

Fig. 26-5 Intramuscular injection using the brachiocephalicus muscle.

attached syringe, is inserted with a quick jab. Some people prefer to tap on the area to be injected a few times with their fist before injecting in an attempt to desensitize the area. When injecting the neck muscles, a fold of skin can be grasped and pulled slightly away from the neck to act as a skin twitch and distract the horse before inserting the needle. Always disconnect the needle from the syringe before inserting it so that if the horse kicks or jumps, the needle will remain in place and not be pulled out by the weight of the syringe. Then the syringe is attached and the plunger is aspirated to ensure that a blood vessel has not been entered. If no blood is visible in the syringe, the medication can be injected safely. The needle and syringe are then removed. No more than 20 ml of solution should be given to mature horses in one IM site.

Intravenous Injections

When administering medication IV, the blood dilutes the medication causing it to become less caustic. The jugular vein is the only appropriate vein for IV injections in horses. The jugular vein runs caudad along the jugular furrow from the head and then enters the thoracic inlet on its way to the heart. The carotid artery runs deep to the jugular vein in the same vicinity, but it courses deeper into the neck and is separated from the jugular vein in the more cranial portion of the neck. This is a very important point to remember. It is safer to attempt venipuncture and IV administration of medications in the cranial one third of the neck, because you are less likely to inadvertently enter the carotid artery when aiming for the jugular vein. If a large-bore needle (18-gauge) is used and the syringe is removed before venipuncture, it should be apparent which blood vessel has been entered. Blood drips out of the hub of an 18-gauge needle if it has been placed in the jugular vein but spurts out of the needle if it is within the high-pressure carotid artery. Smaller-bore needles (20-gauge or smaller) are suitable for obtaining blood samples; however, they do not allow differentiation between arterial

or venous puncture, because in both cases blood drips from the needle. Medications inadvertently injected into the carotid artery pass directly to the brain and can cause severe seizures, collapse, and even death.

When drugs are administered IV, the needle is inserted in the direction of the flow of blood in the jugular vein (pointed caudad, Fig. 26-6, *A*). Some people prefer to insert the needle pointed cranially. Regardless of which direction the needle is placed, it should be well seated into the vein so that there is little chance for perivascular or intraarterial injection. Distend the vein by occluding it with the thumb of one hand; then insert the needle into the vein with the other hand. Blood should drip from the hub of the needle while the vein remains occluded (Fig. 26-6, *B*). Then, attach the syringe to the needle and gently withdraw the plunger to produce a backflow of blood, which confirms that the needle is still in the vein. Then inject the medication slowly.

Medication should *not* be quickly injected as a bolus, because this may cause an adverse reaction. If the medication

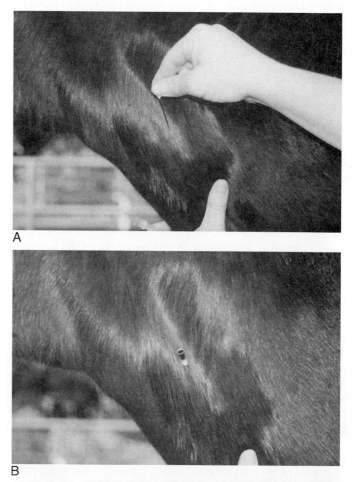

Fig. 26-6 A, Needle insertion for intravenous administration of medication. **B,** Blood should drip, not spurt, from the needle hub when the jugular vein is occluded before an intravenous injection.

is given slowly, administration can be halted if a reaction occurs. Even with good technique, movement of the horse during injection can drive the needle through the jugular vein and into the carotid artery. If the horse moves after connection of the syringe to the needle, the syringe should once again be removed from the needle to check the needle's position. If all is well, the injection can be continued. Remember that it is not reliable to try to distinguish arterial blood from venous blood by color when withdrawn into a syringe filled with a drug. If multiple IV injections are required daily or if large volumes of fluid must be administered, placement of an indwelling catheter is advisable.

Adverse Reactions

Adverse reactions may occur to medications given by any route. In general, however, these reactions occur more rapidly with intravascular injections. Reactions can range from mild sweating, urticaria, and colic, to respiratory distress, collapse, and death. With any reaction, administration of medication should be stopped immediately and, if time allows, the veterinarian should be contacted. Epinephrine 1:1000 given SQ or IM at 3 to 5 ml/ 450 kg of body weight, as well as dexamethasone given IV at 0.02 to 2 mg/kg, may be needed to stop an anaphylactic reaction and save the horse's life. It is always wise to know the appropriate dosage for these drugs and to have them within reach when medication is to be given. The horse's medical record should always be tagged to indicate medications to which the patient has previously reacted.

Intravenous Catheterization

Box 26-1 and Figs. 26-7, 26-8, and 26-9 detail the procedure for intravenous catheterization.

Sites

In adult horses, the jugular vein is preferred for catheter placement. Alternative sites include the lateral thoracic vein, cephalic vein, and, in extreme cases when there are no remaining accessible veins, the saphenous vein. Catheterizing veins in the hind legs of adult horses can be very dangerous and should only be attempted by experienced technicians or veterinarians. The principles of venous catheterization are similar, regardless of the site.

The lateral thoracic vein lies in the ventral one quarter of the thorax on either side. It is visible coursing along the side of the thorax and runs cranially toward the axilla. This vein can be catheterized from its mid to caudal section. The catheter is directed cranially so that it runs with the flow of the blood. It can be secured by suturing in the same manner as for a jugular catheter. The cephalic vein is entered proximal to the carpus and the catheter directed proximally. The saphenous vein is entered proximal to the hock and also directed proximally. It is advisable to wrap the catheter with sterile gauze sponges and an elastic bandage when

using one of these alternative sites for catheterization. If long-term catheterization is anticipated, it is best to use polyurethane or silastic catheters.

Catheter Care

If the insertion site has not been bandaged, clean it gently with povidone-iodine solution. Then apply an antibacterial ointment over the site at least once daily or more often if necessary. Catheters that have been bandaged should have the dressing changed as needed. Foals that spend much time lying down should always have the catheter site bandaged. Bandages covering cephalic catheters usually do not need changing until it is time for the catheter to be removed. Bandages over jugular vein catheters frequently need changing, because the wrap becomes loose and allows bedding material to accumulate under it.

Stent bandages can be used instead of elastic bandages to protect the catheter site (Fig. 26-10). Four sutures are placed around the insertion site to form a rectangle that is smaller than the size of a gauze roll. These sutures are placed loosely so that a loop remains, through which a piece of umbilical tape can be placed. The umbilical tape is threaded through the sutures and then tied to keep a gauze roll in place over the catheter at its insertion site. The insertion site can be cleaned daily and a new gauze roll placed over the insertion site.

Teflon catheters can be left in the vein for 3 to 5 days if the insertion site is kept clean and there is no sign of swelling or thrombophlebitis. Silastic or polyurethane catheters can be left in the vein for up to 2 weeks if adequate care is used in preserving the catheter. This type of catheter is much less thrombogenic than the Teflon type and causes less irritation to the vein. The injection plug and IV tubing should be changed every 24 hours because bacteria may proliferate within the lines. The injection plug should be cleaned with an alcohol swab before administration of medication or fluids through the port. Sterile technique must always be used when handling IV catheters or giving IV infusions because thrombophlebitis can result from bacterial contamination.

Catheter Complications

Teflon catheters can kink, obstructing the flow of IV solutions. The smaller-gauge catheters used in foals (18-gauge) have been known to break off if the catheter is placed where there is much mobility, such as the jugular vein. The catheter first bends and then develops a crease. As the foal continues to move its head, the catheter may become weaker at the kinked site and can eventually break. For this reason, the cephalic vein may be a better site for IV catheter placement in newborn foals.

Catheter sites should be checked frequently to avoid major complications. Local reactions at the insertion site can occur at any time. The swelling may not involve the

BOX 26-1

procedure

Intravenous Catheterization

Materials (Fig. 26-7)

- Gauze sponges, povidone-iodine scrub, povidone-iodine solution, alcohol, water, razor, 2% lidocaine
- For adults, 14- to 16-gauge, 140-mm Teflon catheter or 150-mm polyurethane catheter for the jugular vein
- 2-0 or 0 nonabsorbable suture, such as polypropylene
- Injection plug
- Sterile latex gloves
- Heparinized saline (2500 units in 250 ml saline for adults; 1000 units in 250 ml saline for neonates)
- T-port (optional)
- For foals, elastic tape, sterile gauze sponges and antibacterial ointment. For adults, similar to foal or stent bandage using stretch gauze roll bandage and umbilical tape.

Procedure

1. Shave and aseptically prepare the site to be catheterized.
2. Inject 1 to 5 ml of lidocaine subcutaneously to block the skin.
3. Wearing sterile gloves, take the catheter from the package and place the end of the stylet at the appropriate site. Always insert the catheter with the direction of blood flow.
4. With a sharp and quick jab, insert the catheter through the skin and into the vein. Hold the catheter at about a 45-degree angle to the skin until the vein is penetrated (Fig. 26-8, *A*). Blood should flow freely into the hub if the vein is occluded (jugular), or should flow freely without holding the vein off for other sites. If the horse is severely dehydrated or hypovolemic, backflow of blood may not occur. For the compromised patient, it may be helpful to have the catheter filled with heparinized saline so that once the vein is penetrated, the heparinized saline starts to flow retrograde out the hub of the catheter.
5. After the vein has been entered, orient the catheter and stylet parallel to the vein and advance the catheter ½ inch for adults and ¼ inch for foals. This ensures that both the catheter and stylet are within the lumen of the vein.
6. Hold the stylet in place, and slide the catheter down the stylet and into the vein (Fig. 26-8, *B*). This should be a smooth action; the catheter should easily slide down the stylet; it should not feel like it is sticking. Never advance the stylet into the catheter or pull the catheter onto the stylet once the catheter has been advanced, because this could sever the tip of the catheter off within the vein. If the catheter is not correctly placed with the lumen of the vein, simply remove the entire unit and try again. Always check the tip of the catheter to ensure that it has not been damaged in the

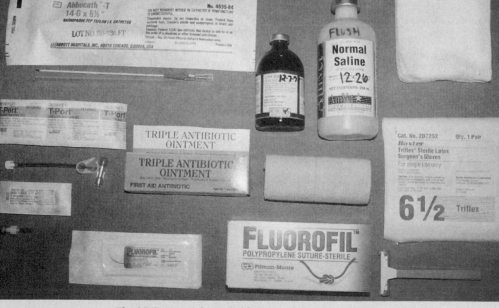

Fig. 26-7 Materials needed for intravenous catheterization.

BOX 26-1

procedure

Intravenous Catheterization—cont'd

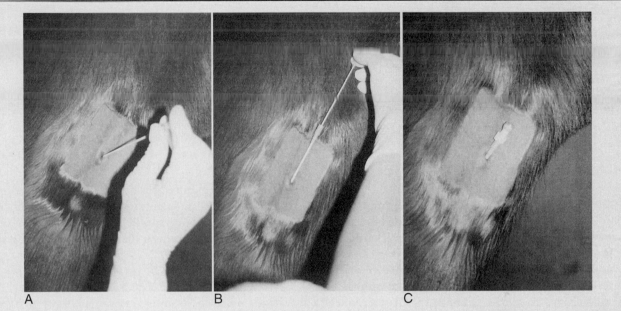

Fig. 26-8 A, Catheterization of the jugular vein. The catheter is placed at about a 45-degree angle to the vein, and the vein is entered with a sharp, quick jab. **B,** Once the vein has been entered, the catheter is oriented parallel to the vein and advanced about ½ inch to ensure that the catheter and stylet are within the lumen. The catheter is then advanced while the stylet is held stationary. **C,** The stylet is removed once the catheter is in place, and an injection plug is used to cap the catheter.

attempt, because this could damage the vein. A new catheter should be used if there is any chance that the original catheter was damaged or contaminated during the procedure.

7. Once the catheter is in place, remove the stylet and place a T-port with injection plug or just an injection plug over the end of the catheter (Fig. 26-8, *C*).

8. The catheter should be sutured in place using the grooves in the hub to mark the site for the first suture, then around the narrow portion of the injection plug or T-port. If a T-port is used, another suture should be placed over the *T* to secure it. In adults, it may be advantageous to also suture the arm of the T-port loosely to add stability without creating tension at the catheter insertion site (Fig. 26-9). The arm of the T-port should slide easily through the loose loop of suture as the horse changes its neck position.

9. Flush the catheter with 3 ml of heparinized saline.

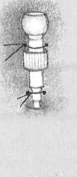

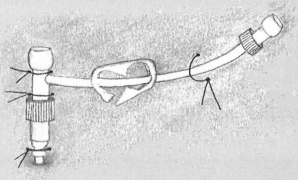

Fig. 26-9 Suture placement for the catheter, showing an injection plug *(top)* and T-port *(bottom)*.

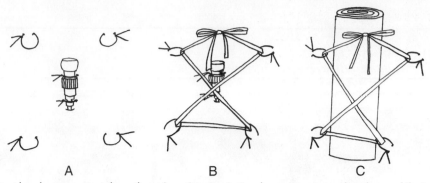

Fig. 26-10 Placement of a stent bandage to protect the catheter insertion site. **A,** Four loose sutures are placed around the insertion site. **B,** Umbilical tape is threaded through the sutures in cruciform pattern. **C,** A roll of gauze is placed over the catheter and held in place by umbilical tape.

vein but only the skin and subcutaneous tissues. This type of swelling may resolve with careful, gentle cleaning of the insertion site. If the swelling persists or progresses, the catheter should be removed and a new catheter inserted at a different site.

Thrombosis can develop secondary to irritation of the vessel walls, with subsequent release of thrombogenic factors that initiate the clotting cascade and platelet adherence. This occurs more frequently with severely compromised patients that may already be prone to coagulation disorders. Horses with endotoxemia, any type of gastrointestinal disorder, or gram-negative infections are at highest risk. A thrombosed vein appears corded and feels firm to the touch, but it may not be painful if it is not infected. It is best to avoid use of the remaining patent jugular vein. This is because if the remaining jugular vein also develops thrombosis, venous return from the head is impaired, and the horse may develop severe swelling of the face and head. This may cause *dyspnea* (difficult breathing) and *dysphagia* (difficulty in eating). If jugular thrombosis develops, the horse should be fed from an elevated position to prevent dependent edema in the head. Softer feed is sometimes beneficial, such as water-soaked hay pellets and mashes. Thrombosed veins can be treated with application of warm compresses two or three times daily and application of dimethyl sulfoxide gel.

Thrombophlebitis is inflammation of a vein. This can occur after administration of irritating substances, such as tetracycline, phenylbutazone, or dimethyl sulfoxide solution at concentrations greater than 10%. Thrombophlebitis can also result from bacterial colonization (infection) of the vein. This can lead to disastrous effects for the horse. The infected vein may be larger than normal size, corded, painful, and warm to the touch. The horse may resent having the vein manipulated. Ultrasound examination may show the vein to be hyperechoic, with or without fluid (blood) centrally. A hyperechoic core may also be present. If the vein is infected, an aspirate can be taken

aseptically and cultured for bacterial growth. Alternatively, the catheter tip can be cultured immediately after catheter removal. Affected horses will require appropriate systemic antibiotics, as well as local therapy consisting of hot compresses.

Intravenous Infusions

Various intravenous infusions can be used to treat sick horses. Crystalloid fluids, such as lactated Ringer's solution or sodium chloride (saline), can be used to combat dehydration and hypovolemia. Colloid solutions, such as plasma or serum, can also be administered to patients requiring protein or antibody supplementation. Large volumes of fluids may be rapidly infused as a bolus in adult horses, but various fluid delivery systems are available to provide continuous fluid drip administration when needed. Care must be taken to change or remove the IV fluid bag when the fluids run out so that blood does not back up from the catheter into the IV line. If blood is allowed to fill the catheter, it may become clotted.

Fluid bags can be hung from a swivel hook and line fixed at the top of the stall (Fig. 26-11). Alternatively, IV fluid administration lines and extension tubes can be attached to rubber tubing that extends from the hook holding the IV fluids and is attached to the horse's halter on the same side as the catheter. The IV line is secured to the rubber tubing so that it forms loops as it travels down the rubber tubing (Fig. 26-12). This allows the horse to move freely in the stall without pulling out the IV line. Horses must be attached so that they do not become entangled in the rubber tubing. If continuous fluid therapy is not necessary, the horse can be restrained in stocks and fluids given as a bolus infusion using a pressure bulb.

Foals require special consideration. Care must be taken not to overhydrate neonates. Special IV delivery pumps can be used to continuously deliver fluids at the desired rate. Administration systems with an in-line reservoir that holds up to 150 ml of fluid can prevent accidental delivery of

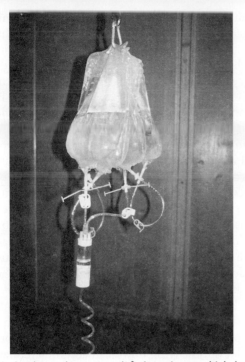

Fig. 26-11 Continuous intravenous infusion using a multiple-bag administration set.

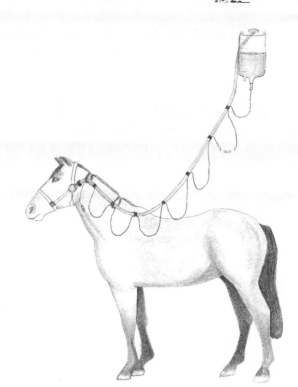

Fig. 26-12 Arrangement for continuous intravenous infusions that allows the horse to move freely in the stall.

excessive fluid volumes. Critically ill neonates are often hypothermic, so IV fluids should be warmed to body temperature before infusion. This can be done by heating the fluids in a bucket of warm water, or by microwaving the fluids (only if they are in plastic bags!). It is important to check the fluids to make sure they have not become too hot. Seriously compromised adult horses may also benefit from warm fluids, although this may not be practical.

Medication may be given through an injection port of the IV line if no other drugs have been added to the fluid bag. Various fluid additives are incompatible with certain medications and form a precipitate in the IV line. If there is any doubt about the compatibility of the medication with the fluids, administration of the fluids should be stopped. The catheter is then flushed with sterile saline and the medication is injected through the injection port. The catheter is flushed again with saline to clear the medication, and fluid administration can be resumed.

The volume of saline needed to flush a catheter depends on the catheter used. In general, 3 ml is sufficient to flush a catheter and T-port. If extension tubing is used, more flush solution may be required. If more than one type of medication is to be given, the catheter must be flushed with saline between injections of each medication. If fluids are not being infused, the final flush should be with heparinized saline to prevent clotting within the catheter. Catheters must be flushed with heparinized saline every 4 to 6 hours when fluids are not being given. As a general rule-of-thumb, most

medications should not be given in IV lines delivering plasma, blood products, or parenteral nutrition.

Horses with protein-losing gastroenteropathies, such as gastric ulcers, colitis, or right dorsal colon ulcers, may require IV plasma therapy. Plasma provides for volume expansion and much-needed protein. Foals with failure of passive transfer of maternal antibodies may also require IV plasma administration to obtain protective antibodies that were not absorbed from the mare's colostrum. Plasma can be harvested directly from an appropriate donor previously screened for compatibility, or more conveniently obtained from commercial sources. Plasma is also available from donors hyperimmunized against *Rhodococcus equi*, *Salmonella*, *Clostridium botulinum*, and the J-5 endotoxin. This plasma contains antibodies directed against specific bacteria or the toxins produced by the bacteria.

Plasma is stored frozen and requires thawing in warm water, *not* in the microwave. This should be done as quickly as possible without overheating the plasma and denaturing the protein. Water that is warm to the touch, but not hot, should be added frequently to facilitate thawing. Special IV administration sets that contain a filter to catch any fibrin clots are necessary when administering plasma or blood products. Some serum products that can be stored in the refrigerator instead of the freezer are also available in concentrated form. These also require warming to body temperature.

Whole-blood transfusions may be needed in cases of severe blood loss or with such conditions as neonatal isoerythrolysis. Blood transfusions should be considered when the hematocrit falls below 12% to 15%. Horses that become anemic or lose blood gradually over a longer period can tolerate relatively lower hematocrits. If a neonate or adult rapidly loses blood to a hematocrit of 15% or less, arrangements should be made to obtain fresh, whole blood. This should be harvested from a donor that has previously been screened for compatibility or, in an emergency, from a gelding that has not received any blood or plasma transfusions. Foals with neonatal isoerythrolysis may be transfused with the dam's red blood cells after they have been separated from the plasma and washed with saline to remove the mare's antibodies that are responsible for lysis of the foal's red blood cells. The mare's washed red blood cells must then be resuspended in saline to a packed cell volume of 50% before administration.

Plasma, serum, and blood should be infused slowly, giving 1 L/hr, if possible, to reduce the chance of an adverse reaction. Plasma or blood is administered very slowly at first to observe for reactions. The speed of the drip can be increased to the desired rate if the horse or foal tolerates it well; however, rapid administration may be necessary if the horse is hemorrhaging. Adverse reactions range from mild *tachypnea* (rapid breathing), shivering, hives, or fever, to severe respiratory distress, colic, hypotension, collapse, and death.

MEDICATION OF THE EYE

Topical ointments or solutions can be applied directly to the eye. Once the horse is adequately restrained, gently pry the eye open with clean fingers, being careful to touch only the outer lids. Apply the medication into the lower conjunctival sac. Take care not to scratch the surface of the cornea. Ointments can be applied by placing a small bead of ointment in the lower conjunctival sac. Ophthalmic drops can be placed in the lower conjunctival sac using the plastic dispenser vial provided or using a sterile tuberculin syringe (no needle!) if the solution is to be used on multiple horses.

Severe corneal ulcers may require topical treatments as often as every 1 to 2 hours. For horses that become head shy and resentful with this frequent treatment schedule, alternative medication delivery systems can be used. Lavage systems can be placed in the upper eyelid (subpalpebral) or inserted into the tear duct (nasolacrimal), and liquid medications can then be delivered easily through either system. Severe corneal ulcers and some other abnormalities may require extra protection for the eye. A protective eyecup can be used to protect the eye and keep the horse from dislodging the lavage system. The black plastic cup also protects the eye from direct sunlight that could cause pain. This may be very important, because many corneal ulcers require treatment with atropine to inhibit ciliary spasm. This makes the horse unable to constrict the pupil when exposed to direct sunlight. Netted fly masks can also be used to provide some protection for the eyes. Horses that spend a lot of time lying down can accumulate shavings or bedding in the eyes. Eye cups or netted fly masks can also be used to help keep the shavings out.

RECOMMENDED READING

Cohen ND et al: Medical management of right dorsal colitis in 5 horses: a retrospective study (1987-1993), *J Vet Intern Med* 9:272-276, 1995.

Getty R: *Sisson and Grossman's the anatomy of the domestic animals*, ed 5, Philadelphia, 1975, WB Saunders.

Madigan JE: *Manual of equine neonatal medicine*, ed 2, Woodland, Calif, 1991, Live Oak Publishing.

Spurlock SL et al: Long-term jugular vein catheterization in horses, *J Am Vet Med Assoc* 196:425-430, 1990.

27

Nursing Care of Food Animals, Camelids, and Ratites

Terry N. Teeple

Learning Objectives

After reviewing this chapter, the reader should understand the following:

- General husbandry terms and techniques used with food animals and ratites
- Methods of sample collection for laboratory analysis
- Routes of administration of medication in cattle, sheep, goats, pigs, and ratites
- Procedures used in intravenous catheterization
- Techniques used in general nursing care of food animals and ratites
- Procedures used in grooming and foot care
- Procedures used in caring for ratites

GENERAL CARE OF CATTLE

The cattle industry can be divided into two distinctly different areas; each with its own set of production goals and management techniques. The beef industry utilizes heavily muscled breeds of cattle that are capable of efficient conversion of hay and grain into skeletal muscle mass for maximum meat production. The dairy industry utilizes other breeds of cattle that are more efficient in converting cattle food into the production of large volumes of saleable milk as the main production goal. Labor expenses in the beef industry are mainly centered on processing and moving the cattle with additional demands around calving time. The labor involved with milking cows in the dairy industry is essentially an all-day, everyday event.

Breeding in the beef industry still occurs by allowing bulls (intact males) to roam the pastures with cows (adult females) seeking those who are in "heat" (estrus). However, many operations are now using artificial insemination (AI) with frozen bull semen as a common method of breeding. The dairy industry uses AI almost exclusively as the preferred method of breeding. The gestation period (pregnancy length) for cattle is about 9 months. The female calf is called a *heifer* (until she has had a calf), and the male calf is called a *bull calf* until he is castrated (at which time he is called a *steer*).

All cattle require various vaccinations and/or blood tests before being sold or transported between states. On behalf of state or federal regulatory departments that require vaccinations and tests, an accredited veterinarian must perform some of the procedures. Private practice veterinarians can become accredited by learning the required laws and rules and by passing a test to demonstrate that knowledge.

COMMON DIAGNOSTIC AND THERAPEUTIC TECHNIQUES

Oral Administration of Medication

Balling gun

Boluses, capsules, or magnets may be given per os (PO) with a balling gun (Fig. 27-1). This instrument is available in various sizes for use in different species. Cattle require a gun with a large head and long handle, with a metal or flexible plastic head. The plastic head produces less trauma to the pharyngeal tissue than a metal head, but it is easily damaged by teeth. Small balling guns are manufactured for use in calves.

The methods of introducing a balling gun, dose syringe, drench bottle, or Frick's speculum are similar in all species.

The authors acknowledge and appreciate the original contributions of Linda R. Kreatovich, Sheila M. Wing-Proctor, Seyedmehdi Mobini, Madonna E. Gemus, Michel Levy, and James T. Blackford, whose work has been incorporated into this chapter.

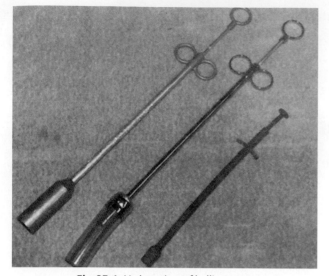

Fig. 27-1 Various sizes of balling guns.

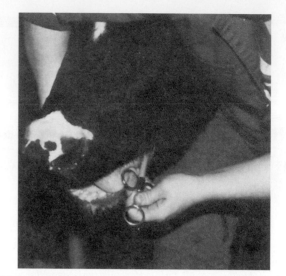

Fig. 27-2 Correct positioning of a cow's head and insertion of the balling gun.

For cattle, stand cranial to the patient's shoulder and face the same direction as the patient. Then place one arm over the patient's head and caudad to the poll, with the patient's head positioned on your hip. This technique may not be possible for people with short arms. In this case, reaching across the bridge of the nose is acceptable. Insert the fingers of this hand into the mouth at the interdental space and apply pressure to the hard palate, which causes the patient to open its mouth.

Insert the balling gun or similar instrument at an upward angle at the interdental space, opposite the restraining hand. Direct the instrument caudad and advance it over the base of the tongue. Once it is over the base, advance the balling gun caudad in a horizontal position until the rings of the handle reach the buccal commissure (corner of the mouth) (Fig. 27-2). This ensures that the gun is back far enough in the mouth to deposit the bolus, forcing the cow to swallow and preventing expulsion of the medication. Depress the plunger to eject the bolus, and remove the instrument. Observe the patient to be sure the medication was swallowed. It is not necessary to elevate the head until the bolus is swallowed if the bolus was deposited correctly.

Frick's speculum

A Frick's speculum may be used to give two or more boluses to cattle (Fig. 27-3). Insert the speculum in the same manner as the balling gun. Once the speculum is placed over the base of the tongue, the boluses are inserted into the speculum. Allow the boluses to travel down the speculum and into the mouth. Remove the speculum and observe for swallowing. This method is used to save time but has the added danger of aspiration of medication.

Orogastric intubation

Orogastric administration, also called stomach tubing, is a quick and relatively painless method to deliver large quantities of liquid medication or fluids. A stomach tube may be passed through the nasal cavity (nasogastric administration), as in horses, but this method is not commonly used in food animals. In food animals, the stomach tube is usually passed through the oral cavity, with the aid of a metal speculum.

An oral speculum is required to prevent damage to the soft stomach tube from the patient's teeth. The Frick's speculum is inserted into the mouth and held in place by an assistant.

Stomach tubes are available in different lengths and diameters. Choose an appropriately sized tube for the individual patient. A tube with an outside diameter of ⅝ to 1 inch is the average size used for adult cattle. A foal stomach tube is often used for "tubing" calves. A stomach pump or a funnel can be used to facilitate administration.

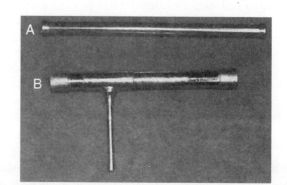

Fig. 27-3 **A,** Regular Frick's speculum. **B,** Modified Frick's speculum.

Measure the distance externally from the mouth to the rumen, and insert the tube approximately this distance. The mouth-rumen distance is then easily estimated. The first 3 feet of the tube should be lubricated with water or water-soluble lubricating jelly before intubation. With an assistant holding an oral speculum in place, insert the tube into the speculum and advance it with gentle pressure. You may feel some resistance when the tube reaches the esophagus. Observe for swallowing, then advance the tube into the esophagus. If passage is difficult, rotate the tube slightly and apply gentle pressure to advance the tube.

Drenching

Giving small volumes of liquids PO is often referred to as drenching. Drenching is done with a dose syringe or a drench bottle (Fig. 27-4). A 60-ml catheter-tipped syringe or a bulb syringe may be used as a dose syringe in calves. The drench bottle, commonly a wine or a soft drink bottle, should be made of strong glass and have a long, tapered neck and smooth mouth.

The technique for drenching is similar to that described for the balling gun. Be certain to insert the drench bottle at the interdental space to prevent the cow from breaking it with its molars. The head should be held slightly elevated so that the nose is level with the patient's eye. If the head is raised excessively, the patient may aspirate some of the medication. Give the medication slowly, allowing the patient to swallow at its own pace.

Dose syringes are also used to give pastes. Commercially prepared syringes containing medication are available, although these are used more often in horses. After inserting the tube the measured distance, check for correct placement in the rumen. If the stomach tube was inadvertently placed in the trachea, the patient may cough, although this should not be used alone to determine correct placement. If the tube has been inadvertently passed down the trachea, air may be felt exiting the tube upon exhalation. Remove

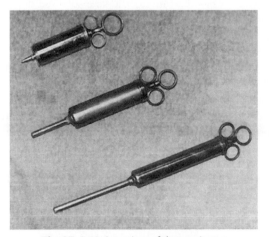

Fig. 27-4 Various sizes of dose syringes.

the tube and reintubate. Another test used to check if the tube has been passed into the rumen is to have one person blow air into the end of the tube while another listens with a stethoscope at the rumen. A gurgling should be heard as air is blown into the tube. The smell of rumen gas may sometimes be detected exiting the tube. In some lightly muscled animals, the tube can be observed progressing caudad down the esophagus. In these patients, one may also palpate the neck for two tubular structures, i.e., the trachea and the stomach tube within the esophagus.

Once the stomach tube is correctly positioned, the medication can be given. After the medication has been infused, rinse the tube with water to flush out remaining medication. Kink the tube or occlude its end and withdraw it quickly. This prevents any fluid remaining in the tube from entering the trachea upon tube removal.

Intravenous Injection

The veins most often used for IV injections in cattle are the jugular veins, coccygeal (tail) vein, and subcutaneous abdominal (milk) veins. The jugular veins are most often used for large-volume IV injections and blood collection. In addition to their accessibility, there is less chance of being kicked when using these veins. The jugular vein is always used for IV injections in calves because it is the largest accessible vessel.

The coccygeal (tail) vein is used for IV injection of small volumes (3 to 5 ml) of drugs and blood-sample collection. Although most cows are more tolerant of tail venipuncture than jugular injections, there is a greater chance of being kicked. This can be minimized with proper restraint. The subcutaneous abdominal vein, also called the mammary or milk vein, is used mainly when the jugular veins are thrombosed (occluded) or cannot be located. There are several disadvantages to milk vein injections. The technician has an increased risk of being kicked. A second person may be required to provide additional restraint. The milk vein rolls easily under the skin, making it hard to puncture the vein and thread the needle. Finally, hematomas are easily formed and may result in thrombosis of the vein.

Preparation for venipuncture is similar for all three veins. A disinfectant, such as 70% alcohol, should be applied to the injection site to remove gross contamination, provide antibacterial activity, and increase visibility of the vein. Venipunctures should not be made through dirt or fecal material, as phlebitis, septicemia, and/or contamination of medication and samples may result.

Intravenous Catheterization

Intravenous catheterization is used primarily for prolonged fluid therapy, but it is also used for administration of injectable anesthetics or repeated IV injections. The jugular vein is most often chosen for IV catheterization in cattle. The caudal auricular vein can be catheterized in cattle, although this vein is used mainly for injection of small volumes of medication. It is difficult to secure a catheter in the ear vein for an extended period because of its location.

Restraint

Restraint required for IV catheterization is identical to that described for IV injection. Restraint needed for catheterizing the auricular vein involves securing the head and possibly use of nose tongs. It may help to cover the patient's eyes with a towel.

Materials

A 10- to 14-gauge catheter is used for adult cattle. Calves require a smaller-gauge catheter (14-, 15-, or 18-gauge).

To catheterize the ear vein of cattle, one can use an 18- to 20-gauge, 1.5- to 2-inch over-the-needle catheter. On large bulls, a 14-gauge, 2-inch catheter may be used if the ear vein is large enough.

Technique

Clip and surgically scrub the site. Local anesthesia is not required. Apply an antiseptic to complete skin preparation. Because of the skin's thickness, attempts to introduce a catheter through it may bend the catheter or damage the tip. To help introduce a catheter, a disposable needle of the same gauge is used to puncture the skin. This enables the catheter to pass through the skin with ease. A No. 15 surgical blade can be used for this purpose also.

For catheterization of the auricular vein, a local anesthetic is useful to decrease ear movement. Skin glue or a suture can be used to secure the catheter. Bandage the catheter site. To give the ear some stability, insert a 4-inch roll of gauze into the ear before bandaging the ear.

Intramuscular Injection

IM injections are commonly used in cattle. Several large muscle masses are available, including the gluteals, semimembranosus, semitendinosus, and lateral cervical muscles. The gluteals are located on the dorsal aspect of the rear legs (Fig. 27-5). The semimembranosus and semitendinosus are located in the rear limbs, between the stifle joint and ischium. The lateral cervical muscles are cranial to the scapula, dorsal to the cervical vertebrae, and ventral to the ligamentum nuchae.

The needle selected for IM injection depends on the viscosity (thickness) of the medication to be administered and the size of the muscle mass selected. A 16-, 18-, or 20-gauge, 1.5-inch needle is commonly used for adults. A smaller-gauge needle is used for calves (18-, 20-, or 22-gauge).

Subcutaneous Injection

SQ injections are given anywhere loose skin can be raised with one's fingers. In cattle, this is easily done on the lateral

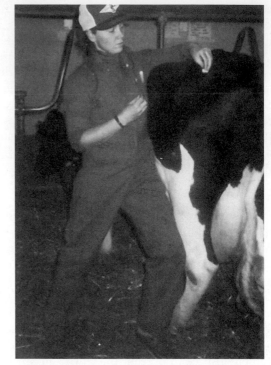

Fig. 27-5 Correct position for IM injection into the gluteal muscle mass on the cow's opposite side.

aspect of the neck and thorax, the axillary region, the fold of the flank, and the brisket.

Restraint

SQ injections generally require minimal restraint. Calves can be cornered in a small area. Adult cattle should have a halter applied in order to be placed in a headgate or stanchion. Aggressive animals may require a chute.

Materials

An 18-, 20-, or 22-gauge, 1.5-inch needle is used for SQ injections in calves. A 14-, 16-, or 18-gauge, 1.5-inch needle is used for cattle. The needle size selected depends on the viscosity of the drug and the thickness of the skin. A syringe is used to inject small quantities. A simplex system may be used to administer larger quantities.

Technique

The site should be cleaned with an antiseptic, such as 70% alcohol. Pinch the skin and raise it to form a "tent," taking care not to penetrate the other side with the needle. After the needle is positioned, aspirate. If blood is not observed upon aspiration, inject the medication. If there is blood present in the needle, withdraw the needle and attempt the injection at a new site. When the injection is completed, withdraw the needle, release the skin fold, and massage the area to enhance spread of the medication and increase its absorption rate.

The volume of medication injected at each SQ site varies according to personal preference and patient size. For cattle, 50 to 100 ml per site is the recommended maximum, although up to 250 ml may be given SQ. When giving large volumes, intermittently direct the needle to prevent depositing large quantities in one site. The amount that can be injected at each SQ site for calves varies from 2 to 30 ml, with a maximum volume of 50 ml.

Intradermal Injection

ID injection is directed into the dermis, the skin layer underlying the most superficial epidermis. Intradermal injections are used mainly to aid in diagnosis of certain diseases. Cattle are tested for tuberculosis using ID injection of bovine tuberculin. ID injections are also used for allergy testing, a procedure usually limited to companion animals. Local anesthetics are injected ID to anesthetize sites for surgery or other invasive procedures.

The caudal tail fold is the site used most often for ID injections of tuberculin. The injections may also be given on the lateral aspect of the neck and abdomen.

Restraint

The restraint required depends on the site chosen, the number of injections to be given, and the patient's temperament. Most patients require minimal restraint. The sites must be free of hair before ID injection is attempted. If a diagnostic test is to be performed, the site should not be cleaned with antiseptics, because the antiseptic may create a skin reaction and interfere with test results. Usually removal of dirt and feces is all that is required for preparation. Antiseptics can be applied to the site if local anesthetics are being deposited before surgery.

Materials

Because of their thick skin, cattle require a large needle, such as a 20- to 22-gauge, 1.5-inch needle. A tuberculin or 3-ml syringe is adequate for injecting small volumes ID.

Technique

The needle, with the syringe attached, is placed parallel to the skin. The free hand is used to pinch the skin. This pulls the skin taut and helps stabilize it. With the bevel directed upward, gently insert the needle into the dermis of the skin. Aspirate if the injection is for local anesthesia over a vessel. A bleb should be visualized as the drug is deposited. If a bleb does not form, the needle is too deep; retract it a small distance and inject the drug. It is not necessary to massage the site, because the goal is to keep the drug localized.

Intramammary Infusion

Veterinarians and dairy farmers often employ intramammary infusions to treat mastitis or to infuse udder quarters when cows are dry (not lactating). The best time to infuse the udder is after the last milking of the day, which allows the medication to remain in the udder overnight. The udder should not be infused before milking, because the beneficial effect of the medication would be lost. Because intramammary antibiotic therapy affects the results of milk culture, obtain milk samples from mastitic quarters *before* treatment.

Restraint

Minimal restraint is required for intramammary infusion. Tail restraint may be necessary for fractious cows. Care must be taken with beef cows, especially if they have been separated from their calves, because they are usually very aggressive.

Technique

To avoid injury from kicking, crouch beside the udder to work; never sit or kneel. Thoroughly clean the udder before treatment, using warm water and antiseptic soap. Use a separate cloth or paper towel to wash each teat so as to decrease the spread of microorganisms among the quarters. Dry each teat with a separate towel to remove contaminated water droplets. Wipe the teat orifice with an alcohol swab and allow to air-dry. If all four quarters are to be infused, swab the far teats before swabbing the near ones, so as to prevent contamination when reaching past the near teats.

Empty the quarter by manually "stripping" out the milk before infusing medication, because residual milk mixes with the medication and dilutes it. Collect the discarded milk in a bucket to prevent contamination of the environment by the bacteria in the milk. After the teat is prepared, grasp it near the base and insert a teat cannula or sterile, disposable mammary infusion cannula into the teat orifice. More commonly, commercially prepared, disposable syringes with an attached cannula are used. Advance the cannula just through the teat sphincter a short distance, and inject the medication slowly. Do not insert the cannula to the hub, because this stretches the teat sphincter and predisposes the quarter to mastitis. As little as 10 to 20 ml or as much as 250 ml may be infused into a quarter. Remove the cannula, and massage the teat and quarter to disseminate the medication. When the procedure is completed, dip the teat in teat dip to prevent invasion of microbes. If the weather is extremely cold (0° C [32° F] or lower), do not let the cow outside until the udder is dry, so as to prevent chapping and frostbite. Mark the cows that were treated so that their milk can be discarded.

Intranasal Insufflation

The intranasal route is used to administer vaccines and local anesthetics. Only vaccines designed for intranasal use should be given in this manner. Other vaccines are not effective when given by this route.

Intranasal anesthetics may be given before potentially painful procedures on the nasal cavity, such as nasogastric intubation, bronchoalveolar lavage, and endoscopy.

Restraint of the head is a necessity. Calves may be manually restrained, whereas adults should be secured with a halter and headgate.

Nasal secretions should be wiped from the nostril with moist cotton before medication administration. A 3- to 5-ml syringe is filled with the vaccine or local anesthetic, with a disposable, blunt tip attached to inject the drug (although the syringe alone may be used). Facing the same direction as the patient, place one hand over the patient's head, pulling it close to your body. Elevate the head slightly to prevent the medication from running out of the nostril. The free hand is used to insert the syringe into the nostril. When the injection is completed, elevate the head for 10 to 15 seconds before releasing it.

Intrauterine Medication

Medication is placed in the uterus to locally treat metritis. Although veterinary technicians may perform this procedure, it is up to the veterinarian to decide as to whether technicians should perform it.

Uterine medication is available as boluses, capsules, and solutions. The form of the drug used depends on the condition of the uterus, stage of the reproductive cycle, types of drugs available, and personal preference.

Cows require minimal restraint for this procedure. Secure the tail away from the perianal region. "Rake" (manually remove) any feces from the rectum before cleaning the vulva, so as to aid in palpation and prevent contamination of the area and equipment. Use an antiseptic soap, warm water, and cotton to wash the vulva and surrounding area. Wipe the vulva, starting at the dorsal commissure of the labia and progressing down to the ventral commissure. Rinse off the soap before treatment.

Intrauterine infusion

A uterine pipette is used to infuse solutions into the uterus, using a syringe to inject the medication through the pipette. An equine nasogastric tube and stomach pump may be used to inject large volumes of medication into the uterus.

To aid passage of the pipette into the uterus, guide it with the opposite hand, placed into the rectum. Grasp the cervix, which lies about 3 to 4 inches cranial to the vulva, with the left hand (for a right-handed person) so that the thumb is dorsal to the cervix and the fingers are located ventrad. Insert the pipette into the vulva, exercising care to avoid touching the pipette's tip to the labia. Advance the pipette at a 30° to 40° angle for 3 to 4 inches. This prevents the pipette from entering the urethral opening, located on the floor of the vagina. Once the tip is past the urethral orifice, advance the pipette in a horizontal position. To aid in passage of the pipette, pull the cervix craniad to straighten the folds of the vagina. As the pipette is advanced, it may become caught in a vaginal fold. If this occurs, do not force the pipette craniad, but simply withdraw and redirect it. Introduce the pipette's tip into the cervical opening, which is usually in the center of the cervix. Gently manipulate the cervix over the pipette. Once the pipette is through the cervix, it slides craniad easily and may be palpated rectally. Beginners commonly deposit the medication in the vagina or cervix rather than in the uterus. Always be certain the tip has passed into the uterus. Inject the medication, and then flush the pipette with air to remove residual medication.

Throughout the entire procedure, it is important never to force the pipette craniad, because this may damage vaginal or cervical tissue. Also, the vaginal and rectal walls may be penetrated if excessive force is used. This may result in such complications as peritonitis, metritis, abscesses, and reproductive disorders.

Intrauterine boluses

Wear a sterile sleeve to insert boluses or capsules into the uterus. Advance the hand into the patient's vulva and vagina until the cervix is located. Form your hand into a wedge, insert it into the patient's dilated os cervix (cervical orifice), and advance it into the uterus, where the medication is deposited. There are fewer complications with this method of intrauterine medication than with infusion. The primary complication is introduction of bacteria into the uterus by using poor sanitary techniques. Also, rough handling can damage vaginal and cervical tissue.

Many farmers medicate their animals with these methods. They should be carefully instructed in use of the proper techniques and informed of possible complications. They should also be informed of drug withdrawal times so that meat or milk from treated animals is not immediately sold.

Jugular Venipuncture

Restraint

Good restraint is necessary when attempting any venipuncture. Ideally, the patient should be restrained in a head gate or stanchion. Injecting medication into the jugular vein of a patient that is not properly restrained is difficult and dangerous. Therefore, never attempt venipuncture on a free-moving large animal. A halter or nose tongs should be applied and the head raised and pulled to one side. A quick-release knot should be used when tying a patient to a stationary object. If the patient should fall during infusion of medication, the head can be released immediately to prevent injury to the patient. If a recumbent cow must be treated, its head can be secured by tying the free end of the halter back above the hock with a quick-release knot. Tying the head to one side secures it, making the vein accessible, but it may also make it more difficult to distend the vein.

Restrain a standing calf by pulling it close to your body, immobilizing its head. Restrain an older calf as you would restrain an adult. It is usually not necessary to apply nose tongs. A recumbent calf should have its head firmly held with the neck extended. If the calf moves excessively, a second person should aid in restraint.

Materials

All required materials should be assembled before attempting venipuncture. The needle selected for IV injection of large volumes of fluids varies according to personal preference and the flow rate desired. A 12- to 14-gauge, 2- to 3-inch needle is best for giving large volumes to adult cattle. Needles less than 2 inches long should not be used. A correctly threaded 3-inch needle is not likely to slip from the vein if the cow thrashes around, decreasing the chances of perivascular infiltration of irritants and hypertonic solutions. For injections of small volumes into the jugular vein, use of a 16-, 18-, or 20-gauge, 1.5-inch needle is recommended for cows and calves. These small-gauge, disposable needles are easier to insert than the reusable, large-bore needles. This is because disposable needles are used only once and are very sharp, whereas reusable needles tend to become dull.

A rubber IV line, referred to as a *simplex*, is used for IV infusions. A syringe may also be used to inject medication. Its size depends on the volume of medication to be injected.

Technique

One should never kneel or stand directly in front of a patient during jugular venipuncture. To distend the jugular vein, apply pressure at the jugular furrow, about two thirds of the way caudad on (down) the neck. Allow time for the vein to fill. Briskly stroking the vein with a finger in a downward motion (toward the heart) helps raise it for easy visualization. Unless the patient is in shock or is severely dehydrated, jugular venipuncture should not be attempted without sufficiently raising the vein. Although the jugular vein is quite large when raised, an inexperienced technician can easily miss it.

Bovine skin is thick and difficult to penetrate with a large-gauge needle; therefore, the needle must be inserted with considerable force. Grasp the needle by the hub, using the thumb and first knuckle of the forefinger. Warn the cow of the impending needle insertion by repeated taps on the neck, *near but not over* the injection site, using the back of the hand holding the needle. These warning strokes may upset the patient more than insertion of the needle. Gradually increasing the intensity of the strokes often prevents this. After two or three warning strokes, flip the hand over and thrust the needle through the skin at a 45- to 90-degree angle to the vessel, with the needle directed toward the heart. Keep the jugular vein occluded to observe for blood flow from the needle, indicating proper placement.

If the vein was entered on the initial attempt and a steady flow of blood exits the needle, keep the vein distended and lay the needle parallel to the skin, then advance it further caudad into the vein. The needle may be directed toward the head for administration of small volumes, but larger volumes should be given with the needle directed toward the heart. If the needle slips out of the vein during insertion, retract it until blood steadily flows from it, then attempt to rethread it. Occasionally, the needle does not enter the vein, but only penetrates the skin. When this occurs, relocate the vein and thrust the needle into it without withdrawing it from the skin. Redirection of the needle may be necessary to find the vein. Once a steady flow of blood is present, the needle should be threaded to its hub. If the needle has been inserted too deeply and has penetrated entirely through the vessel, pull the needle back slowly until the blood flows freely from the hub; at this point the needle can be threaded. Apposition of the bevel of the needle against the vessel wall may also occlude it. This may be corrected by slightly rotating the needle along its long axis. Care must be taken when redirecting the needle to prevent laceration of the vein and consequent hematoma formation.

Small-gauge, disposable hypodermic needles may be inserted as are large-bore needles. However, it is not necessary to use as much force to insert the needles or to strike the patient before insertion, because they are very sharp and easily penetrate the skin. Introduce the needle into the vein at a 30- to 45-degree angle, with or without a syringe attached. The needle may be correctly positioned by attaching a syringe and aspirating blood.

When the needle is correctly threaded, the syringe or simplex is attached. Aspirate (slightly withdraw the syringe barrel), and then inject the medication. If a bottle is used, it should be held in an inverted position. A steady bubbling in the bottle indicates that the medication is flowing into the vein and is being replaced by air in the bottle. If the bubbling becomes irregular or stops, the needle may be occluded or out of the vein. In such cases, lower the bottle, check the needle for correct positioning, and make the appropriate adjustments. When the inverted bottle is lowered, blood flows into the IV line. This can be used to check correct positioning of the needle.

Whether using a simplex or a syringe to administer fluid, observe the jugular furrow for gradual swelling around the needle. This may indicate that medication is flowing into the perivascular space (outside the vein). Correct the needle's position and continue. After IV injection is complete, remove the needle and apply digital (finger) pressure for 15 to 20 seconds over the venipuncture site to prevent hematoma.

Coccygeal Venipuncture

For smaller volumes of medication, the coccygeal (tail) vein is often used rather than the jugular vein. Cattle usually become less agitated when the tail is used for venipuncture. Using the coccygeal vein usually requires less restraint than using the jugular vein.

Restraint

Limited restraint is needed for coccygeal venipuncture. Dairy cattle require a halter or stanchion and a tail jack (see Chapter 16). Beef cattle generally are more fractious and may require restraint in a chute. A tail jack must be used for coccygeal venipuncture, because it is impossible to enter the vein if the tail is not held in a vertical position. Holding the tail in this manner also simultaneously serves as restraint.

Materials

An 18- or 20-gauge, 1.5-inch needle attached to a 3-, 5- or 10-ml syringe is appropriate for coccygeal venipuncture. A needle larger than 18 gauge is too large for the coccygeal vein. A 20-gauge needle is most commonly used.

Technique

The first three coccygeal vertebrae (near the tail base) are the best sites for coccygeal venipuncture. To locate the correct site, apply a tail jack and clean the ventral surface of the tail to remove gross contamination (Fig. 27-6). Palpate the tail for the bony protrusions (hemal arches) of the vertebrae while gently aspirating, directly on the midline at a 45° angle to the tail. If the blood is not withdrawn into the syringe, check the needle for the correct angle and position.

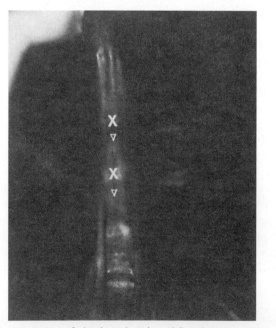

Fig. 27-6 Location of the hemal arches *(X)* and venipuncture sites *(arrowheads)* on the ventral aspect of the bovine tail.

It may be necessary to advance or retreat the needle to locate the vein. Remove the needle, and redirect it if necessary. Inject the medication when the needle is correctly positioned. Periodically aspirate blood into the syringe, and reinject it to clear the needle of residual medication. Either the coccygeal artery or vein may be used for injection. After the injection is completed, remove the needle, lower the tail, and apply digital pressure for 10 to 15 seconds. Hematoma formation is usually not a problem, although digital pressure should be applied if the artery was punctured.

Subcutaneous Abdominal Venipuncture

The milk veins are used when the jugular veins cannot be raised or are inaccessible for other reasons. These veins should be used for administration of large volumes of medication only. It is too dangerous to obtain routine blood samples from them.

Restraint

Tie the patient securely, or restrain in a stanchion. Stand close to the patient's flank, facing the same direction as the patient. One should not face the patient's rear, as it may kick.

Materials

A 14-gauge, 2- to 3-inch needle is used for venipuncture. A syringe may be used to inject medication; however, a simplex system is frequently used. Because blood flows slowly in this vein, administration through a simplex may require more time than anticipated.

Technique

It is not necessary to occlude the milk vein before puncturing it, because it is normally distended. The preferred venipuncture site is immediately caudad to the point where the vessel enters the abdomen; this section of the vein is the most stable. As with jugular venipuncture, it takes some force to introduce the needle through the skin. Insert the needle caudad, and thread it into the vein. If blood does not flow freely from the needle, check the position of the needle and redirect it. Exercise caution when redirecting the needle, for it is easy to create hematomas in this area. Observe the area for perivascular infiltration during administration. When the injection is complete, remove the needle and apply digital pressure for several minutes. Even with digital pressure, hematomas form easily.

GENERAL CARE OF SHEEP

Husbandry terms related to the sheep industry include the following: the *ewe* (adult female) gives birth to one to three young (*lambing*) that are called *ram lambs* (male) or *ewe lambs* (female). The gestation for sheep is about 5 months, and breeding usually occurs in the fall of the year resulting in spring lambs. The intact adult male is called a *ram*, and the castrated male is called a *wether*.

Hoof Trimming

Sheep that are not allowed to graze or that are raised in confinement tend to develop overgrown feet. Typically, the sidewalls and the toes overgrow. Trim the hoofs as needed (Fig. 27-7). Trim the sidewalls to keep the sole flat and the toes pointing forward. Toes are normally squared off. Trimming is done with heavy scissors, hoof rot shears, or a sharp knife (Fig. 27-8). If bleeding occurs, apply hemostatic powder or copper naphthenate solution. Severe bleeding may require bandaging.

Crutching

Ewes close to parturition should be crutched. This procedure removes the wool from around the vulva and the udder. A clean vulval area facilitates passage of the lamb and allows the birthing process to proceed easily. Removing the wool from around the udder assists the lambs in finding and suckling the teats. Lambs suck on anything on the ewe's body, including wool and fecal tags. Trimming this debris from around the vulva and udder areas prevents the lambs from sucking inappropriately.

COMMON DIAGNOSTIC AND THERAPEUTIC TECHNIQUES

Oral Administration of Medication

Stomach tubing

Placement of a stomach tube is a quick and effective method of delivering large volumes of liquid to the rumen or relieving rumen gas bloat. The tube can be passed through a mouth speculum or through the nasal cavity. Equipment should be gathered before attempting to pass a stomach tube. Required equipment includes the following:

- Mouth speculum (swine mouth speculum, Frick's speculum, PVC pipe, or roll of Elastikon)
- Stomach tube (10- to 18-French rubber urinary catheter or 14- to 18-French infant feeding tube for lambs; small to medium foal stomach tube for sheep)
- Dose syringe or funnel

When using the oral route in neonatal lambs, a mouth speculum is usually not required. Measure from the front of the mouth to the rumen for the correct length of tube needed. Lubricate the distal one third of the tube with water, mineral oil, or water-soluble lubricating jelly. Introduce the mouth speculum into the interdental space, being careful not to damage the patient's teeth. Pressing

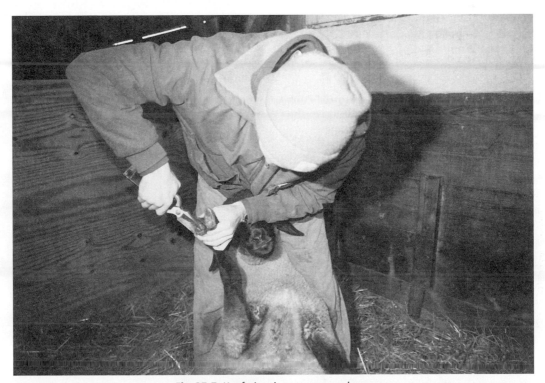

Fig. 27-7 Hoof trimming on a set-up sheep.

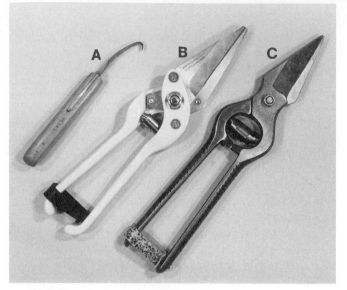

Fig. 27-8 Hoof trimming equipment. **A,** Double-sided narrow knife. **B,** Heavy-duty scissors. **C,** Hoof rot shears.

your thumb against the patient's tongue prompts the sheep to open its mouth. Place the tube into the speculum, and advance steadily with gentle pressure; you may feel resistance at the esophagus. Determine the correct tube placement by watching the patient swallow the tube or by blowing into the tube while someone listens for gurgling sounds in the paralumbar fossa region. Generally, rumen odor is emitted from the tube. An incorrectly placed tube stimulates a cough reflex (tube is in the trachea), and air can be felt on exhalation. Administer fluids or liquid medications through the tube using a funnel or dose syringe. When the treatment is completed, flush the tube with water until it runs clear, then kink or occlude the tube and withdraw it quickly. Failure to occlude the end of the tube can lead to aspiration of fluid into the lungs. Remove the speculum.

Dose syringe

Dose syringes allow oral administration of liquid medications without use of a stomach tube. This technique is simple, but there is always a chance of aspiration into the lungs. Liquid medications should be limited to a volume of 30 ml. The sheep should be standing, with its head parallel to the ground or tilted slightly upward. Insert the tip of a dose syringe/backpack syringe tip into the interdental space, and dispense the medication. Cup the patient's head with your hand during this procedure to keep the patient from spitting the fluid out.

Bolus or pill administration

Boluses are large pills that require a sheep-sized balling gun, either plastic or metal, for administration. The balling gun is introduced into the sheep's mouth at the interdental space. The gun is advanced into the mouth and over the base of the tongue, being careful to avoid injury to the roof of the mouth or the teeth. Push the plunger gently to deliver the bolus. Sheep do not like this method of treatment and begin resisting the procedure if it is performed frequently. It is possible to "pill" a sheep using your fingers to introduce the pill over the base of the tongue, but you can be bitten for your efforts. Remember not to overextend the sheep's neck, because this can cause the bolus to enter the trachea instead of the esophagus.

Rumen inoculation

It is useful to know how to inoculate the rumen of a sick sheep. Without the normal microorganisms in the gut, the sheep is unable to properly digest its food. Rumen contents can be siphoned from a healthy sheep and introduced into the rumen of the debilitated patient through a stomach tube. At least 1 quart of rumen liquid should be administered to the unhealthy patient. Another method is to take a cud from a healthy sheep and place it into the mouth of the sick patient. This does not work well if the patient is debilitated and unable to chew and/or swallow correctly, but the cud can be mixed with water and given via a stomach tube.

Intravenous Injection

The jugular vein is routinely used for administering IV medications and for drawing blood samples. It can be easily accessed in the standing sheep (Fig. 27-9). The cephalic and femoral veins may also be used, with the sheep in a standing or lateral position. Depending on the size of the sheep, an 18- or 20-gauge, 1- to 1½-inch needle is used for IV injection.

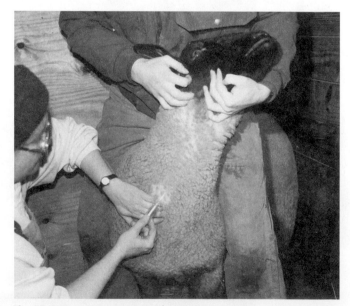

Fig. 27-9 Two-person restraint for intravenous injection or blood sampling using the jugular vein.

Part the wool along the jugular furrow, and wipe the area with an antiseptic. Occlude the vessel at or slightly cranial to the thoracic inlet, stroking or tapping the vessel to help define the borders of the vessel. Insert the needle at a 30° to 45° angle, with or without the needle attached to a syringe. Thread the needle into the vessel. Aspirate and check for blood. If the needle is positioned in the vessel, inject the medication slowly. Redirect the needle if necessary. Withdraw the needle while attached to the syringe, and apply pressure over the injection site to prevent formation of a hematoma. A blood sample may be obtained with a Vacutainer system using this same process. The jugular vein appears deeper in an unshorn sheep, because the wool prevents the technician from resting the syringe/Vacutainer tube against the patient's skin.

Intravenous Catheterization

Intravenous catheters should be placed in patients that require continuous fluid therapy, repeated IV treatments, or administration of irritating medications. The jugular vein is the vessel of choice. The cephalic or femoral veins may be used if the jugular vein is not patent. Catheter dimensions vary, depending on the size of the sheep. In adults, use 14-, 16-, or 18-gauge, 3½- to 5¼-inch catheters. In lambs, use 18-, 20-, or 22-gauge, 1½- to 3½-inch catheters.

Clip and aseptically prepare the skin over the jugular furrow for introduction of the catheter. Local anesthetic may be used at the catheter introduction site. Place an IV catheter in a sterile manner, which includes wearing sterile gloves. Occlude the vein caudad to the insertion site. Puncture the skin at the catheter site with a disposable needle the same diameter as the catheter. This prevents the catheter tip from becoming dull as it passes through the skin. Place the catheter through the needle hole at a 15- to 30-degree angle, and quickly thrust the catheter into the vein and advance it toward the heart. Occlude the vessel to ensure backflow of blood through the catheter; this indicates proper placement of the catheter. Cap the catheter and flush with 10 to 15 ml of heparinized saline.

The catheter should be secured to the neck. Bandaging alone is not sufficient to keep the catheter from slipping out of place. When using a catheter with wings, secure it by placing an 18-gauge, 1½-inch hypodermic needle into the skin near the wing and threading a 2/0 nonabsorbable suture material through the tip of the needle and out the needle hub. Then remove the needle, thread the suture into the hole of the wing, and tie it. Repeat the procedure on the other wing. When using a catheter without wings, secure it by placing the first suture caudad to the hub and a second suture craniad to the hub on the extension or IV line. At least two sutures should be placed to secure the catheter. Suturing the catheter increases the likelihood that the catheter will stay in place. After the catheter is secured,

apply an antibiotic ointment over the catheter exit with a sterile tongue depressor. Place a sterile gauze pad over the ointment, and secure the setup with elastic tape around the sheep's neck. An IV drip line should be looped into or on top of the bandage and held in place with adhesive tape. The loop in the extension line prevents direct tension on the catheter as the patient moves about the stall. The catheter and IV lines should be changed every 3 days to prevent thrombophlebitis and infection. Flushing the catheter every 4 hours with heparinized saline helps keep the catheter patent.

Intramuscular Injection

An IM injection is best done with the patient standing (Fig. 27-10). For adult sheep, use an 18-gauge, 1½-inch needle; for lambs, use a 20-gauge, 1-inch needle. Only the semimembranosus, semitendinosus, and triceps muscles are substantial enough for IM injection.

Part the wool and swab the injection site with an antiseptic. Hold the needle by the hub between your thumb and forefinger, avoiding contact with the sterile shaft. Grasp the muscle near the injection site with the thumb and fingers of the opposite hand, squeeze the muscle, and quickly thrust the needle into the muscle. Attach the syringe and aspirate to check for blood; redirect the needle if necessary. Inject the medication, and withdraw the needle and syringe as a unit.

Subcutaneous Injection

Administer SQ injections with the sheep in a standing, lateral, or set up position. For adult sheep, use an 18-gauge, 1-inch needle; for lambs, use a 20-gauge, 1-inch needle. Any area with loose skin can be used for SQ injection, although using the wool-free areas caudad to the front legs and cranial to the rear legs reduces the chance of pelt damage (see Fig. 27-10). Some caregivers prefer to use the loose skin around the neck, cranial to the scapula, or along the back. Injections in these areas can lead to abscesses, a sore neck (which prevents the patient from eating and drinking), or pelt damage. After wiping the area with an antiseptic, pinch the skin between the fingers to form a tent. Insert the needle into the tent, ensuring that the needle is under the skin. Aspirate to check for blood. If the needle is correctly positioned, inject the medication. Depending on the substance being injected, hold your finger over the puncture site as the needle is withdrawn. This prevents leaking from the injection site and helps control minor skin bleeding.

Intradermal Injection

ID injections are used infrequently in sheep. The main use of ID injection is for tuberculosis testing. The caudal tail fold is the preferred site in sheep. A 25-gauge, ⅝-inch or 26-gauge, ⅜-inch needle is used. The needle with the syringe attached is placed parallel to the skin. The free hand is used

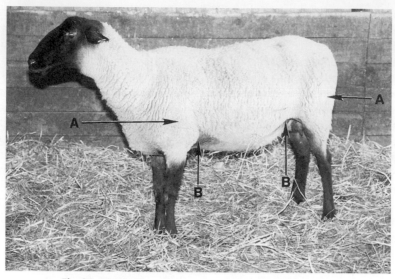

Fig. 27-10 Injection site. **A,** Intramuscular. **B,** Subcutaneous.

to pinch the skin taut and helps stabilize it for the injection. With the bevel directed up, gently insert the needle into the dermis. Aspirate if the injection is for local anesthesia over a vessel. A bleb or wheal should be visualized as the drug is deposited. Tuberculin testing uses only 0.1 ml of testing solution, so care must be taken to deposit material accurately.

Intraperitoneal Injection

The IP route is usually used in neonates when an IV injection is not convenient. The caudoventral abdominal wall cranial to the pubis is the best site for IP injections in sheep. Prepare the site by clipping the area and prepping with a surgical scrub. Restrain the patient in dorsal recumbency with the hindquarters elevated. To avoid puncturing the bladder or injuring the penis in males, insert the needle slightly off midline. Gently insert an 18-gauge, 1- to 1 ½-inch needle, aspirate, and inject the medication. The medication should flow easily if the needle is in the peritoneal cavity. Many problems, such as peritonitis from improper site preparation or puncturing of abdominal organs, can result if improper technique is used in this procedure.

Intramammary Infusion

It may be necessary to check or treat the udder for mastitis. A physical examination is best performed with the sheep in a set up position. Treatments or milk testing in the ewe are usually done with the ewe in a standing position. Thoroughly wash the teats with warm water, an antiseptic soap, and a separate cloth or paper towel. Dry each teat with an individual towel; this decreases the number of contaminating bacteria. Wipe the teat orifices with an alcohol-drenched swab, starting with the far teat and ending with the near. Allow the teats to air-dry. Discard the milk in the streak canal. The teat is now prepared for collecting a milk sample for testing or for infusion of the udder. For testing, collect a midstream squirt of milk into an appropriate container (e.g., strip cup or sterile milk culture tube). Look for flakes or blood in the milk. When treating the udder, grasp the teat near the base and insert the cannula into the teat orifice and deliver the medication into the teat. Remove the cannula, occlude the teat end, and massage the teat to disseminate the medication. Dip the teat in an approved teat dip preparation. If the ewe is to be turned outside and the weather is cold (0° C), allow the udder to dry thoroughly before turning the ewe out. Failure to do this may cause the udder to become chapped, sore, or frostbitten.

Urine Collection

Collecting urine from sheep is easier than with many other patients. Have a specimen cup ready before starting. Hold the sheep in a standing position and pinch the nostrils closed until urination occurs. Generally, the sheep will urinate within 30 seconds. The nostrils may be held off for up to 1 minute. If the sheep does not urinate in that minute, allow the patient to rest for 1 or 2 minutes. Repeat the procedure as necessary to obtain a sample.

GENERAL CARE OF GOATS

The adult female (*doe*) gives birth to *kids* (kidding) following a 5-month gestation. Intact adult males are called *bucks*, and castrated males are called *wethers*. Although there is some demand for goat meat, the major use of goats today is milk production for fluid milk or cheese.

Goats are rising in popularity as an alternative farming enterprise and as pets. They are also used in many teaching and research institutions as models for animal or human diseases. The rise in popularity of goats has increased the need for veterinary team members to familiarize themselves with the nursing care and treatment techniques applicable to goats. Many of the techniques described below are similar to those used for other food animal species, with some adjustments for the species. The importance of the correct method of application of medications and correct dosage for the species cannot be overemphasized. The veterinary technician must be familiar with several basic principles of pharmacology to consider and choose the route of administration.

COMMON DIAGNOSTIC AND THERAPEUTIC TECHNIQUES

Oral Administration of Medication

Oral administration is generally suitable for medications that act on the stomach or intestines or for systemic action after intestinal absorption. Addition of drugs to feed and water can provide therapeutic amounts of drug only if such adulterated feed or water has an acceptable smell or taste, and if the patient's appetite is normal. Mass medication of feed and water is not reliable in goats, because sick goats are likely to have reduced feed and water intake. In addition, goats are very peculiar and may detect a change in odor or flavor and refrain from consuming the altered substance.

Oral liquid medication can be administered as a drench by use of a dosing bottle, drenching gun, or dosing syringe and stomach tube. Small volumes of fluid can be given with a drenching bottle. Stabilize the patient's head, and hold it horizontally at a normal to slightly raised position. With the patient's chin firmly held, the neck of the bottle is inserted into the corner of the mouth and on the back of the tongue, and the liquid medication is poured in the mouth to be swallowed by the goat. If the goat becomes restless or begins to cough, or if fluid runs out of the mouth, treatment must be stopped and the head lowered to prevent inhalation of the fluid. A drenching gun with a short nozzle or a catheter-tip dose syringe is preferred for oral dosing of medications. The tip of the drenching gun or dose syringe is inserted at the commissure of the lips, over the tongue. The nostrils are held off while the liquid medication is quickly dispensed over the tongue.

Boluses (large tablets) can be administered to goats by use of a balling gun. A sheep and goat balling gun is available commercially, or a calf-size gun will work equally well. It is best to have the goat in a corner so that it cannot back up. Fit a bolus snugly into the end of the balling gun. With the goat standing, insert one hand in the interdental space at the commissure of the lips to open the mouth. Insert the balling gun at the opposite corner of the mouth, and direct it carefully over the base of the tongue. Push the gun to the dorsal prominence of the tongue, being careful not to scrape the roof of the mouth. With the head lifted at about a 45-degree angle, push the plunger to "pop" the bolus down the throat. Anything deposited farther rostrally is usually chewed and rejected. Observe the goat for several seconds to be certain that it has swallowed the bolus and does not spit it out.

Orogastric intubation

An orogastric tube (stomach tube) can be used in goats for administration of a large volume of liquid medication or fluids. A 0.54-mm foal stomach tube works well for an adult goat. Restrain the goat appropriately. Use a wood block (with a hole in the middle), a tape roll, or an appropriately sized syringe case (with the end smoothed) as a mouth speculum. Place the speculum in the mouth and pass the lubricated stomach tube through the speculum and over the base of the tongue, into the esophagus and into the rumen. Assess the correct location of the tube by feeling the neck. Passage of the tube into the trachea usually elicits a pronounced cough. You can also smell the end of the tube for rumen gas, which has a characteristic smell. It is also possible to check for correct tube placement by auscultation of the left flank while air is blown into the tube in short, repeated puffs. A stomach pump or a dose syringe may be attached to the stomach tube for administration of the liquid. After fluid administration, flush the tube with some water, blow it free of fluid, kink the free end (to prevent residual fluid from falling into the pharynx or larynx), and withdraw the tube slowly.

In a goat herd, some kids are born very weak or become dehydrated after birth. A feeding probe or stomach tube can be used for administration of colostrum or oral electrolyte solution to save the kid. A commercially available baby lamb probe works very well for kids. This instrument, a stainless-steel ball probe attached to a syringe or dose gun (Fig. 27-11), is designed to prevent accidental entry into the trachea, thus protecting against fluid administration into the lungs. Place the kid on its right side with the head and neck extended. As you insert the probe in the mouth, place one hand around the neck so that you can feed the instrument's end into the esophagus. Do not force the probe. Give the kid a chance to relax and swallow to ease the tube's entry. Attach the syringe, and administer fluid.

A lamb-size probe can be used for kids; however, you can give oral fluids to kids using a small flexible rubber tube (see Fig. 27-11, as in adult goats. These tubes are also available commercially. Hold the tube from the mouth to the end of the last rib (flank area) to estimate the length necessary to reach the rumen. Mark near the top as a guide. Place the kid on its right side with head and neck extended slightly. Open the mouth slightly by pressing on either side of the jaw with your fingers. Slide the tube down the kid's throat as far as the previously marked area. You should feel slight resistance as the tube passes the back of the throat and enters the esophagus. If you feel no resistance, you have probably

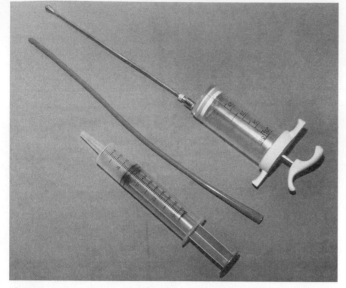

Fig. 27-11 Stainless-steel lamb probe *(top)*, flexible rubber tube *(center)*, and syringe *(bottom)*.

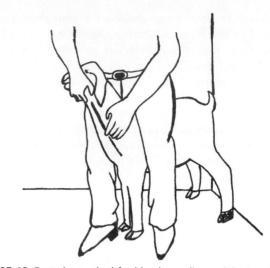

Fig. 27-12 Restraint method for blood sampling or injections into the jugular vein.

entered the trachea. The kid may also cough if the tube is in the trachea. The chance of placing the tube in the trachea is very slim because of the anatomy of a goat's pharynx; the tube almost always passes directly into the esophagus.

Parenteral Injection

Parenteral administration techniques routinely used in goats are SQ, IM, and IV. Whenever the efficacy of treatment is not compromised, drugs and vaccines should be given SQ rather than IM in goats to minimize damage to muscle tissue. It is advisable to use a separate sterile needle for each goat to prevent the spread of caprine arthritis encephalitis (CAE) virus.

Intravenous Injection

The jugular vein is always used for intravenous injections and blood sampling in the goat. To restrain the goat, have an assistant back the patient into a corner. Have the assistant hold the goat between his or her legs, with the goat's neck extended and turned slightly to one side (Fig. 27-12). To make the vein is easier to see, cleanse the upper two thirds of the jugular furrow with a swab soaked in 70% alcohol to remove dust and make the hair lie flat. Occlude the vein about two thirds of the way down the neck, at the jugular furrow or thoracic inlet. Insert the needle at a 45° angle with the tip directed cranially or caudad, with or without the syringe attached. After the needle enters the vein, thread the needle into the vein and aspirate or occlude the vein to ensure that the needle is in the vein before injecting the medication. If the needle comes out of the vein because of the goat's movement, stop injection at once and reposition the needle. It is best to give the injection in the opposite jugular vein if you are unsuccessful in reentering the vein.

Needle size used depends on the viscosity of the drug to be administered. Use the smallest needle possible, because this reduces discomfort to the patient and minimizes trauma. An 18- to 20-gauge, 2- to 3-cm needle is most commonly used.

Jugular Venipuncture and Catheterization

The jugular vein is commonly used to obtain blood samples from goats for various diagnostic tests. The procedure is the same as for IV injection. A Vacutainer needle and needle holder work well in goats for blood sampling.

IV catheterization of the jugular vein is commonly performed in goats for fluid therapy. If properly maintained, an IV catheter may remain functional for several days. An 18-gauge, 5- to 6-cm over-the-needle catheter is most often used in goats. Shorter catheters tend to come out of the vein. The jugular vein area should be clipped and surgically scrubbed as in other species. The vein is located as previously described for IV injection. The catheter is inserted into the vein at a 45° angle, toward the heart. Occlude the vein to ensure a backflow of blood before threading the catheter down the vein. Advance the catheter off of the needle until its entire length is in the vein. Cap the catheter, and flush with heparinized saline. Place butterfly tape around the catheter, and suture it to the skin. Securing a catheter by bandaging alone is not adequate in goats. Place a sterile gauze pad covered with an antiseptic ointment over the site where the catheter enters the skin, and wrap elastic adhesive tape around the neck to secure the suture butterfly.

Intramuscular Injection

Administer IM injections for a goat on the lateral aspect of the neck or semitendinosus/semimembranosus muscle (thigh) (Fig. 27-13). However, the preferred site for IM

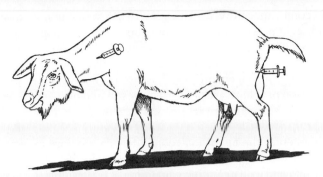

Fig. 27-13 Intramuscular injection sites on a goat.

injections is the lateral aspect of the neck, in a triangular region bounded by the vertebral column ventrally, the ligamentum nuchae dorsally, and the shoulder caudad. Injection into the thigh muscles should be avoided, because the muscle mass is small and sciatic nerve damage is a common complication. This is one of the most valuable parts of a goat carcass, and muscle damage may devalue the marketability of the meat. Gluteal muscles should not be used for injection in goats because of the small mass and the possibility of muscle damage.

For IM injection in an adult goat, use an 18- to 20-gauge, 2- to 3-cm needle. Use a 20- to 22-gauge, 2.5-cm needle for kids. The volume of injection should not be more than 5 ml per site. Use the same cleaning procedure as described for SQ injection. The needle for IM injections should be inserted at a 90-degree angle (perpendicular) to the muscle. Before injecting, aspirate the syringe plunger to ensure that the needle is not in a blood vessel. If blood enters the syringe, withdraw the needle and reinsert in another direction or choose another site. Massage the injection site after completing the injection and removing the needle.

Subcutaneous Injection

SQ injection in the goat is best made into the loose skin of the lateral side of the neck or on the chest wall about 5 cm caudad to the shoulder. Drug absorption is slower after SQ injection than after IM, but tissue tolerance is better. Before injection, vigorously rub the skin of the injection site with a piece of cotton soaked with 70% alcohol to clean and disinfect the skin. Repeat the swabbing process with a new cotton swab until the cotton is no longer dirty after swabbing. A fold of skin should be pinched up to form a tent. Insert a sharp needle by a sudden thrust at a 30- to 45-degree angle to the skin, with or without the syringe attached. Use an 18- to 20-gauge, 2- to 3-cm needle for adult goats and a 20- to 22-gauge, 2- to 3-cm needle for kids. Limit the volume of medication to 5 ml per site. If a large volume is to be injected, divide the dose into several portions injected at different sites. If done correctly, SQ injection should leave a bleb under the skin. After withdrawing the needle, massage

the site to disperse the medication. Avoid SQ injection along the back and dorsal flank if the hide is to be marketed. Vaccines should be injected SQ caudad to the shoulder, because local reactions near the prescapular lymph node may be confused with caseous lymphadenitis (lymph node abscess).

Intradermal Injection

ID injection is used for tuberculosis testing in goats. The injection site is the caudal tail fold. The skin is pinched and stabilized between the thumb and middle finger. A 25-gauge, 1-cm tuberculin needle is used. After cleaning the injection site, direct the needle bevel upward, hold the needle parallel to the skin, and gently insert it into the dermis. A small bleb, called a *wheal*, should be visualized as the drug is deposited. If a wheal is not formed, the needle tip is too deep; retract the needle and inject again.

Intrauterine Infusion

Intrauterine infusion is done in goats to treat retained placenta or metritis. The vulva should be scrubbed and rinsed thoroughly to remove contaminants. A sterile vaginal speculum and a light source are needed. The vaginal speculum, lubricated with sterile, water-soluble jelly, is inserted into the vagina. The light source is inserted inside the speculum, and the speculum is rotated cranially until the cervix is located. A sterile bovine insemination pipette is then inserted into the cervix by applying moderate pressure to penetrate the cervix and enter the uterus. A syringe is attached to the end of the pipette, and the appropriate amount of medicated fluid is infused into the uterus.

Intramammary Infusion

Intramammary infusion is routinely used in dairy goats for treatment of mastitis and before drying off. It consists of introduction of medication through the teat canal. Thoroughly clean the tips of the teats and disinfect them with alcohol swabs to prevent introduction of bacteria with the medication. Intramammary products formulated for cows are usually used in goats. These are available in special plastic syringes with a nozzle suitable for insertion into the teats. The end of the teat is held between two fingers of one hand, and the nozzle is inserted halfway into the teat canal and medication injected. Upon withdrawal of the nozzle, the teat is occluded and massaged, directing the fluid from the teat cistern into the glandular (udder) tissue. For very small teat openings, a sterile tomcat catheter can be used for teat infusion.

Urine and Milk Collection

A female goat generally urinates just after standing. However, urine samples for bacteriologic, chemical, and microscopic testing can be collected directly from the bladder by inserting a catheter using aseptic technique.

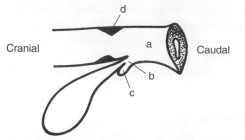

Fig. 27-14 Female goat genitalia. **A,** Vagina. **B,** Urethral orifice. **C,** Suburethral diverticulum. **D,** Cervix.

The doe should be suitably restrained and the vulva cleaned. A double-bladed small animal vaginal speculum is inserted into the vagina. Under visual control with illumination from a light, a sterile curved metal urinary catheter is inserted into the urethra. The tip of the catheter is first pushed a few millimeters into the suburethral diverticulum. Then the tip of the catheter is raised slightly to pass over the fold of mucous membrane at the entrance to the urethral orifice (Fig. 27-14). From this point cranially, no resistance should be encountered. If there is any resistance, the tip of the catheter is probably in the suburethral diverticulum.

Urethral catheterization of a male goat is difficult. Because of the presence of a urethral diverticulum at the level of the ischial arch, it is impossible to introduce a catheter into the urinary bladder of the buck.

Milk samples are commonly collected from dairy goats for bacteriologic examination and somatic cell counts. Disinfect each teat end with an alcohol-soaked cotton swab. Disinfect the teat on the far side of the udder first, then disinfect the one on the near side. Sterile sample tubes are labeled as to the particular quarter, the stopper is removed, and milk is directed into the tube held at a 45-degree angle, rather than held vertically. Milk samples are collected first from the near teat and then from the far one. Before a sample is collected, a small squirt of milk is discarded from each teat to flush out any bacteria present in the teat canal.

GENERAL CARE OF SWINE

The adult female (*sow*) gives birth to piglets (*farrowing*) after a gestation of 3 months, 3 weeks, and 3 days (about 114 days). The intact adult male is called a *boar*, and the castrated male is called a *barrow*. Young females are called *gilts* until they farrow.

Overview of Swine Production

The present trend in swine production is increased use of confinement rearing facilities. These facilities allow producers to raise more pigs per farm and to market pigs in 5 to 6 months. The increase in pig density raises concerns in regard to prevention of disease. If a disease occurs, the herd is affected and the economic loss can be devastating. Pigs become unhealthy because of disease transmission from adjacent pigs or infections from outside sources (e.g., trucking, feed, personnel, wind, or other species of animals). To best prevent disease, ensure good health status, nutrition, housing, management, and husbandry. Diseases and production problems are primarily investigated on a herd level.

Farrowing and piglets

Sows enter the farrowing room a few days before expected parturition. The farrowing room should be clean and disinfected with a solution containing chlorhexidine, formaldehyde solution, phenols, or a quaternary ammonium compound. The area provided for the piglets should be warm (30° to 35° C [86° to 95° F]) and dry to reduce the incidence of chilling and stress in newborn piglets. Litter size ranges from 7 to 12, and the average birth weight is approximately 1.5 kg. Maternal antibodies are transferred to piglets by ingestion of the sow's colostrum. The intestinal epithelial cells absorb the colostral antibodies. Intestinal absorption of colostrum halts by about 24 hours after birth. Therefore, to ensure adequate maternal antibody transfer, it is important that piglets begin nursing within 12 hours after birth.

Hypothermia is also a problem in newborn piglets. The piglet's body temperature at birth is 39° C (102.2° F) but decreases to 37° C (98.6° F) within a few hours. Over the next 24 hours, the piglet's body temperature returns to 39° C (102.2° F). An environmental temperature of 30° to 35° C (86° to 95° F) should be maintained with heat lamps and heat mats during this time of relative hypothermia.

Weaner pigs

This stage of growth is a stressful period. It begins with weaning and placement in a nursery barn. Pigs are approximately 5 to 8 kg at weaning and remain in the nursery until they weigh 25 kg. The diet at the time of weaning changes from predominantly milk to a highly palatable, digestible dry food diet. The level of maternal antibody is declining at this time, and the weaner pig is beginning to produce antibodies stimulated by natural exposure or vaccination. Feed-grade antibiotics are usually added to the diet to improve metabolism of feed. Warm (25° to 30° C [77° to 86° F]), dry housing and a clean, sanitized environment are also important to this group of pigs.

Grower-finisher pigs

This phase includes gilts, and barrows from 25 kg up to market weight at 90 kg to 110 kg. Finisher pigs are fed a mixture of ground corn, soybean meal, and a vitamin-mineral premix.

Breeding Stock

Breeding stock includes gilts, sows, and boars. In addition to the farrowing facility, housing for this phase is provided in the breeding and gestating areas. Breeding stock also require an environment that is clean and dry, with good lighting and minimal stress.

Handling and restraint

A significant animal welfare and production concern is the potential for stress from improper handling of pigs. Proper handling reduces stress during routine production practices, such as moving of hogs, blood sampling, vaccinating, clipping tails and teeth, ear notching, detusking, castration, and administration of therapeutics. Chapter 16 presents information on handling of pigs.

Surgical and processing procedures

Veterinary technicians are often involved in processing procedures as part of the herd health program. Although most producers are skilled in performing these procedures, technicians familiar with these procedures can assist new producers or help train farm employees. Processing includes tooth and umbilical cord clipping, tail docking, ear notching, and castration. Supplies and equipment needed for these practices are a disinfectant (chlorhexidine), tincture of iodine, side cutters, ear notching tool, and a castration knife or scalpel. Place the instruments in the disinfectant between uses.

Clipping teeth

The newborn piglet has eight very sharp canine (wolf) teeth. These teeth arm the piglet against its littermates to establish and maintain teat position on the sow. In large litters, if the needle teeth are left intact, the piglets scratch each other, causing infection. Cutting the teeth in smaller litters may be unnecessary, but many producers clip teeth as a precaution. Using clean, sharp side cutters, position the side cutters parallel to the gumline and clip off the distal half of each tooth. Take care not to cut the pig's gum or tongue. Cutting too short may shatter the teeth, leading to gum infection.

Clipping the umbilical cord. The umbilical cord can act as a portal of entry for bacteria. If the piglet is bleeding from the umbilical cord, tie off the cord immediately using string. Cut the cord 4 to 5 cm from the abdominal wall using disinfected side cutters. Spray with or dip the end of the cord in 2% povidone-iodine.

Tail docking

The tail of piglets is commonly clipped to reduce the incidence of tail biting later in the grower-finisher stage. This behavioral vice may result in stress, lameness, and paralysis. The tail is docked approximately 2 cm from the base using clean, slightly dull side cutters to crush it. Cauterizing clippers tend to reduce the amount of bleeding. Cutting the tail too short may result in anal prolapse.

Castration and inguinal hernia repair

After puberty, male pigs may have an offensive odor or "boar taint" that is evident in pork during cooking. Therefore, marketing of intact males is not allowed in the United States or Canada. There are various techniques of castration, each determined by the age and size of the pig. The best time to castrate is before 3 weeks of age and preferably before 2 weeks.

The disadvantage to early castration is reduced detection of inguinal hernias. A knife blade can be used in boars of any size. A hooked blade (No. 12) works well with pigs weighing less than 15 kg.

Pigs castrated between 2 weeks and 16 weeks of age can be held by the back legs, with the abdomen toward the operator and the back of the pig cradled between the restrainer's legs (Fig. 27-15).

COMMON DIAGNOSTIC AND THERAPEUTIC TECHNIQUES

Oral Administration of Medication

To administer oral medication, restrain the pig as follows: Place the left thumb caudad to the pig's right ear, assuming the handler is right-handed. Place the left index finger in the corner of the left side of the mouth, bringing the lips inside the pig's mouth caudad to the needle teeth to protect the handler from the sharp teeth. Placing the finger inside the mouth also encourages swallowing. Place the remaining fingers under the jaw to support the pig's weight. *Caution:* Piglets can be choked if the remaining fingers are placed around the throat instead of under the jaw.

Intravenous Injection

IV injections are commonly given in the auricular vein (Table 27-1). Pigs less than 15 kg can be held, whereas

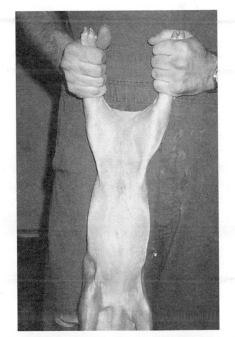

Fig. 27-15 Restraint for subcutaneous injection and castration.

TABLE 27-1

Recommended Needle Sizes, Injection Volumes, and Blood Sample Volumes, Based on Pig Size

	Injections			Blood Sampling					
	IM	SC	IV	Cranial vena cava	Jugular vein	Ear vein	Medial canthus	Tail vein	Cephalic vein
Piglet									
Needle	18-20 gauge, 11 mm	21 gauge, 11 mm		20 gauge, 38 mm	20 gauge, 38 mm		20 gauge, 25 mm		
Quantity	1-2 ml/site			Unlimited			5-10 ml		
Weaner									
Needle	18-20 gauge, 18 mm	21 gauge, 25 mm		20 gauge, 38 mm	20 gauge, 38 mm		20 gauge, 25 mm		20 gauge, 38 mm
Quantity	1-2 ml/site			Unlimited			5-10 ml		5-10 ml
Grower-finisher									
Needle	16 gauge, 18-25 mm	18 gauge, 25 mm		18 gauge, 65 mm	20 gauge, 38 mm	20 gauge, 25 mm	16 gauge, 38 mm		
Quantity	1-3 ml/site			Unlimited		1-2 ml	5-10 ml		
Breeding stock									
Needle	14-16 gauge, 38 mm	18 gauge, 38 mm		16 gauge, 90 mm	20 gauge, 38 mm	20 gauge, 25 mm	14 gauge, 38 mm	20 gauge, 25 mm	
Quantity	1-3 ml/site			Unlimited		1-2 ml	5-10 ml	5-10 ml	

larger pigs should be restrained using a snare. The auricular vein, near the lateral border of the ear, is prominent when held off using a hand or a rubber band as a tourniquet at the base of the ear. After 1 minute, the ear veins become engorged. A butterfly catheter set may be placed for administration of solutions.

Intramuscular Injection

Use the area of the neck muscle caudad to the ear (Fig. 27-16). Avoid injecting pharmaceuticals into the shoulder, loin, or ham so as to prevent contamination of the meat if an abscess should develop at the injection site. Pull the skin back, seat the needle into the neck muscle, inject the substance, and release the skin. Use finger pressure if the injection site is bleeding. Do not inject more than 2 ml of medication into one site (see Table 27-1). Try to use the same injection site for each product. If a particular site shows signs of irritation, you can determine which product is causing the reaction.

Subcutaneous Injection

Some vaccines and anthelmintics are given SQ (see Table 27-1). The lower vascularity of the SQ layer allows for slower release of product into the system. SQ injections in pigs less than 25 kg are given primarily in the loose skin of

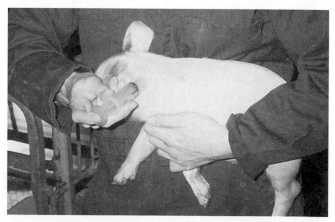

Fig. 27-16 Site for intramuscular injection.

the flank or caudad to the elbow. If injecting into the flank, inject into the folds of the skin and not into the peritoneal cavity. In larger pigs, the preferred injection site is the loose skin caudad to the ear.

Intranasal Injection

Pigs less than 15 kg can be held, whereas larger pigs should be snared and the head elevated. Use a syringe (without a needle) or a special adapter to dispense the medication. Direct the product into the nostril, keeping the pig's head tilted upward during and immediately following administration. To prevent the pig from ejecting the solution by sneezing, time the injection with inspiration.

Blood Collection

Venipuncture is an integral part of blood sampling and administration of solutions. Venipuncture can be achieved using the cranial vena cava, jugular vein, auricular (ear) vein, medial canthus of the eye, or cephalic vein. Techniques for collecting blood from pigs depend on the age and weight of the pigs and restraint techniques available. Table 27-1 shows appropriate blood-collection techniques and needle sizes required for various sizes of pig.

Cranial vena cava and jugular vein

The cranial vena cava and jugular vein venipuncture techniques are most commonly used to retrieve 5 to 20 ml of blood from a large number of pigs. These techniques are cost-effective and expedient; however, some skill is required by the handler and the blood collector. The methods used and anatomy of the area have been described elsewhere. The handler, restraining the pig with a snare, should ensure that the pig is aligned with the shaft of the snare, with the head raised, and neck extended to expose the jugular fossa (Fig. 27-17).

To access the cranial vena cava, the collector should identify the right jugular furrow to the point just cranial to and to the right of the manubrium. The approach is made from the pig's right side, because the right vagus nerve provides less innervation to the heart and diaphragm than the left vagus (accidental puncture of the vagus nerve can cause cyanosis, dyspnea, and convulsive struggling). The needle is directed toward the top of the opposite shoulder blade,

while a slight vacuum is maintained in the syringe. When the vena cava is entered, blood fills the test tube or syringe.

Jugular vein

The collector identifies the deepest hollow in the jugular furrow approximately 5 to 8 cm cranial to and to the right of the manubrium. The needle, usually seated on a Vacutainer, is positioned perpendicular to the skin. The needle and Vacutainer are then directed toward the same shoulder blade of the pig. The advantage of jugular venipuncture is the high degree of safety for the pig. The needle length (38 mm) is unlikely to penetrate the vagus nerve and lymphatics. The jugular vein is not as large as the cranial vena cava, however, and the shorter needle makes the jugular vein more difficult to penetrate in older and overweight pigs.

Auricular vein

This vein is generally used for collecting small samples of only 2 to 5 ml. The procedure is the same as for intravenous injection. An 18- to 20-gauge butterfly catheter can be used for blood collection.

Medial canthus

Blood can be collected from the venous sinus located near the medial canthus of the eye (Fig. 27-18). A small pig can be held in dorsal recumbency on a 45-degree incline, with the head down and the hind end elevated. A larger pig should be restrained with a snare. Position the needle at a 45-degree angle from both the surface of the eye and the nose, and pass it into the medial canthus, just inside (deep to) the nictitating membrane. Direct the needle toward the other side of the jaw until it strikes the lacrimal bone. Rotate the needle until blood flows.

Tail vein

Blood collection from the tail vein is limited to adult pigs without docked tails. The vein is located on the ventral midline of the tail at the junction of the tail with the body.

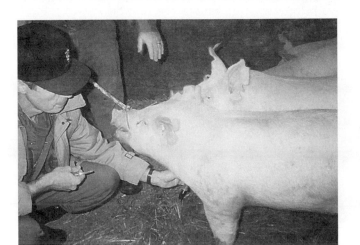

Fig. 27-17 Proper positioning of the pig for blood collection from the cranial vena cava and jugular vein. This pig is being restrained with a hog snare.

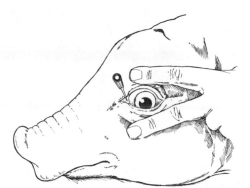

Fig. 27-18 Collection of blood from the medial canthus.

The volume of blood typically obtained is approximately 2 to 5 ml.

GENERAL CARE OF CAMELIDS

Llamas and alpacas are part of a larger group of South American camelids or New World camelids. In recent years, South American camelids have gained popularity, and increasing numbers are now being raised in the United States. Four species of the Lamini tribe are found in South America. The llama (*Lama glama*) and the alpaca (*Lama pacos*) were domesticated about five thousand years ago, whereas the guanaco (*Lama guanicoe*) and the vicuna (*Vicugna vicugna*) are undomesticated.

Anatomic and Physiologic Characteristics

The *llama* is the largest of the four species. The face is usually free of wool, with a long, straight to slightly rounded nose (Fig. 27-19). The ears are also long and erect. The wool covers much of the neck and the body. The back is flat, ending in a tail that curls up and back. The colors are solid black, white, brown, or shaded, but they can also be spotted (Appaloosa), patched, or multicolored.

The *alpaca* is smaller than the llama. It has short ears, a wooly face, a rounded rump, and a straight tail (Fig. 27-20). In the United States, 22 colors are recognized. The *guanaco* is slightly smaller than the llama but of similar conformation. The ears and nose are smaller than those of the llama. All guanacos have the same color pattern: soft brown to rust on the upper body and a white underbelly. Guanacos can be unpredictable and are undomesticated. The *vicuna* is the smallest and the rarest of the four species. They have a small head and a long, thin neck. Their color pattern is consistently golden brown, with a white chest. The vicuna is also undomesticated and in South America is protected from hunting.

A unique feature of camelids is that they have a stomach with three compartments, rather than four like other ruminants. For this reason, they are not considered true ruminants, although they do ruminate, chew their cud, and digest cellulose. The first compartment represents more than 80% of the total stomach in volume and is equivalent to the rumen and reticulum of true ruminants.

A split upper lip facilitates food prehension. Only three pairs of incisors are found in the lower jaw. Together with the upper dental pad, these teeth facilitate browsing and nipping. Eruption of the adult incisors starts at 2 years for the central incisors, 3 years for the middle incisors, and 4 years for the corner incisors. The upper corner incisors and upper and lower canines develop into sharp scimitar-shaped teeth that are used by males in fighting. These teeth erupt in males around 2 to 3 years and are usually removed surgically.

Llamas have two digits on each foot. The second and third phalanges are positioned horizontally and do not bear weight, whereas the first phalanx is in an upright position. A nail (not a hoof) protects the end of the foot, and a digital cushion and a soft pad on the palmar surface supports the remainder of the foot. The nail may need periodic trimming.

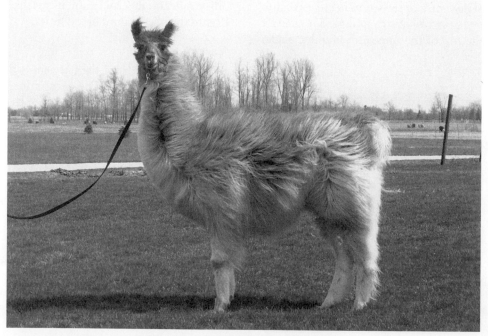

Fig. 27-19 Lateral view of an adult llama.

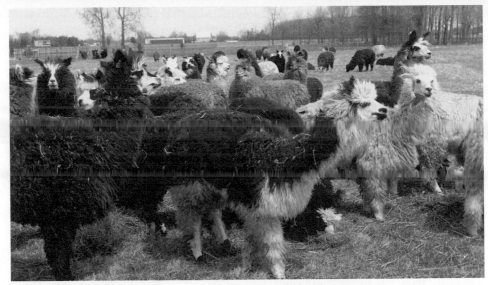

Fig. 27-20 Herd of alpacas. Note the varied coloration.

The skin in the cranial cervical region is very thick (up to 1 cm in adult males). The ventral projection of the transverse processes of the caudal cervical vertebrae forms an inverted *U*, covering the vessel of the neck. The jugular vein is deep in the neck and close to the carotid artery. The location of the jugular vein makes blood sampling and intravenous injection difficult. The uterus of the female llama is bicornuate, with a small uterine body. Most pregnancies occur in the left horn. Although pregnancies have been observed in female llamas as young as six (6) months, it is recommended to delay breeding until 12 months of age. Breeding usually takes place while the female assumes a sternal recumbent position with the male straddling her. Copulation usually lasts about 20 minutes. Ovulation is induced during copulation. Pregnancy is confirmed by rectal palpation at 35 to 40 days, ultrasound findings, or serum progesterone levels above 1 ng/ml at 21 days. The normal gestation period is 335 to 350 days. Most births occur rapidly and typically during daylight hours. Teat enlargement usually occurs 1 to 3 weeks prepartum, with milk letdown 48 to 72 hours before parturition, although the teats can also enlarge after parturition. Table 27-2 lists physical and physiologic characteristics of camelids.

Neonatal Care

At birth, crias are covered by a semitransparent epidermal membrane attached to all mucocutaneous junctions. Within an hour after birth, normal crias can stand and nurse. Average birth weight ranges from 8 to 18 kg. Llama crias weighing less than 8 kg are considered premature or dysmature and may require special attention. Alpaca crias are somewhat smaller; crias weighing less than 5 kg are considered premature.

TABLE 27-2

Physical and Physiologic Characteristics of South American Camelids

	Llama	Alpaca	Guanaco	Vicuna
Height (cm)				
At the withers	115-130	75-95	—	90
At the poll	150-180			
Weight (kg)				
Male	132-244	60-80	100-150	40-65
Female	108-200	55	100-120	30-40
Rectal temperature (°Celsius)	37.2-38.7	37.2-38.7	37.2-38.7	37.2-38.7
Heart rate (beats/min)	60-90	60-90	60-90	60-90
Respiratory rate (resp./min.)	10-30	10-30	10-30	10-30

The first consideration is to make sure the cria can breathe by clearing the membranes and mucus away from the mouth and nostrils. A bulb syringe can be used to carefully suction mucus from the nostril. In addition, lifting and supporting the cria can help clear amniotic fluid from the respiratory tract. Rubbing the back or tickling the nose with a piece of straw can stimulate respiration. Artificial respiration can be done by mouth to nose resuscitation or more effectively by placing a small rubber tube (6 to 7 mm) in the cria's nostril and gently blowing intermittently at about 10 times/minute. Choanal atresia is a frequent congenital abnormality of llamas of which to be aware. Because llamas and alpacas are obligate nasal breathers, crias with these congenital abnormalities show difficulty in breathing, even when fluids have been cleared. Postpartum care of the cria should include dipping the umbilical cord in 7% tincture of iodine or chlorhexidine diluted to a 0.5% solution. This should be done three times within the first 24 hours. Additional care includes drying and weighing the cria and watching for nursing of the colostrum. Normal crias nurse within the first hour following delivery. Crias nurse three or four times per hour, usually for less than 30 seconds each time. If the cria has not been observed nursing for 6 hours, supportive care should be given and llama colostrum should be given in feedings of about 100 to 200 ml every 2 to 3 hours. Goat or cow colostrum can be used as a substitute. Passage of meconium (first bowel movement) should occur within the first 18 to 20 hours.

For compromised crias, oxygen support is provided with a small tube inserted in one nostril and taped to the bridge of the nose. The tube is connected to humidified oxygen and is advanced to the premeasured level of the eye. Initially, the oxygen flow rate is set at 5 L/minute and adjusted to the patient's needs, based on serial evaluations of arterial blood gases. Intravenous fluid is delivered via a 16- to 18-gauge, 5-cm catheter placed aseptically in the jugular vein or, alternatively, in the saphenous vein. The skin of the neonate is usually thin and may not require incision as in the adult, although it may be easier to make a small incision after disinfection and lidocaine desensitization. If long-term catheterization is necessary, a longer, flexible, 14-cm catheter is used. Cyanoacrylate glue is used to bond the hub of the catheter to the skin. Fluid maintenance requirements have not been established for crias. A rate of 60 to 80 ml/kg/day, plus additional fluid requirements to replace ongoing losses, is often used. The efficacy of fluid support is evaluated by frequent weight determination, urine production, and signs of overhydration.

If the cria does not or is not able to nurse, nutritional support can be provided by bottle feeding (soft plastic bottle with a lamb nipple) or orogastric tubing (Fig. 27-21). Tube feeding a cria is easy. A stallion catheter or soft rubber feeding tube is convenient for this use. Before insertion, hold the tube against the patient's side and measure the distance from the mouth to the base of the neck. Water-soluble lubricant (K-Y Jelly) is applied to the tube, which is then slowly passed into the mouth. As the tube is swallowed and advanced to the premeasured length, it should be seen and felt on the side of the neck next to the trachea. To ensure that the tube is in the esophagus and not in the trachea, blow on the tube and watch for the stomach to expand or listen for gurgling sounds. Inject 10 to 15 ml of water into

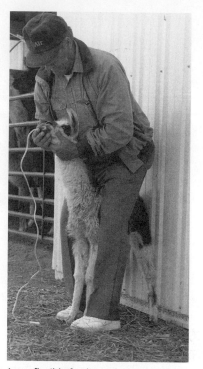

Fig. 27-21 Passing a flexible feeding tube into the nostril of a cria. Note that the cria is restrained by backing against a wall.

the tube before feeding. If the patient gags and/or coughs, the tube is probably in the lungs and should be withdrawn. If a substitute for the dam's milk is necessary, straight goat's milk or a 3:1 volume to volume mixture of goat milk and goat yogurt is recommended.

Behavior, Handling, and Restraint

Llamas and alpacas are shy but curious animals that are usually easy to handle. They are social animals with a strong herd instinct. In a comfortable environment, the ears of the llama are erect and directed rostrally (forward). When a llama is upset, the ears are flattened against the head and the nose is elevated and they begin to vocalize (*orgle*); if they remain agitated, the llama may spit (actually regurgitate stomach contents) and continue to vocalize. Although llamas frequently spit at each other when competing for food or to assess territoriality, they rarely spit at humans. To handle a spitting patient, place a towel or other type of cloth over the muzzle.

Male llamas may bite, charge, or butt with their chest. They may also kick with their rear legs and inflict injury. Llamas rarely charge or bite humans, except for the so-called berserk male syndrome or aberrant male syndrome displayed by some bottle-raised male llamas.

In most cases, a satisfactory approach to working with llamas is to have the client catch and halter the patient before the patient is seen by the veterinarian. If it has not been caught, it is easier to move the whole herd to a smaller enclosure before trying to isolate one patient for examination. Once cornered, the patient can be approached to place a lead rope or an arm around the neck or apply a halter. The person placing the halter should avoid direct eye contact; touching the head of the llama should be minimized. Adult llamas can be easily restrained with a halter and lead rope. Crias (juvenile llamas) can be handled by placing a hand around the front of the neck and grasping around the rump or at the base of the tail. A restraining chute can be very useful for veterinary procedures. Temporary restraint can be achieved using an ear twitch. The base of the ear is encircled with the palm of the hand and squeezed. The ear should not be twisted. Consult the client before using this method.

Herd Health

Immunization

A minimal vaccination program should include Clostridium perfringens C/D and tetanus. Recommendations include annual C/D and tetanus administration for all juveniles (starting at 3 months) and adults. Pregnant females should receive a C/D and tetanus booster 1 month before the anticipated parturition date. Recent information indicates that vaccination of the cria within the first week of age, followed by two monthly boosters, is effective irrespective of colostral immunity. Immunization with a 7- or 8-way clostridial vaccine may cause significant injection site reactions. Other vaccines to consider vary with the area of the country. If leptospirosis is a problem in the region, biannual vaccination of brood females should be considered. No rabies vaccine efficacy testing has been conducted in the llama, yet no adverse reaction following administration of the killed vaccine has been reported.

Parasite control

New World camelids are susceptible to all the nematode parasites that affect ruminants. *Parelophostrongylus tenuis* is a major concern in areas inhabited by white-tailed deer. In enzootic liver fluke areas, llamas should be checked periodically for flukes. Coccidiosis may be a significant cause of diarrhea in young animals. Establishment of a parasite-control program depends on the geographic area, climatic conditions, number of animals, and stocking rate. Fenbendazole and ivermectin have been used successfully to control most nematodes. A minimum of two dewormings (spring and fall) is recommended. In areas with meningeal worms, monthly deworming with ivermectin or daily administration of Strongid C can be used.

Lice are the most common external parasites of llama herds. Topical treatment with organophosphate or carbamate powder is effective. Mange mite infestation is not very common, probably because of extensive use of ivermectin.

Common procedures

Male llamas generally need to have their fighting teeth (incisors and canines) cut by 2 to 2.5 years of age. This procedure can be rapidly done in a restraining chute or under general anesthesia using a surgical wire. Castration is usually performed after 2 years of age but can be done earlier if necessary.

The author is grateful to Kesling's Llamas and Alpacas for their assistance in obtaining the photographs used in this section.

COMMON DIAGNOSTIC AND THERAPEUTIC TECHNIQUES

Oral Administration of Medication

Medication, fluids, or food can be administered with a stomach tube. The technique is fairly similar to the procedure for sheep and cattle. Adult llamas usually resist and may regurgitate, increasing the likelihood of aspiration pneumonia. Restraint is important, and use of a chute with cross-ties is helpful. A speculum is necessary to protect the tube. A Frick's speculum used in cattle is usually too large, except for the largest llamas. A 20-cm segment of PVC pipe, slightly wider than the stomach tube, can be used. The edges must be smoothed or wrapped with adhesive tape. Once the head is secured and slightly flexed, the lubricated tip of the stomach tube is advanced caudad through the speculum to the throat. Gentle pressure and rotation of the tube encourage swallowing. You should feel some resistance as the tube is advanced into the esophagus. The most reliable sign of correct tube placement is palpating it in the left cervical region.

Intravenous Injection

The landmarks and the technique for IV injection are similar to those used for blood collection. The tip of the needle is directed caudad so that the operator is warned of inadvertent carotid artery penetration by high-pressure, bright red blood exiting the hub of the needle. If intravenous catheterization is required, the same technique can be applied in the midcervical area. The right jugular vein is preferred to avoid the esophagus. A large area is clipped and prepared. Except in juveniles or adults with thin skin, the turgid vein is not seen but can occasionally be felt upon percussion. The skin is usually penetrated superficially with a No. 15 scalpel blade. Then a sterile 16- or 14-gauge, 14-cm catheter is inserted and secured to the skin.

Intramuscular Injection

The general rules for giving injections are similar to those for other species, including the need for proper restraint, swabbing of the injection site, and checking for the presence of blood by pulling back on the syringe plunger before injecting the product. IM injections can be done in any large muscle mass using a 22- to 16-gauge, 4-cm needle, depending on the viscosity of the drug. The neck region should be avoided. On most llamas restrained in a chute, the hind legs are most accessible. The semimembranosus and semitendinosus muscles are the sites of choice. If frequent injections are needed, the injection sites should be rotated to avoid soreness. The area of the triceps in the angle formed by the scapula and the humerus may also be used.

Subcutaneous Injection

The technique for SQ injection is similar to that used in other species. The preferred sites include the skin of the thorax and caudad to the elbow, where wool is usually absent.

Blood Collection

Superficial veins are not readily accessible. There is no jugular groove, and visualization of the jugular vein is impossible. Jugular venipuncture can be done at a cranial or caudal location on the neck. The landmark in the cranial location is ventral to a line extending from the ventral border of the mandible to the lateral surface of the neck. Locate the tendon of the sternocephalicus muscle on the neck, and penetrate the vein just caudad to the tendon (Fig. 27-22). Identify the site on the caudal neck by palpating the vertebral process of the fifth or sixth cervical vertebra.

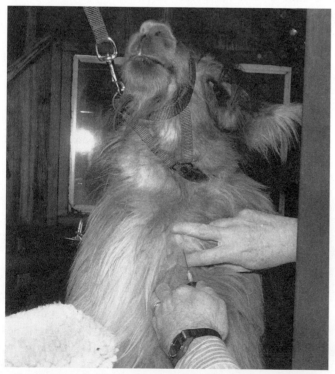

Fig. 27-22 Collecting blood from the jugular vein of an adult llama.

Insert the needle slightly medial to the tip of the process, and direct it toward the center of the neck. This must be done carefully, because the carotid artery is close to the jugular vein. Blood can also be collected from an ear vein near the caudal edge of the pinna. Bend the ear, and insert the needle into the vein. Blood is collected while dripping from the hub. This method is less desirable because llamas are usually head shy. The midventral vein of the tail is located in a similar location as in cattle. The saphenous artery and vein can be used for blood collection in recumbent llamas. The artery and vein can be located on the medial aspect of the stifle. In crias, the cephalic vein can also be used. The location is similar to the position of the cephalic vein in dogs.

Urine Collection

If urine cannot be collected by free catch, bladder catheterization can be performed in female llamas. Free-catch collection of urine is better done in the morning, when llamas go to the dung pile. Bladder catheterization is virtually impossible in the male. In the female llama, catheterization is fairly easy. The external urethral orifice is easily palpated on the floor of the vulva. The ventral suburethral diverticulum complicates catheterization. After the vulva has been thoroughly cleaned, a sterile gloved finger is advanced in the vulva to palpate the meatus. The finger is withdrawn slightly and the catheter (No. 5 French) is advanced into the urethra above the finger to avoid the diverticulum. If the meatus is difficult to palpate, a sterile bitch speculum can be used to visualize it.

GENERAL CARE OF RATITES

Ratites are a group of nonflying birds that include the ostrich *(Struthio casmelus)*, the emu *(Dromaius novaehollandiae)*, and the rhea *(Rhea americana)*. The cassowary *(Casuarius casuarius)* is also included in this group; it is primarily concentrated on the West Coast of the United States.

Visual Evaluation

Visual assessment of the entire flock may provide pertinent information about individual health. The birds' activity level should be noted. The initial response when a stranger approaches and enters a pen is for the birds to run from the intruder. Most will then return out of curiosity. When possible, observe the birds while they are eating. A food bolus can normally be observed as it passes down the cervical esophagus. Unhealthy or sick birds may go through the motions as if they are eating, pecking, and throwing their head upward as if to swallow, but no food bolus is seen passing down the neck. Closer examination should be performed on birds that are inactive, that lag behind, or that are not actively eating.

Note asymmetry of the neck and dorsal spine, and deviations of the appendages. During visual examination, note condition of the integumentary system. Unthrifty plumage may indicate trauma, ectoparasites, nutritional deficiency, or feather plucking by other birds, suggesting overcrowding or boredom.

Physical Examination

The heart rate (60 to 120 beats/min) is most easily determined by auscultation laterally, between the ribs. The respiratory rate (10 to 40 breaths/min) is best determined visually in the unrestrained patient. Temperature (38° to 40° C [100° to 104° F]) can be measured with a rectal or tympanic membrane thermometer. The external ear canal is a large opening caudad to the mandible at the base of the skull. Cloacal temperatures may be 1 or 2 degrees lower than tympanic membrane temperature.

The eye can be superficially examined with a good penlight. The ear canal is easily explored with an otoscope for parasites, hemorrhage, or masses. When the mouth is opened, the mucous membranes are evaluated for color (pink) and capillary refill time (<2.5 sec). Symmetry of the choana (nasopharynx), glottis, and rostral trachea should be noted. Choanal or tracheal swabs can be made for bacterial culture and cytology when a discharge is noted. The neck is palpated for asymmetry of the trachea, right jugular vein, and vertebrae.

The thorax is auscultated and palpated. Auscultation is performed, noting abnormal respiratory sounds associated with the lungs or air sacs. Heart murmurs can also be detected by auscultation of the thorax. There is very little muscle over the thorax, making palpation easy for any signs of asymmetry associated with rib fractures or masses.

The abdomen is easily palpated in the chick. Structures that should be noted include the proventriculus and yolk sac. The proventriculus lies just to the left of the midline, caudad to the rib cage. The structure is firm to the touch and should have feed material within it that is easily compressed with gentle pressure. An empty proventriculus is firm. The yolk sac has the feel of a large bladder, decreasing in size over a 2-week period, when it should be absorbed. As the yolk sac is absorbed, the intestines become more palpable in the young chick.

These structures are not as evident in the adult bird. However, impaction associated with the proventriculus or egg retention can be recognized during careful evaluation of the adult bird's abdomen.

The cloaca should be examined for accumulation of fecal matter and urates on the feathers surrounding the opening. This commonly indicates illness or depression. Mucosal prolapse may be indicative of intestinal obstruction or local trauma. The genitalia can also be evaluated within the cloacal sphincter.

The skin and feathers are evaluated for parasites and trauma. These birds groom themselves, so the feathers should be relatively clean and well separated, unless they have recently given themselves a dust bath. Feather regrowth is a good indicator of adequate nutrition. The wings and limbs of the birds should be examined closely, both visually and by palpation. Ostriches and rheas have well developed wings, whereas the wing of the emu is vestigial and difficult to see when it is held close to the body. Asymmetry is noted, and the structures are palpated for fractures and dislocations.

The thigh and calf regions are well-muscled, making direct palpation of the femur and tibiotarsus difficult. The tarsometatarsus and phalanges are easily palpated, because very little tissue covers these areas. Swollen joints should be noted and the cause explored. The tendons and their sheaths should be examined for pain and swelling. Tendon luxation over the tibiotarsus and the metatarsophalangeal joint are common injuries. The foot should always be examined closely for heat, pain, and swelling. Asymmetry surrounding a phalangeal joint should be carefully explored because of the common incidence of puncture wounds involving these joints. Traumatic avulsion of the toenails may lead to localized infection.

Restraint

Restraining is one of the most important skills to master when working with ratites. Many clients are unable to restrain their birds, and frequently their facilities are less than ideal. The birds have very powerful legs that can inflict severe trauma from kicking. The emu, rhea, and cassowary have sharp claws that can easily lacerate the handler. The danger zone when working on ratites is directly in front of the birds, because they strike forward when they kick. The emu and rhea can also kick to the side, but the most powerful segment of the kick is in front.

Chicks can easily be handled by placing a hand between their legs while cupping the sternum and picking them up, much like holding a football. While in a sitting position, the handler can treat small juvenile birds by placing the bird in the lap, with the bird's legs squeezed between the handler's knees. Larger juveniles can be held standing from the back or from the side, keeping the bird close to the handler's body. When restraining from the back, spread your feet apart to help maintain balance, but hold your knees close together to prevent the bird from backing under you.

Adult birds are more difficult and risky to handle. It is frequently necessary to capture large juveniles or adult ostriches in an open pen. Applying a loose, tubular cloth hood over the head and covering the eyes commonly calms the bird so that evaluation and treatment can be carried out (Fig. 27-23). These birds are generally curious and will approach strangers. Place the hood over the handler's forearm. When the bird is within reach, grasp the neck and pull

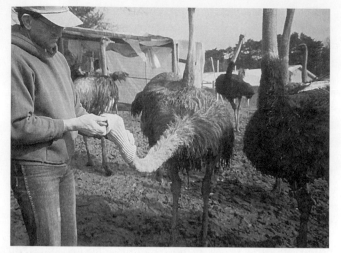

Fig. 27-23 Ostriches can be calmed by applying a cloth hood, such as a sock with the toe cut off.

it down parallel to the ground with the opposite hand. Simultaneously grasp the beak and evert the hood over the head, leaving the nares exposed. If the bird does not approach the handler, a shepherd's hook can be used to capture the head. Then apply the hood as described. To move the bird, have a second handler grasp the tail from behind, pushing forward as gentle traction on the neck steers in the desired direction. Ostriches can also be restrained in stocks or in chutes designed for the birds. When this type of facility is not available, the bird can be restrained by squeezing it between a solid gate and a wall. Caution should be used when working around adult birds, especially males during the breeding season, as these birds can be aggressive.

Emus in general are not aggressive, and males frequently become more docile during the breeding season. Adult emus present more difficulty in handling, because they commonly become very fractious when restrained. Their sharp claws and rough, scaly tarsometatarsus can tear clothing and severely abrade the handler's skin. Many emus do not resist mild restraint. To catch and restrain them, pass an arm around the neck near the sternum and pull the bird firmly into your upper legs and trunk, tilting the bird into an upright position. Low placement of the arm minimizes the chance of injury from kicking. The bird can be moved from this position if you are careful to keep the patient in contact with your body. Sometimes moving the bird backward is easier than moving forward, and it is occasionally necessary to simply pick the bird up to move it.

Male rheas are the most aggressive of the three common species. Two handlers can most easily accomplish restraint. The first handler catches the bird as described for emus. The second handler then grasps the bird's legs and pulls the bird to the ground between the first handler's legs. With the bird's legs held, one individual straddles the recumbent bird on his or her knees, placing gentle pressure on the dorsum of the bird.

A hood can be applied to rheas, but the results are much less predictable than with ostriches. Another option that should be considered, when possible, is working on the birds in a darkened enclosure. This environment has a calming effect on the birds.

COMMON DIAGNOSTIC AND THERAPEUTIC TECHNIQUES

Oral Administration of Medication

Orogastric intubation

Gastric intubation is used to administer fluids, nutrients, and medication. Open the mouth by grasping the upper beak, and direct the tube over the glottis. Once past the glottis, the tube is easily visualized externally, passing down the cervical esophagus. Take care to prevent regurgitation while administering substances through the tube. Esophagostomy tube placement should be considered when long-term enteral nutrition is indicated.

Pill administration

Pills or boluses can be given by grasping the upper beak and gently prying the mouth open. Occasionally, you must insert a finger into the commissure to assist in opening the mouth. Then place the pill over the glottis and use a finger to push it into the cervical esophagus.

Administration of Injections

SQ injections can be given over the lateral thorax caudad to the leg. Lift the skin and insert the needle with care to prevent inadvertent penetration into the chest cavity. IM injections are usually given in the abaxial muscles over the rump and in the proximal thigh. IV injections are administered in the same locations as described for blood sampling, although the metatarsal vein is seldom used for this purpose.

Blood Collection and Catheterization

Blood sampling and catheterization can be performed on the right jugular, cutaneous ulnar, and medial metatarsal veins. The jugular vein is easily distended and visualized in the ostrich and rhea. Watching for feather motion along the course of the distending vein on the neck helps to locate it in the emu. Feathers can be plucked to help visualize the vessel. When this vessel is catheterized, placement is in the upper (cranial) one third of the neck, to prevent the bird from pulling it out. Care is taken not to penetrate the trachea or esophagus.

In the ostrich and rhea, the cutaneous ulnar vein is located on the ventral aspect of the wing, coursing over the distal antebrachium. The vestigial wing in the emu makes this vein impractical for blood sampling and catheterization. Catheters placed in the wing vein should be protected to prevent the bird from pulling them out.

The medial metatarsal vein is located on the medial aspect of the leg, paralleling the metatarsus. Care is taken when collecting blood from this area, because the vessel is easily lacerated if the bird kicks during sampling.

Needles and catheters of 20 to 22 gauge are commonly used in these birds. Larger catheters can be placed in the jugular vein when rapid fluid volume replacement is indicated.

Heparin tubes should be used for collecting ostrich blood, because EDTA adversely affects it. This sample can be used for both hematologic and serum chemistry evaluations. EDTA and clot tubes are suitable for blood collection in emus and rheas.

Fluid Therapy

Fluids can be administered parenterally or enterally. Parenteral administration is performed SQ or IV. Maintenance fluids are administered at 13 ml/kg/hr (range 5 to 28 ml/kg/hr). Enteral fluid administration is performed via an orogastric tube.

RECOMMENDED READING

Cattle

Howard JL: *Current veterinary therapy 3: food animal practice,* Philadelphia, 1993, WB Saunders.
Radostits OM et al: *Herd health: food animal production medicine,* ed 2, Philadelphia, 1994, WB Saunders.
Smith BP: *Large animal internal medicine,* ed 2, St Louis, 1996, Mosby.

Sheep

Pratt PW: *Medical, surgical and anesthetic nursing for veterinary technicians,* ed 2, St Louis, 1994, Mosby.
Pugh DG: *Sheep and goat medicine,* St Louis, 2002, Mosby.
The sheep production handbook, Englewood, Calif, 1988, American Sheep Industry Association.

Thedford TR. *Sheep health handbook,* Morrilton, Ariz, 1983, Winrock International Information Services.

Goats

Ballaglia RA, Mayrose VB: *Handbook of livestock management techniques,* Minneapolis, 1981, Burgess Publishing.
Cebra ML, Cebra CK: Food Animal Medical and Surgical Nursing. In McCurnin DM, Bassert JM: *Clinical textbook for veterinary technicians,* ed 5, St Louis, 2002, WB Saunders.
Pratt PW: *Medical, surgical and anesthesia nursing for veterinary technicians,* ed 2, St Louis, 1994, Mosby.
Pugh DG: *Sheep and goat medicine,* St Louis, 2002, Mosby.
Sinn R: *Raising goats for milk and meat,* Little Rock, Ark, 1985, Heifer Project International.
Smith MC, Sherman DM: *Goat medicine,* Philadelphia, 1994, Lea & Febiger.

Swine

Pond WG, Mersmann HJ: *Biology of the domestic pig,* Ithaca, NY, 2001, Comstock Publishing.
Pond WG, Houpt KA: *The biology of the pig,* London, 1978, Cornell University Press.
Reeves D, ed: *Guidelines for the veterinary practitioner: care and management of miniature pet pigs,* Santa Barbara, Calif, 1993, Veterinary Practice Publishing.
Straw BE: *Diseases of swine,* ed 8, Ames, Iowa, 2000, Iowa State University Press.

Camelids

Alpaca Net, Internet website, address: http://www.alpacanet.com/
Fowler ME: *Medicine and surgery of South American camelids,* Ames, Iowa, 1989, Iowa State University Press.
Johnson LW: *Vet Clin North Am* 5(1), 1989 and 10(2), 1994.
McGee M, Tellington-Jones T: *Llama handling and training,* Dundee, New York, 1992, Zephyr Farm Press.
Llama Banner, monthly magazine, P.O. Box 1968, Manhattan, Kan.
Llamas, bimonthly magazine, P.O. Box 100, Herald, Calif.
Llama Web, Internet website, address: http://www.webcom/com/degraham/

Ratites

Jensen J et al: *Husbandry and medical management of ostriches, emus and rheas,* College Station, Texas, 1996, Wildlife and Exotic Animal Consultants.
Tully TN, Shane SM: *Ratite management, medicine, and surgery,* Malabar, Fla, 1996, Krieger Publishing.

28

Nursing Care of Cage Birds, Reptiles, and Amphibians

Gael L. De Longe and Sarah Okumura

Learning Objectives

After reviewing this chapter, the reader should understand the following:

- Anatomy of birds
- Behavior of birds
- Techniques used in the capture and restraint of birds
- Methods of sample collection for laboratory analysis
- Routes of administration of medication
- Techniques used in general nursing care of birds
- Procedures used in nail, beak, and feather care
- Procedures used in egg incubation and hatching
- Psittacine hand-feeding techniques
- Development of the neonate from hatching to weaning
- Successful weaning
- Common neonatal and pediatric diseases

- GI injuries, infections, and regurgitation
- Common musculoskeletal and beak problems
- Causes of starvation and stunting
- Reasons non-weaned birds should not be sold to inexperienced clients
- Signs of aging in psittacines
- Diseases typically found in geriatric cage birds
- Induction and maintenance of inhalant anesthesia and recognition of anesthetic emergencies
- Positioning used to take plain and contrast radiographs of a bird
- Basic biological characteristics of reptiles and amphibians
- Husbandry techniques for reptile and amphibian pets, including housing and feeding
- Techniques used in restraining snakes, lizards, turtles, and frogs
- General nursing, diagnostic sampling, and treatment techniques for reptiles and amphibians

CAGE BIRDS
Gael L. De Longe

Owners of pet birds are often extremely attached to their companions and seek expert veterinary care. There is a small but growing number of board-certified avian practitioners throughout the United States. Veterinarians in many small-animal practices are interested in treating birds, and some have studied extensively to become more knowledgeable, although they may not be certified. In addition to technical expertise, one of the most important parts of client relations is knowledge about the various species of birds clients will bring to the practice. Technicians must be able to identify the common pet birds. Many descriptive and well-illustrated references are available.

Most young pet birds seen in practice today are domestically bred and hand-raised. These chicks are hatched in captivity, then removed from the parents' care shortly afterwards to be hand-fed formula until weaning. Although birds are not considered domesticated because they are only one or two generations away from the wild, babies raised in this way bond readily to humans and make much more enjoyable family members. They accept humans as part of their flock.

The pet birds seen in practice usually are members of the psittacine or passerine family. These are distinguished by a number of physical characteristics.

Psittacines, or parrots, make up the majority of avian patients. They are more numerous, and clients have usually invested $200 to $2500, with some exotic macaws retailing for up to $15,000. Clients who have purchased a bird of this value are very willing to consult a veterinarian.

Psittacines are also known as *hookbills* because of their highly curved upper beak. Their feet are shaped so that two toes point forward and two toes point to the rear. Many parrots use these agile feet to hold food while they eat or manipulate objects they are interested in exploring. They tend to be good climbers, often moving around their cage using a combination of beak and feet. Many parrots are well socialized and hand-trained, coming out of their cages to spend a portion of their day associating directly with their human families. These birds range in weight from a few grams up to 1700 g. Many of them become accomplished talkers. Most commonly seen in practice are large parrots such as African Greys, Amazons, cockatoos, Eclectus, and large macaws. Occasionally presented for treatment are cockatiels, lovebirds, and budgerigars, or budgies, which are commonly known as parrakeets in the United States.

Passerines are usually small birds with a pointed or slightly curved beak. Their feet are shaped so that three toes point forward and one toe points to the rear. Many species of these birds are very active and tend to hop or fly about their cage. Most are not trained to sit on the client's hand and remain inside their cages. Canaries and finches are the most frequently kept passerines.

ROLE OF THE VETERINARY PRACTICE IN BIRD CARE

Many birds are seen for the first time in practice when they are exhibiting obvious signs of disease. Generally, birds mask their illness until it is far advanced. Clients who recognize a slight difference in behavior, attitude, or physical condition should be asked to bring their bird in for immediate examination.

A knowledgeable veterinarian should examine any new bird within 3 days of purchase, preferably before it is taken to its new home. Many breeders and pet stores offer a limited health guarantee, and it is important for the bird to be seen before this agreement expires. Once at its new home, the new bird should ideally be isolated from any other birds for six weeks. This allows time for all test results to be received and for the bird to show signs of any disease it may have been harboring when purchased. The client must be made aware that he or she can transfer infectious diseases from one bird to another. During the quarantine period, it is important for the client to follow certain procedures after working with a new bird, such as handwashing, wearing a smock, or changing clothing.

In addition to being weighed and thoroughly examined, a new bird should at a minimum be tested for common avian diseases, be swabbed for cultures and/or Gram stains of the choana and cloaca, and have baseline tests including CBC and blood chemistries. Some practices may elect to include a fecal examination and urinalysis. Because the sex of cage birds is impossible to determine in most species by feather coloration or physical appearance, new owners may request DNA sexing using a blood sample.

A regular annual physical examination is important. Because birds often cover up signs of illness and the feathers may hide weight loss, clients should bring their bird in for a physical, a CBC, basic blood chemistries, and possibly screening cultures or swabs of the choana and cloaca yearly. If the bird has been exposed to other birds that were or later

became ill, it may be tested for other specific diseases as well. A few vaccines are available for pet birds. Most veterinarians do not routinely vaccinate cage birds, although a vaccine against polyomavirus is available and sometimes used.

A bird is often presented for routine grooming procedures, such as wing clipping, nail trimming, or beak shaping. Implantation of microchips and application of leg bands for identification are other services performed. Removal of the closed leg band placed on a domestically bred, hand raised baby bird is often requested because of safety concerns.

Specific diagnostic procedures, such as radiography, endoscopy, and ultrasound examination, are common. Surgical procedures, such as sexing, fracture repair, and removal of feather cysts are often done in practice. Anesthesia of birds is similar to that performed in small animals but may actually be used more often for minor procedures for which total restraint is required.

Avian emergencies are not unusual. Birds are curious, fragile, easily startled creatures that can readily be injured. Poisonings, reproductive disorders, gastrointestinal problems, dyspnea, seizures, and traumatic injuries are all common.

Disease related to nutritional problems is one of the primary reasons birds are brought to the veterinary hospital. Discussion of a bird's diet and eating habits is a major part of working with a client. A thorough knowledge of basic bird nutrition and available commercial foods is an essential part of avian practice.

Sick birds must be medicated in the hospital or by the client at home. Hospital staff must be experienced and competent at administering medication and instructing clients in proper techniques.

Client education is an important part of avian practice. Clients considering purchase of a pet bird sometimes consult with a veterinary practice about the characteristics of a given species. They often have questions concerning proper diets, grooming procedures, and behavior. Many practices provide educational materials on these topics to clients.

Basic behavioral counseling should be done only by hospital personnel who are familiar with the nature and needs of both hand-raised and wild-caught parrots. In difficult cases, the client can be referred to an avian behaviorist, several of whom are veterinary technicians. Most behaviorists offer telephone consultations or home-visit services.

Time is an important part of the client-practice relationship. Pet bird appointments take longer than appointments for small animals, generally at least 30 minutes. Taking a complete history, discussing nutrition, observing the bird, completing a physical examination, and performing laboratory procedures are time-consuming. Clients recognize the willingness of a practice to devote the necessary time to their birds and feel confident in the diagnosis and treatment recommended.

BASIC PET BIRD BEHAVIOR

Pet birds retain many behaviors inherent in their wild ancestors. New owners who have not thoroughly researched species characteristics before purchasing their bird may be unpleasantly surprised by some of the traits exhibited by their pet. Veterinary personnel working with birds must also understand some of the expected reactions of their patients to common procedures.

A natural behavior in psittacines is *mouthing* or using the tongue to explore surfaces. Juvenile parrots pass through an innocent "beaking" phase, in which they attempt to taste or chew almost anything, somewhat like puppies do. People who are unfamiliar with this behavior often feel the bird is attempting to bite, so they pull back suddenly, which encourages the bird. Most well adapted young hand-raised birds do not bite humans unless they have been frightened or hurt.

Mature parrots are more likely to bite during handling as a defensive move. Large psittacines, such as macaws, can exert up to 300 pounds of pressure per square inch, inflicting deep bruises and lacerations that require suturing. Puncture wounds from bites may very well become infected. Birds as small as cockatiels have the potential to draw blood. Birds may strike at any portion of the body, so handlers must be alert and cautious when working with them. As with other animals, clients should not be involved in restraint of the bird so they are not injured.

All birds commonly show fear reactions when startled. They may fling themselves about the cage, struggle violently, flap their wings, scream loudly, or take flight in response to sudden movements or unfamiliar sights. Birds may easily be injured in their efforts to get away. Psittacines tend to vocalize in response to discomfort or restraint. Unhappy parrots can scream loudly enough to damage human hearing. Employees at some clinics routinely wear hearing protection when handling birds or working near birds in a boarding facility.

All birds defecate frequently, at least every 15 to 20 minutes, and more often when afraid or stressed. The typical behavior that indicates defecation in a calm bird is a slight wiggle of the tail, followed by a squat and an uplifted tail. Watching for this action can help prevent soiled clothing.

Other common behaviors may be disconcerting to those new to birds. Wagging of the tail back and forth usually indicates a relaxed, happy bird. Beak grinding in a bird that is sitting quietly usually signals readiness to fall asleep. Young hand-fed birds or older birds that are very bonded to their owners may regurgitate food from the crop into the mouth as a sign of affection, which clients may interpret as vomiting and a sign of illness.

Care must be taken when speaking around birds at the clinic. More than one practice has been embarrassed when a talking bird repeats an unsavory word or derogatory phrase after a stay at the clinic. Birds also tend to readily imitate loud, repetitive, or bodily function sounds.

The behavior of pet birds is very different from that of cats or dogs; techniques that work well in those species are often inappropriate for use in birds. The emotional intelligence of many large psittacines is on the level of a 2-year-old child. Some African Greys approach the abilities of a 5-year-old human in problem-solving skills and speech patterns. This high level of intelligence results in a patient that is both entertaining and challenging.

Clients often seek help with such problems as biting, screaming, or destructive feather behavior. Many of the behaviors they wish to modify are the result of instinctive avian reactions or related to the stresses of captivity.

Psittacines attempt to become dominant over their flock, in this case their human family. It is important that all household members use certain techniques to maintain the dominant position in the home. Birds should be taught to consistently step up on or down from the client's hand when asked. Clipping the bird's wings to limit its flying ability will diminish dominance behaviors, such as flying down from a curtain rod to attack a person. When holding the bird, keep it at mid-chest level. Never allowing it to sit on the head or shoulders keeps it from attaining the highest perch, a position of great power. Situating the cage or perches so that the bird is below eye level also discourages dominant behavior.

Biting is a common behavior problem. Birds bite to exhibit dominance, express fear, or exhibit jealousy, or as a result of hormonal fluctuations during puberty or the breeding season. A protective bird may bite the client in an effort to make the person move away from perceived danger. It is important for the client to realize that the bird must not be allowed to bite as a way of controlling any situation.

Vocalization is essential to birds, but it may become a problem in some insecure or dependent birds that call constantly to their owner. Birds tend to be very noisy at dawn and dusk, around feeding time, in response to loud sounds, in an effort to locate flock members, or out of loneliness. Some species are relatively quiet, but all birds make a certain amount of noise. Clients may encourage a bird to make more noise by responding to loud calls with anger or shouting in an effort to quiet the bird.

Feather destructive behavior, also called feather picking or plucking, is a well-known but poorly understood condition. The bird uses its beak to snip off or pull out any feathers that are accessible, including any that start to grow back. Some birds remove all but the feathers on their heads, and some may damage skin as well as muscle. Some affected birds have an underlying physical illness that initiates plucking, but some healthy birds mutilate their feathers in response to stress, such as separation from their owner or change in cage location. This is a difficult problem to solve and may become a chronic condition. It is most common in African Greys and cockatoos.

Correction of behavior problems takes time, an understanding of the underlying cause, and judicious use of behavior modification. Prolonged physical or mental isolation of the bird, withholding food or water, and physical punishment are totally unacceptable methods of dealing with these problems. All may result in permanent emotional or physical damage to the bird.

Unfortunately, many people do not know where to go to receive accurate and helpful advice, often first seeking answers from poorly informed pet store employees. In addition, readily available older books often contain advice that may apply to wild-caught parrots, but is not suitable for hand-raised birds. Many misinformed clients worsen the very behavior they wish to eliminate by using inappropriate techniques. The staff of a veterinary clinic that treats pet birds must know the basics of bird behavior and be prepared to refer problem cases to avian behaviorists. The most current listing of behavioral consultants is found in reputable avian magazines. Practices should provide several references and encourage the client to interview the behaviorists until they find one who is compatible and whose techniques make sense.

AVIAN ANATOMY

Feathers and Skin

Feathers, which are arranged in distinct tracts over the surface of the body, provide warmth and protection. Molting occurs in all species and results in periodic replacement of old feathers. A new growing feather has a vascular supply until it reaches full size. The shafts of these "blood feathers" appear dark and bleed profusely if broken, possibly leading to death.

Birds spend several hours a day preening, or rearranging and conditioning their feathers. Almost all species have a preen gland located at the base of their tail. The oily secretion from this gland is spread over the surface of the feathers to make them more water-resistant.

Birds have several types of feathers (Figs. 28-1 and 28-2). The *contour feathers* cover the body and wings and are identified as *flight feathers* or *body feathers*. The large, *primary flight feathers (remiges)* are found on the outer end of the wing. The *secondary flight feathers* are located on the wing between the body and the primaries. *Body feathers*, also known as *coverts*, provide surface coverage over most of the rest of the bird.

Down feathers insulate the bird and have a soft, fluffy appearance. Cockatoos, cockatiels, and African Greys have powder down, which breaks down to produce a white dusty powder. A healthy bird of these species produces dust that is evident on dark clothing after the bird touches it and on the bird's beak after a grooming session.

The skin is very delicate and has a dry, slightly wrinkled appearance. Underlying muscles and blood give the skin a reddish appearance in some areas. The skin on the legs resembles the scales of reptiles. The *cere* (the area around the nostrils), the beak, and the nails are all modified skin (see Fig. 28-1).

Pet birds often have spectacularly colorful plumage. However, it is important to realize that it is virtually impossible to determine the sex of cage birds by appearance, because males and females of each species look identical. The major exception to this rule is the Eclectus parrot, in which the female is a deep reddish color with a dark beak, and the male is bright green with an orange beak. Some clients attempt to sex their birds using a combination of head and beak shape or size, pelvic bone configuration, and overall size. Blood testing is available to reliably determine the sex of the bird from a small sample. Some veterinarians and clients prefer to have the bird sexed surgically using a laparoscope, which allows the reproductive tract to be evaluated visually for abnormalities.

Musculoskeletal System

The skeleton of birds is highly modified. Some bones are *pneumatized*, or contain air, which results in a lighter skeleton. The bones have thin walls, which makes them lighter but also more fragile. The skull bones are fused, which strengthens the beak structure. The vertebrae of the neck are shaped in such a way as to create a long, flexible neck. The large sternum, or *keel*, supports the pectoral muscles that are needed for flight. A large portion of the caudal vertebrae is fused to form the *synsacrum*, which stabilizes the back during flight.

The largest muscles in the body are the pectorals, which account for approximately 20% of the bird's weight. Because of their mass, they are used to determine the body condition of the bird and are ideal for intramuscular (IM) injections.

Respiratory System

Air enters the respiratory system through the nostrils, travels through the many sinuses in the head, and then enters the oral cavity through the slitlike opening in the roof of the mouth known as the *choana*. It then travels into the opening of the trachea at the base of the tongue and through the *syrinx*, or vocal organ. The air continues into the small lungs, where air exchange takes place. However, the lungs do not have alveoli and therefore do not inflate. Air next flows into the *air sacs*, which are hollow membranous bags

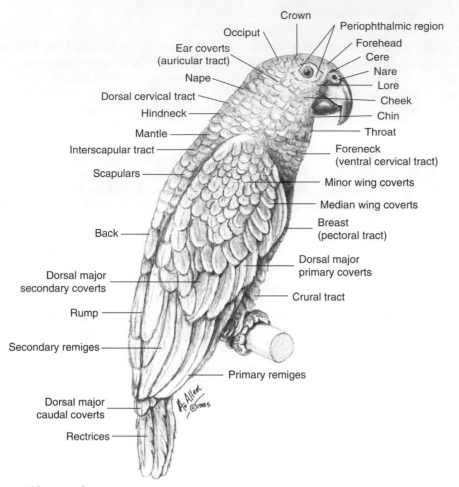

Fig. 28-1 Plumage and external features of an Amazon parrot. *(From Harrison GJ, Harrison LR: Clinical avian medicine and surgery, Philadelphia, 1986, WB Saunders.)*

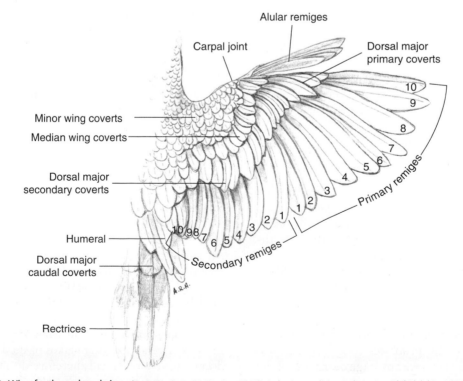

Fig. 28-2 Wing feathers, dorsal view. *(From Harrison GJ, Harrison LR: Clinical avian medicine and surgery, Philadelphia, 1986, WB Saunders.)*

that help move air throughout the respiratory system. Birds have one single and four paired air sacs located within the body cavity. Birds lack a muscular diaphragm and depend on the movement of the rib cage to push air through the respiratory tract. Two complete breath cycles are necessary to move a breath of air completely through the respiratory system.

Digestive System

The high metabolism of birds requires ingestion of large amounts of food. The beak is used to grasp food and crush it with the aid of the tongue. Birds do not have teeth. The mouth is relatively dry, because little saliva is produced. Another avian anatomic variation is the location of the esophagus, which lies on the right side of the neck, as opposed to the left side as in mammals.

When food is swallowed, it travels through the esophagus to the crop at the base of the neck (Fig. 28-3). The *crop*, an enlargement of the esophagus present in most birds, softens food and allows continuous passage of small amounts of food to the proventriculus, or true stomach. In young birds, the crop may become very distended after a meal. The proventriculus is very similar to the stomach of mammals, containing digestive acid and enzymes.

The food next passes into the *ventriculus*, or gizzard. This is a thickly muscled organ that grinds food into smaller particles. Most wild birds need grit, or small pieces of gravel, in the gizzard to break down hard foods. Pet birds do not need to be given grit since most of their diet consists of soft and processed foods. They may even develop an impaction if they have access to grit.

The intestinal tract is very similar to that of mammals. Birds have a pancreas and bilobed liver that produce digestive enzymes and bile. The large intestine terminates at the *cloaca*, which is the chamber into which materials from the digestive, urinary, and reproductive systems pass before release from the body (see Fig. 28-3). The external opening of the cloaca is termed the *vent*, from which the droppings are passed. The droppings, which include feces, urine, and urates, vary in consistency, depending on the diet.

Urinary System

The paired kidneys of birds are closely attached to the vertebrae (see Fig. 28-3). They empty into the ureters, which carry the liquid urine and semisolid urates to the cloaca. Urates, or uric acid, are the major excretion product in birds and comprise the white portion of the droppings. Birds do not have a urinary bladder.

Reproductive System

In the female bird, only the left side of the reproductive tract develops fully. As in mammals, an ovary, oviduct, and vagina are present. Various regions of the oviduct produce the egg white and eggshell. The entire process from ovulation to egg laying takes approximately 15 hours. The female lays eggs even if no male is present. If the hen is bred and produces fertile eggs, she is the one that genetically determines the sex of the offspring.

The male bird has paired testes located internally near the kidneys. During periods of active breeding, they enlarge dramatically in size. Sperm cells travel to the cloaca through the epididymis and then the ductus deferens. Most birds do not have a penis, and mating takes place when the vents of the male and female birds come in contact.

Circulatory System

The heart of birds closely resembles that of mammals, but it is proportionally about 1 ½ times larger (see Fig. 28-3). Heart rates range from 150 to 300 beats per minute in large parrots, and up to 1400 beats per minute in very small species. Blood pressure in birds is higher than in mammals.

The circulatory system of birds differs from that of mammals in several ways. The red blood cells of birds are oval and contain a nucleus (see Chapter 11). Birds do not have lymph nodes, and the lymphatic system is less extensive.

Special Senses

The eyes of birds are relatively large. Their vision is very acute, and they can perceive color. Birds often look closely at something with one eye, tilting their head for a better view. In many species, the color of the iris is often darker in young birds. Birds also have voluntary control of the muscles of the iris and often will rapidly change the size of the circular pupil when excited or intrigued. Blinking is done using the almost transparent nictitating membrane, or third eyelid. Most birds completely close their eyes only when they sleep.

The ears of birds are hidden from view by feathers, which have a slightly different appearance and sometimes are a different color. The external opening is located caudad and ventral to the eye (see Fig. 28-1). The auditory range is similar to that of humans.

Taste and smell are difficult senses to evaluate. Birds have fewer taste buds than humans, and they are located on the roof of the mouth, not on the tongue. Birds can taste, but it is unknown how well. Smell appears to be poorly developed. Many birds enjoy eating highly spiced or sweet foods.

RESTRAINT

A cornerstone of avian practice is proper restraint. Restraint is often required to ensure the safety of the avian patient and the personnel handling the bird during diagnostic and therapeutic procedures. Effective restraint often requires two or more people, so good planning and

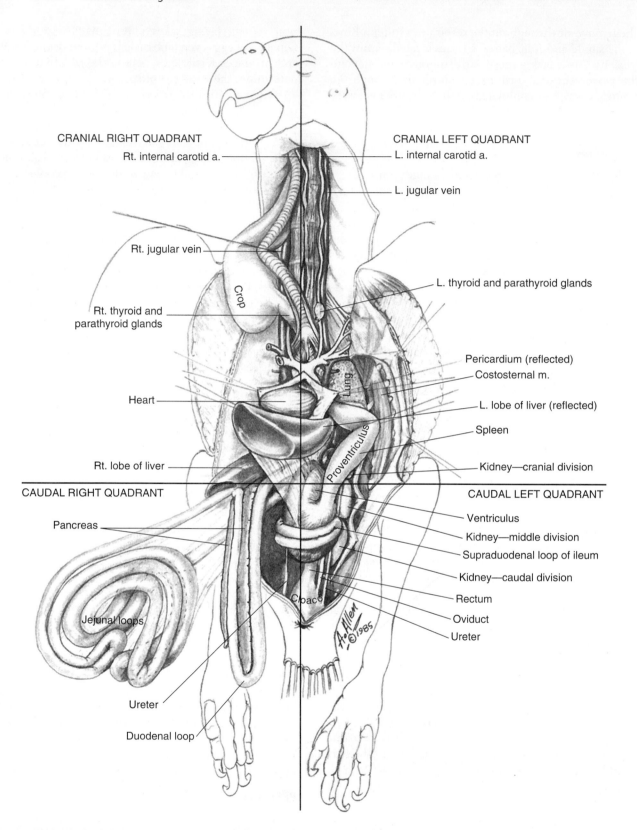

CRANIAL RIGHT QUADRANT

Rt. internal carotid a.

Rt. jugular vein

Crop

Rt. thyroid and
parathyroid glands

Heart

Rt. lobe of liver

CAUDAL RIGHT QUADRANT

Pancreas

Jejunal loops

Ureter

Duodenal loop

CRANIAL LEFT QUADRANT

L. internal carotid a.

L. jugular vein

L. thyroid and parathyroid glands

Pericardium (reflected)

Costosternal m.

L. lobe of liver (reflected)

Spleen

Kidney—cranial division

CAUDAL LEFT QUADRANT

Ventriculus

Kidney—middle division

Supraduodenal loop of ileum

Kidney—caudal division

Rectum

Oviduct

Ureter

Lung

Proventriculus

Cloaca

Fig. 28-3 Internal structures of a bird, ventral view with viscera reflected. *(From Harrison GJ, Harrison LR: Clinical avian medicine and surgery, Philadelphia, 1986, WB Saunders.)*

communication between those involved are vital. This section details many of the techniques commonly used in practice for capture, restraint, and release of pet birds.

Typical reactions to restraint include struggling, vocalizing loudly, flapping of the wings, attempting to bite, and grasping with the feet. Individual birds react differently to being restrained. Their actions depend on their species, previous experiences with restraint, and types of contact with people. Young, hand-fed parrots are often very accepting of human handling, whereas wild-caught birds used for breeding may be extremely difficult to capture and restrain. The speed and agility of small species, such as finches, which are never handled by the client because of their temperament and size, make them challenging to catch and hold.

Restraint Techniques

A terrycloth towel is often useful when capturing and restraining birds ranging in size from the cockatiels or conures to the largest parrots (Fig. 28-4). Paper towels are sometimes used when restraining budgies, cockatiels, or conures. The towel, which is often draped over the hand during capture, is arranged during restraint so that the bird's nares are exposed without uncovering the eyes. The bird should be allowed to chew on the towel if it wishes, which keeps its beak busy and makes it less likely for the holder to be bitten. The smallest birds, such as finches, canaries, and budgerigars, are usually captured using a bare hand. The nails or wings of very small birds may become entangled in a towel, leading to traumatic fractures or other related problems. It is also difficult to evaluate very small patients held in a towel.

The technician should approach any size bird with confidence so that capture is prompt. Once the capture process is initiated, the technician must remain in control of the sit-

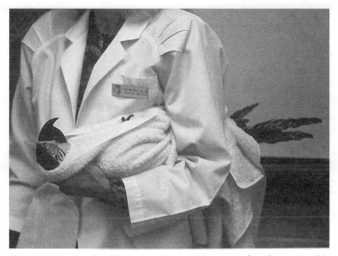

Fig. 28-4 Blue and gold macaw wrapped in a towel and restrained by one person for treatment.

uation and persist until the bird is well secured. Birds are often captured from the back in order to avoid the beak, but some birds are less frightened if approached from the front.

Once the bird is caught, the basic towel-wrapping technique is similar for all sizes of birds. Firmly grip the head from the rear without putting pressure on the eyes. In large birds, the ear openings are convenient positioning areas that are easily felt through the towel. Next, grasp the body and quickly fold the wings close to the body in their natural position. This protects the wings from damage and prevents trauma to the holder from flapping wings. Then tuck the towel around the bird, which is positioned so that its chest is exposed. Restrain the feet to prevent injury by sharp nails as the bird uses its legs and feet to grasp anything in an effort to free itself. A firm grip of the body is necessary, but it is easy to suffocate a bird by squeezing it too tightly.

Correct placement of the technician's hands is essential for proper positioning. When working with small birds, grip the bird's head between your thumb and index finger. The little finger of the same hand restrains the bird's legs, while the remaining fingers circle the trunk. This technique works well for both quiet and struggling birds.

When working with large birds, such as cockatiels and conures, grasp the head, neck, and trunk with one hand. Use the other hand to secure the feet or perform techniques such as administration of medication. Larger birds sometimes require a two-handed restraint method, in which the head is held in one hand and the feet are gripped in the other hand. This allows the bird to be stretched and held very securely so that another person can readily perform procedures.

One person can single-handedly restrain most birds for a majority of procedures. Once the bird is caught and securely wrapped, the handler can control both the head and feet. You can wrap the bird in such a way that the feet are immobilized, allowing the technician to administer medications and vaccinations (see Fig. 28-4).

Restraint can be a very stressful experience for a bird. It is not unusual for it to show signs of extreme distress when released. The bird will typically hyperventilate, have hot feet, hold its wings away from its body, and fluff its feathers to allow air to cool the skin. Birds with naked faces, such as African Greys and macaws, will blush. Occasionally, bruising of the face will be obvious on naked-face birds. Large birds sometimes display sunken eyes if the eye is accidentally compressed during restraint. These problems will disappear within a few hours or days.

Capture Techniques

Small pet birds, such as canaries, budgerigars, and conures, are usually transported to the veterinarian in their own cage. They must be safely and gently removed for a hands-on physical examination. Slow and deliberate movements minimize stress to the bird, accompanied by a quiet tone of voice for reassurance. It may be helpful to dim the room lights before proceeding, because this calms some birds.

Large pet birds are generally brought to the clinic in a carrier, because their cages are usually too large to transport. Allowing the bird to ride freely on the client's hand or shoulder should be discouraged, because the bird may escape after a frightening incident even if its wings have been trimmed to prevent flight.

Large parrots may be caught in the cage, in the carrier, on the floor, or from a tabletop. As with small birds, a slow and deliberate approach works best. A quiet, soothing tone of voice should be used when relating to the bird. In most cases, a towel is used during capture to avoid injury to the bird or technician. It is extremely important to exhibit confidence in the approach to large birds, because they may become aggressive when they detect uncertainty.

The client or technician may place a bird that is easy to remove from a carrier on the floor. Some birds that resist hands-on removal from the carrier will readily walk out of the carrier when it is placed on the floor with the door open. Once on the floor, the bird feels vulnerable, is less likely to fight, and usually is unable to move very quickly. Place a towel over the bird, and pick it up. This technique is often used with Amazons and macaws. A bird that is accustomed to being handled with a towel by the client may sometimes be caught by approaching it from the front, once it is placed on the floor or a tabletop, and gently wrapping the towel from front to back.

A large bird that was caught on the floor or countertop is usually released onto the floor. The holder positions the wrapped patient so that it will be standing when the towel is removed. Keeping a good grip on the head and body, place the bird feet-down on the floor. Then smoothly remove the towel from the body, release the head, and step back to avoid a potential strike.

If a bird is to be released into a cage or carrier, take care to avoid injury by placing it on the floor of the container (never on a perch). Quickly withdraw hands after release to avoid being bitten by an angry bird.

Restraint board

Use the restraint board for procedures that require the awake (not anesthetized) bird to remain completely still, such as for radiographs or implantation of microchips for identification. In other situations, both hands may be needed to perform complicated tasks. Anesthetized birds can be positioned on the restraint board for surgery (Fig. 28-5). The patient is usually secured on the board in dorsal recumbency or in a lateral position.

Two persons are necessary to place an awake bird on a restraint board. The person restraining the bird positions the head and neck, as the second person fastens the neck restraint. The legs are then immobilized by looping gauze strips around the legs proximal to the feet and taping these

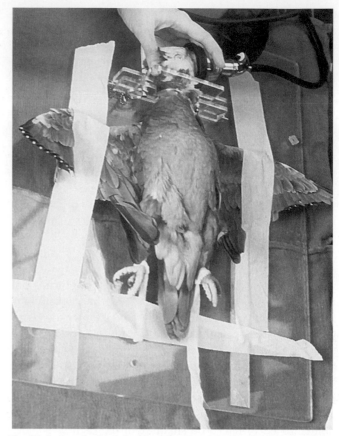

Fig. 28-5 Anesthetized double yellow-head Amazon parrot taped to a restraint board in dorsal recumbency. Note the mask in place over the face to maintain anesthesia.

strips tautly to the board. The wings, which have been held close to the body as the neck and legs are fastened, are restrained by taping them to the board surface using masking tape. Cloth tape should not be used, because it may pull or damage feathers.

Use of gloves

Some practices and textbooks suggest the routine use of leather gloves to protect the handler when catching and restraining large pet birds. Unfortunately, birds may respond to gloves as if they are hands and subsequently become afraid of being handled in any situation. For this reason, use of towels is strongly recommended. Gloves should be avoided if possible.

PHYSICAL EXAMINATION

A physical examination of birds is very similar to that performed on other animals. Because of the unique anatomy of the avian patient, the exam is modified somewhat. The technician must be aware of the anatomic features and differences found in birds.

Physical examination is divided into three parts. First, obtain a thorough history from the client, then carefully observe the bird for signs of health and disease. Finally, capture and examine the bird.

Ask the client the age of the bird, the sex of the bird, how long they have had the bird, where it was obtained, and if it has been exposed to new or visiting birds. Inquire about the bird's diet, including formulated diets, any supplements fed, and how much and what sort of "people" food is offered. Inquire about current signs of illness, medications used to treat the bird, and possible exposure to toxic plants or poisons.

If the bird is transported in its cage, the cage can offer insight into the type of care the bird receives. Pay close attention to whether the size of the cage is appropriate for the species of bird. Note the condition of the cage, the number and type of toys, and the presence of adequate food and water containers. Inspect the cage bedding. If paper is used, evaluate the condition of the droppings. For small flighted birds such as finches and canaries, the cage should be large enough to allow the bird to fly from perch to perch.

When a large bird is presented in a carrier, ask the client to describe the cage they use at home. Important information to obtain includes the following:

- Inside dimensions of the cage
- Material the cage is made of (e.g., stainless steel, powder-coated or painted metal, wrought iron, galvanized steel)
- Type of bedding used
- Type of water containers provided
- Type and number of toys available
- Types of perches in the cage and their location
- Location of the cage in the house

With enough prior notice, a client may be willing and pleased to bring a picture of their bird's cage and surrounding environment to the appointment.

A small bird should be evaluated in its cage, whereas a large bird should be observed in the carrier if practical or out of the carrier in a nonthreatening location. The bird should exhibit normal posture and movement. It should be active, bright, alert, and responsive. Obvious indications of illness, such as difficulty breathing or sitting fluffed up on the bottom of the cage, signal that the bird is extremely sick and should be considered an emergency case.

Special equipment for the avian physical examination includes a pediatric stethoscope and several sizes of metal oral specula used to keep the mouth open for examination. Some practices use a transillumination device that backlights air-filled structures, such as the beak and sinuses, to determine if they contain fluid or other dense materials.

Weighing the bird is generally the first step of the hands-on examination. Avian scales, which are available in a variety of configurations, must be accurate to a gram. It is important to weigh the bird each time it visits the clinic, because clients often do not notice fluctuations in weight. However, most very small birds are not weighed because of the stress associated with handling.

Small birds, such as budgerigars and cockatiels, are often caught by hand and placed in a cloth or paper bag, which is then laid on the scale platform. Some birds weigh only a few grams, and the bag may weigh as much as the bird. To offset the weight of the bag, the scale must first be adjusted to zero with the empty bag on it.

Large birds, such as Amazons and cockatoos, often stand on the scale long enough to be weighed. Some avian scales have a perch attachment on which birds may feel more secure. If necessary, large birds may also be placed in a pillowcase or other large bag for weighing if they refuse to be still when they are put on the scale. The scale must be zeroed with the bag on it before the weight is taken.

Physical examination of larger birds requires two people, one to restrain the bird and the other to examine it. Small birds that can be grasped in one hand may be restrained and evaluated by a single person. The bird is usually wrapped in a cloth or paper towel but may be held in the bare hand if the bird is very small. Take care to avoid restricting chest movement, because the lack of a muscular diaphragm limits the bird's ability to breathe.

Physical examinations generally start with the head. External structures that should be identified and evaluated include the cere, nostrils, beak, ear openings, eyes, and feathers. Evidence of discharge, irritation, or matting of feathers should be noted. The eyes should be clear and bright. The beak should be properly shaped for the species and free of obvious damage. There should be no discharge or odor from the ears. Large parrots can be checked for dehydration by gently lifting the skin above the eyelid and watching to see how long it takes for the skin to return to its normal position.

Use a metal speculum or gauze strips that are looped over the upper and lower beaks to hold the mouth open (Fig. 28-6). The mouth should be fairly dry, with no lesions, discharges, blood, or odors present. The choana should have obvious *papillae*, or fingerlike projections. The tongue shape and coloration should be normal for the species.

Moving down the neck, palpate the crop. This structure may be very obvious in young birds, birds who have eaten recently, or those with digestive problems. It may be impossible to detect a crop in older or very small birds. Examine the skin over the crop for redness or necrosis, which may indicate thermal damage to the crop from feeding overheated formula or other food. Some species do not have a crop.

The breast of the bird should be evaluated for good muscling. The keel, or breastbone, should be palpable as a low ridge surrounded by muscle on about the same level on either side. A bird in poor condition will have a very prominent keel, with low, receding muscles. An overweight bird

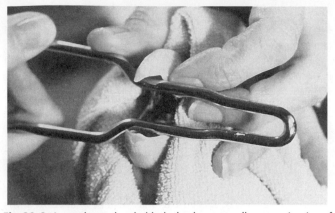

Fig. 28-6 A metal speculum holds the beak open to allow examination of the mouth.

will have a keel buried in a valley between the pectoral muscles.

Evaluation of the abdomen is very limited or impossible in small birds. In large birds, abdominal palpation is used to detect organs that feel hard or unusually shaped. In all birds, the vent should be clean and covered by dry feathers.

A pediatric stethoscope is useful for assessing the heart and respiratory system. The heart and respiratory rates should be within normal limits for the species, but stress may result in unreliable numbers.

The feathers should be clean, symmetric, smooth, and structurally sound. Note evidence of blood feathers (i.e., growing feathers). The presence of the powder down, which is produced by cockatoos, cockatiels, and African Greys, should be evaluated. The delicate skin is usually white, and underlying structures, such as muscle or blood vessels, are somewhat visible. The nails and skin on the legs should be inspected for condition and any abnormal growth. The preen gland, located at the base of the tail in most species, may not be easily found. Swelling or any discharge indicates a problem.

Both wings should be gently examined, with care taken to curve the wing in the direction of the body at all times. Some birds are very sensitive and struggle when their wings are manipulated. Any of the rest of the musculoskeletal system that was not palpated should be checked at this time.

Several procedures typically performed in the examination of domestic animals are omitted in birds. First, the temperature of birds, which ranges from 40° to 44° C (104° to 111° F), is not measured. There is wide variation between individual birds, and the stress associated with the procedure would raise the temperature, resulting in an inaccurate number. Second, the capillary refill time cannot be evaluated using the oral mucosa. Third, birds have no external lymph nodes to palpate.

Hands-on examination should be completed quickly to minimize stress on the patient. A thorough examination should take no longer than 15 minutes. If the patient appears extremely distressed during the examination, it must be released and placed in a quiet location until it has recovered enough to continue.

GROOMING

The health of a bird can depend on several grooming procedures that are routinely performed at the veterinary clinic. Veterinary technicians must be familiar with and competent in these techniques. Effective restraint is often a vital part of these procedures.

Bathing

A very basic technique that many birds enjoy is a bath. There are the several ways to do this. Gently misting the bird with a spray bottle filled with warm water is most common. The warm mist should be directed so that it falls from above the bird, not sprayed directly toward it. The bird may be bathed in this manner either inside or out of the cage, depending on its temperament. Some birds readily bathe in a shallow pan of water. Others like to clean themselves by rolling in wet vegetation, such as lettuce or nonpoisonous houseplants. Many birds enjoy showering with their owners. However the bird takes a bath, soap should *not* be used because of its drying effect on the feathers, and any remaining residue could be toxic.

Nail Trimming

A regularly requested service is trimming of long or sharp nails. The size and temperament of the bird determines the number of people required to perform the trim. Towel restraint is commonly used.

Birds with light-colored nails have easily visible blood vessels, improving the chances of a nail trim without bleeding. In birds with black nails, an understanding of the structure of the nail is important. However, even with extreme care it is not unusual to cut the quick of at least one nail, causing bleeding. Clients should be warned that this may happen.

The most common tools used for nail trims include Resco trimmers, the Dremel (motorized) tool, files, nail scissors, fingernail trimmers, and cautery instruments. These should be disinfected or sterilized after using to prevent the spread of disease between birds. Each clinic and veterinarian prefers certain instruments for nail trims. The typical small-animal practice can easily trim bird nails without purchase of additional equipment.

Resco guillotine clippers are commonly used on birds the size of conures and larger. A pair should be reserved for use in birds to prevent spread of disease. The tool should be cleaned thoroughly before using it on other birds.

The Dremel tool, typically used on large birds, uses a grinding tip to blunt the tips of the nails. This handheld motorized tool is noisy, can overheat nail tissues if applied too long, and may carry contaminants to other birds on which it is used if the grinding head is improperly cleaned.

Flat or rounded fine-toothed files are preferred by some for nail trims of birds of any size. This method slowly blunts the nail tips, causing some birds to become impatient and struggle.

The scissor trimmers used on cat nails work well in birds up to Amazon size. Human fingernail clippers may be used in small birds.

Some veterinarians use electrocautery instruments to trim nails and prevent bleeding at the same time. Many birds exhibit pain reactions, presumably related to the high heat of the instrument.

Small birds, such as budgerigars or finches, can be held in one hand and the nails trimmed with the other. Trimming the nails of Amazons and larger birds generally involves two people, one to restrain the bird and the other to trim the nails. Birds generally grasp at anything that touches their feet, so the toes not being trimmed must be held out of the way of the trimmers.

Closely examine each nail before proceeding. If there is any doubt about how much to remove, only a short tip should be clipped off. More can be removed if necessary.

Any blood loss in birds should be considered serious. In very small birds, loss of what appears to be a minute amount of blood is potentially fatal. When bleeding is noticed, a hemostatic powder must be pressed immediately onto the nail.

Wing Clipping

Most clients have their bird's wings clipped to limit its flying ability. This helps prevent the bird from escaping through an open window or door, or injuring itself by flying through the house. Wing trimming also inhibits development of many dominance behaviors and makes taming and training easier. The wing trim should allow the bird to glide to the floor a short distance from where it began flapping its wings.

Bandage scissors are most often used because of the protected tip. However, any type of scissors can be used if handled carefully. The scissors selected should be suitably sized for the bird to be trimmed.

One person may easily position and trim the smaller species of birds. Two or more handlers are required to trim larger birds. The person performing the wing trim must have a thorough knowledge of wing anatomy and double-check before cutting any feathers. Incorrect trimming procedures may result in accidental wing tip amputation. The wings must be handled carefully to minimize bruising and prevent fractures. They must always be curved toward the body in a natural position, never bent backward. Personnel working with the bird must also be aware that flapping wings can cause bruising and abrasions to human handlers.

Many birds have one or more immature, growing feathers concealed by their mature feathers. These blood feathers can be difficult to locate and identify without inspecting the underside of the wing. When a blood feather is accidentally cut, the hollow shaft bleeds profusely. The bleeding feather must be pulled out immediately using hemostats or a pair of pliers. The wing must be well stabilized in order minimize the chance of breaking a bone. Without intervention, the bird may die of blood loss.

There are several types of wing trims. The standard wing clip, where all primary feathers are trimmed, is most common (Fig. 28-7). Cockatoos and other heavy birds that fly slowly may need trimming of only the tips of the primaries. Cockatiels fly so well that their feathers often must be trimmed to the level of the covert feathers. Other clips involve trimming only a few primaries on each wing to give the bird a more natural look. Some birds still fly quite well after these trims.

Some birds are irritated by very short clips and will chew on the remaining feather shaft. The shaft often splits or frays, leading to more discomfort. If this occurs, any remaining shafts should be removed by pulling them out. This can be a difficult task if the shafts are split, frayed, or bitten to the skin level. General anesthesia may be required

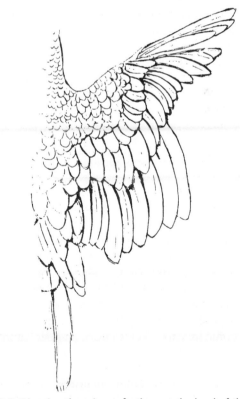

Fig. 28-7 Trimming the primary feathers at the level of the coverts on both wings is not attractive but may be necessary to restrict flight in some species (dorsal view). *(From Harrison GJ, Harrison LR: Clinical avian medicine and surgery, Philadelphia, 1986, WB Saunders.)*

to keep the bird still, to prevent pain, and to allow positioning of the wing so that short, shredded shafts can be grasped effectively.

A newly trimmed bird should be placed on the floor and gently encouraged to fly. In this way, the bird becomes aware of its limited abilities in a safe location. This also reveals whether further trimming is necessary before the bird leaves the clinic.

Beak Trimming

All pet birds, most commonly parrots, may be presented with overgrown, damaged, poorly aligned, flaky, or sharply pointed beaks. Usually only the upper beak requires attention, but the lower beak may need to be smoothed. The majority of healthy birds never need a beak trim if they are provided with plenty of toys to chew on and play with.

The Dremel tool or files are used to shape and modify the beak. Flaky material on the sides of the beak is carefully ground away. If the upper beak is badly overgrown, the tip of the beak may be clipped using nail-trimming instruments, such as Resco clippers. Because the beak has a central blood supply, trimming the tip too short may cause bleeding. A hemostatic powder should be ready. After the beak trim is finished, some practices apply mineral oil to provide an attractive gloss.

One or two people are needed for a beak trim, depending on the size of the bird. For small birds, one person can perform the trim. For large birds, one person restrains the bird while the other does the trim. It is important to keep the bird from mouthing or biting the tools, because they may damage sensitive soft tissue.

IDENTIFICATION TECHNIQUES

Leg Bands

Two types of leg bands are placed on birds for identification purposes. The closed band is a solid ring made of metal or plastic and stamped with numbers, letters, or a combination. The band is designed to fit over the foot for only a few days after hatching, so that only a very young bird can be fitted with one. A breeder bands a domestic hand-fed baby as a means of identification. The open leg band may be found on a wild-caught, imported bird or any bird that has been banded after it is too large for a closed band to fit. The veterinary clinic may be asked to place an open band on an adult bird so that it may be identified quickly. This type of band is always metal and has a small open gap where the edges of the band come together. Identifying letters and/or numbers are also present on the open band.

Two or more people are required to participate in the banding process, one to perform the restraint and another to hold the leg and apply the band. When a large bird is to be banded, a third person is required to steady the leg, as the band application is strenuous enough that it takes two hands to close the crimping instrument. Equipment needed for open band application includes the correct size band and either a hemostat to crimp a small band or a specialized pliers-type of instrument suitable for compressing a larger, heavier band. Restrain the bird, and hold the leg firmly in position; a slip during application may result in trauma to the skin or a fractured leg. Squeezed the band closed until only a small gap between the ends is visible. The bands used on large birds are very stiff and require much effort to close.

Clients may ask to have open or closed leg bands removed, as they have the potential to catch on toys or other objects and cause leg damage. This procedure requires excellent restraint and a steady hand on the part of the person cutting the band. The potential for injury to the bird exists because of the type and size of the tools utilized to cut the band. The small band can be separated using a wire cutter, but the large band demands a heavy, awkward bolt cutter.

Two people can easily remove the open small bird leg band, but three must be involved in large bird open band removal. The leg must be held perfectly still to reduce the chance of injury. Then press the band against the leg; this results in a large gap between the leg and band on the other side. A single cut is needed to open this type of band. The small band will fall harmlessly away, but the large band often springs apart and travels several feet in the air. For this reason, all personnel involved in large open band removal should wear protective goggles. The closed band must be cut in two locations so that it may be removed. This type of band is made of softer material, so the process is less dangerous for the people involved. The general procedure is the same as for the open band.

The number of the band should be recorded in the bird's file and the pieces of the band given to the client for safekeeping.

Microchips

Many owners of large parrots are requesting that microchips be implanted in their birds as a form of permanent identification. Any leg band is easily removed or replaced, so it is not foolproof identification. Several companies provide inch-long ID chips that are nonreactive and can be implanted in muscle. A reader is used to simultaneously activate the microchip and display the serial number assigned to each chip.

The chip implantation may be performed on an awake, restrained bird. An injection device supplied by the manufacturer is used to place the chip deep in the pectoral muscle. The implantation site should be cleaned and swabbed with alcohol. The injection may be placed anywhere in the pectorals, taking care to place the needle between feather follicles. Bleeding may occur, but applying gentle pressure on the site will halt any oozing. A bird may be implanted during anesthesia for another procedure.

The bird's chip number can be registered with the manufacturer or other recording organization. Different companies are striving to produce chip readers that will detect chips made by each manufacturer.

ADMINISTERING MEDICATION

The avian patient may need to be tube-fed to treat a digestive disorder, nebulized to treat pulmonary disease, vaccinated against any of several diseases, given fluid therapy, or medicated topically for an infection. The techniques used for small animals are not always directly applicable to birds.

Parenteral Injection

A bird with a life-threatening disease often refuses to eat and may regurgitate oral medication. Parenteral treatments, or administering medication by injection, can often be quickly accomplished without undue stress to the patient. Injections are usually administered using a 22- to 26-gauge needle. Tuberculin or insulin syringes are used most often, although larger syringes may be needed to administer larger volumes.

Intramuscular injection

The IM route is most commonly used. The large, well-developed pectoral muscles are the site of choice. The bird must be restrained well to prevent struggling during IM injection, because muscle may be damaged if the needle is not held steady. Two people should work together to inject birds of cockatiel size or larger (Fig. 28-8). However, one person with good restraint skills can inject IM medications in almost any bird.

IM injections should be given into the thickest part of the breast muscle. Before inserting the needle, the feathers may be wet down with water (not alcohol, which may increase bleeding at the injection site). Once the needle is in place, pull back the syringe plunger to see if any blood is aspirated into the hub. If blood is present, pull out the needle and placed it in a new site. When a satisfactory location is determined, hold the syringe steady while quickly depressing the plunger. Then remove the needle and apply pressure to the puncture site for several seconds. If relatively large amounts of medication must be given, it should be distributed over several sites. It is important to determine that no surface blood is visible before the bird is released.

Intravenous Injection and Blood Collection

The sites for IV injections include the wing (cutaneous ulnar) vein, the medial metatarsal vein, the brachial vein, and the right jugular vein (Fig. 28-9). Simple restraint is usually adequate for administration of small volumes of a

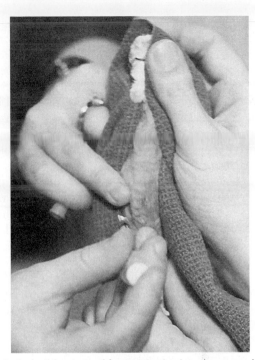

Fig. 28-8 Cockatiel restrained for IM injection into the pectoral muscles. Note the hand placement used to restrain the bird. The injection site is shown *(pointed finger)*.

drug, but a bird requiring a large volume of fluids may be anesthetized to keep it completely still.

Avian veins are extremely delicate, and hematoma formation is common. Use of small-bore, 25- or 26-gauge needles causes the least damage to the vein and minimizes hematomas. The jugular vein is especially fragile, and some practices use it as the last choice, because any hematoma is very visible.

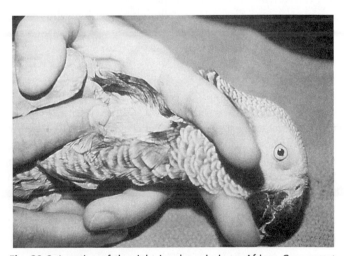

Fig. 28-9 Location of the right jugular vein in an African Grey parrot. Feathers over the area have been plucked. The technician is restraining the head and occluding the vein. *(Courtesy Dr. Heidi Hoefer, Animal Medical Center, New York, N.Y.)*

The person restraining the bird is also responsible for occluding the selected vein and releasing the pressure after the needle is successfully inserted. The injection should be smooth and fast, unless the medication must be given slowly. Once the needle is removed, apply direct pressure to the site for 30 to 60 seconds. A cotton ball soaked in cold water may be used to apply pressure and cause the vessel to constrict somewhat in response to the chilly temperature. The injection site must be evaluated closely for bleeding before releasing the bird.

Blood is usually collected using a 23- or 25-gauge needle. A venous sample may be aspirated into a heparinized syringe and transferred to a microhematocrit tube. The sample can be collected directly into a heparinized microhematocrit tube by holding the tube to the hub of a needle that is in place in the vein. An alternate method is to clip a toenail short enough to induce bleeding and collect the blood into the microhematocrit tube. If the toenail technique is used, the nail should be thoroughly cleaned with alcohol to prevent contaminating the sample with urates from the stool.

Intravenous fluid administration

When a volume of IV fluids must be supplied to a bird, they may be infused using a needle, a butterfly catheter, or a flexible indwelling catheter. A 23- to 25-gauge needle is suitable for large parrots and a 27- to 30-gauge needle is best for the smallest birds, such as budgies. Most birds toy with and destroy IV tubing connected to their catheter, so fluids are often given as a single large-volume injection. A bird in stable condition may be anesthetized to give IV fluids over a more prolonged period.

Before placing a catheter or administering fluids, pluck and surgically prepare the injection site. The fluid usually selected is lactated Ringer's solution, which should be warmed before infusion. A bird that is 10% dehydrated will typically receive replacement fluid volumes of 0.5 ml for a finch, 2 ml for a cockatiel, 8 ml for an Amazon, and 14 ml for a macaw.

Intraosseous injection

When large volumes of fluids must be given to a bird, especially one in shock with collapsed veins, the intraosseous (IO) route is preferred. A needle is inserted directly into the lumen of a long bone that contains marrow. This is because using one of the pneumatic bones, such as the humerus or femur, directs fluids into the respiratory system and can drown the bird. The principal sites are the distal end of the ulna and the proximal end of the tibia. The feathers over the site should be plucked and the skin surgically prepared before the needle is inserted.

Subcutaneous injection

The subcutaneous (SQ) route is not often used, because injected liquid tends to leak readily from the site. However,

if necessary, the dorsal scapular area and the ventrolateral abdomen are used. The most commonly used SQ medications are replacement fluids.

Oral Medication

Most birds reject drugs placed in the mouth, and there are no pilling instruments appropriate for birds. However, certain infections of the intestinal tract must be treated with oral drugs. In exceptional cases, young hand-fed birds may consume medicated food from a syringe or spoon.

One method of treating birds per os (PO) is administering the medication in the food or water. Medicated food or water may have a different taste and not be consumed, or therapeutic levels may never be achieved in the bloodstream. Medicated food allows treatment of large numbers of birds or birds that are impossible to treat in any other manner. Specialized coated feeds and medicated pellets are available commercially. Medicated water is generally used in flock situations.

Tube-feeding

The best way to administer oral medication is the technique known as *gavage*, in which a feeding tube is passed directly into the crop and the medication is injected with a syringe. This is a dangerous and stressful procedure for both patient and technician, because misdirected medication enters the respiratory system, or tube insertion may rupture the esophagus or crop.

A metal feeding tube or red rubber tube may be used. The metal tube is preferable because it is easily palpated to determine correct placement and can be passed without a mouth speculum (Fig. 28-10).

Restrain the bird in a towel in an upright position facing the person passing the tube and hold it as still as possible. One skilled person can usually handle cockatiels and smaller birds, but two experienced people are usually required for larger birds. Insert the tube between the upper and lower mandibles on the bird's left side and is direct it over the tongue and into the esophagus, which lies on the right side of the bird's neck. Placement into the crop is slow and gentle, with palpation of its progress until the crop is reached. Once the medication is infused, slowly withdraw the tube in the same manner. Observe the bird for several minutes for adverse reactions.

Budgies can receive up to approximately 1 ml of medication, cockatiels up to 8 ml, Amazons and cockatoos 15 ml, and the large macaws no more than 30 ml. Slowly inject the proper amount until the crop is full, because excess medication may be regurgitated and aspirated.

Topical Medication

Skin conditions and eye disorders are sometimes treated with topical medication. Feathers that come in contact with topical medications may have to be cleaned with a mild detergent and rinsed well. Birds sometimes ingest medica-

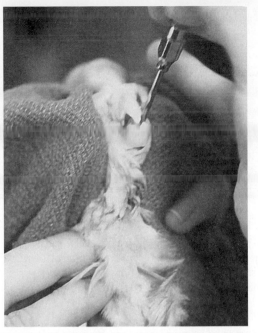

Fig. 28-10 A metal feeding tube is used to administer oral medication to a cockatiel. The tube is passed into the mouth from left to right, and then into the esophagus. The technician is palpating the location of the tube as it is passed. A second person restrains the bird.

tion applied to the skin and may need to be fitted with an Elizabethan collar.

Sinus Flushes

A common problem in pet birds is sinusitis, which may cause signs ranging from sneezing to regional swelling of the head and nasal discharge. Flushing of the sinuses with sterile saline or dilute antibiotic or disinfectant solutions is one method of treatment. Inject the solution directly into the sinus using a needle and syringe, or flush it into the sinus through a nostril using a syringe without a needle.

Nebulization Therapy

In birds with severe or unresponsive respiratory tract infections, nebulization is an effective method of delivering medication directly to the lungs and air sacs. A nebulizer, a machine that creates particles of water minute enough to reach deep into the lung tissue, is required. Nebulization therapy may be done with the bird in a closed chamber or through an anesthetic facemask. A typical treatment regimen is 15 to 30 minutes every 6 to 8 hours using an antimicrobial solution.

CARE OF PEDIATRIC CAGE BIRDS

The psittacines are the most common type of cage birds to be presented for veterinary care during the neonatal and pediatric periods. Most psittacine and passerine species are *altricial*, which means that they have few or no feathers or down when they hatch, they are blind because their eyelids are closed, they cannot hear, and they are helpless. Most neonates cannot stand because of their inadequately developed musculoskeletal system. They are also unable to regulate their body temperature. The skin is very thin at hatching, allowing internal organs to be easily visualized. Their parents or human caretakers must feed them often and provide an environment that is carefully maintained until they are able to see and hear, are feathered, and can eat solid food on their own.

Experienced breeders will seek advice and medical attention when they have a problem in their aviary that is causing higher levels of illness and mortality than usual. Beginning breeders with a number of breeding pairs or individuals who have a single breeding pair may be unfamiliar with the proper techniques required to successfully raise chicks and may consult an avian veterinarian for more basic advice.

Unfortunately, older books and articles that contain incorrect and potentially deadly information are still available for purchase by the client. Some current publications continue to offer advice that is based on outdated ideas or that may have applied to wild caught birds. A practice that sees avian patients should have a list of recommended books and magazines that will educate bird owners.

It is important to have an understanding of the process of raising the domestically bred, hand-raised cage bird from incubation of the egg to the sale of a healthy, well-adjusted young bird to the new owner.

The Avian Neonate

The most common problems encountered in raising cage birds are improper egg incubation, a lack of understanding of the hatching process, poor hand-feeding techniques, improper weaning from formula to a diet of solid food, and unfamiliarity with the phases of development from hatching to weaning.

Incubation of eggs

Eggs may be left with the parents to hatch or placed in an incubator. Eggs tended by parents for 7 to 14 days before being placed in an incubator have a better hatch rate than those incubated soon after they are laid until hatching. In either case, the nest box should replicate conditions in the bird's native environment to increase the number of viable eggs and to prevent inadvertent damage to them by the adults as they move around the nest.

Large breeding facilities generally remove the eggs to an incubator within 24 hours after they are laid to maximize the number of chicks hatched. Incubating eggs need to be turned 5 to 10 times daily, either by the incubator or by hand. This keeps the embryo from sticking to the inside of the egg. Ideally, a temperature of 37.5° C (99.5° F) and humidity of 30% to 45% should be maintained in the incubator for most psittacines. Deviating from these levels will cause many problems for the chick, including high mortality rates. Perform *candling*, or holding a bright light on one side of the egg and inspecting the egg's contents from the other side, every few days to evaluate the embryo's growth. Blood vessels and the growing embryo can be readily seen. Incubation periods range from 30 days for large cockatoos to 18 days for the smallest psittacines. Any eggs that were developing but failed to hatch should be taken to a veterinarian for necropsy to determine the cause of death.

Hatching

Hatching is a complex process that involves several steps. The air pocket present in all eggs will "draw down," or enlarge, 1 to 2 days before the chick emerges. Carbon dioxide levels increase, activating the "hatching muscle" in the neck. During "internal pipping," the egg tooth, a specialized temporary structure located on the tip of the upper beak, breaks through the chorioallantoic membrane and into the air pocket. At this point, the chick breathes air for the first time. The remaining yolk sac contents are drawn into the abdomen and provide nourishment for the hatching process. When CO_2 levels in the air pocket reach 10%, the chick's hatching muscle again begins to twitch and it uses the egg tooth to break through the eggshell in what is known as external "pipping." Some exotic bird breeders will help the chick hatch by removing pieces of shell if the bird seems exhausted before it is completely hatched or is malpositioned within the eggshell and is unable to get out. Others feel the chick must complete the job itself to get a good start in life.

Many aviculturists believe that leaving the chicks with the parents for a while before moving them to a controlled environment will result in larger, healthier chicks.

Hand feeding

Newly hatched psittacine chicks need to be fed every 2 hours for the first 2 days after hatching. On the third day, feedings are scheduled every 3 hours. The number of feedings will be gradually reduced based on the species requirements until the bird is weaned. A syringe, modified spoon, or feeding tube can be used to feed the chick (Fig. 28-11). The crop is relatively large in neonates and is quite visible once the chick has eaten a meal. In some of the larger psittacines, the maxilla is small and the mandible is somewhat enlarged, which helps the parents feed the babies more easily.

Many reputable pet bird food companies make a hand-feeding formula. Typically, water is added to powdered formula. The mixture can be heated in a microwave or prepared with hot water. Microwaved food should be stirred to eliminate any hot spots before feeding. An accurate thermometer

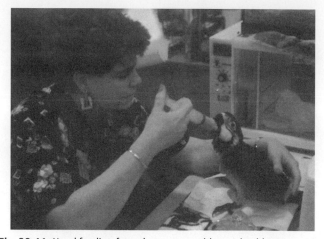

Fig. 28-11 Hand feeding formula to a young blue and gold macaw using a syringe. Note that the syringe enters the beak from the bird's left to right to deposit food near the esophagus. The bird is pumping vigorously during the feeding.

should be used to make sure the formula is between 38° to 40° C (100° and 104° F). Food that is too cold may be refused or may chill the chick, and hot food may cause serious damage to the crop. The consistency of the formula will be very thin (almost watery) for the first feedings. As the bird gets older and larger, a thicker formula is fed.

Breeders may have favorite homemade diets that they have fed to babies for years. Some of these are excellent, but others do not meet the nutritional needs of the chick and lead to stunting or even death.

Weaning

Once the bird is receiving two feedings daily, it can be introduced to solid food. A variety of fresh and cooked foods, as well as formulated diets, should be offered. Weaning is a very stressful period for the bird and may take time to accomplish. Some birds wean themselves by refusing to eat formula, while others beg to be fed formula long after the typical weaning age for the species. The precocious chick that starts eating solid foods on its own before the scheduled time should be allowed to consume what it wants. Weaning must not be rushed or a rigid timeline followed, as the individual bird must be ready both physiologically and mentally to switch to solid food.

A chick should have reached the maximum weight for its species before the weaning process is started. Underweight birds are often more susceptible to disease and may break with a full-blown disease that has been subclinical until weaning stress lowers the immune response. If the weight of the bird is unknown, the age or the amount of feathering can be used to estimate when weaning can begin.

Almost all birds will lose weight during weaning, but will usually regain it in a few weeks or months as they mature. Chicks should be weighed often, preferably daily, to track their progress and to determine when their weight peaks. Weight charts are available in many veterinary avian textbooks or books on psittacine aviculture.

A knowledgeable and experienced person should perform hand feeding. It is easy to feed the bird too quickly or slowly, or to give formula that is too hot or cold. At one time, a majority of breeders believed that the new owner should take the bird home when it was down to one hand feeding per day. The breeders felt that feeding the bird formula would develop a stronger bond between the person and the new bird. It was common to send an unweaned chick home with a new owner with powdered formula and sketchy instructions about the technique of hand feeding. Unfortunately, many young birds died from overfeeding and resulting crop stasis, underfeeding and starvation, inhalation of the formula due to poor technique, and severe crop burns from overheated formula. Conscientious breeders now wean the bird and make sure it is eating solid food well before releasing it to a new owner. The bird will bond just as readily with the new family without the danger of illness, injury, or death due to unskilled and anxious people attempting to learn a difficult technique on their new pet bird. Many avian and veterinary organizations, as well as avian behaviorists, have stated that baby birds must be weaned before they are sold.

Development from hatching to weaning

After hatching, a chick from small species such as the budgie may be left with parents for 1 week to 10 days before starting hand feeding. Species such as the large macaw may be left with parents for up to 3 weeks. If the parents are inattentive or liable to injure the chick due to sudden startle movements, the chicks should be removed sooner.

Once the chick is removed from the nest, it is usually placed in an individual, well-padded container. A flat-bottom plastic cup lined with bunched up paper towels that create a nestlike cavity will help keep the chick upright and clean. As the chick grows, it will be moved to larger plastic containers and bedded on absorbent material such as cloth towels or diapers. Bedding materials such as shavings or ground corncob are very absorbent but may be eaten by curious chicks and lead to intestinal impaction.

Brooders may be used for hatchlings to keep the temperature at 32° to 34° C (90° to 94° F). Once the nestling develops pinfeathers, reduce the temperature to 30° to 32° C (86° to 90° F). When the chick is fully feathered, house it at room temperature (about 21° to 22° C [70° to 72° F]). Keep the humidity at 50%.

The eyes open between the ages of 10 and 26 days, while the ears open from day 2 to day 23. Skin, foot, nail, tongue, and beak pigmentation may be present at hatching or can develop from 2 to 180 days after hatching. The egg tooth will be lost between day 26 and day 44 in most species. The umbilicus heals in 6 to 17 days. Most chicks rest in a sternal position as neonates and will stand up as they mature. The

length of time for each of these phases of development varies with the species of the bird and with each individual.

Common Problems in Neonatal and Pediatric Cage Birds

The most common problems in young birds are infectious diseases; GI injuries, infections, and regurgitation; beak misalignment; musculoskeletal abnormalities; starvation; stunting; and releasing unweaned birds to clients lacking the ability to successfully hand feed the bird.

Infectious diseases

Chlamydiosis. *Chlamydiosis* is caused by the obligate intracellular bacterium, *Chlamydophila psittaci* (formerly *Chlamydia psittaci*). The lungs, air sacs, liver, spleen, CNS, and heart may all be affected. Pneumonia, oculonasal discharge, greenish-yellow diarrhea, dehydration, and weight loss are typical signs. Recovered birds or asymptomatic infected birds may shed the organism. Clinical signs and numerous clinical tests are used to diagnose Chlamydiosis. Unfortunately, no single test will determine whether the bird is acutely ill, a carrier, or uninfected. A 30- to 45-day course of tetracycline is used to treat chlamydiosis and to clear the bird of infection. This disease is zoonotic, so care must be taken to prevent veterinary staff from becoming infected. The health department may need to be notified of documented infections.

Polyomavirus. Polyomavirus is most often characterized by sudden death of young psittacines starting at two weeks of age. It is the most common viral cause of death in breeding facilities. Older affected birds may show lack of blood clotting and GI signs such as vomiting, diarrhea, and crop stasis. Surviving birds grow poorly, have abnormal feather development, and produce excessive and watery feces. Recovered asymptomatic birds shed the virus, keeping the facility contaminated. A test and vaccination are available for polyomavirus. Some veterinarians recommend vaccinating all susceptible birds in a breeding facility, or as soon as possible after purchasing the bird and before it is taken into a new home.

Proventricular dilatation disease. Proventricular dilatation disease, also known as PDD or Macaw Wasting Disease, is a disease first seen as early as 10 weeks of age. Inflammation of the central and peripheral nervous systems are responsible for the characteristic signs of crop stasis, anorexia, cachexia, and incoordination of this fatal disease. Although a virus is suspected to cause the disease, the infectious agent has not been identified. No diagnostic test is available. Treatment trials with the NSAID drug Celebrex (celecoxib, Pfizer) have shown promise in halting the disease.

Psittacine beak and feather disease. Psittacine beak and feather disease (PBFD) is a viral disease that may first be seen in neonates in an infected nursery. Abnormal feather growth is the main sign, and it is easily spread to other birds by feather dust, dander, and feces. The germinal tissues of the beak are also affected, resulting in a misshapen and crumbly beak. Birds are most susceptible up to age 2 or 3 years. Diagnostic testing is available. Young birds that test positive must be isolated and tested again in 90 days, while positive adults must be removed from the flock. All young birds must be tested before they are transferred to new owners or into a breeding situation. New birds are often tested when they receive their postpurchase veterinary examination.

Poxvirus. Poxvirus is most often associated with imported Amazons and macaws, but other species may be infected if housed outside in temperate or subtropical climates.

West Nile virus. West Nile virus is a mosquito-borne disease that primarily infects horses, humans, and birds. It has spread rapidly throughout the United States in the past few years. Psittacines appear to be somewhat resistant, as only a few cases have been reported from endemic areas. However, keeping pet birds inside or in screened areas is suggested to prevent exposure. No avian vaccine is available, but zoo and avian veterinarians are using the equine West Nile virus vaccine produced by the Fort Dodge Company in an attempt to create immunity in exotic species.

Bacterial infections. Bacterial infections commonly affect the gastrointestinal system in psittacine chicks. Birds showing signs of infection such as diarrhea, vomiting, regurgitation, or crop stasis should be treated with antimicrobial and antifungal drugs. Material collected from the crop or cloaca should be cultured and antimicrobial sensitivity determined before treatment begins. Yeast overgrowth is common in birds treated for bacterial infections, so an antifungal medication should be administered during treatment for bacterial infections. Medications are most often given orally, but SC injections are used in birds with crop stasis or regurgitation.

GI injuries, infections, and regurgitation

Crop burns. Crop burns are caused by feeding a young bird formula that is too hot (43° C [110° F] or higher). The burn may affect both the mucosa lining the crop and the skin, but surgery is not performed until a fistula appears. Small burns may heal without surgery. Antimicrobial and antifungal medications are given parenterally, and baseline CBC and blood chemistries are obtained.

Esophageal and pharyngeal punctures. Esophageal and pharyngeal punctures usually occur when a chick is being fed using a tube (red rubber or metal feeding needle) or a catheter-tipped syringe. Birds "pump" as they are fed, becoming more vigorous as weaning approaches. The large macaw chicks are most prone to these punctures. Feeding needles and tubes usually puncture the area where the esophagus enters the crop. The syringe tip penetrates the caudal pharynx slightly to the rear and to the right of the glottis. Emergency surgery is required to repair the tear and remove accumulated food. An endoscope is useful in an anesthetized

bird to locate the tear and flush out the pocket containing the food. Antimicrobials, a short course of corticosteroids, and feeding with a tube will allow healing to occur.

Foreign bodies. Foreign body ingestion is common in young birds. Loose bedding is a favorite for the curious chick. Flushing the crop or removing the material surgically are the most viable options. Surgery may be needed to remove lower GI obstructions.

GI stasis. GI stasis is a common problem in young birds. Crop stasis most often is caused by the yeast infection candidiasis. Other conditions that lead to crop and/or gut stasis are crop burns or punctures, food that is too hot or cold, hypothermia, intestinal foreign bodies, kidney failure, liver failure, and viral infections such as PBFD, PDD, and polyomavirus. Treatment includes SQ or IV fluids, appropriate antimicrobial and antifungal medications, flushing of the crop with saline to remove spoiled food, and support of a very distended crop with a commercial or clinic-made "crop bra."

Regurgitation. Regurgitation is common in birds approaching weaning and indicates that more solid foods should be added to the diet. As the chick increases in size, the crop shrinks in capacity and the number of formula feedings is decreased. If the older chick is overfed formula, it will regurgitate some of the feeding.

Younger birds regurgitate because of crop stasis, crop infection, GI obstruction, overfeeding, and antimicrobial use. Macaws of any age are especially sensitive to sulfa-trimethoprim, doxycycline, and the antifungal nystatin. Young chicks are likely to develop aspiration pneumonia when regurgitated food is inhaled. After a complete physical exam and lab workup, treat the chick with antibacterial and antifungal medications as indicated.

Beak misalignment

Three types of beak malformation are seen in young hand-fed chicks, especially macaws and cockatoos. Scissor beak, the lateral deviation of the maxilla, results in the upper beak slanted to the right or left of the mandible. In the compression deformity, the tips of a shortened maxilla and a normal mandible touch. These two problems affect mostly macaws. Cockatoo chicks may develop an underbite, or mandibular prognathism. Poor feeding technique, stunting, and poorly growing chicks are some of the factors involved. Trimming and physical therapy may be sufficient to correct these deformations in young chicks (Fig. 28-12). The adult bird is able to eat with any of these beak problems, but more frequent trimming may be needed. Surgical repair may be performed in the adult bird if correction of the beak alignment is necessary.

Musculoskeletal abnormalities

Leg problems are often associated with trauma or trying to stand on a slick surface. In splay leg, one or both legs are

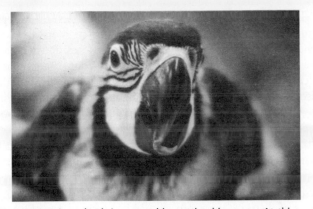

Fig. 28-12 Scissor beak in young blue-and-gold macaw. At this early age, beak misalignment can often be corrected.

deviated laterally so that the chick is unable to stand properly. Chicks may develop an abnormal posture of one leg forward, the other leg back. Young birds respond well to taping the legs in a normal position or using a tape hobble to keep the legs properly aligned. Bedding such as toweling will enable the chick to stand easily without slipping. Some chicks develop a twisted neck. Applying a neckbrace similar to a cervical collar will often straighten the neck into the proper position in a few days. Any bandages or corrective taping must be inspected daily to make sure they are not becoming too tight for a fast-growing chick.

Starvation

Starvation may result from inadequate feeding by the parents, congenital malformation, or underfeeding a hand-fed chick. Inexperienced new bird owners may not be giving the chick enough food at each feeding or may be weaning a chick before the time is right. A new owner may not recognize signs of hunger, begging, or illness exhibited by the chick and can inadvertently starve the young bird.

Stunting

Stunted chicks are very thin and have what appears to be a very large head. The chick grows slowly and may be late in opening its eyes, have dry wrinkled skin, and develop feathers slowly or in irregular patterns. Stress marks that develop on the feathers indicate metabolic irregularities. Subcutaneous fat deposits are minimal. Stunting typically occurs during the first 30 days after hatching. Inadequate feeding, formula that is too watery, environmental temperatures that are too hot or cold, and GI infections are common causes of stunting.

Selling unweaned birds

The Association of Avian Veterinarians, pet bird behaviorists, and knowledgeable breeders oppose releasing unweaned birds to clients lacking the ability to successfully hand feed them. Some breeders promote the false philoso-phy that the client and bird will not bond unless the new owner finishes the weaning process from once daily formula to a diet of solid foods. Many bird behaviorists attribute the majority of behavior problems they are consulted about to weaning techniques that overly stress the bird during the transition to solid food.

Weaning is a time when birds are learning the coordination needed to eat solid food, as well as discovering the social aspects of eating. In some instances, juvenile birds that had been considered weaned entirely to adult food will regress and start begging to be fed by hand. The stress of moving to a new home may trigger this behavior. It is recommended that clients offer warmed food by hand or revert to formula once daily in addition to solid foods. New owners may not know how or whether to feed the bird to satisfy it if they are unfamiliar with the technique of feeding formula and the signs of hunger in a young bird. Some breeders do not respond to calls from frantic new owners once the sale is complete, or they advise them that the bird is weaned and it will eat the solid food in front of it when it becomes hungry enough.

Veterinarians often receive calls from owners of new birds who are unsure what to do. They also see young birds that are starved, begging for food, dehydrated, suffering from aspiration pneumonia, or near death because a well-intentioned but uninformed client did not realize the seriousness of the bird's condition. The bird may die of malnutrition or develop chronic behavioral problems such as constant loud screaming or feather picking.

CARE OF GERIATRIC CAGE BIRDS

Cage birds have only been successfully reared in captivity for about 20 years. Birds acquired before 1980 were wild-caught, often as young nestlings, and tamed before being sold. Captured adult birds were also available, but some never became accustomed to humans as companions. Unless the purchaser obtained a bird that was obviously a juvenile, they never knew how old the bird they brought home was. Poor diets, stress, untreated disease, and lack of knowledge about the intelligence of the most common companion birds also decreased their life span.

The life span of cage birds in captivity has not approached that of birds in the wild. Table 28-1 shows life span differences between birds in the wild and in captivity. The most common life-threatening problem still is feeding a diet that cannot support life. Too many people assume that all a bird needs to consume is seed and water with some snack food. In addition, many people do not understand what bird ownership entails, so they are unprepared for typical avian behaviors such as squawking, destructive chewing, biting, throwing food, and messiness. Behavioral problems lead the list of reasons why people sell their pet

Approximate Life Span of Companion Cage Birds

Species	Potential Life Span in the Wild	Average Life Span in Captivity
Zebra finch	16 years	5 to 6 years
Canary	20 years	7 to 8 years
Budgerigar	18 years	6 years
Cockatiel	30 years	5 to 7 years
Conure	25 years	10 years
African Grey	50 years	15 years
Amazon	75 to 80 years	15 years
Macaw	50 years	15 years

bird. Typically, by the time a bird is 10 years of age, it has passed through a number of homes. A bird that is resilient enough to survive and adapt to these changes may be able to live a longer life if it finally reaches a healthy and compatible home.

Effects of Aging

The oldest documented parrot was an Amazon that lived in Alaska and had numerous owners. She died at the age of 106. She was blind, arthritic, and had a disheveled appearance related to feather loss and lack of preening.

Birds appear to experience most of the same problems that other animals do as they age. The numbers and quality of feathers tend to decrease (Fig. 28-13). Any visible facial skin becomes more wrinkled and thin. The scales on the legs become more pronounced. Swollen, painful joints lead to less activity and stiff movement. Eyesight becomes less keen, cataracts may develop, and some birds lose their hearing. Mental agility often decreases.

Diets lacking in nutrients will affect the liver, kidneys, and other organs (Fig. 28-14). High-fat diets lead to atherosclerosis with narrowing of the arteries and increase the chance of cardiac and cerebral incidents. Neoplasia occurs more often and in more types of tissues. Endocrine disorders such as hypocalcemia and hypothyroidism develop.

A diagnostic workup will include a CBC, blood chemistries to evaluate internal organs, and radiographs or ultrasound if abnormalities are detected or expected from clinical signs. A thorough physical examination is performed. Restraint should be gentle and the exam completed as quickly as possible to minimize stress. If the bird exhibits signs of distress, the exam should be stopped and the bird allowed to rest in a quiet, darkened location.

The life span of hand-fed, hand-raised pet birds provided with a nutritious diet and a stable environment will become evident over the next several decades. The effects of aging will be better understood as the current population of young birds grows older.

ANESTHESIA

Avian anesthesia is common in practice. The veterinary technician must know how birds differ from mammals in their anatomy, response to anesthesia, and recovery. Constant monitoring of the anesthetized avian patient is also extremely important.

Avian Respiratory Tract

The respiratory system of birds is very different than the mammalian tract. The *choana*, a slitlike opening in the roof

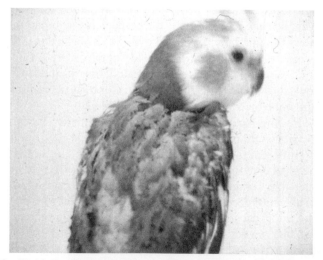

Fig. 28-13 Aged cockatiel with poor feathering. The plumage is rough in appearance, and feather loss is bilateral.

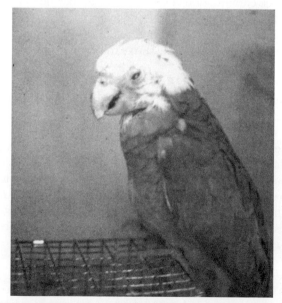

Fig. 28-14 Amazon with vitamin A deficiency from eating a diet exclusively of peanuts. The skin, feathers, and mucous membranes are particularly affected.

of the mouth, opens directly into the nasal cavity. Birds do not have an epiglottis, so they can aspirate crop contents or medications administered by the practitioner. The glottis, located at the base of the tongue, is very visible in many species. The *syrinx*, or vocal organ, located low in the trachea near the thorax, does not interfere with placement of the endotracheal tube. The trachea travels on the right side of the bird's neck adjacent to the esophagus. Air moves down the trachea into the lungs and widely distributed air sacs. The chest should not be restricted during restraint or anesthesia, or suffocation may occur. Birds do not have a muscular diaphragm and use the intercostal and abdominal muscles to move the thorax during the respiratory cycle.

Preanesthesia Evaluation

The veterinarian will usually obtain a weight and perform a thorough physical exam on the bird to be anesthetized. Other tests such as a CBC, blood chemistries, evaluation of swabs from the choana and cloaca, radiographs, and a fecal parasite exam may be performed.

The breathing pattern and rate are closely observed in the bird before proceeding with anesthesia. The bird that exhibits open-mouth breathing or tail bobbing in sync with respirations accompanied by extended wings is not considered a safe anesthetic risk.

The respiratory recovery time (Harrison) will also be tested. After the stress of capture and handling, the respiratory rate should return to normal 3 to 5 minutes after the bird is released. A long recovery time may indicate respiratory system disease, and the bird considered a poor candidate for anesthesia.

Birds are fasted long enough to empty their crop to minimize regurgitation and aspiration of crop contents during anesthesia. Fasting times range from one hour for a budgie to six hours for a macaw. More prolonged fasting may cause hypoglycemia to develop, especially in very small birds.

Birds showing signs of shock, profound anemia, pronounced weight loss, dehydration, crop stasis, respiratory compromise, and noticeable ascites should not be anesthetized until the condition is corrected.

Anesthetic Agents

Isoflurane is the anesthetic agent of choice in birds, as it allows speedy induction, rapid adjustment of the anesthetic level, and fast recovery. Some veterinarians prefer Sevoflurane, but it is much more expensive than isoflurane and should not be used in a vaporizer labeled specifically for halothane or isoflurane. The major advantages of sevoflurane are faster induction and recovery times.

Some practitioners use injectable drugs such as propofol, but the response of individual birds is unpredictable. Many birds will experience cardiac and respiratory depression. Propofol must be injected intravenously, which is painful, and it provides little analgesia. It may be useful for

induction of anesthesia in large birds that respond poorly to mask induction, followed by administration of an inhalant anesthetic. Older injectable drugs such as ketamine are not recommended because they increase the chances of anesthetic death due to the prolonged recovery time and inability to readily reverse the drug.

The isoflurane machine used in small-animal practices is suitable for use with birds. Administer the gas using a semi-open system, which minimizes dead space and allows the bird to breathe easily. The movement of the attached reservoir bag during breathing provides a visual check of the respiratory pattern and is used to bag the patient if its breathing slows or stops. Masks are often used for both induction and maintenance of anesthesia. Depending on the size of the bird, the mask may be placed over the bird's face or head (see Fig. 28-5). Masks used in small-animal or human anesthesia may be suitable for larger birds, but some veterinarians fashion a mask for small birds from a cut-off syringe casing. An induction chamber can be created by positioning a mask completely over the small bird so it forms a tent or by placing a small bird inside a sturdy zipper plastic bag connected to the anesthetic machine tubing (Fig. 28-15).

Types of endotracheal tubes used in birds include uncuffed (or Cole) tubes and cut-off red rubber feeding tubes. Inflatable cuffed tubes may cause tracheal damage and should not be used. Very small birds are rarely intubated because the process is very difficult and the tiny diameter tubes often clog with mucus.

Respiration, heart rate, reflexes, and muscle tone are most commonly monitored during avian anesthesia. The main piece of equipment required is a neonatal stethoscope. Esophageal stethoscopes are rarely placed due to crop anatomy. Some practices utilize ECGs or other electronic monitoring equipment.

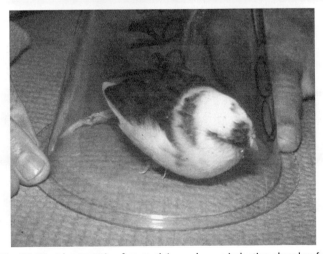

Fig. 28-15 A large canine facemask is used as an induction chamber for a small bird. *(Courtesy Dr. Heidi Hoefer, Animal Medical Center, New York, N.Y.)*

The technician should be familiar with normal reactions to anesthesia and be prepared to act quickly if the bird shows any adverse signs. Epinephrine and doxapram hydrochloride must be available whenever a bird is anesthetized in case of an anesthetic emergency. The dosage and administration of these drugs must be known for any bird anesthetized in the practice.

Induction of Anesthesia

The anesthetic procedure described here is used in many practices, but protocols often differ between clinics. In most cases, no preanesthetic medications are used. Good planning will minimize stress for the patient and veterinary team members.

A mask over the bird's beak and nostrils or entire head will be used to induce anesthesia. The bird's body is well restrained so that it does not struggle unduly and harm itself. A small animal mask is most often used, but small birds may require modified masks.

Induction is accomplished with isoflurane concentrations of 3% to 4%. At the 5% level, some species of birds will hold their breath, resulting in apnea. The oxygen flow rate should minimally be 1 L/min and is usually in the 2- to 3-L/min range for larger birds.

In 1 to 4 minutes, after the bird relaxes, the isoflurane and oxygen levels will be reduced. Most birds will be maintained at 1 to 2 L/min of oxygen and 1% to 2.5% isoflurane. However, macaws are very sensitive to isoflurane and often are maintained at concentrations of 0.5% to 2% to offset respiratory depression.

The facemask is often left in place for the duration of the procedure and is usually secured to the bird's face or head using masking tape or gauze strips tied behind the head. Birds with beak or head injuries must be intubated so repairs can be performed. Most medium to large birds can be easily intubated once they are at maintenance levels of anesthesia. Air sac anesthesia, in which isoflurane is introduced directly into the abdominal air sac, is used in birds that have extensive head or beak trauma or a foreign body in the trachea where continued use of the mask or tracheal intubation would interfere with the repair or surgery.

Monitoring the Anesthetized Bird

The first important parameter to track is the pulse. This is detected by arterial palpation, auscultating the heart with a neonatal stethoscope, or using a cardiac/ECG monitor (Fig. 28-16). If the surgery or procedure prevents hands-on monitoring, an audible cardiac monitor is recommended.

Respiratory rate, rhythm, and depth indicate the plane of anesthesia. Observing the bird prior to anesthesia will allow the respiratory pattern typical to the individual patient to be established. During anesthetic induction, respiration progresses from very irregular to fast and shallow, and finally to the regular breathing of true anesthesia. Shallow, slow breathing indicates a bird that is too deep or has been under anesthesia for a prolonged time. If the respiratory rate is increasing, it is an indication that the bird is too light or that the airway is occluded.

Birds commonly exhibit apnea, especially when induced at the maximum isoflurane concentration of 5%. When this occurs, start positive pressure ventilation (PPV) with pure oxygen, providing enough oxygen to inflate the chest to the normal limits as determined on the awake patient. PPV is also used during normal anesthesia to ensure that the bird is properly ventilated throughout a procedure. A "breath" will be given every few minutes with the isoflurane/gas combination that is being used to maintain anesthesia. Pure oxygen is used only when a bird becomes apneic or is too deeply anesthetized.

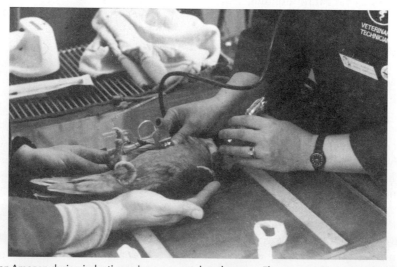

Fig. 28-16 Monitoring an Amazon during induction using a neonatal stethoscope. The next step is to tape the bird to the restraint board.

Accurate assessment of reflexes is difficult in anesthetized birds as compared to small animals. Species differences make the palpebral and corneal reflexes unreliable except during induction. The pupillary reflex is not used because birds have voluntary control of the iris, making any observation questionable.

The loss of muscle tone in the wings and legs, as determined by gently pulling the extremity to check for resistance, indicates the readiness of the bird for basic procedures. Any procedure that causes severe pain will require deeper anesthesia.

Recovery

Recovery after anesthesia with isoflurane is usually rapid and uneventful. As the bird becomes light, muscle tone returns. The bird will move its head, start to right itself, flap its wings, and may vocalize. The bird may be gently held in a towel during recovery or placed in a warm, dark location such as an incubator. The majority of birds will be walking within 10 minutes and fully recovered within 30 minutes.

Some veterinarians inject warm fluids into the anesthetized bird just prior to recovery to increase the fluid volume in the circulatory system and help prevent hypoglycemia. These fluids are administered in both IM and SQ sites. Pure oxygen is sometimes supplied to the bird during the early stages of recovery.

The endotracheal tube must be gently removed as the bird starts to recover muscle tone. The patient may bite the tube in half as it wakes and aspirate the portion left in the trachea.

Potential Anesthesia Problems

Hypothermia may be a life-threatening condition for avian patients. Circulating warm-water pads, bottles filled with warm water, or heated bags of fluids may be used to keep the bird warm. Limb temperature is a commonly used indicator of body temperature, as rectal body temperature is rarely taken in birds.

Bradycardia is common in anesthetized birds. A heart rate below 120 bpm usually indicates a too-deep plane of anesthesia. If the respiratory rate also drops, any procedure underway should be stopped and pure oxygen administered until vital signs improve.

Anesthetic Emergencies

Emergency procedures are started if respiration falls below 25 to 35 bpm for large birds or 35 to 50 bpm for small birds. Pure oxygen is administered, and an injection of doxapram hydrochloride (Dopram) may be given to stimulate respiration. The prognosis is good. When a bird enters respiratory arrest during anesthesia, start emergency procedures immediately. Remove the bird from the anesthesia gases, start it on pure oxygen, and bag several times. If the bird does not start breathing on its own at that time, initiate CPR. Compress the sternum with the fingers at a rate of 30 to 60 times per minute. Doxapram hydrochloride is often injected. The prognosis is good in birds under isoflurane anesthesia.

The prognosis is grave in birds in cardiac arrest. As in respiratory arrest, the bird is placed on pure oxygen, administered sternal CPR, and injected with doxapram hydrochloride. In addition, epinephrine and IV fluids are injected.

AVIAN RADIOGRAPHIC TECHNIQUES

Avian radiography is an easy-to-perform, cost-effective diagnostic tool that results in little radiation exposure for the technician. Restraint is simple in most bird species.

Equipment Used for Avian Radiographs

Any small-animal radiograph machine can readily be used on birds. However, the new generation digital machines provide very close exposure control, resulting in the best quality radiographs. Special radiograph tables are available for exotic pets, which aid in positioning and radiograph control.

The small size of many avian patients, the presence of pneumatic bones, and the internal structure necessitates the use of high-detail film and a high-speed screen system. Special Kevlar cassettes with rare earth screens will yield the best detail. In the absence of a technique chart specific to birds, use of settings for cat extremities of the same thickness should result in satisfactory radiographs.

Proper identification of the patient, hospital, and date of the radiograph are crucial. The position should be marked and special information, such as timing in a barium study, should be clearly indicated on the radiograph.

Adult birds are often immobilized and positioned for radiographs using a restraint board. Once the head is restrained, masking tape is used to hold the patient in position. It is easily removed and reapplied when position changes are made. Baby birds that are still being hand fed may regurgitate when laid flat, so restraint boards must be used cautiously in these birds. Use of the restraint board is stressful for all birds, so materials must be completely assembled and the procedure completed quickly. Even with the best preparations, some birds should be released before the study is completed due to obvious distress.

Large parrots are often anesthetized for even routine radiographs. This eliminates any motion from struggling, decreases the chance of breaking a bone while manipulating the bird, and allows very precise positions to be achieved. The patient must still be taped into position, either on the restraint board or directly to the cassette.

Birds on deficient diets may have fragile bones that fracture under the most gentle handling. Extreme care must be used when positioning any bird for radiographs.

Radiographic Technique

Typical positioning techniques for radiographic studies commonly performed in the clinic are standardized. For the lateral radiograph of the body, place the bird on either side with the wings pulled up and opened away from the body. Arrange the wing closest to the cassette cranial to the upper wing to differentiate between the wings when the radiograph is viewed. Extend both legs caudad. Use masking tape to hold the body, wings, and legs in position directly on the cassette or the restraint board. Fig. 28-17 illustrates a typical lateral radiograph.

Position the bird on its back in a supine position with the wings extended straight out to either side in the ventral-dorsal (VD) view. Use the keel to check for proper positioning. Fig. 28-18 is a typical radiograph in this position.

In both views, the organs are readily visible because they are outlined by the air-filled air sacs. Examine the skeleton closely to estimate density of the bone. Poor contrast indicates insufficient calcification, most often related to a poorly balanced diet.

In order to radiograph the wings or legs without injuring the bird or exposing the technician to the x-ray beam, utilize the restraint board and/or anesthesia. Hold the wings securely in place with masking tape. In small birds, tape the legs down. Place gauze loops on the legs of larger birds just above the feet, and tape the free end to the surface on which the bird is lying to hold the legs in the correct position.

The views taken of the wing are the VD and craniocaudal. The VD view of the wing is positioned exactly like the VD of the body, with the technique adjusted to provide the optimal exposure of the wing structures.

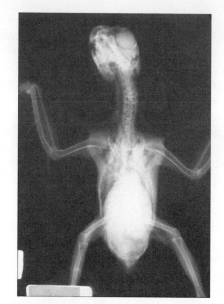

Fig. 28-18 This anesthetized bird is taped directly to the radiograph plate, and the mask has been removed before the radiograph is taken.

Positioning for the craniocaudal view is awkward and somewhat difficult, but the information provided may be impossible to obtain with any other view. Position the cassette perpendicular to the table surface, and rotate the head of the radiograph machine 90° so that the beam is parallel to the table. Place the bird chest-down with the wing fully extended. Hold the front edge of the wing in contact with the cassette. The resulting radiograph is seen in Fig. 28-19.

All joints of the limb should be visible when the leg is radiographed. In a lateral view, the leg under examination rests on the cassette, and the upper leg is pulled caudad to prevent overlap (see Fig. 28-17). Use masking tape to secure the bird on the cassette or restraint board to maintain proper positioning.

The craniocaudal view of the leg is achieved by positioning the bird in dorsal recumbency and extending the leg straight down from the body. The bird is again taped in place during the radiograph (Fig. 28-20).

A variety of radiographic views may be useful if infection of the sinuses or air sacs, or fractures of the head or neck are

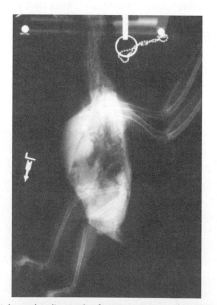

Fig. 28-17 A lateral radiograph of an Amazon. Note that the wings and legs are positioned using masking tape so each can be evaluated individually. The head is held securely by the restraint board.

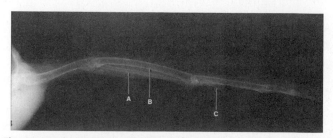

Fig. 28-19 The leading edge of the wing is evaluated using the craniocaudal position. *(From Smith SA, Smith BJ:* Atlas of avian radiographic anatomy, *Philadelphia, 1992, WB Saunders.)*

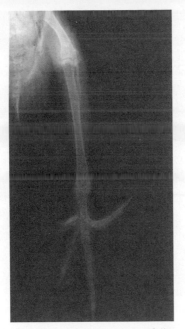

Fig. 28-20 Craniocaudal view of the leg requires full extension of the leg using gauze loops or masking tape for positioning. *(From Smith SA, Smith BJ: Atlas of avian radiographic anatomy, Philadelphia, 1992, WB Saunders.)*

suspected. General anesthesia is generally required in this situation, and the mask or endotracheal tube is removed for most studies. Taping the head and body down will assure proper positioning.

A lateral radiograph is best positioned with the bird on its side. However, the bird is sometimes placed in dorsal recumbency and the head turned into the correct location (Fig. 28-21). The VD view is accomplished by placing the bird on its back in dorsal recumbency with the neck extended and the head rotated back on the cassette

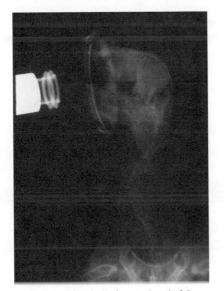

Fig. 28-21 Lateral view of the skull. If more detail of the rostral portion of the head is required, the mask will be briefly removed.

(Fig. 28-22). Masking tape or a nonstretch gauze strip is used to hold the bird's head into position during radiography.

To evaluate the frontal sinuses, the rostrocaudal or skyline view is helpful. For this view, the bird is positioned in dorsal recumbency with the beam directed straight at the beak. Various oblique skull radiographs are useful in determining the extent of lesions.

Gastrointestinal Radiographic Studies

In birds with conditions such as intermittent or chronic diarrhea, suspected GI obstructions, unexplained crop abnormalities, or unusual regurgitation, barium contrast studies may be performed. The bird is fasted for 30 minutes to 4 hours, depending on its size. Recent noncontrast radiographs should be available for comparison with the contrast studies. These radiographs are taken while the bird is awake.

The bird is awake during the entire GI study. Once the fast is finished, pass a stomach tube and infuse warm dilute barium sulfate suspension. Regurgitation and aspiration of the contrast medium may be fatal and should be prevented.

The patient is placed on the restraint board for each VD and lateral radiograph in the series. Radiographs are taken at 1 minute, 30 minutes, 60 minutes, and 2 hours following barium administration. The study is terminated when barium reaches the cloaca, which usually takes about 2 hours. In birds with severe GI involvement, the series is continued until the barium reaches the cloaca or up to 24 hours, whichever is reached first (Fig. 28-23).

Standing Radiograph

A bird with severe respiratory problems may not be able to survive the stress of restraint or may be compromised by the required positions. In this situation, the bird is allowed to rest on a low perch while the wings are gently pulled upward. This provides an unobstructed view of the bird's thorax. Rotate the head of the radiograph machine so the beam is parallel to the tabletop, and hold the radiographic cassette vertically behind the standing bird (Fig. 28-24).

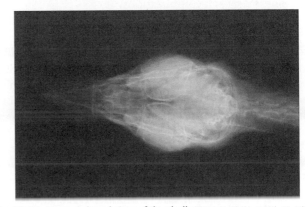

Fig. 28-22 Ventral-dorsal view of the skull. *(From Smith SA, Smith BJ: Atlas of avian radiographic anatomy, Philadelphia, 1992, WB Saunders.)*

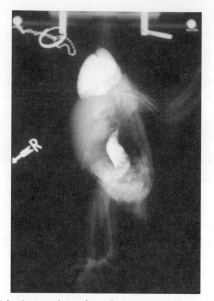

Fig. 28-23 A barium study confirms foreign material in the crop. Lateral view shows high concentration of the barium high in the GI tract after some of it has reached the cecum.

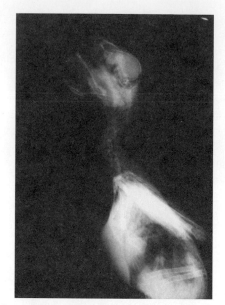

Fig. 28-24 Standing radiograph of a cockatoo in respiratory distress.

Ultrasound Technique

The ultrasound machine is useful in the large parrots and ratites, which includes birds such as ostriches and emus. The systems most commonly evaluated are the liver and female reproductive tract. Visualization of other internal structures is usually impossible, as ultrasound waves are not transmitted by air and most other organs are closely associated with the widely dispersed air sacs.

AVIAN SURGICAL TECHNIQUES

Birds are challenging surgical patients. Anesthesia can be complex. The physical characteristics of birds make hypothermia, hypoglycemia, and blood loss significant factors. Surgeries are carefully planned to minimize time under anesthesia and complications.

Presurgical Evaluations

Birds minimally need to have a thorough physical examination and determination of the respiratory recovery time prior to surgery. If a patient is new or has not been seen by the veterinarian for several months, a fecal exam, CBC, radiographs, blood chemistries, and choanal and cloacal swabs may also be performed.

Birds that are extremely ill or in poor physical condition may have elective surgery delayed until they can be treated medically. Treatments can range from improving the bird's diet to curing underlying infections.

A healthy bird will be fasted prior to surgery for the same period of time as recommended before anesthesia. A large parrot will be fasted for 4 to 6 hours, while a small bird is fasted for 1 to 2 hours. If a bird requires emergency surgery, the crop can be flushed once anesthesia is induced. The bird with a GI disorder that prevents the crop from emptying should have crop contents removed before being anesthetized.

Avian Surgical Equipment

Ophthalmic instruments are commonly used for surgery on the avian patient. Their smaller scale is appropriate for the size of the bird. The veterinarian often uses a magnifying headset to allow visualization of delicate structures.

For internal procedures such as surgical sexing or exploratory laparotomy in which only a small incision is necessary, a rigid or flexible endoscope is widely used. Many practices use electrocautery or electrosurgery units to make incisions and stop bleeding. Other useful devices are heart rate monitors and pulse oximeters.

Nylon or stainless steel suture material is most commonly used in birds and ranges in size from 3-0 to 10-0. Suture should be purchased with swaged-on, or preattached, needles. Some veterinarians make use of internally placed hemostatic clips to control bleeding or for specific surgical procedures.

Surgical Site Preparation and Drapes

The first step in preparation of the surgical site is plucking of feathers in order to provide 2 to 4 cm of bare space surrounding the proposed incision. Once the bird is anesthetized, large feathers are pulled individually in the direction of growth. Groups of 3 or 4 small feathers can be plucked by pulling them opposite the direction they are growing. If possible, removal of flight feathers is avoided. There is the possibility of damage to the feather follicle, resulting in growth of deformed or misdirected feathers.

Feathers adjoining the surgical site are kept away from the incision site by holding them down with nonadhesive stretch tape (Vetrap), masking tape, or sterile water-soluble lubricating gel. A section of Stockinette can be used to encase the bird's body and hold feathers in place.

The surgical site is prepped using dilute chlorhexidine (Nolvasan) or povidone iodine (Betadine) solution. Sterile saline, rather than alcohol, is used to flush the disinfectant solution away. Alcohol is avoided because use may cause hypothermia to develop as it evaporates from the skin.

Transparent adhesive disposable surgical drapes are often used in birds. They adhere directly to the prepped skin, and the incision is made through the plastic drape material. Other advantages include ease of monitoring, conservation of body heat, and low cost. The drape must be removed carefully to minimize trauma to the bird's skin.

Recovery of the Surgical Patient

Awakening birds are often placed in an incubator heated to (86° F) (30° C) and may be given supplemental oxygen. When the bird is alert and exhibiting normal activity, it is often placed in a small cage containing only perches and containers of food and water. Analgesics and antimicrobial medications may be administered after surgery.

Birds often pick at their sutures or bandages. If this occurs, a restraining device such as an Elizabethan collar may be used. Sutures are usually removed 7 days postoperatively.

COMMON SURGICAL PROCEDURES

Endoscopy

The rigid endoscope, which provides superior visualization, is commonly used in avian patients. Many veterinarians use the 2.7-mm scope, as it can be successfully used in almost all size birds.

The endoscope is very delicate and must be picked up by the eyepiece. Following a procedure, rinse the scope rod with distilled water, wipe the lens with lens paper, and rinse the rod portion again with alcohol and allow it to evaporate. The endoscope is then sterilized using ethylene oxide gas or through a timed immersion in a dilute glutaraldehyde solution. It will be stored flat in its protective case between uses. Some bird owners ask that their birds be surgically sexed. Although highly accurate sexing using a blood sample is available, the use of an endoscope to visualize the reproductive tract enables the veterinarian to evaluate the health status of the reproductive organs. Once the bird is anesthetized, prepped, and restrained in right lateral recumbency, a small incision is made between the sternum and last rib. When the tip of the scope is introduced into the incision, it passes into two air sacs and is then positioned so that the reproductive organs are in sight. After careful examination of the tract, the scope is removed. The skin may or may not be sutured.

Other organ systems are evaluated visually using endoscopy. The flank incision location used for surgical sexing is the most common approach. The organs or system to be studied determine whether the right or left side will be the site of entry for the scope. Examples of other conditions that are commonly evaluated using the endoscope are respiratory disorders, systemic disease, and digestive system ailments.

Organs may be sampled using the endoscope's biopsy instrument. Tissues obtained in this manner will be very small and easily lost. After collection, they are often arranged on filter paper or closely woven cloth, which is then immersed in fixative solution. Alternatively, biopsy samples may be placed in fixative in a blood collection tube that does not contain anticoagulant.

Physical interference with the procedure occurs in overweight or ovulating birds, where the organs may be obscured by fat or an enlarged ovary. Complications of exploratory endoscopy include damage to internal organs, infection, and problems with anesthesia.

Reproductive Surgery

Birds that are egg-bound may require surgery to remove the egg that is trapped in the reproductive tract if medical treatment fails. Well-nourished, healthy birds that are treated before the cloaca prolapses often will survive.

Hysterectomies are performed in birds whose health has been threatened by chronic egg laying or egg binding. The uterus and oviduct, but not the ovary, are removed. The bird may still exhibit egg-laying behavior, but the ovary will no longer produce eggs.

Sinus Surgery

Sinus surgery is reserved for birds with refractory sinusitis that is causing pronounced signs that have not responded to medical treatment. These birds often exhibit sneezing, swelling of the face, bulging of the eye, and conjunctivitis. Surgery to remove any cheesy purulent material or foreign bodies is performed through an incision sited between the eye and nostril on each affected side.

COMMON TRAUMATIC INJURIES

Beak Injuries and Repair

Some birds inflict severe injuries to other birds if given the opportunity. They may literally destroy the upper or lower beak of their victim. Fractures of the mandible may occur. Even seemingly minor injuries may lead to permanent damage. After hemorrhage is controlled, the patient is evaluated for the type of repair that will be required.

Injuries that result in minor defects can be filled with acrylic material that hardens and is shaped to match the contours of the rest of the beak. This will eventually be replaced as the beak grows out. Mandibular fractures can be repaired using acrylic with pinning techniques. The fracture will heal in about six weeks.

In cases in which damage is extensive or involves the growth center of the beak, a prosthetic may need to be created. This is fashioned out of acrylic and formed into a "false beak." It is attached somewhat like an artificial fingernail and will need to be replaced regularly. Clients should be informed of the disadvantages, which include pressure necrosis, impaction of food at the attachment site, and development of gaps.

Some developmental beak disorders such as twisting or underbite may need to be corrected surgically if they do not respond to manipulation. For an underbite, the tip of the upper beak is lengthened with acrylic so that the tip is forced into the proper position. This is very successful in young chicks. Removal of a portion of the premaxilla and pinning of the bones may be used in expensive birds to correct beak twisting.

Crop Repair

Timing of surgery on damaged crops will depend on the severity of injury. Birds with extreme trauma from ceiling fans or animal bites must be operated on immediately to save their lives. Surgery on baby birds whose crops were burned with excessively hot formula often is deferred for 7 to 10 days until a fistula develops, and the extent of the injury is obvious. After surgery, the birds are fed small volumes of formula more frequently until healing occurs.

Foreign Bodies

Foreign bodies are often inhaled. Typical, inhalation involves seeds, toys, splinters of wood, and chunks of infected tissue. Removal methods vary with the object and the size of the bird. In large psittacines, an endoscope with grasping forceps may work well. In small birds such as cockatiels or finches, a tracheostomy may be needed to retrieve the object. Other creative methods may be employed.

Potential ingested foreign materials are toys or parts of toys, bedding, metallic items (wire, hairpins), string, fish bones, splinters, and tough plant fibers.

A thorough physical exam and radiographs often determine the problem, but specialized studies may be required. Endoscopic techniques and/or surgical removal may be required to retrieve the objects.

Setting Fractures

The veterinarian should make a number of decisions before proceeding with fracture treatment. The condition, age, and personality of the bird should be considered. The patient should be evaluated for any pre-existing or concurrent medical conditions that prevent immediate repair.

Each individual's fracture is different, and plans for repair may change as the surgery progresses. The client is consulted to determine acceptable outcomes. It is also necessary to access the client's willingness and ability to comply with aftercare of the fracture. Healing time is about 3 to 8 weeks, depending on repair method selected, fracture location and complexity, extent of associated soft tissue injury, and nervous tissue damage. The least invasive, most effective correction method is desired.

Bandages and splints are used when some support of the fracture is all that is necessary. This method will make the bird more comfortable, but may not allow proper healing and return to full function. Fractures commonly stabilized with this treatment are some wing and foot breaks. These techniques are justified in very small birds unsuitable for surgical repair, or if anesthesia and surgery may be fatal.

Long bone fractures, like those of the humerus and femur, require stabilization using mechanical fixation. The large muscles that attach to these bones tend to separate the fracture ends, preventing bony unions. External fixation devices, intramedullary pins, and Doyle devices are all used to repair fractures in birds.

Several types of external fixation devices are used in birds. They produce excellent stabilization of fracture sites and joints. Birds often start using the injured limb within a few days of repair. Most birds tolerate these appliances surprisingly well. Other advantages include their modest price, light weight, and ease of removal. External fixation will provide the best chance for return to full function. Intramedullary pins are used to keep the fracture ends aligned. Used by themselves, they allow rotation of the bony section to occur. Pins may cause damage to internal structures of the bones even when placed correctly. Many surgeons use external fixation with IM pins. Bandages are often applied when fractures of long bones are repaired solely with IM pins. They should be used for up to 3 weeks and result in loss of mobility of the limb, which may be permanent. In extreme cases, a traumatized wing cannot be salvaged. In this instance, amputation may be the only choice. Most psittacines do quite well after losing a leg since they use their beaks to move around. They perch comfortably and rarely develop foot problems. In pet birds, removal of a wing may cause some loss of balance. The majority of birds adapt well to toe amputations.

Feather Cysts

Feather cysts can be found on the wing, back, or body surface. These are a result of ingrown feathers that are surrounded by necrotic tissue, forming a subcutaneous mass. The treatment of choice is surgery, as the cyst will grow back if drained by aspiration or lancing. The cyst may be incidental and associated with trauma, poor nutrition, or infection. Some types of hybrid canaries appear to be genetically predisposed to cyst formation. The entire cyst must be removed, including the involved follicle, and the incision sutured. Care is taken to avoid damage to adjacent feathers or their blood supply. Hemostasis is important. A tourniquet is used on the wing. Stabilization of the wing with a bandage will hasten healing.

Tail feather cysts may require removal of the pygostyle (fusion of the last caudal vertebrae) with the cyst. Cysts found on the body are easy to remove. Entire feather tracts may need to be excised in affected canaries to prevent recurrence.

Tumor Removal

The incidence of tumors varies with the species of bird. Budgies are often referred to as "tumor factories" due to the frequency with which they develop various neoplasias. Other species of birds predisposed to cancer are African Greys, Amazons, cockatiels, and rose-breasted cockatoos. Location, invasiveness, and interference with activities of daily living will determine removal of these growths.

Malignancies in African Greys are increasingly being reported. Many types of tumors have been documented. Of the large psittacines, the Amazons have the highest rate of occurrence of neoplasms. Older birds develop carcinomas, and adenocarcinomas of the liver are common at all ages. Surgical intervention is indicated if neoplasias do not respond to dietary and supportive therapy.

Budgies, even those less than 1 year of age, develop an astonishing number of types of tumors. An overwhelming quantity of lipomas and xanthomas are diagnosed, both of which may respond positively to dietary therapy. Viruses are implicated in production of some growths. Removal of external neoplasia is most successful. Internal tumors often spread to local structures and cannot be excised.

A variety of tumors of the musculature of the wings is common in cockatiels. Surgery can range from removal of the growth to wing amputation.

Rose-breasted cockatoos tend to produce lipomas, especially when they are obese. Weight loss through dietary changes often shrinks this benign tumor. If the lesion is ulcerated, interferes with the bird's daily activities, or is unresponsive to dietary modification, surgical removal is indicated.

EMERGENCIES IN AVIAN PRACTICE

Emergency medicine is one of the most important aspects of dealing with birds in veterinary practice. Decisions must be made without referring to textbooks. Management of the critically ill patient often is the technician's responsibility, and it is imperative that this care be conscientiously handled. Prompt assessment of the bird's physical condition, and obtaining an in-depth history are supremely important. An unanticipated trip to the veterinarian produces much anxiety in both the bird and the client. Immediate physical and emotional cares are indicated. Almost anything out of the ordinary is an emergency with a pet bird. Even if the bird is presented for a grooming appointment or a well bird exam, any noticeable signs indicate trouble.

Patient Evaluation

The pet bird should be closely appraised for signs of illness or injury that may lead to death if the bird is handled. A bird that is dyspneic and sitting on the bottom of the cage is critically ill, and should be placed in an oxygen chamber immediately.

In certain situations, the decision to handle a sick bird immediately depends on the presence of a life-threatening injury or condition.

A bird in a weakened state should be handled carefully. This may mean that a physical exam, bloodwork, cultures, or manipulation are done in stages, allowing the bird to rest in between. Isoflurane gas anesthesia of brief duration is used by some veterinarians to immobilize carefully selected weak, dyspneic, or unruly birds. This allows all the tests to be run expeditiously with little stress. Vigilant monitoring of these anesthetized patients is crucial.

A brief initial history often pinpoints the cause of the immediate problem. An in-depth interview of the client after the bird is stabilized will complete the records and identify any underlying additional problems. A hysterical client is not uncommon. Patience, compassion, and composure are invaluable in calming the client and getting an accurate history.

A weight should be obtained on birds that will not be overly stressed by handling. If this is impossible, drug dosages can be calculated on the average weight for the species.

If no immediate intervention is indicated, the bird can be allowed to rest after sample collection until test results are available. Radiographs are often not taken until the bird is stabilized. If needed for diagnosis, light gas anesthesia is used.

Suggested Emergency Equipment

Besides the emergency equipment commonly found in small-animal practice, other items specific to birds should be on hand (Box 28-1).

Shock and Fluid Therapy Guidelines

A bird that is greater than 10% dehydrated or has lost more than 20% of its blood volume will be in shock when brought to the clinic. It should be given corticosteroids, fluids, and kept warm. Antibiotics and oxygen should be administered if necessary. Bleeding must be stopped using direct pressure or coagulants applied.

Suggested Equipment for Avian Emergencies

- Gram scale
- Intensive care unit
- Gavage equipment
- Red rubber tubes
- Spinal needles for IO fluids
- Leg band cutters
- Fine suture material (5-0, 6-0)
- Injectable calcium
- Antifungal agents
- Assorted bird feeds
- Bandage materials
- Elizabethan collars
- Safe and Warm heating pads
- Isoflurane anesthesia machine
- Butterfly catheters
- Metal feeding tubes
- Insulin syringes and needles
- Electrocautery unit
- Endotracheal tubes
- Drugs-calcium EDTA
- Antibiotics
- Concentrated feeding formula
- Crash cart with emergency drugs
- Wound dressings
- Hemostats for blood feather removal

A severely dehydrated bird will show tenting of the skin of the eyelids. The fluid of choice in shock is lactated Ringer's solution warmed to 38° to 39° C (100.4° to 102.2° F) administered IV or IO.

For IV fluids, a catheter is placed in a leg, wing, or jugular vein. IO fluids are infused by placing a catheter in the distal ulna or proximal tibia. SQ fluids are not recommended, because they absorb slowly and are painful. Oral fluids are only given to an alert bird with no GI impactions.

Since most types of birds will not tolerate IV drip lines and will chew on a catheter or tubing, fluids usually are given as a *bolus* (all at one time). Fluids equal to ¼ to ⅓ of the bird's total blood volume can be given over a 5- to 7-minute period. Only half of the needed fluids should be given the first 24 hours, and the rest of the fluids over the next 48 hours.

COMMON EMERGENCY PROCEDURES

Broken Blood Feathers

Blood feathers are so highly vascular that birds can bleed to death if the shaft breaks. The remaining feather must be pulled to stop the bleeding. Use a hemostat to grasp the feather shaft close to the skin. Stabilize the wing as the feather is gently pulled. This may be difficult, as the flight feathers are embedded in the radius. Any bleeding from the feather site can be stopped using direct pressure.

Clients who call from home about broken feathers should be encouraged to attempt to pull the feather themselves. Give complete and detailed instructions over the telephone. Once the feather is removed, have the client apply peroxide. If bleeding still occurs, flour or cornstarch should be applied. Have the client place the bird in a darkened environment until it can be brought to the clinic.

Wing Fractures

Fractures of the wing usually are immobilized with a figure-8 bandage. This holds the flexed wing snug against the body. If the humerus is fractured, apply a body corset. An open fracture should be flushed and cleaned. Both oral and topical antibiotics are given. Birds that are shocky or have lost blood should be given fluids. Most broken wings will need to be bandaged for three to five weeks with weekly changes. The bandage should be removed as soon as healing is complete.

Complications include stiffness, muscle atrophy from disuse, and loss of flight feathers. Physical therapy will help the bird become limber and recover muscle mass. Some severe fractures are best treated by surgery. The wing will need to be stabilized until surgery can be performed.

Leg Fractures

Some lower leg fractures are stabilized with a splint until healing occurs, usually four to six weeks. Because of the bird's anatomy, splints will worsen fractures of the femur and upper tibiotarsus. These often require prompt surgical repair.

The Schroeder-Thomas splint can used to treat fractures of the lower third of the tibiotarsus and the entire tarsometatarsus. The bandage is changed every one or two weeks and is accompanied by passive physical therapy.

A Robert Jones bandage can be used for simple lower-leg fractures. Although these are heavily padded, additional splinting materials such as tongue depressors may be needed. Change the bandage at least every two weeks.

A Ball bandage is used for broken toes or foot infections. Place a ball formed of gauze sponges so the toes curl around it. Cover the foot with cotton padding and wrap with stretchy self-adherent bandaging.

Very small birds can be difficult to splint. Materials such as pipe cleaners, toothpicks, paper clips, and wooden applicator sticks are used to treat their fractures. Toe fractures can be treated in large birds by taping the broken toe to the neighboring intact toe. With all splints, it is necessary to assess circulation in the foot. Look for swelling of the toes, blue coloration, and coldness. Change the bandage if any of these occur.

Flush and clean open fractures, then apply topical antibiotics. Surgical correction is generally required. Use splints to support the repaired break.

Check bandages often for signs of chewing or moisture. Advise clients to bring the bird to the clinic for a bandage change. It is advisable to remove leg bands, because they may cause fractures when they become caught on a cage or other objects.

Cat Attacks

If the cat does not kill the bird outright, the primary risk is infection of the wound. The sites will need to be thoroughly cleaned and the bird placed on an appropriate antibiotic for 7 days. Advise clients to bring the bird in immediately, even if the wounds seem minor. Most injuries from cat attacks will be found on the back or wings of the bird. The cat stalks the bird so that it cannot be seen and springs on its prey from the rear.

Bird Attacks

Certain types of birds have the reputation of fighting with their mates or others of their species. This may be related to the breeding season, as in cockatoos and Eclectus, or simply aggression, as seen in Australian parakeets and mated pairs of lovebirds. The cockatoo male frequently becomes unpredictable during breeding season and may kill his mate, especially if confined with her in a breeding flight. Typical injuries include beak and head trauma.

The Eclectus hen is the aggressor and may inflict fatal damage on her mate. Injuries are similar to those seen in cockatoos. Lovebirds are known for their quarrelsome marital nature. Arguments and outright fights may lead to various injuries. Some Australian parakeets are totally incompatible and will fight to the finish. Clients must observe these birds closely when they are placed together and separate them if necessary.

Crowded or stressful situations can lead to feather mutilation of cage mates. This is common in finches and may lead to death in the victim.

A veterinarian should see birds that have been injured by others. Antibiotics are commonly prescribed. Severely battered birds may require reconstructive surgery to repair damage. Beaks and feet are typical locations of bird-inflicted trauma.

In general, different species should not be housed together. Larger birds may attack and kill smaller residents. Advise clients to separate any birds that show aggressive tendencies.

POISONING

Exposure to Toxic Fumes

Airborne toxins are very dangerous to birds. They may die within a few minutes of exposure or develop chronic problems. Examples include overheated Teflon pans, hairspray, tobacco smoke, paint fumes, strong cleaning chemicals, carbon monoxide, and dust from leaded paint. Although controversial, there is evidence that newly laid carpet may emit noxious fumes that affect birds and humans.

Treatment for aerosol toxicity includes giving the bird fresh air or placing it on oxygen if signs are particularly acute. Since pulmonary irritation is common, antibiotics are given to prevent infection. Steroids may be used if pulmonary edema (fluid accumulation of the lungs) occurs. Other supportive techniques, such as fluid administration, are used as necessary.

Heavy Metal Poisoning

The two heavy metals most commonly associated with poisoning are lead and zinc. Typically, ingestion of curtain weights, lead clappers from bells, old-style solder, lead-based paints, plaster, foil from wine bottles, and calcium-rich dolomite or bone meal can result in signs of lead poisoning. Galvanized cage wire is the usual source of ingested zinc.

Clinical signs of lead poisoning vary between species. Most birds will show lethargy, loss of weight, polydipsia/polyuria, depression, weakness, wing droop, and neurological signs (head tilt, blindness, circling). Amazon parrots are the only species that will develop hematuria in acute cases. Eclectus will characteristically show biliverdinuria (greenish staining of urine). Other parrots have no urinary color changes.

Diagnosis may be based on signs and radiographic findings of lead or zinc within the body. Both metals may be detected in the digestive system, or lead shot may be found in tissues. Whole blood samples can be sent to an outside lab to analyze for heavy metals. EDTA should not be used as the anticoagulant, as it will interfere with testing. A regenerative anemia is often found in poisoned birds.

Since testing may take days to weeks, treatment should be started before the blood levels are received if radiographs and signs suggest poisoning. Birds are treated with CA EDTA (IM), and/or oral d-penicillamine. If large amounts of metal are present, they need to be removed surgically. Response is usually rapid, and improvement may be seen in a few hours or days.

Ingested Poisons

Birds often explore new items by mouthing them and feeling their texture with their tongues. This exposes them to possible poisoning with lethal effects. It is imperative to prevent contact of a pet bird with any common household cleaners and polishes, prescription drugs not intended for the individual bird, and toiletries such as perfume, shampoo, or deodorant. Cigarettes, matches, and fireworks are potentially fatal. Cleansing agents and detergents may cause skin eruptions, GI upsets (vomiting and diarrhea), respiratory tract irritation, esophageal damage, and coma in extreme cases.

Hydrocarbon-based compounds such as furniture polish and other petroleum products (gasoline, kerosene) lead to central nervous system effects (disorientation, depression), pneumonia (aspiration, lipoid), GI upset, kidney and liver damage, and mucous membrane and skin damage.

Prescription drugs cause a wide variety of signs. The client must bring the container or remaining contents for identification.

Clients often expose birds to toiletries in the bathroom. Perfumes and deodorants may cause damage to the skin and mucous membranes, respiratory tract, kidneys, liver, and CNS. Shampoos lead to diarrhea and irritation of the eyes.

Even small amounts of tobacco products can result in vomiting, diarrhea, convulsions, and sudden death. Eating fireworks or matches can result in vomiting, diarrhea, blood in the stool, and increased respiration. Cyanosis may also occur.

Advise the client to bring the bird in for evaluation as soon as possible after the drug is consumed. To ascertain the correct treatment, consult an up-to-date pharmacology reference book or poison control center.

Affected birds are treated symptomatically. Consult current references for specifics.

Poisonous Plants

Many plants have been blamed for illness in birds, but plant poisoning is actually rare. Birds often will tear leaves without eating them, decreasing the amount ingested. The avian GI tract empties quickly, further reducing chances of poisoning. Clients may unintentionally expose their birds to poisonous plant materials through feeding or use of plants for house decoration.

For the most part, "people food" is safely fed to birds. The one exception is avocado, which can cause nonspecific signs of illness. Typically the bird fluffs its feathers, sits on the bottom of the cage, loses its appetite, and exhibits signs of respiratory distress. Death can occur 15 minutes to 15 hours later. Treatment is symptomatic. Activated charcoal, oxygen, a mild diuretic, and warmth are administered.

Black locust, oak, oleander, and rhododendron branches should not be used for perches as they may cause toxicity. Ornamental plants that may poison birds include clematis, dieffenbachia, foxglove, lily of the valley, lupine, philodendron, poinsettia, and yew. Some clients feed green outdoor plants to their birds. Crown vetch and parsley should be avoided.

If clients call the clinic with a bird showing unusual signs after exposure to any plant, ask them to bring the bird in for evaluation. Have clients bring the offending plant or a sample, and ask them to estimate the amount ingested.

Treatment is supportive. Advise clients that poisonings can be lethal without prompt intervention.

REPRODUCTIVE DISORDERS

Certain reproductive problems are frequently seen in practice.

Egg Binding

This is a commonly seen emergency in budgies, canaries, cockatiels, finches, and lovebirds. The birds typically have been laying eggs for some time, thus depleting their calcium stores. This causes decreased muscle activity in the oviduct, and the egg becomes trapped. Signs can include abdominal distention and straining, depression, sitting on the cage bottom, tail wagging, and walking with widespread legs. Emergency treatment consists of stabilizing the bird if it is shocky. Correction of the problem varies from giving drugs to surgical removal.

Egg Yolk Peritonitis

The disorder is common in budgies, lovebirds, and macaws. Death may occur if treatment is not sought. The cause of this disorder is rupture of a forming egg that has failed to enter the oviduct. The yolk causes inflammation of the lining of the abdomen. Affected birds are anorectic and depressed, presenting with an enlarged abdomen and dyspnea. Immediate treatment includes corticosteroids, antibiotics, a warm location, and fluids. When the patient is stabilized, surgery may be indicated. The prognosis worsens if treatment is delayed.

GASTROINTESTINAL PROBLEMS

Crop Burns

Clients or breeders may bring in a baby bird that has "food leaking from its chest." This is the result of a thermal burn caused most often by too hot food placed in the crop. This is considered an emergency when the resulting hole is so large that the entire feeding leaks out. The bird will become dehydrated and starve to death. Immediate suturing of the region is necessary in these cases to save the bird's life.

Regurgitation

Regurgitation refers to the expulsion of small amounts of crop contents. This may be a breeding behavior or can be pathological. It may be indistinguishable from vomiting. Toxicities, digestive difficulties, or metabolic disease processes may cause abnormal regurgitation. A good history needs to be obtained to determine the type of regurgitation occurring. Birds that have been regurgitating are often dehydrated and will receive fluid therapy. Other treatments include antibiotic or antifungal drugs in infectious cases, toxin neutralizing compounds in poisonings, and removal of any foreign bodies causing the problem.

MISCELLANEOUS PROBLEMS

Acute Dyspnea

Sudden difficulty breathing is most often related to tracheal blockage. The most common causes of this are inhaling foreign material, such as seeds or bedding, exposure to toxic substances, and inhalation of infectious material that has accumulated in the respiratory tract. Diagnosis of the specific cause of respiratory difficulties will determine the course of treatment.

The bird will be anesthetized using isoflurane given through a tube into an air sac. If relief is immediate, the problem is in the upper respiratory tract. Other diagnostic techniques include radiographs, using an endoscope to inspect the trachea directly, and transillumination of the neck in small birds.

To treat a tracheal blockage, suction or forceps are used to remove the material. Cockatiels are often found to have inhaled a seed. In some cases, a tracheostomy must be performed to gain access to the foreign body so that it may be pushed out of the trachea to the mouth.

Seizures

Seizures from exposure to toxins, hyperthermia, liver failure, hypoglycemia, CNS inflammation, hyperglycemia, neoplasia, and cardiac instability all look identical. Diagnostic workups include a complete physical, serological testing, CBC, and a thorough history. Treatment will depend on the findings. If epilepsy is suspected, an EEG may be performed.

NONSPECIFIC ILLNESS

Birds are often presented with nonspecific signs such as "fluffed up," sitting on cage bottom, loss of appetite, untidy appearance, lethargy/weakness, droopy eyelids, and loss of interest in surroundings. The bird that is simply not doing well is a challenge. The patient should be placed in an oxygen cage, handled as little as possible, and allowed to rest between diagnostic procedures to decrease stress that may kill an acutely ill bird.

REPTILES AND AMPHIBIANS
Sarah Okumura

BIOLOGY

Reptiles

Reptiles include snakes, lizards, chelonians (turtles and tortoises), and crocodilians (alligators and crocodiles). Common pet species of snakes include boas and pythons, kingsnakes, corn snakes, and gopher snakes. Common pet species of lizards include iguanas, geckos, monitors, and chameleons. Common pet chelonians include box turtles, red-eared sliders and other water turtles, and various tortoises. Crocodilians are less frequently kept as pets.

Reptiles are *ectothermic* or "cold-blooded," which means they do not generate their own body heat. They instead get body heat from their environment. Each species has a particular environmental temperature at which they do best. The metabolic rate of reptiles depends on their body temperature, so at lower than ideal temperatures their digestive, immune, and other systems do not function well.

All reptiles have protective scales covering their skin. They shed the outermost layer of their skin and scales on a regular basis. Species that shed all at once, such as snakes, are vulnerable to skin injury while they are shedding. They should be handled very gently, if at all, during this time. An interesting feature of the shedding process of snakes is that they will also shed a scale that normally covers the eye. About a week before shedding, the snake's eye will turn cloudy until this scale is shed.

Like birds, reptiles lack a diaphragm to separate the thoracic and abdominal cavities. They have one visceral cavity called the *coelom*.

Most reptiles have a renal portal system, which is a network of blood vessels associated with the kidneys. This is of clinical importance because it may cause medications injected into the caudal part of the body to be carried to the kidneys before being distributed to the rest of the body. This can result in damage to the kidneys or excretion of the drug before it has its desired effect.

Reptile excretions are similar to those of birds, and include solid whitish urates. The cloaca is the common opening through which the urinary, digestive, and reproductive systems empty. Reptiles are adapted to reproduce on land. Their eggs have a tough, leathery covering.

Amphibians

Amphibians include frogs, toads, salamanders, and newts. They are less common pets than reptiles. Frogs and toads are the most popular. Many of the characteristics described for reptiles are also true of amphibians, but there are some important differences. The skin of most amphibians is very soft and tender, and does not have scales. Gases and liquids, including toxins, can be absorbed through this porous body covering.

All amphibians spend at least some portion of their life cycle in water, and reproduction occurs in water. Amphibian eggs are delicate and must be kept wet, similar to fish eggs.

Amphibians do not produces urates. Instead, their urinary waste product is ammonia. Their environment must be kept clean to prevent poisoning from excessive ammonia buildup.

HOUSING

The vast majority of illnesses in pet reptiles and amphibians are related to poor husbandry practices. Therefore, accurate client education on proper housing and feeding of the particular species is the single most effective way that the veterinary team can improve the health of these patients.

Reptiles

Many reptiles can be adequately housed in a simple terrarium that is sized appropriately for the animal. As a rule, the simpler the housing setup, the easier it is to observe the pet and clean the environment.

A terrarium of appropriate size can easily accommodate most pet reptiles. There are many choices of substrates (bedding materials). The substrate should be easy to remove for cleaning or replacement. Artificial turf is most commonly used because it is easy to clean and is attractive. Care should be taken to ensure that the edges do not become frayed. Reptiles may chew on and subsequently ingest this frayed material, causing an impaction in the digestive system.

Other suitable substrates include terrycloth towels, newspaper, and butcher paper. Unacceptable substrates include dirt, sand, cat litter, crushed corncobs, and crushed peanut shells. These substrates are difficult to keep clean, retain moisture that favors the growth of microorganisms, and may be ingested (causing an obstruction).

Water species such as slider turtles should be housed in a modified aquarium that includes a dry area where the animal can leave the water and bask.

Lighting

Lighting is important for reptiles. Many cannot metabolize nutrients, reproduce, or produce vitamin D adequately without the proper type and amount of light. Although species requirements may vary, as a general rule reptiles need approximately 12 hours of light and 12 hours of darkness. The light should be full-spectrum, and the light

source should be within 2 to 3 feet of the animal. Species that have the highest requirements for light are lizards, most notably iguanas.

Heat

Heat is critical for reptiles because they are ectotherms. They should be maintained in their species-specific ideal environmental temperature, also called the *thermoneutral zone*. Iguanas require ambient temperatures between 24° and 37° C (75° and 100° F), box turtles 24° to 29° C (75° to 85° F), and most pythons and boa constrictors 24° to 32° C (75° to 90° F) (Fig. 28-25).

Species requirements vary; consult appropriate texts regarding each species' thermoneutral zone. If animals are not kept in their thermoneutral zone, their metabolism will slow, contributing to anorexia, weight loss, reproductive failure, immune failure, and a host of medical problems.

Most reptiles require a supplemental heat source to remain in their thermoneutral zone. Acceptable sources of heat include heating pads placed beneath the cage or ceramic heating elements hung above or placed within the cage. The heat source must be placed in the animal's enclosure in such a way that the pet is protected from direct contact and burning. Placing the heat source at one end of the enclosure will allow the animal to regulate its body temperature by moving closer to or farther from the heat source as needed. "Hot rocks" are less desirable than other sources, since they often do not adequately warm the entire animal and can become too hot, causing severe burns. Although you may think a reptile would avoid direct contact with something that is too hot, they are relatively insensitive. Therefore, thermal burns are a common type of injury (Fig. 28-26).

Sanitation

Proper sanitation of reptile enclosures is important, as it is with all pets. Enclosures should be thoroughly cleaned and frequently disinfected on a routine basis. This is important

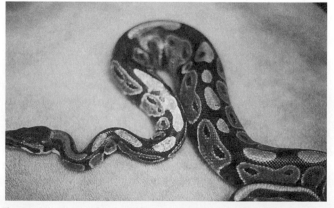

Fig. 28-25 Most pythons and boa constrictors require ambient temperatures between 75° and 90° F (24° to 32° C).

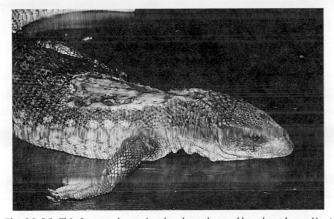

Fig. 28-26 This Savannah monitor has been burned by a heat lamp. Heat sources must be located appropriately to avoid injury. *(Photo courtesy D.R. Mader.)*

to keep the pet healthy and to minimize exposure of clients to bacteria, such as Salmonella, which can make humans ill. Cleaning of reptile enclosures should occur away from places where people eat, drink, and bathe. Emphasize to clients the importance of handwashing after handling pet reptiles or cleaning their enclosures. Some disinfectants may be toxic to pet reptiles, so all equipment should be thoroughly rinsed with water after disinfection.

Humidity

Humidity requirements vary among reptiles. Some species, such as iguanas, are native to tropical areas and need a humid environment to stay healthy. Providing adequate humidity for these species is a challenge that must be taken under consideration before deciding to keep one of these species as a pet.

Amphibians

Most amphibians are kept at cooler temperatures and in a more humid environment than used for reptiles. Although species differences occur, most amphibians do well at an ambient temperature of 21° to 29° C (70° to 85° F) and humidity of 75% to 95%.

Terrestrial amphibians are kept in a moist terrarium that is misted frequently with water. They benefit from having hiding places in their enclosure. Aquatic amphibians, such as frogs, are housed in a typical aquarium with underwater filter. Many aquatic amphibians leave the water at times, so providing a dry resting area is recommended. Amphibian enclosures must be kept very clean. For aquaria, this includes periodic water changes. Amphibians, because of their porous skin, are highly sensitive to poisoning from waste product buildup and disinfectant residues. Hyperthermia and dehydration are other common problems seen in amphibians housed in improper environments.

FEEDING

Improper diet is a common cause of disease in pet reptiles and amphibians. Each species has its own specific requirements, so this chapter does not cover them all in detail. The client prepares most reptile and amphibian diets from raw ingredients. Commercial diets are available for some species, but some of these products are not palatable or adequate. The general dietary needs of common pet species are discussed. Further information is available in texts and journals devoted specifically to reptile and amphibian care.

Water should be constantly available to all species of reptiles and amphibians, but how the water is provided will vary by species. Water bowls of an appropriate size and height are useful for most terrestrial species. Because these animals will often defecate in their water bowls, water should be changed daily. Arboreal species, such as chameleons, primarily drink droplets of water on foliage.

Herbivores

These are animals that eat primarily vegetable matter in the wild, and include iguanas and tortoises. Most herbivores require a wide variety of vegetables and fruits, plus a protein source.

Most of an iguana's diet should consist of edible flowers and leaves and dark green leafy vegetables (not celery or iceberg lettuce, which are low in nutritional value). A small amount of fruits can also be offered. The vegetable and flower "salad" should be chopped into pieces of a size suitable for the iguana's size and offered fresh daily or every other day. A *light* dusting of calcium powder (daily) and vitamin powder (weekly) is often recommended. Fresh water should be available at all times.

There is some controversy among veterinarians as to whether it is acceptable to feed iguanas small amounts of animal protein, such as crickets, moths, or worms. Most veterinarians would probably agree that limiting these animal protein sources to no more than 10% of the diet is safe, although the iguana may not even require these foods (and some iguanas will not eat them). Commercial dog and cat foods are not recommended.

Carnivores

Carnivores are animals that naturally eat small mammals, birds, or fish. Snakes, monitors, and water turtles are examples. Whenever possible, prey animals should be killed before feeding them (with tongs, not hands) to the reptile. This is more humane, and it prevents the reptile from being injured by the prey animal. If an individual animal will only accept live prey, the pet should be supervised while the prey animal is in its enclosure. If the reptile has not killed and eaten the prey within 15 minutes, the prey should be removed and the reptile fed at a later time.

Insectivores

Animals that eat mostly insects include geckos and chameleons. The most readily available insects at pet stores are crickets and mealworms, but a diet of commercially raised insects is usually inadequate. This problem can be minimized by feeding supplements to the reptile or by feeding the insects a rich, nutritionally complete diet before using them as prey.

Omnivores

Omnivores, such as box turtles, eat a varied diet that includes plant material, animals, and insects. As a rule, the diet of box turtles should consist of about 50% plant material (flowers, leaves, dark green leafy vegetables, hay, and fruit) and 50% animal protein. This can include commercial turtle pellets, tofu, sardines, crickets, or worms. Vitamin A deficiency commonly results when turtles are offered only lettuce and fruit or lettuce and crickets. As with iguanas, a *light* daily sprinkling of calcium and weekly sprinkling of vitamins can help supplement the diet of box turtles.

Amphibians

Most amphibians are carnivorous or insectivorous as adults. An improper diet, such as one consisting of only crickets, or only dog and cat food, can cause severe and life-threatening nutritional problems. Consult reference texts regarding the proper diet for the species of amphibian in question.

GENERAL NURSING AND MEDICAL CARE

Reptiles and amphibians, like other wild animals, are good at hiding their illnesses. This enhances survival in nature, but means that it may be difficult for clients to know if their pets are sick. Once signs of illness become apparent, many clients are unsure where to go for advice. They often first try to treat the pet based on information obtained from books, pet stores, or the Internet. As a result of these delays, most of the reptile and amphibian patients presented to the veterinary hospital are already critically ill.

Ideally, reptiles should receive basic preventive medical care on a routine basis. Reptiles and amphibians do not require vaccinations; however, they should receive an annual physical examination and a fecal test for parasites. All new pets should receive an examination and fecal analysis within 48 hours of purchase. Deworming medications can also be given at this time. Clients should be counseled about the likely possibility that their reptile pet may serve as an asymptomatic carrier of *Salmonella* bacteria.

Restraint

As with all veterinary patients, appropriate handling and restraint must be utilized in order to safely and effectively perform any medical procedures or treatments. Because of differences in anatomy, restraint techniques are unique to the type of animal.

Snakes

Snakes will attempt to escape if possible, and may bite if they are unable to escape. Snakes are also more likely to bite if they detect odors resembling those of their prey. For that reason, it is recommended to wash your hands thoroughly before handling snakes. Docile pet snakes may be restrained by grasping the base of the skull gently but firmly with one hand, and supporting the body with the other hand. Very large snakes may require two handlers. It is expected that the snake will attempt to move its body while being held, but it is important to prevent the animal from wrapping itself around the handler or an object.

Lizards

The most common type of lizard encountered in veterinary practice is the iguana. Iguanas use their tail as their primary weapon, but can also bite and scratch. Docile iguanas can be held by supporting the body with one hand between the front legs, holding the rear legs with the other hand, and tucking the tail under the crook of the arm to prevent its whipping action. Aggressive iguanas should have the head restrained to prevent biting. This often requires a second handler. Many other lizard species, such as skinks, geckos, and chameleons, are usually docile and simply need to be held gently but firmly enough to prevent escape. Monitors, on the other hand, are generally aggressive and require special training for safe handling.

Turtles and tortoises

The main defense mechanism for turtles and tortoises is withdrawal into the shell. Occasionally, turtles may bite and can certainly scratch their handlers while attempting to escape. Restraint of chelonians for medical procedures involves encouraging the animal to extend from its shell, and then trapping the required body part by grasping firmly with the thumb and forefinger. This can take some practice. It is important to keep in mind that these animals can be vulnerable to stress, so handlers should aim for success on the first try. If this is impossible, allowing the animal to relax and emerge from its shell again voluntarily is preferable to engaging in a wrestling match.

Amphibians

Amphibians must be handled very gently to avoid injuring them. Because of their porous skin, it in necessary to thoroughly wash and rinse your hands or wear latex gloves before touching an amphibian. Hands should be washed again after handling the animal, because some species secrete toxins from their skin.

Diagnostic Techniques

History and physical examination

A good history and physical examination is key to the proper diagnosis of illness in reptiles and amphibians. In particular, many questions should be asked about husbandry practices, since so many problems are related to improper care. Unlike companion animals, obtaining the body temperature and pulse and respiration rates is generally not part of the technician's duties with reptiles and amphibians. However, obtaining an accurate body weight is essential.

Fecal analysis

Microscopic analysis of fecal samples is used to evaluate animals with diarrhea and any nonspecific complaint (anorexia, lethargy). Sample collection can sometimes be difficult, since some species defecate infrequently and the sample must be fresh. In these cases, the sample is collected via colonic wash (similar to an enema).

The fecal examination procedure is the same as for dogs and cats: a direct smear and fecal flotation should be performed. Gram stains and fecal cultures may be helpful as well, in order to detect abnormal bacteria or yeast.

A parasitology text should be consulted for details on identifying parasites. Most reptiles and amphibians have normal protozoa in the gastrointestinal tract, so care must be taken to differentiate these from actual parasites. Salmonella bacteria are found in the gastrointestinal tract of many normal reptiles. Clients should be counseled to practice good hygiene when handling their pets, since *Salmonella* can cause illness in humans.

Venipuncture and blood collection

Venipuncture is commonly used in reptile patients and is less commonly used in amphibians. Venipuncture is used for withdrawing blood for hematologic and biochemical analysis, administration of certain medications, and intravenous catheterization for administration of fluids. Larger pets, such as large iguanas, usually present little difficulty for venipuncture, other than the need for adequate restraint. Venipuncture is challenging and at times impossible in small reptiles and amphibians.

Anesthesia may be required when performing venipuncture on pets that are difficult to manually restrain. Naturally, anesthesia of reptile patients carries its own risks and challenges. The technician must be thoroughly acquainted with delivery of anesthetic agents and monitoring of anesthesia in reptiles and amphibians.

Although each diagnostic laboratory has specific requirements for the volume of blood required for various tests, most laboratories can perform a mini battery of tests on 0.5 ml of blood collected into a green-top (lithium heparin) tube. To prevent volume depletion in small pets, some clinicians replace the volume of blood withdrawn with an equal volume of balanced electrolyte solution, given intravenously or subcutaneously.

A complete discussion of every method for venipuncture in reptiles and amphibians is beyond the scope of this text. Some of the most common techniques will be outlined, but further study and training are recommended before attempting them on your own.

Snakes. The heart, ventral coccygeal vein, and palatine vessels (on the roof of the mouth) can be used. Cardiac puncture is the most common method for blood collection in snakes (Box 28-2). An alternative site is the ventral coccygeal vein (Box 28-3).

Lizards. The ventral coccygeal vein (tail vein) and ventral abdominal vein can be used. The procedure for venipuncture of the coccygeal vein (Fig. 28-27) is outlined in Box 28-3.

Turtles and tortoises. The following sites can be used: right jugular vein (the left is usually smaller), dorsal coccygeal vein, clipped nail, brachial vein, and the postoccipital vein/venous plexus. Most clinicians prefer the right jugular vein (Fig. 28-28) for blood collection (Box 28-4), although the dorsal tail vein is commonly used in large tortoises. Blood collected from the brachial or postoccipital vein, or by clipping a nail may produce a sample that is contaminated with lymph and/or tissue fluid, so these are less desirable sites. If blood from a clipped nail must be used, it is essential to clean the nail first to avoid contaminating the sample with feces or urates.

BOX 28-2 *procedure*

Cardiac Puncture Technique

Materials

- 23- to 27-gauge needle as appropriate for size of the patient
- Appropriate-sized syringe
- Blood tube
- Alcohol swab

Procedure

1. Gently restrain the patient. If anesthesia is used, have another person monitor the anesthetized animal.
2. Identify the heart by palpation or observing individual beats. Stabilize the heart by placing the thumb and index finger cranial and caudad to it.
3. Clean the area with an alcohol swab.
4. Advance the needle between the scales (scutes) and into the heart. Withdraw the required amount of blood (limited to no more than 5% to 10% of body weight in a 2-week period).
5. Withdraw the needle; apply pressure for 30 to 60 seconds.

procedure

Venipuncture of the Ventral Coccygeal Vein

Materials

- 23- to 25-gauge needle as appropriate for size of the patient
- Appropriate-sized syringe
- Blood tube
- Alcohol swab

Procedure

1. Gently restrain the patient on its back with the ventral aspect of the tail facing upward. If anesthesia is used, have another person monitor the anesthetized animal.
2. Identify the venipuncture site. The vessel lies on the midline caudad to the cloaca.
3. Clean the area with an alcohol swab.
4. Insert the needle between the scales with the needle perpendicular to the patient's tail. Insert the needle to the depth of the vertebral bones. Draw back slightly on the syringe plunger, and slowly back the needle out until blood appears in the syringe. Withdraw the required amount of blood (limited to no more than 5% to 10% of body weight in a 2-week period).
5. Withdraw the needle; apply pressure for 30 to 60 seconds.

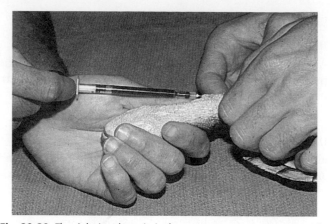

Fig. 28-28 The right jugular vein is the most common venipuncture site in turtles and tortoises. *(Photo courtesy D.R. Mader.)*

procedure

Venipuncture of the Right Jugular Vein

Materials

- 23- to 27-gauge needle as appropriate for size of the patient
- Appropriate-sized syringe
- Blood tube
- Alcohol swab

Procedure

1. Gently restrain the patient with the head extended and the right side of the neck facing up. If anesthesia is used, have another person monitor the anesthetized animal.
2. Identify the venipuncture site. The vessel is very superficial. Visualization may be aided by warming the area.
3. Clean the area with an alcohol swab.
4. Insert the needle into the vein in a cranial to caudad direction. Withdraw the required amount of blood (limited to no more than 5% to 10% of body weight in a 2-week period).
5. Withdraw the needle; apply pressure for 30 to 60 seconds.

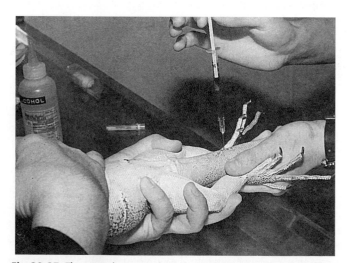
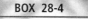

Fig. 28-27 The ventral coccygeal vein is commonly used for venipuncture of lizards and snakes. *(Photo courtesy D.R. Mader.)*

Treatment Techniques

Hospitalization

Although some sick reptiles and amphibians can be treated on an outpatient basis, those that are critically ill must be hospitalized for intensive care. Regular observation, fluid therapy, antibiotics, force-feeding, and proper environment will maximize the chances for successful recovery.

An incubator makes a good hospital enclosure for a sick reptile or amphibian, because maintaining the proper ambient temperature is critical. Human pediatric incubators

Amphibians. The lingual venous plexus, ventral abdominal vein, ventral caudal vein, and heart can be used for blood collection in amphibians.

can be purchased as used units rather inexpensively through medical suppliers or directly from hospitals. Incubators designed specifically for veterinary use are also available. Most reptiles should be maintained at ambient temperatures above 32° C (90° F) while hospitalized, although the preferred optimum temperatures vary between species. Tropical reptiles will benefit from high humidity, whereas desert species do best with drier air. Amphibians have a lower preferred temperature of approximately 21° to 24° C (70° to 75° F) and 75% to 95% humidity.

When necessary, oxygen can be supplemented through a port on most pediatric incubators.

When possible, sick reptiles and amphibians should be isolated from other hospitalized animals and handled only when absolutely necessary. This is not only because of the risk of disease spread but also because these sick pets are extremely stressed. Many reptiles and amphibians are prey in the wild. Housing them near a natural predator (dog or cat) may increase their stress.

Medication administration

Injectable medications are usually preferred over oral medications in hospitalized reptiles and amphibians. This is partially due the difficulty of administering oral medications to these species. However, a more important drawback is the sometimes erratic and unpredictable absorption rates of medications from the gastrointestinal tract. Most clients can be instructed to give injections to their pets. Because most injections need to be given only once daily (and some only once every 48 to 72 hours), the task is not as difficult as it sounds.

Injections can be given SQ, although the IM route is often preferred. Because of the renal portal system in reptiles and amphibians, IM injections should be given in the cranial half (forelimbs) of the body when possible. The epaxial muscles may be used for IM injections on snakes. Injection of certain medications may sting, and injection of some medications given SQ may cause discoloration of the scales. The IO route is preferred for emergency drugs and fluids. IV injections are possible, but often difficult. Intracoelomic injection is another common route of drug administration in reptiles and amphibians.

Injections may be given to amphibians, but injection sites should not be swabbed with alcohol or iodine solutions due to potential toxicity. Chlorhexidine solution is a preferable choice of antiseptic. As an alternative to injection, amphibians can often be treated topically by dripping the medication onto the pet or by immersing it in a bath containing the medication.

Catheterization and fluid therapy

As in other species, rehydration is often necessary for treatment of sick reptiles and amphibians. The simplest method for rehydration of reptiles involves soaking the pet in warm water or electrolyte solution for 5 to 10 minutes several times per day. Tap or bottled drinking water may be used, but *not distilled water*. Baths may be given in the hospital and by clients when the pet is treated at home. The baths often encourage the pet to drink, stimulate elimination, and allow some fluid to be absorbed via the cloaca. Baths for reptiles should be as warm as your hand will comfortably tolerate and deep enough allow the pet to submerge most of its body, but allow its head to remain out of the water. Amphibians can actually "drink" water through their skin. Amphibians should be bathed in cooler water, between 18° and 24° C (64° F and 76° F) in general. To prevent drowning, reptiles and amphibians should be monitored at all times while they are immersed in the bath.

The preferred route for fluid administration in severely dehydrated or ill reptiles and amphibians is via IO catheterization. This route takes the place of IV catheterization, which can be difficult in all but the largest animals. Some pets will require general anesthesia for the catheterization procedure, but those that are gravely ill often require only local anesthesia. IO catheterization is a delicate procedure that should be first attempted only after consulting additional texts and with supervision by someone experienced in the technique.

With IO catheterization, a spinal needle is placed into the medullary (marrow) cavity of a long bone and stabilized as an indwelling catheter. Common sites include the femur, humerus, and tibia. The rate of absorption of a substance injected into the bone marrow is equal to that after injection into a peripheral vein. Most drugs suited for intravenous routes can be safely infused into the marrow, although it is recommended to check with the drug manufacturer if there is any doubt.

IO catheterization may be contraindicated in some cases of sepsis, in which it could cause osteomyelitis. Other potential contraindications include bone diseases and abnormalities, and skin and wound infections in the area of catheter placement.

Much of the information on IO catheterization of reptiles and amphibians has been extrapolated from work in iguanas and other lizards. Naturally, anatomical and physiological differences in other species may require modifications in technique, and may pose greater difficulties. IO catheterization is not performed in snakes or chelonians.

When IO catheterization is not an option, SC or intracoelomic routes of fluid administration can be used. Catheterization of the right jugular vein is an option in chelonians.

Suitable fluid solutions for rehydration of reptiles or amphibians include nonlactated electrolyte solutions such as Normo-Sol-R and Saline, with or without dextrose. There is controversy regarding whether the use of lactated solutions may be detrimental to these species, so many clinicians avoid them. A common maintenance fluid rate used for reptiles is 15 to 25 ml/kg/day.

Force-feeding

Many pet reptiles and amphibians are presented for veterinary care because of anorexia and lethargy. In addition to the need for rehydration, nutritional supplementation is often required. Animals that are not eating are in a *catabolic state*. Decreased food intake results in breakdown of protein and fat for energy. This can contribute to hepatic lipidosis, acidosis, azotemia, muscle wasting, impaired gastrointestinal function, and decreased immunity. To prevent or correct these serious complications, supplementation with food is important. This can be done in the hospital or by the client at home.

The force-feeding procedure is relatively straightforward. The most challenging part of the procedure is opening the animal's mouth. For snakes or lizards, insert a flat, rubber spatula at the rostral extremity of the mouth and use it to open the jaws. Then replace it with an oral speculum. Pass an appropriate-sized red rubber feeding tube orally into the esophagus and into the stomach. On some longer snakes, the tip of the catheter may not reach the stomach but will remain in the esophagus. Semiliquid food is given via the tube, and the tube is withdrawn. Because reptiles have a cranially located glottis (often at the base of the tongue) that is easily visualized upon opening the mouth, it is difficult (if not impossible) to accidentally intubate the trachea. For animals in which force-feeding must be performed repeatedly, a pharyngostomy tube can be placed.

The animal's normal diet can be blended and used for force-feeding. All necessary vitamins and minerals should be included. Alternatively, commercial products such as Emeraid II (Lafeber) or Ensure may be used. For herbivorous and omnivorous species, products designed for humans, such as Ensure, are preferable to products designed for dogs and cats, since the latter tend to be too high in fat.

RECOMMENDED READING

Cage Birds

Beynon PH: *Manual of psittacine birds*, Ames, Iowa, 1996, Iowa State University Press.

Blanchard S: *Companion parrot handbook*, Alameda, Calif, 1999, Pet Bird Information Council.

Gallerstein GA: *The complete bird owner's handbook*, ed 2, New York, 1994, John Wiley & Sons.

Spadafori, G et al: *Birds for dummies*, Hoboken, N.J., 1999, IDG Books.

Zantop D et al: *Avian medicine: principles and application*, abridged, Lake Worth, Fla, 1997, Zoological Education Network.

Companion parrot quarterly, P.O. Box 2428, Alameda, Calif, 94501.

Reptiles and Amphibians

Bennet RA: Reptiles: clinical and diagnostic techniques, *Proceedings of the North American veterinary conference, small animal and exotics, vol. 13*, Orlando, Fla, 1999, Eastern States Veterinary Association.

Bonner B: Chelonian therapeutics, *Veterinary Clinics of North America exotic animal practice, therapeutics*, 3:1, January 2000.

Boyer T: Emergency care of reptiles, *Veterinary Clinics of North America exotic animal practice, critical care*, 1:1, September 1998.

de Vosjoli P: *The general care and maintenance of ball pythons*, Lakeside, Calif, 1990, Advanced Vivarium Systems.

de Vosjoli P: *The general care and maintenance of box turtles*, Lakeside, Calif, 1991, Advanced Vivarium Systems.

de Vosjoli P: *The general care and maintenance of the green iguana*, Lakeside, Calif, 1990, Advanced Vivarium Systems.

Donoghue S: Nutritional support of herbivorous reptiles, *Proceedings of the North American Veterinary Conference, small animal and exotics, vol. 13*, Orlando, Fla, 1999, Eastern States Veterinary Association.

Mader D: *Reptile medicine and surgery*, Philadelphia, 1996, WB Saunders.

Messonnier SP: *Exotic pets: a veterinary guide for owners*, Plano, Tex, 1995, Wordware Publishing.

Messonnier SP: *Common reptile diseases and treatment*, Cambridge, Mass, 1996, Blackwell Science.

Otto C et al: Intraosseous infusion of fluids and therapeutics, *Compend Contin Educ Pract Vet* 4:421-430, 1989.

Walker I, Whitaker B: Amphibian Therapeutics, *Veterinary Clinics of North America exotic animal practice, therapeutics*, 3:1, January 2000.

Wright K: Fluid therapy for amphibians, *Proceedings of the North American Veterinary Conference, small animal and exotics, vol. 13*, Orlando, Fla, 1999, Eastern States Veterinary Association.

Wright K: Fluid therapy for reptiles, *Proceedings of the North American Veterinary Conference, small animal and exotics, vol. 13*, Orlando, Fla, 1999, Eastern States Veterinary Association.

29

Nursing Care of Orphaned and Injured Wild Animals

Stuart L. Porter

Learning Objectives

After reviewing this chapter, the reader should understand the following:
- Techniques used in assessing the condition of orphaned wild animals
- Regulations and laws concerning wildlife care
- Methods of sample collection for laboratory analysis
- Routes of administration of medication
- Principles of rehabilitating orphaned wild animals in captivity
- Techniques used in diagnosing disease in wild animals

GENERAL CONSIDERATIONS

Native wild animals that become injured or orphaned are commonly found by well-meaning individuals. If the veterinary hospital does not accept wild animals as patients, callers should be referred to licensed wildlife rehabilitators, wildlife centers, zoos, or other veterinary hospitals that accept such cases. If only giving advice, the professional staff must provide advice that is medically sound and legal. Because many of these "rescued" animals have no true owners, the practice is often not paid for services rendered. Potential professional liability issues, such as possible zoonoses and staff injuries, must be considered. If the hospital chooses to treat these animals, a wildlife plan should be developed to provide proper diagnostic and supportive care and confirm to local, state, and federal regulations and laws.

History

When a wild animal is presented, it is important to obtain and record as much information as possible from the rescuer including name, address, and phone number. Hospital records should be designed for these wildlife patients. When, where, and under what circumstances the animal was found may be important for diagnostic or prognostic reasons. Since many rescuers make errors in judgment in rescuing and caring for animals, you can use this time to educate them as to what they should have done or not done. This is important because some people may find a number of animals during a year. In some cases, patterns may emerge. This information can be useful as epidemiologic information, or evidence for violations of the law.

PHYSICAL EXAMINATION OF WILDLIFE

Physical examination may be done by a technician or veterinarian. Most of the commonly seen wild animals are easily handled if one pays attention to their offensive and defensive weapons, such as teeth, beaks, claws, antlers, and hooves. These weapons must be neutralized to prevent injury to personnel (Fig. 29-1). Gloves, towels, snares, nets, shields, and other restraint aids may be necessary. These animals are often severely compromised and are poor candidates for general anesthesia. Only vicious animals, such as carnivores, bears, and some rodents, must be anesthetized for this initial examination. A complete physical examination is essential. Because most of these animals are trauma victims, multiple injuries are very common. Do not stop the examination after finding one lesion.

Legal Constraints

There are a number of local, state, and federal regulations and laws that cover native wildlife. Hospitals working with these species should make themselves aware of these

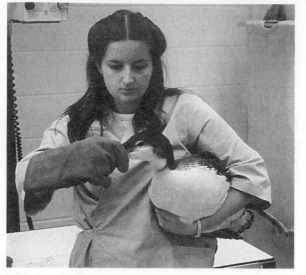

Fig. 29-1 Technician restraining a loon, a heavy-bodied bird with a thick, pointed beak. The technician wears heavy gloves and holds the beak while pressing the bird's wings to its body. When working with birds with a pointed beak, grasp the beak first to prevent injury, and do not release your grip until the bird is placed back in its enclosure.

requirements and ensure that they are obeyed. Every state has an agency that is responsible for regulating possession of native wildlife. Anyone working with threatened or endangered species and most birds must have a permit from this agency. In some states, fees, examinations, facility inspections, and continuing education are required to maintain such a permit. Some states also regulate the possession of mammals and reptiles.

The Fish and Wildlife Service (FWS) of the U.S. Department of Interior (USDI) also regulates the possession of threatened and endangered species and migratory birds (and their parts), which includes most native species except pigeons, house sparrows, and starlings. In order to receive a federal rehabilitation permit, one must first have a permit from his or her state wildlife agency. Both the state agency and the FWS require that people who have a permit submit annual reports detailing all species seen that year.

The least complicated way for a private practitioner to become involved in helping native wildlife is to develop a relationship with a permitted (licensed) rehabilitator. Sometimes an employee of the hospital already has such a permit. Otherwise, the veterinarian should have permits from the state wildlife agency and the (FWS) of the USDI. State wildlife laws vary, and veterinarians should contact their local game wardens for specific information.

Rescuers who do not have wildlife permits should not be allowed to take wild animals from the hospital. These animals should be kept at the hospital and treated or referred to a permitted wildlife rehabilitator.

Releasability

The concept of *releasability* must be considered. The goal of wildlife rehabilitation is to release the animal back to the wild so that it may survive. A totally blind animal or a wild bird with one functional wing or one leg should not be released. Part of the hospital plan should consider the factors that determine whether an animal can be successfully returned to the wild. Unless the unreleasable animal is a threatened or endangered species, it should be humanely euthanized if it cannot be released. Euthanasia may be performed by the same methods used in small animal practice. Birds are readily euthanized by injecting a small amount (0.1 to 0.3 ml) of barbiturate euthanasia solution into the suboccipital sinus at the base of the skull. Small wild animals may be humanely euthanized by placing them in a small, glass chamber containing halothane. The FWS should be contacted prior to the euthanasia of a threatened or endangered species.

Legal placement of unreleasable animals is difficult and time-consuming. Government agencies will not grant permits for individuals to keep unreleasable wildlife, including hand-raised orphans, in their homes. Placement can be arranged through professional wildlife rehabilitation organizations or local zoos or nature centers, but this can be difficult to do for common species.

Diagnostic Testing

After the physical examination, such diagnostic tests as complete blood counts, blood chemistries, radiographs, fecal examination, and toxicologic tests may be required to further evaluate the patient. These procedures are similar to those done on domestic animals. This information is useful for both diagnosis and prognosis.

CARE OF ORPHANED WILDLIFE

During the spring, people find many young wild animals. These animals have fallen from nests, have had their nests destroyed, or are just found on the ground. Many times they call the hospital for information about what to do. If at all possible, the animal should be placed back in the nest or the nest should be rebuilt or replaced. Fledgling birds may be placed in a bush so their parents can still feed them.

If these "orphans" are brought to the veterinary practice, they should be handled like other wild animals. They often are hypothermic and/or dehydrated. Any other medical problems, such as wounds, parasite infestation, and fractures, must be addressed. The diet used varies with the species. There are many milk substitutes on the market, including Esbilac (Pet-Ag, Elgin, Ill.), Unilac (Upjohn, Kalamazoo, Mich.), KMR (Pet-Ag), Zoologic (Pet-Ag), Nurturall (Vet Products Labs, Phoenix, Ariz.), and Just Born (Farnham Pet Products, Phoenix, Ariz.). These can be used to feed baby squirrels, opossums, foxes, raccoons, and other small mammals. Baby rabbits require more fat in their diets; whipping cream is often added to the commercial preparations, or Lamb Milk Replacer (Land O Lakes, Fort Dodge, Iowa) is used. Goat milk or Lamb Milk Replacer is also used for the fawns of white-tailed deer and other ungulates. These formulas may be administered by a variety of means, including dosing needles, eyedroppers, pet nursers, baby bottles, or lamb nipples attached to soda bottles. The amount fed and frequency of administration vary with the size of the animal, but usually 10% to 20% of the body weight is given in divided doses two to four times per day. After the baby mammal opens its eyes, the feeding frequency is decreased, the formula is thickened, and weaning begins.

Bird diets also vary with the species. Commercial diets, such as Nutristart (Lafeber, Odell, Ill.) and Lake's Hand Rearing Formula (Lakes Unlimited) are available. For songbirds, a nonoily canned dog food is mixed 2:1 with chick starter and fed whenever the baby bird gapes for food (Fig. 29-2), or about every 15 to 60 minutes, depending on age of the bird. Insects, such as mealworms, wax worms, and crickets, may be added to the diet at weaning. Young waterfowl and quail may be fed chick or turkey starter. Baby doves and pigeons must be tube-fed formula until weaning. Raptors or birds of prey should be hand-fed chopped rodents or another balanced diet for the first two weeks of life, before they begin eating on their own. Hamburger and organ meat should not be fed, because it is too low in calcium and causes severe bone abnormalities in all young animals. The young of some species, such as wood ducks, killdeer, and chimney swifts, are difficult and time-consuming to raise. Proper training is essential to success with these species.

Before they are released, wild animals must be introduced to natural foods. Predatory species must be given the opportunity to practice killing live prey before release. Various behavioral abnormalities, especially taming, may develop in hand-raised wildlife, so experienced wildlife rehabilitators should be consulted. *Imprinting*, or species identification, occurs at birth or hatching in precocious species, such as deer, ducks, and quail, and later in development in altricial species, such as raptors. Since wild babies are rarely found when they are born or hatch, human imprinting is rarely a problem except in young birds of prey that imprint between 2 and 3 weeks. It is essential that experienced raptor rehabilitators raise young birds of prey to prevent human imprinting from occurring. Human imprinted species should never be released into the wild.

CARE OF INJURED ADULT WILDLIFE

The most common reason adult wild animals are presented to veterinarians is vehicular trauma. These animals suffer the same types of injuries as seen in dogs and cats. Therapy for shock includes fluids and glucocorticoids. Intravenous (IV) fluids are best, but intraperitoneal (IP) fluids work well in small mammals; intraosseous (IO) fluids are commonly used in birds and small mammals. In birds, IO fluids may be administered into the distal ulna or the proximal tibiotarsus. The IO route may also be used in small mammals by placing an 18-gauge needle through the trochanteric fossa into the proximal femur. If the animal is conscious, oral fluids may be administered via a stomach tube (Fig. 29-3).

Because many injured wild animals are hypothermic, warming is an essential part of the treatment. These animals may be placed in an infant incubator, on a warm-water circulating pad, or carefully on a towel-covered heating pad or under a heat lamp. It is important to carefully monitor

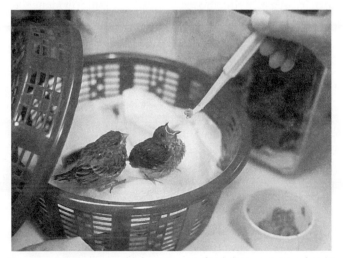

Fig. 29-2 The baby songbird gapes as a food dropper approaches its mouth. These young birds are kept in a simple basket but will be moved to a proper enclosure as they learn to fly.

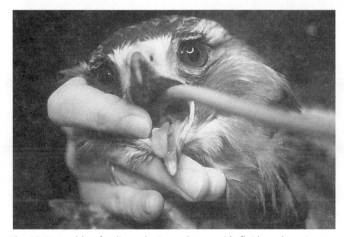

Fig. 29-3 A rubber feeding tube is used to provide fluids and nutrients to this red-tailed hawk. The glottis is visible ventral to the tube.

and frequently move animals placed on electric heating pads or under heat lamps to avoid their becoming burned.

Open wounds require attention, especially in birds in which there is little soft tissue under the skin and the exposed bone or connective tissue may become dry or infected. Wounds should be flushed, debrided, and protected by suturing or bandaging. It is important not to damage a bird's feathers by smearing them with oily topicals or covering them with sticky tape. Masking tape works well to hold bandaging material or immobilize extremities in small animals. Nonstick elastic tape (VetWrap, 3-M Animal Care, St. Paul, Minn.) can be used over or under masking tape.

Traumatized wild animals often exhibit neurologic signs because of brain injury. Signs include ataxia, depression, head tilt, torticollis, or blindness. These animals require supportive therapy to see if they improve over time. Corticosteroids may be used for several days. The condition of these animals may improve within days to weeks, may worsen, or may improve to some extent and then remain static. Euthanasia is indicated if the animal's condition worsens or ceases to improve. Those that appear normal must be permitted to demonstrate the ability to find food and perches and move normally in an enclosure larger than a dog kennel prior to being released.

Eye problems also commonly result from collisions with vehicles. These injuries may be obvious, involving the globe, cornea, iris, or lens, or they may be obscure, involving the posterior segment. A complete eye examination should include observing if the animal can visually follow a finger moved near its face, pupillary light reflex, and ophthalmoscopy. An animal that is totally blind should never be released into the wild. Most animals with vision in only one eye, however, can survive in the wild and may be released once they have demonstrated that they have otherwise recovered.

Fractures are common in traumatized wild animals and require at least stabilization initially. Many fractures in smaller animals can be treated only with external immobilization by taping the extremity to the body, or splinting it in extension using aluminum rods, tongue depressors, syringe casings, finger splints, or casting material. Some fractures may require surgery, but surgery should be performed after the patient's condition has stabilized. It is wise to combine internal fixation with external fixation to provide additional support. Because contracture of connective tissue is a common problem in birds, extremities should not be immobilized longer than 3 to 4 weeks. Physical therapy involving joint massage, flexing and extending joints, and exercise in a flight pen is essential for birds that have had their wings immobilized.

Chemical Restraint and Anesthesia

General anesthesia is most rapidly and safely induced with isoflurane or sevoflurane. Other inhalation agents may be used, but they are generally not as safe (see Chapters 19 and 28). If the patient can be physically restrained, induction by mask works well (Fig. 29-4). Endotracheal intubation is usually performed except for quick procedures or in species that are difficult to intubate, such as rodents, rabbits, and deer. Injectable agents alone, or in combination, may also be used as they are in domestic animals. The products most commonly used include ketamine, Telazol, xylazine, and Propofol. All anesthetized wild animals should be monitored as in domestic animals. Since many of these animals are small, it is very important to prevent hypothermia.

It is important to allow the patient to recover from general anesthesia in a dark, quiet, warm space to prevent it from injuring itself. With isoflurane or sevoflurane anesthesia, patients are physically restrained until they are standing, usually within 5 to 10 minutes. Some injectable drugs such as xylazine may be reversed, otherwise these patients should be carefully monitored during the recovery process.

CARE OF POISONED WILDLIFE

Although trauma is the most common cause of neurologic signs, poisonings also commonly affect the nervous system. The poisonings may be intentional or accidental. Birds are most commonly involved, but mammals are sometimes affected. Nonspecific clinical signs include convulsions, ataxia, depression, diarrhea, salivation, nystagmus, and opisthotonos. Usually one patient is presented at a time, but if many animals are affected, state or federal wildlife officials should be contacted immediately.

The two most common types of poisonings seen are lead toxicity and organophosphate/carbamate toxicity. Lead toxicity may be diagnosed by radiographic evidence of

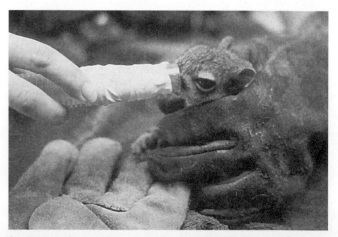

Fig. 29-4 A plastic syringe casing has been modified to serve as a mask for induction of anesthesia in an immature gray squirrel.

lead shot in the gastrointestinal tract or by elevated lead levels in the blood. The most common treatment for lead toxicity is calcium disodium edentate (Calcium Disodium Versenate, Riker Labs, St. Paul, Minn.) IM at 35 mg/kg BID for 5 days. Organophosphate or carbamate toxicity is diagnosed by finding depressed levels of cholinesterase in the blood or by identifying the chemical in the crop or stomach contents. The treatment for organophosphate poisoning is atropine at 0.5 to 5.0 mg/kg IV or IM. Atropine only alleviates clinical signs and does not affect cholinesterase levels. Affected birds may require several weeks to fully recover.

Botulism, also called *limberneck*, is a major cause of death in wild birds. It is frequently seen in waterfowl; many birds may be affected at one time. Affected birds exhibit an inability to control their neck or wings and a prolapsed nictitans (third eyelid). Treatment is primarily supportive, although neostigmine (Prostigmin, Roche, Nutley, N.J.) may increase neuromuscular function.

CARE OF WILDLIFE IN CAPTIVITY

Diagnosis and treatment of injury or illness in wildlife can be relatively easy, but coaxing the patient to eat while in captivity may be more of a challenge. It is not unusual for a wild animal to become debilitated or even to starve to death while in captivity. Providing a proper diet is essential for maintaining a wild animal in captivity. Canned dog food is used as a base diet for a variety of species, including songbirds, opossums, raccoons, skunks, foxes, and bears. Commercial diets are also available. The diet can be made more appealing by adding mealworms for insectivores, honey for bears, and banana for other species. Rabbits, squirrels, and other rodents are fed sweet feed, sweet potato, dark green leafy vegetables, and rodent or rabbit pellets. Owls, hawks, vultures, and eagles may be fed laboratory rodents, chopped chicken, carrion, or prepared, supplemented horse meat (Bird of Prey Diet, Animal Spectrum, North Platte, Neb.).

Some species will not eat in a small cage but readily accept the same food in a quiet, larger pen. If the patient will not eat on its own, then nourishment must be provided. Various hyperalimentation formulas, such as Isocal (Mead Johnson, Evansville, Ind.), Emeraid II (Lafeber, Odell, Ill.), and Clinical Care (Pet-Ag, Elgin, Ill.), are administered by stomach tube.

In addition to an adequate diet, proper management of captive wild animals also includes housing so that the patient does not injure its feathers, wings, legs, or head. Birds often destroy feathers or break their legs when kept in wire cages. Excessive noise and activity often excite the animal, causing it to bang its head or wings against the sides of the enclosure. Deer readily panic due to strange sights and sounds and will run into the sides of their enclosures or slip and break their legs and/or backs. Carnivores subject to environmental stress may self-mutilate. Birds of prey in particular are subject to infections on the bottoms of their feet from inadequate perches or substrate. The veterinary hospital is not an ideal place to house wild animals unless they can be kept in an isolated, quiet area.

Return to the Wild

A major consideration in wildlife rehabilitation is determination of when the patient is ready for release. Criteria used must be aimed at ensuring the survival of the animal in the wild. These may include healed injuries, normal blood values, ability to fly or run, and ability to obtain food.

Once the patient has been judged ready for release, then thought must be given to proper release sites. It is not acceptable to just open the door and let the patient go anywhere. In most cases, it is best to release the patient where it was found; however, this may be contraindicated, such as if the animal was found near a busy highway. Some animals, such as groundhogs, deer, and beavers, are considered pests, and should be released only where permission has been granted by the landowner. Ideally the animal should be released into a suitable habitat, away from people, pets, and motor vehicles. It is not uncommon for a family to work hard to raise a songbird, release it in their backyard, and then watch in horror as it is killed by their cat. Some captive raised orphans, such as Canada geese and wood ducks, imprint on their release site and return there to nest. Consideration should also be given to the weather and time of year. Animals should not be turned out during or just preceding inclement weather. Releasing reptiles and adolescent mammals in winter is also not a good idea. Migrating birds should not be released after the migration has finished. Some birds are transported to Florida for release during winter.

RECOMMENDED READING

Mammals, Birds, and Raptors

Benyon P, ed.: *Manual of raptors, pigeons, and waterfowl*, Ames, Iowa, 1996, Iowa State University Press.

Davidson WR, Nettles VF: *Field manual of wildlife diseases in the southeast United States*, ed 2, Athens, Ga, 1997, Southeast Cooperative Wildlife Disease Study.

Fairbrother A, Locke L, and Hoff G: Noninfectious diseases of wildlife, ed 2, Ames, Iowa, 1996, Iowa State University Press.

Fowler M: *Restraint and handling of wild and domestic animals*, ed 2, Ames, Iowa, 1995, Iowa State University Press.

Fowler M, and Miller E, eds: *Zoo and wild animal medicine: current therapy 4*, Philadelphia, 1999, WB Saunders.

Friend M, Franson J, eds: *Field manual of wildlife diseases*, Washington, DC, 1999, USGS, NWHC.

Kreeger T: *Handbook of wildlife chemical immobilization*, Laramie, Wyo, 1996, International Wildlife Veterinary Services.

McKeever K: *Care and rehabilitation of injured owls*, Vineland, Ontario, Can, 1987, WF Rannie.

Moore AT, Joosten S: *NWRA principles of wildlife rehabilitation*, St Cloud, Minn, 1997, National Wildlife Rehabilitators' Association.

Redig PT et al, eds: *Raptor biomedicine*, Minneapolis, 1993, University of Minnesota Press.

Ritchie BW, Harrison GJ, Harrison LR: *Avian medicine: principles and application*, Lake Worth, Fla, 1994, Wingers Publishing.

Samuel W, Pybus, M, and Kocan A, eds: *Parasitic diseases of wild mammals*, ed 2, Ames, Iowa, 2001, Iowa State University Press.

Williams E, Barker I, eds: *Infectious diseases of wild mammals*, ed 3, Ames, Iowa, 2001, Iowa State University Press.

Wildlife Rehabilitation Today Magazine, Coconut Creek Publishing, 2201 NW 40th Terrace, Coconut Creek, Fla.

National Wildlife Rehabilitators Association (NWRA)
14 North 7th Avenue
St. Cloud, Minn 56303-4766
www.nwrawildlife.org

International Wildlife Rehabilitation Council
829 Bancroft Way
Berkeley, Calif 94710
www.iwrc-on-line.org

30

Nursing Care of Small Mammals

Karen Hrapkiewicz

Learning Objectives

After reviewing this chapter, the reader should understand the following:

- General characteristics of mice, rats, hamsters, gerbils, guinea pigs, chinchillas, rabbits, and ferrets
- Use of rodents, rabbits, and ferrets as pets and in research
- Husbandry and principles of sanitation

- General nursing care of rodents, rabbits, and ferrets
- Techniques used in diagnosing and treating disease in small mammals
- Methods of sample collection for laboratory analysis
- Routes of administration of medication
- Identification methods used in research animals
- Anesthesia of rodents, rabbits, and ferrets

GENERAL CONSIDERATIONS

Small mammals are popular pets. These include ferrets, rabbits, mice, rats, hamsters, gerbils, guinea pigs, and chinchillas. They are frequently referred to as "pocket pets" due to their small size. Although small mammals are easy to care for, they require care different from that of dogs and cats.

Small mammals are often purchased as first pets for children. Small mammals can make acceptable pets for children, but children should always be supervised when handling these delicate creatures. Small mammals can bite. Children should be made aware of this and told that these pets are "real live creatures" and not stuffed animals. All pets should be handled with care. Small mammals should not be allowed free run of the house, because this can prove fatal. Because the life span of most small mammals is only 2 to 4 years, children should be counseled so that an "early" death is not unexpected. Allergies to animal dander, saliva, and urinary proteins occur commonly in humans. Cutaneous and upper respiratory allergies to small mammals especially rats and guinea pigs are very common.

Small mammals are also utilized as research animals. Rodents, particularly the mouse and rat, are most commonly used. Commercial breeders produce most of these rodents specifically for research. The animals are defined genetically and microbiologically and may have specific traits to mimic certain diseases. They are reared in special environments, pathogen-free barriers that prevent the introduction of disease agents. Animals are used to study drug effects, toxicity, neoplasia, embryology, diabetes, infectious diseases, parasitology, the heart, and high blood pressure, to name a few. These animals have made valuable contributions to science and have advanced the medical care of humans and animals alike.

HOUSING

Caging must be escape-proof to prevent injury or fatality. Rodents can be housed in plastic or metal cages with slotted bar or wire mesh lids. Shoebox-type cages made of plastic materials are popular for housing rodents (Fig. 30-1, *A*). Cages hung from a supporting frame are frequently seen in research settings (Fig. 30-1, *B*). Several individual cages can be placed on a shelving unit called a *rack* (Fig. 30-1, *C*). Cage flooring can be either solid-bottom or wire mesh. Solid flooring with bedding material is generally preferred. If mesh flooring is used, care must be taken to prevent foot injury and loss of neonates through the flooring. Aquariums are adequate to house pet rodents, but should have a screen-type top with a locking device. This type of housing unit allows easy access to the pet, but it is heavy and can be difficult to clean. When aquariums are used for housing, care should be taken to ensure that rodents have access to food and water. Conventional cages such as those purchased from pet stores should have a large door to facilitate easy removal of the animal and be easy to disassemble and clean. Rabbits, chinchillas, and ferrets can be housed in wire or front-opening cages with catch pans to collect urine and feces (Fig. 30-1, *D*). Pet ferrets and rabbits can also be housed in large cat or dog carriers with a litter box. Some clients build rather elaborate "condos" for their pet rabbits and ferrets. Rabbits and ferrets can be housed outdoors, but care must be taken to prevent heat stroke, myiasis (fly strike) and dog and cat attacks. Animals maintained outdoors should be provided with shelter from direct sunlight, rain, snow, and wind.

In a research setting, different species are housed in separate rooms to meet experimental requirements, prevent interspecies disease transmission, and reduce anxiety because of interspecies conflict. In addition, special housing may be required. Immunocompromised rodents are housed in micro-isolator cages or other protective cages to reduce their exposure to viruses or bacteria. Metabolism cages allow for collection of urine and feces, and inhalation chambers provide a way to expose an animal to various agents.

Animals should be housed in caging that is appropriate for the animal's size and weight and in accordance with current regulations or guidelines. Some animals like chinchillas are very acrobatic and active and should be provided with a large cage to allow for exercise. Cage height should allow an animal to make normal postural adjustments. For example, gerbils frequently sit upright, so the height of their caging should allow them to do so. The cage should be located in an area protected from climatic extremes. Care should be taken not to house pet rodent cages in direct sunlight as they will overheat. Changes in temperature and humidity and/or drafty conditions should be avoided, because they can be stressful and predispose the animal to disease. The recommended housing temperature is 18° to 26° C (64° to 79° F) for mice, rats, hamsters, gerbils, and guinea pigs, 16° to 22° C (61° to 72° F) for rabbits and chinchillas, and 4° to 18° C (39° to 64° F) for ferrets. The acceptable range of relative humidity is 30% to 70%. The guideline for ventilation in an animal housing room is 10 to 15 air changes per hour. A light cycle of 12 hours of light to 12 hours of darkness is most commonly used in animal housing rooms. Albino rodents are susceptible to phototoxicity, so care should be taken to ensure safe illumination levels in their housing area. Noise should be minimized in animal housing areas, because excessive sound exposure can be stressful and produce untoward effects. It is important to remember that many species can hear frequencies of sound that are inaudible to humans. Some rodents are prone to sound-induced seizures.

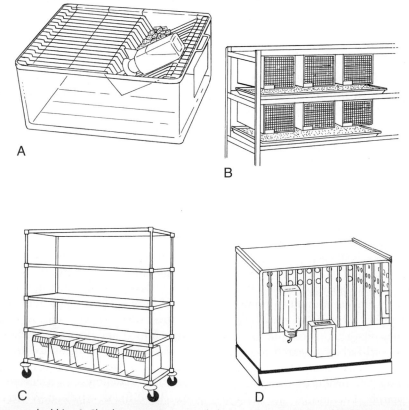

Fig. 30-1 Caging used for rodents and rabbits. **A,** Shoebox cage. **B,** Suspended cages. **C,** Rack holding shoebox cages. **D,** Rabbit cage with J feeder. *(From McBride DF: Learning veterinary terminology, ed 2, St Louis, 2002, Mosby.)*

Bedding used for solid-bottom caging should be absorbent, comfortable, nonnutritive, nontoxic, and disposable. A variety of bedding material can be used including paper, sawdust and soft pine, aspen, cedar, corncob, or hardwood chips. Cedar and soft pine shavings are frequently used for pet rodent bedding because of their pleasant aroma. These should be avoided in a research setting because they emit aromatic hydrocarbons that induce liver changes and cytotoxicity. Burrowing rodents such as the rat and gerbil should be provided with deeper bedding to allow for this behavior.

Cage toys can provide psychological stimulation as well as exercise for small mammals. Tubes, mazes, and exercise wheels are popular. Timid animals such as guinea pigs and chinchillas are more comfortable if they are given a place to hide. Polyvinyl chloride plumbing pipes, especially elbows and *Y* and *T* sections make ideal hiding places. These pipes can be sanitized in the dishwasher. Cardboard tubes, softwood pieces, and small Nylabones can be given to rodents to gnaw on. Paper tissues or towels can be given to rodents who build nests such as mice, gerbils, and hamsters. Metallic items such as washers can be suspended in a rabbit's cage to encourage nudging, playing, and investigative behaviors. Paper bags, hard plastic or metal toys, or cloth toys made for cats or babies are safe for ferrets. Ferrets love to run through cylindrical objects like large mailing tubes and dryer vent tubing. Latex rubber toys that are intended for dogs or cats should not be given to ferrets.

SANITATION

Sanitation involves bedding changes, cleaning to remove dirt and debris, and disinfection to reduce or eliminate microorganisms. All animal caging and bedding must be cleaned or changed as often as necessary to prevent accumulation of odor and waste, and to keep the animal clean and dry. A major cause of respiratory disease in small mammal pets is poor environmental ventilation, which allows ammonia from accumulation of urine to irritate the pet's airways. Caging should be cleaned once or twice per week. After removal of gross dirt, urine, and feces, cages should be disinfected by washing all surfaces with hot water (82° C) or by applying a disinfectant solution. A good, safe, readily available disinfectant for animal cages is laundry bleach (5% sodium hypochlorite), prepared by mixing 30 ml bleach in 1 L of water. A fresh mixture should be prepared prior to using, because it deteriorates upon standing. Rabbit, guinea pig, and hamster urine is alkaline and contains crystals. Urine crystals accumulate forming a scale on the cage that can be difficult to remove. Acidic products available commercially or white vinegar can be used to remove the scale. It is important to thoroughly rinse detergents and disinfectants from cleaned cages and feeders, because residues may cause health problems. Deodorizers should not be used to mask animal odors, because they can be toxic to the animal or add a variable to a research study.

DIET

The rat and mouse are omnivorous, whereas the guinea pig, chinchilla, and gerbil are herbivorous. The hamster is primarily graminivorous. Ferrets are carnivorous and depend on meat protein and fats for their dietary requirements. Animals should be fed a clean, wholesome, and nutritious diet *ad libitum*, free choice. It is important to feed a balanced diet, freshly milled and formulated for that particular species. Pelleted foods are available commercially. These diets are complete and do not require supplementation. Block-style pellets work well for rodents such as mice, rats, hamsters, and gerbils. Much of the rodent feed found in pet stores and sold as seed mixes or treats are inadequate in protein for these species. Smaller pelleted foods work well for guinea pigs, chinchillas, and rabbits. Rabbits should be fed a high-fiber rabbit chow to prevent obesity and hairball formation. Rabbits, guinea pigs, and chinchillas can be fed small amounts of grass or alfalfa hay. Hay provides them with fiber and helps reduce boredom. Ferrets can be fed ferret chow or commercial cat food. As with dogs and cats, periodontal disease is common in ferrets. Feeding dry food can help reduce tartar accumulation. In most instances, the food should be placed in a feeder hung in the animal's cage. This prevents soiling of the food with urine and feces, keeping it dry and clean. If vegetables or fruit are offered to supplement the diet, they should be fresh and washed before feeding them. Any uneaten vegetables or fruits should be removed daily. Supplements should not make up more than 10% of the animal's daily food ration. Animals should have access to fresh water via an automatic watering system or water bottles with sipper tubes.

RODENTS

Mice, rats, gerbils, hamsters, guinea pigs, and chinchillas are rodents. The word *rodent* is derived from a Latin verb that means "to gnaw." Rodents have continuously erupting chisel-like incisors and powerful jaw muscles that contribute to their gnawing ability. They are for the most part *nocturnal*, being more active at night. The sex of most rodents can be determined by *anogenital* distance, the distance being longer in males and shorter in females (Fig. 30-2). Rodents are usually prolific breeders. Clients should be aware of the potential for overpopulation when housing animals of the opposite sex together. The term *murine* specifically refers to mice and rats. Guinea pigs and

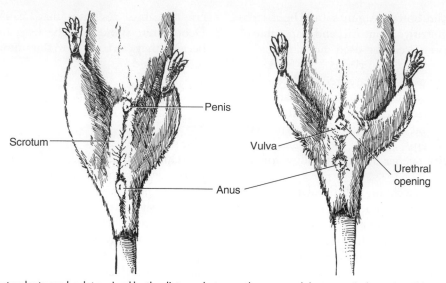

Fig. 30-2 The gender of most rodents can be determined by the distance between the anus and the urogenital opening. This anogenital distance is greater in males *(left)* than in females *(right)*. *(Adapted from* American Association for Laboratory Animal Science training manual series, vol 1: assistant laboratory animal technician, *Cordova, Tenn, AALAS.)*

chinchillas are *hystricomorph*, or hedgehog-like, rodents related to porcupines.

Although rodents do not require annual vaccinations, an annual examination is recommended to ensure good health and husbandry. Clients should be encouraged to bring their new pet in for a visit to the veterinarian. The patient can be examined to ensure health, maintain the "health guarantee" that may accompany the purchase, and allow the technician and veterinarian to educate the client on proper feeding, housing, and handling of the species.

Mice

The mouse (*Mus musculus*) is a small rodent, easily housed and handled, and relatively inexpensive to purchase and maintain as a pet. It is the animal most commonly used in research. *Balb/c* (albino), *C57BL* (black), and *C3H* (agouti) are common inbred strains of mice. *Swiss* and *ICR* are outbred stocks of mice. Mutant and genetically engineered strains of inbred mice provide researchers with a wide variety of animal models to study diseases. Scientific technology has made it possible to add or remove genetic material. A mouse that results from the introduction of genetic material from one animal into the fertilized egg of a different animal is *transgenic. Knockout* mice result from the removal of one or more genes from the fertilized egg.

Mice can live up to 3 years. They weigh 20 to 40 g and have a rapid heart rate (approximately 500 to 600 beats/min). Their body temperature is 36.5° to 38° C. Mice have a high metabolic rate and are constantly active. They spend much of their time grooming and keeping their environment organized. Their mammary glands are extensive, reaching from the ventral midline to the back and neck.

Like most rodents, mice are sexed by anogenital distance. Mice are continuously polyestrous, with an estrous cycle of 4 days. Mating can be confirmed by the presence of a white, waxy vaginal plug 12 to 24 hours after breeding. The gestation length is 21 days, with pups born hairless and helpless. Pups are weaned at 21 days of age.

Mice can be caught and safely picked up by grasping the scruff of the neck with forceps or by grasping the base of the tail with the fingers (Fig. 30-3, *A*). For manipulation or examination, the patient is caught by the base of the tail and placed on a surface it can grasp, such as the cage lid. The thumb and forefinger grasp the scruff of the neck (Fig. 30-3, *B*), and the mouse is inverted to lie on its back with the tail positioned between the palm of the hand and the little finger. Clear plastic restraint devices can also be used for restraint and manipulation.

A dominant mouse sometimes chews the fur off a subordinate mouse in the facial area. This harmless behavior is called *barbering*. Unlike female mice, male mice housed together frequently fight. Bite wounds are inflicted on the back and rump. This can be differentiated from mite infestation, which is evident by the presence of areas of alopecia around the facial area and accompanied by pruritus. *Syphacia* and *Aspicularis* are common endoparasites. These pinworms are generally considered nonpathogenic. Diarrhea is often of viral origin. Mouse Hepatitis Virus (MHV) infection is widespread and highly contagious. It can produce respiratory and/or gastrointestinal disease.

Rats

The common rat (*Rattus norvegicus*), found in pet stores or in research laboratories, was developed from the wild

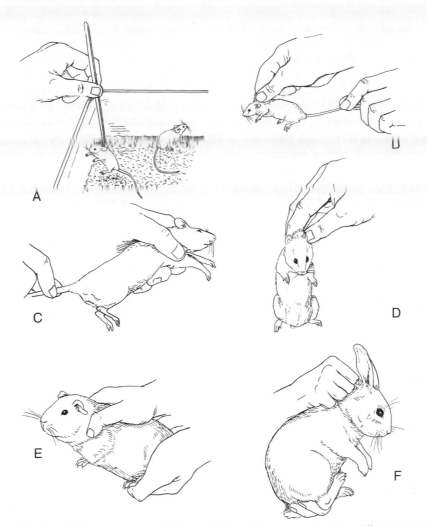

Fig. 30-3 Handling laboratory animals. **A,** Picking up a mouse with forceps. **B,** Restraining a mouse by the scruff. **C,** Restraining a rat. **D,** Picking up a hamster by the scruff. **E,** Restraining a guinea pig. **F,** Lifting a rabbit by the scruff while supporting the hindquarters. *(From McBride DF: Learning veterinary terminology, ed 2, St Louis, 2002, Mosby.)*

brown Norway rat. Rats are easily maintained and make excellent pets if handled gently. They are burrowers and communal critters. Several females and males may be housed together, because fighting rarely occurs among adults. They are the second most commonly used laboratory animal. Hooded or Long-Evans rats have pigmented eyes and are white with darker hair (tan to black) over portions of the head and back. They tend to be smaller than albino rats, such as Sprague-Dawley and Wistar.

The life span of the rat is 2 ½ to 3 ½ years. Rats weigh 250 to 500 g, with females being smaller than males. Their body temperature is 36° to 37.5° C. Rats have continuously erupting incisors and cheeks that close into the *diastema*, a space that separates the incisors from the oral cavity. They have no gallbladder. The Harderian gland, a lacrimal gland located caudal to the eyeball, secretes a red porphyrin-rich secretion that lubricates the eye. In times of stress or illness, red tears overflow and stain the face and nose. The stomach

is divided into two parts, a nonglandular forestomach and a glandular pyloric portion. The esophagus enters through a fold of the ridge that separates the two parts of the stomach. This fold is responsible for the rat's inability to vomit.

Rats are continuously polyestrous, with an estrous cycle of 4 to 5 days. Mating can be confirmed by the presence of a vaginal plug 12 to 24 hours after breeding. The vaginal plug can also be discharged in the cage or litter pan. Females are usually separated from the male before parturition. The gestation length is 21 days, with pups born hairless and helpless. Pups are weaned at 21 days of age.

Rats can be caught and safely picked up by grasping the base of the tail to transport them a short distance such as when changing cages. When rats are held upside down, they are more interested in righting themselves rather than in biting the handler. To restrain for manipulation or examination, pick up the rat by placing the hand firmly over the back and rib cage and restraining the rat's head and shoulders with the thumb and forefinger. If additional control is needed, the base of the tail may be restrained with the other hand (Fig. 30-3, *C*). An alternative method is to pin the rat with your free hand while pulling on the base of the tail. Position your index and third fingers to firmly grasp either side of the rat's neck caudal to the mandible; the thumb and other fingers are used to gently restrain the chest.

Overgrowth of the incisors can occur when the jaw is maloccluded or if the diet is too soft. If rat pups are housed in low humidity, *ringtail* can occur. Ringtail is characterized by annular constrictions that may progress to necrosis and spontaneous amputation of a portion of the tail. Nonspecific signs of illness in rats include rough hair coat, weight loss, and red ocular discharge. Rats are susceptible to respiratory disease caused by *Mycoplasma pulmonis* and cilia-associated respiratory bacillus. Mammary gland tumors are common. Aged rats are frequently affected by chronic renal disease.

Hamsters

The Syrian or golden hamster *(Mesocricetus auratus)* originated in the Middle East. It is the most common hamster in the pet trade and in research. It is noted for its ease of taming, low waste production, and lack of odor. The golden hamster is stocky and short-tailed, weighs approximately 120 g, and has a reddish golden-brown body color with a gray ventrum. Other color varieties, such as cinnamon, cream, white, piebald, albino, and the longhaired teddy bears, are popular as pets. The Chinese or striped hamster *(Cricetulus griseus)* is gray-brown with a dark strip down its back and is smaller than the golden hamster, weighing 35 g. It tends to be more difficult to handle and thus is not as popular as a pet. Female Chinese hamsters are belligerent and must be housed individually. Several dwarf species are being seen as pets. Caging should be selected with the knowledge that hamsters are adept cage chewers and escape artists. Hamsters easily chew through the plastic tubes frequently sold as cage extensions. Hamsters seem to enjoy running on exercise wheels placed in their cages.

Hamsters usually have a life span of 1½ to 2 years. They have cheek pouches that can transport an amazing amount of food and bedding. A female hamster sometimes packs her whole newborn litter in her pouches to move them to another location. Hamsters have extremely loose skin. Marking glands called *flank* or *hip* glands are located in the skin of both flanks and are more prominent in males. At temperatures below 8° C (46° F), some hamsters become inactive for periods of 2 to 3 days. During this transient state of hibernation, they have a reduced body temperature and reduced heart and respiratory rates. Hamster urine is normally turbid and milky because it contains a large amount of crystals.

Hamsters are sexed by anogenital distance. Females have an estrous cycle length of 4 days. They are commonly belligerent toward males unless sexually receptive. During the winter, hamsters have a normal seasonal breeding quiescence. Hamsters have a gestation length of 16 days, the shortest of the laboratory animals. Cannibalism is common during the first pregnancy and in the first week postpartum. Care should be taken not to disturb a new litter during this period. Providing nest material such as paper tissue several days prior to delivery of young helps the female feel more secure. Newborn hamsters have fully erupted incisor teeth. Hamsters are weaned at 21 days of age. Hamsters are sound sleepers and on casual observation may appear dead. An important point to remember when handling a hamster is to avoid surprising it. Ensure that the hamster is awake and knows that the handler intends to pick it up. Startled or awakened hamsters often bite. Hamsters are most easily moved by grasping the loose skin across the shoulders or by using the hands as a scoop to transfer the hamster from one cage to another. They can also be picked up in a small can or cup. To restrain a hamster, gently grasp the loose skin across the back by curling the fingers and thumb around opposite sides of the animal to gather in as much loose skin as possible. Grasp the skin, not the body, of the hamster (Fig. 30-3, *D*). An alternative method is to reverse your hand so that your thumb and forefinger hold the skin at the base of the tail.

Proliferative ileitis, or *wet tail*, is caused by a bacterial infection and is the most common spontaneous disease of hamsters. Young animals are affected most often and produce foul-smelling, watery diarrhea, hence the term wet tail. Aged hamsters are frequently affected with cardiomyopathy and amyloidosis, a metabolic disease. Lymphocytic choriomeningitis virus (LCMV) can infect hamsters. LCMV is zoonotic and of public health concern.

Gerbils

The Mongolian gerbil *(Meriones unguiculatus)* is a native to desert regions of Mongolia and northeastern China. It is an active, burrowing, social animal that tends to be more exploratory than other rodents. The gerbil is clean and produces little waste, making it one of the simplest laboratory animals to maintain. It is relatively odorless, nonaggressive, and easy to handle, making it a good pet. The agouti or mixed-brown gerbil is the color variety most commonly seen, but black and other colors, such as piebald, white, and cinnamon, are available.

The gerbil, or *jird*, as it is sometimes referred to, has an average life span of 3 years and weighs less than 100 g when mature. It has long hind limbs adapted for leaping and, unlike most other rodents, has a hair-covered tail. When threatened or excited, gerbils will drum their hind legs on the cage flooring. They have large adrenal glands, adaptive mechanisms for temperature extremes, and a unique ability to conserve water. Gerbils have high cholesterol levels and lipemic serum. These can be accentuated by feeding sunflower seeds. Both sexes have a distinct dark orange midventral sebaceous gland, which is used for territorial marking. Gerbils form stable lifelong monogamous arrangements and breed throughout the year. The female is polyestrous and has an estrous cycle of 4 to 6 days. Gestation normally lasts 24 days but can be as long as 48 days. The male participates in care of the young and can be left in the cage. Gerbils are weaned at 21 days of age.

A gerbil can be safely picked up by cupping both hands under it or by grasping the base of the tail to lift it from its cage. To restrain the gerbil for examination or injection, grasp the loose skin at the nape of the neck with one hand and grasp the base of the tail with the other hand. Extreme care must be taken not to grasp the tip of the tail because the skin may tear and slip off, exposing the underlying muscle and vertebrae. Alternatively, an over-the-back grip can be used. Gerbils resist being placed on their back.

Spontaneous seizures frequently occur when gerbils are stimulated by loud noises, rough handling, or a novel environment. The seizure is usually short, lasting from a few seconds to more than a minute. During a seizure, the gerbil freezes and holds its legs stiffly extended, while the body trembles. No treatment is necessary. Humidity in excess of 50% will cause a gerbil's coat to matt. *Sorenose*, or rednose, is common in gerbils. This nasal dermatitis is associated with excessive burrowing activity, porphyrin secretion, and staphylococcal infection. Gerbils are very susceptible to Tyzzer's disease caused by *Clostridium piliforme*.

Guinea Pigs

The guinea pig *(Cavia porcellus)* is tailless, with a compact, stocky body and short legs. It originated in South America and is a hystricomorph rodent related to chinchillas and porcupines. The guinea pig is a good children's pet, because it is docile and seldom bites or scratches. Guinea pigs have a variety of vocalizations and will frequently whistle and squeak when a caregiver approaches their cage. They are messy housekeepers and commonly scatter food and bedding. The guinea pig has been associated with research for so long that a human volunteer for an experiment is often called a "guinea pig." Guinea pigs can be monocolored, bicolored, or tricolored. The most common pet and laboratory variety is the English, American, or shorthaired guinea pig. The Abyssinian has short, rough hair arranged in whorls or rosettes; the Peruvian or "rag mop" variety has long, silky hair.

The guinea pig, or *cavy* as it is commonly called, weighs 700 to 1200 g as an adult. It has a normal body temperature of 37.2° to 39.5° C and a life span of 4 to 5 years. Guinea pigs have four digits on their front limbs and three digits on their hind limbs. All teeth are open-rooted and erupt continuously. They have a large cecum and a long colon. Guinea pigs are actively coprophagic. Their urine is normally opaque and creamy yellow, and contains crystals.

Large, mononuclear lymphocytes called *Kurloff cells* are seen in the blood especially during times of estrogen stimulation. Marking glands are located around the anus and on the rump. Both male and female guinea pigs have inguinal nipples. Sexing is difficult because, unlike other rodents, there is little difference in the anogenital distance in males and females. The female has a *Y*-shaped anogenital opening and vaginal membrane that remains intact and closed except during the few days of estrus and at parturition. Males have scrotal pouches lateral to the anogenital line and a penis that can be protruded by manual pressure.

Female guinea pigs are called *sows*, males are called *boars*, and the act of giving birth is called *farrowing*. The sow is polyestrous throughout the year and has an estrous cycle of 15 to 17 days. A sow should be bred for the first time prior to 7 months of age, before fusion of the pubic bones, to prevent dystocia. The gestation period is lengthy, averaging 68 days. Neonates are precocious and nearly self-sufficient. They are born fully furred, with eyes and ears open and teeth erupted. Young guinea pigs eat solid food within the first few days postpartum and can be weaned at 14 to 21 days.

To restrain a guinea pig, lift the animal by grasping under the trunk with one hand while supporting the rear quarters with the other hand (Fig. 30-3, *E*). It is especially important to use a two-hand support method with adult and pregnant animals. An alternative method is to place one hand over the shoulder area, with the thumb and forefingers just caudal to the front legs, while the other hand supports the rear quarters. Use care not to overly compress the chest with this method. Like the rabbit, the guinea pig is herbivorous. Food preferences are established very early in life. Guinea pigs have rigid eating habits, and any change in food or water may cause them to stop eating. Dietary vitamin C must be provided to guinea pigs because, like primates, they cannot synthesize their own vitamin C. Lack of vitamin C causes *scurvy*. Guinea pigs with scurvy have swollen joints and are reluctant to move. Even under ideal storage conditions, the vitamin C content of food deteriorates rapidly, so it is important to use freshly milled food. Commercial rabbit and guinea pig foods look alike; both are small pelleted chows, but they differ in vitamin C content. Citrus fruits, cabbage, peppers, and kale can be fed to supplement vitamin C. Guinea pigs are notorious for playing with sipper tubes of their water bottle causing the bottle to empty. They will also blow chewed food through the sipper tube and block it or foul the water supply.

Lower premolar teeth are frequently maloccluded and overgrown and can cause excessive salivation or *slobbers*. Pododermatitis, also called *bumblefoot*, is found in obese animals housed on wire. Animals have pressure sores on the palmar and plantar surfaces of their feet. Subcutaneous abscesses or cervical "lumps" caused by *Streptococcus zooepidemicus* are common in guinea pigs. Respiratory disease is frequently accompanied by nasal and ocular discharge. Guinea pigs are susceptible to *Bordetella bronchiseptica* and should not be housed with rabbits, dogs, cats, or other species that carry the bacteria subclinically. Conjunctivitis is commonly due to bacterial infection. Guinea pigs are sensitive to antibiotics that change their gastrointestinal flora. Penicillin should not be used in guinea pigs, because it often induces fatal reactions in this species.

Chinchillas

The chinchilla *(Chinchilla laniger)* has a compact body, delicate limbs, large eyes, large round ears, long whiskers, and a bushy tail. It has a soft, very dense haircoat that is normally bluish-gray with yellow-white under parts. It originated in South America like its relative the guinea pig. Chinchillas are quiet, shy animals that adapt well to humans when handled at a young age. They rarely bite and are virtually odorless. Chinchillas are very active, agile, and like to climb and jump. They require a larger cage than do guinea pigs, which tend to be less active.

The chinchilla weighs 400 to 600 g as an adult. It has a normal body temperature of 37° to 38° C (99° to 100.4° F) and a life span of 10 years. Its life span is much longer than that of other pet rodents. Chinchillas have four toes on their front and rear feet. Like the guinea pig, all their teeth are open-rooted and ever growing. They have a long gastrointestinal tract and are coprophagic. The female has a vaginal closure membrane that remains intact and closed except during a few days of estrus and at parturition. The anogenital distance is the best criterion for sexing. The female has a large urinary papilla that can be confused with a penis. The penis can be protruded by manual pressure to confirm the sex. Males do not have a true scrotum. The testes are contained within the open inguinal canal or abdomen.

Chinchillas can be housed in pairs or in larger units. Females tend to be highly selective in their choice of mate and can be aggressive. If housed in pairs, the male can remain with the female if she tolerates him during parturition and raising of the young. Chinchillas are seasonally polyestrus and have a lengthy gestation period of 111 days. Unlike the guinea pig, dystocias are uncommon. The young are precocious being fully furred with teeth and eyes open at birth. The female chinchilla stands rather than lying on her side when nursing young. Young chinchillas begin to eat solid foods at a week of age and can be weaned at 6 to 8 weeks of age. They are sexually mature at 8 months of age.

A tamed chinchilla will willingly come out of its cage. To restrain it, place one hand under the abdomen or around the scruff of the neck and hold it by the base of the tail with the other hand. If the chinchilla escapes from its cage, you must quickly catch it. Use care, as a frightened chinchilla can loose a patch of fur where it is grasped. This condition is called *fur-slip* and is a predator avoidance mechanism. It takes 6 to 8 weeks for the hairless patch to fill in.

Access to a dust bath should be provided for one hour daily to prevent matted fur. Commercial chinchilla dust or a mixture of silver sand and Fuller's earth can be used. One inch of dust is placed in a pan that is big enough for the chinchilla to roll around in and fluff its fur. Chinchillas are susceptible to many of the same bacterial diseases as guinea pigs. The bones of chinchillas are thin and fragile. It is common to see traumatic fractures. The tibia is particularly fragile being longer than the femur and has little soft tissue covering it. Chinchillas are prone to heat stroke at environmental temperature exceeding 28° to 30° C (82° to 86° F), especially when coupled with high humidity.

Rabbits

The domestic rabbit *(Oryctolagus cuniculus)* is a descendant of the wild rabbit of Europe. The Flemish Giant is a large breed weighing 6 to 7 kg, the New Zealand and Californian are medium-size breeds weighing 2 to 5 kg, and the Dutch and Polish are small breeds weighing 1 to 2 kg. The albino New Zealand is popularly used for meat production and research. The smaller breeds are used as pets and in research. Rabbits make good pets. They are mild-tempered, seldom bite, and can be housetrained.

Rabbits are *lagomorphs*, differentiated from rodents by the presence of two upper pairs of incisors that continuously grow. The rabbit has a life span of 5 to 6 years or more, body temperature of (101° to 104° F) 38.5° to 40° C, heart rate 130 to 325 beats per minute, and respiratory rate of 30 to 60 breaths per minute. Rabbits have a wide field of vision, can readily detect motion, and see well in dim light. Their ears are highly vascular and function in heat regulation. They have a small skeletal mass as compared with similar-sized animals and large hindquarter muscles that make them prone to back fractures.

Rabbits have several unusual features to their intestinal tract, including a sacculus rotundus located at the terminal end of the ileum, a large cecum that terminates in a vermiform process or appendix, and a colon with regular sacculations called *haustra*. Rabbits are coprophagic and pass two types of feces. Soft, moist "night feces" are rich in vitamins and protein and are eaten directly from the anus. Firm, dry pellets are passed during the daytime. The color of rabbit urine varies from orange-red to brown.

Male rabbits are called *bucks*, and female rabbits are called *does*. Sexing can be accomplished by gently pressing the skin back from the genital opening. Females have an elongated vulva, with a slit opening; males have a rounded, protruding penile sheath. The *dewlap*, a heavy fold of skin at the throat, is more prominent in females. Rabbits do not have a true estrous cycle but have periods of sexual receptivity. They are induced ovulators. Because the doe is territorial, she is taken to the buck's cage for breeding. Mating usually occurs within minutes. Gestation is approximately 31 days. Parturition in the rabbit is called *kindling*. The young are called *kits* or, more commonly, *bunnies*. Young rabbits are born hairless and helpless, yet they require little maternal care. Does nurse young rabbits only for a few minutes once or twice daily. Weaning occurs at 6 to 8 weeks of age.

To remove a rabbit from a cage or to carry it a short distance, grasp the scruff of the rabbit's neck with one hand and support the hindquarters and back with the other (Fig. 30-3, *F*). When carrying a rabbit longer distances, its head should be tucked into the crook of the arm that is supporting the hindquarters (Fig. 30-4, *A*). Rabbits that are incorrectly handled can injure themselves by struggling and fracturing their back or their handler by scratching him or her. A towel wrapped around the rabbit works well for restraint, especially if the eyes are covered. Mechanical devices made of plastic or metal are frequently used for restraint during minor procedures, such as blood collection from an ear vein, IV injections, or treatments. The restraining device holds the head in place and has a sliding partition that fits snugly against the rabbit's rump (Fig. 30-4, *B*). Rabbits should never be lifted or restrained by grabbing their ears, because the ears are sensitive and fragile. When returning a rabbit to its cage, place it in the cage rump first to prevent injury to the rabbit or handler. A rabbit has a tendency to leap toward the cage if allowed to enter the cage headfirst.

Malocclusion can result in overgrown incisors that may need to be trimmed every 2 to 3 weeks. Ear mite infections with *Psoroptes* are common in pet rabbits. The mites characteristically cause a dry, brown, crusty material to accumulate on the inner surface of the ears. Pododermatitis, a pressure necrosis of the plantar surface of the metatarsal area, commonly called *sore hocks*, is seen in heavy, obese rabbits. Rabbits are susceptible to infection with *Pasteurella multocida*. Several clinical forms of the disease occur; the most common are rhinitis (*"snuffles"*) and pneumonia. Stressed or recently weaned rabbits frequently are affected with coccidia.

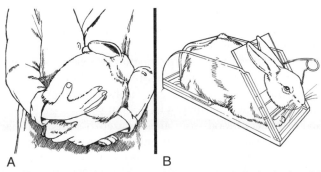

Fig. 30-4 A, Rabbits can be carried by supporting the body while directing the head into the crook of the elbow. **B,** Device to restrain rabbits. *(Adapted from American Association for Laboratory Animal Science training manual series, vol 2: laboratory animal technician, Cordova, Tenn., 2000 AALAS.)*

Ferrets

The domestic ferret (*Mustela putorius furo*) belongs to the same family as the weasel, mink, otter, and skunk. Ferrets were initially used as hunting animals for the control of rabbits and rodents and raised for their pelts. They have become popular pets due to their small size, ease of care, and comical engaging personalities. Keeping domestic ferrets as pets is not legal in all states and/or cities. Thus, it is important to be aware of legislation in your locality regarding the keeping of ferrets as pets. The natural color of ferrets is *fitch*, also as known as sable. Fitch-colored ferrets have black guard hair with a cream-colored undercoat, black feet and tail, and a black mask on the face. Two other natural colors that are seen are albino and cinnamon. In addition, there are more than 30 color variations recognized. Ferrets have long tubular bodies with short legs and very flexible spines. This allows them to get into small openings and turn around easily. Ferrets leap, jump, and can climb. Pet owners need to keep a ferret in a secure, escape-proof cage. If a ferret is allowed to run loose, the house should be "ferret proofed" to close up any holes or areas from which a ferret cannot be retrieved.

Ferrets that are neutered early weigh 0.8 and 1.2 kg when adult. Non-neutered animals are larger, especially males. The ferret has a life span of 5 to 8 years, a body temperature of 37.8° to 40° C, a heart rate 180 to 250 beats per minute, and a respiratory rate of 33 to 36 breathes per minute. A ferret's skin is remarkably thick, especially over the neck and shoulders. Ferrets experience a seasonal change in body fat, losing weight in the summer and gaining it back in the winter. They also molt in the spring and fall. Ferrets do not have sweat glands in their skin and thus are prone to heat stroke. Their claws are not retractable as in cats and need to be trimmed. The canine teeth are prominent as they are in other carnivorous animals. Ferrets have a simple stomach and short small intestine. They do not have a cecum. Ferrets have well-developed anal glands that produce a foul smelling liquid when they are frightened. The anal gland secretion, however, is not responsible for the musky body odor of ferrets. The sebaceous secretions of their skin produce the odor. Ferrets originating from large breeding farms are routinely descented and neutered when they are 5 to 6 weeks of age, prior to entering the pet market.

Female ferrets are called *jills*, and males are called *hobs*. Young ferrets are called *kits*. A neutered female is called a *sprite* and a neutered male a *gib*. It is easy to sex a ferret. The preputial opening in male ferrets is located on the ventral abdomen as in male dogs, and the os penis is readily palpable. The urogenital opening in female ferrets is located in the perineal region ventral to the anus. The breeding season for ferrets is from March to August in most climates. Females are seasonally polyestrous. During estrus, the vulva becomes swollen and protuberant. Gestation is 42 days, and young ferrets are weaned at 6 to 8 weeks of age.

Most ferrets are quite docile and can be easily examined without undo restraint. Assistance is usually needed to give medications. Tractable ferrets can be lightly restrained on the exam table. An active ferret can be restrained by scruffing the loose skin on the back of the neck and suspending it off the table. Many animals can be distracted by feeding Nutri-Cal with a syringe or placing a small amount of it on their fur for them to lick.

Ferrets are highly susceptible to canine distemper. They must be vaccinated against this virus as canine distemper is typically a fatal disease in ferrets. Ear mites are very common in ferrets. Ferrets are very susceptible to human influenza virus. Influenza causes upper respiratory disease in ferrets as it does in humans. Adrenal gland disease and insulinomas are common conditions seen in older pet ferrets. If female ferrets are not spayed, they frequently remain in estrus if they are not bred. They can develop estrogen toxicity with bone marrow suppression and severe anemia.

GENERAL NURSING CARE

Because of the cost involved in hospitalization and intensive care, most pet rodents are treated on an outpatient basis, whereas rabbits and ferrets are often hospitalized. As with any other sick pet, proper nursing care is vital to maximize the chances for full recovery.

Pet rodents that must be hospitalized are usually critically ill. Fluid therapy, antibiotics, force-feeding, and proper environment are important. These patients should be handled as little as possible. The proper ambient temperature must be maintained. Incubators serve this function well, but care must be taken not to overheat small mammals to extremes in heat. The temperature should be kept no warmer than 27° C (80° F). Temperatures above this often result in death from heat stroke. When necessary, oxygen can be supplemented through a port on the incubator. Food and water should be offered even if force-feeding is needed.

When possible, small mammals should be isolated from other hospitalized animals. This is due to the risk of disease (e.g., *Bordetella* passed from dogs, cats, or rabbits to guinea pigs) and the fact that these sick pets are extremely stressed. Remember that most small mammals are prey in the wild. Housing them near a natural predator such as a dog or cat may increase their stress levels.

DIAGNOSTIC AND TREATMENT TECHNIQUES

Techniques used to diagnose disease in companion and food animals are used in small mammals. Some techniques such as skin scrapings can be more challenging in rodents because they are very mobile and can be difficult to restrain. Diagnostic testing is important as many of these pets are presented with vague complaints such as lethargy and lack of appetite. Although certain syndromes are more common in certain species, diagnostic testing can help determine a definitive diagnosis and proper treatment plan. Unfortunately, many owners of some less expensive small mammals, particularly rodents, may not allow diagnostic testing because of the cost involved. In addition, the small size of these animals makes it more difficult to obtain adequate laboratory samples. In the research setting, the health status of the rodent colony is often more important that the health status of an individual animal. Health status is frequently monitored by serologic testing of sentinel animals that are placed in the colony.

Venipuncture

Venipuncture is a technique commonly used in ferrets and rabbits and infrequently used in pet rodents. Venipuncture is used for withdrawing blood for hematologic and biochemical analysis, administration of certain medications, and catheterization for administration of fluids. Anesthesia may be required when performing venipuncture on small mammals. Although each diagnostic laboratory has specific requirements for the volume of blood required for various tests, most laboratories can perform a mini-battery of tests (CBC, chemistries, electrolytes) on 0.5 ml of blood collected in a green-top (lithium heparin) tube. Special blood-collection tubes (Microvette) that hold a maximum of 300 L (0.3 ml) are available commercially. These are particularly useful when collecting samples from small rodents. Except for mice and gerbils, 0.5 ml is a realistic amount of blood to collect from a small mammal. 0.2 ml of blood can be routinely collected from a mouse or gerbil. To prevent volume depletion in pet rodents, some clinicians replace the volume of blood withdrawn with an equal volume of balanced electrolyte solution.

Rodents

Small blood samples can be collected from rodents by toe-nail clip or superficial venipuncture. The lateral saphenous vein is a good superficial vessel to utilize. Other superficial vessels that can be utilized include the cephalic vein, jugular vein, and tail vessels in rodents that have long tails. The central vena cava of guinea pigs is easily accessible, but they must be anesthetized first. The orbital sinus is frequently used to collect blood from anesthetized rodents. Cardiac puncture can also be used in an anesthetized rodent, but it is not recommended except for collection before euthanasia.

Rabbits

The marginal ear veins and central ear artery of the rabbit are easily visualized and can be used to collect blood (Fig. 30-5). Blood can be collected with a syringe and needle or

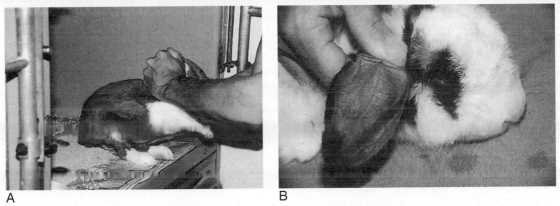

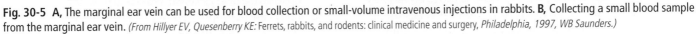

Fig. 30-5 A, The marginal ear vein can be used for blood collection or small-volume intravenous injections in rabbits. **B,** Collecting a small blood sample from the marginal ear vein. *(From Hillyer EV, Quesenberry KE: Ferrets, rabbits, and rodents: clinical medicine and surgery, Philadelphia, 1997, WB Saunders.)*

by cannulating the vessel and collecting the blood in a blood tube or heparinized microhematocrit tube as it drips freely from the vessel. Jugular venipuncture is also fairly easy. The rabbit is placed in ventral recumbency, and the blood is collected in a similar manner to dogs and cats. The cephalic vein tends to be a more difficult vessel from which to collect blood.

Ferrets

The cephalic vein, jugular vein, cranial vena cava, and lateral saphenous vein can be used to collect blood samples in ferrets. Venipuncture is most easily performed under isoflurane anesthesia maintained by facemask. When obtaining a jugular sample, the ferret is placed in dorsal recumbency, with the legs pulled caudad while the head and neck are extended dorsally. Venipuncture can be done in an awake cooperative ferret. Obtaining a small volume of blood from a larger ferret is possible using the central artery of the tail.

Force-Feeding

Many small mammals are presented for veterinary care because of anorexia and lethargy. In addition to the need for rehydration, nutritional supplementation is often required but overlooked. Small mammals such as rodents have high metabolic rates and thus high energy requirements. Animals that are not eating are in a *catabolic state*. Decreased food intake results in breakdown of protein and fat for energy. This can contribute to hepatic lipidosis (especially in rabbits), acidosis, azotemia, muscle wasting, impaired gastrointestinal function, and decreased immunity. To prevent or correct these complications, supplementation with food is important. Force-feeding can be done in the hospital or by the client at home if the pet will be treated on an outpatient basis.

High-energy paste supplements such as Nutri-Cal can be given to all small mammals on a short-term basis. Sick

rabbits often eat hay or greens, such as carrot tops and parsley, even if they refuse pellets. These can be offered free choice. Apples and yogurt can also be used. A nasogastric or gastric tube can be used to deliver a mixture of powdered pellets and water. Rodents can be supplemented with apples and peanut butter. Sweetened condensed milk is also a favorite. Pedialyte or Gatorade can be fed via small syringe for hydration along with water. Hospitalized ferrets can be force-fed any of the diets suitable for cats including Hill's a/d or CliniCare. Meat-based baby foods can also be used. The food can be offered to the ferret to eat voluntarily or given with a syringe or through a tube. Warming the food slightly may increase the appetite of ferrets.

Administration of Medications

With the exception of ferrets, small mammals are difficult to medicate with pills. The pet will usually accept a liquid oral medication given with an eyedropper or small syringe. Because of the small size of rodents, medications usually have to be diluted. For increased accuracy of dosing, it is important to have an accurate body weight and use a tuberculin syringe. Medication can also be administered orally by mixing the medication in the water or feed, and by gavage needle. Rodents often do not drink medicated water because of its unpleasant taste.

Injectable medications are usually preferred over oral medications in hospitalized small mammals. Extremely ill pets may have reduced intestinal function, making absorption of oral medication erratic and unpredictable. Using the parenteral rather than oral route of administration also decreases the possibility of gastrointestinal problems in these small mammals.

The standard routes of injection (intravenous [IV], intramuscular [IM], subcutaneous [SC or SQ], intradermal [ID], and intraperitoneal [IP]) are used in laboratory animals. Rodents have few readily accessible veins, making it difficult to administer drugs IV. Tail veins can be used in the mouse and rat. The margin ear veins located on the lateral sides of the pinna in the rabbit are accessible and can be used for IV injections. Because it is difficult to do venous catheterization in small mammals, some doctors and technicians prefer intraosseous (IO) catheterization to administer fluids to critically ill exotic pets. The trochanteric fossa of the femur is the preferred site for IO catheterization. The SQ route is frequently used for fluid supplementation. SQ fluids are given over the dorsal neck, back, and flank of small mammals. Fluids can also be given IP in rodents. The small-muscle mass of rodents makes it difficult to inject drugs IM. For this reason, the IP route is more commonly used in rodents. When giving IP injections, it is best to use the caudal left abdominal quadrant and tilt the animal's head and forequarters ventrally. This helps to avoid accidental puncture of the large cecum.

Antibiotics

Caution must be utilized when administering antibiotics to rodents and rabbits. These animals have a predominantly gram-positive gastrointestinal flora and are very sensitive to antibiotics that change the balance of the flora. Guinea pigs and rabbits are particularly prone to antibiotic-associated enterotoxemia. Drugs such as ampicillin and penicillin will destroy susceptible gram-positive organisms and allow overgrowth of *Clostridium difficile* and production of its toxin. Safe antibacterials for use in rabbits and rodents include enrofloxacin, ciprofloxacin, trimethoprim-sulfas, and chloramphenicol. If diarrhea develops, drug administration should be stopped immediately and the animal should be examined. Ferrets can safely be treated with most antibacterials used in cats.

Vaccines

Rodents and rabbits do not currently require annual vaccines. Ferrets must be vaccinated against canine distemper virus with an appropriate vaccine. Never use canine combination vaccines or vaccines of ferret cell origin because of the possibility of vaccine-induced disease. Give ferrets a series of vaccines at 6 to 8 weeks, 10 to 12 weeks, and 14 weeks of age, then annually. Vaccination against rabies is highly recommended for ferrets, especially in rabies-endemic areas. An inactivated rabies vaccine approved for use in ferrets should be given SQ at 3 months of age and annually.

Fecal Analysis

Microscopic fecal analysis is used to evaluate animals with diarrhea and any nonspecific complaint. The method is similar to that used in dogs and cats. A fresh fecal smear and flotation should be performed. A cellophane tape test can be used on the anal region to check for the presence of pinworms in rodents.

Urine Collection

Urine samples can be obtained by gentle digital pressure or cystocentesis. Rodents can be placed on a cold surface or in a cooled plastic bag until urine is voided.

IDENTIFICATION METHODS USED IN RESEARCH ANIMALS

Identification of individual animals is important in a research setting, as many animals appear identical. The researcher frequently needs to tell individual animals apart. Rodents are identified by ear tag or by an ear notch or punch pattern. Ear tags or ear tattoos are used in rabbits. A microchip can be implanted SQ in laboratory animals for quick electronic identification.

ANESTHESIA

Many factors, such as species, strain, ingesta content, weight, and nutritional and health status, affect the response of rabbits and rodents to anesthesia. Small rodents are not fasted before inducing anesthesia. Food, but not water, should be withheld for 3 to 6 hours from guinea pigs, chinchillas, and rabbits before inducing anesthesia. Young ferrets like dogs and cats are fasted for 8 hours. Food is withheld from older ferrets for no more than 4 hours. A small scale should be used to obtain an accurate weight of the animal to calculate the dose when using injectable anesthetic agents. Inhalation agents, such as isoflurane and halothane, can also be used; however, they should be delivered using a calibrated vaporizer to prevent anesthetic overdose. Inhalation agents are commonly administered via chamber, facemask, or nose cone, because it is difficult to intubate most small mammals. Ferrets can be intubated in a similar fashion to cats. It is essential to monitor the animal closely and keep it warm to prevent hypothermia. Hydration, nutritional support, and analgesia are important postoperative considerations.

RECOMMENDED READING

American Association for Laboratory Animal Science training manual series, vol. 1, assistant laboratory animal technician, Cordova, Tenn, 1998, AALAS.

American Association for Laboratory Animal Science training manual series, vol. 2, assistant laboratory animal technician, Cordova, Tenn, 2000, AALAS.

Harkness JE, Wagner JE: *The biology and medicine of rabbits and rodents*, ed 4, Media, Penn, 1995, Williams & Wilkins.

Hillyer EV, Quesenberry KE: *Ferrets, rabbits, rodents: clinical medicine and surgery*, Philadelphia, 1997, WB Saunders.

Hrapkiewicz K, Medina L, Homes D: *Clinical laboratory animal medicine, an introduction*, ed 2, Ames, Iowa, 1998, Iowa State University Press.

Index